ENDOVASCULAR AND PERCUTANEOUS THERAPY OF THE BRAIN AND SPINE

ENDOVASCULAR AND PERCUTANEOUS THERAPY OF THE BRAIN AND SPINE

EDITORS

MICHAEL P. MARKS, M.D.

Associate Professor of Radiology and Neurosurgery
Stanford University School of Medicine
Chief of Interventional Neuroradiology
Stanford University Medical Center
Stanford, California

HUY M. DO, M.D.

Assistant Professor of Radiology and Neurosurgery
Stanford University School of Medicine
Stanford, California

LIPPINCOTT WILLIAMS & WILKINS
A **Wolters Kluwer** Company
Philadelphia • Baltimore • New York • London
Buenos Aires • Hong Kong • Sydney • Tokyo

Acquisitions Editor: Joyce-Rachel John
Developmental Editor: Grace Caputo
Production Manager: Toni Ann Scaramuzzo
Production Editor: Michael Mallard
Manufacturing Manager: Tim Reynolds
Cover Designer: Joan Greenfield
Compositor: Maryland Composition
Printer: Maple Press

530 Walnut Street
Philadelphia, PA 19106 USA
LWW.com

Printed in the USA

Library of Congress Cataloging-in-Publication Data

Endovascular and percutaneous therapy of the brain and spine / editors, Michael P. Marks, Huy M. Do.
p. ; cm.
Includes bibliographical references and index.
ISBN 0-7817-3035-X
1. Cerebrovascular disease—Surgery. 2. Brain—Cancer—Surgery. 3. Spinal cord—Surgery. 4. Intravenous catheterization. I. Marks, Michael P., 1953- II. Do, Huy M.
[DNLM: 1. Cerebrovascular Disorders—surgery. 2. Brain Neoplasms—surgery. 3. Catheterization. 4. Spinal Cord Diseases—surgery. 5. Vascular Surgical Procedures. WL 355 E558 2002]
RD594.2 .E526 2002
617.4′81—dc21

2002016283

---

10 9 8 7 6 5 4 3 2 1

To Susan, Ethan, and Eliana

M.P.M.

To my parents

H.M.D.

TABLE OF CONTENTS

CONTRIBUTORS

Stanley L. Barnwell, M.D., Ph.D. Associate Professor of Neurosurgery, Dotter Interventional Institute, Oregon Health Sciences University, Portland, Oregon

Patricia E. Burrows, M.D. Chief, Division of Cardiovascular and Interventional Neuroradiology; Professor of Radiology, Children's Hospital, Boston, Massachusetts

John C. Chaloupka, M.D. Chief, Section of Interventional Neuroradiology, Director, Custom Stent and Interventional Neuroradiology Center, Professor of Radiology and Neurosurgery, University of Iowa Hospitals and Clinics, Iowa City, Iowa

Ram Chavali, M.D. Department of Interventional Neuroradiology, Lahey Clinic Medical Center, Burlington, Massachusetts

In Sup Choi, M.D. Professor of Radiology, Tufts University School of Medicine, Boston, Massachusetts; Chair, Department of Interventional Neuroradiology, Lahey Clinic Medical Center, Burlington, Massachusetts

Harry J. Cloft, M.D., Ph.D. Associate Professor of Radiology and Neurosurgery, Mayo Clinic; Senior Associate Consultant, Department of Radiology, Saint Mary's Hospital, Rochester, Minnesota

Huy M. Do, M.D. Assistant Professor of Radiology and Neurosurgery, Stanford University School of Medicine; Interventional Neuroradiologist, Department of Radiology, Stanford University Medical Center, Stanford, California

Christopher F. Dowd, M.D. Associate Clinical Professor of Radiology and Neurological Surgery, University of California, San Francisco, San Francisco, California

Ian G. Fleetwood, M.D., F.R.C.S.C. Cerebrovascular Surgery Fellow, Department of Neurosurgery and Stanford Stroke Center, Stanford University, Stanford, California

Raymond R. Gaeta, M.D. Associate Professor of Anesthesia, Director, Pain Management Center, Stanford University School of Medicine, Stanford, California

Van V. Halbach, M.D. Clinical Professor of Radiology and Neurological Surgery, University of California, San Francisco, San Francisco, California

Randall T. Higashida, M.D. Clinical Professor, Departments of Radiology, Neurological Surgery, Neurology, and Anesthesiology, University of California, San Francisco San Francisco, California

Mary E. Jensen, M.D. Associate Professor, Departments of Radiology and Neurosurgery, University of Virginia Health Sciences Center, Charlottesville, Virginia

Chelsea Kidwell, M.D. Assistant Professor of Neurology, UCLA School of Medicine; Neurology Co-Director, UCLA Stroke Center, UCLA Medical Center, Los Angeles, California

Todd A. Kuether, M.D. Assistant Professor, Dotter Interventional Institute, Oregon Health Sciences University, Microneurosurgical Consultants, St. Vincent's/Providence, Portland, Oregon

James E. Lefler, M.D. Radiology Associates of Tampa, Interventional and Therapeutic Neuroradiology, Tampa General Hospital, Tampa, Florida

Adel M. Malek, M.D., Ph.D. Instructor, Department of Surgery, Harvard Medical School; Cerebrovascular and Endovascular Neurosurgery, Department of Surgery, Beth Israel Deaconess Medical Center, Boston, Massachusetts

Michael P. Marks, M.D. Associate Professor of Radiology and Neurosurgery, Stanford University School of Medicine; Chief of Interventional Neuroradiology, Stanford University Medical Center, Stanford, California

Philip M. Meyers, M.D. Assistant Professor of Radiology and Neurosurgery, Columbia University; Interventional Neuroradiologist, New York Presbyterian Hospitals, New York, New York

Yuichi Murayama, M.D. Assistant Professor, Division of Interventional Neuroradiology, Department of Radiological Sciences, UCLA School of Medicine and Medical Center, Los Angeles, California

Gary M. Nesbit, M.D. Associate Professor, Dotter Interventional Institute, Oregon Health Sciences University, Portland, Oregon

Constantine C. Phatouros, M.B.B.S., F.R.A.N.Z.C.R. Consultant Interventional Neuroradiologist, Neurointerventional Service, Royal Perth and Sir Charles Gairdner Hospitals, Perth, Australia

Jeffrey L. Saver, M.D. Neurology Director, UCLA Stroke Center; Attending, Neurobehavior Program; Associate Professor of Neurology, UCLA School of Medicine, Los Angeles, California

Gary K. Steinberg, M.D., Ph.D. Lacroute-Hearst Professor and Chairman, Department of Neurosurgery, Stanford University; Chief, Department of Neurosurgery, Stanford University Medical Center, Stanford, California

Marcus A. Stoodley, Ph.D., F.R.A.C.S. Senior Lecturer, Clinical School, University of New South Wales, Sydney, Australia; Neurosurgeon, Institute of Neurological Sciences, Prince of Wales Hospital, Randwick, Australia

Thomas A. Tomsick, M.D., F.A.C.R. Professor of Radiology and Adjunct Professor of Neurosurgery, University of Cincinnati; Director, Section of Neuroradiology, University Hospital, Cincinnati, Ohio

Fernando Viñuela, M.D., Ph.D. Professor of Radiological Sciences; Chief, Division of Interventional Neuroradiology, Department of Radiological Sciences, UCLA School of Medicine and Medical Center, Los Angeles, California

Bryce K. A. Weir, M.D. Maurice Goldblatt Professor of Surgery and Neurology, Vice-President for Medical Affairs, University of Chicago, Chicago, Illinois

Robert A. Willinsky, M.D., F.R.C.P.C. Associate Professor, Medical Imaging, University of Toronto, Neuroradiologist, Toronto Western Hospital, Toronto, Ontario, Canada

PREFACE

This textbook comes at an exciting time in the use of endovascular and percutaneous therapy for the brain and spine. We have been witness to the birth and growth of a whole host of techniques for this treatment. Technical developments in imaging, delivery systems, and embolic implantable devices and materials have paced this evolution and fueled continued and inexorable improvements in our field. We are truly able to reach farther, proceed more safely, and, in the end, do far more than we could previously. As physicians, this is the most heartening change we have witnessed: being able to offer more to our patients.

In considering this project, we felt that no textbook provided an accurate, comprehensive, and up-to-date review of endovascular and percutaneous therapy of the brain and spine. We hoped to accomplish two major goals with this undertaking. The first was to provide the reader with a well-referenced, comprehensive understanding of the diseases for which these therapies are used. The second goal was to provide technical guidance in a kind of "how I do it" section, imparting details about the workup and treatment of patients undergoing these therapies. We therefore sought out recognized and highly experienced contributors who could speak with both academic and clinical authority about their subjects.

To address these goals, we asked the contributing authors to structure their chapters into two major sections. The first part of the chapter is designed to provide a basic understanding of these disease processes, including their etiology, pathophysiology, and natural history. Authors were also asked to review treatment alternatives and outcomes, as well as to review the pertinent literature. The second portion of the chapter describes the application of endovascular and percutaneous therapy, along with a discussion of the pitfalls and complications of treatment. Individual chapters address the vascular, neoplastic, and developmental diseases treated with these techniques. In addition, because some subjects were more exhaustive, overview chapters have been included for ischemic disease, aneurysms, and arteriovenous malformations.

We believe that *Endovascular and Percutaneous Therapy of the Brain and Spine* will be useful to physicians performing these procedures in neuroradiology, neurosurgery, neurology, and allied fields. We hope that other physicians and health care professionals interested in the diseases discussed in this text will also find this book useful as a reference and that for any reader it will provide insight into the capabilities and limitations of this exciting field.

Michael P. Marks, M.D.
Huy M. Do, M.D.

ACKNOWLEDGMENTS

We would like to thank Joyce-Rachel John at Lippincott Willams & Wilkins, who provided the invitation and impetus for writing this book. We also thank Grace Caputo at LWW for her invaluable help with the organization of the chapters and communication with contributors. We thank our secretary, Barbara Hargis, for her calm and steady preparation of the edited chapter manuscripts. And we are indebted to our nurse coordinator, Mary Marcellus, the heart of our interventional service, who helped us with case material and organized our clinical time so that we could accomplish our goal of completing this project during these many months.

ENDOVASCULAR AND PERCUTANEOUS THERAPY OF THE BRAIN AND SPINE

1

ISCHEMIC STROKE: OVERVIEW

CHELSEA KIDWELL
JEFFREY L. SAVER

EPIDEMIOLOGY

Incidence

Ischemic stroke is a common, crippling, and deadly disease. Stroke is the third leading cause of death and the leading cause of adult disability in the United States. More than 750,000 symptomatic strokes and more than 11 million silent strokes occur each year in the United States [1–3]. Ischemic cerebral infarction accounts for 80% to 85% of all strokes, intracerebral hemorrhage about 10%, and subarachnoid hemorrhage about 7% [4]. Consequently, it is estimated that more than 600,000 symptomatic ischemic strokes and over 9 million silent ischemic strokes occur each year in the United States.

Mortality and Morbidity

Stroke is frequently fatal. The 1-month mortality after ischemic stroke is 15%, and the 1-year mortality approaches 30% [5,6]. Thirty-day mortality varies by ischemic stroke subtype, with cardioembolic stroke and strokes of undetermined cause producing higher fatality rates than lacunar strokes and large-vessel atherothromboembolic strokes. Altogether, more than 150,000 individuals die each year in the United States directly from stroke.

When not fatal, stroke is often disabling. Currently, there are more than 4.5 million survivors of symptomatic stroke in the United States [7]. More than 70% of stroke survivors are unable to return fully to their prior occupations [6]. Thirty-one percent of stroke survivors require assistance with activities of daily living, 20% need help walking, and 16% are chronically institutionalized [6]. The financial toll exacted by stroke is immense—in 1998, more than $40 billion. The personal toll, on affected patients and families, is even greater. Nearly one-half of older Americans consider a major stroke a fate worse than death [8].

C. Kidwell: Department of Neurology, UCLA School of Medicine, and UCLA Stroke Center, UCLA Medical Center, Los Angeles, California.

J.L. Saver: Department of Neurology, UCLA School of Medicine, and UCLA Stroke Research Center, UCLA Medical Center, Los Angeles, California.

Risk Factors

Risk factors for ischemic stroke may be broadly divided into nonmodifiable and modifiable categories. Leading nonmodifiable risk factors are age, sex, ethnicity, and heredity.

Stroke is an age-related disease. About two-thirds of strokes occur in individuals over the age of 65. The incidence of symptomatic stroke approximately doubles in every age decade over 45, climbing from 104 per 100,000 at ages 45 to 54, to 1,837 per 100,000 over age 85 [9]. Men are more prone to cerebral infarction than women, with an incidence ratio of 1.4:1. However, stroke-related case-fatality rates are higher in women than in men, likely because women tend to have strokes at an older, more vulnerable age than men. The influence of sex on ischemic stroke incidence varies by stroke subtype. Although the age-adjusted incidence of large-artery atherothromboembolic stroke is almost fourfold greater in men than women, lacunar stroke is only 1.3-fold more common, and cardioembolic stroke occurs with roughly equal frequency between the sexes [10]. Blacks have twice the incidence of stroke compared to whites, adjusting for age, sex, and place of residence [11].

Single-gene disorders strongly disposing to stroke are numerous, but collectively they account for only a small fraction of affected patients. Over 110 heritable disorders, 175 genetic loci, and 2,000 unique mutations increasing susceptibility to stroke have been identified [12]. In general, however, heredity exerts a modest influence on stroke risk. A family history of an affected first-degree relative increases the risk of stroke 1.2- to 2.0-fold.

The modifiable risk factors for ischemic stroke include predisposing conditions, predisposing behaviors, and herald events. Leading predisposing conditions for ischemic stroke identified in case-control and prospective cohort studies include hypertension, diabetes, hypercholesterolemia, atrial fibrillation, recent myocardial infarction, and carotid artery stenosis (Table 1-1) [13]. Leading predisposing behaviors include tobacco use, alcohol abuse, and physical inactivity. The number of excess strokes caused by these risk factors, the population attributable risk, can be calculated from the strength of their association with stroke and their prevalence in the population (Table 1-2) [14]. Fully 75% to 80% of all strokes

TABLE 1-1. MODIFIABLE RISK FACTORS FOR STROKE

Risk Factor	Relative Risk	Prevalence (%)[a]
Hypertension	4.0–5.0	25–40
Tobacco use	2.0–4.0	20–40
Hyperlipidemia	1.0–2.0	6–50
Alcohol abuse	1.0–2.0	5–30
Diabetes mellitus	1.5–3.0	4–8
Asymptomatic carotid stenosis	2.0–3.0	1–5
Atrial fibrillation	5.6–17.6	1

[a] Prevalence varies by age, sex, ethnicity, and definition of stroke risk factor.

would be avoided if current recommendations for healthy lifestyles and preventive treatments were universally followed. Stroke is among the most preventable of all catastrophic medical conditions.

Herald events are episodes of cerebral ischemia that indicate the presence of active, stroke-causing conditions, and represent important opportunities for initiation of secondary stroke prevention treatment. Patients who experience transient ischemic attack (TIA) are at substantially increased risk of stroke, with an incidence of 24% to 29% over the 5 years following the TIA. Patients who experience a first ischemic stroke have an even higher incidence of subsequent ischemic stroke, 25% to 40% over the next 5 years. TIAs precede ischemic stroke in 10% to 20% of patients. TIA frequency varies by ischemic stroke subtype. TIAs are most common in large-vessel atherothromboembolic strokes, preceding 40% of events, and less common in lacunar stroke, preceding 20%, and in cardioembolic stroke, preceding 10%. The risk of stroke after a TIA is greatest immediately after the event. Ten percent of patients who have had a TIA experience ischemic stroke within 90 days, and one-half of these occur within the first 2 days after the TIA [15].

TABLE 1-2. POPULATION LEVEL IMPACT OF SELECTED MODIFIABLE RISK FACTORS FOR STROKE

Risk Factor	Population Attributable Risk (%)[a]	Number of Strokes that Could be Prevented Annually in U.S.[b]
Hypertension	49	390,000
Obesity	20	150,000
Hypercholesterolemia	20	150,000
Tobacco use	12	92,000
Alcohol abuse	5	35,000

[a] The population attributable risk estimates the percentage of excess stroke attributable to a given risk factor. The provided estimates do not take into account interactions between risk factors.
[b] The number of strokes that would be prevented if the given risk factor were completely controlled in the U.S. population, derived by multiplying the population attributable risk by the annual number of strokes (750,000).

Individuals with cervicocephalic atherosclerosis may be stratified into different risk levels based on the manifestations of their disease. Patients with a first major ischemic stroke have a higher risk of subsequent ischemic stroke than those with a first minor ischemic stroke, whose risk is higher in turn than those with transient hemispheric ischemic attack, followed by patients with transient monocular blindness and patients with asymptomatic cervical carotid artery stenosis [16,17]. A hierarchy of vascular event risk is presented in Table 1-3.

PATHOPHYSIOLOGY OF ISCHEMIC STROKE

Cerebral Blood Flow and Metabolism

Cerebral ischemia occurs when reduction in cerebral blood flow deprives tissue of the nutrients required for normal cell function and homeostasis. Within minutes of an ischemic insult, a core region of tissue experiences profound blood flow reduction and becomes irreversibly injured, even if blood flow is rapidly restored. However, surrounding this core is a zone of moderate blood flow reduction and ischemic tissue that may still be rescued for several hours or more from symptom onset. This zone has been called the ischemic penumbra and constitutes the target of acute stroke therapy. A variety of definitions have been proposed to demarcate the ischemic penumbra. A straightforward operational approach is to consider the penumbra the zone of tissue that is at risk of infarction, but still salvageable if adequate blood flow is restored.

Changes in cerebral blood flow result in a continuum of metabolic and ionic disturbances that occur in a predictable order (Fig. 1-1) [18]. Studies in animal models of focal stroke suggest that, as blood flow declines, inhibition of protein synthesis begins at values that are mildly below normal (40 to 50 ml/100 g per minute), followed by anaerobic glycolysis (35 ml/100 g per minute), loss of synaptic transmission (20 ml/100 g per minute), and finally anoxic depolarization of cell membranes (15 ml/100 g per minute) [19]. These observations in stroke animal models have been supported by human positron emission tomography (PET) studies. Regional cerebral blood flow (rCBF) below 12 ml/100 g per minute results in tissue necrosis, while only transient deficits occur when rCBF remains above 22 ml/100 g per minute [20]. Tissue with rCBF between 12 ml/100 g and 22 ml/100 g per minute represents the ischemic penumbra, an area of stunned parenchyma surrounding the ischemic core, which has the potential for recovery, but only if reperfusion is rapidly established. New magnetic resonance imaging (MRI) techniques, such as diffusion-perfusion MRI show promise as a practical and clinically useful means to identify the ischemic penumbra in patients with acute stroke (see Workup of the Patient with Stroke and Transient Ischemic Attack section).

In addition to the magnitude of blood flow reduction, the length of time cells are ischemic also determines viabil-

TABLE 1-3. ANNUAL VASCULAR EVENT RATES FOR INDIVIDUALS WITH VARIOUS CLINICAL MANIFESTATIONS OF CERVICOCEPHALIC ATHEROSCLEROTIC DISEASE

Clinical Features	Stroke	Vascular Death	All Death
General elderly population	0.6	1.0	—
Asymptomatic stenosis	1.3	3.4	5.4
Transient monocular blindness	2.2	3.5	4.3
Transient hemispheric ischemic attack	3.7	2.3	4.0
Minor stroke	6.1	3.2	4.9
Major stroke	9.0	3.5	7.6

From Wilterdink J, Easton J. Vascular event rates in patients with atherosclerotic cerebrovascular disease. *Arch Neurol* 1992;49:857–863, with permission.

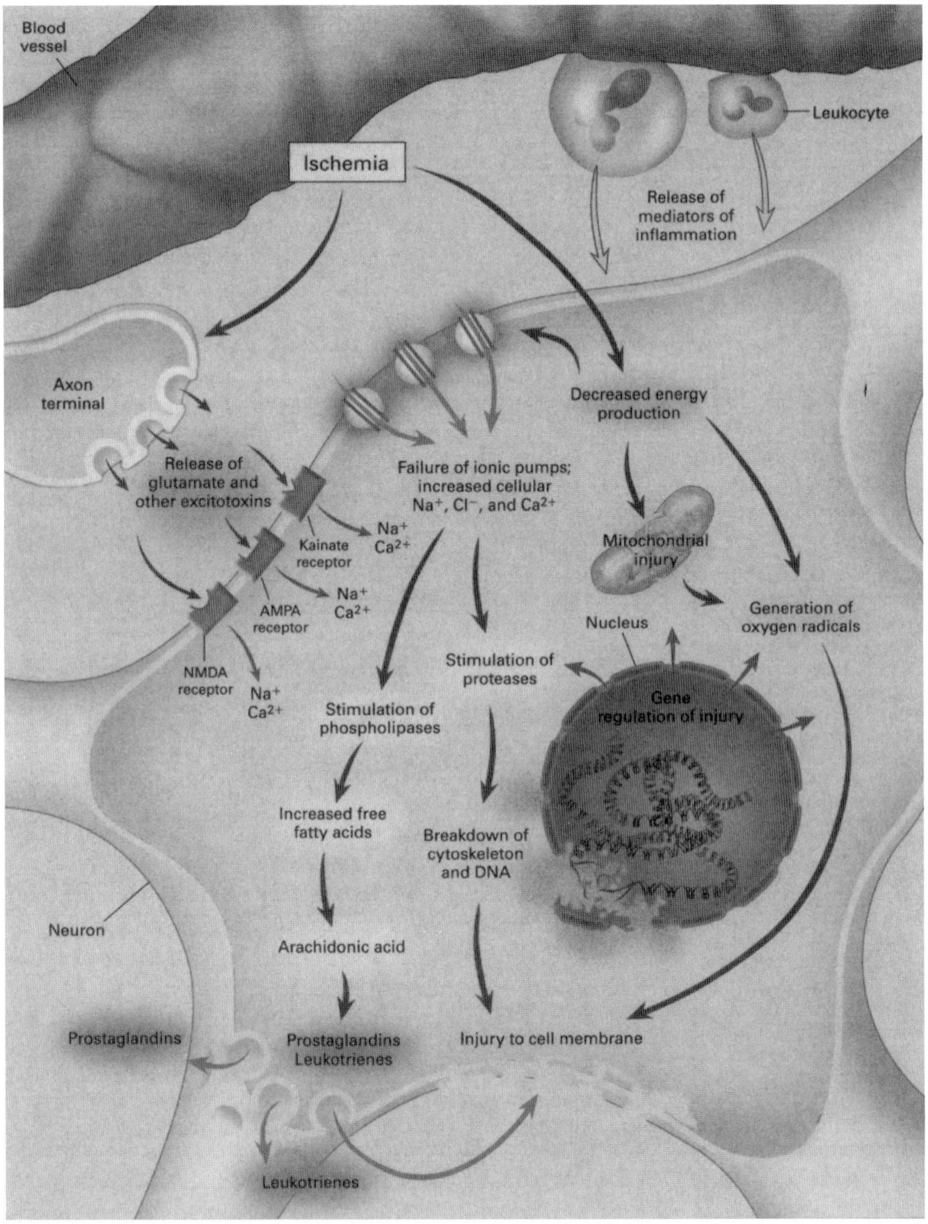

FIGURE 1-1. The ischemic cascade. (From Brott T, Bogousslavsky J. Treatment of acute ischemic stroke. *N Engl J Med* 2000;343:710–722, with permission.) (See Color Figure 1-1.)

ity. Numerous studies indicate the threshold for metabolic and ionic disturbance increases as the duration of ischemia increases [19]. For example, studies have shown that during the first 2 hours of vascular occlusion, the threshold for irreversible suppression of spontaneous neuronal unit activity rises from 5 ml/100 g to 12 ml/100 g per minute [21]. Other studies have shown that when ischemia lasts only a few hours, brain tissue is able to survive flows as low as 12 ml/100 g per minute. However, if the ischemia is permanent, brain necrosis occurs in regions with flows as high as 24 mg/100 g per minute [19]. Thus, the viability of the ischemic area is in flux during the first few hours after stroke onset, its fate determined by the extent and duration of impaired blood flow. However, this dynamic period of potential reversibility is evanescent. Studies in a large number of rodent and nonhuman primate stroke models demonstrate that, in general, significant volumes of neuronal tissue can be salvaged by reperfusion only within the first several hours of ischemia onset [22].

Atherosclerosis

Atherogenesis begins in childhood and progresses throughout the lifespan. The earliest lesions are fibroblastic intimal thickening and deposition of lipids as fatty streaks, evident within the first two decades of life [23]. Fatty streaks are grossly visible as regions of yellowish discoloration of the arterial intimal surface, and microscopically consist of foam cells (lipid-laden macrophages) and extracellular lipids. Fatty streaks are widely distributed throughout the vasculature and do not show the strong focal predilections of more advanced atherosclerotic lesions [24]. Over many years, at arterial branch points or opposite arterial bifurcations, fatty streaks progress to fibrous plaques. Fibrous plaques consist of a central necrotic core of cellular debris and free extracellular lipid and cholesterol crystals, a fibrous cap of foam cells, transformed smooth muscle cells, lymphocytes, and connective tissue matrix, and an overlying, intact endothelial lining. Fibrous plaques progress to complicated plaques, which additionally contain hemosiderin and areas of intraplaque calcification, and demonstrate disruption of the endothelial lining.

Atherogenesis is likely the result of both a response to injury and a lipid dysregulation process, acting synergistically [24]. The response to injury hypothesis suggests that atherogenesis is the result of inflammatory, reparative responses of the vessel wall to various injurious stimuli, including hypertension, hyperlipidemia, tobacco, hemodynamic shear stress, radiation, and homocysteine. Sustained exposure of the vessel wall to local shear factors and additional risk factors insidiously overcomes defensive mechanisms that maintain vascular integrity. Key mediators of this process are adhesion and intimal migration of circulating monocytes due to endothelial disruption and upregulation of cellular adhesion molecules and selectins; smooth muscle cell migration from the adventitia into the intima; cytokine release by macrophages, smooth muscle cells, endothelial cells, and T lymphocytes; and cell death of lipid-laden cells generating a liquid core. The lipid hypothesis suggests that a crucial atherogenic mechanism is production of oxidized low-density lipoprotein (LDL) from increased serum concentrations of LDL, resulting from dietary factors and variations in the lipoprotein receptors that mediate cholesterol trafficking in the liver, the serum, the bile, and vessel plaques. Oxidized LDLs are chemotactic to blood monocytes, cytotoxic to endothelial cells, and promote smooth muscle cell migration and proliferation. The oxidation of LDL is influenced by the balance of prooxidant and antioxidant activity from cellular and molecular elements in the serum and the vessel wall.

Serial ultrasonographic studies of progression of carotid artery atherosclerosis have identified two distinct patterns that occur independently. Diffuse dilative atherosclerosis is slow and continuous, and focal stenotic atherosclerosis is nonlinear, rapid, and unpredictable [25,26]. Plaque stability is determined by the relative proportions of cellular elements, extracellular lipid, and collagen matrix in plaques. Stable atheromas are characterized by a dense fibrous cap with a high content of smooth muscle cells and connective tissue and a relatively small lipid core. Unstable plaques, susceptible to rupture, are characterized by a thin fibrous cap, large lipid core, and inflammation within the cap with activation of macrophages and T lymphocytes. Plaque disruptions preferentially occur in the plaque shoulder region, where inflammatory cells secrete matrix metalloproteinases and other tissue-degrading enzymes, a process that can be accelerated by systemic inflammatory states [27]. Disruption of the plaque surface promotes luminal thrombosis and local vessel occlusion or artery-to-artery embolization [28].

CLINICAL PROFILES AND COURSE

The clinical picture of ischemic stroke depends on both the site and etiology of vessel occlusion. Table 1-4 provides a synopsis of topographic stroke syndromes. Among the different vascular mechanisms producing cerebral infarction, large-artery atherothromboembolism accounts for 35% to 45%, cardioembolism for 30% to 40%, and small-vessel penetrator (lacunar) stroke for 25% to 30%, with the remainder due to hypercoagulable states, vasculitis, migraine, dissection, and other less common causes (Fig. 1-2). Because therapy varies according to ischemic stroke subtype, it is important to recognize the distinctive clinical profiles of the diverse vascular causes of ischemic stroke.

Cervicocephalic Atherosclerosis

Large-vessel atherosclerosis is responsible for 35% to 45% of all ischemic strokes. Whites are prone to develop extracranial carotid atherosclerosis while Asians and African-Ameri-

TABLE 1-4. COMMON NEUROVASCULAR SYNDROMES

Cerebral Artery	Symptoms
Middle cerebral artery (MCA)	Contralateral hemiparesis (face and arm weaker than leg) Contralateral hemisensory loss (face and arm denser than leg) Contralateral visual field deficit Dominant hemisphere Aphasia—global (complete MCA), Broca (superior division), or Wernicke (inferior division) Gerstmann syndrome Nondominant hemisphere Contralateral neglect Constructional apraxia
Anterior choroidal	Contralateral hemiparesis Contralateral hemisensory loss Contralateral visual field defect
Anterior cerebral artery (ACA)	Contralateral leg paresis Contralateral leg hypoesthesia Language dysfunction (mutism, transcortical motor aphasia) Unilateral ideomotor apraxia, alien hand syndrome Primitive reflexes (paratonia, grasp) Abulia
Posterior cerebral artery (PCA)	Contralateral homonymous hemianopsia (occipital) Memory loss (mesial temporal) Contralateral hemisensory loss (thalamus) Alexia without agraphia (dominant hemisphere)
Medial medullary penetrators	Contralateral hemiparesis Contralateral loss of vibration and position sense Ipsilateral CN XII palsy
Lateral medullary circumferential arteries (Wallenberg)	Contralateral loss of pain and temperature sensation Ipsilateral loss of pain and temperature sensation on face Ipsilateral Horner syndrome Dysphagia and dysarthria Ipsilateral dysmetria Vertigo Hiccoughs
Anterior inferior cerebellar artery (AICA)	Ipsilateral deafness Ipsilateral facial palsy and/or gaze palsy or skew deviation Ipsilateral facial sensory loss Contralateral sensory loss
Medial pontine penetrators	Contralateral hemiparesis Ipsilateral CN VI palsy
Lateral pontine circumferential arteries	Ipsilateral CN VIII injury with deafness or tinnitus
Midbrain penetrators	Contralateral hemiparesis Ipsilateral CN III palsy
Superior cerebellar artery (SCA)	Ipsilateral dysmetria and limb movement disorders Ipsilateral Horner syndrome Contralateral pain and temperature sensory loss Contralateral CN IV palsy
Distal basilar artery ("top of the basilar")	Oculomotor—Parinaud syndrome (vertical gaze paresis, lid retraction, skew deviation, impaired convergence) Unilateral or bilateral CN III palsy Pupils: small reactive pupils and ptosis (sympathetic involvement) Behavioral changes: delirium, somnolence, coma Visual field defects: hemianopia, cortical blindness, Balint syndrome
Anterior watershed	Proximal bibrachial paresis (man-in-barrel syndrome) Transcortical motor aphasia
Posterior watershed	Cortical blindness with macular sparing (Anton syndrome—deny deficits) Transcortical sensory aphasia Balint syndrome (simultagnosia, optic ataxia, ocular apraxia)
Lacunar syndromes	
Pure motor hemiparesis	Contralateral face, arm, and leg weakness
Pure sensory stroke	Face, arm, and leg numbness, paresthesias, or pain
Sensorimotor stroke	Contralateral face, arm, and leg weakness and hypoesthesia
Clumsy hand/dysarthria	Dysarthria, dysphagia, facial weakness, tongue deviation, clumsy hand
Ataxic hemiparesis	Ataxia and contralateral weakness

CN, cranial nerve.

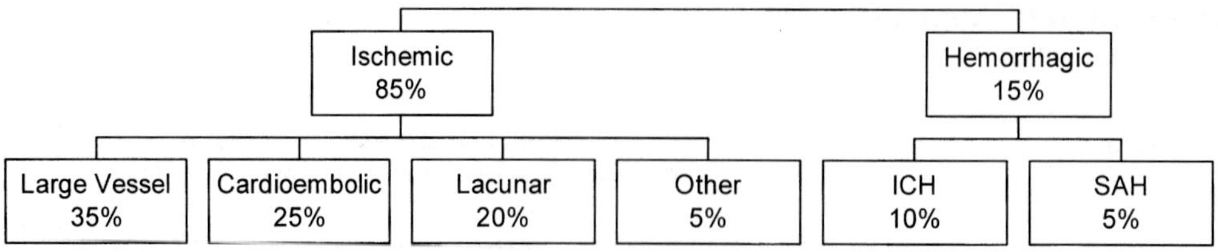

FIGURE 1-2. Frequencies of stroke subtypes among all cases of stroke. Data are approximations based on numerous population-based studies and large hospital stroke registry cohorts in U.S. and European populations.

cans are more disposed to develop intracranial disease [29]. Ischemia related to cervicocephalic atherosclerosis may be caused by one of two principal mechanisms, (a) thromboembolism with obstruction of blood flow due to an embolus arising from the atheroma surface (artery-to-artery embolism, responsible for approximately 80% to 90% of events), and (b) hypoperfusion across a fixed stenosis or occlusion (occurring in isolation in approximately 10% to 20% of events). Frequently, these two mechanisms interact, with hypoperfusion causing inefficient clearing of emboli and poor collateral flow around embolic occlusions [30].

Extracranial Carotid Artery Atherosclerosis

The bifurcation of the common carotid artery is the most frequent site for development of extracranial cervicocephalic atherosclerosis. Plaque structure and characteristics are important determinants of stroke risk. Ulceration and hemorrhage into a plaque represent high-risk sources for distal embolization (Fig. 1-3) [31].

In some cases, carotid stenosis and even eventual occlusion may remain asymptomatic, particularly when progression is gradual, allowing sufficient time for development of adequate collateral circulation. On physical examination, a carotid bruit may provide a clue to the presence of asymptomatic cervical internal carotid stenosis [32]. The differential diagnosis of a cervical bruit includes transmitted cardiac murmurs, hyperdynamic circulatory states, tortuosity without carotid stenosis, and stenoses in the subclavian, vertebral, or external carotid arteries rather than in the common or internal carotid arteries. In various series, 20% to 85% of patients with cervical bruits are found to have hemodynamically significant carotid stenosis, and 25% to 40% of patients with known hemodynamically significant stenosis exhibit a bruit on physical examination.

Clinically important carotid atherosclerosis generally occurs in the most distal portion of the common carotid artery and the most proximal portion of the internal carotid artery, at the level of the carotid bifurcation. In most people, the carotid bifurcation lies high in the neck, near the angle of the jaw. Bruits caused by focal constriction of the internal carotid artery are usually high pitched, very focal, loudest high in the neck, and often not audible at the base.

In contrast, most cervical bruits due to transmitted cardiac murmurs and hyperdynamic circulatory states are low pitched, heard over the entire length of the neck, louder at the base than near the jaw, and even better appreciated over the supraclavicular fossa. With transmitted cardiac murmurs, of course, the murmur will also be detected near its origin over the precordium. One common cause of a hyperdynamic state is when one carotid artery is occluded and flow in the contralateral carotid increases, giving rise to a bruit on the side opposite the disease. Subclavian stenoses are better appreciated over the supraclavicular fossa than the neck.

Bruit amplitude, frequency, and duration provide important clues to severity of stenosis. When stenosis is less than

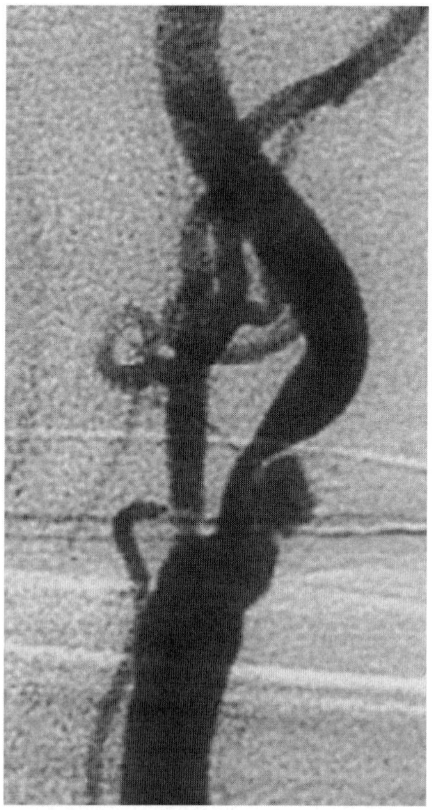

FIGURE 1-3. Cerebral angiogram demonstrating internal carotid artery stenosis. Complex, ulcerated, irregular plaque producing approximately 80% stenosis is demonstrated at the origin of internal carotid artery.

50%, bruits are soft. Loudness grows progressively as arterial narrowing increases up to 90%, but at greater degrees of narrowing, bruit loudness typically diminishes again, becoming soft or inaudible, reflecting diminished flow. Bruit pitch correlates with residual vessel diameter. Low-grade stenoses usually produce relatively low-pitched sounds, with the predominant frequency less than 175 Hz. As the lumen becomes more stenotic, pitch increases. The duration of a carotid bruit increases as the artery narrows, lengthening to throughout systole and then into diastole as stenosis increases.

Findings from palpation of the carotid artery must be interpreted cautiously. The common carotid artery can be palpated in the low and midportions of the neck and the external carotid artery in the high portion of the neck. But the internal carotid artery, the vessel of greatest interest, proceeds posteriorly from the bifurcation and generally cannot be palpated directly. Severe internal carotid stenosis can sometimes lead to slow flow in the feeding common carotid, resulting in a diminished palpable pulse. Increased flow in the external carotid artery, however, can cause a bounding palpable pulse even with severe stenosis or occlusion of the internal carotid artery. Accordingly, carotid artery palpation does not provide reliable information on carotid stenosis.

When symptomatic, internal carotid artery bifurcation atherosclerosis produces ischemia through distal emboli (approximately 50% of cases), sudden local thrombotic occlusion with distal emboli (approximately 25%), sudden local thrombotic occlusion with hemodynamic low flow (approximately 15%), or low-flow hemodynamic insufficiency across a fixed stenosis or occlusion (approximately 10% of cases). Hemispheric embolic ischemic events most frequently localize to the middle cerebral artery and less commonly to the anterior cerebral artery. The exact symptomatology depends on the ultimate destination of an embolus (see Table 1-4) [33,34]. Motor and sensory symptoms most commonly occur together in a contralateral faciobrachial distribution, although isolated face, isolated arm, isolated leg, and combined face and arm motor or sensory loss or both are also not infrequent [35]. Dysarthria is common. Visual symptoms may include loss or distortion of vision in the ipsilateral eye or contralateral hemifield. Aphasia occurs with dominant and neglect with nondominant hemispheric lesions.

Transient monocular visual loss (amaurosis fugax) is an important clue to the presence of underlying carotid disease, although less than one-half of patients with transient monocular visual loss will demonstrate more than 50% carotid stenosis at imaging [33,34]. The pattern of visual loss provides additional information. An altitudinal or lateralized loss in the monocular field, like a descending, ascending, or side-closing curtain, is most strongly predictive of carotid disease, reflecting the focal effects of an artery-to-artery embolus appearing in the retinal circulation [36]. Other patterns, such as diffuse loss of vision simultaneously throughout the monocular visual field or concentric constriction inward from the periphery, less frequently reflect carotid lesions. Episodes in the same patient of transient monocular blindness and ipsilateral hemispheral TIAs are highly suggestion of extracranial carotid disease.

A less-common manifestation of carotid distribution TIA is loss of vision precipitated by exposure to sunlight [37]. The visual loss is diffuse rather than altitudinal or sectorial. Recovery occurs when the patient returns to a darker environment, over minutes to hours. These episodes have been associated with severe obstructive carotid disease ipsilateral to the affected eye. The presumed mechanism is slowed regeneration of retinal pigment due to energetic compromise from chronic borderline ischemia.

Rarely, positive motor phenomena—transient limb-shaking episodes—may be attributed to ischemia in the distribution of the carotid arteries [38]. These episodes are commonly confused with simple partial motor seizures. However, they are characteristically precipitated by postural changes, walking, or neck hyperextension. Also, while the movements are involuntary, coarse, and often unilateral, they are nonrhythmic. Spell duration is seconds to minutes, and movement frequencies approximate 3 to 12 Hz. During the episode there is no alteration in consciousness. Limb shaking during ischemic episodes appears to be caused by disinhibition of subcortical motor circuitry. These spells almost invariably represent hemodynamic, rather than embolic, TIAs and are often associated with ipsilateral carotid occlusion.

Extracranial Vertebral Artery Atherosclerosis

Atherosclerosis in the proximal extracranial vertebral artery (V1 segment) occurs in 25% of patients with cerebrovascular symptoms, and is the sole identifiable cause of stroke in up to 10% of patients with posterior circulation cerebral infarction [39]. Infarcts most often are due to artery-to-artery embolism, with the most common recipient vessels being the posterior inferior cerebellar artery and the posterior cerebral artery. Preceding TIAs or dizziness and visual disturbance may occur. Strokes are abrupt in onset. Dizziness and ataxia are the most common symptoms, but some patients with posterior cerebral artery infarction have isolated hemianopia. Hemodynamic cerebral ischemia is uncommon due to the convergence of the vertebral arteries to form the basilar artery, allowing compensatory flow for an interrupted vessel. However, patients with bilateral vertebral artery disease may have frequent TIAs and stroke, with symptoms of faintness, blurred vision, dizziness, and bilateral weakness [39,40].

Intracranial Atherosclerosis

Although large-vessel intracranial atherosclerotic disease is less common than extracranial carotid stenosis, it remains an important cause of ischemic stroke. In one series of 438 patients undergoing stroke evaluation, intracranial atherosclerosis was found in 8% of cases [41]. Recent technologic advances, including refined angiography as well as noninvasive imaging techniques (e.g., magnetic resonance angiography [MRA], computerized tomographic angiography [CTA], and transcranial Doppler [TCD] ultrasonography) have provided detailed characterization of these lesions not routinely available 20 or 30 years ago. Stereotyped recurrent TIAs often provide clues to the presence of an underlying intracranial stenosis.

Atherosclerosis may develop within the carotid siphon, usually distal to the ophthalmic artery origin. Ischemic symptoms due to carotid siphon disease most commonly involve the middle cerebral artery territory and, less commonly, the anterior cerebral artery and border-zone territories (see Table 1-4).

Atherosclerosis of the middle cerebral artery most commonly involves the M1 stem, often proximal to the takeoff of the lenticulostriate arteries [42]. Ischemic events may result from complete occlusion at the site of the stenosis, emboli to distal middle cerebral artery branches, border-zone ischemia in the setting of low perfusion, or less commonly lacunar syndromes due to blockage of the origins of the lenticulostriate vessels. Over 60% of infarcts seen in the presence of middle cerebral artery atherosclerosis are confined to the superficial middle cerebral artery territory, sparing the deep penetrators [43]. TIAs precede more than 50% of atherosclerotic middle cerebral artery infarcts and have a mean duration of 1 to 2 hours, decidedly longer than that typical of extracranial internal carotid artery disease. When infarction occurs, the onset is often stuttering, with progression occurring over days or weeks [44]. The anterior cerebral artery is less commonly affected by *in situ* atherosclerosis. Infarctions in this territory often lead to leg weakness, language dysfunction, and occasionally disconnection syndromes.

Atherosclerosis of the intracranial posterior circulation most commonly involves the vertebral artery at the origin of the posterior inferior cerebellar artery, the vertebrobasilar junction, or the proximal or middle basilar artery. Atherosclerotic disease of the intracranial vertebral artery may be a source of distal emboli to the distal basilar artery, cerebellar arteries, or the posterior cerebral arteries. Complete occlusion or tight stenosis of one vertebral artery may be asymptomatic if there is sufficient flow through the other vertebral artery.

Basilar artery occlusive syndromes depend on the site of the lesion and time course [45]. The proximal and middle thirds of the basilar artery are more susceptible to atherosclerotic change than the distal basilar, but only slightly so. In a review of 412 reported cases of basilar artery atherostenotic disease, the proximal segment was affected in 48%, the middle in 56%, and the distal in 40% [46]. Patterns of vessel injury include intrinsic atherosclerosis confined to the basilar artery, complex plaques arising in a distal intracranial vertebral artery extending into the proximal basilar artery, and diffuse, disseminated vertebral and basilar atherosclerosis. Unilateral or bilateral pontine dysfunction and, less often, cerebellar, midbrain, occipital, or temporal ischemia are typical manifestations. Large-vessel pontine ischemia commonly is associated with long-tract motor dysfunction, alteration in the level of consciousness, and oculomotor abnormalities, especially disordered horizontal eye movement. The most characteristic motor manifestation is an asymmetric quadriparesis, although hemiparesis, hemiplegia, and quadriplegia do occur. Proximal basilar syndromes may be limited to pontine ischemia if there is adequate retrograde flow from the anterior circulation to the distal basilar through the posterior communicating arteries.

Infarcts due to proximal and middle basilar artery stenosis or occlusion are preceded by TIAs in three-fourths of cases. Often one or more TIAs culminate in infarction over a 3- to 6-month period. Infarcts often progress with a stuttering course of stepwise worsening over minutes, hours, or days, although abrupt onset of a maximal deficit may occur. Outcomes in recent series suggest that about one-half of patients have severe or moderate residual deficits, an occasional patient has a fatal outcome, and the remainder show minimal or no impairment. Distal basilar occlusion may lead to a "top of the basilar" syndrome (see Table 1-4), with involvement of the midbrain, thalami, superior cerebellar hemispheres, or occipital lobes, singly or in combination [45].

Aortic Arch Atherosclerosis

Atherosclerosis of the ascending aorta and aortic arch is increasingly recognized as an important source of cerebral embolism [47]. The French Study of Aortic Plaques in Stroke Group found atherosclerotic plaques 4 mm or thicker in 14.4% of patients with ischemic stroke compared with 2% of controls. This study demonstrated that aortic plaques 4 mm or thicker were independent predictors of recurrent brain infarction and other vascular events [48]. Protruding, complex, and freely mobile plaques carry a particularly high embolic potential. Dislodging of atherosclerotic material during manipulation of the ascending and transverse aorta during cardiopulmonary bypass is an important mechanism of intraoperative stroke [49].

Nonatherosclerotic Arteriopathies

Dissection

Cervicocephalic cerebral dissections account for approximately 1% to 2% of all ischemic strokes [50–52]. However, dissections are a common and important cause of stroke in younger patients, with pediatric and young adult stroke series showing an incidence of 10% to 25% [53]. Dissections, or tears in the arterial wall, are defined by the occurrence of an intramural hematoma. Seventy-five percent of dissections involve the cervical internal carotid artery and 15% the cervical vertebral arteries [50]. Less common locations include the intracranial carotid arteries, middle cerebral arteries, intracranial vertebral arteries, and the basilar artery. Approximately 15% of patients will have multiple vessels involved (Fig. 1-4).

Up to one-half of patients have a history of some form of precipitating minor or major trauma, such as a sports or whiplash injury or chiropractic neck manipulation. Cerebral dissection has also been associated with a variety of disorders including fibromuscular dysplasia, connective tissue disorders such as Marfan's syndrome, and migraine headaches [50,54].

Typically, a dissection alters vascular anatomy in one of two ways. With an intimal-medial tear, the inner vessel wall protrudes inward causing narrowing and compromise of the vessel lumen. If the tear is between the medial and adventitial layers, an outpouching dissecting aneurysm may occur.

The clinical features and neurologic symptoms of cerebral dissections are generally due to either local effects of the dissecting hemorrhage or consequent cerebral ischemia. Local effects caused by a dissecting intramural hematoma include headache or neck pain, which occurs in up to 75% of patients with dissections. Horner syndrome may develop as a result of stretching of sympathetic fibers that travel along the internal carotid artery in the neck or because of an infarct in the medulla in a vertebral artery dissection. Cranial neuropathies, particularly involving cranial nerves XI and XII, are caused by dissecting aneurysms expanding outward and compressing adjacent structures. Pulsatile tinnitus can occur from abnormal or turbulent blood flow patterns. A lateral medullary infarct (Wallenberg syndrome) is particularly common in patients with vertebral artery dissections due to involvement of the posterior inferior cerebellar artery.

Ischemic symptoms may be due to low-flow hemodynamic insufficiency caused by significant local lumen compromise, or more often to distal embolization of clots formed at the site of the dissection. If the dissection occurs intracranially, subarachnoid hemorrhage may occur. Cerebral ischemia in association with head pain, neck pain, with or without Horner syndrome, should always raise the suspicion of possible dissection.

Migraine

Epidemiologic studies have shown an association between migraine and stroke [55,56]. The annual incidence of stroke among adults with migraine has been estimated to be 3.36 in 100,000 [57]. Several studies have suggested an especially strong association between migraine and stroke in women under the age of 45 [58]. In one series, women with migraine with aura had a sixfold increase in stroke risk, with further increases among those with a history of tobacco or oral contraceptive use [59].

Migraine headaches may be associated with stroke in one of the three following ways: (a) a patient may have an unrelated migraine disorder—chance association likely occurs frequently due to the high incidence of migraine in the general population, (b) an ischemic stroke may provoke a migraine event [60], or (c) a migraine may be the actual cause of a cerebral infarct.

True migrainous infarction is relatively rare, being responsible for less than 1% of ischemic strokes overall. In various pediatric and young adult stroke series, migraine-induced stroke accounts for 2% to 33% of ischemic strokes, with a clustering at approximately 10%. Migrainous stroke is usually ischemic rather than hemorrhagic. Specific criteria to make the diagnosis of migraine-induced stroke have been proposed [61]. To meet these criteria, a patient must have the following:

1. Migraine occurs with aura (although cases of apparent migrainous stroke have also been reported in patients with migraine without aura) [59,62].
2. The migraine attack appearing to provoke the stroke must be phenomenologically identical to prior migraine attacks.

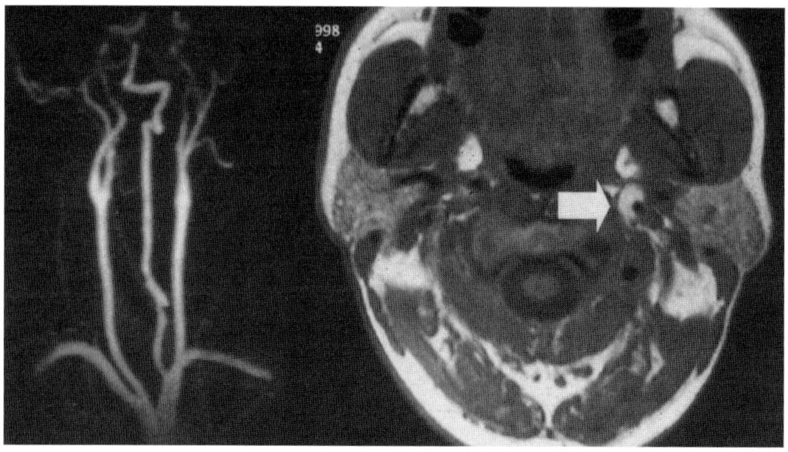

FIGURE 1-4. Patient with simultaneous dissection of four cervicocerebral vessels. **Left:** Contrast-enhanced magnetic resonance angiogram demonstrates dissecting aneurysm in proximal left vertebral artery; narrowed, irregular right vertebral artery from origin upward; and tapering stenoses in both internal carotid arteries distally. **Right:** Axial T1 MR image shows pathognomonic crescent sign *(arrow)* with stenotic lumen *(small flow void)* and surrounding crescent of high signal indicating intramural hematoma.

3. Neurologic deficit must persist for longer than 7 days or neuroimaging must confirm infarction or both.
4. Finally, other causes must be excluded.

The pathogenesis of migrainous stroke is still not well understood. It has been suggested that the frequency and duration of migraine episodes are significant factors. Theories include vasospasm, dissection, endothelial hyperplasia, and hypercoagulability. Some investigators have reported an association between patent foramen ovale, migraine, and stroke [63,64]. Others have suggested an association between antiphospholipid antibodies and migrainous stroke in young patients [65]. When migrainous infarction does occur, there is a propensity for involvement of the occipital lobes in the territory of the posterior cerebral artery [66].

The long-term recurrence rate for patients with migrainous stroke is unclear. Some series report a low frequency of further stroke [66,67], while others have reported that one-third of patients had subsequent recurrent events [68].

Cerebral autosomal arteriopathy associated with subcortical infarcts and leukoencephalopathy (CADASIL) is an inherited disorder characterized by progressive subcortical ischemic infarcts and dementia, often associated with migraine-like headaches. CADASIL is caused by mutations in the notch 3 gene on chromosome 19, which encodes a transmembrane receptor protein [12,69].

Fibromuscular Dysplasia

Fibromuscular dysplasia (FMD) is caused by a poorly understood nonatherosclerotic abnormality of the smooth muscle, fibrous, or elastic tissue within vessel walls. The renal arteries are most often affected, with cervicocerebral vessels involved in 25% of cases, the internal carotid and vertebral arteries being the most frequent sites. Multivessel involvement is common.

FMD is a disorder with a high female predominance that in some cases is familial [12]. Cervicocephalic FMD is often asymptomatic and discovered incidentally. Neurologic symptoms may include headaches, pulsatile tinnitus, TIAs, or stroke. These symptoms may be due to direct, compressive effects of the disrupted vessel wall, or may be due to global or focal ischemia. Ischemic events may result from thromboemboli originating from the irregular vessel wall, spontaneous vessel dissection, or hemodynamic insufficiency due to progressive stenosis [70]. The diagnosis is generally made by magnetic resonance (MR), computed tomography (CT), or catheter angiography, which demonstrate a characteristic string-of-beads appearance with intermittent areas or narrowing and dilation.

Vasculitis

Vasculitis affecting the central nervous system (CNS) remains an intriguing but poorly understood entity that poses diagnostic and treatment challenges for physicians and patients alike. Vasculitis (or angiitis) is defined as an inflammation of blood vessels. Most experts distinguish primary (or isolated) angiitis of the CNS from secondary causes (systemic vasculitides, connective tissue disorders, drugs or toxins, malignancy, or infections) [71]. CNS vasculitis can be classified by the size and the type of vessels affected or more commonly by the underlying pathogenic mechanism (Table 1-5).

TABLE 1-5. DIFFERENTIAL DIAGNOSIS AND CLASSIFICATION OF CENTRAL NERVOUS SYSTEM VASCULITIDES

Primary CNS Vasculitides	Primary angiitis of the central nervous system Cogan syndrome Eales disease
Secondary CNS Vasculitides	
Systemic vasculitides	Polyarteritis nodosa Giant cell arteritis (temporal arteritis) Takayasu arteritis Wegener granulomatosis Henoch-Schönlein purpura Mixed essential cryoglobulinemia Churg-Strauss syndrome Other hypersensitivity vasculitides Bechets disease Neurosarcoidosis
Connective tissue diseases	Systemic lupus erythematosus Rheumatoid arthritis Scleroderma Mixed connective tissue disease Sjögren syndrome Ankylosing spondylitis Reiter syndrome
Malignancy	Hodgkin lymphoma Non-Hodgkin lymphoma Leukemia Metastatic small cell lung cancer Lymphomatoid granulomatosis
Infections	Bacterial meningoencephalitis Basilar meningitis—fungal, AFB Syphilis Lyme disease Viral, retroviral Protozoal Mycoplasmal Rickettsial
Drug induced or toxins	Cocaine Amphetamine Ephedrine Allopurinol Phenylpropanolamine Ergotamine Heroin
Other	Inflammatory bowel disease Acute posterior multifocal placoid pigment Epitheliopathy Cerebral amyloid angiopathy

CNS, central nervous system; AFB, acid-fast bacteria.

CNS vasculitis, either primary or secondary to other disease states, is relatively rare, although it is an important entity to consider in the differential diagnosis of stroke in the young. Clinical manifestations of CNS vasculitis are varied and often nonspecific, including ischemic or hemorrhagic stroke, encephalopathy, headache, cranial neuropathies, and occasionally myelopathy. The onset may be acute, subacute, or insidious and the course self-limiting, indolent, or fulminant. The clinical picture generally depends on the size, distribution, extent, and location of vessels involved. Other systemic signs or symptoms (fever, arthritis, arthralgias, rash, pulmonary or renal dysfunction) may provide clues to secondary causes (rheumatologic syndromes, infections).

On histologic analysis, involved vessels demonstrate infiltration of one or more layers by inflammatory cells including polymorphonuclear cells, mononuclear cells, giant cells, and occasionally eosinophils. The inflammatory response causes structural injury within the vessel wall, often with fibrinoid necrosis. Luminal narrowing or obstruction results in ischemia; wall injury may lead to aneurysm formation with resultant hemorrhage.

Diagnosis of CNS vasculitis relies on a high index of suspicion based on the symptomatology, combined with thorough laboratory, radiographic, and tissue evaluation (Table 1-6). The diagnosis is often difficult to make, and no single test is both highly sensitive and specific. In 50% to 90% of patients, cerebral spinal fluid (CSF) analysis reveals nonspecific inflammatory changes [72,73]. CSF analyses should include viral, fungal, and bacterial cultures, bacterial antigen assays, viral PCR (polymerized chain reaction) testing (varicella zoster virus [VZV], herpes simplex virus [HSV]), and cytology to search for an underlying infectious or neoplastic process.

Brain CT and MRI demonstrate areas of ischemia or, less commonly, hemorrhage in up to 65% of patients [72, 74]. MRA and CTA may demonstrate abnormalities (vessel narrowings or occlusions) in patients with vasculitic involvement of the large basal vessels; however, these findings may be nonspecific.

Cerebral angiography should be routinely performed in suspected cases of CNS vasculitis. Abnormalities suggestive of a vasculitic or vasculopathic process occur in 70% to 75% of patients [75,76]. These abnormalities include segmental narrowings and dilations that create a "beading" appearance (seen in 30% of cases). The vascular narrowings may be caused by vessel wall infiltration and inflammation, compression by meningeal or parenchymal infiltration of inflammatory cells, or possibly vasospasm [77]. The study may be negative if the vasculitis primarily affects small vessels beyond the resolution of angiography. It is important to recognize that a specific diagnosis of CNS vasculitis can not be made by angiography alone, because a variety of noninflammatory vasculopathies may mimic the radiographic appearance of vasculitis.

TABLE 1-6. DIAGNOSTIC WORKUP FOR CENTRAL NERVOUS SYSTEM VASCULITIDES

- Serum
  - CBC with platelets
  - Chemistry panel
  - Lipid panel[a]
  - PT/PTT
  - ESR
  - ANA, dsDNA
  - RNP[a]
  - Rheumatoid factor
  - Cryocrit/cryoglobulins[a]
  - ANCA
  - C3/C4, CH-50
  - C reactive protein[a]
  - Cold agglutinins[a]
  - SCL70[a]
  - Anti-Smith antibody[a]
  - Anti-Ro and anti-La antibodies (SSA, SSB)[a]
  - Circulating immunocomplexes (Raji test)[a]
  - ACE[a]
  - VDRL
  - HIV
  - HTLV-I[a]
  - Serum protein electropheresis/immunoelectropheresis[a]
  - Hepatitis serology
  - Cocci titers[a]
  - PEG (immune complex)[a]
  - Hypercoagulable workup, including antiphospholipid antibodies (DRVVT, aCL antibody)[a]
  - Lyme titers
  - Blood cultures
- Urine
  - Urinalysis
  - Cultures
- Chest radiograph
- Lumbar puncture
  - Cell count, glucose, protein
  - VDRL
  - Cytology
  - Angiotensin-converting enzyme
  - IgG synthesis, oligoclonal bands
  - Cultures
  - Viral titers and PCRs (VZV)
- MRI with gadolinium
- Angiogram
- Brain biopsy[a]
- MRA or CTA
- Ophthalmologic examination, including fluorescein angiography
- Transthoracic or transesophageal echocardiography or both
- Indium-labeled white blood cell scanning[a]

CBC, complete blood count; PT, prothrombin time; PTT, partial thromboplastin time; ESR, erythrocyte sedimentation rate; ANA, antinuclear antibodies; dsDNA, double-stranded DNA; RNP, ribonucleoprotein; ANCA, anti-neutrophil cytoplasmic autoantibodies; C3, esterase inhibitor; C4, complement; CH-50, total functional hemolytic complement; SCL70, anti-scl70 antibodies; ACE, angiotensin-converting enzyme; VDRL, Venereal Disease Research Laboratory (test); HIV, human immunodeficiency virus; HTLV-I, human T-cell lymphocytotrophic virus-I; DRVVT, dilute Russell's viper venom titer; aCL, anticardiolipin; IgG, immunoglobulin G; VZV, varicella zoster virus; MRI, magnetic resonance imaging; MRA, magnetic resonance angiography; CTA, computed tomographic angiography.

[a] Select patients.

In general, histopathologic examination is required for a definitive diagnosis. However, even biopsy (combined leptomeningeal and cortical biopsy has the highest yield) is positive in only 70% of cases due to the patchy nature of the disease [78–80].

Cardioembolic Stroke

General Profile

Intracardiac thrombi arise in conditions of blood stasis (atrial fibrillation, acute myocardial infarction, cardiomyopathy), endothelial disruption (acute myocardial infarction, prosthetic cardiac valve), and systemic coagulopathy (nonbacterial thrombotic endocarditis). Infectious debris, tumors, fibrin strands, bland vegetations, and valvular calcific material also may embolize from heart to brain [81]. Transcardiac emboli arise when a venous embolus traverses an intracardiac shunt, avoiding filtering by the pulmonary circulation, to gain access to the arterial system. In the past, travel of embolic material from the heart to the cerebral circulation was thought to be a rare event that was almost invariably symptomatic. Transcranial Doppler ultrasonographic cerebral monitoring studies, however, have shown that high-risk cardiac sources often shed microembolic particles several times a day, even several times an hour [82, 83]. Fortunately, brain collateral micro circulation copes with this constant barrage remarkably well, preventing symptomatic ischemia in the preponderance of embolic episodes, and failing only when larger macroemboli compromise a greater volume of the cerebral circulation.

Emboli of cardiac origin tend to lodge at discrete sites in the cerebral circulation: at the terminal portion of arteries just prior to arterial branching, at foci of atheroma, and in distal intracranial arterial branches [84]. Small, deep, penetrating vessels are rarely recipients of cardiac emboli [85]. The distal basilar artery ("top of the basilar"), the terminus of the supraclinoid internal carotid artery ("carotid T"), and the terminus of the middle cerebral artery stem are favored recipient sites, where emboli too large to enter smaller branch vessels tend to arrest. Among distal intracranial vessels, the distribution of cardiac emboli is influenced by the tendency of symptom-causing embolic particles of cardiac origin to be larger than symptom-causing embolic particles of arterial origin [86]. Larger particle size and solid particle composition interact with recipient vessel lumen size acuity of branching angle, and position relative to gravity to dispose entry of cardiac emboli into the inferior rather than superior division of the middle cerebral artery, and the superior rather than inferior branches of the posterior cerebral artery [87].

Cardioembolism is characterized by large emboli traveling from a proximal site to lodge in a circulation unprepared by chronic ischemia to tolerate blood flow reduction. These pathophysiologic factors determine the distinctive clinical profile of cardioembolic stroke. Cerebral infarcts due to emboli of cardiac origin are usually abrupt in onset, with a deficit that is maximal from the start [88,89]. Progressive worsening generally does not occur. Sometimes, however, marked improvement transpires after a delay when an embolus spontaneously fragments, a phenomenon that has been christened the *spectacular shrinking deficit* [90]. Early diminished level of consciousness is more common in cardioembolic than in noncardioembolic stroke [88]. Neurologic deficits suggesting cortical compromise, rather than isolated subcortical insult, are common, including aphasia, neglect, and visual field defects [91,92].

Cardioembolic strokes are preceded by TIAs infre-

TABLE 1-7. SELECTED CARDIAC SOURCES OF EMBOLI

Arrhythmias
Atrial fibrillation[a]
Atrial flutter
Sick sinus syndrome[a]
Myocardial Infarction
Recent anterior wall myocardial infarction[a]
Ventricular aneurysm[a]
Mural thrombi[a]
Recent inferior wall myocardial infarction
Akinetic left ventricular segment[a]
Cardiomyopathies
Severe dilated cardiomyopathy[a]
Mild-to-moderate dilated cardiomyopathy
Valvular Disease
Native Valves
Rheumatic mitral stenosis[a]
Rheumatic aortic stenosis[a]
Bacterial endocarditis[a]
Nonbacterial thrombotic endocarditis[a]
Mitral valve prolapse
Mitral annulus calcification
Mitral valve strands
Mitral stenosis
Bicuspid aortic valve
Calcific aortic stenosis
Prosthetic Valves
Mechanical[a]
Bioprosthetic
Intracardiac Lesions
Myxomas[a]
Malignant cardiac tumors
Fibroelastomas
Metastatic tumors
Septal Abnormalities (Paradoxical Embolism)
Patent foramen ovale (PFO)
Other large atrial septal defect (ASD)[a]
Ventricular septal defect[a]
Atrial septal aneurysm[a]

[a] Indicates high-risk cardioembolic sources. Remainder are low-to-medium risk.

quently, perhaps in 10% of cases. When TIAs do occur, they may involve different vascular distributions in different episodes (as opposed to the more stereotyped TIAs of large-vessel atherosclerotic or small-vessel disease, occurring in the same vascular bed each time). Cardioembolic TIAs also tend to be of long duration, often 1 hour or more.

Causes

Cardiac sources of embolism may be classified by mechanism and embolic risk (Table 1-7). Atrial fibrillation is the most common cause of cardioembolism, accounting for 45% of cardioembolic strokes. Wall motion abnormalities following acute myocardial infarction account for 15%, chronic dilated cardiomyopathy and ventricular aneurysm for 7.5%, rheumatic valvular disease for 7.5%, prosthetic cardiac valves for 10%, and patent foramen ovale, atrial septal aneurysm, endocarditis, and other rarer causes for the remaining 15% [93].

Lacunar and Long Pial Penetrator Stroke

Lacunar Infarct

Lacunes are small infarcts, generally 1 to 15 mm in diameter, occurring in the territory of single, deep, penetrating arteries. These vessels arise at right angles to much larger parent arteries and penetrate the brain parenchyma, with few collateral connections between one penetrating vessel and the next. Lacunar infarcts most commonly occur in the internal capsule, centrum semiovale, basal ganglia, thalamus, pons, and deep cerebellar nuclei (Fig. 1-5).

Intracranial atheromatous branch disease is the vascular lesion usually responsible for symptomatic lacunar infarcts. Subtypes of intracranial atheromatous branch disease include microatheromas arising in the penetrating arteries themselves, parent-artery atheroma occluding the orifices of penetrating branches, and junctional plaques in which atheroma originating in the parent artery extends into the penetrating vessel [94,95]. Lipohyalinosis is a frequently coexisting process in which penetrating arteries show fibrinoid degeneration without atheroma. Lipohyalinosis tends to produce very small infarcts, smaller than 5 mm, that are individually asymptomatic [96]. Embolism, from a proximal arterial, cardiac, or transcardiac source, is an uncommon cause of lacunar infarcts, because embolic particles typically flow along the parent artery without diverting perpendicularly into small penetrators.

Several clinical syndromes have been described that suggest lacunar infarcts, because they localize to deep fiber tracts or nuclei commonly affected by discrete penetrator vessels [97]. Over 70 lacunar infarct syndromes have been recorded [98], but five classic syndromes account for 75% of cases [99]. Pure motor hemiparesis is characterized by isolated face, arm, or leg weakness on one side of the body. The causative lesion is in the pyramidal tract, two-thirds of the time at the level of the internal capsule or corona radiata, and one-third of the time at the level of the basis pontis.

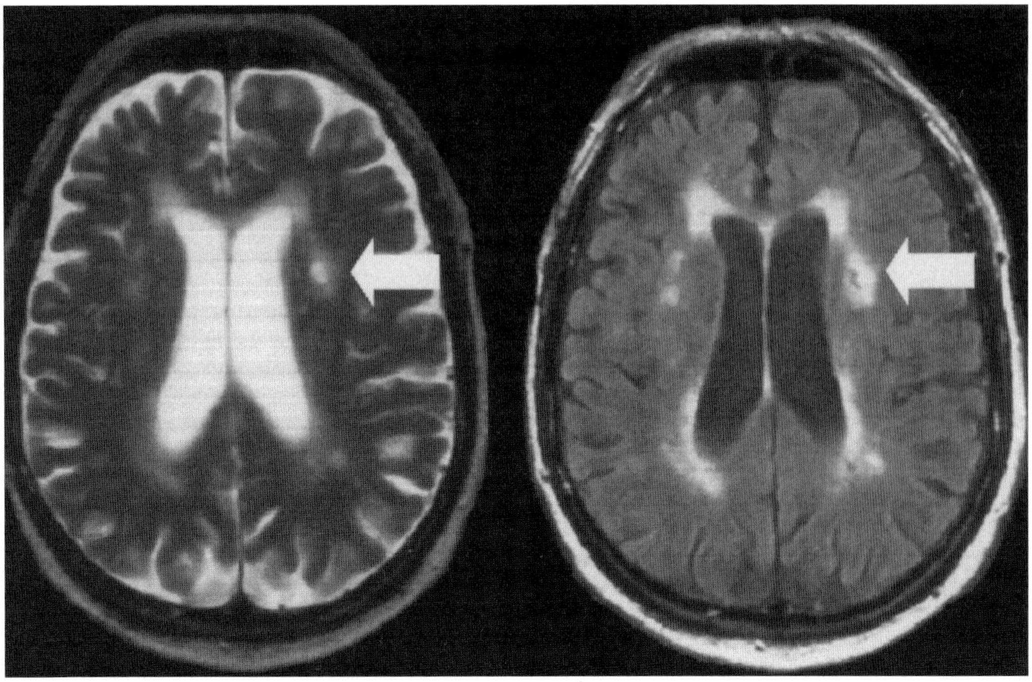

FIGURE 1-5. MRI demonstrating lacunar infarct. **Left:** T2-weighted image shows focus of hyperintensity in the left centrum semiovale *(arrow)*. **Right:** FLAIR image demonstrates central hypointensity and surrounding hyperintensity at this site *(arrow)*.

Pure sensory stroke is manifested as hypoesthesia of the face, arm, or leg. Most cases are due to an infarct in the ventroposterolateral thalamus, with lateral medullary, other brainstem, and thalamoparietal radiation lesions seen infrequently. Pure sensorimotor stroke is characterized by combined motor and sensory deficits of the face, arm, or leg, without aphasia, neglect, or other deficits. The most common lesion is in the internal capsule and corona radiata trespassing upon the thalamus, with pontine sites also described. Ataxic hemiparesis is characterized by homolateral ataxia and hemiparesis, and it reflects a small lesion disrupting both the pyramidal tract to produce the weakness and the adjoining frontopontocerebellar tracts to produce disproportionate incoordination. Common causative sites are pericapsular and pontine. Dysarthria–clumsy hand syndrome has the features its name announces, and also is most frequently due to pericapsular and pontine lesions.

Lacunar infarcts most commonly show a rapid onset of near-maximal deficit, but 10% to 30% evolve slowly or in stepwise fashion over hours to days [96,100]. About 20% are preceded by TIAs.

Long Pial Penetrator Infarct

Long pial penetrator infarcts are closely allied in pathophysiology and clinical profiles to lacunar infarcts. Central regions of the cerebral white matter at the level of the top of the ventricles are supplied by long, penetrating arteries, arising perpendicularly from substantially larger pial surface arteries coursing over the convexity of the brain. The pial penetrators are subject to branch atheromatous disease, lipohyalinosis, marked tortuosity, and artery-to-artery embolism from arterial sources. Occlusion of a pial penetrator may produce a discrete infarct in the centrum semiovale [101]. Symptom onset is often slow or stuttering. Because of the more expansive spatial distribution of fiber systems at this level of the brain, the resulting clinical deficits may be more fractionated than with deep infarcts, and include pure motor hemiparesis, pure sensory stroke, and ataxic hemiparesis.

WORKUP OF THE PATIENT WITH STROKE AND TRANSIENT ISCHEMIC ATTACK

The goals of the evaluation of a patient with TIA or ischemic stroke are to (a) determine whether an immediate complication is likely, (b) confirm that ischemic stroke, and not a mimic, is the cause of the focal deficit, (c) assess the reversibility of the pathology, (d) obtain clues to the likely vascular mechanism and etiology, and (e) institute appropriate treatment.

History

If the patient is a candidate for acute interventions, establishing the time of stroke onset is especially important. When onset cannot be specified precisely, the ischemia duration clock is started from the time the patient was last known to be well. This convention applies to patients who awaken with their deficits, who are found down and uncommunicative, or who simply are unable to communicate clearly when their deficit started.

Other essential history questions focus on ruling out stroke mimics (seizures, intoxications, head trauma, complicated migraine headaches, and acute systemic infections) and provisionally characterizing the stroke mechanism. The presence of cervical trauma and neck pain may point toward a diagnosis of dissection. Headaches and nausea raise the possibility of intracerebral hemorrhage or brainstem infarction. The tempo of deficit onset is ascertained. Registry studies suggest that strokes with maximal disability at onset but without headache are most often found to be embolic, either cardiac or artery-to-artery, while those with a fluctuating course are more likely due to thrombosis [102,103]. A history of multiple prior TIAs in the same circulation suggests an atherothrombotic mechanism. A steadily expanding deficit over 5 to 20 minutes is typical of intracerebral hemorrhage.

Inquiring about previous medical conditions also can shed light on the stroke mechanism. Patients suffering from cardiac disease including arrhythmia, valvular disease, ventricular aneurysm, patent foramen ovale, and congestive heart failure are prone to cardioembolic events. A history of hypertension, coronary artery disease, tobacco use, diabetes, or claudication is associated with large-vessel atherothrombosis. Hypertension and, to a lesser degree, tobacco use and diabetes also are often seen in patients with lacunar infarcts.

Physical Examination

The goals of the initial exam are to determine patient level of consciousness, stroke severity, stroke localization, and stroke etiology [18,104]. Careful neurovascular examination includes auscultating the heart for the presence of gallops, murmurs, or arrhythmias. The peripheral vascular system is examined by palpating the radial, femoral, and pedal pulses to determine strength and regularity. The carotid artery is palpated and the neck auscultated for bruits. The funduscopic examination provides a unique opportunity to visualize blood vessels directly. Signs of internal carotid artery disease include cholesterol crystals, retinal infarctions, and venous stasis retinopathy. Unexplained fever or nuchal rigidity raise the possibility of other diagnoses such as meningitis or other infection, or subarachnoid hemorrhage. Coma is extremely uncommon in acute ischemic stroke, and it suggests intracerebral or subarachnoid hemorrhage, or metabolic causes and processes other than stroke.

The neurologic examination includes screening of mental state, including tests of aphasia and neglect; cranial nerve evaluation including visual field and ocular motility testing;

motor, coordination, sensory, reflex, and gait examination. The pattern of findings permits localization to the anterior or posterior circulations and their subdivisions. Use of a formalized examination scale permits quantification of stroke severity. In widest use is the National Institutes of Health Stroke Scale (NIHSS), which has been incorporated into formal guidelines for thrombolytic therapy decision making [105].

Laboratory Evaluation

Table 1-8 lists recommended tests that should be ordered on all patients with stroke on an emergent basis. The frequent coexistence of heart disease with ischemic stroke mandates concern in all patients for acute myocardial infarction, congestive heart failure, arrhythmias, and sudden death, dictating the need to draw blood for cardiac enzyme levels, for electrocardiography, and for chest radiographic evaluation. The possibility of early aspiration and pneumonitis also supports chest radiography. Cardiac monitoring should be maintained continuously throughout the first 24 hours to detect potentially lethal arrhythmias and to document episodes of atrial fibrillation. Glucose measurement is essential, because hypo- and hyperglycemia may mimic or exacerbate stroke deficits. Electrolyte and renal dysfunction may also exacerbate stroke impairments. Tests of blood cell counts, platelet count, and the clotting system identify coagulation abnormalities that may have contributed to the acute stroke and that will influence urgent management. Table 1-9 lists tests to be performed in patients with suspected hypercoagulable states as a cause of ischemic stroke.

TABLE 1-8. LABORATORY EVALUATION FOR PATIENTS WITH ACUTE ISCHEMIC STROKE

Initial Tests for All Patients
Electrocardiogram and initiation of continuous cardiac monitoring
Chest radiograph
Complete blood count
Platelet count
Prothrombin time
Partial thromboplastin time
Electrolytes
Blood glucose
Troponin or CK/MB
Blood urea nitrogen and creatinine
Pulse oximetry
Additional Tests in Select Patients
Lateral cervical spine radiograph (if trauma is suspected)
Lumbar puncture (if subarachnoid hemorrhage suspected and CT results are negative)
Electroencephalogram (if seizure suspected)
Pregnancy test (in women of childbearing age)
Liver function tests (if altered level of consciousness)
Arterial blood gas (if hypoxia suspected)
Urine toxicology (if substance abuse suspected)
Blood cultures and ESR (if endocarditis or other infection suspected)

CK, creatine kinase; MB, myocardial bands; CT, computed tomography; ESR, erythrocyte sedimentation rate.

TABLE 1-9. HYPERCOAGULABLE STATE WORKUP

Protein C
Protein S
Antithrombin III
Anticardiolipin antibody
Lupus anticoagulant (DRVVT)
β-2-Glycoprotein I antibodies
Activated protein C resistance/factor V Leiden mutation
Prothrombin gene mutation
Homocysteine (fasting, serum)
Fibrinogen
Factor VIII level
Screen for underlying malignancy

DRVVT, dilute Russell's viper venom titer.

Neuroimaging

As therapeutic options for treatment of acute stroke evolve, neuroimaging strategies are assuming an increasingly important role in the initial evaluation and management of patients. There is a recognized need for objective neuroimaging methods to identify the best candidates for early intervention. Both acute and long-term treatment decisions for stroke patients are optimally guided by neuroimaging information regarding tissue status (size, location, vascular distribution, and degree of reversibility of ischemic injury, as well as presence of hemorrhage), vessel status (site and severity of stenoses and occlusions), and cerebral perfusion (size, location, and severity of hypoperfusion). The ability to acutely identify the ischemic penumbra and use this information to steer treatment decisions may be within reach, particularly with the multimodal data provided by magnetic resonance techniques. All patients with suspected ischemic stroke should undergo imaging of the brain parenchyma and of the cervicocephalic vasculature. In addition, cerebral perfusion imaging is often useful, especially in the acute setting.

Brain Parenchymal Imaging

Noncontrast Computed Tomography

Noncontrast CT of the head is routinely employed as the initial imaging study in patients with suspected acute ischemic stroke. It is used as a screening tool to exclude hemorrhage and other nonischemic causes of acute neurologic deficits (tumor, infection) and has the advantages of being rapid and inexpensive with widespread availability. With the advent of intravenous tissue plasminogen activator (t-PA), there has been growing interest in employing CT to

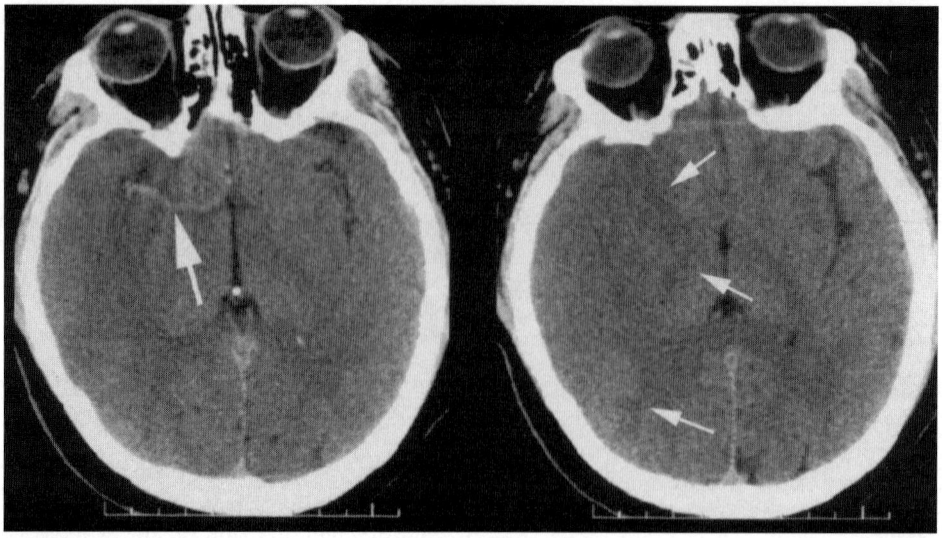

FIGURE 1-6. Early infarct signs on noncontrast CT. **Left:** Hyperdensity of the right middle cerebral artery (hyperdense MCA sign) indicating acute thrombus *(large arrow).* Images show hypodensity and loss of gray-white cortical ribbon in the right temporal lobe *(smaller arrows).* **Right:** Loss of sulcal markings indicating edema in the right temporal lobe.

identify early infarct signs (hyperdense middle cerebral artery sign, loss of gray-white differentiation, hypodensity, and sulcal effacement; Fig. 1-6). These signs may be seen in up to 82% of patients within 6 hours from symptom onset [106]. Pathophysiologic studies suggest that parenchymal CT early infarct signs represent early cytotoxic edema and that they are only rarely reversible.

Several studies have demonstrated that early infarct signs are associated with a poorer outcome [107,108]. However, the utility of using these early signs in selecting candidates for thrombolysis has been controversial. In the NINDS (National Institutes of Neurological Disorders and Stroke) study, early edema and mass effect on CT were associated with an eightfold increased risk of symptomatic intracerebral hemorrhage, yet patients with these findings who were treated were more likely to have a normal or nearly normal 3-month outcome [109]. In the first European Cooperative Acute Stroke Study (ECASS), patients with involvement of greater than 33% of the middle cerebral artery territory had an increased risk of intracerebral hemorrhage, and those with involvement of less than 33% benefited most from treatment [108]. Haring et al. reported a recent study showing that the presence of widespread attenuated corticomedullary contrast within the middle cerebral artery territory as visualized on early CT (performed within 18 hours of stroke onset) is both highly sensitive and specific for malignant middle cerebral artery infarction, suggesting that CT can help select patients for aggressive craniectomy or hypothermia [110].

However, the ability of physicians to reliably and reproducibly identify early infarct signs on CT has not been demonstrated consistently [111,112]. Marks et al. found that neuroradiologists detected hypodensity in greater than one-third of the middle cerebral artery territory with sensitivity ranging from 60% to 87% and interrater correlation coefficients ranging from 0.44 to 0.65 [113]. Similarly, Kalafut et al. found that emergency physicians, neurologists, and general radiologists detected any infarct signs in 78% of patients with greater than one-third middle cerebral artery hypodensity on CT [112]. In a study of CT scans from the NINDS Stroke Trial, interrater correlation statistics remained modest, even for physicians experienced in selecting and treating patients with acute stroke with t-PA [114].

Magnetic Resonance Imaging

Within the first few hours of ischemia onset, standard MRI sequences (T1-, T2-, and proton density–weighted) are relatively insensitive to ischemia, showing abnormalities in under 50% of cases [115]. The earliest changes, seen as increased signal on T2-weighted and fluid-attenuated inversion recovery (FLAIR) sequences, are due to a net increase in overall tissue water content primarily due to vasogenic edema—a process which takes several hours to develop to levels visible on MRI. Although the preponderance of ischemic lesions are evident on both CT and conventional MRI by 24 hours, standard MRI is superior to CT in identifying posterior fossa and subcortical lesions.

Diffusion-weighted imaging (DWI) allows visualization of regions of ischemia within minutes of symptom onset [116]. When strong diffusion-weighted sensitizing gradients are applied during a standard spin-echo sequence, the random movement of water protons within a tissue can be detected. During ischemia, there is decreased free-water diffusion in brain tissue related to the flux of water from the extracellular to intracellular space leading to early cytotoxic edema. This impaired water motion causes an increased (bright) signal on DWI sequences. The decrease in diffusion can be quantitatively measured on the apparent diffusion coefficient (ADC) maps, with darker areas representing decreased diffusion. The increase in signal on DWI may persist for several weeks or longer, partially due to a T2 effect. The ADC, however, returns to normal or supranormal levels within 7 to 10 days from onset of ischemia [117]. Early reperfusion, as from thrombolytic therapy, may reverse cytotoxic edema and normalize DWI images [118]. DWI sequences are sensitive to regional magnetic susceptibility effects and chemical shift artifacts, which may lead to erroneous interpretations. Diffusion imaging is optimally obtained with echo-planar imaging (EPI) techniques, which are not universally available.

An increasing number of studies have provided data demonstrating the clinical utility of diffusion MRI in current practice [119–121]. Diffusion imaging allows early identification of lesion size, lesion age, neuroanatomic site, and vascular territory involved (Fig. 1-7). DWI has a high degree of sensitivity (88% to 100%) and specificity (95% to 100%) for acute ischemia, even at very early time points [122–125]. In the study of Ay et al., of 782 consecutive patients presenting with stroke-like deficits, DWI was positive in 99% of patients with cerebral infarction. The 27

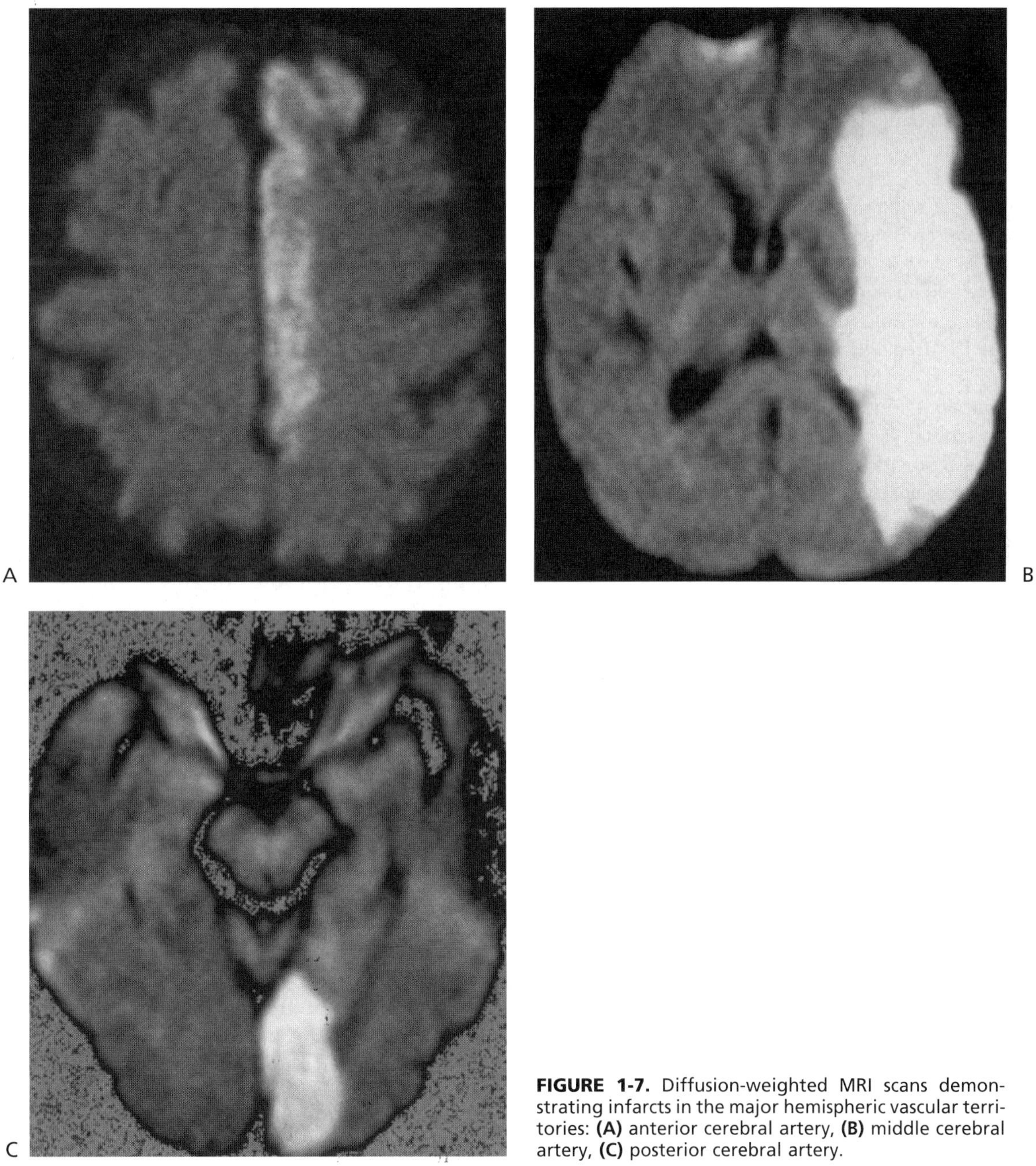

A B C

FIGURE 1-7. Diffusion-weighted MRI scans demonstrating infarcts in the major hemispheric vascular territories: **(A)** anterior cerebral artery, **(B)** middle cerebral artery, **(C)** posterior cerebral artery.

negative studies included 10 patients with etiologies other than stroke for their deficits and 10 patients with reversible deficits. DWI hyperintensity may occasionally be seen in diverse other cerebral disorders including status epilepticus, tumors, Creutzfeldt-Jakob disease, and hyperthermia. Examination of the T2-weighted and ADC sequences generally allows these entities to be differentiated from acute ischemia.

Numerous studies have shown that initial diffusion lesion volume correlates well with final infarct volume as well as neurologic and functional outcomes in stroke patients, suggesting that diffusion MRI can provide important early prognostic information [120,126,127]. These strong clinicoradiographic correlations indicate that diffusion imaging is superior to CT as a reliable surrogate or auxiliary outcome marker in stroke clinical trials [128]. MRI demonstration of decreased lesion growth over the first hours and days provides physiologic evidence of drug efficacy, and it may demonstrate treatment effects in smaller samples of patients than use of standard clinical rating scale end points would mandate.

A distinctive advantage of DWI is its ability to distinguish acute from chronic ischemia, allowing new lesions to be identified in patients even when these are near or within areas of prior ischemic injury [119,129,130]. Another important insight into stroke pathophysiology offered by diffusion MRI is the frequent visualization of multiple acute lesions in different vascular territories in patients who have only one clinically symptomatic acute insult, providing evidence of an embolic stroke mechanism [131]. Diffusion imaging can also provide important localizing and etiologic information in patients with TIAs. In a study of 42 patients with TIA, almost one-half demonstrated early DWI abnormalities [132]. Presence of a diffusion lesion correlated with longer duration of symptoms.

Currently, the main limitation preventing MRI from being widely adopted as the sole imaging modality in patients with acute stroke symptoms is concern about its ability to accurately detect hyperacute hemorrhage. Recently, several reports have suggested that hyperacute parenchymal blood can be reliably detected employing gradient-recalled echo (GRE) or echo-planar susceptibility-weighted MRI [133–135]. Large, multicenter studies to prospectively validate the accuracy of these sequences in detecting acute intracerebral hemorrhage are under way.

Cerebral Perfusion Imaging

Xenon Computed Tomography

Xenon-enhanced CT provides an absolute quantitative measurement of cerebral blood flow (CBF). As the patient inhales a 33% mixture of inert xenon gas, a steady state of xenon is achieved in the brain parenchyma. The density changes within the brain parenchyma following xenon gas inhalation can be equated to CBF. Several studies have suggested that thresholds of reversible and irreversible ischemia in patients with acute stroke may be identified using xenon CT [136,137]. Kaufmann et al. reported that a CBF of 6 $cm^3/100\ g^{-1}/min^{-1}$ or less correlated with regions of irreversible infarction in patients with acute middle cerebral artery stroke [137], while Firlik et al. reported that very low CBFs were predictive of subsequent edema and herniation [138]. This same group also found that patients with neurologic deficits but CBFs in the mildly reduced or normal range were likely to have subsequent resolution of their symptoms, suggesting that xenon-enhanced CT can be used to triage acutely symptomatic patients among conservative and thrombolytic therapeutic regimens [139]. Xenon-enhanced CT is currently limited by a sensitivity to patient motion, and the requirement for rigorous adherence to protocol.

Perfusion Computed Tomography

Perfusion CT is an emerging method used to assess the relative cerebral blood flow (rCBF) in the acute stroke setting. The technique uses rapid CT scanning to track the first pass of a bolus of contrast material delivered intravenously. Recent reports demonstrate a high degree of sensitivity and specificity for detecting cerebral ischemia with this technique. A preliminary study suggests that perfusion CT may be able to differentiate rCBF thresholds of reversible and irreversible ischemia [140]. In addition, several reports suggest that perfusion CT can provide useful information regarding the status of collateral circulation [141–143]. Perfusion CT has the advantage of rapid data acquisition and rapid postprocessing, and can be performed in conjunction with the baseline CT of the head and CT angiography scans (Fig. 1-8). Future studies are required to validate the CBF measurements and to further explore the ability of this technique to detect ischemic thresholds.

Magnetic Resonance Perfusion Imaging

Perfusion-weighted imaging (PWI) is most commonly performed by the rapid injection of an intravenous paramagnetic contrast agent. The temporal passage of the contrast agent through contiguous slices of brain tissue is tracked with a sequence of rapid MRI scans. This signal intensity information is then used to derive a concentration time curve. Perfusion measures that can be derived from this technique include mean transit time (MTT), relative cerebral blood volume (rCBV), and rCBF. Currently, the principal disadvantage of this type of MR perfusion imaging is that it provides a relative, rather than quantitative, measure of cerebral tissue perfusion. While MR arterial spin labeling techniques offer promise as a means to quantify cerebral perfusion without the need for injection of a contrast agent, these techniques are still in the early stages of investigation for application in the acute stroke setting [144,145].

Several studies have demonstrated that baseline MR perfusion lesion volumes correlate well with final infarct vol-

A 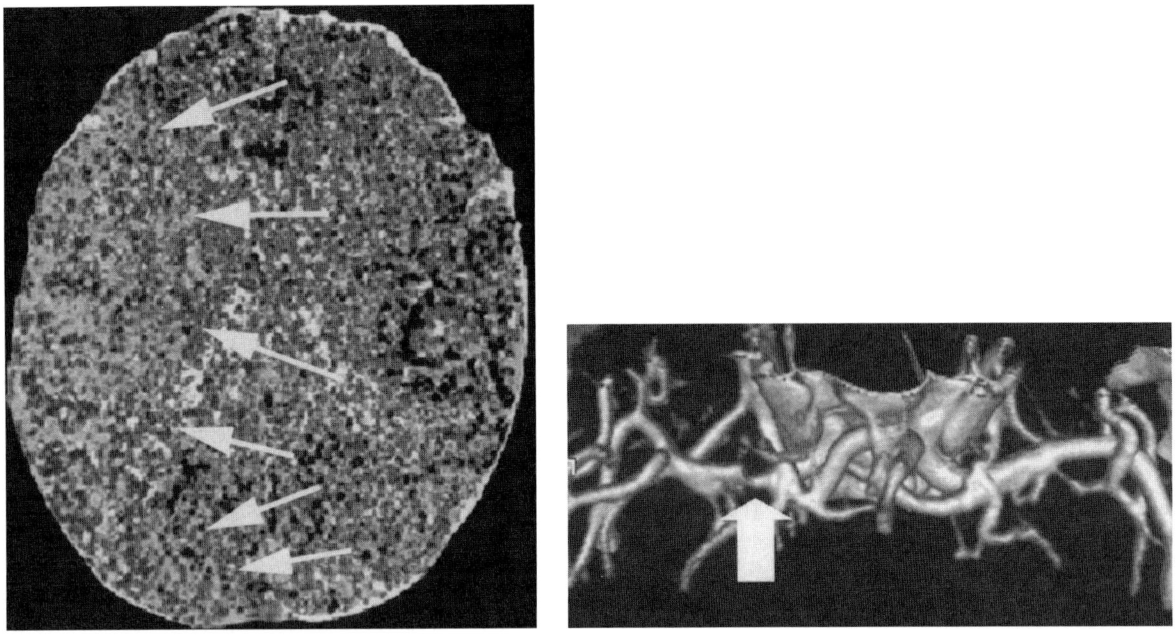 B

FIGURE 1-8. The multimodal CT strategy in acute stroke neuroimaging. **A:** Perfusion CT scan mean transit time image shows reduced regional perfusion throughout the right middle cerebral artery territory *(arrows)*. **B:** CT angiogram demonstrates severe stenosis of the right middle cerebral artery trunk *(arrow)*.

ume as well as neurologic and functional outcome, and in fact correlate somewhat better than the baseline diffusion lesion volumes [127]. Perfusion lesion volume likely identifies all tissue at risk of infarction if vessel recanalization does not occur, while diffusion imaging identifies only tissue that has already sustained advanced bioenergetic failure.

Recent diffusion and perfusion MR studies have begun to elucidate the evolution of ischemic lesions in humans, providing important insights into MRI of the ischemic penumbra. It has been suggested that early MRI can characterize the ischemic penumbra as regions of perfusion but not diffusion abnormality (diffusion–perfusion mismatch). These are regions in which blood flow is reduced but in which tissue bioenergetic failure, as evidenced by cytotoxic edema, has not yet developed. This hypothesis is supported by studies demonstrating that the natural history of diffusion MRI abnormalities is to grow over time, particularly in patients evaluated early after symptom onset [146,147]. This growth occurs primarily in patients with large regions of mismatch [120,148–150], suggesting gradual failure of the ischemic penumbra within the region of mismatch as it is incorporated into the infarct core. However, prior animal studies and a recent case series in humans undergoing intraarterial thrombolytic therapy have shown that diffusion abnormalities can be partially reversed with early reperfusion [118,151]. This data suggests that early after onset of ischemia, the penumbra likely includes not only regions of diffusion–perfusion mismatch, but also portions of the region of diffusion abnormality.

Several groups have also reported that an altered evolution of infarction can be visualized on serial diffusion and perfusion imaging studies in patients undergoing intravenous thrombolytic therapy. Jansen et al. found inhibition of lesion growth in patients experiencing reperfusion compared with patients with persistent perfusion deficits [152]. Marks et al. found regions of higher ADC within the initial ischemic field on follow-up imaging in patients undergoing reperfusion within 36 hours of onset compared to nonreperfusers [153].

These studies suggest that it is feasible and potentially advantageous to use diffusion-perfusion MRI to select patients for thrombolytic therapy, employing MRI to characterize the degree of perfusion impairment and amount of remaining salvageable tissue (Fig. 1-9). Efforts are under way to identify specific MR signatures and criteria to identify regions of reversible versus irreversible infarction. Schlaug et al. used a logistical regression model to differentiate regions of ultimate infarction versus noninfarction based on the baseline perfusion measures [154]. MRI may provide the means of assessing acutely the results of thrombolytic therapy (Fig. 1-10). Kidwell et al. used automated image registration techniques to analyze diffusion-perfusion MRI data on patients treated with intraarterial thrombolytic therapy. A stepwise discriminant analysis was performed using baseline ADC, MTT, rCBV, and rCBF values to identify tissue that was labeled as infarcted versus normal at day 7. In this preliminary model, baseline diffusion-perfusion MRI variables predicted ultimate tissue infarction versus noninfarction to a high degree [155]. Further characterization of the MR signatures of penumbra and core infarction

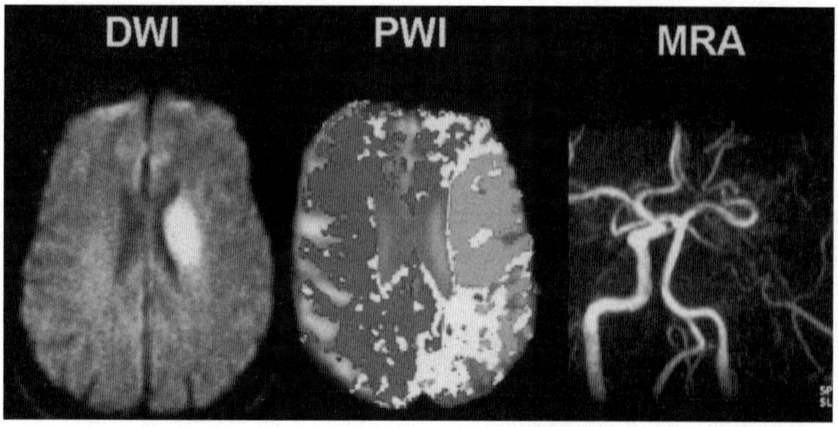

FIGURE 1-9. The multimodal MR strategy in acute stroke neuroimaging. **Left:** Diffusion-weighted sequence showing early diffusion injury (hyperintensity) in the deep left periventricular white matter. **Center:** Perfusion-weighted MR showing reduced perfusion throughout the middle cerebral artery territory. The large extent of the perfusion than diffusion lesion (perfusion–diffusion mismatch) suggests a large volume of potentially salvageable penumbral tissue. **Right:** MR angiogram showing absence of signal from the left internal carotid and left middle cerebral arteries.

may allow extension of the time window for treatment beyond current standards, basing treatment decisions on individual patient pathophysiology rather than rigid time windows [156].

Positron Emission Tomography

Oxygen-15 positron emission tomography (PET) is the gold standard for quantifying cerebral perfusion and oxygen consumption. PET studies provided the first documentation of a probable existing penumbra in humans by identifying regions of decreased cerebral blood flow and increased oxygen extraction fraction (OEF) with relatively preserved oxygen metabolism (misery perfusion) [157,158]. Various studies have demonstrated that this state can be detected up to 16 to 48 hours after symptom onset in humans [20,159].

Heiss et al. recently performed serial oxygen-15–labeled water in PET studies to measure rCBF without arterial sampling in patients undergoing intravenous thrombolysis. They reported that the volume of severe hypoperfusion predicted the development of subsequent infarction and long-term clinical outcome. They also found a significant correlation between clinical course and extent of reperfusion. Because PET provides absolute rather than relative CBF values, it is also well suited to evaluating postischemia hyperperfusion, a condition that may be important to recognize as a target for neuroprotective strategies [160]. Other minimally invasive methods to identify the ischemic penumbra with PET have been described that employ radioligands to molecules such as flumazenil and fluoromisonidazole that are preferentially trapped in penumbral fields [161, 162].

Although PET remains the gold standard for cerebral perfusion measurements, logistical and practical considerations limit its application in the emergent stroke setting. Moreover, arterial sampling techniques required for absolute, quantitative CBF values are relatively contraindicated with standard systemic thrombolysis.

Single Photon Emission Computed Tomography

Single photon emission computed tomography (SPECT) provides a noninvasive evaluation of rCBF by measuring

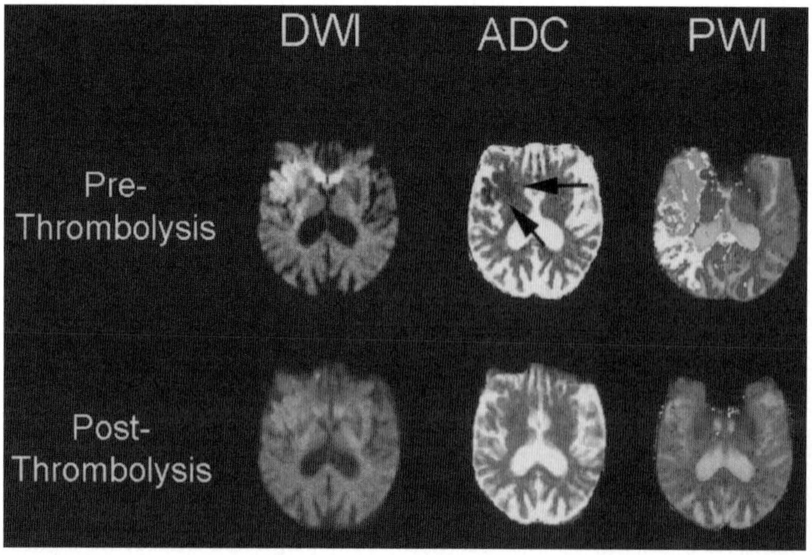

FIGURE 1-10. Reversal of diffusion-weighted abnormality. Top row are pretreatment images in patient presenting with acute left hemiparesis, left hemisensory loss, left hemianopia, and left hemineglect. Diffusion-weighted image (DWI) **(left)** shows early abnormal hyperintensity in the right inferior frontal lobe. Apparent diffusion coefficient (ADC) image **(center)** shows correlative hypointensity in the same region *(arrows).* Perfusion-weighted image (PWI) **(right)** demonstrates reduced perfusion throughout the right MCA field, worse anteriorly at the site of diffusion change. Bottom row shows images obtained 4 hours after successful recanalization was achieved by intraarterial thrombolysis with tissue plasminogen activator. DWI **(left)** and ADC **(center)** show normalization of previously abnormal signal. PWI sequence **(right)** shows restoration of normal perfusion.

the concentration of a radioactive tracer trapped within the brain parenchyma. Several studies have suggested that SPECT may be able to identify thresholds for reversible ischemia and may be useful in predicting clinical outcome and monitoring response to therapy. Ueda et al. found that tissue with rCBF greater than 55% of cerebellar flow may still be salvageable up to 12 hours from symptom onset, while tissue with rCBF less than 35% of cerebellar flow may be at risk for hemorrhagic transformation [163]. Grotta and Alexandrov demonstrated perfusion defects in patients with large hemispheric infarcts and found reperfusion was greater in patients treated with standard intravenous t-PA versus placebo [164]. Berrouschot et al. reported that technetium-99m ethyl cysteinate dimer SPECT performed within 6 hours of symptom onset is highly accurate for predicting fatal ischemic brain edema [165] and for differentiating transient ischemic symptoms from stroke [166]. Although SPECT is less invasive than oxygen-15 PET, limitations include availability, expense, tracer preparation, and that it provides relative, not absolute, measures of CBF.

Cervicocephalic Vessel Imaging

A wide variety of imaging techniques are now available to assess the status of large- and medium-caliber cervicocephalic vessels. Choice of imaging modality in a particular clinical setting depends on availability, individual patient characteristics, and type of information sought. It is widely recognized that performance of at least one of these techniques is mandatory in the standard evaluation of anterior circulation ischemia to assess for cervical carotid artery stenosis, because the presence of moderate-to-severe symptomatic carotid stenosis warrants evaluation for carotid endarterectomy [167,168].

Magnetic Resonance Angiography

In recent years, MRA has become an increasingly useful tool for noninvasive screening of supraaortic vessels. When compared to digital subtraction angiography for detection of cervical and intracranial stenoses, sensitivity and specificity have ranged from 70% to 100% in various studies [169–172]. In the intracranial vasculature, MRA is useful in identifying acute proximal large-vessel occlusions, but it does not reliably identify distal or branch occlusions. Combined with data from DWI, MRA substantially improves acute diagnosis of stroke mechanism. Lee et al. found that in patients who undergo imaging within 24 hours of admission, the combined data from DWI and MRA improved correct stroke subtype classification from 48% to 94% [121].

Although advances in MR technology have led to new and improved MRA sequences, information employed to generate time-of-flight MRA scans is derived from blood flow rather than vessel anatomy. Standard MRA is therefore susceptible to a number of flow artifacts including in-plane flow saturation, susceptibility to turbulent or complex flow, and flowlike effects from adjacent short T1 substances such as thrombus and fat. A resulting disadvantage of MRA is a tendency to overestimate the degree of stenosis, making the technique inadequate for the identification of near occlusions [173]. Newer power-injector, contrast-enhanced techniques may mitigate some of the limitations of standard MRA [170,174,175].

Computed Tomography Angiography

Helical CT angiography is performed by rapid administration of an intravenous contrast agent followed by data acquisition over the time of passage of the bolus within large vessels of the target vascular system. The method relies on continuous scanning as the patient is moved through the x-ray beam, allowing for volumetric rather than conventional tomographic data acquisition. In addition to acquisition of axial cuts, image postprocessing permits the data to be visualized using multiplanar reformatting, surface or 3-dimensional volume rendering, and maximal intensity projection (MIP) techniques [176].

Helical CT angiography offers promise as a means to rapidly and noninvasively evaluate the neurovasculature of patients with suspected cerebrovascular disease, providing potentially important information about the presence of vessel occlusions or stenoses in both the intra- and extracranial circulations [177]. Disadvantages of CTA include requirement for intravenous contrast dosing, use of ionizing radiation, and simultaneous arterial and venous phase imaging.

Ultrasonographic Procedures

Carotid and transcranial Doppler ultrasonographic techniques offer another noninvasive method to assess the neurovasculature acutely. Ultrasonographic studies of the carotid bifurcation are a well-established noninvasive test used for the diagnosis of stroke. A full carotid ultrasonographic battery includes continuous-wave Doppler measurement of blood velocity, B-mode imaging of vessel anatomy, and color-flow imaging of flow direction and lumen caliber. Carotid ultrasonography visualizes only the proximal cervical carotid arteries and very limited segments of the cervical vertebral arteries. TCD ultrasonography employs a low-frequency probe to penetrate the skull and interrogate the major basal intracranial arteries [178]. The TCD approach offers a practical, noninvasive assessment of intracranial vessel status that provides early diagnostic and prognostic information in patients with acute stroke [179]. In addition, TCD ultrasonography can be used to monitor cerebral hemodynamic status and response to recanalization therapy [180]. Ultrasonographic procedures have the advantage that they can be performed at the bedside in a timely fashion. The costs are minimal and patient cooperation is not essential. Disadvantages of ultrasonography include that it is highly operator dependent, and distinguishing high-grade stenosis from complete occlusion is difficult.

Catheter Angiography

Digital subtraction angiography remains the gold standard imaging modality to assess vessel anatomy and pathology while providing important collateral flow information. Although the 0.5% to 1% permanent neurologic complication risk makes other noninvasive vessel imaging techniques, such as CTA and MRA, very attractive, it is likely that catheter angiography will continue to play an important role in stroke evaluation. Advantages include better visualization of medium and small vessels than with noninvasive techniques, and the ability to proceed directly to an endovascular intervention after diagnostic imaging. Catheter angiography can detect arterial dissection with high sensitivity and can define the route and, to some degree, the adequacy of collateral circulation. It remains the only way to confidently make a diagnosis of diseases affecting small-caliber vessels, such as vasculitis. It is also often of help in the rapidly deteriorating patient, the patient with conflicting or unrevealing noninvasive vascular imaging, the patient with suspected dissection, and the young stroke patient. Disadvantages include periprocedural risks of stroke, exposure to nephrotoxic iodinated contrast and potential for allergic response, and lack of around-the-clock availability outside of large medical centers.

Cardiac Imaging

An electrocardiogram and blood tests (troponin or creatine kinase isoenzymes) to assess for arrhythmias and cardiac ischemia should be performed routinely in all patients admitted with suspected cerebral ischemic symptoms.

In addition, echocardiography should be considered in all patients to identify potential cardiac sources of cerebral embolism. Transthoracic echocardiography (TTE) is superior for evaluating the left ventricle and cardiac apex, while transesophageal echocardiography (TEE) is excellent for investigating the atrium and atrial appendage, the interatrial septum, and the aorta. The yield of TTE in patients with no clinical history of heart disease, normal cardiac physical examination, and normal electrocardiogram is quite low. In patients with such an apparently benign clinical cardiac status, ordering routine TTE is not cost effective. However, such patients may harbor patent foramen ovale or aortic arch atherosclerosis detectable by TEE. One reasonable strategy is to start with a transthoracic echocardiogram in any patient with a history or findings of prior heart disease. In patients with lacunar stroke, no further cardiac imaging is pursued. However, in patients with large-vessel stroke, if TTE is negative and the stroke mechanism remains unclear after cervicocephalic arterial imaging, TEE is obtained to screen for patent foramen ovale and aortic arch atheroma. In young or healthy patients without any cardiac history, it is reasonable to proceed directly to TEE, bypassing TTE.

MEDICAL AND SURGICAL THERAPY FOR PREVENTION OF STROKE

Risk Factor Modification

Hypertension

Treatment of hypertension is effective both in preventing first stroke (primary prevention) and preventing recurrent stroke (secondary prevention). A metaanalysis of 14 early trials of antihypertensive drugs, chiefly diuretics and β-blockers, enrolling over 37,000 individuals showed that a 5- to 6-mm Hg reduction in diastolic blood pressure was associated with a 34% to 40% reduction in first stroke [181]. More recent trials have demonstrated that treatment of isolated systolic hypertension also dramatically reduces first ischemic stroke risk, especially lacunar stroke [182–184]. For example, in the Systolic Hypertension in the Elderly Program, treatment of isolated systolic hypertension reduced stroke incidence by 36% over 5 years [185].

Initiating long-term antihypertensive therapy after a first stroke to prevent recurrent stroke was suggested to be beneficial in four early trials. More recently, the Perindopril Protection Against Recurrent Stroke Study (PROGRESS) definitively demonstrated that institution of combined long-term therapy with an angiotensin-converting enzyme (ACE) inhibitor and a diuretic after stroke substantially reduces recurrence, among high-normotensive as well as hypertensive patients (277). Similarly, in the Heart Outcomes Prevention Evaluation (HOPE) trial, among patients with vascular risk factors and average entry blood pressure in high-normal range at 139/79, adding an ACE inhibitor reduced stroke events by 31% [186]. Less than one-half of this reduction could be attributed to observed blood pressure–lowering effects of treatment, suggesting that ACE inhibitors exert some of their benefits through additional, non–blood pressure mechanisms, including effects on endothelial function, platelet function, and fibrinolytic state.

The optimal timing of antihypertensive therapy after stroke is uncertain. Certainly during the first few hours after onset, precipitous lowering of blood pressure is to be avoided, because it may reduce cerebral perfusion and produce stroke extension. One reasonable strategy is to wait until the patient has been neurologically stable for 24 to 48 hours and then initiate blood pressure–lowering therapy cautiously, aiming to achieve full control over the next several days to weeks rather than hours.

Diabetes

Intensive treatment of both type 1 and type 2 diabetes, targeting near-normal levels of serum glucose, has not yet been conclusively demonstrated to reduce macrovascular complications, including stroke. However, measures to achieve tight glycemic control do substantially reduce the risk of microvascular complications, including retinopathy, nephropathy, and neuropathy, and are indicated in diabetic patients on this basis alone [187,188].

Tobacco

Tobacco abstinence substantially reduces the risk of stroke. Convergent data from the Framingham Study and Nurses' Health Study indicate that the risk of ischemic stroke nearly reverts to that of nonsmokers 2 to 5 years after smoking cessation [189]. Nicotine replacement therapy, with gum, patches, or nasal spray, and bupropion hydrochloride are effective adjuncts to smoking cessation programs.

Alcohol

Alcohol alters the risk of ischemic stroke in a J-shaped manner, and increases the risk of hemorrhagic stroke in a dose-dependent fashion [190,191]. Light and moderate drinkers of alcohol (up to two drinks a day) have reduced incidence of ischemic stroke compared to abstinent individuals, likely related to decreased platelet aggregation, decreased fibrinogen levels, and increased high-density lipoprotein cholesterol levels. Heavy drinkers have increased risk of both ischemic and hemorrhagic stroke compared to abstainers. The increase in ischemic stroke risk at high alcohol intake levels is likely due to induction of hypertension, hypercoagulable states, cardiac arrhythmias, and reduced cerebral blood flow. Based on these observations, individuals with atherosclerotic cerebrovascular disease who drink alcohol to excess should be advised to moderate their intake or cease alcohol consumption, and those who drink in moderation should be advised to continue. However, consensus guidelines caution that those who do not customarily drink alcohol should not be encouraged to begin regular intake [191].

Obesity, Physical Inactivity, Diet

Although weight loss has not yet been demonstrated to reduce stroke risk, abdominal obesity in men and obesity and weight gain in women are independent risk factors for stroke. Accordingly, weight reduction in overweight individuals is indicated in a stroke prevention program [188]. Several large-scale epidemiologic studies have demonstrated a protective effect of physical activity against stroke. The antistroke effect is likely mediated, at least in part, through beneficial effects on comorbid conditions, including hypertension, cardiovascular disease, diabetes, and body weight. Regular exercise, consisting of at least 30 minutes of moderate-intensity activity daily, is recommended to reduce the risk of comorbid conditions that predispose to stroke [192]. With regard to nutrition and diet, epidemiologic observations support recommendations to limit intake of saturated fat and sodium, replace vitamin B_{12}, B_6, and folic acid when deficiencies are identified, and consume at least five daily servings of fruits and vegetables [188,191].

Hyperlipidemia and Statins

Observational, epidemiologic studies have been able to document only a weak association between total serum cholesterol and increased risk of ischemic stroke [193]. An inverse relationship between high-density lipoprotein levels and stroke risk has also been found [194]. Ultrasonographic studies have established an association between lipid levels and extracranial internal carotid artery atherosclerosis [195].

In contrast, interventional clinical trials employing statin agents have shown consistent benefits in the primary prevention of stroke among individuals with coronary artery disease and cholesterol levels that are borderline elevated or higher. Metaanalyses of more than 13 trials enrolling more than 20,000 patients demonstrate that statin therapy reduces the risk of stroke by 20% to 35% [196–198]. These clinical end point observations are supported by surrogate end point clinical trials demonstrating that statins can slow the progression, or cause regression, of carotid artery intimal-medial thickening (medical recanalization) [199]. These observations support the aggressive use of statin agents in all patients with cervicocephalic atherosclerosis. In the most recent National Cholesterol Education Panel III guidelines regarding cholesterol therapy, symptomatic carotid artery disease is recognized as a risk equivalent to symptomatic coronary artery disease, meriting aggressive lipid-lowering therapy with a target fasting low-density lipoprotein level less than 100 mg/dl [200].

Atrial Fibrillation

The annual risk of stroke in patients with atrial fibrillation not on antithrombotic therapy is 3% to 5%. Convergent evidence from 14 randomized trials demonstrates that warfarin is highly effective, and aspirin modestly effective, in reducing stroke events in patients with atrial fibrillation [201]. Warfarin reduces the relative risk of stroke by two-thirds. A variety of stratification schemes have been proposed to distinguish the great preponderance of patients with atrial fibrillation who are at high risk of stroke and merit warfarin therapy and a small subgroup of patients with atrial fibrillation at low risk of stroke who are adequately treated with aspirin. National consensus guidelines from the American College of Chest Physicians indicate that warfarin is preferred in any patient with atrial fibrillation who has any one of the following additional risk factors: hypertension, age over 75, poor left ventricular systolic function, prior stroke or TIA, rheumatic mitral valve disease, prosthetic cardiac valves, or any combination of age 65 to 75, diabetes mellitus, and coronary artery disease [202].

Antithrombotic Therapy after Noncardioembolic Stroke or Transient Ischemic Attack

Antiplatelet therapy is of clear benefit in reducing recurrent stroke after a first cerebral ischemic event due to large-artery atherothromboembolism or intrinsic small-vessel disease. Current oral antiplatelet agents modulate platelet function via three different pathways. Aspirin irreversibly inhibits platelet cyclooxygenase, preventing generation of the proaggregant metabolite thromboxane. The thienopyridines, ticlopidine and clopidogrel, block adenosine diphosphate (ADP)-induced platelet aggregation. Dipyridamole inhibits phosphodiesterase, which leads to increased cyclic adenosine monophosphate (AMP) levels and impaired platelet adhesion. The combination of sustained-release dipyridamole plus aspirin and the thienopyridines clopidogrel and ticlopidine are superior to aspirin alone in preventing major vascular events [203–205]. Ticlopidine is generally avoided because of bone marrow suppression side effects.

Additional combinations of antithrombotic agents besides dipyridamole plus aspirin show promise in patients with ischemic stroke but await definitive clinical trial testing [206,207]. Patients with stroke are at increased risk of hemorrhagic side effects from combination therapy because of older age and cervicocephalic arteriopathy, so that beneficial effects of combination therapy observed in other circulatory beds cannot be assumed to apply to the cerebrovascular bed [208–210].

As a general secondary prevention treatment strategy for noncardioembolic stroke, long-term anticoagulation therapy is inferior to long-term antiplatelet therapy. Randomized clinical trials have demonstrated that warfarin at high dose is less effective, and at moderate dose not more effective, than aspirin for broadly selected patients with noncardioembolic stroke [211]. In small subgroups, including patients with antiphospholipid antibody syndrome and other hypercoagulable states, warfarin is preferred [47,212]. In patients with symptomatic intracranial atherosclerosis, the relative merits of warfarin versus aspirin are still being defined by ongoing clinical trials [213].

Preventive Therapy in Nonatherosclerotic Arteriopathies

Optimal antithrombotic management is uncertain in patients with cerebral ischemia due to cervicocerebral dissection because controlled trials to guide therapy are lacking. Anticoagulation is often recommended, because angiographic studies suggest that neurologic worsening most frequently results from embolization of thrombotic fragments or propagation of *in situ* thrombus [50]. However, anticoagulation is contraindicated in intracranial dissections associated with subarachnoid hemorrhage. A reasonable strategy is anticoagulation for 3 months, at which time an imaging study is repeated. Approximately 70% of dissections will heal within this 3-month period. If the dissected vessel has fully healed, remains fully occluded, or has a smooth residual stenosis, the patient is then switched to long-term antiplatelet therapy, or antithrombotic therapy is halted. If a severe, irregular stenosis persists, anticoagulation is continued for at least 3 more months. In patients with expanding dissecting aneurysms causing cranial neuropathy, or with recurring ischemic events on medical therapy, interventional procedures or surgery may be pursued, including angioplasty, stenting, and vessel reconstruction or bypass procedures. Recurrent dissections occur at a rate of 1% per year, afflicting the initial or a different cervicocephalic vessel [214–216].

The optimal antithrombotic regimen for patients with migrainous stroke is unknown. Additive risk factors should be minimized (cessation of tobacco use or oral contraceptive use). Treatment with antiplatelet agents and migraine prophylactic agents such as calcium-channel blockers is a reasonable first-line strategy [68]. Vasoconstrictors such as triptans and ergotamines should be avoided in patients with a history of migrainous infarction, due to the theoretical concern of precipitating vasoconstriction or vasospasm with these medications.

In most cases of symptomatic cervicocephalic FMD, antiplatelet therapy is preferred, because the irregular vessel surface and only modest degree of stenosis suggest that patients are most at risk for forming high-flow, shear-induced, white clots. In patients with progressive vessel narrowing, angioplasty or surgical reconstruction may be considered. Intracranial aneurysms in FMD are usually treated with clipping or coiling. The prognosis for cerebrovascular FMD is generally benign, with progression of lesions or subsequent ischemic events occurring in only a minority of untreated patients.

Because cerebral vasculitis is generally linked to autoimmune mechanisms, corticosteroids and other immunosuppressive agents are the mainstays of therapy [71]. Corticosteroids may, however, augment vessel constriction and platelet aggregation [217]. Treatment with corticosteroids and a cytotoxic agent may be more effective than steroids alone and allows minimization of steroid dosage. Steroid and additional immunosuppressive therapy can, in turn, lead to a new set of medical problems including infection or delayed malignancy. In patients with an underlying secondary cause, treatment is aimed at eliminating any offending agent (drug) or the underlying disorder (infection or malignancy). Until the 1980s, most forms of CNS vasculitis, especially primary angiitis of the CNS, were frequently fatal. More recently, improved understanding of the underlying pathophysiologic processes combined with aggressive treatment have resulted in a more favorable prognosis for some patients.

Carotid Endarterectomy, Angioplasty, and Stenting

Therapeutic recommendations for treatment of carotid stenosis depend on the presence of ischemic symptoms and the degree of stenosis. Recommendations for the treatment of symptomatic stenosis are based on the results of the

North American Symptomatic Carotid Endarterectomy Trial (NASCET) and European Carotid Surgery Trial (ECST) [218,219]. Both of these trials demonstrated a clear benefit of carotid endarterectomy (CEA) compared to best medical management for patients with hemispheric or retinal symptoms and severe stenosis, defined as 70% or more reduction in lumen diameter as measured by NASCET criteria. In NASCET, after 2 years of follow-up, the rate of combined perioperative complications and ipsilateral stroke in the surgical group was 9%, compared with 26% for the medically treated group.

The NASCET trial also demonstrated a modest benefit in favor of CEA for patients with moderate degrees of stenosis, 50% to 69% by NASCET criteria. In the surgical group, the 5-year event rate was 15.7% compared with 22.7% in the medical group ($p = 0.04$). Subgroups that derived a greater benefit from surgery included males and patients with hemispheric rather than retinal symptoms. No benefit from surgery was seen for stenosis less than 50%. It is important to note that the NASCET results were based on angiographically proven stenosis defined by NASCET measurement methods and surgeons whose perioperative morbidity and mortality rates were less than 6%.

Optimal treatment recommendations for asymptomatic carotid stenosis remain controversial. From large-scale natural history studies and the medical arms of endarterectomy trials, event rates in patients with asymptomatic carotid stenosis greater than 50% to 60% are generally as follows: risk of ipsilateral carotid stroke—2.0% per year; risk of stroke in other distribution—0.9% per year; risk of ipsilateral carotid disabling stroke—1.2% per year; risk of TIA—4.0% per year; risk of myocardial infarction—2.3% per year; and risk of vascular death—1.1% per year. All patients with carotid atherosclerosis, whether managed medically or surgically, should be considered for statin therapy, ACE inhibitors, and aggressive vascular risk factor control. Carotid atherosclerosis is as strong a predictor of myocardial infarction as is the presence of stable angina.

In 1995, the results of the Asymptomatic Carotid Atherosclerosis Study (ACAS) were reported suggesting a modest benefit of CEA for patients with asymptomatic stenosis greater than 60% [220]. Two metaanalyses of asymptomatic trials confirm that the overall benefits of endarterectomy for asymptomatic disease are quite small [221,222]. In ACAS, over 5 years, the combined perioperative complication and ipsilateral stroke rate was 5.1% in the surgical group and 11% in the medical group. Although this is an impressive-sounding 54% reduction in terms of relative risk, the reduction in absolute risk is just 5.9% over 5 years, or 1.2% per year. A patient goes from a 2.2%-per-year risk with medical therapy to a 1%-per-year risk with surgical therapy, with much of the surgical risk occurring at the time of surgery. The benefits were greatest in men and younger patients. The surgical morbidity and mortality rate of the surgeons in ACAS was remarkably low, less than 1.1%.

One reasonable current strategy in managing asymptomatic carotid artery disease is to lean toward CEA if the patient has 80% to 99% asymptomatic carotid stenosis, and to lean toward medical management with annual follow-up carotid imaging if the patient has 60% to 79% stenosis [32]. These leanings are modified by patient-specific factors. Parameters favoring surgery are being male, having a highly ulcerated plaque, being young, and being free of cardiac or multiorgan disease. Parameters favoring medical therapy are being female, having a smooth plaque, being older, and having cardiac or multiorgan disease.

More specialized, physiologic tests may help to further grade the risk of the asymptomatic carotid disease. Transcranial Doppler embolus detection studies detect clinically silent microemboli passing under the ultrasonographic probe in up to 10% of patients with asymptomatic carotid stenosis, and this subgroup is at substantially higher risk for stroke if managed medically [223]. Patients with intracranial hemodynamic insufficiency due to the carotid stenosis are also at higher risk for stroke and can be identified with any of several perfusion tests, including TCD carbon dioxide reactivity testing, xenon-enhanced CT with acetazolamide challenge, and PET with acetazolamide challenge.

Because the advantage of surgery over medical therapy in the ACAS trial was so slight, endarterectomy should be considered only if the surgeon can match the excellent perioperative morbidity and mortality rates attained by the surgeons in that study. Patients whose surgeons have even slightly higher complication rates obtain no net benefit, and patients whose surgeons have moderately higher complication rates obtain net harm from surgery. CEA is recommended over medical management for asymptomatic disease only when the combined arteriographic and surgical mortality and morbidity rates are less than 3%.

Following carotid endarterectomy, appropriate risk factor management and antithrombotic therapy should be initiated. Antiplatelet therapy should be employed to reduce the risk of early rethrombosis at the endarterectomy site. The ASA and Carotid Endarterectomy (ACE) trial investigators found that the risk of stroke, myocardial infarction, and death within 30 days and 3 months of endarterectomy was lower for patients taking low-dose (81 mg or 325 mg) aspirin daily than for those taking a high dose (650 mg or 1,300 mg) [224].

Extracranial-to-intracranial Bypass

Observational studies have suggested that patients with internal carotid artery occlusion are at high risk of subsequent stroke, with estimates ranging from 2% to 6% per year for ipsilateral stroke [225,226]. The role of extracranial-to-intracranial (EC-IC) bypass for the prevention of stroke in patients with symptomatic anterior-circulation occlusive disease was evaluated in a large clinical trial in the 1980s [227]. The study failed to demonstrate a benefit from surgery for the overall cohort or for the subgroup of patients with internal carotid artery occlusion. However, this trial did not distinguish between patients with an embolic versus low-flow hemodynamic etiology for their symptoms. It has been suggested that patients with poor collateral circulation and hemodynamic impairment from significant occlusions may still benefit from a bypass procedure. Grubb et al. demonstrated that increased oxygen extraction fraction measured by PET distal to a symptomatic internal carotid artery occlusion identifies a subgroup of patients at particularly high risk for subsequent stroke when treated medically [228]. Based on these findings, a National Institutes of Health randomized trial evaluating surgical revascularization for patients with carotid occlusion and hemodynamic impairment documented by PET is under way.

MEDICAL THERAPY FOR ACUTE ISCHEMIC STROKE

Early Supportive Therapy

Oxygenation

Systemic oxygen desaturation will exacerbate and extend brain injury originating from focal cerebral hypoxia. Patients with acute stroke are at risk for respiratory compromise due to aspiration, hypoventilation, upper airway obstruction, atelectasis, or, rarely, a reduction in the ventilatory drive or neurogenic pulmonary edema. One-third of patients with acute ischemic stroke exhibit overt or silent aspiration [229]. Pneumonia complicates acute stroke in 5% to 12% of cases [230,231]. All patients with acute stroke should be monitored for hypoxia with a goal of maintaining serum oxygen saturation levels of greater than 95%. If this cannot be achieved on room air, supplemental oxygen should be used. No evidence supports the routine use of supplemental oxygen for patients with adequate blood oxygen saturation when breathing room air [104,232]. If ventilatory assistance is required to achieve adequate oxygenation, or if the upper airway is threatened because of obtundation or laryngeal dysfunction, endotracheal intubation and mechanical ventilation should be instituted with dispatch.

Blood Pressure Management

The treatment of hypertension in the patient with acute stroke has long been the subject of debate [233,234]. Although it is well known that chronic hypertension is an independent risk factor for the occurrence of ischemic stroke, lowering elevated blood pressure during an episode of cerebral ischemia has the potential to extend the area of hypoperfusion.

Elevated blood pressures occur naturally in the first few hours of ischemic stroke for a variety of reasons, including response to stress, full bladder, pain, underlying hypertension, physiologic compensation for hypoxia, and increased intracranial pressure. Untreated, pressures will usually spontaneously decline substantially within 24 hours of onset, and return to the patient's likely baseline by 4 to 7 days after the event [235,236]. This observation underlies the adage that the most effective treatment of hypertension in the patient with stroke is to wait 5 minutes and recheck it.

In the normal brain, to ensure adequate oxygenation, cerebral blood flow is maintained at a constant level over a wide range of systemic perfusion pressures through cerebrovascular autoregulation. When systemic blood pressure rises, cerebral arterioles constrict, increasing vascular resistance, and net cerebral blood flow remains unchanged. In contrast, a drop in blood pressure results in dilation of cerebral arterioles to reduce resistance and avoid a fall in blood flow. Patients who have a background history of hypertension will have chronically shifted their autoregulatory range upward, so that cerebral blood flow declines at a higher mean arterial pressure than in normotensive individuals.

Autoregulation is impaired in the ischemic field of patients with acute ischemic stroke. The cerebrovascular endothelium in these regions is, itself, experiencing ischemia and loses the ability to respond fully to autoregulatory signals. As a consequence, in the ischemic field cerebral blood flow varies directly with systemic blood pressure [237]. Reducing the systemic blood pressure may diminish blood flow to the ischemic penumbra and promote extension of the infarct. On the other hand, although it makes sense to prevent precipitous drops in blood pressure in patients with stroke, it is also possible that markedly elevated blood pressures could cause further damage by promoting edema formation, increasing the risk of hemorrhagic transformation, and exacerbating vascular damage.

Against this theoretical background largely based on observations in animal models, data on the efficacy of alternative blood pressure management strategies in acute human ischemic stroke is sparse. Suggestive data against active lowering of blood pressure have come from large observational series [238,239]. For example, among 868 consecutive patients with acute ischemic stroke in whom initial blood pressure was recorded, for every 20-mm Hg drop in systolic blood pressure, the relative risk of worsening condition within 36 hours of stroke onset increased by a factor of 0.66 [239].

Conversely, the strategy of actively raising the blood pressure in all patients with ischemic stroke has also not been tested directly in major clinical trials. Indirect observations from randomized clinical trials of hemodilution (sometimes associated with volume expansion and blood pressure elevation) suggest that many elderly stroke patients with coexisting cardiac morbidities do not tolerate induced hypertension well, and congestive heart failure, myocardial infarction, and other complications of therapy negate possible gains in cerebral perfusion. In select patients carefully managed in the intensive care unit, induced hypertension with phenylephrine has been shown to improve cerebral perfusion and possibly favorably influence the clinical course [240].

Based on these data, it is recommended that antihypertensive therapy should be withheld during the first few hours after ischemic stroke onset, unless blood pressure is in hypertensive encephalopathy–range on two consecutive measurements at least 5 minutes apart, with systolic blood pressure above 220 mm Hg or mean arterial pressure greater than 130 mm Hg [241–243]. This recommendation is modified if a patient has a concurrent condition that independently requires moderation of blood pressure, including acute myocardial infarction, aortic dissection, acute renal failure due to accelerated hypertension, or early hemorrhagic transformation of cerebral infarct. In these circumstances, a compromise must be struck between the need to maintain systemic blood pressure to maximize cerebral perfusion and the need to lower blood pressure to avoid extension of visceral injury. Another exceptional case is during the first 24 hours after thrombolytic therapy administration when, to minimize the risk of cerebral hemorrhagic transformation, the systolic blood pressure should be maintained at less than 180 mm Hg and diastolic blood pressure less than 105 mm Hg.

The choice of antihypertensive medications must take into account the effect of drugs on the cerebrovascular as well as the systemic circulation [237]. Nitroglycerin, sodium nitroprusside, calcium-channel blockers, and hydralazine are cerebral vasodilators that increase cerebral blood volume and may thereby increase intracerebral pressure and impair autoregulation. In contrast, α- and β-adrenergic blockers, ganglion blockers, and ACE inhibitors have little effect on cerebral blood volume. Parenteral agents that allow rapid, controlled titration to target pressures are often useful in the hyperacute setting and include enalapril, labetalol, and nitroprusside. Regimens for management of blood pressure in both thrombolytic and nonthrombolytic stroke adapted from the NINDS t-PA trialists approach are shown in Table 1-10 [18,244].

TABLE 1-10. BLOOD PRESSURE MANAGEMENT ALGORITHMS FOR PATIENTS WITH ACUTE ISCHEMIC STROKE

For Patients not Treated with Thrombolysis
Monitor BP q 15 min for 1 hr after ER arrival
Then q 1 hr $\times$ 3 for 3 hr
Then q 2 hr $\times$ 2 for 4 hr
Then q 4 hr $\times$ 4 for 16 hr
For SBP >220 mm Hg or DBP 120–140 mm Hg on two readings 5–10 min apart
Give labetalol 10 mg IV every 1–2 min
May repeat or double every 10–20 min, up to 150 mg
If response not satisfactory, use nitroprusside 0.5–10 μg/kg per min
Monitor BP at least every 15 min
Observe for hypotension
For DBP >140 mm Hg
Nitroprusside 0.5–10 μg/kg/min
Monitor BP at least every 15 min
Observe for hypotension
For Patients Treated with Thrombolytics
Monitor BP q 15 min for 2 hr after initiation of t-PA
Then q 30 min $\times$ 12 (for 6 hr)
Then q 60 min $\times$ 16 (for 16 hr)
For SBP >230 mm Hg or DBP 121–140 mm Hg on two readings 5–10 min apart
Give labetalol 10 mg IV every 1–2 min
May repeat or double every 10–20 min, up to 150 mg
If response not satisfactory, use nitroprusside 0.5–10 μg/kg per min
Monitor BP at least every 15 min
Observe for hypotension
For SBP 180–230 mm Hg and/or DBP 105–120 mm Hg
Give labetalol 10 mg IV
May be repeated or doubled every 10–20 min, up to 1,500 mg
For DBP >140 mm Hg
Nitroprusside 0.5–10 μg/kg per min
Monitor BP at least every 15 min
Observe for hypotension

BP, blood pressure; ER, emergency room; SBP, systolic blood pressure; DBP, diastolic blood pressure; t-PA, tissue plasminogen activator; IV, intravenous.

Hypotension is uncommon in ischemic stroke but, when present, vigorous treatment is warranted. First a treatable cause, such as decreased volume status (e.g., dehydration or hemorrhage), pump failure (e.g., arrhythmia, myocardial infarction, or congestive heart failure), or decreased peripheral vascular resistance (e.g., sepsis) should be sought, and corrected if identified. If the pressure falls below 90/60 mm Hg, or if blood pressure is in low-normal range and collateral insufficiency appears to be producing stroke progression, colloid solutions, hypervolemic therapy, and vasopressor agents should be administered. Often in these circumstances central venous or Swan-Ganz catheter monitoring should be employed because coexisting cardiac disease is common in the elderly population with ischemic stroke. Raising blood pressure to the patient's baseline level is a reasonable initial target.

Fluid Management

The majority of strokes occur in the elderly, who are liable to fluid and electrolyte disturbance. Decades ago it was common to restrict fluid intake in patients with acute ischemic stroke because of concern about cerebral edema. However, diminished fluid input decreases intravascular volume, promoting collateral failure, and increases blood viscosity, promoting recurrent arterial and venous thrombosis. Patients with ischemic stroke are often dehydrated upon hospital arrival. Large cohort studies have demonstrated that only 10% to 20% of patients with ischemic stroke develop edema that produces clinical deterioration. Edema generally peaks

3 to 5 days after stroke onset and is essentially never a concern during the first few hours *post ictus.*

Careful management of fluids is mandatory in patients with acute cerebral ischemia. Because of the frequency of aspiration, oral feedings should be avoided or minimized during the first few hours. All patients with acute stroke require an intravenous access line. Although cerebral edema is rarely a concern in the acute setting, hypotonic intravenous fluids are best avoided. Most patients should receive normal saline at full-maintenance volume, with infusion rates of 75 to 125 ml/hr to maintain intravascular volume and optimize brain perfusion [18,104,243].

Glucose Management

Hyperglycemia is the most common metabolic derangement in acute ischemic stroke. Many patients have a background history of diabetes that predisposed them to stroke. Even in nondiabetic patients, the physiologic stress of stroke frequently evokes a systemic sympathetic nervous system response that elevates blood sugar acutely.

Studies in animal models of focal and global ischemia have suggested that acute hyperglycemia may increase infarct size. Oxygen deprivation forces ischemic neuronal tissues to convert from aerobic to anaerobic metabolism. In ischemic regions, serum glucose is metabolized to lactate by anaerobic glycolysis. The greater the glucose level in the blood entering an ischemic neuronal field, the greater the resulting lactic acidosis. Lactic acid is neurotoxic. Consequently, avoidance of hyperglycemia during the acute stage might improve stroke outcome. However, overaggressive lowering of serum glucose levels to produce symptomatic hypoglycemia may also adversely affect patient course.

Several large observational studies have demonstrated that elevated blood glucose upon admission in acute ischemic stroke correlates with poor outcome [245,246]. However, it has not been demonstrated whether this association reflects a direct adverse effect of hyperglycemia upon outcome, or an epiphenomenon of severe initial brain injury producing a secondary rise in blood sugar. In patients undergoing intravenous thrombolysis, acute hyperglycemia is a risk factor for hemorrhagic transformation [247,248].

Although definitive studies are pending, current basic science and clinical observations suggest that hyperglycemia should be treated promptly in acute stroke. Employing a sliding insulin scale to maintain a glucose level of <200 mg/dl is a reasonable strategy [18,241]. In patients with profound hyperglycemia, glucose reduction should be limited to 75 to 100 mg/dl per hour to reduce the risk of osmotic injury to the brain [249]. Dextrose-containing intravenous solutions in general should be avoided during the first several hours after stroke onset, except in symptomatic hypoglycemia.

Temperature Management

Hyperthermia markedly worsens ischemic and traumatic brain injury in animal models [250]. Several mechanisms have been proposed to explain the deleterious effects of hyperthermia. Enhanced release of neurotransmitters, increased numbers of potentially damaging ischemic depolarizations in the focal ischemic penumbra, impaired recovery of energy metabolism, enhanced inhibition of protein kinases, and worsening of cytoskeletal proteolysis have all been implicated. A few large acute ischemic stroke cohort studies have found hyperthermia on admission to be an independent risk factor for poor outcome. These observations are intriguing, but they cannot exclude the possibility that early hyperthermia is a consequence of severe stroke, rather than a promoter of increased injury. Induced hypothermia is a promising neuroprotective strategy in human stroke. Conventional hypothermic therapy, however, requires intubation and paralysis of musculature to prevent shivering, steps which may pose risks to patients, especially those with milder strokes. Large-scale interventional trials are needed to determine whether systemic or selective cerebral hypothermic treatment can improve stroke outcome. A strategy of maintaining normothermia by administering prophylactic, standing-order antipyretics, such as acetaminophen, for the first 24 to 72 hours after stroke onset has shown promise in pilot trials, but it is likely to have only mild effects on clinical outcome [251,252].

Acute stroke patients with fever should be investigated for a source of infection and treated. In addition, the fever should be reduced promptly with antipyretics and cooling blankets if necessary.

Intravenous Fibrinolytic Therapy

Fibrinolytic agents activate plasminogen to form plasmin, which actively digests fibrin strands. The fibrinolytic agents that have been most extensively investigated in ischemic stroke are recombinant t-PA and streptokinase. t-PA is a serine protease endogenously released in human tissues from vascular endothelium. Unlike urokinase and streptokinase, t-PA preferentially activates plasminogen that is bound to fibrin. It has been proposed that this specificity results in fibrinolysis somewhat confined to localized thrombus, minimizing systemic fibrinolytic activation. Streptokinase is a protein synthesized by streptococci that forms complexes with and activates both circulating plasminogen and bound plasminogen.

By promoting early recanalization of occluded vessels and early reperfusion of ischemic fields, pharmacologic thrombolysis has the potential to salvage penumbral neuronal tissue. However, by exposing injured brain to lytic agents, thrombolytic therapy also increases the risk of hemorrhagic transformation of infarct with worsening of clinical deficit. Only large-scale clinical trials can determine whether, and

TABLE 1-11. CLINICAL TRIALS OF INTRAVENOUS THROMBOLYTICS IN ACUTE ISCHEMIC STROKE

Trial	Agent	Dose (% of MI Dose)	Time Window (Mean Time)	Ischemic Stroke Type	Sample Size	Hematoma/Symptomatic Hemorrhage (%)		Good Outcome[a]	
						Drug	Placebo	Drug	Placebo
NINDS Trial 1	t-PA	75	<3 hr (~2.2 hr)	All	291	6	0	47	27
NINDS Trial 2	t-PA	75	<3 hr (~2.2 hr)	All	333	7	1	39	26
ECASS I	t-PA	85	<6 hr (4.4 hr)	Mod–sev MCA	620	20	7	36	29
ECASS II	t-PA	75	<6 hr (NA)	Mod–sev MCA	800	8.8	3.4	40	37
ATLANTIS	t-PA	75	3–5 hr (4.4 hr)	All	613	6.7	1.3	42	40
MAST-E	SK	100	<6 hr (4.6 hr)	Mod–sev MCA	310	21	3	20	18
MAST-I	SK	100	<6 hr (NA)	All	622	8	1	37	35
ASK	SK	100	<4 hr (3.5 hr)	All	340	13	2	34	35

MI, myocardial infarction; NINDS, National Institute of Neurologic Diseases and Stroke; t-PA, tissue plasminogen activator; ECASS, European-Australasian Cooperative Acute Stroke Study; MCA, middle cerebral artery; NA, not available; ATLANTIS, Alteplase Thrombolysis for Acute Noninterventional Therapy in Ischemic Stroke; MAST-E, Multicenter Acute Stroke Trial—Europe; MAST-I, Multicenter Acute Stroke Trial—Italy; SK, streptokinase; ASK, Australian Streptokinase Trial.
Good outcome measures: NINDS Trials 1 and 2, ATLANTIS, Rankin disability score <2; ECASS I and II, MAST-E, and MAST-I, Rankin <3; ASK, Barthel Index 95–100. [a]Number shown represents %.

when, intravenous thrombolytic therapy confers overall benefit (or harm) in acute ischemic stroke.

Nine large-scale clinical trials of intravenous fibrinolytic therapy have been completed. Trial features and results are summarized in Table 1-11.

The findings of the two NINDS t-PA companion trials provided the foundation for U.S. Food and Drug Administration (FDA) approval of ischemic stroke as an added indication for t-PA administration. Patients were enrolled within 3 hours of stroke onset (one-half within 90 minutes of onset) and the total dose administered was 0.9 mg/kg [109]. The only CT exclusion criterion was hemorrhage; enrollment of patients with early signs of infarction was permitted.

In trial 1, the primary end point was a measure of early drug effect, the percentage of patients who improved by 4 points or more at 24 hours on a neurologic deficit scale, the NIHSS. Trial 1 enrolled 291 patients. In the t-PA group 47% of patients improved by the 4-point threshold versus 39% of the placebo group, a difference that did not reach statistical significance ($p = 0.21$). Other measures of early activity were positive. For example, both the control and the t-PA groups had an NIHSS score of 14 upon admission. At 24 hours the t-PA group's neurologic deficit score had improved to 8 versus 12 in the placebo group, a statistically significant group difference ($p > 0.02$) [253]. Also, 3-month secondary end points were positive, including statistically significant differences in Barthel, Rankin, and NIHSS scores.

Trial 2 was alike in all design and dose-regimen respects to trial 1, differing only in the prespecified primary end point. This consisted of a global statistic combining 3-month scores on the Barthel, Rankin, and NIHSS scales, and the Glasgow Outcome Scale. A total of 333 patients were enrolled. The primary end point and each of its component outcome measures were significantly favorable for the t-PA arm. For example, no or minimal disability on the Barthel Index was present in 50% of the t-PA group versus 38% of the placebo group. No or minimal residual neurologic deficits measured on the NIHSS were present in 31% of the t-PA group versus 20% of the placebo group. The absolute risk difference of 12% in the Barthel outcome translates into a number needed to treat of 8.3, that is, for every 8.3 patients treated with intravenous t-PA, one more patient will have no or minimal disability at 3 months. Patients at all degrees of initial stroke severity and with all stroke subtypes, including large-vessel atherothrombotic, small-vessel lacunar, and cardioembolic, appeared to benefit from t-PA in subgroup analysis. Safety data in the NINDS t-PA trials demonstrated a tenfold increased incidence of symptomatic intracerebral hemorrhage with t-PA, 6.4% versus 0.6%. However, no difference was noted in overall 3-month mortality, 17% in the t-PA group versus 21% with placebo, because deaths from herniation and systemic medical complications of large cerebral infarcts in the placebo group more than offset deaths from intracerebral hemorrhage in the t-PA group.

In multifactorial analysis, two variables independently predicted the development of symptomatic hemorrhage with t-PA therapy in the combined NINDS t-PA trials. Early signs of mass effect, hypodensity, and edema on the pretreatment CT scan increased the risk of symptomatic hemorrhage 7.8-fold, and severe neurologic deficit at baseline (NIHSS score > 20) increased the risk 1.8-fold [109]. For this reason, some authorities have recommended caution or avoidance of t-PA in patients with these features. However, patients with early hypodensity on CT and patients with baseline NIHSS score > 20 tended to fare better if assigned to thrombolytic therapy [253]. The overall prognosis is guarded for both sets of patients, who have evidence of severe ischemia at time of therapeutic decision making. For example, of those patients with an NIHSS score > 20, 10% of the t-PA group had a favorable outcome compared to 4% of the control group. An analysis of the combined trial populations, analyzing 26 patient variables with 90% power to detect an influence on treatment response, found no single variable or combination of variables that identified nonresponders to therapy, suggesting a generalized efficacy of t-PA for patients who met trial inclusion and exclusion criteria [254].

Three randomized placebo-controlled trials of intravenous streptokinase were conducted in the mid-1990s and showed no clear benefit, with significant risk of major hemorrhage and only minimal beneficial trends in final outcome. The disparate findings among clinical trials of intravenous thrombolysis occasioned a great deal of controversy [253,255]. The positive findings of the two NINDS t-PA trials, however, can be fully explained by several distinctive, biologically salient aspects of their conduct (see Table 1-11). Perhaps most crucially, the time window for entry and the median time poststroke at treatment were markedly shorter in the NINDS trials than in the remaining studies. Also, based on preliminary dose-escalation safety trials, the NINDS investigators employed a thrombolytic dose approximately 75% of the standard myocardial infarction dose, versus 100% in the streptokinase and other studies. Additionally, management of blood pressure and other supportive care may have been more uniform and intensive in the smaller number of centers participating in the NINDS studies than in the geographically more diverse comparator trials. The combination of shorter time to treatment, lower dose, agent type, and intensive supportive care are fully adequate to account for differences in trial results.

Extending the time window of the 0.9 mg/kg dose of t-PA beyond 3 hours was the focus of two more recent clinical trials. The second European-Australasian Cooperative Acute Stroke Study (ECASS II) enrolled 800 patients within 0 to 6 hours of symptom onset, randomized to 0.9 mg/kg of t-PA or placebo. In contrast to the NINDS t-PA trial, a substantial majority (80%) of the patients enrolled in ECASS II were treated during the 3- to 6-hour time window [256]. The primary end point of a favorable outcome as determined by the modified Rankin scale at 90 days was achieved by 40.3% of patients receiving t-PA versus 36.6% of patients receiving placebo. This 3.7% difference was not statistically significant. A *post hoc* analysis using the modified Rankin scale found a difference between the groups if outcome was classified according to independence (Rankin 0 to 2 versus 3 to 5, respectively). This analysis revealed an absolute difference of 8.3% in favor of the t-PA group in reaching independence.

The Alteplase Thrombolysis for Acute Noninterventional Therapy in Ischemic Stroke (ATLANTIS) trial randomized patients who were 3- to 5-hours post stroke onset to 0.9 mg/kg t-PA or placebo. The study was stopped early when an interim analysis showed no major difference in the primary end point between treatment arms, and futility analysis suggested little chance of an important difference emerging. These data suggest that 3 hours post onset is a critical time point for intravenous t-PA therapy. Under 3 hours, therapy confers substantial benefit on average, while beyond 3 hours intravenous t-PA offers little overall gain to unselected patients. These findings are reinforced by a time-of-treatment analysis of the NINDS t-PA trial data, which shows that the earlier thrombolysis was initiated, the greater the differential benefit in the t-PA arm versus placebo, with outcomes converging upon unity at the 3-hour mark [257].

Important additional information regarding the use of intravenous t-PA comes from observations in a large cohort of patients treated in actual clinical practice after it reached the market [248,258]. For example, among 960 patients treated according to FDA-approved criteria, symptomatic hemorrhages occurred in only 6%. However, in 57 patients in whom treatment deviated from FDA-approved criteria, symptomatic hemorrhages occurred in 10.7% [248]. These data suggest that strict adherence to FDA-approved criteria is required to maximize the safety of therapy.

Substantial clinical trial evidence supports the use of intravenous t-PA in patients who meet the inclusion and exclusion criteria of the NINDS t-PA trials. Patients are candidates for thrombolysis if they have an acute neurologic deficit that is potentially disabling and thought to be caused by cerebral ischemia, their CT scan shows no hemorrhage, and therapy can be started within 3 hours of symptom onset. (A detailed checklist for determining eligibility is provided in Table 1-12.) As with any potentially harmful treatment, the risks and benefits of thrombolytic therapy must be discussed with the patient or the patient's representative or both, or two-physician consent employed if no legally authorized representative is available. t-PA is administered at a dose of 0.9 mg/kg with a maximum dose of 90 mg. Ten percent of the total dose is given as a bolus over 1 to 2 minutes and the remainder is infused over 1 hour. Anticoagulants and antiplatelet agents are not to be administered within the first 24 hours following thrombolytic treatment.

After infusion, close monitoring of blood pressure and neurologic status is mandatory and is best carried out in a neurologic intensive care unit or stroke unit (see Table 1-10). Neurologic deterioration, new-onset headache, acute hypertension, nausea, or vomiting may be signs of intracranial hemorrhage and must be investigated immediately. An acute rise in blood pressure may be the first indication of intracerebral hemorrhage. If the patient is still receiving t-PA, the infusion should be discontinued and a CT scan obtained immediately. A blood sample for prothrombin time (PT), partial thromboplastin time (PTT), platelet count, and fibrinogen level should be sent for stat analysis.

TABLE 1-12. ALGORITHM FOR INTRAVENOUS FIBRINOLYTIC THERAPY

Inclusion Criteria

Ischemic stroke with a defined onset of <3 hr from time t-PA is to be started.

Ascertain last time patient known to be awake and deficit free.

Measurable deficit on NIH Stroke Scale.

Neurologic deficit > minimal weakness, isolated ataxia, isolated sensory, or isolated dysarthria.

CT scan shows no evidence of intracranial hemorrhage.

If early signs of new major hemisphere infarct are present (e.g., edema, mass effect, sulcal effacement) reassess time of onset. The presence of these CT findings may be associated with an increased risk of hemorrhage.

Exclusion Criteria

History

Stroke or serious head trauma within past 3 mo

Major surgery or serious trauma within past 14 d

History of intracranial hemorrhage, AVM, or aneurysm

GI or urinary tract hemorrhage within previous 21 d

Arterial puncture at a noncompressible site OR LP within previous 7 d

Clinical

Rapidly improving neurologic signs or minor symptoms

SBP >185 mm Hg OR DBP >110 mm Hg OR aggressive (IV) treatment required to reduce patient's BP to specified limits

Seizure at onset

Symptoms suggestive of subarachnoid hemorrhage

Recent myocardial infarction–induced pericarditis

Laboratory

PT >15 sec (INR >1.7)

Patient received heparin within 48 hr preceding stroke onset AND has an elevated PTT

Platelet count <100,000 per mm^3

Glucose concentration <50 mg/dl (2.7 mmol/L) OR >400 mg/dl (22.2 mmol/L)

Women with a positive pregnancy test

Discuss the risks and benefits of thrombolytic therapy with the patient and family (if possible) and document the discussion in the medical record.

Before Administering t-PA

Review checklist to confirm inclusion and exclusion criteria.

Confirm patient is not spontaneously improving.

Treatment and Management

Administer t-PA 0.9 mg/kg total or maximum 90 mg.

Administer 10% of t-PA dose as a bolus.

Administer remaining 90% of t-PA as a constant infusion over 1 hr.

DO NOT give anticoagulants for 24 hr from start of t-PA administration.

DO NOT give antiplatelet agents for 24 hr from start of t-PA administration.

Admit to ICU OR acute stroke unit.

Maintain SBP UNDER 180 mm Hg and DBP UNDER 115 mm Hg.

Restrict central venous line placement OR arterial puncture for 24 hr.

DO NOT insert indwelling bladder catheter for >30 min after t-PA administration.

AVOID insertion of NG tube for 24 hr after t-PA administration.

t-PA, tissue plasminogen activator; NIH, National Institutes of Health; CT, computed tomography; AVM, arteriovenous malformation; GI, gastrointestinal; LP, lumbar puncture; IV, intravenous; SBP, systolic blood pressure; DBP, diastolic BP; PT, prothrombin time; INR, international normalized ratio; PTT, partial thromboplastin time; ICU, intensive care unit; NG, nasogastric.

If the CT scan shows hemorrhage, then the laboratory results should be evaluated for abnormalities and corrected with fibrinogen, cryoprecipitate, or platelets, or a combination. A neurosurgical consultation may be warranted for hematoma evacuation or intervention to relieve increased intracranial pressure. If the guidelines for intravenous t-PA are rigorously adhered to, this therapy is effective in treating patients with acute ischemic stroke.

Combined Intravenous and Intraarterial Thrombolytic Therapy

Intraarterial fibrinolysis possesses several theoretical advantages over intravenous fibrinolysis. Higher concentrations of fibrinolytic agent are delivered to the clot, increasing the likelihood of recanalization. Conversely, lower concentrations of fibrinolytic agent escape into the systemic circulation, potentially decreasing the risk of systemic hemorrhagic complications. Gentle mechanical disruption may be employed to potentiate the pharmacologic thrombolytic intervention. The diagnostic angiogram that immediately precedes intervention provides precise information regarding stroke pathophysiology not available from noninvasive testing (Fig. 1-11). The time at which recanalization is achieved is known with certainty, and supportive therapy such as fluid and blood pressure management can immediately be adjusted for a reopened rather than occluded vessel.

These benefits must be weighed against several theoretical disadvantages of intraarterial fibrinolysis versus intravenous fibrinolysis. The start of fibrinolytic therapy is substantially delayed by the need to move the patient to an angiography suite, prep the patient for the procedure, mobilize the interventional team, and catheterize the involved vessel. In controlled trials, the time delay from completion of CT scan to catheter placed on clot and start of fibrinolytic infusion has generally ranged from 70 to 120 minutes. Intraarterial therapy requires manipulation of a catheter in the ischemic bed and injured vessels, possibly increasing the risk of cerebral hemorrhage. Intraarterial treatment is both labor and capital intensive, and requires highly experienced interventionists. Consequently it is likely, even if beneficial, to remain an intervention confined to tertiary stroke critical care centers.

Intraarterial fibrinolytic therapy techniques and results are discussed in detail in Chapter 4. Combined intravenous and intraarterial fibrinolysis strategies have evolved in an attempt to combine the advantages of rapid start of treatment of intravenous therapy and the eventual more definitive recanalization of intraarterial therapy. Intravenous fibrinolytic therapy is begun immediately upon the completion of CT scan, within 3 hours of symptom onset. Simultaneously the patient is transported to the angiography suite and catheterization begun. When the catheter arrives on clot, intravenous infusion is ended (or it has ended

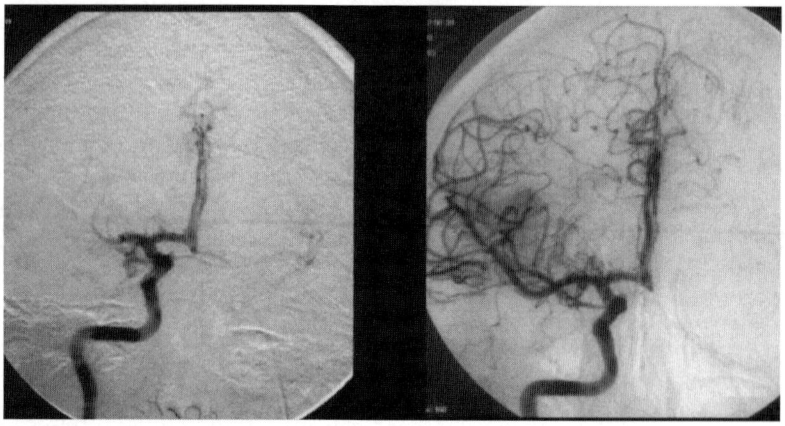

FIGURE 1-11. Thrombolytic recanalization. Patient presents with left hemiparesis, hemisensory deficit, hemianopia, and hemineglect and initial angiogram demonstrates right middle cerebral artery trunk occlusion **(left).** Intraarterial thrombolysis with tissue plasminogen activator is performed. End of procedure angiogram **(right)** shows full recanalization of MCA and good filling of distal sylvian MCA branches.

earlier after reaching a prespecified maximal dose) and intraarterial infusion begun.

The feasibility and safety of combined intravenous and intraarterial t-PA therapy has been investigated in open series and the Emergency Management of Stroke (EMS) Bridging Trial [259–261]. These studies have demonstrated that combined therapy is feasible, yields good recanalization rates, and appears to have acceptable hemorrhagic adverse event rates. Larger, definitive trials comparing combined intravenous and intraarterial thrombolysis with pure intravenous and pure intraarterial strategies are needed.

Acute Antiplatelet Therapy

Antiplatelet agents are of potential benefit in acute ischemic stroke by reducing the formation of *white thrombi,* platelet and fibrin aggregates that form in fast-moving arterial streams upon damaged endothelial surfaces. Antiplatelet therapy may discourage propagation of the initial thrombus to block additional vessels and recurrent embolization. However, antiplatelet therapy may also increase the risk of hemorrhagic transformation of an infarct. Several clinical trials have examined the use of antiplatelet therapy in the setting of acute ischemic stroke.

Two megatrials examined the efficacy of aspirin therapy within 48 hours of ischemic stroke onset. The Chinese Acute Stroke Trial (CAST) enrolled 21,106 patients within 48 hours of stroke onset and randomized patients to 160 mg of aspirin a day or placebo [262]. Treatment was administered daily for 4 weeks. Ninety-seven percent of the patients completed the 4 weeks of medication, whether they remained hospitalized for 4 weeks or were discharged before that time. The primary end points for the study were death from any cause during the first 4 weeks following stroke and death or dependence at discharge. Secondary end points included fatal or nonfatal recurrent stroke and death or nonfatal stroke within 4 weeks. Study results for the primary end point demonstrated a significant reduction in death at 4 weeks from 3.9% in the control group to 3.3% in the aspirin group. Secondary analyses demonstrated modest but statistically significant reductions with aspirin in recurrent ischemic strokes at 4 weeks and 4-week mortality.

The International Stroke Trial (IST) employed a 3 × 2 factorial design to investigate whether aspirin, low-dose unfractionated heparin, high-dose unfractionated heparin, or a combination of aspirin and unfractionated heparin are safe and efficacious in the treatment of ischemic stroke [263]. There were 19,435 patients enrolled within 48 hours of symptom onset with an average time to randomization of 19 hours. Sixteen percent of patients were enrolled within 6 hours of symptom onset. Subjects were randomized to one of the six following groups: unfractionated heparin 5,000 IU s.c. b.i.d., unfractionated heparin 12,500 IU s.c. b.i.d., aspirin 300 mg q.d., aspirin 300 mg q.d. plus unfractionated heparin 5,000 IU s.c. b.i.d., aspirin 300 mg q.d. plus unfractionated heparin 12,500 IU s.c. b.i.d., or avoid aspirin and unfractionated heparin. Subjects were treated for 14 days or until time of discharge. The average duration of treatment was 11 days with the main reason for early discontinuation being hospital discharge. The primary outcomes for the study were death within 14 days and death or dependency at 6 months.

Aspirin-treated patients had significantly fewer recurrent ischemic strokes with no significant increase in hemorrhagic strokes within 14 days. The recurrent ischemic stroke rate declined from 3.9% to 2.8% with aspirin therapy. A nonsignificant decrease in mortality within 14 days was observed. At 6 months there was a nonsignificant trend towards a smaller percentage of the aspirin group being dead or dependent, 62.2% versus 63.5%.

A metaanalysis combining the results in 40,397 randomized subjects from the IST, CAST, and one additional small trial demonstrates the following statistically significant effects of aspirin: early recurrent ischemic stroke is reduced from 3.2% to 2.4%, symptomatic hemorrhagic transformation is increased from 0.8% to 1.0%, and overall death or nonfatal stroke at 6 months is reduced from 9.1% to 8.2%. These findings indicate that aspirin confers a statistically significant, but biologically quite small, benefit upon patients with acute ischemic stroke. Use of aspirin during the first weeks after onset yields a reduction of 9 deaths or recurrent strokes per 1,000 patients treated. Thus the number needed to treat with aspirin to prevent one death or recurrent stroke in the first few weeks is 111. It is unclear from these trials to what, if any, degree this small treatment effect of aspirin reflects beneficial actions during the first hours after stroke onset, versus prevention of secondary stroke on subsequent days.

Other antiplatelet agents have not been systematically investigated in the acute stroke setting. Ticlopidine takes 4 to 5 days to reach maximal effectiveness at standard dosage, limiting its theoretical utility in the first few hours. Loading doses of clopidogrel are well tolerated, yield rapid onset of antiplatelet effect, and have been shown to be beneficial in acute coronary syndromes. Trials of intravenous glycoprotein IIa/IIIb platelet antagonists in acute ischemic stroke are under way.

These data support the use of aspirin during the first 2 weeks after ischemic stroke onset, and provide some support for the use of aspirin at a dose of 160 to 325 mg during the first few hours. All patients not receiving thrombolytic or anticoagulant therapy should be treated with aspirin, unless there is a history of hypersensitivity to aspirin, active peptic ulcer disease, recent gastrointestinal bleeding, or other contraindication. To promote rapid therapeutic effect, patients able to take pills orally should be instructed to chew the aspirin tablet prior to swallowing. Patients unable to swallow safely should receive therapy either by nasogastric tube or rectal suppository. Loading-dose clopidogrel, 300 to 375 mg, is an attractive strategy in the patient with acute ischemic stroke who is intolerant of aspirin.

Acute Anticoagulation

Administering anticoagulation therapy for acute stroke is a time-honored, but until recently essentially untested, therapeutic practice. Theoretically anticoagulation is most effective on red thrombi, which tend to form in areas of low flow or stagnation. It has been hypothesized that anticoagulation may prevent embolism from the site of stenosis, clot propagation, and thrombotic occlusion of a stenotic lesion. Conversely, acute anticoagulation may increase the risk of hemorrhagic transformation. More than 22 trials enrolling more than 24,000 patients have now been performed testing anticoagulation in acute ischemic stroke, and no net benefit has been identified [264].

Unfractionated Heparin

Unfractionated heparin has been employed in acute ischemic stroke for over 40 years. Unfractionated heparin is a mixture of glycosaminoglycans isolated from porcine intestinal mucosa. Heparin binds to endothelial cell surfaces and works by binding and accelerating 1,000-fold the actions of antithrombin III. Antithrombin III forms stable complexes with and inhibits several clotting factor proteases. Heparin catalyzes this reaction without being consumed. Once an antithrombin–protease complex is formed, heparin is released intact for binding to another antithrombin molecule.

Unfractionated heparin was initially tested in several small clinical trials, some in the pre-CT era when some enrolled patients may have had hemorrhage present on entry. A metaanalysis of all trials of acute anticoagulation (chiefly with unfractionated heparin) reported through 1993 identified ten trials enrolling a total of only 1,047 patients. Across all studies of ischemic stroke, anticoagulation in the acute phase showed a nonsignificant trend toward reduction in the odds of death.

The IST examined the effects of aspirin, subcutaneous unfractionated heparin, and a combination of these two drugs in patients with ischemic stroke who sought treatment within 48 hours of stroke onset [263]. As noted above, subjects were randomized to six treatment arms in a 3 × 2 factorial design, including high subcutaneous dose, low subcutaneous dose, and avoid unfractionated heparin arms. Treatment was continued for 14 days or until time of discharge, and the average duration of treatment was 11 days.

Patients treated with unfractionated heparin had significantly fewer recurrent ischemic strokes within 14 days (2.9% versus 3.8%), but this benefit was offset by a similar increase in hemorrhagic strokes (1.2% versus 0.4%). Treatment groups showed no difference in the incidence of death and disability at 6 months. No net benefit of anticoagulation given during the acute period was seen when analysis was confined to the subgroup of 3,169 patients who had atrial fibrillation and likely cardioembolic stroke. Considering each of the six treatment group subarms across the entire trial population, there was a trend to best outcome in patients assigned to aspirin plus low-dose unfractionated heparin given daily.

The results of the IST argue against a policy of fixed, high-dose, subcutaneously administered unfractionated heparin for all comers with acute ischemic stroke. Whether these findings can be generalized to the more common U.S. practice of adjusted-dose, intravenous unfractionated heparin for selected patients is uncertain. Avoiding treatment of acutely ill patients with risk factors for hemorrhagic transformation might improve the benefit-to-risk ratio. Large

TABLE 1-13. ALGORITHM FOR ANTITHROMBOTIC THERAPY IN ACUTE ISCHEMIC STROKE

Initial IV heparin (using loading bolus if worsening during last 30 min), aim PTT 50–60 sec for:
- Suspected critical, symptomatic carotid artery stenosis, when exam suggests infarct size is small to moderate (<4 cm)
- Suspected basilar artery thrombosis

Initial aspirin 325 mg, crush and chew, for all others (substitute clopidogrel 300 mg for patients intolerant of aspirin)

Initial subcutaneous unfractionated heparin, 5,000 units b.i.d. or low-dose LMWH, for:
- All nonambulatory patients not on full-dose anticoagulation

Subsequent IV heparin with a bolus, aim PTT 50–60 sec, for:
- Large-vessel atherothrombotic stroke in progression despite aspirin, when the physician believes the progression may be due to clot propagation or recurrent embolism
- Lacunar stroke in progression despite aspirin, when the physician believes the progression may be due to clot propagation

Subsequent arterial dose LMWH (e.g., enoxaparin 1 mg/kg s.c. b.i.d.) for:
- Cardioembolic stroke after 24–48-hr delay, when infarct size is small (<3 cm)

IV, intravenous; PTT, partial thromboplastin time; LMWH, low–molecular-weight heparin.

series have suggested that large infarct size, severely elevated blood pressures, and older age increase the risk of hemorrhage [265].

At present, clinical trial data do not suggest major net benefit or harm of intravenous, dose-adjusted unfractionated heparin in acute ischemic stroke. Because aspirin and t-PA are of proven benefit, these agents should in general be preferred over anticoagulation in the acute setting except in select situations. Our own current algorithm for the use of antiplatelet and anticoagulant therapy is provided in Table 1-13.

Low–molecular-weight Heparins and Heparinoids

Heparin can be fractionated by either chemical or enzymatic depolymerization to yield fragments about one-third the size of the average molecular component of unfractionated heparin. Purified low–molecular-weight heparins (LMWHs) also work by binding to antithrombin III. LMWHs differ in several important respects, however, from unfractionated heparin. They exert relatively less effect on clotting factor IIa, which has been associated with hemorrhagic complications in animal models, but equal effect on factor Xa, associated with beneficial antithrombotic activity. They are much less likely than unfractionated heparin to provoke an antibody response and the syndrome of heparin-induced thrombocytopenia with *in vivo* thrombosis. They have high bioavailability and a more prolonged half-life, yielding a more predictable anticoagulant response, and consequently can be administered at arterial disease treatment levels with once- or twice-daily subcutaneous injections without requiring laboratory monitoring and dose adjustment.

Heparinoids are mixtures of LMWH, dermatan sulphate, and chondroitin sulphate. Their mode of action and relative advantages compared with unfractionated heparin are comparable to LMWHs, although their half-lives are considerably longer.

Several double-blinded placebo-controlled trials of LMWHs in acute ischemic stroke have been performed. The first, studying nadroparin, found a benefit [266]. These promising results, however, were not replicated in a second, larger confirmatory trial of nadroparin [267]. A trial of tinzaparin also demonstrated no advantage of acute LMWH over control given acutely. Another prospective trial compared the LMWH dalteparin with aspirin given within 30 hours of atrial fibrillation–associated stroke. There were no statistically significant differences between treatment groups in death and physical dependency at 3 months [268].

Perhaps the most detailed information regarding the effect of novel anticoagulants in acute ischemic stroke comes from a trial of a heparinoid in acute ischemic stroke, TOAST [269]. This randomized, double-blind trial compared danaparoid to placebo for 7 days in 1,281 patients enrolled within 24 hours of stroke onset. Danaparoid was administered by continuous intravenous infusion, dose adjusted by laboratory monitoring of factor Xa. On the primary outcome measure of favorable Barthel activities-of-daily-living score at 3 months, no difference between the treatment groups was observed. Subgroup analysis did suggest a beneficial effect in patients with large-vessel (primarily carotid) atherothrombotic stroke mechanisms, with very favorable 3-month outcomes in 43.3% of the danaparoid group versus 29.1% of the placebo group. No benefit at all was detected in patients with cardioembolic and lacunar stroke mechanisms.

It is instructive to consider event rates observed in the control arms in recent trials of anticoagulant therapy. In the TOAST trial, progression or recurrence of infarct was observed in only 1.3% of placebo-treated patients over the first 7 days, despite the absence of antiplatelet or anticoagulant therapy. In the cardioembolic TOAST placebo subgroup, recurrent infarct occurred in only 1.6% of patients not receiving anticoagulant therapy. Similarly, in patients with atrial fibrillation enrolled in the IST and assigned to the avoid aspirin and avoid unfractionated heparin arm, recurrent infarct occurred in only 1.1% of patients over 14 days. These observations suggest that with modern fluid management and general supportive care, progression or recurrence of infarct occurs very infrequently in patients with acute ischemic stroke even in the absence of antithrombotic therapy. As a result, opportunities for anticoagulation therapy to be beneficial are circumscribed.

Clinical trial data provide no firm evidence of net benefit

or net harm of LMWHs or heparinoids in acute ischemic stroke. Therefore, no firm recommendation can be given, and their use remains at the discretion of the treating physician. The TOAST trial suggests that patients with large-vessel atherothrombotic stroke may benefit from heparinoid treatment, but this subgroup analysis requires prospective confirmation in a new trial. The risk-to-benefit ratio of these agents may be improved by avoiding their use during the first 5 to 7 days in patients with large cerebral infarcts (e.g., those involving greater than 4 cm of tissue in longest dimension). In patients with subacute stroke requiring bridging parenteral anticoagulation to long-term warfarin, one cohort study has suggested that LMWHs, used both in the hospital and on an outpatient basis, may be safer and more cost effective than intravenous unfractionated heparin [270]. One approach to antithrombotic therapy is outlined in Table 1-13.

REHABILITATION OF PATIENTS WITH ISCHEMIC STROKE

Mechanisms of Recovery and Rehabilitative Therapies

The majority of functional recovery following a stroke occurs during the first 3 to 6 months, with lesser degrees of improvement up to 18 months or more [271]. Data from the Framingham Study showed that 80% of long-term stroke survivors regain independence in ambulation and 66% independence in activities of daily living. Fundamental mechanisms of recovery include the following [272]:

- Recovery of neuronal excitability by stunned parenchyma
- Activity in partially spared pathways
- Unmasking dormant parallel pathways
- Alteration in neuronal networks to recruit cells not ordinarily involved in an activity
- Synaptic sprouting
- Remyelination
- Axonal and dendritic regeneration
- Repopulation from neural stem cell progenitors
- Alternative behavioral strategies

Important prognostic factors for recovery include severity of initial neurologic impairment, age, and available family and social support systems. Neurorehabilitation using a multidisciplinary team approach increases the likelihood of attaining functional independence.

Initial measures that help prevent development of medical complications of stroke include deep venous thrombosis prophylaxis, appropriate evaluation of swallowing function and nutrition, and early mobility. Physical, occupational, and speech therapy should be initiated during the acute hospitalization period for most patients and continued through the subacute to chronic period as needed.

Neurotransplantation

Cell transplantation is a promising approach to restoring function in patients with chronic disabilities due to stroke. Basic scientific studies have demonstrated that cells derived from a variety of precursor or progenitor cells can develop the capacity to function as mature neuronal cells, expressing neurotransmitters and forming synapses. Studies in animal models of focal ischemia have suggested that cell transplantation is feasible in ischemic stroke and can improve long-term functional outcome [273–275]. Clinical trials are currently under way to test the efficacy of these techniques in humans [276].

CONCLUSION

Our concepts of the pathophysiology and treatment of stroke have changed dramatically over the past 20 years. In acute cerebral ischemia, basic scientific and clinical studies have emphasized the importance of rapid intervention to restore blood flow and prevent permanent ischemic damage. With the recent development of effective thrombolytic acute stroke therapy, the era of therapeutic nihilism is at an end. Now stroke is recognized as an eminently treatable medical emergency, and every minute counts when caring for a patient with an acute stroke. In addition to these dramatic advances in acute ischemic stroke therapy, tremendous progress has occurred in stroke prevention. Clinical trial–validated treatments to prevent ischemic stroke are numerous and could avert more than three-quarters of all strokes if widely applied. Care according to the principles outlined in this chapter will help to reduce the personal, familial, and societal burden of this devastating disease.

REFERENCES

1. Williams GR, Jiang JG, Matchar DB, et al. Incidence and occurrence of total (first-ever and recurrent) stroke. *Stroke* 1999;30: 2523–2528.
2. Broderick J, Miller R, Khoury J, et al. Incidence rates of stroke for blacks and whites: preliminary results from the Greater Cincinnati/Northern Kentucky Stroke Study. *Stroke* 2001;32:320.
3. Leary M, Saver J. Incidence of silent stroke in the United States. *Stroke* 2001;32:363.
4. Rosamond W, Folsom A, Chambless L, et al. Stroke incidence and survival among middle-aged adults: 9-year follow-up of the Atherosclerosis Risk in Communities (ARIC) cohort. *Stroke* 1999;30:736–743.
5. Sacco R, Wolf P, Kannel W, et al. Survival and recurrence following stroke: the Framingham Study. *Stroke* 1982;13: 290–305.
6. American Heart Association. 1999 Heart and Stroke Statistical Update. Dallas, TX: American Heart Association, 1998.
7. American Heart Association. 2001 Heart and Stroke Statistical Update. Dallas, TX: American Heart Association, 2000.
8. Samsa G, Matchar D, Goldstein L, et al. Utilities for major stroke: results from a survey of preferences among persons at increased risk for stroke. *Am Heart J* 1998;136:703–713.

9. Broderick J, Phillips S, Whisnant J, et al. Incidence rates of stroke in the eighties: the end of the decline in stroke? *Stroke* 1989;20:577–582.
10. Petty G, Brown R, Whisnant J, et al. Ischemic stroke subtypes: a population-based study of incidence and risk factors. *Stroke* 1999;30:2513–2516.
11. Sacco R. Frequency and determinants of stroke. In: Fisher M, ed. *Clinical atlas of cerebrovascular disorders.* St Louis: Mosby–Year Book, 1994:1.2–1.16.
12. Saver J, Tamburi T. Genetics of cerebrovascular disease. In: Pulst SM, ed. *Neurogenetics.* New York: Oxford University Press, 2000:403–431.
13. Sacco R, Benjamin E, Broderick J, et al. Risk factors. *Stroke* 1997;28:1507–1517.
14. Gorelick PB. Stroke prevention: windows of opportunity and failed expectations? A discussion of modifiable cardiovascular risk factors and a prevention proposal. *Neuroepidemiology* 1999; 16:163–173.
15. Johnston S, Gress D, Browner W, et al. Short-term prognosis after emergency department diagnosis of TIA. *JAMA* 2000;284: 2901–2906.
16. Wilterdink J, Easton J. Vascular event rates in patients with atherosclerotic cerebrovascular disease. *Arch Neurol* 1992;49: 857–863.
17. Streifler JY, Eliasziw M, Benavente OR, et al. The risk of stroke in patients with first-ever retinal vs hemispheric transient ischemic attacks and high-grade carotid stenosis. North American Symptomatic Carotid Endarterectomy Trial. *Arch Neurol* 1995; 52:246–249.
18. Kalafut MA, Saver JL. The acute stroke patient: the first six hours. In: Cohen SN, ed. *Management of ischemic stroke.* New York: McGraw-Hill, 2000:17–52.
19. Hossmann KA. Viability thresholds and the penumbra of focal ischemia. *Ann Neurol* 1994;36:557–565.
20. Heiss WD, Huber M, Fink GR, et al. Progressive derangement of periinfarct viable tissue in ischemic stroke. *J Cereb Blood Flow Metab* 1992;12:193–203.
21. Heiss WD, Graf R, Wienhard K, et al. Dynamic penumbra demonstrated by sequential multitracer PET after middle cerebral artery occlusion in cats. *J Cereb Blood Flow Metab* 1994; 14:892–902.
22. Zivin JA. Factors determining the therapeutic window for stroke. *Neurology* 1998;50:559–603.
23. Willeit J, Kiechl S. Biology of arterial atheroma. *Cerebrovasc Dis* 2000;20[Suppl 5]:1–8.
24. DeGraba TJ, Fisher M, Yatsu FM. Atherogenesis and strokes. In: Barnett HJM, Mohr JP, Stein BM, et al., eds. *Stroke: pathophysiology, diagnosis, and management,* 2nd ed. New York: Churchill Livingstone, 1992:29–48.
25. Kiechl S, Willeit J. The natural course of atherosclerosis. Part I: incidence and progression. *Arterioscler Thromb Vasc Biol* 1999; 19:1484–1490.
26. Kiechl S, Willeit J. The natural course of atherosclerosis. II. Vascular remodeling. *Arterioscler Thromb Vasc Biol* 1999;19: 1491–1498.
27. Rothwell PM, Villagra R, Gibson R, et al. Evidence of a chronic systemic cause of instability of atherosclerotic plaques. *Lancet* 2000;355:19–24.
28. Rauch U, Osende JI, Fuster V, et al. Thrombus formation on atherosclerotic plaques: pathogenesis and clinical consequences. *Ann Intern Med* 2001;134:224–238.
29. Moossy J. Pathology of cerebral atherosclerosis. Influence of age, race, and gender. *Stroke* 1993;24[Suppl 12]:I22–23, I31–32.
30. Caplan LR, Hennerici M. Impaired clearance of emboli (washout) is an important link between hypoperfusion, embolism, and ischemic stroke. *Arch Neurol* 1998;55:1475–1482.
31. Eliasziw M, Streifler JY, Fox AJ, et al. Significance of plaque ulceration in symptomatic patients with high-grade carotid stenosis. North American Symptomatic Carotid Endarterectomy Trial. *Stroke* 1994;25:304–308.
32. Saver JL. Consultant's corner: a 68-year-old woman with a loud left carotid bruit. *Fam Pract Recert* 2000;22:11–20.
33. Cohen M, Biller J, Saver JL. Advances in the management of carotid disease. *Curr Probl Cardiol* 1994;19:473–530.
34. Fernandez-Beer E, Saver JL. Symptomatic internal carotid artery stenosis. In: Feldmann E, ed. *Current diagnosis in neurologic disease.* St Louis: Mosby, 1994:29–34.
35. Harrison MJ, Iansek R, Marshall J. Clinical identification of TIAs due to carotid stenosis. *Stroke* 1986;17:391–392.
36. Bruno A, Corbett JJ, Biller J, et al. Transient monocular visual loss patterns and associated vascular abnormalities. *Stroke* 1990; 21:34–39.
37. Kaiboriboon K, Piriyawat P, Selhorst JB. Light-induced amaurosis fugax. *Am J Ophthalmol* 2001;131:674–676.
38. Baumgartner RW, Baumgartner I. Vasomotor reactivity is exhausted in transient ischaemic attacks with limb shaking. *J Neurol Neurosurg Psychiatry* 1998;65:561–564.
39. Wityk RJ, Chang HM, Rosengart A, et al. Proximal extracranial vertebral artery disease in the New England Medical Center Posterior Circulation Registry. *Arch Neurol* 1998;55:470–478.
40. Fisher CM. Occlusion of the vertebral arteries. Causing transient basilar symptoms. *Arch Neurol* 1970;22:13–19.
41. Sacco RL, Kargman DE, Gu Q, et al. Race-ethnicity and determinants of intracranial atherosclerotic cerebral infarction. The Northern Manhattan Stroke Study. *Stroke* 1995;26:14–20.
42. Saver JL, Biller J. Superficial middle cerebral artery. In: Bogousslavsky J, Caplan LR, eds. *Stroke syndromes.* New York: Cambridge University Press, 1996:247–258.
43. Bogousslavsky J, Barnett HJ, Fox AJ, et al. Atherosclerotic disease of the middle cerebral artery. *Stroke* 1986;17:1112–1120.
44. Caplan L, Babikian V, Helgason C, et al. Occlusive disease of the middle cerebral artery. *Neurology* 1985;35:975–982.
45. Kalafut M, Saver JL. Basilar artery strokes. In: Gilman S, ed. *MedLink neurology.* San Diego: MedLink Corporation, 2001.
46. Caplan LR. *Posterior circulation disease: clinical findings, diagnosis, and management.* Cambridge, MA: Blackwell Science, 1996.
47. Saver JL. Emerging risk factors for stroke: patent foramen ovale, aortic arch atherosclerosis, antiphospholipid antibodies, and activated protein C resistance. *J Stroke Cerebrovasc Dis* 1997;6: 167–172.
48. Atherosclerotic disease of the aortic arch as a risk factor for recurrent ischemic stroke. The French Study of Aortic Plaques in Stroke Group. *N Engl J Med* 1996;334:1216–1221.
49. Tunick PA, Kronzon I. Atheromas of the thoracic aorta: clinical and therapeutic update. *J Am Coll Cardiol* 2000;35:545–554.
50. Saver JL, Easton JD. Dissections and trauma of the cervicocerebral arteries. In: Barnett HJ, Mohr JP, Stein BM, et al., eds. *Stroke: pathophysiology, diagnosis, and management,* 3rd ed. Philadelphia: Churchill Livingstone, 1998:769–786.
51. Giroud M, Fayolle H, Andre N, et al. Incidence of internal carotid artery dissection in the community of Dijon. *J Neurol Neurosurg Psychiatry* 1994;57:1443.
52. Schievink WI, Mokri B, Whisnant JP. Internal carotid artery dissection in a community. Rochester, Minnesota, 1987–1992. *Stroke* 1993;24:1678–1680.
53. Schievink WI. Spontaneous dissection of the carotid and vertebral arteries. *N Engl J Med* 2001;344:898–906.
54. Schievink WI, Wijdicks EF, Michels VV, et al. Heritable connective tissue disorders in cervical artery dissections: a prospective study. *Neurology* 1998;50:1166–1169.
55. Buring JE, Hebert P, Romero J, et al. Migraine and subsequent

risk of stroke in the Physicians' Health Study. *Arch Neurol* 1995; 52:129–134.
56. Merikangas KR, Fenton BT, Cheng SH, et al. Association between migraine and stroke in a large-scale epidemiological study of the United States. *Arch Neurol* 1997;54:362–368.
57. Henrich JB, Horwitz RI. A controlled study of ischemic stroke risk in migraine patients. *J Clin Epidemiol* 1989;42:773–780.
58. Carolei A, Marini C, De Matteis G. History of migraine and risk of cerebral ischaemia in young adults. The Italian National Research Council Study Group on Stroke in the Young. *Lancet* 1996;347:1503–1506.
59. Tzourio C, Tehindrazanarivelo A, Iglesias S, et al. Case-control study of migraine and risk of ischaemic stroke in young women. *BMJ* 1995;310:830–833.
60. Olesen J, Friberg L, Olsen TS, et al. Ischaemia-induced (symptomatic) migraine attacks may be more frequent than migraine-induced ischaemic insults. *Brain* 1993;116(pt 1):187–202.
61. Welch KM, Levine SR. Migraine-related stroke in the context of the International Headache Society classification of head pain. *Arch Neurol* 1990;47:458–462.
62. Narbone MC, Leggiadro N, La Spina P, et al. Migraine stroke: a possible complication of both migraine with and without aura. *Headache* 1996;36:481–483.
63. Del Sette M, Angeli S, Leandri M, et al. Migraine with aura and right-to-left shunt on transcranial Doppler: a case-control study. *Cerebrovasc Dis* 1998;8:327–330.
64. Wilmshurst PT, Nightingale S, Walsh KP, et al. Effect on migraine of closure of cardiac right-to-left shunts to prevent recurrence of decompression illness or stroke or for haemodynamic reasons. *Lancet* 2000;356:1648–1651.
65. Tietjen GE. The relationship of migraine and stroke. *Neuroepidemiology* 2000;19:13–19.
66. Hoekstra-van Dalen RA, Cillessen JP, Kappelle LJ, et al. Cerebral infarcts associated with migraine: clinical features, risk factors and follow-up. *J Neurol* 1996;243:511–515.
67. Lanzino G, Andreoli A, Di Pasquale G, et al. Etiopathogenesis and prognosis of cerebral ischemia in young adults. A survey of 155 treated patients. *Acta Neurol Scand* 1991;84:321–325.
68. Rothrock J, North J, Madden K, et al. Migraine and migrainous stroke: risk factors and prognosis. *Neurology* 1993;43: 2473–2476.
69. Joutel A, Corpechot C, Ducros A, et al. Notch3 mutations in CADASIL, a hereditary adult-onset condition causing stroke and dementia. *Nature* 1996;383:707–710.
70. Healton EB, Mohr JP. Cerebrovascular fibromuscular dysplasia. In: Barnett HJM, Mohr JP, Stein BM, et al., eds. *Stroke: pathophysiology, diagnosis, and management,* 3rd ed. Philadelphia: Harcourt Brace and Company, 1998.
71. Kidwell CS, Liebeskind DS, Saver JL. Diagnosis and management of central nervous system vasculitis. In: Cohen SN, ed. *Management of ischemic stroke.* New York: McGraw-Hill, 2000: 329–358.
72. Stone JH, Pomper MG, Roubenoff R, et al. Sensitivities of noninvasive tests for central nervous system vasculitis: a comparison of lumbar puncture, computed tomography, and magnetic resonance imaging. *J Rheumatol* 1994;21:1277–1282.
73. Calabrese LH, Duna GF. Evaluation and treatment of central nervous system vasculitis. *Curr Opin Rheumatol* 1995;7:37–44.
74. Younger DS, Kass RM. Vasculitis and the nervous system. Historical perspective and overview. *Neurol Clin* 1997;15: 737–758.
75. Harris KG, Tran DD, Sickels WJ, et al. Diagnosing intracranial vasculitis: the roles of MR and angiography. *AJNR Am J Neuroradiol* 1994;15:317–330.
76. Calabrese LH, Mallek JA. Primary angiitis of the central nervous system. Report of 8 new cases, review of the literature, and proposal for diagnostic criteria. *Medicine (Baltimore)* 1988;67: 20–39.
77. Greenan TJ, Grossman RI, Goldberg HI. Cerebral vasculitis: MR imaging and angiographic correlation. *Radiology* 1992;182: 65–72.
78. Hankey GJ. Isolated angiitis/angiopathy of the central nervous system. *Cerebrovasc Dis* 1991;1:2–15.
79. Calabrese LH, Furlan AJ, Gragg LA, et al. Primary angiitis of the central nervous system: diagnostic criteria and clinical approach. *Cleve Clin J Med* 1992;59:293–306.
80. Moore PM. Diagnosis and management of isolated angiitis of the central nervous system. *Neurology* 1989;39:167–173.
81. Caplan LR. Of birds and nests and brain emboli. *Rev Neurol* 1991;147:265–273.
82. Georgiadis D, Lindner A, Manz M, et al. Intracranial microembolic signals in 500 patients with potential cardiac or carotid embolic source and in normal controls. *Stroke* 1997;28: 1203–1207.
83. Babikian VL, Caplan LR. Brain embolism is a dynamic process with variable characteristics. *Neurology* 2000;54:797–801.
84. Minematsu K. Cardioembolic stroke. In: Fisher M, ed. *Clinical atlas of cerebrovascular disorders.* London: Mosby–Year Book, 1994:7.1–7.21.
85. Jung DK, Devuyst G, Maeder P, et al. Atrial fibrillation with small subcortical infarcts. *J Neurol Neurosurg Psychiatry* 2001; 70:344–349.
86. Timsit SG, Sacco RL, Mohr JP, et al. Brain infarction severity differs according to cardiac or arterial embolic source. *Neurology* 1993;43:728–733.
87. Liebeskind DS, Saver JL, Lim SR, et al. CT angiography of the middle cerebral artery elucidates the association of Wernicke's aphasia with cardioembolic stroke. *Stroke* 2000;31:294.
88. Kittner SJ, Sharkness CM, Price TR, et al. Infarcts with a cardiac source of embolism in the NINCDS Stroke Data Bank: historical features. *Neurology* 1990;40:281–284.
89. Arboix A, Oliveres M, Massons J, et al. Early differentiation of cardioembolic from atherothrombotic cerebral infarction: a multivariate analysis. *Eur J Neurol* 1999;6:677–683.
90. Minematsu K, Yamaguchi T, Omae T. 'Spectacular shrinking deficit': rapid recovery from a major hemispheric syndrome by migration of an embolus. *Neurology* 1992;42:157–162.
91. Kittner SJ, Sharkness CM, Sloan MA, et al. Features on initial computed tomography scan of infarcts with a cardiac source of embolism in the NINDS Stroke Data Bank. *Stroke* 1992;23: 1748–1751.
92. Worrall BB, Farace E, Hillis AE, et al. Correlation of aphasia and/or neglect with cortical infarction in a subpopulation of RANTTAS. *Cerebrovasc Dis* 2001;11:257–264.
93. Woolfenden AR, Albers GW. Cardioembolic stroke. In: Fisher M, Bogousslavsky J, eds. *Current review of cerebrovascular disease.* Philadelphia: Current Medicine, 2001:123–136.
94. Caplan LR. Intracranial branch atheromatous disease: a neglected, understudied, and underused concept. *Neurology* 1989; 39:1246–1250.
95. Sweeny R, Cheng E, Kidwell CS, et al. Incidence of intracranial large vessel disease in patients with radiologic lacunar stroke. *Neurology* 1999;52[Suppl 2]:A557.
96. Fisher CM. Lacunar strokes and infarcts: a review. *Neurology* 1982;32:871–876.
97. Bamford JM. Lacunar syndromes—are they still worth diagnosing? In: Donnan GA, Norrving B, Bamford JM, et al., eds. *Lacunar and other subcortical infarctions.* New York: Oxford Medical Publications, 1995:32–43.
98. Fisher CM. Lacunar infarcts: a review. *Cerebrovasc Dis* 1991;1: 311–320.
99. Gan R, Sacco RL, Kargman DE, et al. Testing the validity of

the lacunar hypothesis: the Northern Manhattan Stroke Study experience. *Neurology* 1997;48:1204–1211.
100. Orgogozo JM, Bogousslavsky J. Lacunar syndromes. In: Vinken PJ, Buruyn GW, Klawans HL, eds. *Handbook of clinical neurology. Vascular diseases.* 1989:235–269.
101. Bogousslavsky J, Regli F. Centrum ovale infarcts: subcortical infarction in the superficial territory of the middle cerebral artery. *Neurology* 1992;42:1992–1998.
102. Foulkes MA, Wolf PA, Price TR, et al. The Stroke Data Bank: design, methods, and baseline characteristics. *Stroke* 1988;19: 547–554.
103. Caplan LR, Hier DB, D'Cruz I. Cerebral embolism in the Michael Reese Stroke Registry. *Stroke* 1983;14:530–536.
104. Adams HP Jr. Guidelines for the management of patients with acute ischemic stroke: a synopsis. A Special Writing Group of the Stroke Council, American Heart Association. *Heart Dis Stroke* 1994;3:407–411.
105. Brott T, Adams HP Jr, Olinger CP, et al. Measurements of acute cerebral infarction: a clinical examination scale. *Stroke* 1989;20:864–870.
106. von Kummer R, Nolte PN, Schnittger H, et al. Detectability of cerebral hemisphere ischaemic infarcts by CT within 6 h of stroke. *Neuroradiology* 1996;38:31–33.
107. von Kummer R, Allen KL, Holle R, et al. Acute stroke: usefulness of early CT findings before thrombolytic therapy. *Radiology* 1997;205:327–333.
108. Hacke W, Kaste M, Fieschi C, et al. Intravenous thrombolysis with recombinant tissue plasminogen activator for acute hemispheric stroke. The European Cooperative Acute Stroke Study (ECASS). *JAMA* 1995;274:1017–1025.
109. Tissue plasminogen activator for acute ischemic stroke. The National Institute of Neurological Disorders and Stroke rt-PA Stroke Study Group. *N Engl J Med* 1995;333:1581–1587.
110. Haring HP, Dilitz E, Pallua A, et al. Attenuated corticomedullary contrast: an early cerebral computed tomography sign indicating malignant middle cerebral artery infarction. A case-control study. *Stroke* 1999;30:1076–1082.
111. Schriger DL, Kalafut M, Starkman S, et al. Cranial computed tomography interpretation in acute stroke: physician accuracy in determining eligibility for thrombolytic therapy. *JAMA* 1998; 279:1293–1297.
112. Kalafut MA, Schriger DL, Saver JL, et al. Detection of early CT signs of >1/3 middle cerebral artery infarctions: interrater reliability and sensitivity of CT interpretation by physicians involved in acute stroke care. *Stroke* 2000;31:1667–1671.
113. Marks MP, Holmgren EB, Fox AJ, et al. Evaluation of early computed tomographic findings in acute ischemic stroke. *Stroke* 1999;30:389–392.
114. Grotta JC, Chiu D, Lu M, et al. Agreement and variability in the interpretation of early CT changes in stroke patients qualifying for intravenous rtPA therapy. *Stroke* 1999;30:1528–1533.
115. Mohr JP, Biller J, Hilal SK, et al. Magnetic resonance versus computed tomographic imaging in acute stroke. *Stroke* 1995; 26:807–812.
116. Baird AE, Warach S. Magnetic resonance imaging of acute stroke. *J Cereb Blood Flow Metab* 1998;18:583–609.
117. Schlaug G, Siewert B, Benfield A, et al. Time course of the apparent diffusion coefficient (ADC) abnormality in human stroke. *Neurology* 1997;49:113–119.
118. Kidwell CS, Saver JL, Mattiello J, et al. Thrombolytic reversal of acute human cerebral ischemic injury shown by diffusion/perfusion magnetic resonance imaging. *Ann Neurol* 2000;47: 462–469.
119. Lutsep HL, Albers GW, DeCrespigny A, et al. Clinical utility of diffusion-weighted magnetic resonance imaging in the assessment of ischemic stroke. *Ann Neurol* 1997;41:574–580.
120. Barber PA, Darby DG, Desmond PM, et al. Prediction of stroke outcome with echoplanar perfusion- and diffusion-weighted MRI. *Neurology* 1998;51:418–426.
121. Lee LJ, Kidwell CS, Alger J, et al. Impact on stroke subtype diagnosis of early diffusion-weighted magnetic resonance imaging and magnetic resonance angiography. *Stroke* 2000;31: 1081–1089.
122. Lövblad KO, Laubach HJ, Baird AE, et al. Clinical experience with diffusion-weighted MR in patients with acute stroke. *AJNR Am J Neuroradiol* 1998;19:1061–1066.
123. Ay H, Buonanno FS, Rordorf G, et al. Normal diffusion-weighted MRI during stroke-like deficits. *Neurology* 1999;52: 1784–1792.
124. van Everdingen KJ, van der Grond J, Kappelle LJ, et al. Diffusion-weighted magnetic resonance imaging in acute stroke. *Stroke* 1998;29:1783–1790.
125. Gonzalez RG, Schaefer PW, Buonanno FS, et al. Diffusion-weighted MR imaging: diagnostic accuracy in patients imaged within 6 hours of stroke symptom onset. *Radiology* 1999;210: 155–162.
126. Lövblad KO, Baird AE, Schlaug G, et al. Ischemic lesion volumes in acute stroke by diffusion-weighted magnetic resonance imaging correlate with clinical outcome. *Ann Neurol* 1997;42: 164–170.
127. Tong DC, Yenari MA, Albers GW, et al. Correlation of perfusion- and diffusion-weighted MRI with NIHSS score in acute (<6.5 hour) ischemic stroke. *Neurology* 1998;50:864–870.
128. Saver JL, Johnston KC, Homer D, et al. Infarct volume as a surrogate or auxiliary outcome measure in ischemic stroke clinical trials. The RANTTAS Investigators. *Stroke* 1999;30: 293–298.
129. Schonewille WJ, Tuhrim S, Singer MB, et al. Diffusion-weighted MRI in acute lacunar syndromes: a clinical-radiological correlation study. *Stroke* 1999;30:2066–2069.
130. Fitzek C, Tintera J, Müller-Forell W, et al. Differentiation of recent and old cerebral infarcts by diffusion-weighted MRI. *Neuroradiology* 1998;40:778–782.
131. Baird AE, Lövblad KO, Schlaug G, et al. Multiple acute stroke syndrome: marker of embolic disease? *Neurology* 2000;54: 674–678.
132. Kidwell CS, Alger JR, Di Salle F, et al. Diffusion MRI in patients with transient ischemic attacks. *Stroke* 1999;30: 1174–1180.
133. Linfante I, Llinas RH, Caplan LR, et al. MRI features of intracerebral hemorrhage within 2 hours from symptom onset. *Stroke* 1999;30:2263–2267.
134. Schellinger PD, Jansen O, Fiebach JB, et al. A standardized MRI stroke protocol: comparison with CT in hyperacute intracerebral hemorrhage. *Stroke* 1999;30:765–768.
135. Saver JL, Kidwell CS, Liebeskind DS, et al. Diffusion-perfusion MRI evaluation of peri-hematomal ischemia in hyperacute intracerebral hemorrhage. *Neurology* 2000;54[Suppl 3]:A262.
136. Touho H, Karasawa J. Evaluation of time-dependent thresholds of cerebral blood flow and transit time during the acute stage of cerebral embolism: a retrospective study. *Surg Neurol* 1996; 46:135–146.
137. Kaufmann AM, Firlik AD, Fukui MB, et al. Ischemic core and penumbra in human stroke. *Stroke* 1999;30:93–99.
138. Firlik AD, Yonas H, Kaufmann AM, et al. Relationship between cerebral blood flow and the development of swelling and life-threatening herniation in acute ischemic stroke. *J Neurosurg* 1998;89:243–249.
139. Firlik AD, Rubin G, Yonas H, et al. Relation between cerebral blood flow and neurologic deficit resolution in acute ischemic stroke. *Neurology* 1998;51:177–182.
140. Klotz E, Konig M. Perfusion measurements of the brain: using

dynamic CT for the quantitative assessment of cerebral ischemia in acute stroke. *Eur J Radiol* 1999;30:170–184.
141. Knauth M, von Kummer R, Jansen O, et al. Potential of CT angiography in acute ischemic stroke. *AJNR Am J Neuroradiol* 1997;18:1001–1010.
142. Hunter GJ, Hamberg LM, Ponzo JA, et al. Assessment of cerebral perfusion and arterial anatomy in hyperacute stroke with three-dimensional functional CT: early clinical results. *AJNR Am J Neuroradiol* 1998;19:29–37.
143. Wildermuth S, Knauth M, Brandt T, et al. Role of CT angiography in patient selection for thrombolytic therapy in acute hemispheric stroke. *Stroke* 1998;29:935–938.
144. Alsop DC, Detre JA. Multisection cerebral blood flow MR imaging with continuous arterial spin labeling. *Radiology* 1998; 208:410–416.
145. Detre JA, Alsop DC, Vives LR, et al. Noninvasive MRI evaluation of cerebral blood flow in cerebrovascular disease. *Neurology* 1998;50:633–641.
146. Schwamm LH, Koroshetz WJ, Sorensen AG, et al. Time course of lesion development in patients with acute stroke: serial diffusion- and hemodynamic-weighted magnetic resonance imaging. *Stroke* 1998;29:2268–2276.
147. Neumann-Haefelin T, Wittsack HJ, Wenserski F, et al. Diffusion- and perfusion-weighted MRI. The DWI/PWI mismatch region in acute stroke. *Stroke* 1999;30:1591–1597.
148. Karonen JO, Vanninen RL, Liu Y, et al. Combined diffusion and perfusion MRI with correlation to single-photon emission CT in acute ischemic stroke. Ischemic penumbra predicts infarct growth. *Stroke* 1999;30:1583–1590.
149. Sorensen AG, Copen WA, Ostergaard L, et al. Hyperacute stroke: simultaneous measurement of relative cerebral blood volume, relative cerebral blood flow, and mean tissue transit time. *Radiology* 1999;210:519–527.
150. Beaulieu C, de Crespigny A, Tong DC, et al. Longitudinal magnetic resonance imaging study of perfusion and diffusion in stroke: evolution of lesion volume and correlation with clinical outcome. *Ann Neurol* 1999;46:568–578.
151. Hasegawa Y, Fisher M, Latour LL, et al. MRI diffusion mapping of reversible and irreversible ischemic injury in focal brain ischemia. *Neurology* 1994;44:1484–1490.
152. Jansen O, Schellinger P, Fiebach J, et al. Early recanalisation in acute ischaemic stroke saves tissue at risk defined by MRI. *Lancet* 1999;353:2036–2037.
153. Marks MP, Tong DC, Beaulieu C, et al. Evaluation of early reperfusion and i.v. tPA therapy using diffusion- and perfusion-weighted MRI. *Neurology* 1999;52:1792–1798.
154. Schlaug G, Benfield A, Baird AE, et al. The ischemic penumbra: operationally defined by diffusion and perfusion MRI. *Neurology* 1999;53:1528–1537.
155. Kidwell CS, Alger JR, Saver JL, et al. MR signatures of infarction vs. salvageable penumbra in acute human stroke: a preliminary model. *Stroke* 2000;31:285(abst).
156. Koroshetz WJ, Gonzalez G. Diffusion-weighted MRI: an ECG for "brain attack"? *Ann Neurol* 1997;41:565–566.
157. Baron JC, Bousser MG, Rey A, et al. Reversal of focal "misery-perfusion syndrome" by extra-intracranial arterial bypass in hemodynamic cerebral ischemia. A case study with ^{15}O positron emission tomography. *Stroke* 1981;12:454–459.
158. Furlan M, Marchal G, Viader F, et al. Spontaneous neurological recovery after stroke and the fate of the ischemic penumbra. *Ann Neurol* 1996;40:216–226.
159. Marchal G, Beaudouin V, Rioux P, et al. Prolonged persistence of substantial volumes of potentially viable brain tissue after stroke: a correlative PET-CT study with voxel-based data analysis. *Stroke* 1996;27:599–606.
160. Marchal G, Young AR, Baron JC. Early postischemic hyperperfusion: pathophysiologic insights from positron emission tomography. *J Cereb Blood Flow Metab* 1999;19:467–482.
161. Read SJ, Hirano T, Abbott DF, et al. Identifying hypoxic tissue after acute ischemic stroke using PET and 18F-fluoromisonidazole. *Neurology* 1998;51:1617–1621.
162. Heiss WD, Grond M, Thiel A, et al. Permanent cortical damage detected by flumazenil positron emission tomography in acute stroke. *Stroke* 1998;29:454–461.
163. Ueda T, Sakaki S, Yuh WT, et al. Outcome in acute stroke with successful intra-arterial thrombolysis and predictive value of initial single-photon emission-computed tomography. *J Cereb Blood Flow Metab* 1999;19:99–108.
164. Grotta JC, Alexandrov AV. tPA-associated reperfusion after acute stroke demonstrated by SPECT. *Stroke* 1998;29: 429–432.
165. Berrouschot J, Barthel H, von Kummer R, et al. 99m technetium-ethyl-cysteinate-dimer single-photon emission CT can predict fatal ischemic brain edema. *Stroke* 1998;29:2556–2562.
166. Berrouschot J, Barthel H, Hesse S, et al. Differentiation between transient ischemic attack and ischemic stroke within the first six hours after onset of symptoms by using 99mTc-ECD-SPECT. *J Cereb Blood Flow Metab* 1998;18:921–929.
167. Barnett HJM, Taylor DW, Eliasziw M, et al. Benefit of carotid endarterectomy in patients with symptomatic moderate or severe stenosis. *New Engl J Med* 1998;339:1415–1425.
168. Brott T, Bogousslavsky J. Treatment of acute ischemic stroke. *N Engl J Med* 2000;343:710–722.
169. Qureshi AI, Isa A, Cinnamon J, et al. Magnetic resonance angiography in patients with brain infarction. *J Neuroimaging* 1998; 8:65–70.
170. Scarabino T, Carriero A, Giannatempo GM, et al. Contrast-enhanced MR angiography (CE MRA) in the study of the carotid stenosis: comparison with digital subtraction angiography (DSA). *J Neuroradiol* 1999;26:87–91.
171. Rasanen HT, Manninen HI, Vanninen RL, et al. Mild carotid artery atherosclerosis: assessment by 3-dimensional time-of-flight magnetic resonance angiography, with reference to intravascular ultrasound imaging and contrast angiography. *Stroke* 1999;30:827–833.
172. Jackson MR, Chang AS, Robles HA, et al. Determination of 60% or greater carotid stenosis: a prospective comparison of magnetic resonance angiography and duplex ultrasound with conventional angiography. *Vasc Surg* 1998;12:236–243.
173. Furst G, Saleh A, Wenserski F, et al. Reliability and validity of noninvasive imaging of internal carotid artery pseudo-occlusion. *Stroke* 1999;30:1444–1449.
174. Mathews VP, Ulmer JL, White ML, et al. Depiction of intracranial vessels with MRA: utility of magnetization transfer saturation and gadolinium. *J Comput Assist Tomogr* 1999;23: 597–602.
175. Leclerc X, Pruvo JP. Recent advances in magnetic resonance angiography of carotid and vertebral arteries. *Curr Opin Neurol* 2000;13:75–82.
176. Villablanca JP, Martin N, Jahan R, et al. Volume-rendered helical computerized tomography angiography in the detection and characterization of intracranial aneurysms. *J Neurosurg* 2000; 93:254–264.
177. Leclerc X, Gauvrit JY, Pruvo JP. Usefulness of CT angiography with volume rendering after carotid angioplasty and stenting. *AJR Am J Roentgenol* 2000;174:820–822.
178. Saver JL, Feldmann E. The basic transcranial Doppler examination: technique and anatomy. In: Babikian VL, Wechsler L, eds. *Transcranial Doppler sonography: clinical and research applications.* Philadelphia: BC Decker, 1992:11–28.
179. Toni D, Fiorelli M, Zanette EM, et al. Early spontaneous improvement and deterioration of ischemic stroke patients. A serial

study with transcranial Doppler ultrasonography. *Stroke* 1998; 29:1144–1148.
180. Demchuk AM, Burgin WS, Christou I, et al. Thrombolysis in brain ischemia (TIBI) transcranial Doppler flow grades predict clinical severity, early recovery, and mortality in patients treated with intravenous tissue plasminogen activator. *Stroke* 2001;32: 89–93.
181. Collins R, Peto R, MacMahon S, et al. Blood pressure, stroke, and coronary heart disease. Part 2. Short-term reductions in blood pressure: overview of randomised drug trials in their epidemiological context. *Lancet* 1990;335:827–838.
182. Staessen JA, Fagard R, Thijs L, et al. Randomised double-blind comparison of placebo and active treatment for older patients with isolated systolic hypertension. The Systolic Hypertension in Europe (Syst-Eur) Trial Investigators. *Lancet* 1997;350: 757–764.
183. Gasowski J, Wang JG, Staessen JA. Clinical trials in isolated systolic hypertension. *Curr Hypertens Rep* 1999;1:387–393.
184. Perry HM Jr, Davis BR, Price TR, et al. Effect of treating isolated systolic hypertension on the risk of developing various types and subtypes of stroke: the Systolic Hypertension in the Elderly Program (SHEP). *JAMA* 2000;284:465–471.
185. Prevention of stroke by antihypertensive drug treatment in older persons with isolated systolic hypertension. Final results of the Systolic Hypertension in the Elderly Program (SHEP). SHEP Cooperative Research Group. *JAMA* 1991;265:3255–3264.
186. Yusuf S, Sleight P, Pogue J, et al. Effects of an angiotensin-converting-enzyme inhibitor, ramipril, on cardiovascular events in high-risk patients. The Heart Outcomes Prevention Evaluation Study Investigators [published errata appear in *N Engl J Med* 2000;342:748 and 2000;342:1376]. *N Engl J Med* 2000; 342:145–153.
187. Wolf PA, Clagett GP, Easton JD, et al. Preventing ischemic stroke in patients with prior stroke and transient ischemic attack: a statement for healthcare professionals from the Stroke Council of the American Heart Association. *Stroke* 1999;30:1991–1994.
188. Goldstein LB, Adams R, Becker K, et al. Primary prevention of ischemic stroke: a statement for healthcare professionals from the Stroke Council of the American Heart Association. *Stroke* 2001;32:280–299.
189. Kawachi I, Colditz GA, Stampfer MJ, et al. Smoking cessation and decreased risk of stroke in women. *JAMA* 1993;269: 232–236.
190. Sacco RL, Elkind M, Boden-Albala B, et al. The protective effect of moderate alcohol consumption on ischemic stroke. *JAMA* 1999;281:53–60.
191. Gorelick PB, Sacco RL, Smith DB, et al. Prevention of a first stroke: a review of guidelines and a multidisciplinary consensus statement from the National Stroke Association. *JAMA* 1999; 281:1112–1120.
192. Pate RR, Pratt M, Blair SN, et al. Physical activity and public health. A recommendation from the Centers for Disease Control and Prevention and the American College of Sports Medicine. *JAMA* 1995;273:402–407.
193. Cholesterol, diastolic blood pressure, and stroke: 13,000 strokes in 450,000 people in 45 prospective cohorts. Prospective studies collaboration. *Lancet* 1995;346:1647–1653.
194. Sacco RL, Benson RT, Kargman DE, et al. High-density lipoprotein cholesterol and ischemic stroke in the elderly: the Northern Manhattan Stroke Study. *JAMA* 2001;285: 2729–2735.
195. Dobs AS, Nieto FJ, Szklo M, et al. Risk factors for popliteal and carotid wall thicknesses in the Atherosclerosis Risk in Communities (ARIC) Study. *Am J Epidemiol* 1999;150:1055–1067.
196. Blauw GJ, Lagaay AM, Smelt AH, et al. Stroke, statins, and cholesterol. A meta-analysis of randomized, placebo-controlled, double-blind trials with HMG-CoA reductase inhibitors. *Stroke* 1997;28:946–950.
197. Warshafsky S, Packard D, Marks SJ, et al. Efficacy of 3-hydroxy-3-methylglutaryl coenzyme A reductase inhibitors for prevention of stroke. *J Gen Intern Med* 1999;14:763–774.
198. Di Mascio R, Marchioli R, Tognoni G. Cholesterol reduction and stroke occurrence: an overview of randomized clinical trials. *Cerebrovasc Dis* 2000;10:85–92.
199. Ballantyne CM, Herd JA, Dunn JK, et al. Effects of lipid lowering therapy on progression of coronary and carotid artery disease. *Curr Opin Lipidol* 1997;8:354–361.
200. Executive Summary of The Third Report of The National Cholesterol Education Program (NCEP) Expert Panel on Detection, Evaluation, and Treatment of High Blood Cholesterol in Adults (Adult Treatment Panel III). *JAMA* 2001;285:2486–2497.
201. Segal JB, McNamara RL, Miller MR, et al. Anticoagulants or antiplatelet therapy for non-rheumatic atrial fibrillation and flutter. *Cochrane Database Syst Rev* 2001;1:CD001938.
202. Albers GW, Dalen JE, Laupacis A, et al. Antithrombotic therapy in atrial fibrillation. *Chest* 2001;119[Suppl 1]:194S–206S.
203. Hass WK, Easton JD, Adams HP Jr, et al. A randomized trial comparing ticlopidine hydrochloride with aspirin for the prevention of stroke in high-risk patients. Ticlopidine Aspirin Stroke Study Group. *N Engl J Med* 1989;321:501–507.
204. CAPRIE Steering Committee CI. A randomised, blinded, trial of clopidogrel versus aspirin in patients at risk of ischemic events. *Lancet* 1996;348:1329–1339.
205. Diener HC, Cunha L, Forbes C, et al. European Stroke Prevention Study. 2. Dipyridamole and acetylsalicylic acid in the secondary prevention of stroke. *J Neurol Sci* 1996;143:1–13.
206. Bekavac I, Hanna JP, Sila CA, et al. Warfarin and low-dose aspirin for stroke prevention from severe intracranial stenosis. *J Stroke Cerebrovasc Dis* 1999;8:33–37.
207. Easton JD. Future perspectives for optimizing oral antiplatelet therapy. *Cerebrovasc Dis* 2001;11 Suppl 2:23–28.
208. Hart RG, Benavente O, Pearce LA. Increased risk of intracranial hemorrhage when aspirin is combined with warfarin: a meta-analysis and hypothesis. *Cerebrovasc Dis* 1999;9:215–217.
209. Mitka M. Results of CURE trial for acute coronary syndrome. *JAMA* 2001;285:1828–1829.
210. Saver JL, Kalafut M. Combination therapies and the theoretical limits of evidence-based medicine. *Neuroepidemiology* 2001;20: 57–64.
211. A randomized trial of anticoagulants versus aspirin after cerebral ischemia of presumed arterial origin. The Stroke Prevention in Reversible Ischemia Trial (SPIRIT) Study Group. *Ann Neurol* 1997;42:857–865.
212. Rosove MH, Brewer PM. Antiphospholipid thrombosis: clinical course after the first thrombotic event in 70 patients. *Ann Intern Med* 1992;117:303–308.
213. Benesch CG, Chimowitz MI. Best treatment for intracranial arterial stenosis? 50 years of uncertainty. The WASID Investigators. *Neurology* 2000;55:465–466.
214. Saver JL, Jannatti P. Cervicocerebral dissections. In: Gilchrist JP, ed. *Prognosis in Neurology*. Philadelphia: Butterworth-Heinemann Medical, 1998.
215. Bassetti C, Carruzzo A, Sturzenegger M, et al. Recurrence of cervical artery dissection. A prospective study of 81 patients. *Stroke* 1996;27:1804–1807.
216. Schievink WI, Mokri B, O'Fallon WM. Recurrent spontaneous cervical-artery dissection. *N Engl J Med* 1994;330:393–397.
217. Villringer A, Moore P. *Vasculitides and other nonatherosclerotic vasculopathies of the nervous system*. New York: Academic Press, 1996.
218. Barnett HJ, Taylor DW, Eliasziw M, et al. Benefit of carotid endarterectomy in patients with symptomatic moderate or se-

vere stenosis. North American Symptomatic Carotid Endarterectomy Trial Collaborators. *N Engl J Med* 1998;339: 1415–1425.
219. Randomised trial of endarterectomy for recently symptomatic carotid stenosis: final results of the MRC European Carotid Surgery Trial (ECST). *Lancet* 1998;351:1379–1387.
220. Endarterectomy for asymptomatic carotid artery stenosis. Executive Committee for the Asymptomatic Carotid Atherosclerosis Study. *JAMA* 1995;273:1421–1428.
221. Benavente O, Moher D, Pham B. Carotid endarterectomy for asymptomatic carotid stenosis: a meta-analysis. *BMJ* 1998;317: 1477–1480.
222. Chambers BR, You RX, Donnan GA. Carotid endarterectomy for asymptomatic carotid stenosis. *Cochrane Database Syst Rev* 2000;2:CD001923.
223. Siebler M, Nachtmann A, Sitzer M, et al. Cerebral microembolism and the risk of ischemia in asymptomatic high-grade internal carotid artery stenosis. *Stroke* 1995;26:2184–2186.
224. Taylor DW, Barnett HJ, Haynes RB, et al. Low-dose and high-dose acetylsalicylic acid for patients undergoing carotid endarterectomy: a randomised controlled trial. ASA and Carotid Endarterectomy (ACE) Trial Collaborators. *Lancet* 1999;353: 2179–2184.
225. Klijn CJ, Kappelle LJ, Tulleken CA, et al. Symptomatic carotid artery occlusion. A reappraisal of hemodynamic factors. *Stroke* 1997;28:2084–2093.
226. Hankey GJ, Warlow CP. Prognosis of symptomatic carotid occlusion: an overview. *Cerebrovasc Dis* 1991;1:245–256.
227. Failure of extracranial-intracranial arterial bypass to reduce the risk of ischemic stroke. Results of an international randomized trial. The EC/IC Bypass Study Group. *N Engl J Med* 1985; 313:1191–1200.
228. Grubb RL Jr, Derdeyn CP, Fritsch SM, et al. Importance of hemodynamic factors in the prognosis of symptomatic carotid occlusion. *JAMA* 1998;280:1055–1060.
229. Daniels SK, Brailey K, Priestly DH, et al. Aspiration in patients with acute stroke. *Arch Phys Med Rehabil* 1998;79:14–19.
230. Johnston KC, Li JY, Lyden PD, et al. Medical and neurological complications of ischemic stroke: experience from the RANTTAS trial. RANTTAS Investigators. *Stroke* 1998;29:447–453.
231. del Zoppo GJ, Higashida RT, Furlan AJ, et al. PROACT: a phase II randomized trial of recombinant pro-urokinase by direct arterial delivery in acute middle cerebral artery stroke. PROACT Investigators. Prolase in acute cerebral thromboembolism. *Stroke* 1998;29:4–11.
232. Ronning OM, Guldvog B. Should stroke victims routinely receive supplemental oxygen? A quasi-randomized controlled trial. *Stroke* 1999;30:2033–2037.
233. Yatsu FM, Zivin J. Hypertension in acute ischemic strokes. Not to treat. *Arch Neurol* 1985;42:999–1000.
234. Spence JD, Del Maestro RF. Hypertension in acute ischemic strokes. Treat. *Arch Neurol* 1985;42:1000–1002.
235. Broderick J, Brott T, Barsan W, et al. Blood pressure during the first minutes of focal cerebral ischemia. *Ann Emerg Med* 1993;22:1438–1443.
236. Carlsberg B, Asplun DK, Hagg E. Course of blood pressure in different subsets of patients after acute stroke. *Cerebrovasc Dis* 1991;1:281.
237. Powers WJ. Acute hypertension after stroke: the scientific basis for treatment decisions. *Neurology* 1993;43(pt 1):461–467.
238. Bratina P, Greenberg L, Pasteur W, et al. Current emergency department management of stroke in Houston, Texas. *Stroke* 1995;26:409–414.
239. Jorgensen HS, Nakayama H, Raaschou HO, et al. Effect of blood pressure and diabetes on stroke in progression. *Lancet* 1994;344:156–159.
240. Rordorf G, Koroshetz WJ, Ezzeddine MA, et al. A pilot study of drug-induced hypertension for treatment of acute stroke. *Neurology* 2001;56:1210–1213.
241. Adams HP Jr, Brott TG, Crowell RM, et al. Guidelines for the management of patients with acute ischemic stroke. A statement for healthcare professionals from a special writing group of the Stroke Council, American Heart Association. *Stroke* 1994;25: 1901–1914.
242. Saver JL, Starkman S. State of the art medical management of acute ischemic stroke. *J Stroke Cerebrovasc Dis* 1997;4:189–194.
243. The European Ad Hoc Consensus Group. Optimizing intensive care in stroke: a European perspective. *Cerebrovasc Dis* 1997;7: 113.
244. Brott T, Lu M, Kothari R, et al. Hypertension and its treatment in the NINDS rt-PA Stroke Trial. *Stroke* 1998;29:1504–1509.
245. Weir CJ, Murray GD, Dyker AG, et al. Is hyperglycaemia an independent predictor of poor outcome after acute stroke? Results of a long-term follow up study. *BMJ* 1997;314: 1303–1306.
246. Mankovsky BN, Patrick JT, Metzger BE, et al. The size of subcortical ischemic infarction in patients with and without diabetes mellitus. *Clin Neurol Neurosurg* 1996;98:137–141.
247. Demchuk AM, Morgenstern LB, Krieger DW, et al. Serum glucose level and diabetes predict tissue plasminogen activator-related intracerebral hemorrhage in acute ischemic stroke. *Stroke* 1999;30:34–39.
248. Tanne D, Bates VE, Verro P, et al. Initial clinical experience with IV tissue plasminogen activator for acute ischemic stroke: a multicenter survey. The t-PA Stroke Survey Group. *Neurology* 1999;53:424–427.
249. Wass CT, Lanier WL. Glucose modulation of ischemic brain injury: review and clinical recommendations. *Mayo Clin Proc* 1996;71:801–812.
250. Ginsberg MD, Busto R. Combating hyperthermia in acute stroke: a significant clinical concern. *Stroke* 1998;29:529–534.
251. Kalafut MA, Llanes J, Kidwell CS, et al. Can prophylactic acetaminophen prevent hyperthermia in acute stroke? Results of the Normothermia and Stroke Outcome (NOTHOT) Pilot clinical trial. *Stroke* 2001;32:381.
252. Kasner SE, Wein TH, Piriyawat P, et al. Acetaminophen for altering body temperature in acute stroke. *Neurology* 2001; 2001[Suppl 3]:A78.
253. Haley EC Jr, Lewandowski C, Tilley BC. Myths regarding the NINDS rt-PA Stroke Trial: setting the record straight. *Ann Emerg Med* 1997;30:676–682.
254. Generalized efficacy of t-PA for acute stroke. Subgroup analysis of the NINDS t-PA Stroke Trial. *Stroke* 1997;28:2119–2125.
255. Wardlaw JM, Warlow CP, Counsell C. Systematic review of evidence on thrombolytic therapy for acute ischaemic stroke. *Lancet* 1997;350:607–614.
256. Hacke W, Kaste M, Fieschi C, et al. Randomised double-blind placebo-controlled trial of thrombolytic therapy with intravenous alteplase in acute ischaemic stroke (ECASS II). Second European-Australasian Acute Stroke Study Investigators. *Lancet* 1998;352:1245–1251.
257. Marler JR, Tilley BC, Lu M, et al. Early stroke treatment associated with better outcome: the NINDS rt-PA stroke study. *Neurology* 2000;55:1649–1655.
258. Katzan IL, Furlan AJ, Lloyd LE, et al. Use of tissue-type plasminogen activator for acute ischemic stroke: the Cleveland area experience. *JAMA* 2000;283:1151–1158.
259. Lewandowski CA, Frankel M, Tomsick TA, et al. Combined intravenous and intra-arterial r-TPA versus intra-arterial therapy of acute ischemic stroke: Emergency Management of Stroke (EMS) Bridging Trial. *Stroke* 1999;30:2598–2605.
260. Ernst R, Pancioli A, Tomsick T, et al. Combined intravenous

and intra-arterial recombinant tissue plasminogen activator in acute ischemic stroke. *Stroke* 2000;31:2552–2557.

261. Saver JL, Kidwell CS, Starkman S, et al. Combined intravenous and intra-arterial tissue plasminogen activator for acute ischemic stroke: recanalization, safety, and early clinical outcome. *Neurology* 2001;56[Suppl 3]:A150.
262. CAST: randomised placebo-controlled trial of early aspirin use in 20,000 patients with acute ischaemic stroke. CAST (Chinese Acute Stroke Trial) Collaborative Group. *Lancet* 1997;349: 1641–1649.
263. The International Stroke Trial (IST): a randomised trial of aspirin, subcutaneous heparin, both, or neither among 19435 patients with acute ischaemic stroke. International Stroke Trial Collaborative Group. *Lancet* 1997;349:1569–1581.
264. Gubitz G, Counsell C, Sandercock P, et al. Anticoagulants for acute ischaemic stroke. *Cochrane Database Syst Rev* 2000;2: CD000024.
265. Chamorro A, Vila N, Saiz A, et al. Early anticoagulation after large cerebral embolic infarction: a safety study. *Neurology* 1995; 45:861–865.
266. Kay R, Wong KS, Yu YL, et al. Low-molecular-weight heparin for the treatment of acute ischemic stroke. *N Engl J Med* 1995; 333:1588–1593.
267. Hommel M. Fraxiparine in ischemic stroke study. *Cerebrovasc Dis* 1998;8[Suppl 4]:19A.
268. Berge E, Abdelnoor M, Nakstad PH, et al. Low molecular-weight heparin versus aspirin in patients with acute ischaemic stroke and atrial fibrillation: a double-blind randomised study. HAEST Study Group. Heparin in Acute Embolic Stroke Trial. *Lancet* 2000;355:1205–1210.
269. Low molecular weight heparinoid, ORG 10172 (danaparoid), and outcome after acute ischemic stroke: a randomized controlled trial. The Publications Committee for the Trial of ORG 10172 in Acute Stroke Treatment (TOAST) Investigators. *JAMA* 1998;279:1265–1272.
270. Kalafut MA, Gandhi R, Kidwell CS, et al. Safety and cost of low-molecular-weight heparin as bridging anticoagulant therapy in subacute cerebral ischemia. *Stroke* 2000;31:2563–2568.
271. Jorgensen HS, Nakayama H, Raaschou HO, et al. Stroke. Neurologic and functional recovery the Copenhagen Stroke Study. *Phys Med Rehabil Clin North Am* 1999;10:887–906.
272. Dobkin BH. *Neurological rehabilitation.* Philadelphia: FA Davis, 1996.
273. Borlongan CV, Tajima Y, Trojanowski JQ, et al. Transplantation of cryopreserved human embryonal carcinoma-derived neurons (NT2N cells) promotes functional recovery in ischemic rats. *Exp Neurol* 1998;149:310–321.
274. Li Y, Chopp M, Chen J, et al. Intrastriatal transplantation of bone marrow nonhematopoietic cells improves functional recovery after stroke in adult mice. *J Cereb Blood Flow Metab* 2000;20:1311–1319.
275. Mattsson B, Sorensen JC, Zimmer J, et al. Neural grafting to experimental neocortical infarcts improves behavioral outcome and reduces thalamic atrophy in rats housed in enriched but not in standard environments. *Stroke* 1997;28:1225–1232.
276. Kondziolka D, Wechsler L, Goldstein S, et al. Transplantation of cultured human neuronal cells for patients with stroke. *Neurology* 2000;55:565–569.
277. PROGRESS Collaborative Group. Randomized trials of a perindopril-based blood-pressure-lowering regimen among 6,105 individuals with previous stroke or transient ischaemic attack. *Lancet* 2001;358:1033–1041.

Endovascular and Percutaneous Therapy of the Brain and Spine, edited by Michael P. Marks and Huy M. Do.

2

ANGIOPLASTY AND STENT PLACEMENT IN THE EXTRACRANIAL CIRCULATION

CONSTANTINE C. PHATOUROS
RANDALL T. HIGASHIDA
JAMES E. LEFLER
ADEL M. MALEK
PHILIP M. MEYERS
CHRISTOPHER F. DOWD
VAN V. HALBACH

The past two decades have witnessed an increasing application of endovascular techniques for the treatment of atherosclerotic disease of the extracranial carotid arteries, vertebral arteries, subclavian arteries, and brachiocephalic artery. Beginning with balloon angioplasty, these minimally invasive techniques have now progressed to the use of stent-supported angioplasty. Stent-supported angioplasty is currently providing a therapeutic alternative to traditional methods of open surgery for revascularization of these vessels and increasing the therapeutic options available for patients who have failed maximal medical therapy. Additionally, endovascular techniques are also being used successfully to treat a variety of nonatherosclerotic disease affecting the extracranial arteries such as inflammatory, radiation, and anastomotic graft strictures, acute intimal dissection, traumatic and spontaneous arteriovenous fistulas, and aneurysms or pseudoaneurysms. In some cases, endovascular procedures are now considered the preferred therapeutic modality. Continued innovation and refinement of endovascular devices and techniques will inevitably improve technical success rates, reduce procedure-related complications, and broaden the endovascular therapeutic spectrum for extracranial cerebrovascular disease. In this chapter we examine the current indications, protocols, and benefits for the use of endovascular techniques in the extracranial circulation.

C.C. Phatouros: Neurointerventional Service, Royal Perth and Sir Charles Gairdner Hospitals, Perth, Australia.
R.T. Higashida: Department of Radiology and Neurosurgery, UCSF Medical Center, San Francisco, California.
J.E. Lefler: Radiology Associates of Tampa, Tampa General Hospital, Tampa, Florida.
A.M. Malek: Department of Surgery, Harvard Medical School and Beth Israel Deaconess Medical Center, Boston, Massachusetts.
P.M. Meyers: Departments of Radiology and Neurosurgery, Columbia University, New York Presbyterian Hospitals, New York, New York.
C.F. Dowd and V.V. Halbach: Departments of Radiology and Neurosurgery, University of California at San Francisco, San Francisco, California.

BACKGROUND

Atheromatous Carotid Artery Disease

Cerebrovascular disease is the third leading cause of mortality in the United States [1,2]. Approximately 700,000 people suffer a stroke annually, costing an estimated $45 billion in treatment and lost productivity [3,4]. Carotid occlusive disease is responsible for up to 25% of these strokes [5]. Large population-based studies indicate the prevalence of carotid stenosis is approximately 0.5% in the sixth decade and increases to 10% in those over 80 years of age. The vast majority of cases are asymptomatic [6–8]. Surgical carotid endarterectomy has traditionally represented the principal method for revascularization of carotid occlusive disease and is currently the accepted standard of treatment [9]. However, this status is being challenged by rapid improvements in percutaneous endovascular techniques using catheter-based stent technology. To date, more than 5,000 carotid stenting procedures have been performed in North America, Europe, South America, and Asia, with excellent preliminary results that appear comparable to surgical carotid endarterectomy [10]. Endovascular carotid stenting is providing an alternative therapeutic option for patients with atherosclerotic carotid stenosis who pose a high surgical risk because of significant comorbidities, as well as those with surgically inaccessible or tandem carotid lesions, contralateral carotid occlusion, or postendarterectomy restenosis.

The efficacy of surgical carotid endarterectomy for treatment of symptomatic carotid stenosis has been proven by multiple, large, well-constructed, randomized, controlled trials [11–16]. The North American Symptomatic Carotid Endarterectomy Trial (NASCET) conducted at 106 centers in the United States, Canada, Europe, and Australia randomized 2,885 patients with symptomatic carotid stenosis stratified into two groups—30% to 69% (2,226 patients) and 70% to 99% (659 patients). The NASCET demonstrated unequivocal benefit of surgery over best medical management in symptomatic patients with carotid stenosis of at least 70% [11]. Endarterectomy reduced the 2-year risk of any ipsilateral stroke in the medical group from 26% (annual event rate of 13%) to 9% in the surgical group, an absolute risk reduction of 17%. In other words, for every 100 patients undergoing surgery, 17 nonfatal strokes or deaths were prevented over a 2-year period.

These rates of risk reduction are directly contingent upon the surgical complication rates. In the NASCET, the full rate of risk-reduction benefit for patients with a stenosis of at least 70% was obtained, assuming a 30-day perioperative complication rate (nonfatal strokes and death) of no greater than 6% [11]. In symptomatic stenoses of 50% to 69% the requisite complication rate falls to 2% [12]. The patient inclusion criteria for the NASCET were very strictly defined. Patients were excluded for a previous ipsilateral endarterectomy, an intracranial lesion that was more severe than the surgically accessible lesion, no angiographic visualization of both carotid arteries and their intracranial branches, and lung, liver, or renal failure. Temporary exclusion criteria included uncontrolled diabetes mellitus, hypertension, unstable angina pectoris, myocardial infarction within the previous six months, contralateral carotid endarterectomy within the previous 4 months, signs of progressive neurologic dysfunction, or a major surgical procedure within the previous 30 days. These patients could be included if the disorder responsible for their ineligibility resolved within 120 days of their qualifying cerebrovascular event. In the NASCET, the incidence of major stroke, myocardial infarction, or death in the surgical group was 3.1%. The inclusion of minor strokes (defined as a stroke with functional recovery within 90 days) increased the complication rate to 6.7%.

The NASCET investigators recently reported the 8-year follow-up results for patients who underwent endarterectomy for symptomatic high-grade stenosis of at least 70%. In these patients, the 8-year risk of an ipsilateral disabling stroke was 6.7%, of any ipsilateral stroke was 15.2%, of any stroke was 29.4%, and of any stroke or death was 46.6%. Therefore, despite the durability of endarterectomy in preventing an ipsilateral disabling stroke, the risk of any stroke or death over the ensuing 8 years was nearly 50% [12].

The NASCET results examining the benefit of carotid endarterectomy in patients with symptomatic moderate stenoses of 30% to 69% over a mean follow-up of 5 years have now been published [12]. Among patients with a stenosis of 50% to 69%, the 5-year rate of any ipsilateral stroke was 15.7% in the surgical group versus 22.2% in the medical group, an absolute risk reduction from any stroke or death of 6.5% (1.3% per annum). However, among patients with 30% to 49% stenosis, the 5-year rate of any ipsilateral stroke was 14.9% for surgical patients versus 18.7% for medically treated patients, an insignificant risk reduction. The perioperative major stroke or death rate was 2.1%. Univariate analysis of all baseline characteristics identified seven factors that doubled the risk of perioperative stroke or death, namely contralateral carotid occlusion, left-sided carotid disease, less than 650 mg of aspirin per day, no history of angina or myocardial infarction, an ipsilateral lesion present on brain computed tomography (CT) or magnetic resonance imaging (MRI), diabetes mellitus, and diastolic blood pressure above 90 mm Hg.

Recently, the surgical and medical complication rates for all patients (n = 1,415) undergoing carotid endarterectomy as part of the NASCET (30% to 99% symptomatic stenosis) have been reported [17,18]. The overall rate of perioperative stroke and death was 6.5%. The mortality rate was 1.1%. Five baseline variables were predictive of statistically significant increased surgical risk: hemispheric versus retinal transient ischemic attack as the qualifying event, left-sided procedure, contralateral carotid occlusion, ipsilateral ischemic lesion on CT scan, and irregular or ulcerated ipsilateral plaque. The incidence of perioperative wound complications was 9.3% and cranial nerve damage was 8.6% [17]. Medical complications occurred in 8.1% of patients undergoing endarterectomy. All of these patients experienced a cardiovascular complication and approximately one-fourth had attendant noncardiovascular medical complications. Cardiovascular complications included myocardial infarction (1.2%), congestive heart failure (1.2%), and hypotension (2.1%). Patients with a history of myocardial infarction, angina pectoris, or hypertension were at a significantly higher risk. Medical complications resulted in a prolonged hospitalization in approximately 30% of cases [18].

The European Carotid Surgery Trial (ECST), another large, randomized, controlled trial, demonstrated similar benefits and results to the NASCET after appropriate adjustment for the different methods used to determine the degree of angiographic stenosis [13–15]. The ECST method used an estimation of the normal carotid bulb diameter as the reference denominator rather than the distal cervical internal carotid artery diameter used in the NASCET. This resulted in a higher degree of angiographic stenosis for any given lesion compared to the NASCET [19]. The ECST enrolled 3,024 patients stratified into three groups: 0 to 29%, 30% to 69%, and 70% to 99% carotid stenosis with a mean follow-up of 6.1 years. The final ECST results demonstrated that endarterectomy reduced the risk of major stroke or death in patients with a symptomatic stenosis of at least 80% (at least 60% as measured by the NASCET method) from 26.5% in the control group (an annual event rate of 8.8%) to 14.9% in the surgical group [15]. This reflects an absolute risk reduction of 11.6% over 3 years. The rate of nonfatal stroke (symptoms lasting more than 7 days) or death from surgery was 7%. The ECST did not specify rates of nonstroke surgical complications such as cranial nerve injury or cardiac events.

The Veterans Affairs Cooperative Symptomatic Carotid Stenosis Trial (VA-CSP-309), a third large, randomized trial examining endarterectomy in symptomatic carotid stenosis, was prematurely terminated when the NASCET and ECST data were released [16]. VA-CSP-309 enrolled 189 male patients, with a mean follow-up of 11.9 months, demonstrating an absolute risk reduction for stroke or crescendo transient ischemic attacks of 11.7% in patients with carotid stenosis of at least 70% who underwent endarterectomy. The authors reported a perioperative surgical stroke and death rate of 5.5%. Among the three perioperative deaths, none was due to ischemic stroke.

The only large, well-constructed, randomized, controlled trial published to date comparing surgical endarterectomy with medical therapy in asymptomatic carotid stenosis is the Asymptomatic Carotid Atherosclerosis Study (ACAS), which enrolled 1,662 patients at 39 centers with a median follow-up of 2.7 years [20]. As in the NASCET, the inclusion criteria for the ACAS were stringent. Patients were excluded from the ACAS because of previous cerebral infarction, previous endarterectomy with restenosis, previous extracranial-to-intracranial bypass, any disorder that could seriously complicate surgery or prevent continuing participation over 5 years, long-term anticoagulation therapy, or a surgically inaccessible lesion. Patients in the medical control group received 325 mg of aspirin per day. The ACAS reported an actuarial estimated 5-year risk (mean follow-up was only 2.7 years) for any stroke or death in patients with a carotid stenosis of 60% or greater, of 5.1% for surgical patients versus 11% (annual event rate of 2.2%) for medically treated patients, yielding an absolute risk reduction of 5.9% (1.2% per annum). Therefore, over a 5-year period, approximately one stroke per year was prevented for every 85 patients undergoing endarterectomy. This result was obtained with a low 30-day perioperative stroke or death (0.1%) rate of 2.3%, 52% of these complications attributable to strokes caused by diagnostic cerebral angiography (arteriography stroke rate of 1.2%). Stratification of data revealed no significant reduction in risk of stroke or death in females undergoing endarterectomy. Furthermore, no correlation between benefit and degree of stenosis was demonstrated. Given these results, the cost effectiveness of performing surgical endarterectomy for asymptomatic carotid stenosis has been questioned [21]. The results of a second large, multicenter, randomized trial examining endarterectomy in asymptomatic carotid stenosis, the Asymptomatic Carotid Surgery Trial (ACST), currently in progress, are awaited [22].

The benefit of surgical endarterectomy over medical therapy has therefore been clearly demonstrated for patients with symptomatic lesions of at least 70%. However, this stroke-reduction benefit is reduced, albeit still significant, in symptomatic patients with lesions of 50% to 69% [12], and reduced further in asymptomatic patients with lesions of at least 60%. This stroke-reduction benefit is also heavily contingent upon appropriate and strict patient selection and established, low surgical complication rates. The requisite surgical complication rate falls from 6% for symptomatic patients with lesions of at least 70%, to 2% for symptomatic patients with lesions of 50% to 69% and asymptomatic patients with lesions of at least 60% stenosis.

Carotid Artery Angioplasty

Percutaneous transluminal balloon angioplasty for carotid artery stenosis was first reported by Kerber et al. in 1980 [23]. In 1987, Theron et al. published the first large series of internal carotid angioplasty in 48 patients with *de novo* atherosclerosis or postsurgical restenosis. Technical success was achieved in 94% of cases, with a 4.1% rate of serious morbidity [24]. In Kachel's review of the literature through 1995, 523 carotid angioplasty procedures had subsequently been reported [25]. The overall technical success rate was 96.2% with a 2.1% rate of morbidity, 6.3% rate of transient minor complications, and no deaths. In one of the largest single-institution series, Gil-Peralta et al. (1996) performed 85 balloon angioplasties in 82 patients with symptomatic carotid stenoses of greater than 70% over a 4-year period [26]. They reported a technical success rate of 92% (residual stenosis of less than 50%), with a 30-day mortality rate of 0 and a major morbidity rate of 4.9%, which compares very favorably with the ECST and NASCET results. The rate of recurrent stenosis (all of which was asymptomatic) was 6.7% at a mean follow-up of 18.7 months, with almost all of these occurring between the third and sixth months. Rates of restenosis (less than 2 years) reported in other large angioplasty series are between 0 and 16% [25,27–30], and in carotid endarterectomy series approximately 10% in the first year [31–34].

Despite ostensibly favorable results, simple balloon angioplasty has a number of potential drawbacks including vessel wall recoil, angiographically evident intimal dissection, and plaque dislodgement with particulate embolization (Fig. 2-1). Angioplasty of atherosclerotic lesions has been reported to generate emboli composed of atheroma, cholesterol crystals, thrombus, and platelet aggregates [35–38]. Embolization of microparticles has been demonstrated both during and after carotid endarterectomy and has been shown to correlate with complex plaque morphology [39] and with clinical postoperative cerebral ischemia [40–43]. However, studies examining the frequency of emboli during carotid balloon angioplasty using transcranial Doppler (TCD) have failed to show a clearcut correlation between embolism frequency and neurologic sequelae [36–38]. Crawley et al., in an analysis of 14 patients undergoing carotid balloon angioplasty versus 14 endarterectomy patients with shunt placement, reported an average of 202 embolic signals during carotid balloon angioplasty compared with 52 during carotid endarterectomy [37]. During the recovery period of 20 minutes, however, the average number of embolic signals was lower for balloon angioplasty than endarterectomy (5 versus 19). There was no correlation between the number of TCD-detected em-

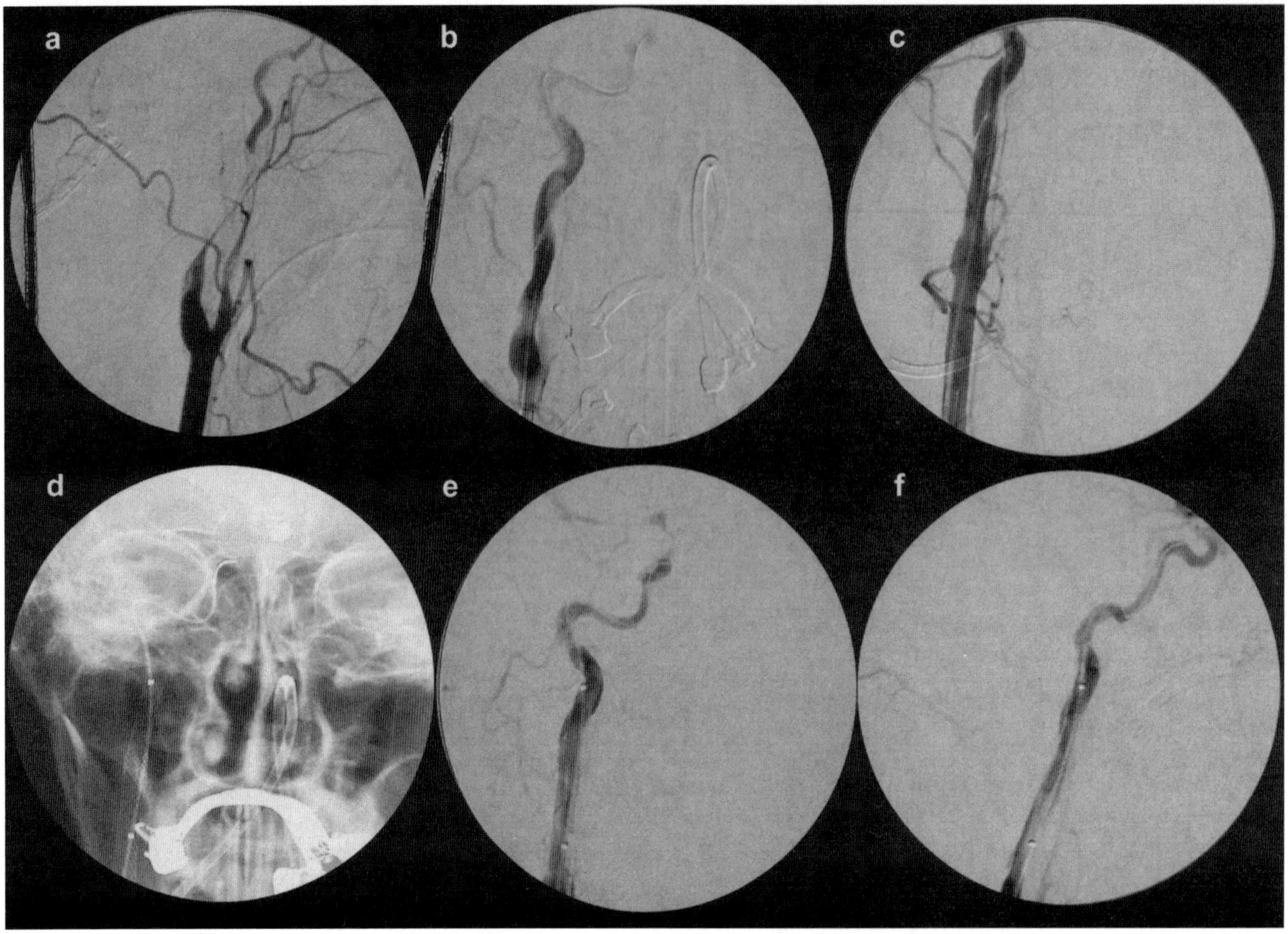

FIGURE 2-1. Angioplasty followed by stent placement for iatrogenic carotid dissection. The patient is a 47-year-old man 9 days after hemorrhage from a ruptured anterior communicating artery aneurysm (status postcoil occlusion) for diagnostic angiogram to rule out vasospasm. **a:** Routine diagnostic angiogram of the right common carotid artery demonstrates severe long-segment dissection involving the cervical segment of the right internal carotid artery. **b:** After angioplasty with Cordis Powerflex 5-mm × 20-mm balloon dilation catheter, angiogram of the carotid artery in the anteroposterior projection demonstrates better patency of the internal carotid artery. However, continued spiral dissection extends into the petrous segment of the damaged artery. **c:** After stenting with 8-mm × 40-mm Schneider Wallstent, the majority of the spiral dissection flap is treated. There still remains a short-segment dissection flap just cephalad to the stent. **d:** Deployment of a second stent (Schneider 6-mm × 20-mm Wallstent) for treatment of the distal dissection flap can be seen on this anteroposterior scout film of the skull. **e,f:** Right common carotid injection in the anteroposterior and lateral projections, respectively, after angioplasty and placement of the two vascular stents but prior to removal of the exchange wire, demonstrates good patency of the internal carotid artery and little evidence of remaining dissection. Note the vasospasm involving the supraclinoid internal carotid artery and M1 segment of the middle cerebral artery (treated with intracranial balloon angioplasty).

boli and the periprocedural stroke rate [37]. Furthermore, Crawley et al. compared the neuropsychological outcomes after surgical endarterectomy and balloon angioplasty in two matched groups of patients with severe symptomatic carotid stenosis, 96% of whom had been randomized in the Carotid and Vertebral Artery Transluminal Angioplasty Study (CAVATAS), at a single center. They reported that at 6 weeks, five patients in each group showed a similar decline in neuropsychological performance; global measures showed no significant difference between the two procedures, despite a significantly higher incidence of microemboli during balloon angioplasty [44].

The risk of cerebral damage is thought to depend upon the size and composition of the embolic material as well as the extent and location of brain involvement. Since it is difficult to distinguish accurately between air and particulate emboli using TCD [45], the lack of correlation between emboli and clinical sequelae has led to the suggestion that the large majority of emboli detected during balloon angioplasty are either gaseous or small platelet aggregates less than

200 μm in diameter, all of which correlate with a more benign outcome [35–37]. This underscores the importance of premedication with antiplatelet agents. A recent study examining the rate of cerebral microembolic signals in nine patients following transient ischemic attacks or minor strokes showed a rapid decline in seven patients, starting 30 minutes after an intravenous acetylsalicylic acid (antiplatelet) bolus injection [46].

Endovascular revascularization of carotid occlusive disease may result in cerebral hypoperfusion from luminal compromise by catheters and guidewires crossing the stenotic lesion or during balloon inflation. This is of even greater relevance in the presence of contralateral carotid artery occlusion or stenosis. Eckert et al. monitored 22 patients undergoing carotid balloon angioplasty using TCD, noting that a greater than 50% reduction of middle cerebral artery mean blood flow velocity compared with baseline values represented a critical threshold for the development of ischemic symptoms (transient ischemic attacks in five and minor stroke in one) in conscious patients, even with short occlusion times (10 to 40 seconds) [47]. However, Crawley et al. reported hemodynamic ischemia was significantly greater with endarterectomy than balloon angioplasty and was not predictive of adverse neurologic outcome [37]. It is recommended to keep balloon inflation and occlusion times to a minimum of less than 30 seconds to avoid potential cerebral ischemia. If there is attendant compromise of the contralateral carotid artery, establishing the adequacy of the cerebral collateral circulation becomes even more important, and the procedure should be performed with as little sedation as possible to facilitate neurologic monitoring. Tsurutani et al. described the successful use of a continuous perfusion-dilation catheter in a conscious patient with a contralateral carotid occlusion and poor collaterals, who on two separate occasions developed loss of consciousness and convulsions when a conventional balloon angioplasty catheter was inflated for only 10 seconds [48].

Carotid Artery Stenting

Data from coronary artery trials of stent-assisted balloon angioplasty versus simple balloon angioplasty have demonstrated a benefit in event-free survival at 1 year and a lower rate of repeat angioplasty with stenting. This evidence provided the initial impetus for primary stenting of atherosclerotic lesions of the carotid artery [49–51]. Since 1996 there have been at least 11 large, individual, carotid stent series published, in which the total number of patients treated with carotid artery stenting is approximately 1,000 [52–62]. Comparative analysis of these reports is made difficult by inconsistencies in the sample populations, lesion characteristics, endovascular techniques, and outcome data. Nonetheless, the overall reported rate of technical success is over 95%. Procedure-related mortality rates (including cardiac deaths) are 0.6% to 4.5%, major stroke rates are 0 to 4.5%, minor stroke rates are 0 to 6.5%, and a 6-month restenosis rate is less than 5% (excluding the studies by Teitlebaum, Gross, Malek, and their colleagues [59,61,62], which represented very–high-risk cohorts).

NASCET criteria were applied to the patient cohorts in six of these carotid stenting series, demonstrating that 81% of these 637 patients would have failed eligibility because of comorbidities [52,56–58,61,62]. In spite of this, morbidity rates of 2.0% to 7.9% and mortality rates of 0.6% to 2.0% for these carotid stenting reports compare favorably with those in the NASCET and the ECST. However, it should be noted that 41% (n = 263) of these patients had asymptomatic carotid stenosis for which lower endarterectomy morbidity and mortality rates would be expected. Mathur et al. retrospectively analyzed the risk factors for stroke in 231 patients undergoing elective stenting of the extracranial carotid arteries, 14% of which were NASCET eligible [63]. The overall 30-day stroke rate was 6.9%; however, by stratifying for the NASCET-eligible group the stroke rate dropped to 2.7%. Advanced age (more than 80 years) and long or multiple stenoses were found to be independent predictors of periprocedural strokes. However, contralateral carotid occlusion, prior carotid endarterectomy, and combined carotid and coronary procedures, all of which are associated with a higher incidence of complications in carotid endarterectomy, were not found to confer an increased risk of adverse outcome in patients who received stents [32, 63–66]. Mericle et al. also reported on 23 patients with high-grade carotid stenosis and a contralateral carotid occlusion undergoing elective carotid stenting [67]. The 30-day perioperative stroke or death rate was zero. This is in contrast to the NASCET, which reported a perioperative stroke or death rate for patients with contralateral occlusions of 14.3% [11]. Increasing age was also identified as a predictor of increased risk for carotid stenting procedures by Chastain et al., who stratified 182 patients undergoing elective carotid artery stenting into three age groups—over 80 years, 75 to 79 years, and under 75 years [68]. The overall rate of major stroke and death (0.5%) was 1.6%, with a 0.5% rate of myocardial infarction. Neurologic complications (mostly minor strokes) were significantly more frequent in patients more than 80 years old than for those less than 75 years of age—25% versus 8.6%, respectively [68].

Wholey et al. recently published the results of a worldwide stent survey in which 5,210 endovascular cervical carotid artery stent procedures are reported from 36 centers in North and South America, Europe, and Asia [10]. They reported a 30-day procedure-related mortality rate of 0.86%, major stroke rate of 1.49%, minor stroke rate of 2.72%, and restenosis rate at 6 and 12 months of 1.99% and 3.46%, respectively. Previously, Wholey et al. had reported that centers where fewer than 50 cases were performed had a 6.4% rate of major stroke and death, compared with 2.3% for centers where between 50 and 100 cases had been performed [69]. They thus suggested a learning curve of at least 50 cases for carotid stenting.

It should also be noted that carotid stenting carries no risk of cranial nerve palsies. In a recent prospective review of 200 consecutive carotid endarterectomies, Ballotta et al. reported a 12.5% incidence of nonpermanent cranial nerve and cervical nerve dysfunction: hypoglossal (5.5%), recurrent laryngeal (4%), superior laryngeal (1%), marginal mandibular and greater auricular (2%) [70]. The mean recovery time was 5.8 months. Two patients (8%) with recurrent laryngeal nerve palsies had prolonged recovery times of 31 and 37 months.

Given that the evidence to date supporting the use of carotid stenting is largely derived from retrospective series using disparate sample populations, comparison with the far superior endarterectomy data should be undertaken with caution. Nonetheless, it appears that carotid stenting may present advantages over surgical endarterectomy in specific clinical subgroups such as patients with significant comorbidities, contralateral carotid occlusion [62,67], postendarterectomy restenosis [71,72], or surgically inaccessible or tandem lesions (Fig. 2-2). Yadav et al. reported on 22 patients with angioplasty and stenting for postendarterectomy carotid stenosis with no major and only one minor stroke (4.5%) [71]. Lanzino et al. also reported similar favorable results in 18 patients undergoing angioplasty and stenting for recurrent carotid stenosis following endarterectomy, with no periprocedural strokes and one transient ischemic attack [72]. Meyer et al. reported a perioperative morbidity and mortality rate of 10.8% in their series of 82 patients undergoing carotid endarterectomy for recurrent stenoses—5 times the risk of a routine endarterectomy at the author's institution [32]. A North American multicenter, randomized, controlled trial directly comparing stent-supported angioplasty with endarterectomy in patients with symptomatic stenosis of at least 50% is currently in progress (Carotid Revascularization Endarterectomy versus Stent Trial [CREST]) [73]. CAVATAS, which compared surgical endarterectomy and balloon angioplasty, has recently concluded. Patients with symptomatic stenoses (at least 30%

A,B 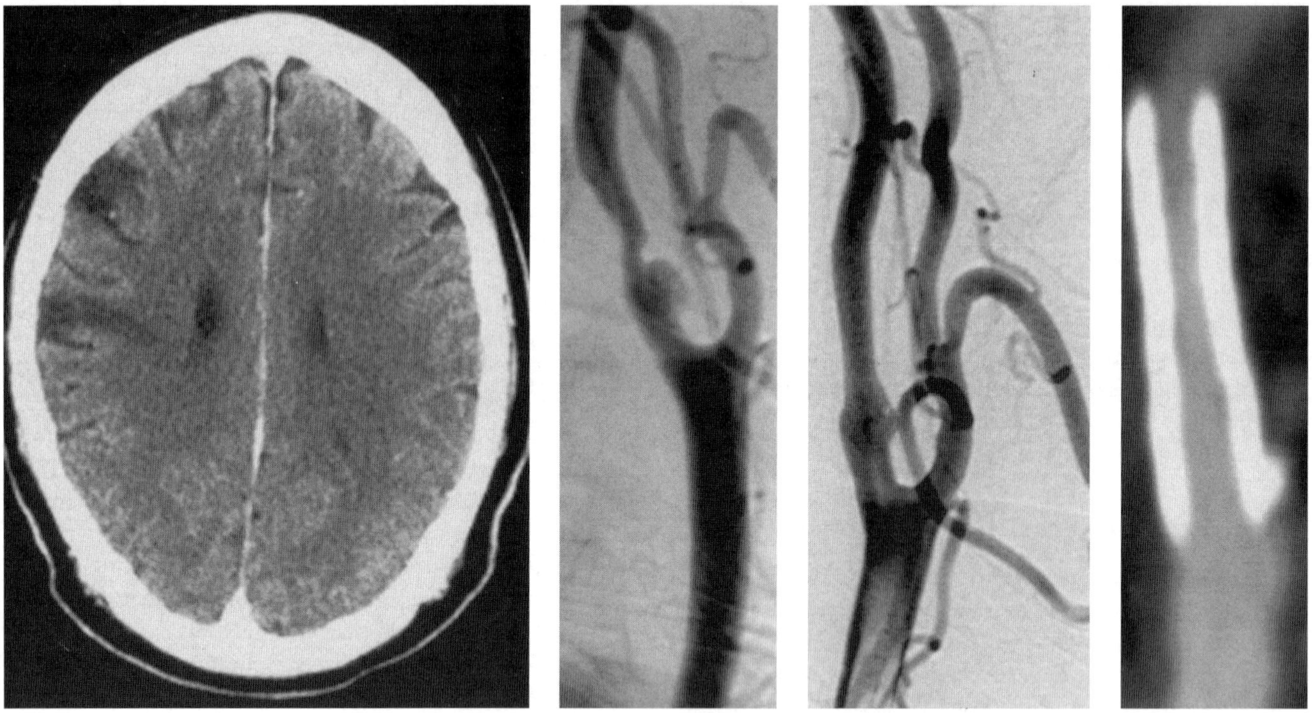 C,D

FIGURE 2-2. Stenting of internal carotid artery with high bifurcation of common carotid artery. This is a 63-year-old man with a history of right hemispheric transient ischemic attacks and infarction. Right common carotid bifurcation is at the C2 to C3 level. The patient underwent attempted carotid endarterectomy with nasal intubation, splitting of the digastric musculature, and extensive retraction. These maneuvers did not result in the ability to obtain adequate control of flow distal to the endarterectomy target. The patient was referred for endovascular revascularization. **A:** Axial contrast-enhanced CT image reveals old strokes in the right MCA territory. **B:** Right CCA angiogram lateral view shows 60% stenosis by NASCET criteria of the proximal ICA. Note high bifurcation of CCA at the level of C2. **C:** Right CCA angiogram lateral view following stent placement demonstrates resolution of stenosis. **D:** Sagittal reformatted maximal intensity projection CT image obtained at follow-up 14 months following stent placement demonstrates patency of stent with no restenosis. The patient remained asymptomatic with no recurrent TIAs. (Courtesy Huy M. Do and Michael P. Marks.)

luminal diameter reduction) suitable for surgery were randomized to either angioplasty or surgery [74]. Patients unsuitable for endarterectomy were randomized between percutaneous transluminal techniques and medical treatment alone. The CAVATAS randomized 504 patients between surgery and angioplasty over 5 years. There was no significant difference in the risk of stroke or death related to the procedure between carotid endarterectomy or angioplasty. The rate of any stroke lasting more than 7 days or death within 30 days of first treatment was approximately 10% in both the surgery and angioplasty groups. The rate of disabling stroke or death within 30 days of first treatment was 6% in both groups. Preliminary analysis of long-term survival showed no difference in the rate of ipsilateral stroke or any disabling stroke in patients up to 3 years after randomization. The rates of stroke or death within 30 days in the CAVATAS in both groups are higher than in many previous reports but not significantly different to the ECST rate of 7%. Cranial nerve injury and myocardial ischemia were reported at the time of treatment only in the surgical group. Long-term follow up is not yet available [75]. The CAVATAS II, which will compare surgical endarterectomy with carotid stenting, is planned.

Carotid Artery Dissection

Acute dissection of the cervical carotid artery may occur spontaneously (atraumatic or minor trauma) or result from more severe trauma which may be blunt, penetrating, or iatrogenic. Acute carotid dissection may result in luminal stenosis or occlusion, distal thromboembolism, or acute pseudoaneurysm formation. In asymptomatic patients, management is usually conservative using antiplatelet agents or systemic anticoagulation or both to prevent thromboembolic sequelae. In symptomatic cases, more aggressive therapy may be warranted, especially in patients whose symptoms or angiographic abnormalities (vessel narrowing or pseudoaneurysm) are progressing or in whom anticoagulation is contraindicated. The presence of established cerebral infarction is a relative contraindication to revascularization because of the increased risk of hemorrhagic transformation. If cerebral infarction is in a watershed distribution and cerebral collateral flow is poor, however, acute revascularization may be necessary. Traditionally, open surgery in the form of arterial ligation with or without extracranial-to-intracranial bypass, endarterectomy and thrombectomy, or arterial reconstruction with autologous vein or synthetic grafts has been performed in these instances [76–78]. Generally, these surgical procedures are technically demanding and may yield disappointing results, particularly if performed during an acute ischemic episode. Endovascular revascularization involving the use of stents may prove to be a potential alternative. The endovascular approach allows concurrent thrombolysis or mechanical disruption of an associated intracranial thromboembolus. An occluded carotid artery is not a contraindication to therapy, particularly if the clinical event, or any clinical change, is recent.

At present there are only isolated published reports describing the use of stents in this clinical setting [79–87]. DeOcampo et al. successfully reestablished flow in an occluded left carotid artery using stent-supported angioplasty in a patient with fibromuscular dysplasia and bilateral carotid artery occlusions from acute dissections [81]. Despite medical therapy, the patient experienced progressive neurologic deficits with bilateral cerebral infarctions. Following carotid stenting these neurologic deficits resolved. Duke et al. reported using endovascular stent placement to treat six patients with nonpenetrating carotid artery injuries [83]. They reported immediate reconstruction of the injured vessel in all cases and noted that, compared with medical therapy, only temporary anticoagulation was required and the risk of future pseudoaneurysm formation and distal embolization was eliminated. Bejjani et al. reported their experience in treating five patients with symptomatic acute carotid dissection [79]. Watershed infarction depicted by CT or MRI was present in four out of five patients, and one patient had a complete carotid occlusion. All patients experienced significant initial clinical improvement and complete long-term recovery. Malek et al. treated ten patients with dissection of the extracranial artery using stents [87]. All patients had either failed maximal medical therapy or possessed a contraindication to anticoagulation. There were no procedural transient ischemic attacks or strokes. Clinical follow-up at a mean of 16.5 months revealed significant improvement in pretreatment neurologic status. One delayed stroke occurred in a patient with a contralateral carotid occlusion following a uterine hemorrhage. The long-term durability of stenting for carotid artery dissection in seven patients was reported upon by Liu et al. [88]. One patient exhibited progression to asymptomatic occlusion 3 months after stenting. The remaining six patients exhibited no significant changes in luminal diameters (mean radiologic follow-up period of 17.7 months). All patients remained in clinically stable condition, with no ischemic symptoms, during more than 3.5 years (mean period) of follow-up monitoring (Fig. 2-3).

In recent years there have been increasing reports of stents used for treatment of wide-necked or fusiform aneurysms and pseudoaneurysms of the cervical carotid artery. Aneurysms in this location are most frequently seen as a complication of dissection. Conventional endovascular treatment of these aneurysms using electrolytically detachable coils is often unsuccessful because of coil loop herniation through the broad neck into the parent artery. In 1994, Marks et al. reported on two patients with cervical carotid pseudoaneurysms secondary to dissection treated by endovascular stent placement across the aneurysmal neck. In both cases there was progressive aneurysm thrombosis [89]. This is in accordance with experimental data in which surgically created lateral carotid aneurysms in dogs were obliter-

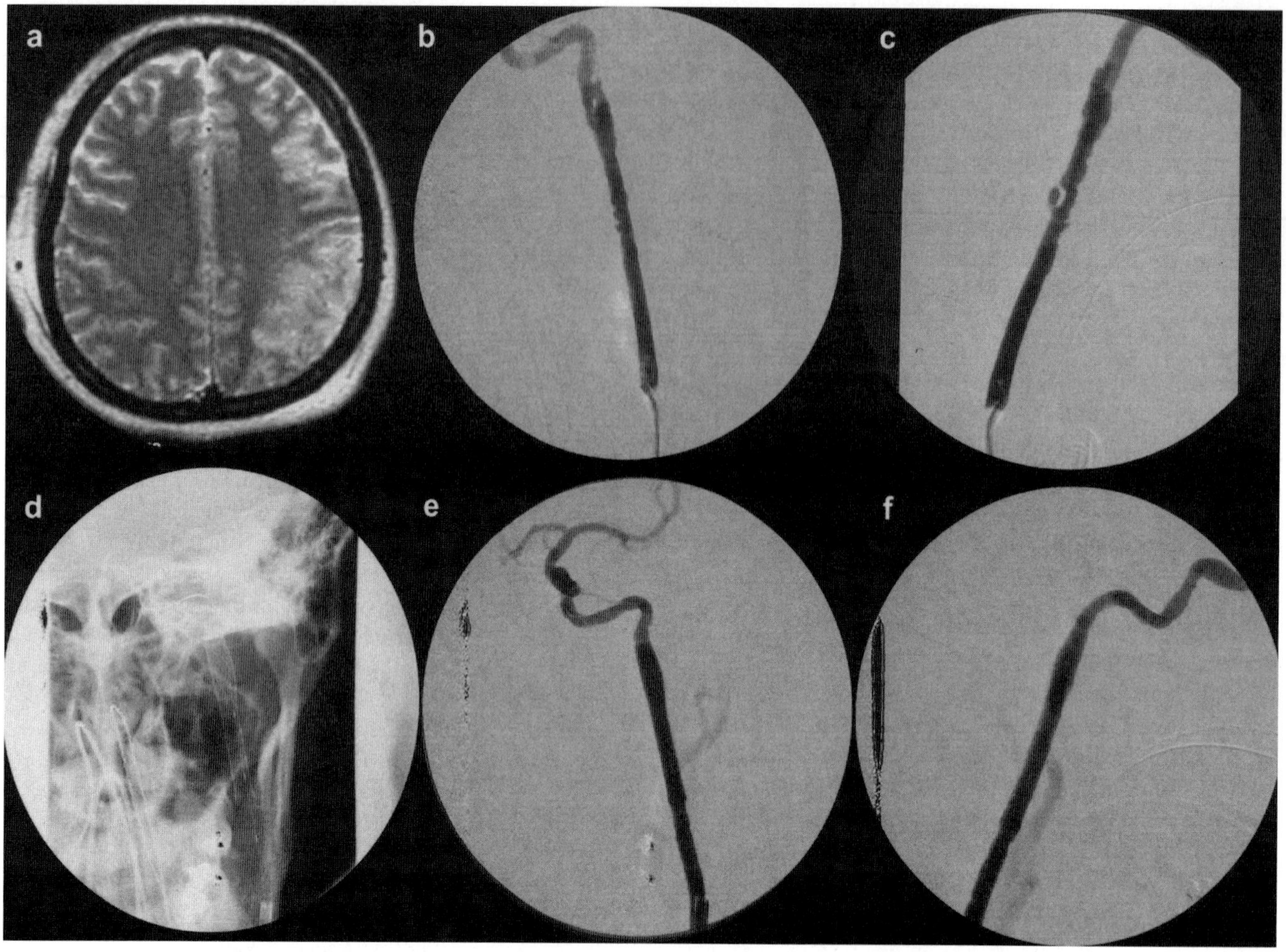

FIGURE 2-3. Extracranial carotid artery dissection treated with primary stenting. The patient is a 24-year-old woman status post motor vehicle accident, found to have left hemispheric strokes. Workup revealed a long-segment left internal carotid artery dissection as the embolic source. **a:** Axial T2-weighted image demonstrates areas of T2 prolongation in the frontal lobe as well as in the parietal lobes consistent with acute infarcts (no evidence of hemorrhage on the T1-weighted images—not shown). **b,c:** Left internal carotid artery angiogram in the anteroposterior and lateral projections, respectively, demonstrates long-segment internal carotid artery dissection with two associated pseudoaneurysms. **d:** Scout film was taken after deployment of a Cordis 8-mm × 40-mm S.M.A.R.T. stent mounted on an 0.014-inch 300-cm stabilizer exchange wire. **e,f:** Digital subtraction angiography of the left internal carotid artery in the anteroposterior and lateral projections, respectively, demonstrates a good angiographic result without evidence of filling of either pseudoaneurysm. Angiography of the intracranial circulation (not shown) both prior to and after stent deployment did not demonstrate any evidence of branch occlusion.

ated using endovascular stents [90–92]. The successful thrombosis of the aneurysms is attributed to stent-related alterations in aneurysmal lumen mechanical flow dynamics as described by Graves et al. [93]. Increased high-flow resistance into the aneurysm through the stent interstices, combined with a preexistent low-pressure gradient between the parent artery and aneurysm, results in reduced intraaneurysmal flow vortices or intraaneurysmal stasis [94]. Similar favorable outcomes using stents in isolation to treat cervical pseudoaneurysms have since been reported by a number of authors [95–100].

Alternatively, the stent may be used as a scaffold to support electrolytically detachable coils used to then occlude the aneurysm. Following deployment of the stent across the aneurysm neck, the coils are delivered into the aneurysmal lumen via a microcatheter passed through the stent interstices. An additional benefit of this combined approach may be a reduced likelihood of future coil compaction—a phenomenon observed particularly in wide-necked aneurysms. The technical feasibility of this approach has been validated by experimental studies performed in canines and swine [101–104]. Three case reports describe the successful clinical application of this technique for cervical carotid artery pseudoaneurysms [105–107]. Phatouros et al., in their series of seven patients who underwent stent-assisted coil embolization, described three cases in the extracranial carotid artery—all pseudoaneurysms [108]. In these patients there were no procedural complications, and angiographic follow-up (mean of 6 months) showed complete aneurysmal occlusion (Fig. 2-4). A potential problem with this technique, particularly in fusiform aneurysms, is reliable fluoroscopic detection of coil-loop herniation through the stent interstices into the parent artery lumen. Intravascular ultrasonography (IVUS) or three-dimensional rotational angiography may prove to be useful adjunctive imaging modalities in this situation.

Covered stents using synthetic materials, such as Dacron, polytetrafluoroethylene (PTFE), polyester, or autologous venous grafts, may in the future also prove useful in this clinical situation. Covered stents have been used successfully in the peripheral circulation to treat penetrating arterial injury and pseudoaneurysm formation [109], and their successful use in the carotid artery for similar indications has also been reported [110–112]. Poor long-term patency rates of covered-stent grafts remains a potential problem. Link et al. reported thrombotic occlusion occurring in seven of eight Dacron-covered stent grafts used to treat surgically created common carotid artery aneurysms in swine at 2-week angiographic follow-up [113].

Miscellaneous Conditions of the Carotid Artery

Radiation-induced strictures of the cervical carotid artery are difficult surgical lesions because of the long lesion length, periarterial scarring with ill-defined planes of resection, and a higher rate of wound complications [114,115]. Endovascular stent placement offers clear advantages for patients in this subset (Fig. 2-5). Al-Mubarak et al. treated 14 patients with severe radiation-induced extracranial carotid artery stenoses using stents [116]. In two patients, ipsilateral vertebral artery lesions were stented concomitantly. Technical success was achieved in all patients. One patient had a minor stroke after the procedure but recovered fully in 2 days. No other complications were encountered. Nine (64%) patients had 6-month follow-up imaging (angiography or duplex scanning) that showed no evidence of restenosis [116]. Bali et al. reported on six patients with inflammatory strictures of

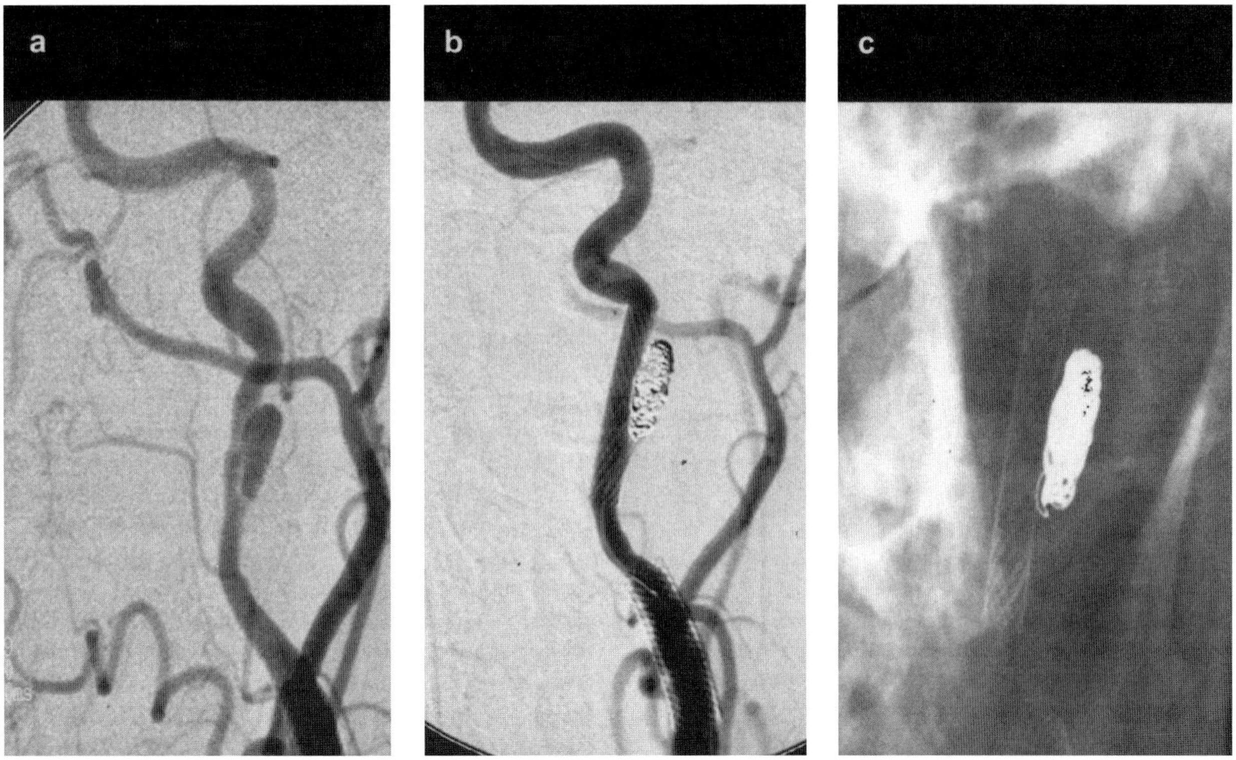

FIGURE 2-4. Stent-supported coil embolization in the extracranial carotid circulation. This is a 42-year-old woman who has had embolization of a ruptured anterior communicating artery aneurysm with iatrogenic guiding catheter, left internal carotid artery dissection, and pseudoaneurysm formation. **a:** Follow-up left common carotid artery injection in the anteroposterior projection demonstrates an enlarging dissection and pseudoaneurysm of the cervical segment of the internal carotid artery. **b:** Status post stent-supported coil embolization with a 6-mm × 24-mm Magic Wallstent and multiple Guglielmi-Detachable Coils demonstrates no evidence of residual filling of the pseudoaneurysm. **c:** Scout film better delineates the relationship of the stent to the coils.

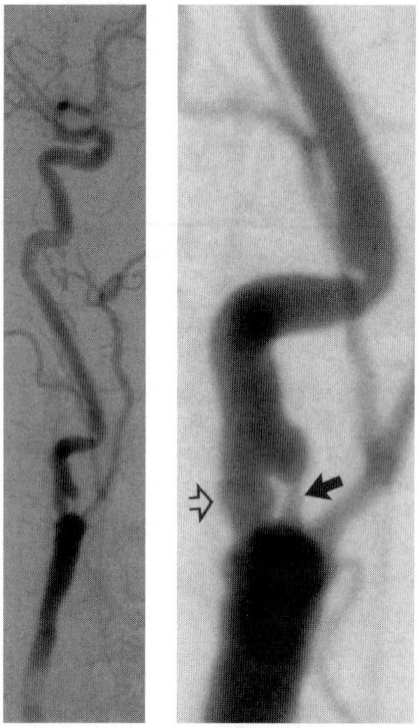

A,B

FIGURE 2-5. Stent placement of left ICA for radiation therapy–induced stenosis. The patient is a 66-year-old woman with history of head and neck squamous cell carcinoma. The patient has undergone surgery with left radical neck dissection and radiotherapy of the neck. She sought treatment for transient ischemic attacks manifesting as transient left monocular blindness that were refractory to antiplatelet medications. Left CCA angiogram normal **(A)** and magnified **(B)** lateral views show severe stenosis *(closed arrow)* of the proximal ICA with large atherosclerotic outpouching posteriorly *(open arrow).* **B,C:** Spot images demonstrate sequential *(from left to right)* stent deployment and postplacement balloon dilation of the stent. **D:** Posttreatment angiographic images demonstrate good angiographic results with stasis of contrast in posterior outpouching *(arrow).* (Courtesy Huy M. Do and Michael P. Marks.)

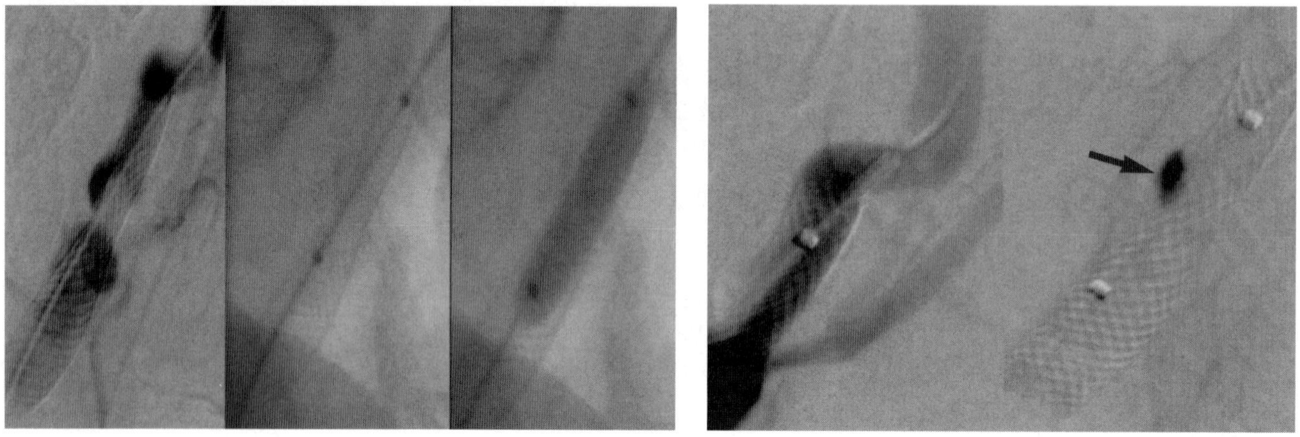

C D

the carotid arteries secondary to Takayasu arteritis treated successfully by endovascular stent placement [117]. Stent placement has also been used to successfully treat two cases of carotid artery vein graft strictures caused by intimal hyperplasia.

Atheromatous Vertebral Artery Disease

Atherosclerotic occlusive disease is the most frequent pathology affecting the extracranial portion of the vertebral artery. The data concerning the overall frequency and sites of predilection for vertebral artery atherosclerosis are derived from pathologic [118–122] and angiographic studies [123–126]. The incidence of vertebral artery atherosclerosis has been variously reported. Fisher et al., in their series of 178 unselected autopsies, reported the frequency and severity of atherosclerosis in the vertebral arteries as somewhat less than in the carotid arteries and about equal to that of the cerebral arteries [119]. The authors also noted that in contradistinction to the focal nature of atheroma deposition in the carotid arteries, atherosclerotic plaques in the vertebral artery were distributed in a relatively diffuse manner along the length of the artery. However, Hutchinson and Yates, in a series of 83 autopsies selected for cerebrovascular disease, reported the incidence of lesions involving the carotid and vertebral systems to be about equal [120], and Schwartz and Mitchell, in their series of 93 unselected autopsies, reported finding atherosclerotic stenosis more commonly in the vertebral arteries than in the carotid arteries [122]. The Joint Study of Extracranial Arterial Occlusion as a Cause of Stroke, which angiographically examined 4,478 patients with cerebrovascular insufficiency, reported the frequency of atherosclerotic plaques was highest at the carotid bifurcation and the vertebral artery origin in a ratio of approximately 2:1 [123].

The large majority of these reports identify the origin or first segment of the vertebral artery as the most frequent site of atherosclerotic stenosis and atherothrombotic occlusion. However, in their series of 44 autopsies with arterial occlusions of the vertebrobasilar system, Castaigne et al. identified the intradural segment of the vertebral artery as the most frequent site for atherothrombotic occlusion and found coexistent brain infarcts in 50% of patients with vertebral artery occlusion [118]. Fisher et al., in their series of 178 unselected autopsies, identified the vertebral artery origin as the most frequent site of occlusion, noting however that all of these patients were probably asymptomatic [119]. In accordance with the data of Castaigne et al. [118], they found evidence of brain infarction in all patients with distal vertebral artery occlusion, thus suggesting intracranial vertebral artery lesions are more commonly symptomatic [119].

The morphologic and pathologic characteristics of atherosclerotic plaque at the vertebral artery origin differ from those of internal carotid artery disease. Vertebral artery plaques are usually annular and concentric, fibrous (hard) and smooth, with a very low incidence of ulceration or intramural hemorrhage [119,127]. Atherosclerotic plaque at the vertebral artery origin may extend to involve the adjacent subclavian artery. Vertebral artery–origin atherosclerotic stenosis has thus been likened to renal artery ostial stenosis [128]. This has important implications for the implementation of endovascular therapy. Theoretically, plaque dislodgment and particulate embolization during endovascular manipulations may be less frequent than encountered with carotid plaque; however, increased vessel recoil may adversely influence long-term patency rates.

Other less frequent causes of luminal stenosis include intimal dissection, osteophytic encroachment, and head extension or rotation or both.

Although the first descriptions of vertebrobasilar insufficiency were reported in the late 1940s and early 1950s, there exists little published data pertaining to the natural history of extracranial vertebral artery occlusive disease [129–131]. Moufarrij et al. (1984) followed up on 96 patients with at least 50% unilateral vertebral artery stenosis for an average of 4.6 years. In 93% of cases, the stenosis was at the vertebral artery origin, with 3% occurring intracranially. During follow-up no patient had a definite vertebrobasilar ischemic attack. Two patients (2%) suffered brainstem strokes (both of which were fatal); however both patients had coexistent basilar artery stenosis. Forty-two percent of patients died during follow-up, with 50% of these deaths due to cardiac causes and 15% due to anterior cranial circulation strokes. The authors concluded that stenosis of the vertebral artery origin is a relatively benign lesion when not associated with basilar artery stenosis [132]. Wityk et al. (1998), however, reported that of 407 patients with signs and symptoms of posterior circulation ischemia, 20% had an occlusive lesion of the V1 segment of the vertebral artery, and in 9% this lesion was the only detected cause of stroke [133]. They noted that patients with vertebral artery origin plaque share common risk factors for stroke that include hypertension, diabetes, coronary artery disease, and cigarette smoking.

In another study, Moufarrij et al. (1986) followed 44 patients with 50% or greater stenosis of the distal vertebral or basilar artery for an average of 6.1 years [134]. During follow-up 23% of patients had definite or possible vertebrobasilar transient ischemic attacks. Five patients (11%) suffered posterior circulation strokes, two of which were fatal. Overall, 27% of patients developed vertebrobasilar ischemia (transient ischemic attacks or stroke) during follow-up. The authors concluded that distal vertebral artery lesions are more dangerous than origin stenosis [134]. Similar results were reported by the Warfarin-Aspirin Symptomatic Intracranial Disease (WASID) Study Group (1998) [135]. The authors reported on 68 patients with symptomatic stenosis of the intracranial posterior circulation of 50% or higher severity, treated with warfarin (n = 42) or aspirin (n = 12), followed for a median period of 13.8 months. During follow-up 16% of patients had nonfatal and 6% had fatal strokes. The calculated stroke rate for patients with intracranial vertebral stenosis was 13.7 per 100 patient-years of follow-up.

The symptoms of vertebrobasilar ischemia have been defined by the National Institute of Neurologic and Communicative Diseases [136]. Symptoms include vertigo, ataxia, dizziness, syncope, drop attacks, visual disturbances, and motor and sensory changes—sometimes bilateral. The pathophysiologic mechanisms for vertebrobasilar ischemia resulting from atherosclerotic lesions include embolism, hemodynamic compromise, and propagation of thrombus from a recent occlusion [137,138]. Vertebrobasilar ischemic stroke is thought to account for 20% of all intracranial ischemic strokes [139]. Embolism from distant sites is responsible for at least 50% of these strokes, with vertebrobasilar atherosclerotic disease the primary etiologic factor in the remainder [140,141].

However, it remains unclear as to whether embolism or hemodynamic impairment is the predominant mechanism of vertebrobasilar ischemia related to vertebral occlusive disease [142]. In the aforementioned posterior circulation registry review by Wityk et al. (1998), ischemia associated with V1 lesions was more frequently caused by artery-to-artery embolism than hemodynamic compromise associated with bilateral disease [133]. However, the largest group of symptomatic patients were those in whom V1 lesions were associated with coexistent lesions of the intracranial vertebral and basilar arteries [133]. In this group of patients ischemia may have been due to either thrombosis or hemodynamic effects of the intracranial lesion, but the potential contribution of the V1 segment lesion to either artery-to-artery embolism or hemodynamic compromise was uncertain.

The relative infrequency of clinically symptomatic hemodynamic compromise associated with V1 lesions is partially explained by the unique anatomical arrangement and patterns of collateral circulation in the vertebrobasilar system. The basilar artery is the only large artery in humans where two flows merge; hence attenuation of flow in one vessel may be compensated for by flow from the other. In approximately 8% of human subjects, however, one or both of the vertebral arteries is hypoplastic (less than 2 mm in diameter) or, as previously mentioned, the distal vertebral artery on one side is either hypoplastic or terminates as the ipsilateral posterior inferior cerebellar artery (PICA) [119]. Occlusive lesions in the extracranial vertebral artery may result in the development of collateral vessels arising from the ipsilateral external carotid artery and subclavian arteries that reconstitute distal flow. The posterior communicating arteries also provide collateral flow to the vertebrobasilar system via the circle of Willis, although hypoplasia of the posterior communicating arteries occurs with a frequency of approximately 32% [143].

Radiographic angiography is still required for definitive anatomical evaluation of the extracranial vertebral artery. The vertebral artery origin is usually best demonstrated with mild cranial and contralateral oblique tube angulation using a subclavian artery contrast injection (8 ml/sec for a total volume of 16 ml) with an inflated pressure cuff on the ipsilateral arm. Doppler ultrasonography is insensitive due to the presence of surrounding bone, and because the most frequent site for occlusive disease is at the vessel origin, a nonsuperficial location not readily insonated. The proximal vertebral artery is frequently tortuous or kinked, making accurate diagnosis and assessment of stenotic lesions difficult using magnetic resonance angiography (MRA) because of spin dephasing caused by turbulent flow and out-of-plane signal loss.

The vertebral artery is usually the first and largest branch of the subclavian artery arising from the posterior aspect of the first part of the subclavian artery. It is characterized by its small diameter (0.5 to 5.5 mm) relative to its long length (15 to 35 cm). In approximately 75% of cases the left vertebral artery is of equal size or larger than the right [144–146]. In approximately 6% of cases, the left vertebral artery arises directly from the aorta, usually between the left common carotid and left subclavian arteries. In this case it may be of smaller caliber and terminate intracranially as the ipsilateral PICA without contributing to the basilar artery. A so-called vertebral artery-PICA termination occurs in approximately 0.2% of cases [147]. Rarely, the right vertebral artery may arise directly from the aorta or right common carotid artery.

The vertebral artery is anatomically divided into an extracranial and an intracranial portion. From its origin it courses superiorly and posteriorly between the longus colli muscle medially and scalenus anterior muscle laterally to most commonly enter the foramen transversarium of C6. In the case of a direct origin from the aorta, the vertebral artery usually has a longer extraspinal segment entering the C4 transverse foramen [148]. The vertebral artery then ascends through the foramina transversaria of the cervical spine anterior to the cervical nerve roots, surrounded by the vertebral venous plexus, giving rise to small segmental cervical branches subdivided into muscular and spinal categories. The muscular branches may anastomose with branches of the ipsilateral external carotid or subclavian arteries including the occipital artery, inferior thyroid artery, and ascending and deep cervical arteries. The spinal branches enter the vertebral canal through the intervertebral foramen to reinforce the anterior and posterior spinal arteries. A dominant spinal artery supplying the cervical anterior spinal artery may arise, often bilaterally, at the C4 to C6 level and is referred to as the artery of cervical enlargement.

After traversing the C2 transverse foramen, the vertebral artery courses laterally and posteriorly before turning sharply upward to pass through the C1 transverse foramen, which is the most laterally positioned. It then passes backward, horizontally grooving the posterior arch of C1 where, at the posterior margin, it turns sharply anteromedially to pierce the atlantooccipital membrane and dura. This point is marked angiographically by a characteristic mild waistlike constriction of the vessel and the origin of the posterior meningeal artery, which is angiographically visible in 30% to 40% of cases [149]. The vertebral arteries then pass through the ventral foramen magnum to unite at or near the ventral pontomedullary junction to form the basilar artery. Duplication of the vertebral artery can occur at any level.

A commonly used angiographic classification is that of Krayenbuhl and Yasargil (1957) in which the vertebral artery is divided into four segments [150]. V1, or the soft tissue segment, is between the origin and the foramen transversarium of C6; V2, or the intraosseous segment, is between the foramina transversaria of C2 and C6; V3 is between the foramen transversarium of C2 and the point of dural entry; and V4 is the intradural segment.

Medical treatment of extracranial vertebral artery occlusive disease remains largely empirical consisting of antiplatelet agents, systemic anticoagulation, increasing mean arterial blood pressure and blood volume, and avoidance of orthostatic hypotension. The data supporting the efficacy of anticoagulation is limited. Whisnant et al. (1978) reported on a 15-year follow-up of 199 patients with carotid or vertebrobasilar transient ischemic attacks [151]. They found that patients commenced on anticoagulant therapy within 2 months of diagnosis had a significantly lower probability of stroke at 3 months through 5 years. However, in patients who began therapy at 6 months, no significant difference was present. This study however had significant limitations including small sample size, lack of randomization, and no imaging correlation to support the clinical diagnosis of vertebrobasilar ischemia. The WASID Study was a retrospective, multicenter trial comparing the efficacy of warfarin with aspirin for the prevention of major vascular events (ischemic stroke, myocardial infarction, or sudden death) in 151 patients with a symptomatic stenosis of a major intracranial artery, followed for a median period of 14.7 months (warfarin group) or 19.3 months (aspirin group) [152]. The stroke rate for patients treated with warfarin was 3.6 per 100 patient-years versus 10.4 per 100 patient-years for the aspirin group, a statistically significant risk reduction. Although this study included only patients with intracranial lesions, the results are often extrapolated to justify systemic anticoagulation in patients with clinically symptomatic extracranial vertebral artery occlusive disease.

Vertebral Artery Angioplasty and Stenting

Revascularization procedures are reserved for patients with symptoms recalcitrant to maximal medical therapy or in whom anticoagulation is contraindicated. Traditionally, open surgery has been performed in this group of patients. In 1957, Cate and Scott performed the first successful vertebral and subclavian artery endarterectomy in a patient with disabling vertebrobasilar insufficiency [153]. Since that time, three basic surgical revascularization procedures have been performed for vertebral artery occlusive disease: endarterectomy, bypass grafting, and direct arterial anastomosis (transposition) [154]. However, due to the small size of the vertebral artery and relative surgical inaccessibility of this region, these surgical procedures are technically demanding with perioperative combined morbidity and mortality rates of up to 20% [155]. Endovascular access of the extracranial vertebral artery is comparatively straightforward.

Balloon angioplasty for the treatment of vertebral artery occlusive disease was first reported in 1981 [156,157]. Over the following decade numerous investigators reported favorable short-term results using this technique [158–165]. Higashida et al. (1993) reported treating 34 proximal vertebral atherosclerotic lesions in 33 patients with vertebrobasilar ischemic symptoms or stroke in whom medical therapy had failed [166]. Technical success (less than 30% residual stenosis) was achieved in all cases. They reported a 9% incidence of transient intraprocedural complications and no permanent complications. Follow-up radiography revealed a 9% incidence of restenosis within 5 months [166]. Clinical follow-up at 12 months disclosed improvement of symptoms in all but one patient, who died from a rupture of an unrelated contralateral vertebral artery aneurysm. In Kachel's review of the endovascular literature up to 1996, 268 vertebral balloon angioplasty procedures had been attempted with an overall technical success rate of 95.1%, morbidity rate of 0.7%, minor complication rate of 3.3%, and no procedure-related mortality [25]. Although the consequences of vertebrobasilar embolism are potentially disastrous, transcranial Doppler studies show that frequency of emboli occurring during balloon angioplasty of vertebral ostial plaque is lower than seen in carotid bifurcation lesions [167]. This is explained by the histopathologic and surface differences between vertebral and carotid plaque (see pathologic considerations above).

Endovascular therapy of extracranial vertebral artery strictures has evolved from simple balloon angioplasty to stent-supported angioplasty, principally to overcome the problems of elastic recoil and early restenosis [168,169]. In 1996, Storey et al. first reported the successful use of stents to treat vertebral ostial strictures in three patients who developed symptomatic recurrent stenosis within 3 months of angioplasty. Angiographic follow-up at 12 months in two patients revealed stent patency [170]. Fessler et al. reported on six patients with symptomatic vertebral artery stenosis (five proximal lesions and one distal lesion) undergoing stent placement [155]. Technical success was achieved in all cases, although one patient required the use of three additional stents to treat an iatrogenic dissection. One patient (17%) had a transient neurologic event. There was no permanent morbidity or mortality. All patients experienced resolution of symptoms at an average 8.4 months of follow-up. Angiographic follow-up in four cases at a minimum of 3 months revealed stent patency. Malek et al. treated 21 patients with symptomatic occlusive subclavian (n = 13) or vertebral artery stenosis (n = 8) refractory to medical therapy using stents [171]. Technical success was achieved in all cases, with the mean degree of overall stenosis reduced from 75% to 4.5%. There were no periprocedural vertebrobasilar strokes. One patient (4.8%) experienced a periprocedural transient ischemic attack. At a mean clinical follow-up of 21 months, 90.5% of surviving patients had experienced resolution or improvement of symptoms. One patient died from a carotid artery territory stroke. Similarly, Chastain et al. treated 55 extracranial vertebral artery stenoses in 50 patients with vertebrobasilar insufficiency [172]. Technical success was achieved in 54 (98%) of 55 vessels, with no procedure-related complications. Clinical follow-up performed at a mean of 25 ± 10 months revealed two patients (4%) with recurrence of symptoms. Six-month angiographic follow-up was performed in 90% of eligible patients, with a 10% incidence of restenosis [172] (Fig. 2-6).

Despite the limited published data, stent-supported angioplasty is emerging as a viable therapeutic option for medically refractive vertebral artery occlusive disease, offering improved rates of technical success and better long-term patency over balloon angioplasty alone.

Dissections and Arteriovenous Fistulas of the Vertebral Artery

Extracranial dissections of the vertebral artery may occur spontaneously (atraumatic or minor trauma) or result from more severe trauma which may be blunt, penetrating, or

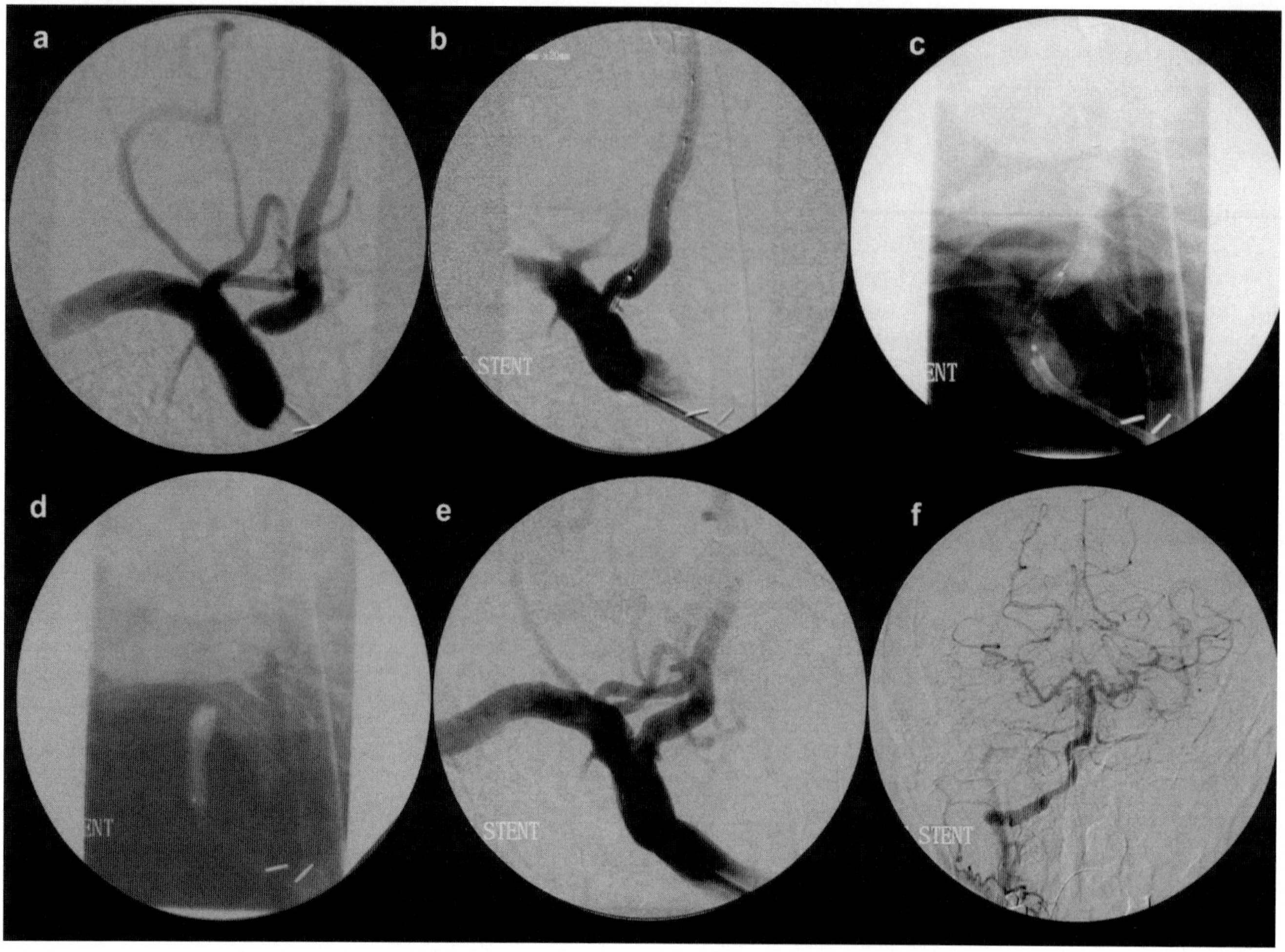

FIGURE 2-6. Extracranial vertebral origin stent angioplasty. This patient is a 66-year-old man with a history of vertebrobasilar insufficiency manifested by temporary inferior quadrant hemianopsia in the setting of alcohol withdrawal. **a:** Right subclavian angiography in the anteroposterior projection demonstrates a high-grade stenosis involving the right vertebral origin. **b:** Right subclavian angiogram after angioplasty with Jupiter PTA 6-mm × 20-mm balloon is shown. The lesion was initially crossed with a Stabilizer 300-cm 0.014-inch exchange wire. **c:** Right subclavian angiogram through a 7-Fr. Cordis Vista Brite Tip guiding catheter with a Cordis Corinthian PQ124B stent mounted on a 6-mm × 20-mm Jupiter balloon dilation catheter prior to stent deployment demonstrates good positioning of the stent across the stenosis. **d:** Stent deployment shown with the Jupiter balloon inflated. **e:** Right subclavian angiography after stent deployment demonstrates good angiographic result with no recurrent stenosis. **f:** Right subclavian injection centered over the head in the Townes projection demonstrates no evidence of major branch occlusions.

iatrogenic. Acute dissection may result in luminal stenosis or occlusion, distal thromboembolism, or acute pseudoaneurysm formation [173]. Additionally, traumatic dissecting aneurysms or pseudoaneurysms of the extradural vertebral artery can be associated with massive external hemorrhage or neck hematomas [174,175]. In asymptomatic patients, current management is usually conservative using antiplatelet agents or systemic anticoagulation or both to prevent thromboembolic sequelae. In symptomatic cases, more aggressive therapy may be warranted, especially in patients whose symptoms persist despite anticoagulation or in whom anticoagulation is contraindicated. Because vertebral artery dissection is bilateral in only one-fifth of cases coupled with the excellent collateralization potential in the vertebrobasilar circulation, revascularization of an occlusive lesion is rarely required on the basis of hemodynamic compromise [176].

There is scant published data on the use of endovascular techniques to treat spontaneous extracranial vertebral dissections [99,177,178]. Halbach et al. reported successful use of balloon occlusion of a vertebral artery proximal to a dissection containing a large intraluminal thrombus, in a patient experiencing ongoing embolic events despite systemic anticoagulation and antiplatelet agents [177]. They also reported the use of endovascular techniques to treat three traumatic extradural vertebral artery dissecting aneurysms with external bleeding. Detachable balloons or coils were used to occlude the vertebral artery just proximal to the lesion in two cases following successful balloon test occlusion. In the last case, coil embolization of a traumatic pseudoaneurysm was achieved with preservation of the parent artery lumen [177]. Price et al. used local thrombolysis followed by stenting to treat a critically ill patient with propagating vertebrobasilar thrombosis secondary to a traumatic extracranial vertebral artery dissection [178]. The patient subsequently made a full recovery.

Aneurysms or pseudoaneurysms of the extracranial vertebral artery are uncommon, usually resulting from trauma or dissection. Indications for treatment include thromboembolic symptoms despite medical therapy, aneurysm enlargement, or local mass effect. Previously, endovascular treatment options have included deconstructive procedures resulting in parent vessel sacrifice, such as aneurysm trapping using detachable balloons or coils. Currently, aneurysms possessing a narrow neck or favorable geometry may be successfully treated using electrolytically detachable coils deployed within the aneurysm with preservation of the parent artery. However, many pseudoaneurysms have wide necks or fusiform morphology, making conventional coil embolization difficult because of the tendency for coil-loop herniation through the broad neck into the parent vessel. The use of intravascular stents may be a potential solution to this problem. Experimental data in dogs demonstrates that surgically created lateral carotid aneurysms can be obliterated using endovascular stents [90–92]. The successful thrombosis of the aneurysms is attributed to stent-related alterations in aneurysmal lumen mechanical flow dynamics [91]. Increased high-flow resistance into the aneurysm through the stent interstices combined with a preexistent low–pressure gradient between the parent artery and aneurysm results in reduced intraaneurysmal flow vortices or intraaneurysmal stasis [94]. Similar favorable outcomes using stents in isolation to treat cervical pseudoaneurysms have been reported by a number of authors [89,95, 97–100]. Horowitz et al. reported using this technique successfully for the treatment of an extracranial vertebral aneurysm [96].

Alternatively, the stent may be used as a scaffold to support electrolytically detachable coils used to then occlude the aneurysm. Following deployment of the stent across the aneurysm neck, the coils are delivered into the aneurysmal lumen via a microcatheter passed through the stent interstices (stent-supported coil embolization). The technical feasibility of this approach has been validated by experimental studies performed in canines and swine [101–104]. Several case reports describe the successful clinical application of this technique for aneurysms and pseudoaneurysms: three in the cervical carotid artery [105–107], one in the intracranial carotid artery [179], and three in the intracranial vertebral artery [180–182]. Phatouros et al. reported treating a patient with a pseudoaneurysm of the extracranial vertebral artery using this technique with an excellent angiographic result (obliteration of the aneurysm with preservation of the parent artery) and without complication [108].

Stents covered with synthetic materials, such as Dacron, PTFE, or polyester, or autologous venous grafts, have also proven useful for treatment of subclavian pseudoaneurysms or arteriovenous fistulas, usually traumatic in etiology [109, 112,183–186]. Despite concerns regarding the long-term patency of covered grafts, most studies [112,183,185,186] indicate durable stent patency at medium-term (mean duration of 10 to 19 months) follow-up. However, stent disruption has been reported in the postvertebral (mobile) segment of the subclavian artery [185].

Vertebral arteriovenous fistulas are uncommon lesions comprising abnormal connections between the extracranial vertebral artery or its branches and neighboring veins. The most frequent cause of these lesions is penetrating neck trauma (with or without vertebral artery transection). Other less frequent causes include inadvertent vertebral damage during insertion of long lines and venous catheters [187, 188], anterior interbody cervical fusion [189], and blunt trauma resulting in cervical spine fracture [190]. Many are spontaneous and are often thought to be congenital. Neurofibromatosis [191] and fibromuscular dysplasia [192] are predisposing diseases. Neck pain and bruit are common symptoms; however, neural dysfunction can occur due to venous hypertension or arterial steal [193,199]. Additionally, traumatic fistulas may have associated expanding hematomas or enlarging pseudoaneurysms that can result in massive hemorrhage or symptoms related to local mass effect.

Endovascular techniques provide an effective method of treatment in most cases [175,194–200]. In cases of spontaneous fistula or traumatic etiology without vessel transection, occlusion of the fistula using detachable balloons or coils with preservation of the parent artery is usually possible. In cases of traumatic transection, fistula closure without sacrifice of the parent artery is usually not possible. Higashida et al. reported treating 21 patients with traumatic vertebral arteriovenous fistulas using detachable balloon embolization therapy [197]. All cases of vertebral transection ($n = 16$) required vertebral artery occlusion. In all other cases vertebral artery flow was preserved [197]. The only significant complication consisted in one patient of mild cerebellar dysfunction from delayed ischemia to a posterior inferior cerebellar artery associated with ipsilateral vertebral occlusion.

Halbach et al. used detachable balloon embolization to treat eight patients with spontaneous fistulas, achieving fistula closure with preservation of vertebral flow in all cases [175]. Three patients developed transient neurologic deficits. The authors postulated that the normal perfusion pressure breakthrough phenomenon was the responsible mechanism [201,202]. Stents may provide a useful treatment option in the future for closure of vertebral arteriovenous fistulas while maintaining vessel patency.

Atheromatous Disease of the Subclavian and Innominate Arteries

Subclavian artery stenosis occurs in approximately 0.5% to 2% of cases and is usually found in patients with widespread vascular disease [203]. Atheromatous occlusive disease most commonly involves the first part of the subclavian artery proximal to the vertebral artery origin. The left side is more often affected than the right [125]. Indications for treatment include brachial ischemia, vertebrobasilar ischemia caused by subclavian steal syndrome, and reduced inflow to internal mammary–to–coronary artery grafts, axillofemoral grafts, or hemodialysis fistulas. Open surgery, usually in the form of trans- or extrathoracic bypass grafting, is associated with complication rates up to 23%, including Horner syndrome, phrenic nerve palsy, pleural effusion, pneumothorax, chylothorax, cervical lymph fistulas, infection, and hemorrhage [204]. A retrospective review of 52 surgical reports (2,496 patients) identified an average overall complication rate of 16%, stroke rate of 3%, and mortality rate of 2% [205].

Percutaneous balloon angioplasty for subclavian artery stenosis was first reported in 1980 [206]. For patients with proximal stenosis of the subclavian artery, review of the literature indicates balloon angioplasty results in improved symptomatology in 72% to 100% of patients and is associated with technical success rates of 90% to 100%, periprocedural complication rates of 0 to 10%, major stroke and death rates of 0 to 4%, and restenosis rates of 0 to 4% at approximately 2-year follow-up [207–212]. Some authors argue the incidence of vertebrobasilar embolic stroke is reduced in cases of balloon angioplasty for subclavian steal syndrome, because reversal of vertebral artery flow to an anterograde direction usually occurs after a variable period of time (20 seconds to more than 20 minutes) following successful angioplasty [213].

Percutaneous balloon angioplasty for the treatment of subclavian artery occlusions is generally associated with lower rates of technical success and long-term patency [169, 214,215]. Mathias et al. attempted recanalization of proximal subclavian artery occlusions in 46 patients and were successful in 38 (83%) [215]; however, seven patients required the immediate use of a stent to treat residual stenosis or acute *in situ* thrombus formation. No significant complications occurred. At a mean follow-up of 33 months, the restenosis (n = 5) or occlusion rate (n = 1) was 16%.

Endovascular therapy of subclavian artery stenosis has evolved from simple balloon angioplasty to stent-supported angioplasty, principally to overcome the problems of elastic recoil with residual stenosis, intimal dissection, acute *in situ* thrombosis, and restenosis [214,216]. Al-Mubarak et al. recently reported the use of primary stenting to treat 38 patients with subclavian artery stenosis (n = 34) or occlusion (n = 4) [206]. Technical success was achieved in 92% of patients (stenosis reduced from mean of 86% to 8%) without complications. All technical failures occurred in occluded arteries. One of these patients suffered a guidewire-induced dissection of the subclavian and axillary artery which was managed conservatively. At a mean follow-up of 20 months, 89% of patients had experienced durable relief of symptoms. Angiographic follow-up was performed in the three patients with recurrent symptoms demonstrating two cases of restenosis (6%).

In one of the largest single-center series, Henry et al. treated 113 patients with subclavian artery stenosis (n = 94) or occlusion (n = 19) using balloon angioplasty (n = 57) or stenting (n = 46) over a 9-year period [209]. Stents were initially used in a "bail-out" role for failed balloon angioplasty but became routine (primary stenting) during the final 3 years of the study. Symptoms were associated with vertebrobasilar ischemia, brachial ischemia, coronary steal, and anticipated coronary artery bypass grafting using the internal mammary artery in 12 asymptomatic patients. The authors reported an overall technical success rate of 91%; however, only 47% of occlusions were successfully recanalized. The major complication rate was 2.6% with a major stroke and a death rate of 0.9%. Over a mean follow-up of 4.3 years, the restenosis rate was 16%; all of these cases occurred in stenotic rather than occluded arteries. Interestingly, 75% of all restenoses occurred in unstented arteries. Martinez et al. used primary stenting to treat 17 patients with total occlusion of the subclavian artery and reported a 94% success rate with no neurologic morbidity or mortality, and only one (6%) procedural complication of acute axillary artery thrombosis successfully treated with local fibrinolysis. One asymptomatic restenosis (6%) occurred during a mean follow-up of 19.4 months [217] (Fig. 2-7).

However, isolated cases of subclavian artery and vein stent breakage and disruption have been reported [185,218, 219]. This is unlikely to be a problem within the prevertebral or first part of the subclavian artery; however, more distally positioned stents may undergo compression between the clavicle and first rib, particularly during arm abduction. The use of Nitinol self-expanding stents, which are crush recoverable, may therefore be indicated in this location.

Occlusive disease of the innominate artery is rare. Operative repair in the form of endarterectomy or bypass grafting is associated with significant morbidity [261]. The results of balloon angioplasty are similar to those obtained in the proximal subclavian artery [169,220]. In his review of the endovascular literature until 1996, Kachel reported 44 attempted innominate balloon angioplasty procedures, in which a 97.7% technical success rate was achieved with no major or minor complications [25]. There are few published

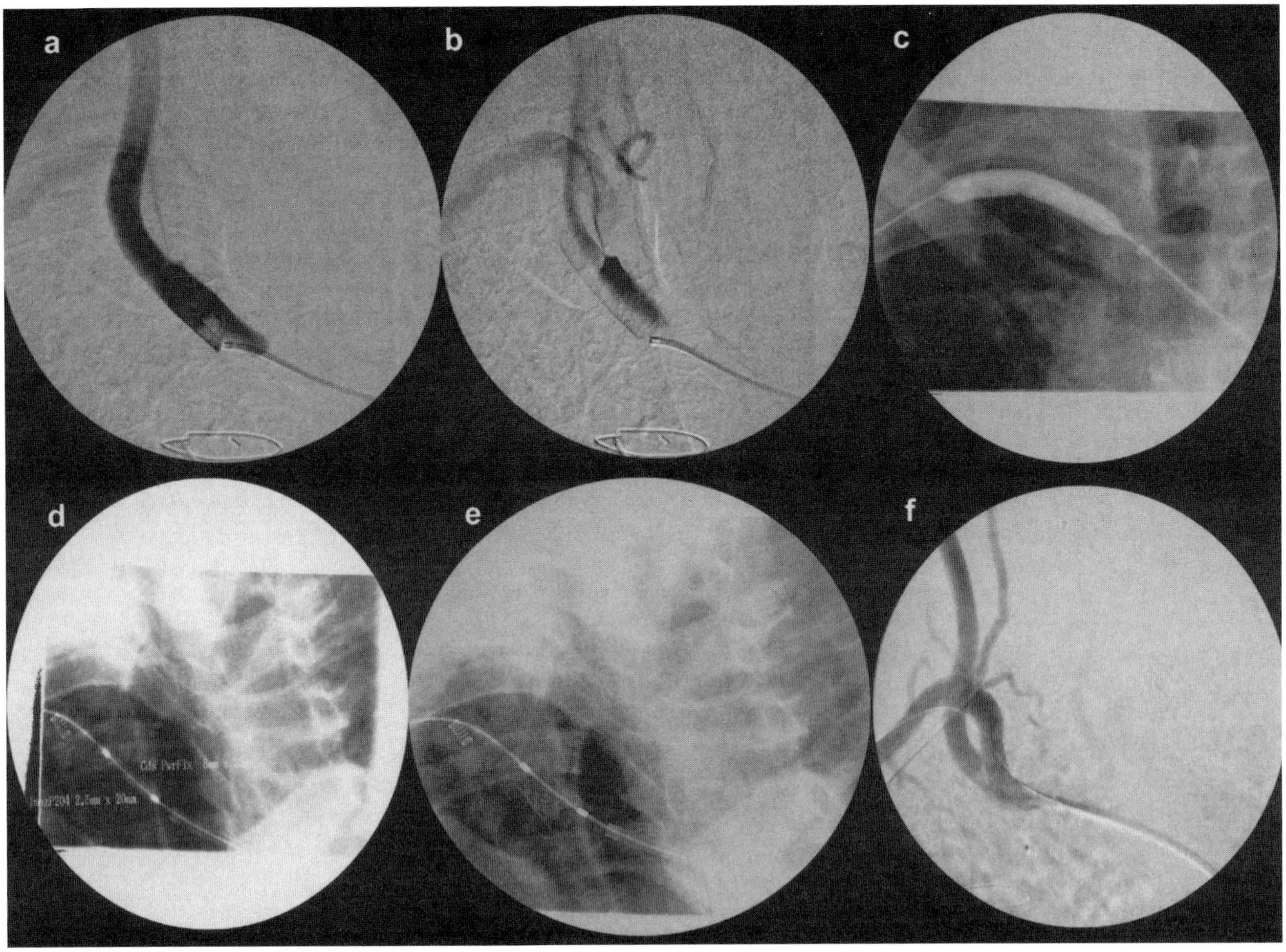

FIGURE 2-7. Subclavian artery origin stent angioplasty. A 56-year-old man sought treatment for numbness and tingling in the right upper extremity. Physical examination revealed an 80-mm Hg pressure gradient difference between the two upper extremities and decreased pulses in the right arm. **a,b:** Right innominate artery angiography demonstrates preocclusive stenosis involving the origin to the right subclavian artery. Only a subtle amount of contrast opacifies the subclavian artery. **c:** Angioplasty was performed with a Cordis Powerflex 7-mm × 40-mm balloon dilation catheter primed with a Storq 0.035-inch 300-cm exchange wire. **d:** Palmaz P204 stent mounted on a Cordis Powerflex 2-mm × 20-mm balloon dilation catheter is seen crossing the lesion over the Storq exchange. **e:** Unsubtracted scout film after stent deployment. **f:** Posttherapy innominate artery injection demonstrates good angiographic result and no evidence of restenosis.

reports specifically describing the use of percutaneous stenting for treatment of innominate artery stenosis. Hadjipetrou et al. performed primary stent placement to treat three patients with symptomatic obstruction of the innominate artery [205]. They reported technical success without major complications in all cases. At a mean follow-up of 17 months, all patients were asymptomatic without evidence of stent restenosis. At the University of California at San Francisco we have treated three high-grade lesions of the innominate artery using stents. In all cases there was an excellent technical result without complications. Because the innominate artery is nonexposed and accurate positioning is desirable (to prevent stent protrusion into the aortic arch), the balloon-expandable Palmaz stent is well suited to this location (Fig. 2-8).

Miscellaneous Conditions of the Subclavian and Innominate Arteries

A number of reports describe the successful use of balloon angioplasty and stenting for the treatment of axillary, subclavian, and innominate artery lesions in Takayasu and giant cell arteritis [117,221–225]. Tyagi et al. reported the immediate and long-term results of balloon angioplasty for subcla-

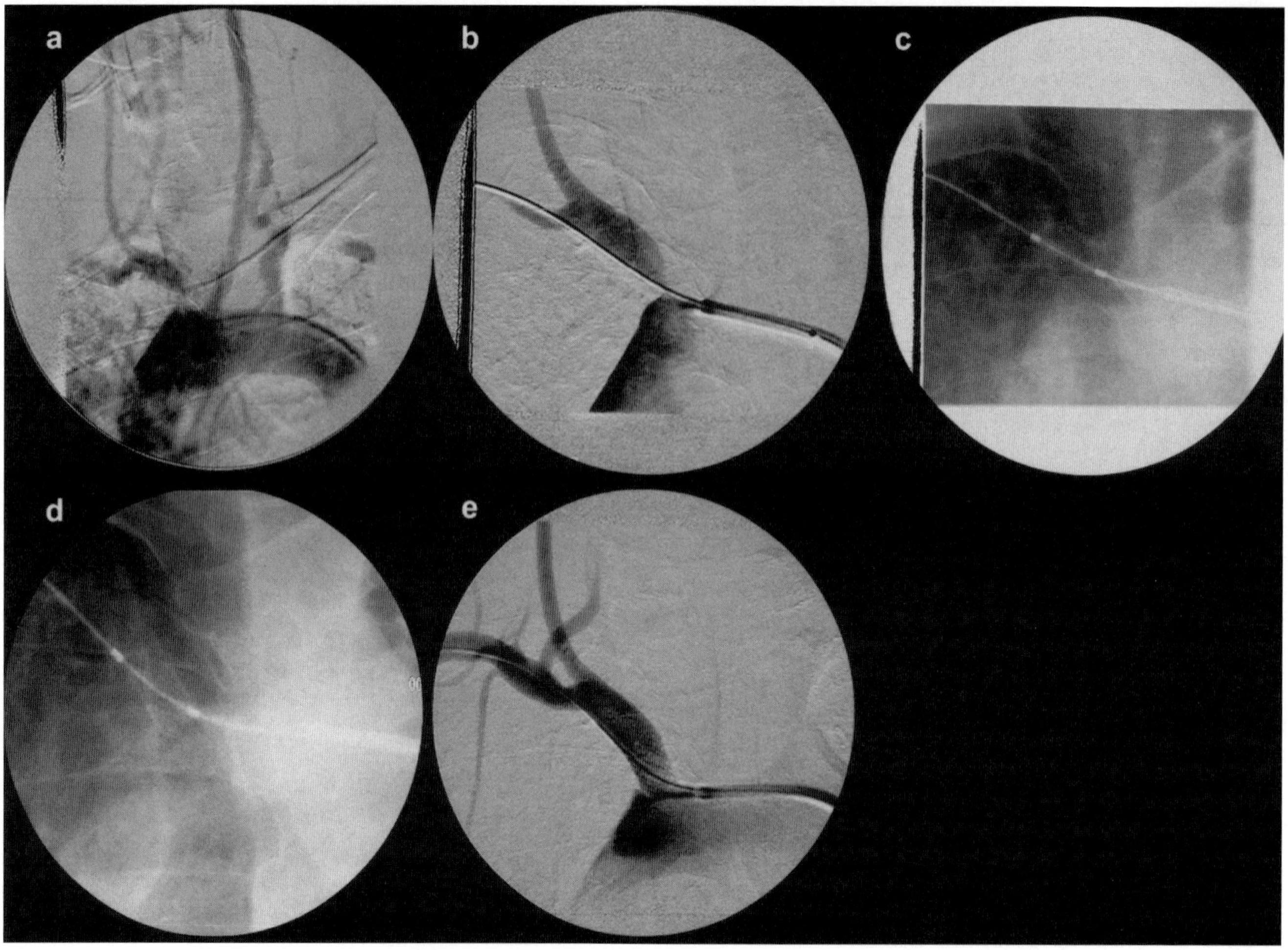

FIGURE 2-8. Innominate artery stent angioplasty. The patient is a 52-year-old man who underwent recent arm surgical thrombectomy for arm ischemia. **a:** Arch aortogram in the left anterior oblique projection demonstrates critical stenosis involving the innominate artery origin. **b:** Angiogram after primary angioplasty with Cordis Powerflex 4-mm × 20-mm balloon dilation catheter demonstrates mild decrease in the degree of stenosis. Note the Storq 0.035-inch 300-cm exchange wire across the lesion and a 9-Fr. Cordis Vista Brite Tip guiding catheter at the origin of the innominate artery. **c:** Prior to stent deployment in this unsubtracted scout view of the right upper thorax demonstrating correct positioning of a Palmaz P204 stent mounted on a Cordis Powerflex 8-mm × 10-mm balloon dilation catheter. **d:** Scout view after stent deployment. **e:** Angiogram through the guiding catheter after stent deployment demonstrates excellent angiographic result without evidence of dissection or restenosis.

vian stenosis or occlusion in atherosclerotic disease (n = 23) versus Takayasu arteritis (n = 32) [225]. Compared with atherosclerosis, patients with Takayasu arteritis were younger, more often were female, gangrene was less common, and diffuse involvement was more frequent. The degree of narrowing was similar in both groups, although higher balloon inflation pressures were required in the arteritis group (average 10 versus 5.5 atmospheres [atm]), which also had a higher degree of residual stenosis. The complication rate of 5.4% did not significantly differ between the two groups. There were no neurologic complications. Clinical symptoms in both groups showed marked improvement following successful revascularization. Restenosis was more frequently observed in patients with arteritis, particularly those with diffuse arterial narrowing. However, these lesions could be effectively redilated. Other authors have similarly reported excellent long-term patency for focal lesions but less durable patency for diffuse disease [222]. Bali et al. reported using stents to successfully revascularize two occluded subclavian arteries in patients with Takayasu arteritis [117]. Dellaripa and Eisenhauer reported the successful use of balloon angioplasty to treat symptomatic bilateral axillary artery stenosis in a 68-year-old female patient with giant cell arteritis [222]. Balloon angioplasty has also been used successfully to treat a subclavian artery stenosis secondary to neurofibromatosis type 1 [226].

The successful use of balloon angioplasty and stenting for radiation-induced strictures of the subclavian and axillary arteries that has been reported by a number of authors [227–231]. Radiation-induced strictures are difficult surgical lesions because of the long lesion length, periarterial scarring with ill-defined planes of resection, and a higher rate of wound complications [114,115,230]. Endovascular treatment offers clear advantages in this subset of patients. Similarly, endovascular therapy may be used to treat innominate, subclavian, or vertebral bypass graft strictures secondary to fibrointimal hyperplasia.

TECHNIQUE FOR ANGIOPLASTY AND STENTING

Patient Workup

The following descriptions represent a guide to the technique we employ for carotid artery angioplasty. Although this discussion is specific to the carotid artery, many of the aspects and principles of the technique are applied to the other extracranial arteries. It should also be noted that significant diversity exists in the current technique, and technologic changes will continue to alter this technique.

A complete neurologic history and examination is requisite prior to any carotid stent procedure. Ideally, this should be performed and documented by both the interventionist and the cerebrovascular neurology team. A baseline brain CT or MRI scan should be obtained to document preexistent infarction and exclude nonvascular neuropathology, such as tumor that may mimic transient ischemic attacks. Baseline laboratory values, including hemoglobin and hematocrit, serum creatinine, blood urea and electrolytes, and prothrombin and activated partial thromboplastin (aPTT) times, as well as a preprocedural electrocardiogram and chest radiograph, are obtained. Patients fast before the procedure from midnight but are permitted to take any regular medications (particularly antihypertensives) orally with a sip of water. Patients on long-term anticoagulation should discontinue warfarin 3 days prior to the procedure and are admitted the day before for intravenous heparinization. Similarly, patients with preexistent renal disease are admitted on the prior day for intravenous hydration. Oral enteric-coated aspirin, 325 mg/day, and clopidogrel, 75 mg/day, are recommended for at least 3 days before the procedure to reduce periprocedural platelet emboli. Experimental data suggests aspirin and clopidogrel have a synergistic effect on platelet aggregation inhibition, antithrombotic activity, and in preventing myointimal proliferation (restenosis) [232,233].

Preliminary diagnostic angiography of both carotid arteries in a minimum of two planes, including the intracranial circulation, should be performed. Selective catheterization of the common carotid arteries in persons less than 40 years of age can usually be accomplished using small-diameter catheters (5 or 5.5 French [Fr.]) with simple shapes (a short, angled tip), such as 5-Fr. UCSF II (Cordis, Miami Lakes, FL) or 5.5-Fr. Norman (Cook, Bloomington, IN), in combination with soft-tipped guidewires such as an 0.035-inch Bentson (Cook, Bloomington, IN) with a long floppy (and shapeable) tip that is relatively atraumatic. In older patients, vessel elongation, tortuosity, and dilation may require the use of larger-diameter and hence stiffer catheters in combination with stiffer guidewires, such as hydrophilic-coated 0.035-inch Terumo Glidewire (Medi-tech, Watertown, MA). Alternatively, a reverse-curve catheter such as a Simmons type may be used. The Simmons catheter may be preferred for evaluation of carotid bifurcation disease because only a short length of leading guidewire is required, thus reducing the likelihood of guidewire impingement against atherosclerotic plaque.

Standard angiographic projections for demonstrating the carotid bifurcation are anteroposterior, lateral, and an ipsilateral anterior oblique (30 to 45 degrees). The internal carotid artery (ICA) invariably arises posterior to the external carotid artery and, in most cases, laterally. Thus an ipsilateral anterior oblique or lateral view is usually optimal for displaying the bifurcation; however, pinhole or weblike high-grade stenoses may be underestimated unless multiple oblique projections are performed [234]. A contrast injection rate of 5 to 8 ml/sec, for a total volume of 5 to 8 ml, can be used for the carotid bifurcation, and 6 to 8 ml/sec for a total volume of 7 to 10 ml for the intracranial circulation. A filming rate of three to five images per second for 4 to 5 seconds, followed by one image per second for 7 or 8 seconds, is usually employed [235]. In the case of presumed ICA occlusion, prolonged filming is necessary, because otherwise delayed, faint, anterograde opacification of the cervical ICA may be missed ("string sign" of critical ICA stenosis) [236]. Standard anteroposterior and lateral intracranial views should be obtained in all cases to establish the adequacy of the intracranial collateral circulation via the external carotid and anterior communicating arteries, and also to document any intracranial stenotic lesions. Many experienced operators also advocate routine vertebral angiography to assess collateral flow via the posterior communicating arteries and document any extracranial or intracranial vertebrobasilar stenoses. Certainly, in cases of contralateral carotid occlusion, bilateral severe stenosis, or deficient anterior collateral pathways, evaluation of the adequacy of collateral flow via the posterior circulation becomes even more important.

Angioplasty and Stenting Procedure

The procedure is usually performed under conscious sedation using local anesthesia of the femoral artery region. The pedal pulses are examined (by Doppler if not palpable) and marked for later reference. A urinary catheter is inserted and external cardiac pacemaker leads are attached to the patient prior to sterile draping. A sheath is inserted into the common femoral artery and a baseline activated clotting time (ACT) is obtained. The groin sheath size is dependent upon the type of stent used and the sheath length: the current self-expanding Wallstent (Schneider, Minneapolis, MN) requiring the minimal use of a 7- to 9-Fr. guiding catheter (Cordis Brite Tip: Cordis Endovascular, Miami Lakes, FL) or a 90-cm long 6- to 8-Fr. sheath (Arrow Interventional, Reading, PA).

Prior to stenting, the patient is fully heparinized using an intravenous loading dose (70 to 100 units/kg) to a target therapeutic ACT of 2- to 2.5-times baseline or 250 to 300 seconds. This is followed by a continuous intravenous heparin infusion (15 to 20 units/kg per hour) or hourly boluses of one-half the initial dose. Some operators are now reporting the prophylactic use of glycoprotein IIb/IIIa inhibitors such as abciximab following initial heparinization instead of further administration of heparin [237]. These agents, which have been shown to decrease mortality and morbidity in a number of coronary stent studies and also potentially improve long-term patency rates [238–240], also have a potential role in the uncommon event of acute stent thrombosis, because platelet aggregation (white thrombus) represents the primary mechanism [241]. Tong et al. have reported using abciximab to successfully treat an acute occlusion of an internal carotid artery stent immediately following stent placement [242].

Self-expanding stents, such as the Wallstent, are currently the most frequently used type for internal carotid artery–origin disease and hence this technique will be primarily described. Generally, a 300-cm exchange guidewire (Storq: Cordis Endovascular, Miami Lakes, FL) is placed in the ipsilateral external carotid artery and the guiding catheter advanced over this into the distal common carotid artery, using a coaxial system: a 90-cm, 7- to 9-Fr. guide catheter primed with an inner 110-cm, 5- to 7-Fr. diagnostic catheter. In younger patients (less than 50 years) and those with nontortuous great vessels, primary selection of the common carotid artery with the coaxial guiding catheter system or long sheath may be attempted. The guiding catheter is then connected to a continuous pressurized heparinized saline flush (1 unit of heparin/ml normal saline at 100 ml/hr) via a large-bore Tuohy-Borst–type rotating hemostatic valve (Big Easy: Microvena, White Bear Lake, MN). One inch of topical 2% nitroglycerine ointment may be applied prior to guide and catheter positioning to reduce the likelihood of mechanically induced arterial vasospasm [243].

If the minimal internal carotid artery diameter is less than 2.5 mm, it is initially traversed under digital roadmap guidance with a 2.3-Fr. microcatheter (Rapid Transit: Cordis Endovascular, Miami Lakes, FL) and 0.014-inch guidewire (Transend: Scimed, Maple Grove, MN) to reduce the risk of embolism. The microcatheter tip is positioned within the petrocavernous segment of the internal carotid artery and the Transend guidewire is exchanged for a 300-cm, 0.014-inch exchange-length guidewire (Balance: Advanced Cardiovascular Systems Inc., Santa Clara, CA). Alternatively, the lesion can be crossed initially using the 0.014-inch exchange guidewire alone. Carotid stenoses of lesser severity may be initially traversed under roadmap guidance using a 0.018- or 0.035-inch guidewire; however, these larger-diameter and hence stiffer guidewires have an increased risk of plaque dislodgement and should not generally be advanced beyond the cervical segment of the internal carotid artery because of the risk of intimal dissection or vessel spasm. Newer "monorail" carotid stent delivery catheters may be used without the need for exchange-length guidewires.

The decision to predilate the lesion using balloon angioplasty depends upon the type and size of stent being used, the narrowest lumen diameter, and the morphological configuration of the stenotic segment. Many operators perform routine predilation to approximately 4-mm diameter. However, others suggest that the risk of embolism is highest during this part of the procedure, and if atraumatic crossing of the lesion with the stent delivery catheter is possible without predilation it may be attempted. However, if any resistance to advancement is encountered then the stent delivery catheter is removed and predilation performed. Certainly, if the smallest-lumen diameter is less than 2.5 mm, predilation to approximately 3.5 to 4 mm in diameter is recommended (Titan: Cordis Endovascular, Miami Lakes, FL). Ideally a single, brief (less than 30 seconds) balloon inflation is performed. Prior to balloon inflation, 0.5 mg of atropine or 0.1 to 0.2 mg of glycopyrrolate is administered intravenously to prevent reflex bradycardia or asystole, which may occur in 5% to 10% of patients. A roadmap image is obtained and the stent delivery catheter advanced over the immobilized guidewire. The interventionist should also note the bony landmarks delineating the desired stent position, because patient movement may degrade the roadmap image. Advancement of the stent delivery catheter can also straighten and distort the internal carotid artery, rendering such landmarks inaccurate. The stent is carefully advanced across the lesion and, when satisfactorily positioned, deployed by immobilizing the delivery catheter and retracting the outer sleeve for a self-expanding stent, or inflating the balloon to deploy the balloon-expandable stent. Following stent deployment, the delivery catheter or balloon may be gently rotated to aid in stent separation and then carefully withdrawn while ensuring the stent remains stationary.

Postdeployment angioplasty using a high-pressure (12 to 20 atm), semicompliant balloon (Jupiter: Cordis Endovascular, Miami Lakes, FL) may then be performed to closely appose the stent and intima and, moreover, expand regions of residual stent narrowing. This may require the use of varying diameter balloons, particularly if the stent extends into the common carotid artery. Obvious gaps between the stent circumference and endoluminal surface should be avoided, because this potentially increases the risk of acute or delayed thromboembolism [244]. The balloon should be inflated for no longer than 30 seconds at a time using 12 to 20 atm, with sufficient pause between inflations to allow restoration of cerebral perfusion. Generally, postdeployment stent balloon angioplasty is performed from distal to proximal. Residual minor ulceration external to the stent is usually of no clinical significance. Some operators do not advocate routine postdeployment angioplasty of the stent other than for obvious gaps between the stent and vessel wall and regions of residual stenosis, suggesting this reduces the risk of embolic complications and improves restenosis rates because of reduced intimal injury (Fig. 2-9). Iatrogenic vasospasm usually resolves shortly after removal of the guidewire from the internal carotid artery. Some investigators describe the use of injectable nimodipine (200 μg diluted in 10 ml injected slowly as a 2- to 3-ml bolus) [244] or nitroglycerin (100 μg) [57] into the carotid artery to treat mechanically induced vasospasm. Recalcitrant iatrogenic vasospasm usually responds well to low-pressure balloon angioplasty (less than 3 atm) (Endeavor: Target Therapeutics, Fremont, CA).

Anteroposterior and lateral cerebral angiograms should be obtained after stenting in all cases to exclude any embolic branch occlusion and document new patterns of flow. The patient is carefully examined neurologically. Neurologic

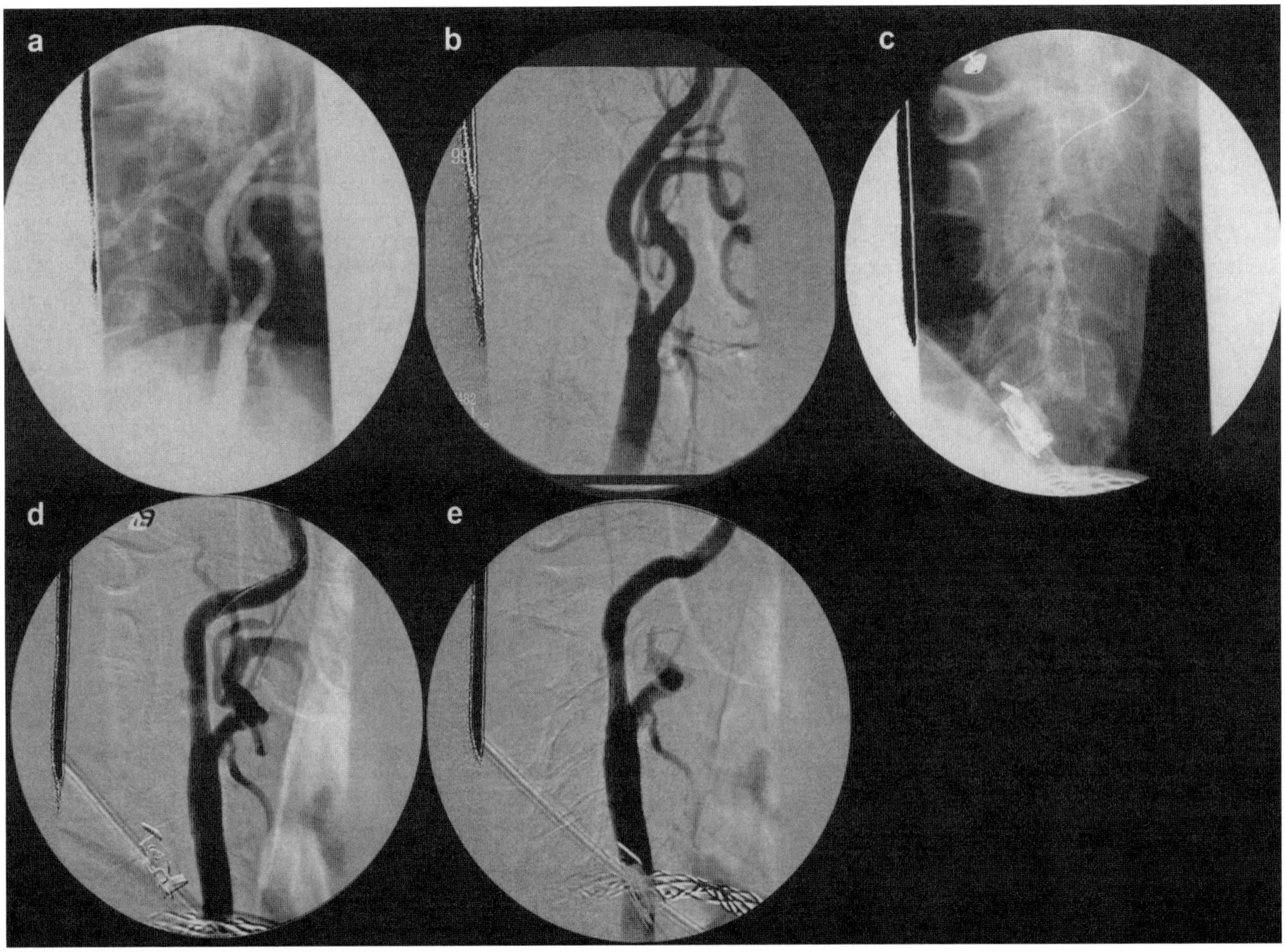

FIGURE 2-9. Extracranial carotid stent angioplasty. An 85-year-old woman with a history of atrial fibrillation, on warfarin, comes in with epistaxis. To prevent right hemispheric transient ischemic attacks while off warfarin, stenting angioplasty was performed. **a:** Right common carotid angiogram in the lateral projection demonstrates long-segment severe stenosis at the C3 level. **b:** Subtracted view from the right common carotid injection in the lateral projection better delineates the stenosis. **c:** Scout film in the lateral projection using a Storq 0.035-inch 300-cm exchange wire followed by Stabilizer 0.014-inch 300-cm exchange wire after primary angioplasty with 3.5-mm × 18-mm Powerflex balloon dilation catheter, stent deployment with a 8-mm × 20-mm Schneider Wallstent, and postangioplasty with a 5-mm × 20-mm Jupiter balloon dilation catheter. **d:** Posttreatment angiogram of the common carotid bifurcation prior to removal of the exchange wire demonstrates excellent angiographic result. **e:** After removal of the exchange wire there is no evidence of restenosis or dissection.

deficits may be due to intracranial embolism, hemorrhage, or reperfusion injury [245]. The phenomenon of reperfusion hemorrhage following surgical endarterectomy is well described. Ouriel et al., in a review of 1,471 patients undergoing surgical endarterectomy, reported an 0.75% incidence of intracerebral hemorrhage [246]. Hemorrhage occurred at a median of 3 days postoperatively and accounted for 35% of the total perioperative neurologic events. Death from massive hemorrhage and herniation occurred in 36% of cases. Factors correlating with an increased hemorrhage risk were hypertension, high-grade ipsilateral stenosis, high-grade contralateral stenosis or occlusion, and younger age. Schoser et al. reported on two patients with reperfusion hemorrhage—one intraparenchymal hemorrhage and one subarachnoid hemorrhage—following balloon angioplasty for carotid and vertebral artery stenosis [245]. Meyers et al. reported a 5% incidence of clinical or radiologic manifestations of cerebral hyperperfusion syndrome following craniocervical stenting procedures on 140 patients [247]. Morrish et al. reported a 4.4% incidence of cerebral hemorrhage following extracranial carotid artery stenting in 90 patients—75% of these hemorrhages being fatal [248]. These early studies suggest the incidence of cerebral hyperperfusion syndrome and intracranial hemorrhage may be increased in carotid stenting procedures because of factors such as increased severity of treated lesion, higher incidence of compromised collateral flow pathways, and more aggressive use of anticoagulation (Fig. 2-10). Prior to stent deployment, the mean arterial blood pressure should be maintained at or above baseline. However, following successful revascularization, lowering of the mean arterial pressure to 10% to 20% below baseline may be desirable to prevent cerebral reperfusion injury. Intravenous diltiazem may be used postprocedurally to control elevated blood pressure (5-mg/kg per minute loading dose followed by a continuous intravenous infusion of 5 to15 μg/kg per minute), particularly if associated with headache or neurologic sequelae, because it has minimal cerebral vasodilatory effects [249].

Alternatively, postprocedural prolonged bradycardia or hypotension, or both, may occur as a result of carotid sinus dysfunction, necessitating the use of intravenous vasopressors or inotropic agents [250]. Dangas et al. reported a 19% incidence of post–carotid artery stenting hypotension—defined as a greater than 40-mm Hg decrease in arterial pressure without evidence of hypovolemia, with a systolic pressure lower than 90 mm Hg at the end of the stenting procedure and lasting at least 1 hour—in 133 consecutive patients [251]. The incidence was higher when balloon-expandable (34%) versus self-expandable stents (14%) were used. Additionally, poststenting hypotension was correlated with an increased rate of postprocedural minor strokes and long-term risk of death [251].

Heparinization is generally allowed to taper physiologically rather than reversed using protamine sulphate. The femoral sheath is removed when the aPTT has returned to baseline. Alternatively, the femoral sheath may be removed immediately after the procedure, without the need for heparin reversal or groin pressure, using either a percutaneous suture closure (Perclose Inc., Redwood City, CA), or collagen plug delivery (VasoSeal, AngioSeal) device. Postprocedural hematocrit values are obtained, because the likelihood of a retroperitoneal hematoma is increased by the use of large-diameter sheaths in conjunction with high levels of anticoagulation. The patient is usually monitored in the intensive care unit for 12 to 24 hours after treatment. Clopidogrel, 75 mg/day, is continued for 4 to 6 weeks and enteric-coated aspirin, 325 mg/day, indefinitely. The patient is advised to avoid vigorous neck manipulation or deep massage. A follow-up ultrasonographic examination of the neck is obtained at 6 months to document continued patency, because restenosis usually occurs within the first 6 months after treatment.

In terms of stent sizing, the stent margins should optimally extend 1 centimeter beyond the proximal and distal margins of the stenotic plaque. This may necessitate crossing the external carotid artery origin, which does not usually result in significant clinical sequelae. Prominent carotid artery curves or kinks should also be taken into account when determining the appropriate stent length. It is not desirable to position the stent margins within an acute bend or kink in the carotid artery because this risks luminal obstruction by the stent. This is less of a problem (although not eliminated) with more conformable, self-expanding Nitinol stents (S.M.A.R.T. stent: Cordis Endovascular, Miami Lakes, FL). Phatouros et al. reported using five S.M.A.R.T. stents in four consecutive patients with carotid stenosis of at least 70% [252]. Technical success was achieved in all cases without any procedural complications specifically related to use of the S.M.A.R.T. stent (Fig. 2-11). Another potential problem that may be encountered is relocation of carotid artery redundancies or kinks adjacent to the stent margins. In our experience, these "nouveau" kinks have not usually been flow limiting and thus have not required further intervention.

The stent diameter should be 1 to 2 mm larger than the largest vessel diameter the stent will need to appose. Stent oversizing leads to a greater metallic coverage of the lesion per unit area, which is theoretically advantageous in preventing distal embolism, reducing tissue prolapse, and is not necessarily associated with a higher rate of restenosis [253,254]. Occasionally more than one stent will be required, in which case an approximate 20% stent overlap is desirable without incongruity of the opposing stent circumferences (the second stent diameter should be greater than the *in situ* stent diameter it is to contact). Accurate stent positioning can be problematic using self-expanding stents due to stent foreshortening with deployment. The Wallstent may notably foreshorten, the precise amount dependent upon the diameter to which the stent expands [255]. The S.M.A.R.T. stent foreshortens by 8% or less at the hub end.

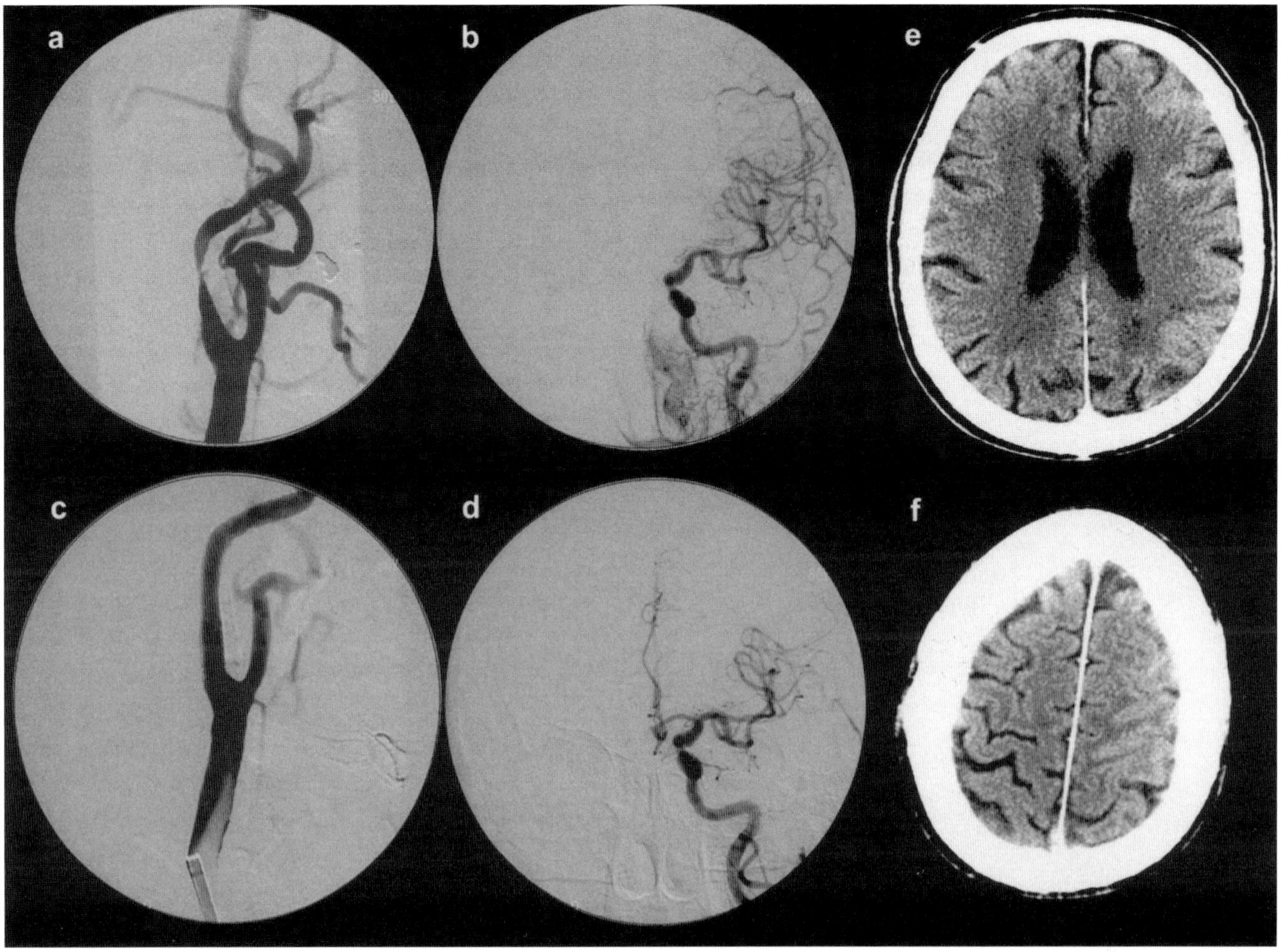

FIGURE 2-10. Cerebral hyperperfusion after extracranial carotid stent/angioplasty. An 80-year-old man has a left carotid bruit found on workup for open heart surgery. **a:** Left common carotid injection in the lateral projection demonstrates severe stenosis of the left internal carotid artery. **b:** Left common carotid injection centered over the head (anteroposterior projection) demonstrates antegrade flow in the internal carotid artery and middle cerebral artery but absence of filling of the anterior cerebral artery. **c:** Left common carotid injection status postangioplasty (4-mm × 20-mm Jupiter balloon dilation catheter) and stent deployment (Schneider 7-mm × 20-mm Wallstent) demonstrates good angiographic result and no evidence of restenosis. **d:** Left common carotid arteriography centered over the head (anteroposterior projection) demonstrates antegrade flow in the internal carotid, anterior cerebral, and middle cerebral arteries without evidence of branch occlusions. **e,f:** After stent deployment, the patient developed mixed aphasia and right arm paresis. CT scan following the procedure demonstrates swollen gyri in the frontal and parietal lobes on the left suspicious for hyperperfusion injury.

Early reports of carotid stenting mainly used balloon-expandable stents such as the Palmaz stent (Johnson & Johnson Interventional Systems, Warren, NJ), which can usually be positioned with greater precision than self-expandable types [52–55,57,256]. However, reports of a 2% to 16% rate of Palmaz stent collapse on follow-up imaging has led to increased use of self-expandable types [52,69, 257]. Mathur et al. reported Palmaz stent collapse in 11 of 70 patients (16%) at 6-month angiographic follow-up, attributing this to probable external compression. Furthermore, carotid Doppler ultrasonography, performed retrospectively in seven patients with stent compression, was only 29% sensitive [257]. Compression of balloon-expandable stents has been found to be a significant cause of restenosis in the superficial femoral arteries and hemodialysis grafts [258]. The 1999 global survey of 3,047 carotid stenting procedures by Wholey et al. reported 3,033 endovascular carotid stents placed [69]. Balloon-expandable Palmaz stents were used in 47% of cases, self-expandable Wallstents in 46%, and other stents including Strecker (Medi-tech, Watertown, MA), Integra (Medi-tech), Symphony (Medi-tech), and S.M.A.R.T. stents (Cordis Endovascular, Miami Lakes, FL) in the remaining 7% of cases. In this series, 28 stent deformations occurred exclusively with the Palmaz

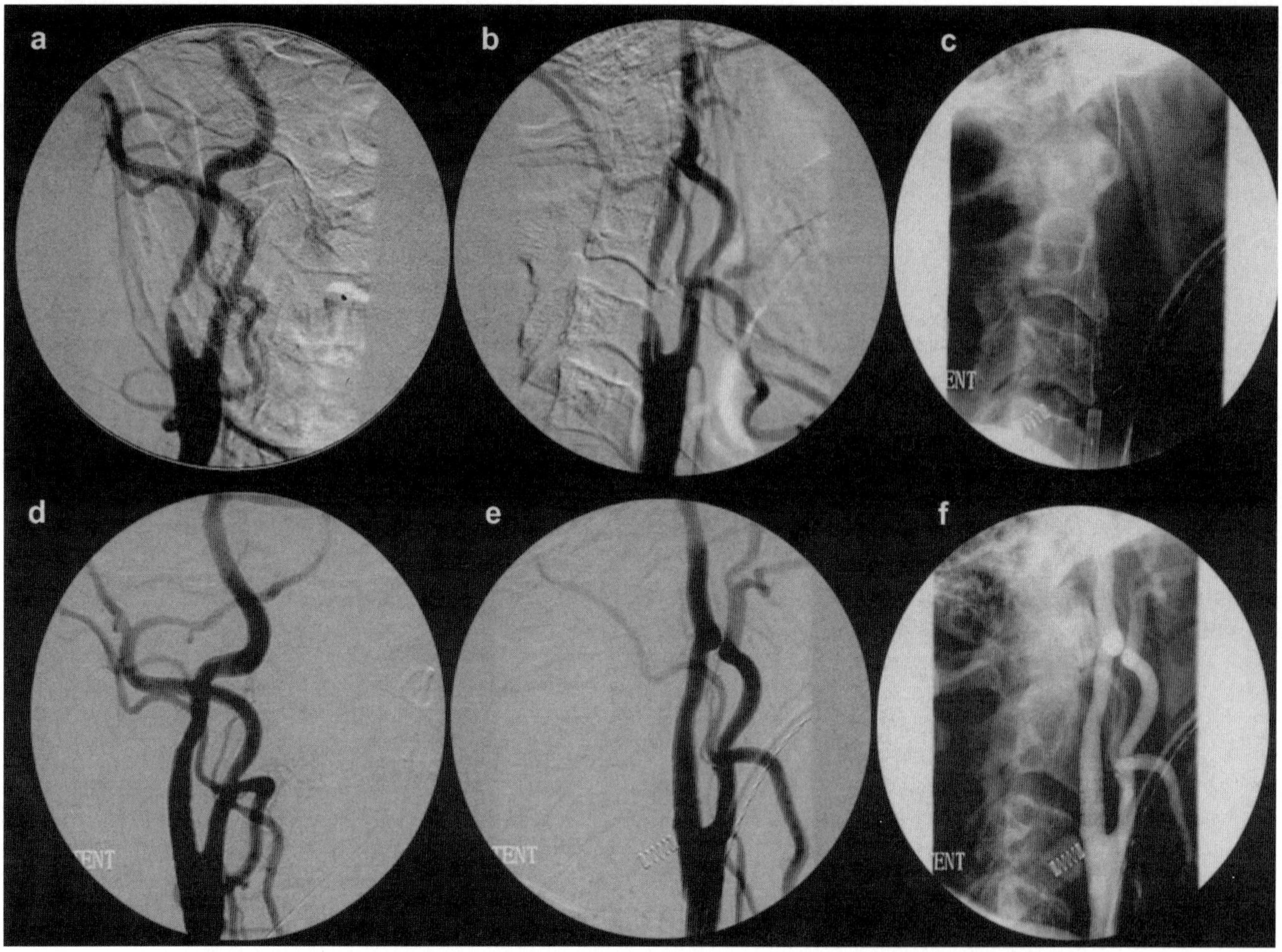

FIGURE 2-11. Extracranial carotid artery stenosis treated with a S.M.A.R.T. stent. A 75-year-old man with a history of hypertension, IDDM, prior left hemispheric stroke status post bilateral carotid endarterectomies in the past, now has symptomatic recurrent right internal carotid artery restenosis. **a,b:** Right common carotid angiography in the anteroposterior and lateral projections, respectively, demonstrates focal high-grade stenosis of the right internal carotid artery at the C2 to C3 level. **c:** Status post primary angioplasty (3.5-mm × 18-mm Titan balloon dilation catheter) and secondary stent placement (S.M.A.R.T. 6 mm × 20 mm). Residual stenosis treated with a Jupiter 5.5-mm × 20-mm PTA dilation catheter. This was performed over an 0.014-inch Stabilizer 300-cm exchange wire. Scout film in the lateral projection demonstrates the stent from the C2 to C3 level. **d,e:** Digital subtraction angiography of the right carotid bifurcation in the anteroposterior and lateral projections, respectively, demonstrates placement of the stent across the lesion within the internal carotid artery without evidence of restenosis or dissection. **f:** Unsubtracted angiography in the lateral projection demonstrates location of the stent within the internal carotid artery.

stent (2%). However, Bergeron et al. reported no instances of compression at a mean 13-month follow-up among 96 patients with carotid stenosis all treated with Palmaz stents [60]. Nevertheless, the Palmaz stent may not be an ideal choice for superficially exposed arteries such as the internal carotid. However, in nonexposed locations, such as the vertebral artery or great vessel origins, the superior positional accuracy of deployment may be advantageous. Self-expanding Nitinol stents offer the purported advantage of crush recoverability or springlike behavior. If an external force compresses or deforms a Nitinol stent, it will reassume its expanded shape upon removal of the external stress.

Future Technical Developments

The potential for further improvement in endovascular equipment and hence technique remains immense. Currently carotid stents are mainly adaptations of coronary or peripheral stent designs. Dedicated carotid stent designs that taper in diameter distally to accommodate the size discrepancy between the common and internal carotid artery may be advantageous, particularly with Nitinol stents which, in time, fully expand to their shape-memory diameter. Other potential areas of innovation include methods of providing cerebral protection using intravascular filters or balloons; smaller diameter, more flexible and hence less traumatic delivery systems; lowering rates of restenosis secondary to intimal hyperplasia by using local catheter brachytherapy or radiation-emitting stents [259–261]; and improved adjuvant pharmacological regimes using antiplatelet agents such as the glycoprotein IIb/IIIa inhibitors that could potentially reduce the incidence of acute thromboembolism and improve long-term patency [262]. This genuine potential for improvement has prompted some authors to suggest that a direct comparison with carotid endarterectomy is premature [263–266].

It remains unclear whether carotid artery stent placement helps reduce the number of particulate emboli by trapping them beneath the metallic meshwork. Current stent designs may trap larger fragments but not efficiently prevent microemboli because the interstices are too large [244]. A recent prospective study, in which patients undergoing carotid artery stenting were examined pre- and postprocedurally with MRI, failed to show evidence of brain signal abnormality referable to emboli [267]; however, a similar prospective study examining 19 patients with diffusion-weighted MRI showed new lesions in three cases, two of which were clinically silent [268]. Indeed, a study in which balloon angioplasty was performed in one carotid artery and stent placement within the contralateral side in ten cadavers with severe atherosclerosis demonstrated no difference in the severity of distal embolization between angioplasty and stenting. Furthermore, MRI accurately depicted postinterventional changes, and the findings correlated closely with those of intravascular ultrasonographic and histopathologic analysis [269]. A number of commercial devices aimed at reducing the microembolic burden associated with carotid angioplasty and stenting, using filters or guidewire-attached balloons, are currently available. These include a low-profile embolic filter deployed and retrieved on an 0.014-inch shaft that serves as the guidewire for balloon and stent-delivery catheters. Studies in *ex vivo* models have shown 88% capture of particles released during angioplasty and stenting of the carotid plaque lesion [270] (Fig. 2-12). Alternatively, an 0.014-inch guidewire with a protection balloon incorporated into the tip has been used. Following angioplasty and stenting with the protection balloon inflated, an over-the-wire aspiration catheter is passed through the dilated area to clear debris. This balloon-protection method has the disadvantage of temporary occlusion of carotid flow, whereas filter devices allow constant cerebral perfusion. Henry et al. reported mean cerebral flow occlusion times of 346 ± 153 seconds during predilation and 303 ± 143 seconds during stent placement in 48 patients undergoing carotid artery angioplasty and stenting [271]. Total mean flow occlusion time was 542 ± 243 seconds. A third device (Parodi Anti-Embolic System: ArteriA, San Francisco, CA) employs a dual-lumen guiding catheter with an external balloon cuff that is inflated within the common carotid artery. A guidewire incorporating a distal balloon is then passed through the guiding catheter and positioned within the external carotid artery where the balloon is inflated. This results in flow reversal of the ipsilateral internal carotid artery after the proximal end of the guiding catheter is connected to the femoral vein. Carotid angioplasty and stenting is then performed via the guiding catheter.

A

B

C

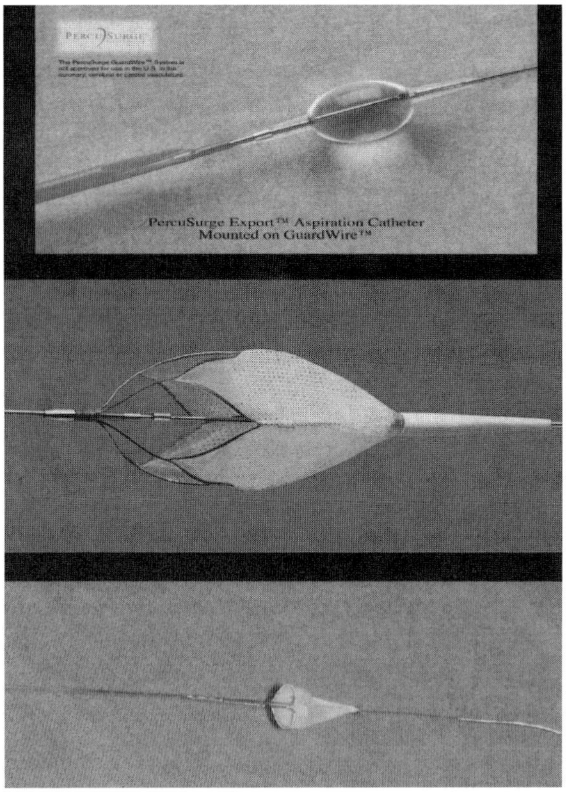

FIGURE 2-12. Carotid protection devices. **A:** PercuSurge Export Aspiration Catheter mounted on a GuardWire. **B:** Accunet filter. **C:** E-Trap filter.

REFERENCES

1. The National Advisory Neurological Disorders and Stroke Council. Stroke and cerebrovascular disease. In: *Status report: decade of the brain.* Bethesda, MD: National Institutes of Health, 1992:26–27.
2. Bonita R, Beaglehole R. Stroke: populations, cohorts, and clinical trials. In: Whisnant JP, ed. *Stroke mortality.* Oxford, UK: Butterworth-Heinemann, 1993:59–79.
3. American Heart Association. 1999 heart and stroke statistical update. Dallas, TX: American Heart Association, 1998:13–15.
4. Matchar D, Duncan P. Cost of stroke. *Stroke Clin Updates* 1994;3:9–12.
5. Dyken M. Stroke risk factors. In: Norris JW, Hachinski VC, eds. *Prevention of stroke.* New York: Springer-Verlag, 1991: 83–102.
6. Ricci S, Flamini FO, Celani MG, et al. Prevalence of internal carotid artery stenosis in subjects older than 49 years: a population study. *Cerebrovasc Dis* 1991;1:16–19.
7. Prati P, Vanuzzo D, Casaroli M, et al. Prevalence and determi-

nants of carotid atherosclerosis in a general population. *Stroke* 1992;23:1705–1711.

8. O'Leary DH, Polak JF, Kronmal RA, et al. Distribution and correlates of sonographically detected carotid artery disease in the Cardiovascular Health Study. The CHS Collaborative Research Group. *Stroke* 1992;23:1752–1760.
9. Zarins CK. Carotid endarterectomy: the gold standard. *J Endovasc Surg* 1996;3:10–15.
10. Wholey MH, Wholey M, Mathias K, et al. Global experience in cervical carotid artery stent placement. *Catheter Cardiovasc Interv* 2000;50:160–167.
11. North American Symptomatic Carotid Endarterectomy Trial Collaborators. Beneficial effect of carotid endarterectomy in symptomatic patients with high-grade carotid stenosis. *N Engl J Med* 1991;325:445–453.
12. Barnett HJ, Taylor DW, Eliasziw M, et al. Benefit of carotid endarterectomy in patients with symptomatic moderate or severe stenosis. North American Symptomatic Carotid Endarterectomy Trial Collaborators. *N Engl J Med* 1998;339: 1415–1425.
13. European Carotid Surgery Trialists' Collaborative Group. MRC European Carotid Surgery Trial: interim results for symptomatic patients with severe (70-99%) or with mild (0-29%) carotid stenosis. *Lancet* 1991;337:1235–1243.
14. European Carotid Surgery Trialists' Collaborative Group. Endarterectomy for moderate symptomatic carotid stenosis: interim results from the MRC European Carotid Surgery Trial. *Lancet* 1996;347:1591–1593.
15. European Carotid Surgery Trialists' Collaborative Group. Randomised trial of endarterectomy for recently symptomatic carotid stenosis: final results of the MRC European Carotid Surgery Trial (ECST). *Lancet* 1998;351:1379–1387.
16. Mayberg MR, Wilson SE, Yatsu F, et al. Carotid endarterectomy and prevention of cerebral ischemia in symptomatic carotid stenosis. Veterans Affairs Cooperative Studies Program 309 Trialist Group. *JAMA* 1991;266:3289–3294.
17. Ferguson GG, Eliasziw M, Barr HW, et al. The North American Symptomatic Carotid Endarterectomy Trial: surgical results in 1415 patients. *Stroke* 1999;30:1751–1758.
18. Paciaroni M, Eliasziw M, Kappelle LJ, et al. Medical complications associated with carotid endarterectomy. *Stroke* 1999;30: 1759–1763.
19. Donnan GA, Davis SM, Chambers BR, et al. Surgery for prevention of stroke. *Lancet* 1998;351:1372–1373.
20. Executive Committee for the Asymptomatic Carotid Atherosclerosis Study. Endarterectomy for asymptomatic carotid artery stenosis. *JAMA* 1995;273:1421–1428.
21. Warlow C. Endarterectomy for asymptomatic carotid stenosis? *Lancet* 1995;345:1254–1255.
22. Halliday AW, Thomas D, Mansfield A. The Asymptomatic Carotid Surgery Trial (ACST): rationale and design. Steering committee. *Eur J Vasc Surg* 1994;8:703–710.
23. Kerber CW, Hornwell LD, Loeden OL. Catheter dilatation of proximal carotid stenosis during distal bifurcation endarterectomy. *AJNR Am J Neuroradiol* 1980;1:348–349.
24. Theron J, Raymond J, Casasco A, et al. Percutaneous angioplasty of atherosclerotic and postsurgical stenosis of carotid arteries. *AJNR Am J Neuroradiol* 1987;8:495–500.
25. Kachel R. Results of balloon angioplasty in the carotid arteries. *J Endovasc Surg* 1996;3:22–30.
26. Gil-Peralta A, Mayol A, Marcos JR, et al. Percutaneous transluminal angioplasty of the symptomatic atherosclerotic carotid arteries: results, complications, and follow-up. *Stroke* 1996;27: 2271–2273.
27. Munari LM, Belloni G, Perretti A, et al. Carotid percutaneous angioplasty. *Neurol Res* 1992;14:156–158.
28. Eckert B, Zanella FE, Thie A, et al. Angioplasty of the internal carotid artery: results, complications and follow up in 61 cases. *Cerebrovasc Dis* 1996;27:2271–2273.
29. Higashida RT, Tsai FY, Halbach VV, et al. Transluminal angioplasty, thrombolysis, and stenting for extracranial and intracranial cerebral vascular disease. *J Interv Cardiol* 1996;9:245–255.
30. Theron JG, Payelle GG, Coskun O, et al. Carotid artery stenosis: treatment with protected balloon angioplasty and stent placement. *Radiology* 1996;201:627–636.
31. Sundt TM Jr, Whisnant JP, Houser OW, et al. Prospective study of the effectiveness and durability of carotid endarterectomy. *Mayo Clin Proc* 1990;65:625–635.
32. Meyer FB, Piepgras DG, Fode NC. Surgical treatment of recurrent carotid artery stenosis. *J Neurosurg* 1994;80:781–787.
33. Frericks H, Kievit J, van Baalen JM, et al. Carotid recurrent stenosis and risk of ipsilateral stroke: a systematic review of the literature. *Stroke* 1998;29:244–250.
34. Moore WS, Kempczinski RF, Nelson JJ, et al. Recurrent carotid stenosis: results of the asymptomatic carotid atherosclerosis study. *Stroke* 1998;29:2018–2025.
35. Bladin CF, Bingham L, Grigg L, et al. Transcranial Doppler detection of microemboli during percutaneous transluminal coronary angioplasty. *Stroke* 1998;29:2367–2370.
36. Markus HS, Clifton A, Buckenham T, et al. Carotid angioplasty: detection of embolic signals during and after the procedure. *Stroke* 1994;25:2403–2406.
37. Crawley F, Clifton A, Buckenham T, et al. Comparison of hemodynamic cerebral ischemia and microembolic signals detected during carotid endarterectomy and carotid angioplasty. *Stroke* 1997;28:2460–2464.
38. McCleary AJ, Nelson M, Dearden NM, et al. Cerebral haemodynamics and embolization during carotid angioplasty in high-risk patients. *Br J Surg* 1998;85:771–774.
39. Gaunt ME, Brown L, Hartshorne T, et al. Unstable carotid plaques: preoperative identification and association with intraoperative embolisation detected by transcranial Doppler. *Eur J Vasc Endovasc Surg* 1996;11:78–82.
40. Levi CR, O'Malley HM, Fell G, et al. Transcranial Doppler detected cerebral microembolism following carotid endarterectomy: high microembolic signal loads predict postoperative cerebral ischaemia. *Brain* 1997;120:621–629.
41. Spencer MP. Transcranial Doppler monitoring and causes of stroke from carotid endarterectomy. *Stroke* 1997;28:685–691.
42. Gaunt ME, Martin PJ, Smith JL, et al. Clinical relevance of intraoperative embolization detected by transcranial Doppler ultrasonography during carotid endarterectomy: a prospective study of 100 patients. *Br J Surg* 1994;81:1435–1439.
43. Muller M, Behnke S, Walter P, et al. Microembolic signals and intraoperative stroke in carotid endarterectomy. *Acta Neurol Scand* 1998;97:110–117.
44. Crawley F, Stygall J, Lunn S, et al. Comparison of microembolism detected by transcranial Doppler and neuropsychological sequelae of carotid surgery and percutaneous transluminal angioplasty. *Stroke* 2000;21:1329–1334.
45. Ringelstein EB, Droste DW, Babikian VL, et al. Consensus on microembolus detection by TCD. International Consensus Group on Microembolus Detection. *Stroke* 1998;29:725–729.
46. Goertler M, Baeumer M, Kross R, et al. Rapid decline of cerebral microemboli of arterial origin after intravenous acetylsalicylic acid. *Stroke* 1999;30:66–69.
47. Eckert B, Thie A, Valdueza J, et al. Transcranial Doppler sonographic monitoring during percutaneous transluminal angioplasty of the internal carotid artery. *Neuroradiology* 1997;39: 229–234.
48. Tsurutani T, Orita T, Kitahara T. Percutaneous transluminal angioplasty of the internal carotid artery with a continuous-

perfusion dilatation catheter. *AJNR Am J Neuroradiol* 1997;18: 696–698.
49. Serruys PW, de Jaegere P, Kiemeneij F, et al. A comparison of balloon-expandable-stent implantation with balloon angioplasty in patients with coronary artery disease. Benestent Study Group. *N Engl J Med* 1994;331:489–495.
50. Macaya C, Serruys PW, Ruygrok P, et al. Continued benefit of coronary stenting versus balloon angioplasty: one-year clinical follow-up of Benestent trial. Benestent Study Group. *J Am Coll Cardiol* 1996;27:255–261.
51. Serruys PW, van Hout B, Bonnier H, et al. Randomised comparison of implantation of heparin-coated stents with balloon angioplasty in selected patients with coronary artery disease (Benestent II) [published erratum appears in *Lancet* 1998;352: 1478]. *Lancet* 1998;352:673–681.
52. Roubin GS, Yadav S, Iyer SS, et al. Carotid stent-supported angioplasty: a neurovascular intervention to prevent stroke. *Am J Cardiol* 1996;78:8–12.
53. Diethrich EB, Ndiaye M, Reid DB. Stenting in the carotid artery: initial experience in 110 patients. *J Endovasc Surg* 1996; 3:42–62.
54. Criado FJ, Wellons E, Clark NS. Evolving indications for and early results of carotid artery stenting. *Am J Surg* 1997;174: 111–114.
55. Vozzi CR, Rodriguez AO, Paolantonio D, et al. Extracranial carotid angioplasty and stenting: initial results and short-term follow-up. *Tex Heart Inst J* 1997;24:167–172.
56. Yadav JS, Roubin GS, Iyer S, et al. Elective stenting of the extracranial carotid arteries. *Circulation* 1997;95:376–381.
57. Wholey MH, Jarmolowski CR, Eles G, et al. Endovascular stents for carotid artery occlusive disease. *J Endovasc Surg* 1997; 4:326–338.
58. Henry M, Amor M, Masson I, et al. Angioplasty and stenting of the extracranial carotid arteries. *J Endovasc Surg* 1998;5: 293–304.
59. Teitelbaum GP, Lefkowitz MA, Giannotta SL. Carotid angioplasty and stenting in high-risk patients. *Surg Neurol* 1998;50: 300–312.
60. Bergeron P, Becquemin JP, Jausseran JM, et al. Percutaneous stenting of the internal carotid artery: the European CAST I Study. Carotid Artery Stent Trial. *J Endovasc Surg* 1999;6: 155–159.
61. Gross CM, Kramer J, Uhlich F. Treatment of carotid artery stenosis by elective stent placement instead of carotid endarterectomy in patients with severe coronary artery disease. *Thromb Haemost* 1999;82[Suppl 1]:176–180.
62. Malek AM, Higashida RT, Phatouros CC, et al. Stent angioplasty for cervical carotid artery stenosis in high-risk symptomatic NASCET-ineligible patients. *Stroke* 2000;31:3029–3033.
63. Mathur A, Roubin GS, Iyer SS, et al. Predictors of stroke complicating carotid artery stenting. *Circulation* 1998;97: 1239–1245.
64. Das MB, Hertzer NR, Ratliff NB, et al. Recurrent carotid stenosis: a five-year series of 65 reoperations. *Ann Surg* 1985;202: 28–35.
65. McCrory DC, Goldstein LB, Samsa GP, et al. Predicting complications of carotid endarterectomy. *Stroke* 1993;24: 1285–1291.
66. Vassilidze TV, Cernaianu AC, Gaprindashvili T, et al. Simultaneous coronary artery bypass and carotid endarterectomy: determinants of outcome. *Tex Heart Inst J* 1994;21:119–124.
67. Mericle RA, Kim SH, Lanzino G, et al. Carotid artery angioplasty and use of stents in high-risk patients with contralateral occlusions. *J Neurosurg* 1999;90:1031–1036.
68. Chastain HD II, Gomez CR, Iyer S, et al. Influence of age upon complications of carotid artery stenting. *J Endovasc Surg* 1999;6:217–222.
69. Wholey MH, Wholey MH, Eles G. Clinical experience in cervical carotid artery stent placement. *Carotid Neurovasc Interv* 1998;1:2–9.
70. Ballotta E, Da Giau G, Renon L, et al. Cranial and cervical nerve injuries after carotid endarterectomy: a prospective study. *Surgery* 1999;125:85–91.
71. Yadav JS, Roubin GS, King P, et al. Angioplasty and stenting for restenosis after carotid endarterectomy: initial experience. *Stroke* 1996;27:2075–2079.
72. Lanzino G, Mericle RA, Lopes DK, et al. Percutaneous transluminal angioplasty and stent placement for recurrent carotid artery stenosis. *J Neurosurg* 1999;90:688–694.
73. Hobson RW II. CREST (Carotid Revascularization Endarterectomy versus Stent Trial): background, design, and current status. *Semin Vasc Surg* 2000;13:138–143.
74. Sivaguru A, Venables GS, Beard JD, et al. European carotid angioplasty trial. *J Endovasc Surg* 1996;3:16–20.
75. Brown MM. Vascular surgical society of Great Britain and Ireland: results of the carotid and vertebral artery transluminal angioplasty study. *Br J Surg* 1999;86:710–711.
76. Miyamoto S, Kikuchi H, Karasawa J, et al. Surgical treatment for spontaneous carotid dissection with impending stroke: case report. *J Neurosurg* 1984;61:382–386.
77. Morgan MK, Sekhon LH. Extracranial-intracranial saphenous vein bypass for carotid or vertebral artery dissections: a report of six cases. *J Neurosurg* 1994;80:237–246.
78. Schievink WI, Piepgras DG, McCaffrey TV, et al. Surgical treatment of extracranial internal carotid artery dissecting aneurysms. *Neurosurgery* 1994;35:809–816.
79. Bejjani GK, Monsein LH, Laird JR, et al. Treatment of symptomatic cervical carotid dissections with endovascular stents. *Neurosurgery* 1999;44:755–761.
80. Coric D, Wilson JA, Regan JD, et al. Primary stenting of the extracranial internal carotid artery in a patient with multiple cervical dissections: technical case report. *Neurosurgery* 1998; 43:956–959.
81. DeOcampo J, Brillman J, Levy DI. Stenting: a new approach to carotid dissection. *J Neuroimaging* 1997;7:187–190.
82. Dorros G, Cohn JM, Palmer LE. Stent deployment resolves a petrous carotid artery angioplasty dissection. *AJNR Am J Neuroradiol* 1998;19:392–394.
83. Duke BJ, Ryu RK, Coldwell DM, et al. Treatment of blunt injury to the carotid artery by using endovascular stents: an early experience. *J Neurosurg* 1997;87:825–829.
84. Hong MK, Satler LF, Gallino R, et al. Intravascular stenting as a definitive treatment of spontaneous carotid artery dissection. *Am J Cardiol* 1997;79:538.
85. Yamashita K, Okamoto S, Kim C, et al. Emergent treatment of iatrogenic dissection of the internal carotid artery with the Palmaz-Schatz stent: case report. *Neurol Med Chir (Tokyo)* 1997; 37:336–339.
86. Malek AM, Higashida RT, Halbach VV, et al. Patient presentation, angiographic features, and treatment of strangulation-induced bilateral dissection of the cervical internal carotid artery. *J Neurosurg* 2000;92:481–487.
87. Malek AM, Higashida RT, Phatouros CC, et al. Endovascular management of extracranial carotid artery dissection achieved using stent angioplasty. *AJNR Am J Neuroradiol* 2000;21: 1280–1292.
88. Liu AY, Paulsen RD, Marcellus ML, et al. Long-term outcomes after carotid stent placement treatment of carotid artery dissection. *Neurosurgery* 1999;45:1368–1373.
89. Marks MP, Dake MD, Steinberg GK, et al. Stent placement

for arterial and venous cerebrovascular disease: preliminary experience. *Radiology* 1994;191:441–446.

90. Geremia G, Haklin M, Brennecke L. Embolization of experimentally created aneurysms with intravascular stent devices. *AJNR Am J Neuroradiol* 1994;15:1223–1231.
91. Turjman F, Acevedo G, Moll T, et al. Treatment of experimental carotid aneurysms by endoprosthesis implantation: preliminary report. *Neurol Res* 1993;15:181–184.
92. Wakhloo AK, Schellhammer F, de Vries J, et al. Self-expanding and balloon-expandable stents in the treatment of carotid aneurysms: an experimental study in a canine model. *AJNR Am J Neuroradiol* 1994;15:493–502.
93. Graves VB, Strother CM, Partington CR, et al. Flow dynamics of lateral carotid artery aneurysms and their effects on coils and balloons: an experimental study in dogs. *AJNR Am J Neuroradiol* 1992;13:189–196.
94. Aenis M, Stancampiano AP, Wakhloo AK, et al. Modeling of flow in a straight stented and nonstented side wall aneurysm model. *J Biomech Eng* 1997;119:206–212.
95. Bernstein SM, Coldwell DM, Prall JA, et al. Treatment of traumatic carotid pseudoaneurysm with endovascular stent placement. *J Vasc Interv Radiol* 1997;8:1065–1068.
96. Horowitz MB, Miller G III, Meyer Y, et al. Use of intravascular stents in the treatment of internal carotid and extracranial vertebral artery pseudoaneurysms. *AJNR Am J Neuroradiol* 1996;17:693–696.
97. Huang A, Baker DM, al-Kutoubi A, et al. Endovascular stenting of internal carotid artery false aneurysm. *Eur J Vasc Endovasc Surg* 1996;12:375–377.
98. Hurst RW, Haskal ZJ, Zager E, et al. Endovascular stent treatment of cervical internal carotid artery aneurysms with parent vessel preservation. *Surg Neurol* 1998;50:313–317.
99. Manninen HI, Koivisto T, Saari T, et al. Dissecting aneurysms of all four cervicocranial arteries in fibromuscular dysplasia: treatment with self-expanding endovascular stents, coil embolization, and surgical ligation. *AJNR Am J Neuroradiol* 1997;18:1216–1220.
100. Mase M, Banno T, Yamada K, et al. Endovascular stent placement for multiple aneurysms of the extracranial internal carotid artery: technical case report. *Neurosurgery* 1995;37:832–835.
101. Massoud TF, Turjman F, Ji C, et al. Endovascular treatment of fusiform aneurysms with stents and coils: technical feasibility in a swine model *AJNR Am J Neuroradiol* 1995;16:1953–1963.
102. Szikora I, Guterman LR, Wells KM, et al. Combined use of stents and coils to treat experimental wide-necked carotid aneurysms: preliminary results. *AJNR Am J Neuroradiol* 1994;15:1091–1102.
103. Turjman F, Acevedo G, Massoud TF, et al. An experimental study of the treatment of aneurysms using an intravascular prosthesis. *J Neuroradiol* 1997;24:205–211.
104. Turjman F, Massoud TF, Ji C, et al. Combined stent implantation and endosaccular coil placement for treatment of experimental wide-necked aneurysms: a feasibility study in swine. *AJNR Am J Neuroradiol* 1994;15:1087–1090.
105. Klein GE, Szolar DH, Raith J, et al. Posttraumatic extracranial aneurysm of the internal carotid artery: combined endovascular treatment with coils and stents. *AJNR Am J Neuroradiol* 1997;18:1261–1264.
106. Matsuura JH, Rosenthal D, Jerius H, et al. Traumatic carotid artery dissection and pseudoaneurysm treated with endovascular coils and stent. *J Endovasc Surg* 1997;4:339–343.
107. Perez-Cruet MJ, Patwardhan RV, Mawad ME, et al. Treatment of dissecting pseudoaneurysm of the cervical internal carotid artery using a wall stent and detachable coils: case report. *Neurosurgery* 1997;40:622–626.
108. Phatouros CC, Sasaki TYJ, Higashida RT, et al. Stent-supported coil embolization: the treatment of wide-neck aneurysms and pseudoaneurysms. *Neurosurgery* 2000;47:107–115.
109. Parodi JC, Schonholz C, Ferreira LM, et al. Endovascular stent-graft treatment of traumatic arterial lesions. *Ann Vasc Surg* 1999;13:121–129.
110. Marotta TR, Buller C, Taylor D, et al. Autologous vein-covered stent repair of a cervical internal carotid artery pseudoaneurysm: technical case report. *Neurosurgery* 1998;42:408–413.
111. Ruebben A, Merlo M, Verri A, et al. Exclusion of an internal carotid aneurysm by a covered stent. *J Cardiovasc Surg (Torino)* 1997;38:301–303.
112. du Toit DF, Strauus DC, Blaszczyk M, et al. Endovascular treatment of penetrating thoracic outlet arterial injuries. *Eur J Vasc Endovasc Surg* 2000;19:489–495.
113. Link J, Feyerabend B, Grabener M, et al. Dacron-covered stent-grafts for the percutaneous treatment of carotid aneurysms: effectiveness and biocompatibility-experimental study in swine. *Radiology* 1996;200:397–401.
114. Loftus CM, Biller J, Hart MN, et al. Management of radiation-induced accelerated carotid atherosclerosis. *Arch Neurol* 1987;44:711–714.
115. Murros KE, Toole JF. The effect of radiation on carotid arteries: a review article. *Arch Neurol* 1989;46:449–455.
116. Al-Mubarak N, Roubin GS, Iyer SS, et al. Carotid stenting for severe radiation-induced extracranial carotid artery occlusive disease. *J Endovasc Ther* 2000;7:36–40.
117. Bali HK, Jain S, Jain A, et al. Stent supported angioplasty in Takayasu arteritis. *Int J Cardiol* 1998;66[Suppl 1]:S213–S220.
118. Castaigne P, Lhermitte F, Gautier JC, et al. Arterial occlusions in the vertebro-basilar system: a study of 44 patients with post-mortem data. *Brain* 1973;96:133–154.
119. Fisher CM, Gore I, Okabe N, et al. Atherosclerosis of the carotid and vertebral arteries: extracranial and intracranial. *J Neuropathol Exp Neurol* 1965;24:455–476.
120. Hutchinson EC, Yates PO. Carotico-vertebral stenosis. *Lancet* 1957;1:2–8.
121. Martin MJ, Whisnant JP, Sayre GP. Occlusive vascular disease in the extracranial cerebral circulation. *Arch Neurol* 1960;3:530–537.
122. Schwartz CJ, Mitchell JR. Atheroma of the carotid and vertebral arterial systems. *BMJ* 1961;2:1057–1063.
123. Hass WK, Fields WS, North RR, et al. Joint study of extracranial arterial occlusion. II. Arteriography, techniques, sites, and complications. *JAMA* 1968;203:961–968.
124. Meyer JS, Sheehan S, Bauer RB. An arteriographic study of cerebrovascular disease in man. I. Stenosis and occlusion of the vertebral-basilar arterial system. *Arch Neurol* 1960;2:27–45.
125. Staikov IN, Do DD, Remonda L, et al. The site of atheromatosis in the subclavian and vertebral arteries and its implication for angioplasty. *Neuroradiology* 1999;41:537–542.
126. Stein BM, McCormick W, Rodriquez JN, et al. Incidence and significance of occlusive vascular disease of the extracranial arteries as demonstrated by post-mortem angiography. *Trans Am Neurol Assoc* 1961;86:60–66.
127. Imparato AM, Riles TS, Kim GE. Cervical vertebral angioplasty for brain stem ischemia. *Surgery* 1981;90:842–852.
128. Crawley F, Brown MM, Clifton AG. Angioplasty and stenting in the carotid and vertebral arteries. *Postgrad Med J* 1998;74:7–10.
129. Biemond A. Thrombosis of the basilar artery and vascularization for the brain stem. *Brain* 1951;74:300–317.
130. Kubik CS, Adams RD. Occlusion of the basilar artery: a clinical and pathological study. *Brain* 1946;68:73–121.
131. Millikan CH, Siekert RG. The syndrome of intermittent insufficiency of the basilar arterial system. *Mayo Clin Proc* 1955;30:61–68.

132. Moufarrij NA, Little JR, Furlan AJ, et al. Vertebral artery stenosis: long-term follow-up. *Stroke* 1984;15:260–263.
133. Wityk RJ, Chang HM, Rosengart A, et al. Proximal extracranial vertebral artery disease in the New England Medical Center Posterior Circulation Registry. *Arch Neurol* 1998;55:470–478.
134. Moufarrij NA, Little JR, Furlan AJ, et al. Basilar and distal vertebral artery stenosis: long-term follow-up. *Stroke* 1986;17:938–942.
135. WASID Investigators. Prognosis of patients with symptomatic vertebral or basilar artery stenosis. The Warfarin-Aspirin Symptomatic Intracranial Disease (WASID) Study Group. *Stroke* 1998;29:1389–1392.
136. Heyman A, Leviton A, Millikan CH, et al. Transient focal cerebral ischemia: epidemiological and clinical aspects. *Stroke* 1974;5:277–287.
137. Caplan LR, Amarenco P, Rosengart A, et al. Embolism from vertebral artery origin occlusive disease. *Neurology* 1992;42:1505–1512.
138. Caplan LR, Tettenborn B. Vertebrobasilar occlusive disease: review of certain aspects. *Cerebrovasc Dis* 1992;2:256–265.
139. Turney TM, Garraway WM, Whisnant JP. The natural history of hemispheric and brainstem infarction in Rochester, Minnesota. *Stroke* 1984;15:790–794.
140. Caplan LR. *Posterior circulation disease: clinical findings, diagnosis and management.* Cambridge, MA: Blackwell Science, 1996.
141. Koennecke HC, Mast H, Trocio SS Jr, et al. Microemboli in patients with vertebrobasilar ischemia: association with vertebrobasilar and cardiac lesions. *Stroke* 1997;28:593–596.
142. Caplan LR, Hennerici M. Impaired clearance of emboli (washout) is an important link between hypoperfusion, embolism, and ischemic stroke. *Arch Neurol* 1998;55:1475–1482.
143. Saeki N, Rhoton AL Jr. Microsurgical anatomy of the upper basilar artery and the posterior circle of Willis. *J Neurosurg* 1977;46:563–578.
144. Bosniak MA. An analysis of some anatomic-roentgenologic aspects of the brachiocephalic vessels. *Am J Roentgenol Radium Ther Nucl Med* 1964;91:1222–1231.
145. Osborn AG. *Introduction to cerebral angiography.* Philadelphia: Harper & Row, 1980:33–48.
146. Thomas LM, Hardy WG, Lindner DW, et al. Retrograde brachial angiography in cerebrovascular disease. *Arch Neurol* 1962;7:339–346.
147. Newton TH, Mani RL. The vertebral artery. In: Newton TH, Potts DG, eds. *Radiology of the skull and brain. Vol 2. Angiography.* St Louis: Mosby, 1974:1659–1709.
148. Lippert H, Pabst R. *Arterial variations in man: classification and frequency.* Munich: JF Bergmann-Verlag, 1985:3–9.
149. Dilenge D, David M. La branch meningee de l'artere vertebrale. *Neurochirurgie* 1965:8:121–126.
150. Krayenbuhl H, Yasargil MG. *Die vaskularen erkrankungen im giebert der arteria vertebralis und arteria basilaris.* Stuttgart: Thieme, 1957.
151. Whisnant JP, Cartlidge NE, Elveback LR. Carotid and vertebral-basilar transient ischemic attacks: effect of anticoagulants, hypertension, and cardiac disorders on survival and stroke occurrence—a population study. *Ann Neurol* 1978;3:107–115.
152. Chimowitz MI, Kokkinos J, Strong J, et al. The Warfarin-Aspirin Symptomatic Intracranial Disease Study. *Neurology* 1995;45:1488–1493.
153. Cate WR, Scott HW. Cerebral ischemia of central origin: relief by subclavian-vertebral artery thromboendarterectomy. *Surgery* 1959;45:19–31.
154. Edwards WH Sr. Vertebral basilar insufficiency: a 25-year experience with proximal subclavian and vertebral artery lesions. In: Calligaro KD, DeLaurentis DA, Baker WH, eds. *Management of extracranial cerebrovascular disease.* Philadelphia: Lippincott–Raven Publishers, 1997:151–160.
155. Fessler RD, Wakhloo AK, Lanzino G, et al. Stent placement for vertebral artery occlusive disease: preliminary clinical experience. *Neurosurg Focus* 1998;5:Article 15.
156. Motarjeme A, Keifer JW, Zuska AJ. Percutaneous transluminal angioplasty of the vertebral arteries. *Radiology* 1981;139:715–717.
157. Schutz H, Yeung HP, Chiu MC, et al. Dilatation of vertebral-artery stenosis [Letter]. *N Engl J Med* 1981;304:732.
158. Bruckmann H, Ringelstein EB, Buchner H, et al. Percutaneous transluminal angioplasty of the vertebral artery: a therapeutic alternative to operative reconstruction of proximal vertebral artery stenoses. *J Neurol* 1986;233:336–339.
159. Courtheoux P, Tournade A, Theron J, et al. Transcutaneous angioplasty of vertebral artery atheromatous ostial stricture. *Neuroradiology* 1985;27:259–264.
160. Higashida RT, Hieshima GB, Tsai FY, et al. Percutaneous transluminal angioplasty of the subclavian and vertebral arteries. *Acta Radiol Suppl* 1986;369:124–126.
161. Higashida RT, Hieshima GB, Tsai FY, et al. Transluminal angioplasty of the vertebral and basilar artery. *AJNR Am J Neuroradiol* 1987;8:745–749.
162. Kachel R, Endert G, Basche S, et al. Percutaneous transluminal angioplasty (dilatation) of carotid, vertebral, and innominate artery stenoses. *Cardiovasc Intervent Radiol* 1987;10:142–146.
163. Motarjeme A, Keifer JW, Zuska AJ. Percutaneous transluminal angioplasty of the brachiocephalic arteries. *AJR Am J Roentgenol* 1982;138:457–462.
164. Theron J, Courtheoux P, Henriet JP, et al. Angioplasty of supraaortic arteries. *J Neuroradiol* 1984;11:187–200.
165. Tournade A, Zenglein JP, Braun JP, et al. Percutaneous transluminal angioplasty of the vertebral and subclavian arteries: an angiographic-velocimetry comparison. *J Neuroradiol* 1986;13:95–110.
166. Higashida RT, Tsai FY, Halbach VV, et al. Transluminal angioplasty for atherosclerotic disease of the vertebral and basilar arteries. *J Neurosurg* 1993;78:192–198.
167. Sawada M, Hashimoto N, Nishi S, et al. Detection of embolic signals during and after percutaneous transluminal angioplasty of subclavian and vertebral arteries using transcranial Doppler ultrasonography. *Neurosurgery* 1997;41:535–541.
168. Feldman RL, Rubin JJ, Kuykendall RC. Use of coronary Palmaz-Schatz stent in the percutaneous treatment of vertebral artery stenoses. *Cathet Cardiovasc Diagn* 1996;38:312–315.
169. Motarjeme A. Percutaneous transluminal angioplasty of supra-aortic vessels. *J Endovasc Surg* 1996;3:171–181.
170. Storey GS, Marks MP, Dake M, et al. Vertebral artery stenting following percutaneous transluminal angioplasty: technical note. *J Neurosurg* 1996;84:883–887.
171. Malek AM, Higashida RT, Phatouros CC, et al. Treatment of posterior circulation ischemia with extracranial percutaneous balloon angioplasty and stent placement. *Stroke* 1999;30:2073–2085.
172. Chastain HD II, Campbell MS, Iyer S, et al. Extracranial vertebral artery stent placement: in-hospital and follow-up results. *J Neurosurg* 1999;91:547–552.
173. Mas JL, Bousser MG, Hasboun D, et al. Extracranial vertebral artery dissections: a review of 13 cases. *Stroke* 1987;18:1037–1047.
174. Friedman AH. Traumatic injury of neck and intracranial vessels. *Contemp Neurosurg* 1990;12:26.
175. Halbach VV, Higashida RT, Hieshima GB. Treatment of vertebral arteriovenous fistulas. *AJR Am J Roentgenol* 1988;150:405–412.

176. Mokri B, Houser OW, Sandok BA, et al. Spontaneous dissections of the vertebral arteries. *Neurology* 1988;38:880–885.
177. Halbach VV, Higashida RT, Dowd CF, et al. Endovascular treatment of vertebral artery dissections and pseudoaneurysms. *J Neurosurg* 1993;79:183–191.
178. Price RF, Sellar R, Leung C, et al. Traumatic vertebral arterial dissection and vertebrobasilar arterial thrombosis successfully treated with endovascular thrombolysis and stenting. *AJNR Am J Neuroradiol* 1998;19:1677–1680.
179. Mericle RA, Lanzino G, Wakhloo AK, et al. Stenting and secondary coiling of intracranial internal carotid artery aneurysm: technical case report. *Neurosurgery* 1998;43:1229–1234.
180. Higashida RT, Smith W, Gress D, et al: Intravascular stent and endovascular coil placement for a ruptured fusiform aneurysm of the basilar artery: case report and review of the literature. *J Neurosurg* 1997;87:944–949.
181. Lylyk P, Ceratto R, Hurvitz D, et al. Treatment of a vertebral dissecting aneurysm with stents and coils: technical case report. *Neurosurgery* 1998;43:385–388.
182. Sekhon LH, Morgan MK, Sorby W, et al: Combined endovascular stent implantation and endosaccular coil placement for the treatment of a wide-necked vertebral artery aneurysm: technical case report. *Neurosurgery* 1998;43:380–384.
183. Criado E, Marston WA, Ligush J, et al. Endovascular repair of peripheral aneurysms, pseudoaneurysms, and arteriovenous fistulas. *Ann Vasc Surg* 1997;11:256–263.
184. Pastores SM, Marin ML, Veith FJ, et al. Endovascular stented graft repair of a pseudoaneurysm of the subclavian artery caused by percutaneous internal jugular vein cannulation: case report. *Am J Crit Care* 1995;4:472–475.
185. Patel AV, Marin ML, Veith FJ, et al. Endovascular graft repair of penetrating subclavian artery injuries. *J Endovasc Surg* 1996; 3:382–388.
186. Szeimies U, Kueffer G, Stoeckelhuber B, et al. Successful exclusion of subclavian aneurysms with covered nitinol stents. *Cardiovasc Intervent Radiol* 1998;21:246–249.
187. Colley DP. Vertebral arteriovenous fistula: an unusual complication of Swan-Ganz catheter insertion. *AJNR Am J Neuroradiol* 1985;6:103–104.
188. Robinson PN, Jewkes DA, Kendall B. Vertebrovertebral arteriovenous fistula: a complication of internal jugular catheterisation. *Anaesthesia* 1984;39:46–47.
189. Weinberg PE, Flom RA. Traumatic vertebral arteriovenous fistula. *Surg Neurol* 1973;1:162–167.
190. Avellanosa AM, Glasauer FE, Oh YS. Traumatic vertebral arteriovenous fistula associated with cervical spine fracture. *J Trauma* 1977;17:885–888.
191. Kamiyama K, Endo S, Horie Y, et al. Neurofibromatosis associated with intra- and extracranial aneurysms and extracranial vertebral arteriovenous fistula. *No Shinkei Geka* 1985;13: 875–880.
192. Bahar S, Chiras J, Carpena JP, et al. Spontaneous vertebrovertebral arterio-venous fistula associated with fibro-muscular dysplasia: report of two cases. *Neuroradiology* 1984;26:45–49.
193. Nagashima C, Iwasaki T, Kawanuma S, et al. Traumatic arteriovenous fistula of the vertebral artery with spinal cord symptoms: case report. *J Neurosurg* 1977;46:681–687.
194. Reizine D, Laouiti M, Guimaraens L, et al. Vertebral arteriovenous fistula: clinical presentation, angiographical appearance and endovascular treatment. A review of twenty-five cases. *Ann Radiol (Paris)* 1985;28:425–438.
195. Debrun G, Legre J, Kasbarian M, et al. Endovascular occlusion of vertebral fistulae by detachable balloons with conservation of the vertebral blood flow. *Radiology* 1979;130:141–147.
196. Goodman SJ, Hasso A, Kirkpatrick D. Treatment of vertebrojugular fistula by balloon occlusion: case report. *J Neurosurg* 1975; 43:362–367.
197. Higashida RT, Halbach VV, Tsai FY, et al. Interventional neurovascular treatment of traumatic carotid and vertebral artery lesions: results in 234 cases. *AJR Am J Roentgenol* 1989;153: 577–582.
198. Hungerford GD, Perot PL. Detachable balloon treatment of carotid-cavernous and vertebro-vertebral fistulas. *J S C Med Assoc* 1982;78:479–483.
199. Scialfa G, Vaghi A, Valsecchi F, et al. Neuroradiological treatment of carotid and vertebral fistulas and intracavernous aneurysms: technical problems and results. *Neuroradiology* 1982;24: 13–25.
200. Vinuela F, Fox AJ. Interventional neuroradiology and the management of arteriovenous malformations and fistulas. *Neurol Clin* 1983;1:131–154.
201. Halbach VV, Higashida RT, Hieshima GB, et al. Normal perfusion pressure breakthrough occurring during treatment of carotid and vertebral fistulas. *AJNR Am J Neuroradiol* 1987;8: 751–756.
202. Spetzler RF, Wilson CB, Weinstein P, et al. Normal perfusion pressure breakthrough theory. *Clin Neurosurg* 1978;25: 651–672.
203. Harjola PT, Valle M. The importance of aortic arch or subclavian angiography before coronary reconstruction. *Chest* 1974; 66:436–438.
204. Young JR, Graor RA, Olin JW, et al. *Peripheral vascular diseases.* St Louis: Mosby–Year Book, 1991:111–133.
205. Hadjipetrou P, Cox S, Piemonte T, et al. Percutaneous revascularization of atherosclerotic obstruction of aortic arch vessels. *J Am Coll Cardiol* 1999;33:1238–1245.
206. Al-Mubarak N, Liu MW, Dean LS, et al. Immediate and late outcomes of subclavian artery stenting. *Catheter Cardiovasc Interv* 1999;46:169–172.
207. Dorros G, Lewin RF, Jamnadas P, et al. Peripheral transluminal angioplasty of the subclavian and innominate arteries utilizing the brachial approach: acute outcome and follow-up. *Cathet Cardiovasc Diagn* 1990;19:71–76.
208. Hebrang A, Maskovic J, Tomac B. Percutaneous transluminal angioplasty of the subclavian arteries: long-term results in 52 patients. *AJR Am J Roentgenol* 1991;156:1091–1094.
209. Henry M, Amor M, Henry I, et al. Percutaneous transluminal angioplasty of the subclavian arteries. *J Endovasc Surg* 1999;6: 33–41.
210. Millaire A, Trinca M, Marache P, et al. Subclavian angioplasty: immediate and late results in 50 patients. *Cathet Cardiovasc Diagn* 1993;29:8–17.
211. Motarjeme A, Keifer JW, Zuska AJ, et al. Percutaneous transluminal angioplasty for treatment of subclavian steal. *Radiology* 1985;155:611–613.
212. Vitek JJ. Subclavian artery angioplasty and the origin of the vertebral artery. *Radiology* 1989;170:407–409.
213. Ringelstein EB, Zeumer H. Delayed reversal of vertebral artery blood flow following percutaneous transluminal angioplasty for subclavian steal syndrome. *Neuroradiology* 1984;26:189–198.
214. Duber C, Klose KJ, Kopp H, et al. Percutaneous transluminal angioplasty for occlusion of the subclavian artery: short- and long-term results. *Cardiovasc Intervent Radiol* 1992;15: 205–210.
215. Mathias KD, Luth I, Haarmann P. Percutaneous transluminal angioplasty of proximal subclavian artery occlusions. *Cardiovasc Intervent Radiol* 1993;16:214–218.
216. Kumar K, Dorros G, Bates MC, et al. Primary stent deployment in occlusive subclavian artery disease. *Cathet Cardiovasc Diagn* 1995;34:281–285.
217. Martinez R, Rodriguez-Lopez J, Torruella L, et al. Stenting for

occlusion of the subclavian arteries: technical aspects and follow-up results. *Tex Heart Inst J* 1997;24:23–27.
218. Kessel D, Robertson I, Scott J, et al. Re: successful exclusion of subclavian aneurysm with covered nitinol stents [Letter]. *Cardiovasc Intervent Radiol* 1999;22:86–87.
219. Meier GH, Pollak JS, Rosenblatt M, et al. Initial experience with venous stents in exertional axillary-subclavian vein thrombosis. *J Vasc Surg* 1996;24:974–983.
220. Ligush J Jr, Criado E, Keagy BA. Innominate artery occlusive disease: management with central reconstructive techniques. *Surgery* 1997;121:556–562.
221. Vitek JJ, Raymon BC, Oh SJ. Innominate artery angioplasty. *AJNR Am J Neuroradiol* 1984;5:113–114.
222. Dellaripa PF, Eisenhauer AC. Bilateral percutaneous balloon angioplasty of the axillary arteries in a patient with giant cell arteritis and upper extremity ischemic symptoms not responsive to corticosteroids. *J Rheumatol* 1998;25:1429–1433.
223. Joseph S, Mandalam KR, Rao VR, et al. Percutaneous transluminal angioplasty of the subclavian artery in nonspecific aortoarteritis: results of long-term follow-up. *J Vasc Interv Radiol* 1994;5:573–580.
224. Kumar S, Mandalam KR, Rao VR, et al. Percutaneous transluminal angioplasty in nonspecific aortoarteritis (Takayasu's disease): experience of 16 cases. *Cardiovasc Intervent Radiol* 1989; 12:321–325.224a. Staller BJ, Maleki M. Percutaneous transluminal angioplasty for innominate artery stenosis and total occlusion of subclavian artery in Takayasu's-type arteritis. *Cathet Cardiovasc Diagn* 1989;16:91–94.
225. Tyagi S, Verma PK, Gambhir DS, et al. Early and long-term results of subclavian angioplasty in aortoarteritis (Takayasu disease): comparison with atherosclerosis. *Cardiovasc Intervent Radiol* 1998;21:219–224.
226. Smith TP, Halbach VV, Fraser KW, et al. Percutaneous transluminal angioplasty of subclavian stenosis from neurofibromatosis. *AJNR Am J Neuroradiol* 1995;16:872–874.
227. Guthaner DF, Schmitz L. Percutaneous transluminal angioplasty of radiation-induced arterial stenoses. *Radiology* 1982; 144:77–78.
228. Hinchcliffe M, Ruttley MS, Carolan-Rees G. Case report: percutaneous transluminal angioplasty of irradiation induced bilateral subclavian artery occlusions. *Clin Radiol* 1995;50:804–807.
229. McBride KD, Beard JD, Gaines PA. Percutaneous intervention for radiation damage to axillary arteries. *Clin Radiol* 1994;49: 630–633.
230. Melliere D, Becquemin JP, Berrahal D, et al. Management of radiation-induced occlusive arterial disease: a reassessment. *J Cardiovasc Surg (Torino)* 1997;38:261–269.
231. Piedbois P, Becquemin JP, Blanc I, et al. Arterial occlusive disease after radiotherapy: a report of fourteen cases. *Radiother Oncol* 1990;17:133–140.
232. Herbert JM, Dol F, Bernat A, et al. The antiaggregating and antithrombotic activity of clopidogrel is potentiated by aspirin in several experimental models in the rabbit. *Thromb Haemost* 1998;80:512–518.
233. Makkar RR, Eigler NL, Kaul S, et al. Effects of clopidogrel, aspirin and combined therapy in a porcine ex vivo model of high-shear induced stent thrombosis. *Eur Heart J* 1998;19: 1538–1546.
234. Trigaux JP, Delchambre F, Van Beers B. Anatomical variations of the carotid bifurcation: implications for digital subtraction angiography and ultrasonography. *Br J Radiol* 1990;63: 181–185.
235. Phatouros CC, Higashida RT. Diagnostic cerebral angiography: carotid and neurovascular intervention. 1998;1:10–20.
236. Mehigan JT, Olcott CT. The carotid "string" sign: differential diagnosis and management. *Am J Surg* 1980;140:137–143.
237. Qureshi A, Suri MF, Khan J, et al. Abciximab as an adjunct to high-risk carotid or vertebrobasilar angioplasty: preliminary experience. *Neurosurgery* 2000;46:1316–1325.
238. EPILOG Investigators. Platelet glycoprotein IIb/IIIa receptor blockade and low-dose heparin during percutaneous coronary revascularization. The EPILOG Investigators. *N Engl J Med* 1997;336:1689–1696.
239. CAPTURE Investigators. Randomised placebo-controlled trial of abciximab before and during coronary intervention in refractory unstable angina: the CAPTURE Study [published erratum appears in *Lancet* 1997;350:744]. *Lancet* 1997;349:1429–1435.
240. Chronos N, Vahanian A, Betriu A, et al. Use of abciximab in interventional cardiology. *Eur Heart J* 1998;19[Suppl D]: D31–D39.
241. Jeong MH, Owen WG, Staab ME, et al. Porcine model of stent thrombosis: platelets are the primary component of acute stent closure. *Cathet Cardiovasc Diagn* 1996;38:38–43.
242. Tong FC, Cloft HJ, Joseph GJ, et al. Abciximab rescue in acute carotid stent thrombosis. *AJNR Am J Neuroradiol* 2000;21: 1750–1752.
243. Erba M, Jungreis CA, Horton JA. Nitropaste for prevention and relief of vascular spasm. *AJNR Am J Neuroradiol* 1989;10: 155–156.
244. Theron J, Guimaraens L, Coskun O, et al. Complications of carotid angioplasty and stenting. *Neurosurg Focus* 1998;5:1–19.
245. Schoser BG, Heesen C, Eckert B, et al. Cerebral hyperperfusion injury after percutaneous transluminal angioplasty of extracranial arteries. *J Neurol* 1997;244:101–104.
246. Ouriel K, Shortell CK, Illig KA, et al. Intracerebral hemorrhage after carotid endarterectomy: incidence, contribution to neurologic morbidity, and predictive factors. *J Vasc Surg* 1999;29: 82–89.
247. Meyers PM, Higashida RT, Phatouros CC, et al. Cerebral hyperperfusion syndrome after percutaneous transluminal stenting of the craniocervical arteries. *Neurosurgery* 2000;47:335–345.
248. Morrish W, Grahovac S, Douen A, et al. Intracranial hemorrhage after stenting and angioplasty of extracranial carotid stenosis. *AJNR Am J Neuroradiol* 2000;21:1911–1916.
249. Hirayama T, Katayama Y, Kano T, et al. Control of systemic hypertension with diltiazem, a calcium-antagonist, in patients with a mildly elevated intracranial pressure: a comparative study. *Neurol Res* 1994;16:97–99.
250. Qureshi AP, Luft AR, Lopes DK, et al. Postoperative hypotension after carotid angioplasty and stenting: report of three cases. *Neurosurgery* 1999;44:1320–1324.
251. Dangas G, Laird JR Jr, Satler LF, et al. Postprocedural hypotension after carotid artery stent placement: predictors and short- and long-term clinical outcomes. *Radiology* 2000;215:677–683.
252. Phatouros CC, Higashida RT, Malek AM, et al. Endovascular stenting for carotid artery stenosis: preliminary experience using the shape-memory-alloy-recoverable-technology (SMART) stent. *AJNR Am J Neuroradiol* 2000;21:732–738.
253. Piamsomboon C, Roubin GS, Liu MW, et al. Relationship between oversizing of self-expanding stents and late loss index in carotid stenting. *Cathet Cardiovasc Diagn* 1998;45:139–143.
254. Izzat MB, Mehta D, Bryan AJ, et al. Influence of external stent size on early medial and neointimal thickening in a pig model of saphenous vein bypass grafting. *Circulation* 1996;94: 1741–1745.
255. Watkinson AF. Metallic stents: individual designs and characteristics. In: Adam A, Mueller P, Dondelinger R, eds. *Textbook of metallic stents.* Oxfordshire, UK: Isis Medical Media, 1997: 207–233.
256. Bergeron P, Chambran P, Hartung O, et al. Cervical carotid artery stenosis: which technique, balloon angioplasty or surgery? *J Cardiovasc Surg (Torino)* 1996;37:73–75.

257. Mathur A, Dorros G, Iyer SS, et al. Palmaz stent compression in patients following carotid artery stenting. *Cathet Cardiovasc Diagn* 1997;41:137–140.
258. Rosenfield K, Schainfeld R, Pieczek A, et al. Restenosis of endovascular stents from stent compression. *J Am Coll Cardiol* 1997; 29:328–338.
259. Teirstein PS, Massullo V, Jani S, et al. Catheter-based radiotherapy to inhibit restenosis after coronary stenting. *N Engl J Med* 1997;336:1697–1703.
260. Fischell TA, Carter AJ, Laird JR. The beta-particle-emitting radioisotope stent (isostent): animal studies and planned clinical trials. *Am J Cardiol* 1996;78:45–50.
261. Laird JR, Carter AJ, Kufs WM, et al. Inhibition of neointimal proliferation with low-dose irradiation from a beta-particle-emitting stent. *Circulation* 1996;93:529–536.
262. Oesterle SN, Whitbourn R, Fitzgerald PJ, et al. The stent decade: 1987 to 1997. Stanford Stent Summit faculty. *Am Heart J* 1998;136:578–599.
263. Dorros G. Stent-supported carotid angioplasty: should it be done, and, if so, by whom? A 1998 perspective. *Circulation* 1998;98:927–930.
264. Hobson RW II, Brott T, Ferguson R, et al. Regarding "Statement regarding carotid angioplasty and stenting" [Letter]. *J Vasc Surg* 1997;25:1117.
265. Heuser RR. Success with carotid stenting: a stroke of good luck or the wave of the future? *Cathet Cardiovasc Diagn* 1998;44: 7–8.
266. Wholey MH. Randomizing carotid endarterectomy to carotid stenting? *J Endovasc Surg* 1999;6:127–130.
267. Esselink RAJ, Ernst JMPG, Overtoom TTC, et al. Neurological transcranial Doppler and MRI monitoring in carotid stenting. *Stroke* 1998;29:2235(abst).
268. Lovblad KO, Pluschke W, Remonda L, et al. Diffusion-weighted MRI for monitoring neurovascular interventions. *Neuroradiology* 2000;42:134–138.
269. Manninen HI, Rasanen HT, Vanninen RL, et al. Stent placement versus percutaneous transluminal angioplasty of human carotid arteries in cadavers in situ: distal embolization and findings at intravascular US, MR imaging and histopathologic analysis. *Radiology* 1999;212:483–492.
270. Ohki T, Roubin GS, Veith FJ, et al. Efficacy of a filter device in the prevention of embolic events during carotid angioplasty and stenting: an *ex vivo* analysis. *J Vasc Surg* 1999;30: 1034–1044.
271. Henry M, Amor M, Henry I, et al. Carotid stenting with cerebral protection: first clinical experience using the PercuSurge GuardWire system. *J Endovasc Surg* 1999;6:321–331.

3

ENDOVASCULAR THERAPY FOR INTRACRANIAL ATHEROSCLEROTIC DISEASE

MICHAEL P. MARKS

Endovascular treatment of intracranial atherosclerotic stenosis in the form of angioplasty and stent placement has undergone rapid evolution during the past several years. These techniques have been much more widely applied to the coronary and peripheral circulations and have only more recently been used in the cerebrovascular circulation. In the cerebrovascular circulation, extracranial angioplasty and stent placement have seen wider use. In the intracranial circulation, apprehension about perforation of the smaller diameter arteries being treated, fear of thromboembolic complications, and concern relating to the accessibility of the intracranial circulation all played a role in limiting the use of endovascular techniques earlier. Recently, with the development of easily trackable angioplasty balloon systems and the refinement of stenting technology, intracranial angioplasty, and stenting is being done with greater frequency. This chapter will focus on the treatment of atherosclerotic disease, as it is the etiology for almost all stenotic lesions being treated. Chapter 8 will discuss endovascular techniques such as angioplasty in the intracranial circulation as they apply to the treatment of vasospasm.

EPIDEMIOLOGY

Extracranial atherosclerosis is a far more common cause of ischemic disease in the cerebrovascular circulation than intracranial atherosclerosis. Nevertheless, approximately 8% to 10% of ischemic strokes are likely to have as their etiology an intracranial atherosclerotic stenosis [1–3]. This accounts for approximately 40,000 strokes per year in the United States alone [4]. In an interventional neuroradiology practice population, patients with intracranial atherosclerotic stenosis also may make up a greater percentage of those patients with ischemic disease because we are able to offer a therapeutic alternative for this disease.

M.P. Marks: Departments of Radiology and Neurosurgery, Stanford University Medical Center, Stanford, California.

It is difficult to determine the exact incidence of intracranial atherosclerotic disease. Angiographic studies provide one possible source for this type of information. A commonly cited study in which cerebral angiography was performed in 4,478 patients describes the incidence of atherosclerosis in the individual right and left segments of all the intracranial arteries [5]. However this study reported on a group of patients with cerebrovascular symptoms and therefore is not likely to be representative of a true incidence of the disease. Nevertheless, a relative incidence of intracranial atherosclerosis for individual arteries as compared to the incidence in the extracranial circulation can be gleaned from this data. For example, stenosis or occlusion was seen at the carotid bifurcation in 42.3% of the right carotid arteries studied and 42.6% of the left carotid arteries studied, whereas stenosis or occlusion was seen in cavernous carotid segment in 7.0% of the right carotid arteries studied and 7.7% of the left carotid arteries studied.

Information obtained from pathologic examinations also provides a relative incidence of intracranial atherosclerosis as compared to extracranial disease, but still it does not provide conclusive incidence data. As an example Samuel evaluated a consecutive series of 82 patients over the age of 45 who came to autopsy [6]. The carotid artery system showed definite atherosclerotic narrowing at the origin of the carotid artery in 34 of 82 patients (41.5%), while involvement of the cavernous carotid with atherosclerotic narrowing was seen in 18 of 82 patients (21.9%).

Risk factors such as diabetes and hypertension may increase the likelihood of the patient developing intracranial atherosclerotic lesions [7–10]. Age also plays a significant role in the development of intracranial atherosclerosis. Fisher et al. evaluated 178 cases of routine postmortem examination in which a detailed analysis of the cerebrovascular circulation was made [11]. Precise incidences of intracranial atherosclerosis cannot be obtained from this data, because the authors used a complicated grading system for atherosclerosis. However the severity of atherosclerosis in the intracranial arteries was observed to parallel that of the aorta, and the coronary and extracranial carotid arteries, showing similar influences from risk factors such as age, blood pressure, and diabetes.

Race also affects the incidence of intracranial atherosclerosis. It has been observed that black patients, as well as Asians of Japanese and Chinese descent, have significantly higher incidences of large-vessel intracranial atherosclerotic disease than do white patients. Gorelick et al. found higher incidences of intracranial atherosclerotic lesions in black patients with anterior circulation symptoms than in white patients with similar symptoms [12]. In a later study by the same group, higher incidences of intracranial atherosclerotic stenoses were also found in blacks than in whites when evaluating asymptomatic anterior circulations [7]. They also documented similar changes in the posterior circulation when comparing black patients with white patients. White patients in their study were found to have proximal or extracranial vertebral artery disease more commonly in this study [8].

The incidence of cerebrovascular atherosclerosis in Japanese patients with transient ischemic attacks (TIAs) of the carotid artery system has been compared to American whites with the same symptoms in study populations matched for age and sex [13]. It was found that 84.4% of the Japanese patients and 93.7% of American patients had atherosclerotic stenoses within the carotid circulation. However, 83.3% of the severe stenoses were located intracranially in the Japanese patients, while 85% of the severe stenoses were located in the extracranial carotid artery in the American white patients [13]. Similarly higher rates of intracranial atherosclerosis have been shown in Chinese patients [3]. The Extracranial-Intracranial (EC-IC) Bypass Study evaluated a large subgroup of 352 patients with atherosclerotic disease of the middle cerebral artery and also found that race influenced the incidence of intracranial disease [14]. Eighteen percent of the white patients in the EC-IC bypass study had middle cerebral artery disease, while 34.1% of the black patients enrolled and 58% of the Asian patients enrolled had middle cerebral artery disease. In addition, when studies have controlled for cerebrovascular risk factors such as diabetes and hypertension, race appears to be independently associated with intracranial lesions as a site of atherosclerosis [3,7].

Where are the common sites of atherosclerosis when it does affect the intracranial circulation? Again, precise incidence is difficult to glean from available data, but a relative frequency of atherosclerotic involvement in the various regions of the intracranial circulation can be ascertained. In the anterior circulation the two most common sites are the carotid siphon and the M1 segment of the middle cerebral artery. The previously cited angiographic study by Hass et al. demonstrated approximately a 7% to 8% incidence of atherosclerotic lesions in the cavernous region and approximately a 5% to 6% incidence of atherosclerotic disease in the M1 segment of the middle cerebral artery in the anterior circulation [5]. Atherosclerotic disease of the carotid siphon is the second most common site in the carotid artery circulation after the internal carotid artery origin. The incidence of tandem disease involving both the origin and the siphon may be quite high when one considers those patients with evidence of siphon disease. Marzewski et al. reported that 55% of patients with siphon disease had tandem lesions involving the internal carotid artery [15]. Atherosclerotic disease in the middle cerebral artery usually involves the more proximal portion of the M1 segment at either the origin of the middle cerebral artery or in the lenticulostriate segment, but it can involve the more distal regions in the area of the bifurcation or trifurcation of the middle cerebral artery [16]. In the anterior circulation, the anterior cerebral artery is less commonly affected by atherosclerosis, and infarcts in this territory are often caused by cardiac or artery-to-artery emboli [17].

In the posterior circulation the most common sites are the distal portion of the vertebral artery and the basilar artery. In the angiographic study performed by Hass et al. the distal vertebral artery was involved approximately 7% to 8% of the time and the basilar artery 8% of the time [5]. Intracranial atherosclerosis involving the vertebral arteries tends to occur in the distal segment near the vertebral basilar junction [18,19]. The proximal basilar artery has been said to be more commonly involved with atherosclerosis than the more distal segments [11]. However, atherosclerotic lesions of the basilar artery can occur throughout the length of this vessel [20].

NATURAL HISTORY

Many of the available studies providing prognosis or outcome data for patients with intracranial atherosclerosis are retrospective series. In general, these series are location specific and do provide some insight into the frequency of strokes in these patients. In addition, some prospective data is available which comes from the EC-IC bypass study [21].

Craig et al. performed a retrospective evaluation of 58 patients with both symptomatic and asymptomatic intracranial carotid atherosclerotic stenoses [22]. Patients were followed for a mean of 30 months. During the follow-up period 25 patients (43%) died. Nine of these deaths were due to stroke and 16 were due to coronary artery disease or other causes. In the entire group of 58 patients, 17 patients (29%) had a stroke. Eleven of these strokes were ipsilateral, yielding an annual ipsilateral stroke rate of 7.6% per year. Marzewski et al. did a retrospective evaluation of 66 patients with intracranial carotid atherosclerotic stenoses exceeding 50% [15]. Mean follow-up was 3.9 years for the study patients, and during that period ten patients (15.2%) suffered a stroke and 33 patients (50%) died. Eight of the ten patients who had stroke suffered these in the hemisphere ipsilateral to the intracranial stenosis. However, data from this study is complicated by the fact that a high percentage of patients (55%) had tandem extracranial carotid artery stenoses.

Borozan et al. reported on 93 patients with carotid siphon stenosis in a retrospective study [23]. Because a number of the patients had bilateral lesions, the investigators considered there to be 115 vascular territories at risk in the study population. Data was reported separately for those patients who had symptomatic versus asymptomatic lesions. The entire group of patients was followed for a mean time of 22.5 months. During this follow-up period 4.3% of the patients with asymptomatic lesions developed strokes, while 9.1% of the patients who were initially symptomatic developed strokes. These differences in stroke rate were not statistically significant, however. One contrasting retrospective study by Wechsler et al. showed a low stroke rate in patients with carotid siphon stenosis [24]. The study reported similar stroke and TIA rates during the average 51-month follow-up as did previous studies. Despite this, only one of the strokes was directly attributable to the intracranial carotid artery atherosclerotic stenosis. The study only included 15 patients, however.

The EC-IC bypass study provides the only available prospective data estimating the stroke rate in intracranial carotid atherosclerosis [21]. A subgroup in this study was defined with severe stenosis (≥70%) at or above the C2 level of the carotid artery. Seventy-two patients were in this subgroup. These patients were included in the study because they were not candidates for endarterectomy. It is likely that due to the distribution of atherosclerosis in the internal carotid artery previously discussed, most of these lesions were intracranial; most of the lesions were in the petrous, cavernous, or supraclinoid carotid and not at the C1 to C2 level. Mean follow-up for all the patients in the study was 55.8 months. The mean follow-up of the carotid artery subgroup was not specified. Twenty-six (36%) of these patients had a stroke. Assuming the mean follow-up for this subgroup was similar to that of the entire study group, this represents an annual stroke rate of approximately 7% to 8%.

The presence of tandem lesions with involvement of the extracranial carotid is not an uncommon occurrence and may affect the overall prognosis of patients with carotid siphon disease. Marzewski et al. reported that 22% of the patients in their study with tandem stenoses had a stroke during the 3.9-year follow-up period, while only 7% of the patients without tandem lesions had a stroke [15]. In a more recent study evaluating patients enrolled in the North American Symptomatic Carotid Endarterectomy Trial (NASCET), intracranial atherosclerotic disease was found to be an independent risk factor predicting subsequent stroke in conservatively treated patients [25]. The NASCET trial primarily evaluated patients with atherosclerotic stenoses at the origin of the internal carotid artery, and the NASCET protocol excluded patients with severe intracranial atherosclerotic disease. Therefore, most of the patients described as having intracranial atherosclerotic disease in this study had stenoses of less than 50% or mild irregularities without a significant stenosis. Nevertheless, the 3-year risk of ipsilateral stroke in patients with 70% to 84% stenosis at the carotid bifurcation and evidence of intracranial atherosclerotic disease was 28.8%, while this risk was reduced to 23.3% if there was no intracranial disease seen. Similarly, when patients had an 85% to 99% stenosis at the bifurcation region and intracranial atherosclerosis the 3-year stroke risk was 45.7%, which was reduced to 25.3% if no intracranial disease was present.

Retrospective studies of patients with isolated middle cerebral artery stenoses have been even more limited than those studies in patients with intracranial carotid lesions. These retrospective studies have suggested a low rate of stroke in the middle cerebral artery territory [9,16,26]. However the EC-IC bypass study group does provide prospective data on the outcome of patients with atherosclerotic stenoses in the middle cerebral artery [14,21]. A subgroup of 352 patients with atherosclerotic disease of the middle cerebral artery were randomized to bypass surgery versus medical treatment (325 mg aspirin 4 times a day) in the study. These patients had either occlusion or stenosis of the middle cerebral artery. In the medically treated arm of the study 164 patients were followed for a mean of 42 months. Those patients with middle cerebral artery occlusion had an annual stroke rate of 10.1% and an ipsilateral infarct rate of 7.1%, while those patients with middle cerebral artery stenosis had an overall annual stroke rate of 9.5% and an ipsilateral stroke rate of 7.8%.

Limited natural history data for posterior circulation lesions is also available. Moufarrij et al. evaluated 44 patients with greater than 50% stenosis of the distal vertebral or basilar artery or both [27]. Patients were followed for an average of 6.1 years. During the follow-up period 12 patients (27%) had symptomatic vertebrobasilar ischemia, with seven having TIAs and five completed strokes. Pessin et al. evaluated a small series of nine patients with symptomatic basilar artery stenosis [20]. They found that only one patient of nine (11%) had a stroke in the 2-year median follow-up period.

A more recent publication has selectively evaluated outcome in 75 patients seeking treatment for severe intracranial vertebral artery occlusive disease [18]. Sixty-five patients in this series were available for follow-up and were followed for a mean of 36 months. Six had recurrent vertebrobasilar symptoms, with two having TIAs and four having recurrent strokes. Many of the patients in this series had occlusions at the time of study, so determining the stroke incidence for those with stenoses is not possible. These somewhat limited retrospective studies suggest lower risks of stroke than seen with the stenoses encountered in the anterior circulation. However, a more recent report from the Warfarin-Aspirin Symptomatic Intracranial Disease (WASID) study group suggests a much higher rate of stroke in symptomatic patients with intracranial vertebral or basilar artery stenoses [28]. In this study 68 patients with greater than 50% stenosis of the vertebral, basilar, posterior, or posterior-inferior cerebellar arteries were followed for a median of 13.8 months. The majority of patients (87%) had either vertebral or basilar stenoses, while 13% had stenoses of the posterior cerebral and posterior-inferior cerebellar arteries. During the follow-up period, 15 patients (22%) had an ischemic stroke and four of these were fatal strokes. This translates to overall stroke rates of 15% per year of follow-up in patients with basilar artery stenosis and 13.7% per year of follow-up in patients with vertebral artery stenosis. If only strokes involving the artery in question are considered, the rates were 10.7% per year of follow-up in the basilar artery and 7.8% per year of follow-up in the vertebral artery. There is no clear explanation for the discrepancy between this study and the prior retrospective reports; however, possible explanations may include a difference in the age of the patients in the studies, differences in the number of patients with severe stenoses, and in some of the earlier studies inclusion of asymptomatic as well as symptomatic patients.

Although exact stroke incidence in patients with intracranial stenosis is not available, this data does provide some estimates for an annual incidence. It is important to consider that when data has been available for symptomatic versus asymptomatic patients, it suggests there is a higher stroke rate in those patients with symptomatic lesions. This has certainly been true in prospective studies that have followed conservatively treated patients with extracranial cerebrovascular disease involving the carotid artery [29,30]. Available prospective data suggest annual stroke rates of 7% to 8% for stenoses involving the carotid siphon and the middle cerebral artery with conservative treatment [14,21]. This is for strokes appropriate to the stenotic artery. In the posterior circulation prospective data is not available, but retrospective data suggest the stroke rate may be 7 to 8% in patients with symptomatic vertebral artery stenosis and 10% to 11% in patients with symptomatic basilar artery stenosis [28].

MEDICAL AND SURGICAL THERAPY

The previously mentioned EC-IC bypass study is the only study to follow patients with middle cerebral and intracranial carotid artery disease using a medical therapy arm of aspirin (325 mg qid) [14,21]. There have been no prospective trials comparing the efficacy of medical therapies. Antiplatelet agents and anticoagulation with warfarin is, however, widely employed in the treatment of this disease. Aspirin has certainly been shown to be effective in lowering the risk of stroke in symptomatic patients who have a TIA or minor stroke [31–35]. These studies have not required delineation of anatomic lesion for enrollment, however. Two other agents, ticlopidine and clopidogrel, prevent platelet aggregation and have also been used in stroke prevention. In randomized trials of ticlopidine versus aspirin, ticlopidine has been shown to be more effective than aspirin in reducing the rate of stroke [36,37]. Clopidogrel has also been compared with aspirin in a trial evaluating its effectiveness in preventing ischemic events, such as stroke, myocardial infarction, and vascular death, and has been shown to have a slightly more beneficial effect when compared with aspirin at preventing these end points [38]. Again, these studies have not required imaging evaluation of the cerebrovascular circulation, and as such it is impossible to know if any of these therapies are effective against intracranial atherosclerotic disease.

Warfarin has been shown in multiple randomized studies to be effective at reducing the stroke rate in the presence of cardioembolic disease such as atrial fibrillation [39]. There has, however, been no prospective study to date evaluating the efficacy of warfarin in the treatment of intra- or extracranial atherosclerotic disease of the cerebrovascular system.

One retrospective study compared aspirin with warfarin in the treatment of symptomatic intracranial atherosclerosis [40]. In this study 151 patients with angiographically proven stenoses of greater than 50% in the anterior and posterior circulation were followed after treatment with either aspirin or warfarin. Sixty-three of the patients were treated with aspirin and followed for a mean of 19.3 months, while 88 patients were treated with warfarin and followed for a mean of 14.7 months. The rate of major vascular events was 18.1 per 100 patient-years of follow-up in the aspirin group, while it was 8.4 per 100 patient-years of follow-up in the warfarin group. The stroke rate was 10.4 per 100 patient-years in the aspirin group and 3.6 per 100 patient-years in the warfarin group. Major hemorrhagic complications did occur more frequently in the warfarin group; however, this did not eclipse the overall benefit for warfarin when compared with aspirin in the prevention of major vascular events. In a later study from the WASID study group, 68 patients with symptomatic intracranial stenoses involving exclusively the posterior circulation were reported [28]. In this study, differences in stroke rates between the aspirin and warfarin group were found to be even greater. Here the stroke rate for patients on aspirin was 21.5 per 100 patient-years of follow-up while it was 6.3 on warfarin ($p = 0.02$).

Many neurologists use warfarin in the setting of symptomatic large-artery intracranial stenotic disease on the basis of these uncontrolled and retrospective study data [41]. In a number of patients an antiplatelet agent is added to warfarin, particularly when those patients continue to be symptomatic with warfarin alone. There is currently a prospective randomized, double-blind trial examining whether warfarin alone is more effective at reducing the stroke incidence when compared with aspirin in patients with symptomatic intracranial stenosis [42]. One of the hoped-for outcomes of this trial may be to identify which patients continue to have a high stroke rate, and this population could be used to compare endovascular therapy with best medical therapy [4].

One recent study evaluated the outcome in patients with symptomatic intracranial stenosis who initially fail antithrombotic therapy [43]. Fifty-two patients with intracranial stenosis felt to be atherosclerotic in nature were included in the study. Twenty-nine of these patients had evidence of a cerebral ischemic event (TIA or stroke) while on antiplatelet agents, warfarin, or heparin. Fifteen of these 29 (51.7%) patients failed antithrombotic therapy, then went on to have recurrent ischemia events. These included recurrent TIA (seven patients), stroke (seven patients), or death (one patient). The median time for these recurrent events was only 36 days. This study suggests that patients who fail antithrombotic therapy have an extremely high rate of recurrent TIA, stroke, or death. Moreover the time to failure is quite short.

Interest in bypass surgery for the treatment of intracranial large-artery stenoocclusive disease has waned since the publication of the EC-IC bypass study [21]. In this study patients randomized to bypass surgery had higher rates of fatal and nonfatal strokes when compared to patients treated medically. Analysis of the subgroup of patients with exclusively intracranial disease in the middle cerebral artery distribution showed that this group fared even worse when compared with the entire study population. Despite the unequivocally poor results for bypass surgery, there still remains an interest that a subgroup of patients with persistent hypoperfusion identified by blood flow reactivity studies may benefit from surgical bypass [44].

ENDOVASCULAR TREATMENT

Angioplasty

In 1980, Sundt et al. were the first to describe intracranial angioplasty in the treatment of a basilar stenosis, achieving operative access from the vertebral artery [45]. Following this report, percutaneous transluminal angioplasty (PTA) of the intracranial arteries did not begin to be reported until the latter portion of the 1980s and the first half of the 1990s, when case reports and limited small series began to appear [46–51]. Since then, reports in the literature have still been limited to single-center series; however, there has been a significant growth in the clinical experience and additional follow-up information has become available.

The largest of these series through the mid-1990s was reported by Clark et al. in 1995 [52]. This series involved 17 patients in whom 22 vascular sites were treated by intracranial angioplasty. Immediately following angioplasty the mean stenosis went from 72% ± 8% to 51% ± 18%. In eight of the patients representing 12 angioplasty sites, repeat angiography was done at 6 months postangioplasty to evaluate for restenosis. In these cases the mean stenosis improved from the immediate postangioplasty study, going from 51% ± 10% to 37% ± 21% ($p = 0.5$). There were two strokes during angioplasty. All the patients in the series had a resolution of their neurologic symptoms and no further neurologic events at 3 and 6 months follow-up. In longer-term follow-up of 8 to 54 months (mean 22 ± 16 months) there were no neurologic events in the territories of the angioplasty vessels.

Additional single-center experiences in which intracranial angioplasty was performed in atherosclerotic lesions in 10 to 20 patients were reported around this time [53–57]. Touho reported an experience in 13 patients who had angioplasty [57]. In this series, 19 total patients were initially described, but angioplasty was not performed in six of the patients because the author described severe atherosclerotic changes proximal to the lesions that made access to the lesions with the angioplasty balloon impossible. In the 13 patients treated with an angioplasty balloon, the mean degree of stenosis went from 83.1% ± 8.6% before percutaneous treatment to 35.8% ± 17.3%. All of the patients in this series had fixed neurologic deficits at the time of treatment. In addition, four of the patients had repetitive TIAs. The author reported that three of the patients with repetitive TIAs showed complete resolution, although one continued to have TIAs after angioplasty. In addition, in four patients with persistent and fluctuating neurologic deficit, the author reported improvement, although the deficits did not disappear completely. All of the patients in this series were evaluated for cerebral perfusion before and 6 months after angioplasty using technetium-99m-hexamethyl-propyleneamine-oxime (HMPAO) single-photon emission computed tomography (SPECT). Prior to PTA, those patients who experienced improvement in their neurologic condition showed low levels of cerebral perfusion in the affected areas and subnormal vasodilatory responses to administration with acetazolamide. In contradistinction, five of the six patients (83.3%) who did not show improvement in baseline neurologic condition had either normal perfusion or a normal vasodilatory response to acetazolamide prior to angioplasty.

Terada et al. reported experience in the treatment of 12 patients with posterior circulation stenoses involving either the distal vertebral or basilar arteries [53]. Stenosis went from 84% pretreatment to 44% after angioplasty in this group of patients. Two patients in this series had permanent complications as a result of the angioplasty procedure, both due to dissection. In both instances complications resulted in strokes, with one being fatal. One patient experienced recurrent TIAs and restenosis. The remainder of the patients was symptom free following PTA. McKenzie et al. reported the treatment of 12 intracranial atherosclerotic lesions [54]. Five additional patients were reported in this series, who underwent intracranial angioplasty for vasculitis. In these five patients with vasculitis there was an initial improvement in the stenosis, but the lesions eventually progressed to occlusion despite endovascular treatment. Eleven of the 12 patients with atherosclerotic disease were described as clinically improved at 12-month follow-up in this report. Callahan et al. reported the results in the treatment of 15 patients [55]. There were two complications in the series. In one case a small-vessel brainstem stroke occurred, and in the second case an artery ruptured resulting in the death of the patient. A single-center experience reported by Takis et al. involved the treatment of ten patients with intracranial atherosclerotic lesions [56]. In two patients the angioplasty site could not be accessed, leaving eight patients in whom the angioplasty balloon was used to dilate the vessel. These authors reported vasospasm in five patients following treatment, and in two of the patients this was reported to lead to a stroke at the time of the procedure. It is unclear why the authors experienced this unusual complication of angioplasty with such frequency.

More recently, a series of reports have analyzed a larger clinical experience or provided more extensive follow-up after angioplasty [58–61]. Mori et al. reported on the follow-up of 42 patients with hemodynamically significant lesions treated by angioplasty during a 4-year period [58]. Using a standard derived from the treatment of coronary arteries, the authors divided treated lesions into three categories on the basis of the pretreatment cerebral angiogram as follows: Type A, short (less than 5 mm long) stenotic lesion; Type B, tubular (5 to 10 mm long), extremely eccentric or totally occluded lesion less than 3 months old; Type C, diffuse lesions (more than 10 mm long), extremely angulated (over 90 degrees), with proximal tortuosity or totally occluded lesions more than 3 months old. In 10 of the 42 patients angioplasty attempts were not successful. In most of these cases this was due to the difficulty accessing the lesion or achieving patency in the setting of chronic total occlusion. In the 32 patients in whom dilation could be performed successfully, treatment stenosis went from 82% ± 10% to 30% ± 10% on the immediate posttreatment angiogram. Angiographic follow-up was available in all patients at 1 year and the rate of restenosis observed in Types A, B, and C was 0% (0 of 11), 33% (6 of 18), and 100% (3 of 3), respectively. Including the initial complications experienced, the cumulative risk of fatal or nonfatal ipsilateral ischemic stroke in Types A, B, and C was 8%, 12%, and 56%, respectively, at 1 and 2 years.

Eckard et al. reported the long-term results of the intracranial angioplasty of the internal carotid artery [59]. This was a small series (eight patients), but it did concentrate on long clinical follow-up. In this series all eight patients were successfully treated with angioplasty and followed for 30 to 64 months (mean 53 months). Six patients sought treatment for TIAs while on aspirin therapy, and two had completed strokes. Two of the patients in the series had symptoms in another vascular territory during follow-up. None of the remaining patients experienced additional cerebrovascular symptoms, and there were no symptoms experienced by patients in the territory of treatment during this period of follow-up.

Marks et al. reported results of 23 patients treated over a 5-year period [60]. Twenty-one of 23 patients (91.3%) were successfully treated by angioplasty. In one patient the lesion could not be accessed and, in another, balloon dilation resulted in vessel rupture which caused the one periprocedural death in the series. Patients who underwent successful angioplasty were followed for 16 to 74 months (mean 35.4 months). There was one stroke in the same vascular territory as the angioplasty and two strokes in the series overall. This yielded an annual stroke rate of 3.2% for strokes in the territory appropriate to the angioplasty site.

Connors and Wojack reported a 9-year experience in the treatment of 70 patients [61]. They describe an evolution in their technique with three distinct periods of treatment, an earlier period in which angioplasty balloon size approximated the vessel size, a middle period in which the angioplasty balloon was oversized and angioplasty was rapid and brief, and a current period in which the balloon is always undersized and they use a slow balloon dilation. Their most recent period of treatment reports the results in 50 patients. One patient in the series suffered a guidewire perforation resulting in the single intraprocedural patient death in this group. Dissections were observed following seven of the angioplasties and in two cases thrombolysis was required. No strokes were associated with these events. Two hemorrhagic strokes were observed in the periprocedural period, one due to a hemorrhagic conversion of a prior subacute infarction, and a second patient developed a hematoma in the territory of angioplasty. The authors were not able to provide long-term follow-up data for this patient population.

Stent Placement

Metallic stents have been used extensively in the treatment of the coronary and peripheral circulation, and recently they have become widely used in the treatment of extracranial cerebral vascular disease (see Chapter 2). Only a short time ago has the use of metallic stents in the intracranial circulation begun to be reported. In 1999 a series of case reports involving either primary stenting or secondary stenting following the development of dissection began to appear in the literature [62–66]. Following this, limited single-center experiences have also appeared in the literature [67–69]. Mori et al. reported on treatment of 12 atherosclerotic lesions in ten patients [67]. These lesions involved the vertebral circulation or the distal internal carotid artery. In two patients stents could not be placed because of an inability to access the site of stenosis. Ten lesions were therefore treated in eight patients. No complications occurred before or after the procedure. Mean follow-up has been 11 months in this series of cases and no recurrent episodes of TIA or stroke have occurred in this patient group. Rasmussen et al. reported on the treatment of vertebral basilar atherosclerosis in eight patients with four distal vertebral lesions and four basilar lesions treated with stent placement [68]. Patients in this series underwent heparinization and 12-hour infusions of abciximab. One of the patients developed transient encephalopathy, and one patient died the evening of the procedure due to a massive subarachnoid hemorrhage. Finally, Gomez et al. also reported on a series of 12 patients who underwent elective stenting of the basilar artery after episodes of vertebral basilar insufficiency [69]. Stent placement was successful in all cases. One patient developed diplopia after the procedure, which cleared within a few days, and one patient developed sixth and seventh cranial nerve pareses which resolved in 8 weeks. Follow-up was limited to 0.5 to 16 months (mean 5.9 months). One patient developed an episode of visual disturbances at 4 months, and an angiogram done on this patient disclosed occlusion of the basilar artery proximal to the stent. This was successfully recanalized with balloon angioplasty, and the patient was placed on long-term anticoagulation with warfarin following the procedure.

It is too early to assess the relative role of primary stenting versus angioplasty based upon the retrospective single-center reports available. Angioplasty alone has a longer track record, and available information suggests there is a low rate of subsequent ischemic events (TIAs or strokes) following angioplasty. However, stenting may be advantageous if there is a significant rate of restenosis following angioplasty alone that is reduced by stenting. Any advantage would have to outweigh any added risk that comes from additional difficulties that may be incurred with stent placement.

TECHNIQUE FOR INTRACRANIAL ANGIOPLASTY

Patient Selection

Previously discussed Natural history data suggests there is approximately a 7%- to 8%-per-year stroke rate for symptomatic patients with hemodynamically significant intracranial stenoses using conservative management. This data had been obtained in patients who are on some form of antithrombotic medication. Additional data (which was also previously discussed) suggests that patients who fail medical therapy are at even greater risk for stroke [43]. These data are not prospective but do provide a general understanding of the natural history of this patient population.

In addition there is limited outcome data available from PTA and stent series. We are therefore generally conservative in our use of endovascular therapy in the intracranial circulation. Only those stenoses that are hemodynamically significant are treated. In general this means a stenosis that measures greater than 70%. Treatment is currently limited to those patients who have had ischemic symptoms before angioplasty in a territory appropriate to the stenosed artery. We are not currently treating asymptomatic patients. Treatment patients have also failed antithrombotic therapy. This means that the patient has suffered a TIA or stroke while on adequate doses of antithrombotic medication. Usually these patients have been treated with heparin or warfarin, with laboratory adjustment of dosage to maintain adequate anticoagulation levels. For heparin the dosage is adjusted to keep the partial thromboplastin time (PTT) at 1.5- to 2.0-times normal, and for warfarin the international normalized ratio (INR) is maintained at 2.0 to 3.0 or the prothrombin time (PT) at 1.3- to 1.5-times normal. We do consider treating a patient who has failed antiplatelet therapy alone. Usually this therapy is aspirin, although it may be one of the other antiplatelet agents such as ticlopidine or clopidogrel. As mentioned before, there are retrospective data suggesting that anticoagulation may be of greater benefit in preventing stroke than antiplatelet therapy. Often we ask that patients be placed upon adequate anticoagulation in concert with antiplatelet therapy before medical therapy is considered a failure. In cases in which access to the lesion is relatively clear cut and the lesion appears to be one that would morphologically lend itself well to intervention, we may treat a patient who has failed single-drug therapy (either anticoagulant or antiplatelet therapy alone) (Fig. 3-1). This has become easier to consider as we have gained more experience with intracranial angioplasty. Endovascular therapy may be used before the patient has failed anticoagulation if there is a relative contraindication to using anticoagulation, such as in a patient a history of gastrointestinal bleeding, a patient with unsteady gait, or a patient for whom compliance with anticoagulation therapy may be difficult. On the other hand, if access to the lesion to be treated appears to be more difficult or the lesion does not appear to be one morphologically that lends itself well to treatment, we would be more inclined to try a course of combined antiplatelet therapy and anticoagulation before considering a relatively higher-risk endovascular intervention (Fig. 3-2).

Patient Workup

A decision to treat an intracranial atherosclerotic lesion using endovascular means depends on imaging that accurately depicts the morphology of the lesion as well as the degree of stenosis. In addition, imaging studies are needed to identify vascular irregularities proximal and distal to the atherosclerotic stenosis that may influence the way the lesion is accessed or treated. Currently we believe this can be ac-

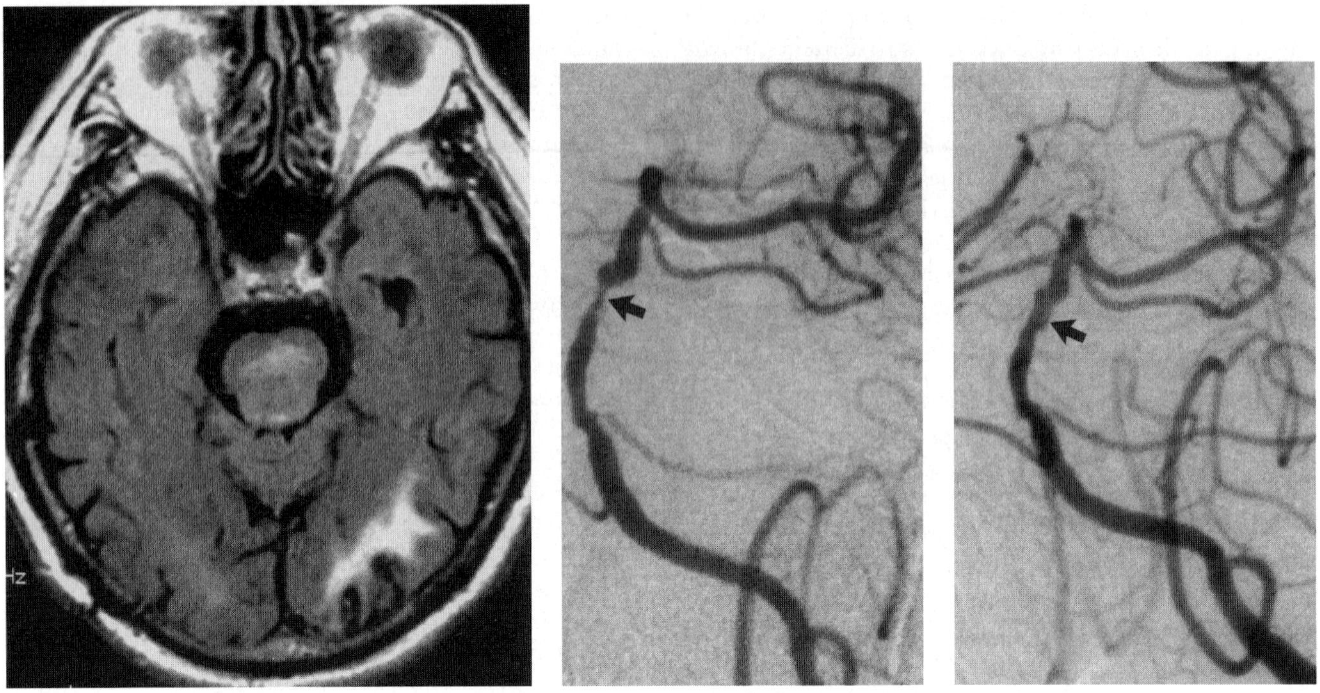

A,B C

FIGURE 3-1. This 74-year-old man experienced frequent episodes of vertebrobasilar TIAs. These were manifest as blurred vision and bilateral lower extremity weakness with accompanying gait unsteadiness. Their frequency had increased over the prior 2 months. At the time he was seen they were occurring almost daily. He had been placed on therapeutic doses of warfarin but continued having these symptoms despite medical treatment. **A:** Axial FLAIR MRI demonstrates ischemic changes in the brainstem and left occipital lobe. **B:** An oblique anterior projection of a left vertebral artery angiogram demonstrates multiple areas of irregularity in the basilar artery. One area in the midbasilar is a short-segment flow-limiting stenosis *(arrow).* **C:** Because the patient was having repeated symptoms on warfarin and the stenosis was a short-segment lesion, the patient was treated without the addition of antiplatelet therapy. This postangioplasty angiogram demonstrates reversal of the stenosis *(arrow).* The patient was switched to aspirin at discharge and at last follow-up (14 months following angioplasty) the patient has had no repeated symptoms.

complished only with cerebral angiography. Most patients will have noninvasive imaging, which may include transcranial Doppler (TCD) ultrasonography, computed tomographic angiography (CTA), and magnetic resonance angiography (MRA). None of these modalities presently has exhibited adequate sensitivity and specificity for the detection of stenosis and accuracy in the grading of stenosis. In addition, these modalities cannot accurately depict the morphology of the intracranial stenosis and may not clearly demonstrate irregularities in the surrounding vasculature.

MRA and CTA have both been employed for the investigation of intracranial vascular stenosis and occlusions. Three-dimensional (3-D) time-of-flight MRA has been the most widely used MRA sequence [70]. When 3-D time-of-flight MRA is optimized using modifications, such as magnetization transfer and variable flip angles, it will correctly grade normal arteries and occlusions with a high degree of sensitivity and specificity [71]. However, when evaluating stenotic disease the technique is less accurate for a variety of reasons. The actual length and degree of stenosis can be exaggerated by the complex flow within the stenosis. In addition, flow-related artifacts and susceptibility artifacts may create false-positive stenosis readings. Contrast-enhanced MRA has been suggested as a possible solution to some of these imaging limitations [72,73]. However, significant concerns include limited spatial resolution as well as signal dropout and artifacts at the margin of the acquisition volume [74]. CTA has also been proposed for the noninvasive evaluation of intracranial vasculature [75–77]. However, CTA has limitations based on the variability of the amount of contrast reaching the image volume, movement artifacts, and beam-hardening artifacts. In one study comparing CTA to 3-D time-of-flight MRA, the MRA proved more reliable than CTA in grading middle artery stenosis [77]. Because of these limitations with noninvasive imaging, we base treatment decisions on catheter-based angiography (Fig. 3-3).

The smaller size of intracranial vessels has raised concerns as to how accurate the measurement of intracranial stenosis is, even with a technique that has excellent spatial resolution such as cerebral angiography. We use a previously described technique that has been shown to have good interobserver and intraobserver reliability [78]. The view that shows the artery in question at its most severely stenosed is used for

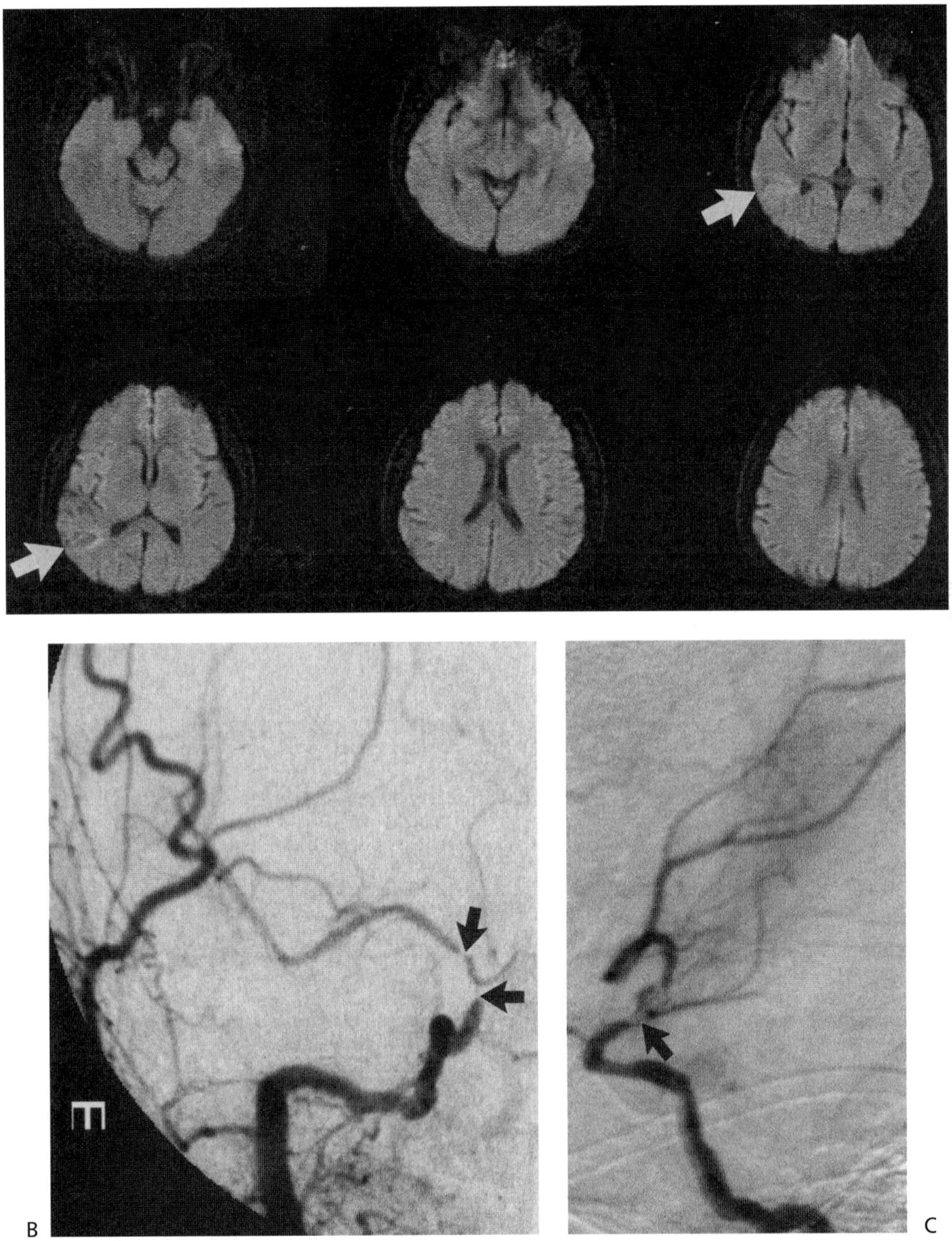

A B C

FIGURE 3-2. This 66-year-old woman with a history of hypertension and diabetes developed transient episodes of aphasia and left-sided weakness while on aspirin. Workup demonstrated stenoses involving the distal right internal carotid artery and the proximal middle cerebral artery. Because of the morphology of these lesions, it was initially decided to add anticoagulation to the patient's treatment regimen rather than perform angioplasty, which was felt to be a higher-risk procedure. However the patient developed continued episodes of aphasia and left-sided weakness and demonstrated new evidence of infarction while on both therapeutic warfarin and antiplatelet therapy. Following this, angioplasty was performed. **A:** Serial slices from diffusion-weighted images at the time of patient's initial visit following an episode of acute transient aphasia and left-sided weakness. The diffusion-weighted image demonstrated no evidence of an acute infarct. There was an older infarction *(arrows)* seen in the right posterior temporal lobe region. This was better seen on T2-weighted imaging. **B,C:** Anteroposterior and lateral views, respectively, from a right common carotid artery angiogram demonstrate slow flow within the intracranial carotid circulation and severe stenoses involving the supraclinoid segments of the carotid and the proximal M1 segment of the middle cerebral artery *(arrows)*. Because of the severe stenoses and tandem lesions, the patient was felt to be at high risk for angioplasty, and maximal medical therapy in the form of both antiplatelet and anticoagulation was used. *(Figure continues.)*

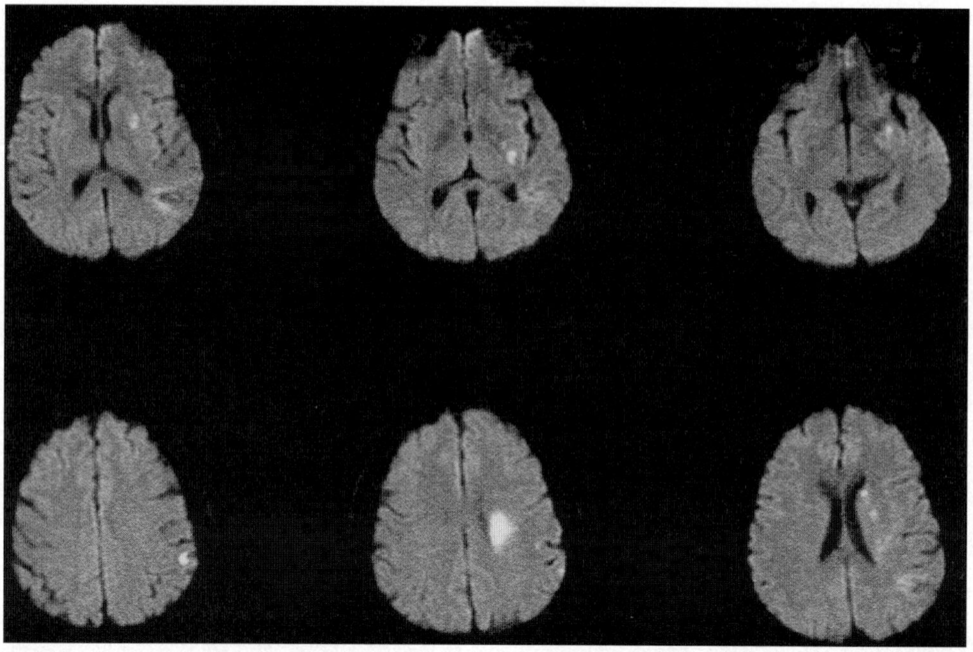

D

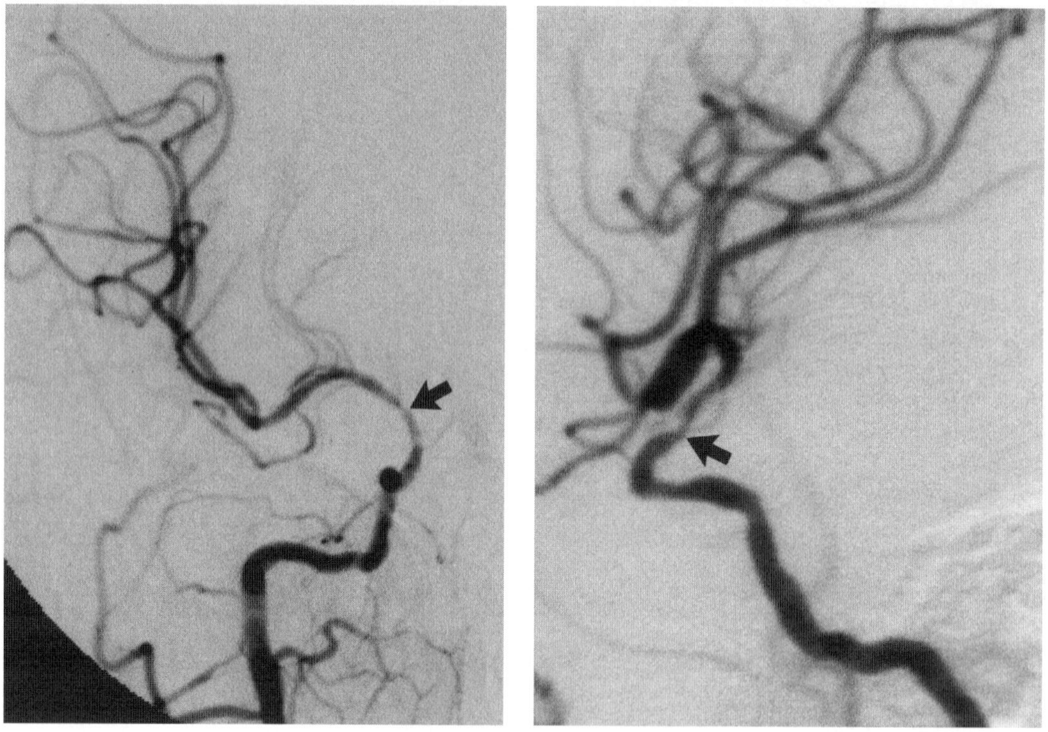

E F

FIGURE 3-2. *Continued.* **D:** These are diffusion-weighted MR images obtained approximately 2 weeks after the initial angiogram following a repeated episode of transient aphasia and left-sided weakness. The patient was slower to recover from this episode of weakness and aphasia. The diffusion-weighted MRI demonstrates multiple infarctions in the deep gray matter and deep white matter of the right hemisphere as well as in the cortex, suggesting watershed or hemodynamic infarction. These are seen as areas of high signal (white regions) on the DWI maps. Because the patient was having repeated symptoms while on maximal medical therapy, it was decided angioplasty would be performed despite the morphology of the lesions. **E,F:** Anteroposterior and lateral views, respectively, from a right carotid artery angiogram following angioplasty of the supraclinoid and middle cerebral artery stenoses with a l.5-mm angioplasty balloon are shown. Note the improvement in the degree of stenoses in the supraclinoid and M1 segments as compared to the prior angiogram *(arrows).* Compare to **(B,C).** Also note the significantly improved intracranial flow with filling of the lenticulostriate vessels and middle cerebral artery opercular vessels not seen on the prior angiogram.

A,B

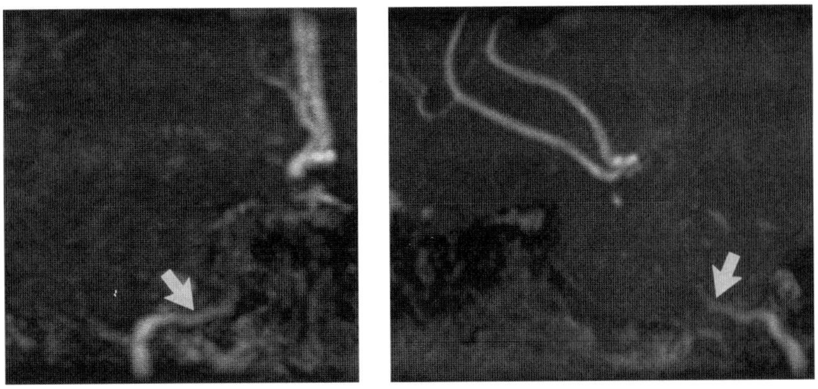

FIGURE 3-3. This is a 3-D time-of-flight MRA from the same patient seen in Fig. 3-2 preangioplasty. Anteroposterior **(A)** and lateral **(B)** views, respectively, from the time-of-flight MRA done as selective regions of interest for the right carotid artery circulation. Portions of the petrous carotid artery circulations are visible *(arrows),* but the cavernous and supraclinoid carotid artery circulation cannot be seen on either of these views, nor can the middle cerebral artery flow be seen. This poor visualization of the stenoses in an otherwise open artery is an example of the flow dropout that can be seen in the areas of complex flow or slow flow when intracranial stenoses are present.

measurements. The percentage of stenosis is determined using the equation: percentage of stenosis = (1 − D stenosis ÷ D normal) × 100, where D stenosis = the diameter of the artery at the point of most severe stenosis and D normal = the diameter of the normal artery. The diameter of the artery proximal to the stenosis where the artery is judged to be normal is the first choice for D normal. If the stenosis is in the proximal part of the artery or the proximal part of the artery is diseased, we use the more distal portion of the artery beyond the stenosis. Rarely, no segment of the artery in question can be used because disease extends throughout the length of the artery in question. We then use the nearest normal segment of artery feeding the artery with the stenosis.

Technique

Patients being considered for intracranial angioplasty or stent placement are often on a combination of anticoagulation (warfarin) and antiplatelet therapy as outpatients prior to procedure. If this is the case, they are generally converted to heparin and left on antiplatelet therapy prior to the start of the procedure. If they are not already on antithrombotic medications, patients are premedicated with antiplatelet therapy, either aspirin or clopidogrel. Systemic heparinization is used during the procedure.

In advance of angioplasty, a complete cerebral angiogram is obtained. This is done to understand the state of the circle of Willis, the remainder of the possible collateral supply, and to know whether additional stenoocclusive disease exists in the cerebrovascular circulation. This information may prove helpful both in the decision to treat the patient and in dealing with complications should they arise. Diagnostic angiography is usually done with a 5-French (Fr.) (0.35-inch inner diameter) catheter. Following the diagnostic angiogram a 6-Fr. or 7-Fr. guide catheter is introduced into the cervical segment of the appropriate artery. We then measure the degree of stenosis of the vessel. We also measure the size of the vessel in which the angioplasty or stenting, are going to be performed. We rely on calibration measurements using the guide catheter as a reference. The guide catheter has been placed in the distal cervical segment of the carotid or vertebral artery, and a magnified view is obtained showing both the guide catheter and the artery to be treated. The diameter of a normal segment of artery adjacent to the stenosis is measured, and the length of the stenosis is also measured.

To access and dilate the lesion we use a 2- to 4-mm × 10- to 20-mm angioplasty balloon. These are usually coronary PTA catheters used to perform the dilation. A 0.014-inch microguidewire, which has a hydrophilic coating, is used to cross the lesion. The area of stenosis is gently crossed by the guidewire, followed by the balloon. The balloon is slowly inflated to its nominal pressure. The inflation is usually done over approximately 15 seconds and the balloon is maintained at nominal pressure for approximately 30 to 45 seconds. A waist is initially visible in many cases and we inflate the balloon until there is no visible waist present. In some cases this may mean we exceed the nominal pressure. Care is taken to ensure we stay below the rated burst pressure of the balloon. With smaller balloons (2 to 2.5 mm) it is often difficult to visualize the waist and the balloon is dilated using nominal pressure as a guide. The balloon is then deflated and, with the balloon still in position across the region of the stenosis, an angiogram is obtained. If an acceptable result has been achieved, the balloon is withdrawn proximal to the region of stenosis, with the wire left across the stenosis, and a repeat check angiogram is performed to more fully evaluate the lumen in the region of stenosis (Fig. 3-4).

The choice of the size of the angioplasty balloon is predicated on the angiographic measurement of the length of the stenosis and the diameter of the vessel adjacent to the region of the stenosis. We choose the shortest balloon possible to cross the stenosis, because a shorter balloon is more easily trackable in the intracranial circulation. We also deliberately undersize the angioplasty balloon by about 0.5 mm (bal-

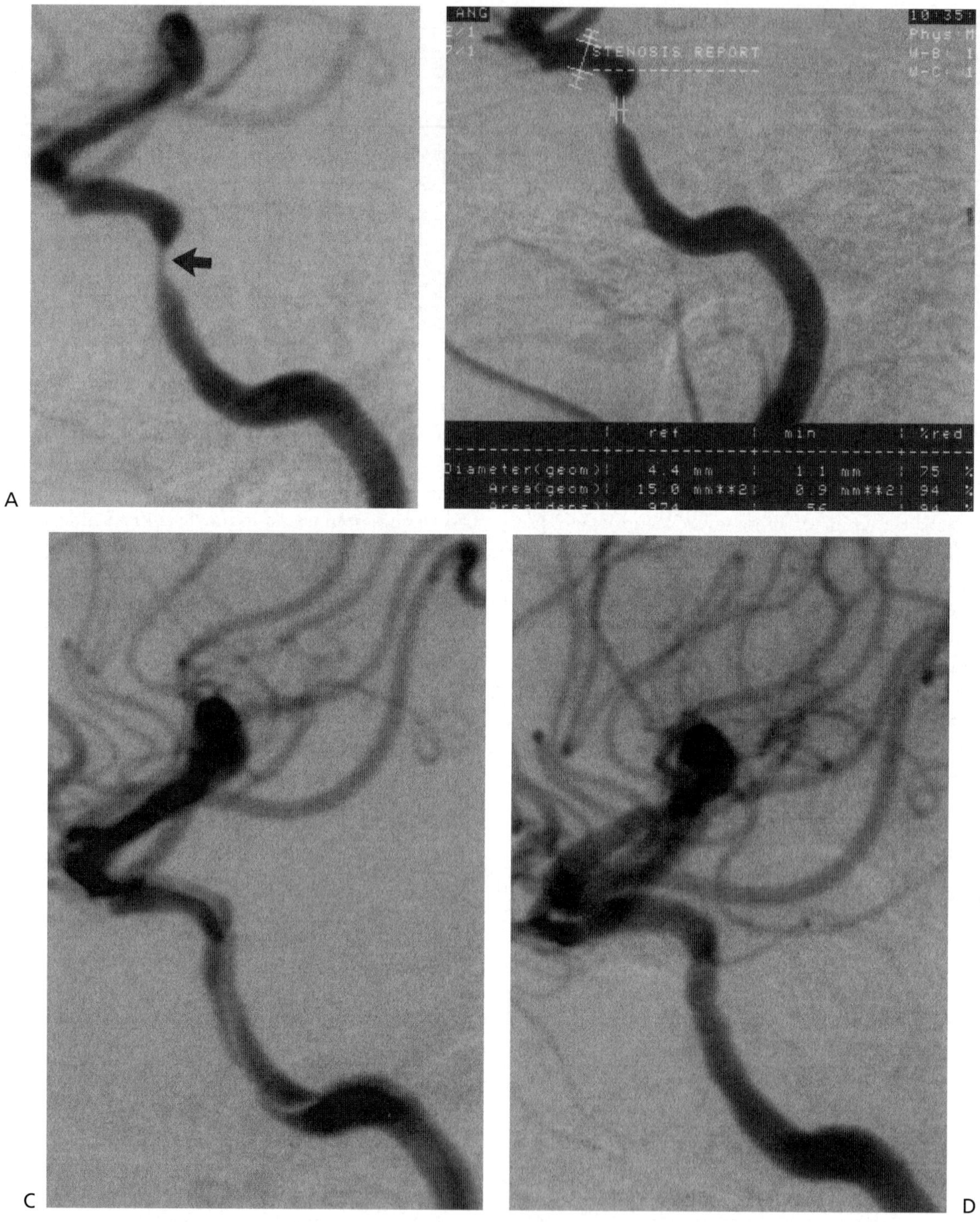

FIGURE 3-4. This 69-year-old man with a history of hypertension and diabetes had undergone a prior left carotid endarterectomy following a left hemispheric ischemic event. The ischemic event and carotid endarterectomy had occurred several years prior. More recently he had a series of TIAs manifest as right hemiparesis and slurred speech while on antiplatelet therapy. **A,B:** Lateral and anterior projections, respectively, from a left carotid artery angiogram demonstrate a severe stenosis *(arrow)* involving the petrous carotid. In **B,** an overlying stenosis report demonstrates that this is approximately a 75% stenosis relative to the normal vessel just distal to the area of stenosis. **C:** Lateral carotid artery angiogram following a balloon dilation with the balloon deflated and the wire remaining across the lesion, demonstrating reversal of the stenosis. This view is obtained prior to removing the wire to see if adequate luminal patency has been achieved and to ascertain if there is a dissection post angioplasty. **D:** Lateral carotid artery angiogram following removal of the wire from across the lesion shows good luminal patency without residual stenosis. This patient was followed for 2 years after this procedure and had no additional symptoms.

loons come in 0.5-mm increments). We feel this minimizes the risk of vessel perforation. Prior experimental work on the intracranial vessels suggests they will not rupture until dilated to 120% to 200% of the initial unstretched diameter of the vessel [79]. These experiments were performed on undiseased vessels, however, and the presence of atherosclerotic plaque may greatly alter results such as this. Early in our experience we found that some of these lesions could be eccentric, and using a balloon that achieved full dilation may well increase the risk of vessel perforation (Fig. 3-5). Angioplasty may result in a small intimal flap or dissection despite gentle balloon dilation and an undersized balloon. It has been our experience, however, that these iatrogenic dissections in general do well and do not result in thromboembolic complications. If the dissection is not significantly flow limiting, we do not at the present time use stenting

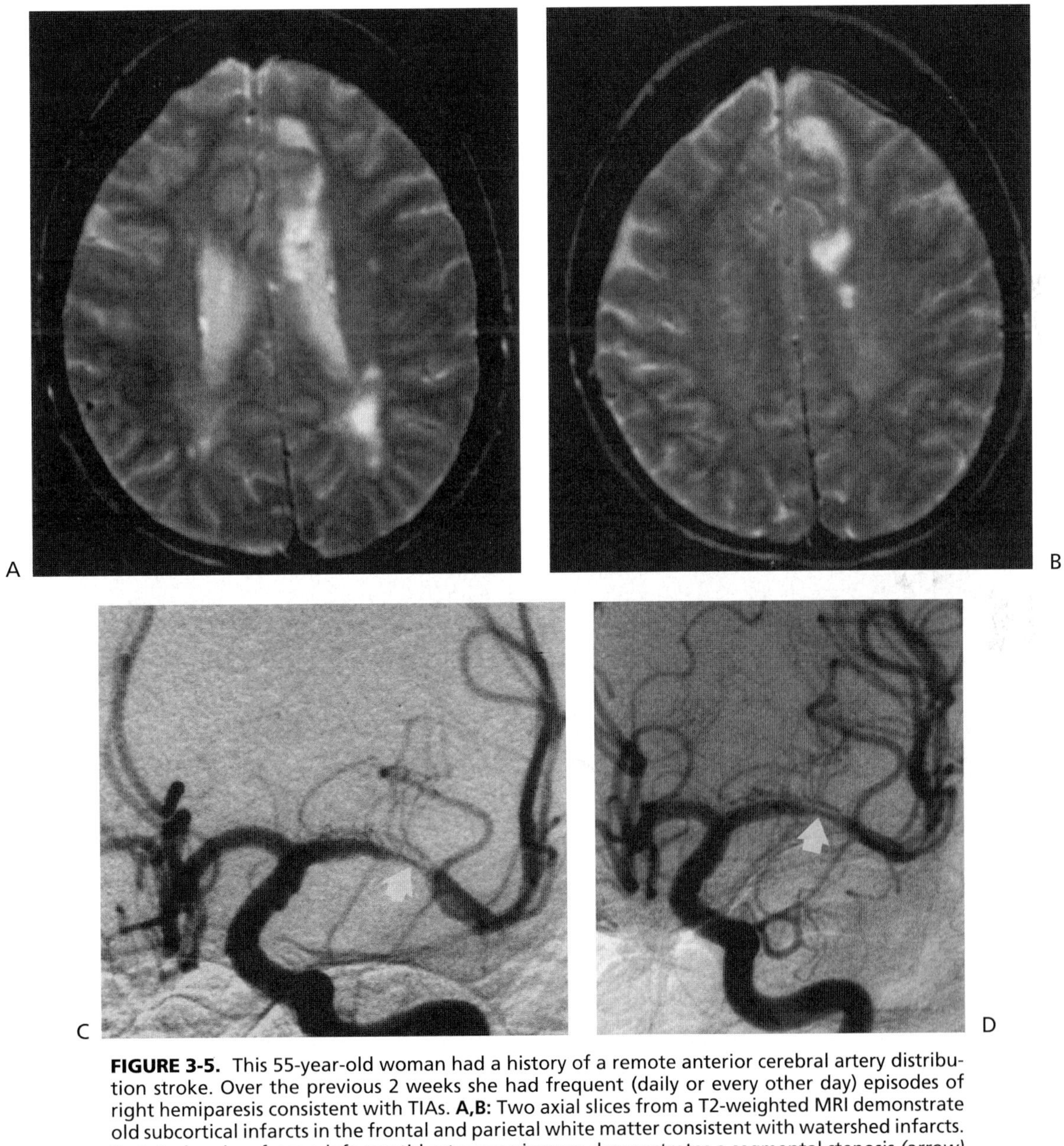

FIGURE 3-5. This 55-year-old woman had a history of a remote anterior cerebral artery distribution stroke. Over the previous 2 weeks she had frequent (daily or every other day) episodes of right hemiparesis consistent with TIAs. **A,B:** Two axial slices from a T2-weighted MRI demonstrate old subcortical infarcts in the frontal and parietal white matter consistent with watershed infarcts. **C:** Anterior view from a left carotid artery angiogram demonstrates a segmental stenosis *(arrow)* involving the left middle cerebral artery. The stenosis measured approximately 70%, and the middle cerebral artery just proximal to the stenosis was 3 mm. A 2.5-mm balloon was initially introduced to dilate this segmental stenosis. **D:** Anterior view of a left carotid artery angiogram immediately following angioplasty with a 2.5-mm balloon. This angiogram demonstrated a minimal response at the site of angioplasty *(arrow)* and it was decided to used a 3-mm balloon to dilate the lesion. The lesion was crossed without difficulty and predilation fluoroscopy showed normal antegrade flow in the vessel. *(Figure continues.)*

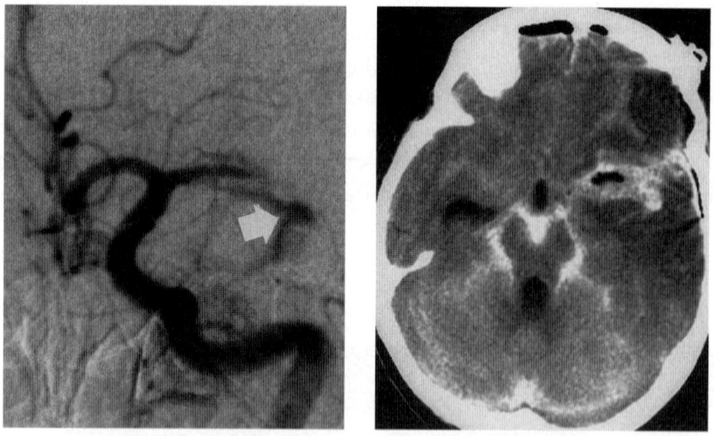

E,F

FIGURE 3-5. *Continued.* **E:** Left carotid artery angiogram immediately following dilation with the 3-mm balloon. This demonstrates cutoff of the contrast column and extravasation *(arrow)* into the subarachnoid space. The patient was immediately taken to the operating room to attempt repair of the artery. At surgery the middle cerebral artery was found to be lacerated at the site of angioplasty and the atherosclerotic plaque within the middle cerebral artery was markedly eccentric. The vascular perforation occurred on the side of the vessel that did not contain extensive plaque. An endarterectomy was performed and the artery was repaired. **F:** Axial CT slice obtained several hours after angioplasty and surgery demonstrates extensive subarachnoid blood and a large developing middle cerebral infarct. The patient eventually succumbed as a result of this event.

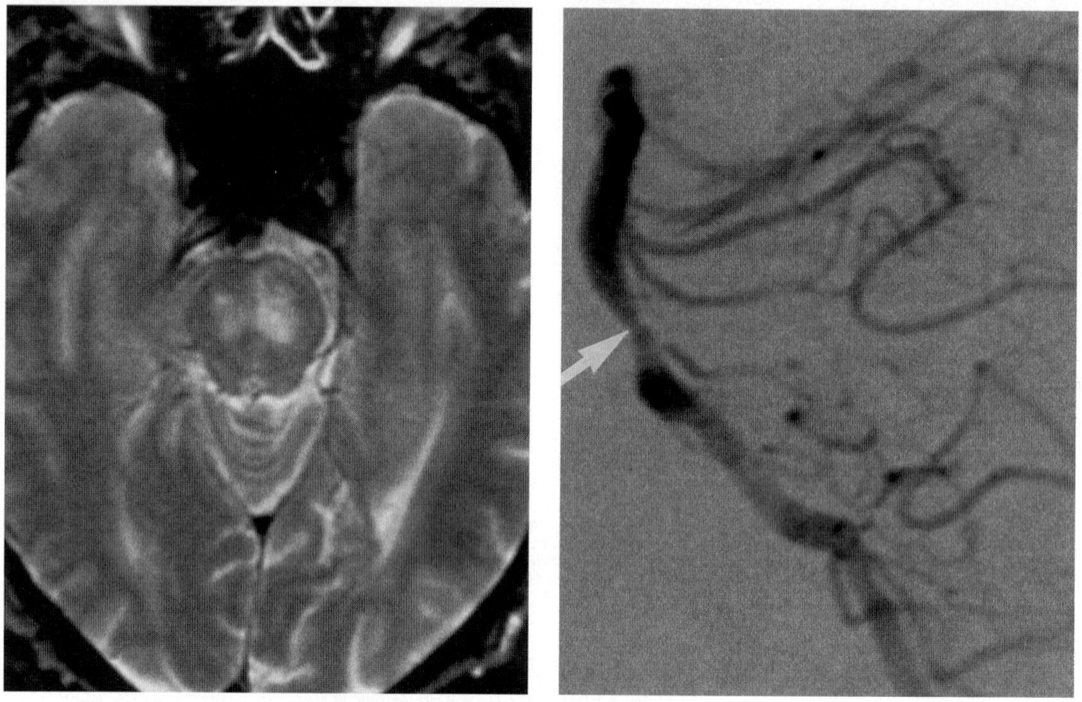

A B

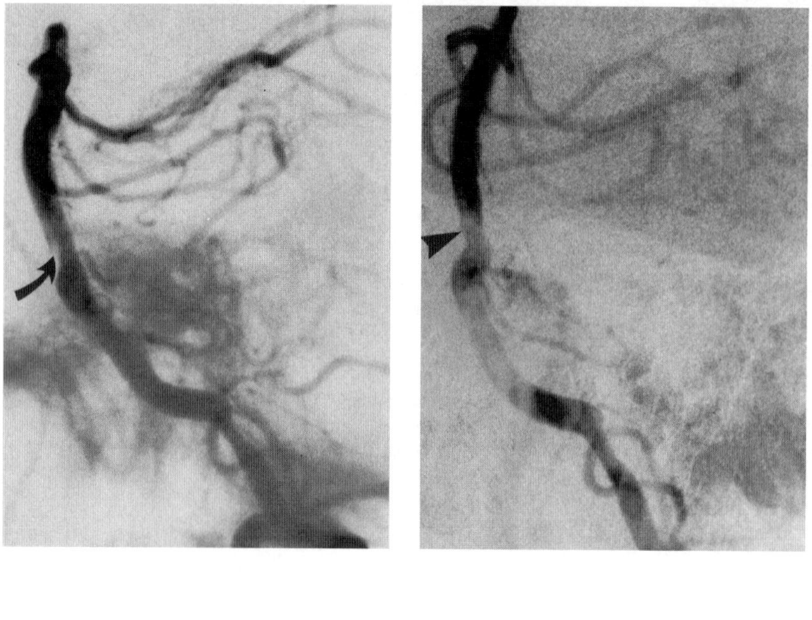

C,D

FIGURE 3-6. This 63-year-old man had vertebrobasilar TIAs several times per week despite therapeutic doses of warfarin. **A:** T2-weighted axial scan through the brainstem shows ischemic changes at the pontomesencephalic junction. **B:** Lateral projection from a right vertebral artery angiogram demonstrates a severe proximal basilar artery stenosis *(arrow).* **C:** Lateral projection from an angiogram done immediately after balloon angioplasty. A 3.5-mm x 10-mm balloon was used for the angioplasty. Lucency located anteriorly suggests a small intimal tear *(curved arrow).* Because the true lumen was widely patent and the dissection was not flow limiting, no further intervention was pursued. **D:** Lateral projection from an angiogram 3 months later shows healing at the angioplasty site with a minimal residual stenosis *(arrowhead).* (From Marks MP, Marcellus M, Norbash AM, et al. Outcome of angioplasty for atherosclerotic intracranial stenosis. *Stroke* 1999;30:1065–1069, with permission.)

to correct the dissection. It has been our experience that most of these iatrogenic dissections heal without sequelae (Fig. 3-6). On the other hand, if the dissection flap results in severe stenosis we may consider stenting (Fig. 3-7).

The initial or immediate postangioplasty angiogram may show only slight improvement in the degree of stenosis. Because we have had the opportunity to follow many patients beyond this period, we have found that even small corrections in the degree of stenosis appear to improve the patient's symptoms. In addition, it has been our experience that follow-up angiography shows continued improvement in the degree of stenosis beyond the immediate postangioplasty angiogram (Fig. 3-8). Other researchers have also found this to be true [52]. The aim of angioplasty is not to obtain complete or even near complete reversal of the patient's angiographically apparent stenosis but to improve blood flow. It is important to keep in mind that flow is directly proportional to the fourth power of the radius of a vessel. Stated another way, blood flow is doubled when the radius is increased by approximately 20% or the diameter by approximately 10%. In addition, we believe those patients who have suffered chronically low blood flows in the capillary bed beyond the stenosis site are at risk of perfusion breakthrough bleeding. This may create an additional risk to opening the stenosis fully. These patients may have impaired autoregulation and manifest a hyperperfusion syndrome following angioplasty [80] (Fig. 3-9).

Stenting in the intracranial circulation is in a relative nascent period. In general we do not employ primary stenting, because only small increases in the luminal diameter appear necessary to improve the patients' symptoms and because we have found that dissection does not result in a common clinical complication of our procedure. As stent technology becomes more refined we may in the future move to primary stenting. It is important that the added benefit of stenting outweigh any additional risks that may come with stent placement. In addition, it is not at all clear that stenting provides a better outcome in the cerebrovascular circulation. Issues such as intimal hyperplasia and poststent restenosis have yet to be addressed.

Following angioplasty, patients are kept on long-term antiplatelet therapy regardless of the results of the proce-

A,B 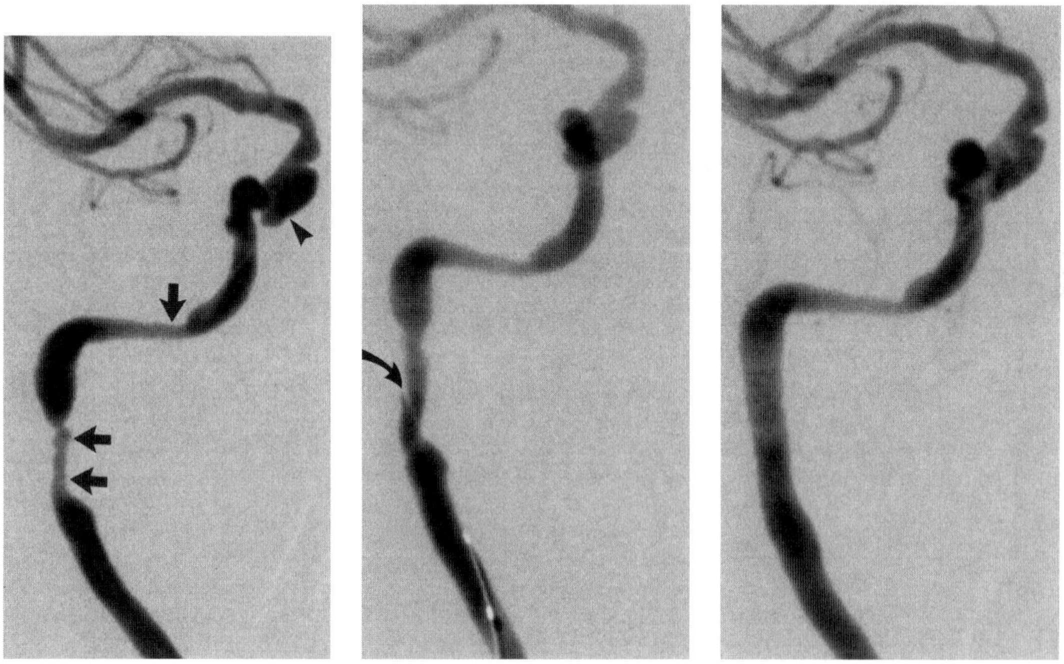 C

FIGURE 3-7. This 87-year-old man had multiple episodes of transient weakness involving the left upper and lower extremities, despite being on therapeutic doses of anticoagulant and antiplatelet medication. **A:** Anterior view of a right internal carotid artery angiogram demonstrates a severe stenosis of the distal cervical carotid artery *(two arrows)* and an additional stenosis involving the horizontal petrous segment of the carotid artery *(single arrow).* Extensive plaques and ulceration are also noted in the area of the cavernous carotid artery *(arrowhead).* **B:** Anterior view of a right internal carotid artery angiogram immediately following balloon angioplasty. The normal cervical carotid artery just proximal to the stenosis measured 4 mm, so a 3-mm balloon was used to dilate the distal cervical segment. This angiogram obtained immediately after balloon angioplasty demonstrates a postangioplasty dissection with a rather severe flow-limiting stenosis at the base of the dissection flap *(curved arrow).* Because this stenosis was a severe flow-limiting lesion, a 4-mm stent was introduced into the carotid artery at this location. **C:** Anterior view of a right internal carotid angiogram following stent placement shows that normal luminal diameter has been achieved.

A,B 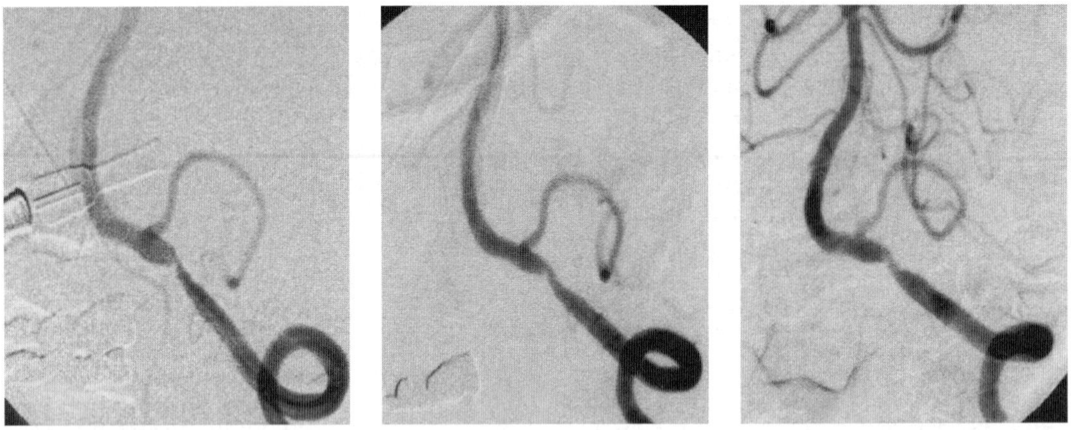 C

D,E 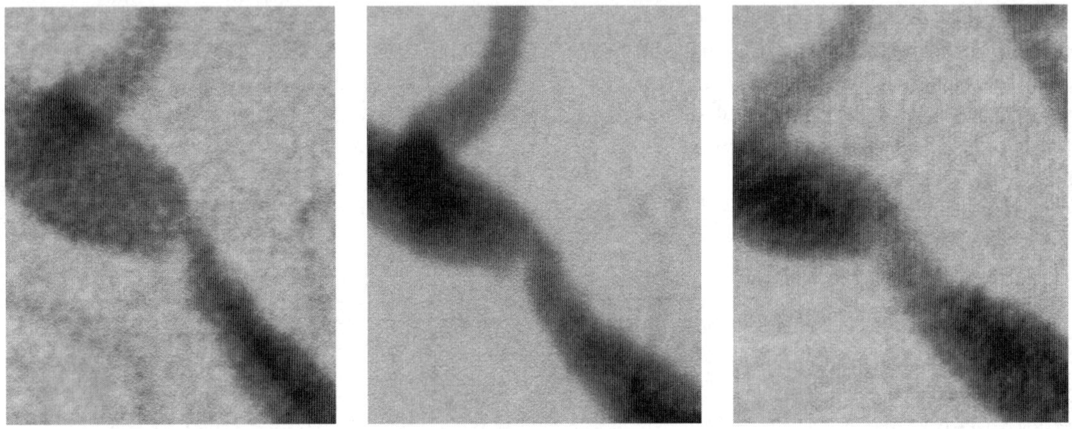 F

FIGURE 3-8. This 73-year-old man had several episodes of vertebrobasilar TIAs despite being on therapeutic doses of warfarin. These TIAs were manifest as episodic vertigo and double vision. Workup demonstrated an isolated posterior fossa circulation without significant flow from posterior communicating arteries. The left vertebral artery was occluded, and angiographic study of his right vertebral artery demonstrated a severe stenosis in the distal vertebral artery just proximal to the takeoff of the posterior inferior cerebellar artery (PICA). **A–C:** Oblique lateral projections from the right vertebral artery angiogram were done **(A)** preangioplasty, **(B)** immediately postangioplasty, and **(C)** 5 months following angioplasty. **D–F:** Magnified views from the same angiograms shown in **(A–C)** demonstrate **(D)** the site of stenosis before angioplasty, **(E)** immediately after angioplasty, and **(F)** 5 months afterward. These angiograms demonstrate a slight increase in the luminal diameter immediately after angioplasty and a moderate increase following healing at 5 months. There was also improvement seen in the flow to the intracranial circulation on the angiogram at 5-months. The patient is now more than 24 months postangioplasty. He remains on anticoagulant therapy; however, he has had no further ischemic events.

FIGURE 3-9. This 81-year-old woman had left hemispheric TIAs despite therapeutic levels of anticoagulation with warfarin. These were manifest as periods of dysphasia. **A:** Noncontrast head CT—two contiguous slices at the level of the basal ganglia 6 days prior to left M2-segment balloon angioplasty demonstrate left frontal and subinsular small-vessel disease. **B:** Left internal carotid artery angiogram (anterior projection) at the time of initial evaluation reveals a severe, approximately 95% focal stenosis of the proximal M2 segment *(arrow)* of the left middle cerebral artery. **C,D:** Xenon-CT with axial CT and blood-flow map images are shown on two contiguous slices before **(C)** and after **(D)** acetazolamide challenge 1 day prior to balloon angioplasty. Loss of cerebrovascular autoregulation is most notable in the left frontal lobe as demonstrated by paradoxically low cerebral blood flow after acetazolamide administration. Note *arrows* between areas on the postacetazolamide scans. The coding scale is defined in units of ml/100 g tissue per minute. (See Fig. 3-9C,D.) **E,F:** Left internal carotid artery angiogram (anterior projection) followed left M2-segment balloon angioplasty *(arrow)*. The focal stenosis was reduced to approximately 55% with no evidence of vessel dissection, perforation, or thrombus formation. **F:** CT of the head was made 2 hours following angioplasty, at the time of acute-onset right hemiparesis and aphasia. A massive left frontal intraparenchymal hemorrhage is seen with subfalcine herniation. (From Liu AY, Do HM, Alpers GW, et al. Hyperperfusion syndrome with hemorrhage after angioplasty for middle cerebral artery stenosis. *AJNR Am J Neuroradiol* 2001;22:1597–1601, with permission.) (See Color Figure 3-9C,D.)

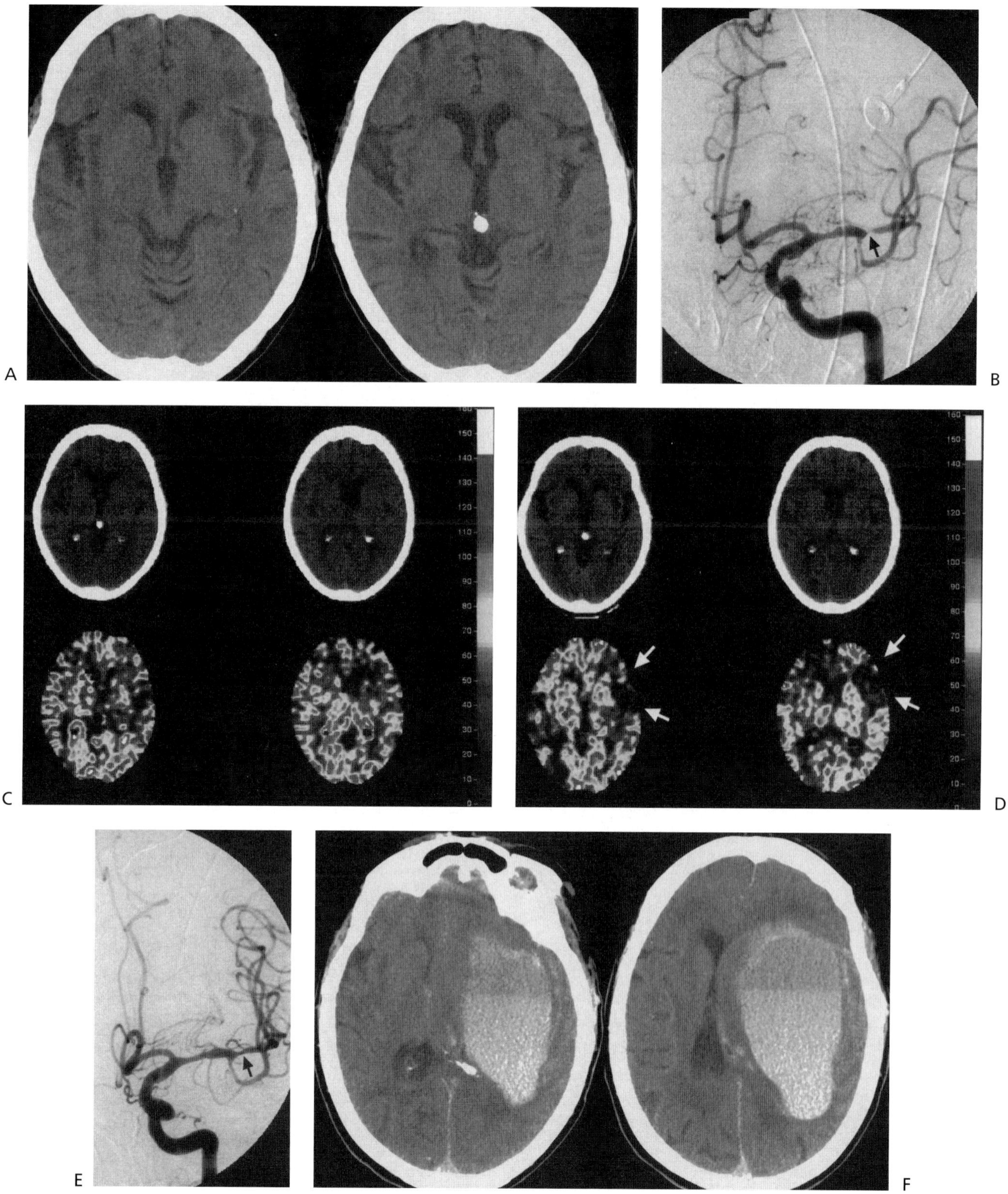
A
B
C
D
E
F

dure. It has been shown that angioplasty causes intimal injury and this injury promotes a rapid platelet aggregation [81]. We often use both aspirin and clopidogrel in the periprocedural period and switch to a single agent (usually aspirin) approximately 6 to 8 weeks after angioplasty. Beyond this subacute period we feel there may be a benefit of maintaining a patient on antiplatelet therapy. In addition, when the residual stenosis is greater than 50%, patients may be continued on anticoagulation.

Angioplasty in the Setting of Acute Infarction

Many patients with acute infarcts present outside of the first several hours following the infarct, beyond the time when fibrinolytic therapy has been shown to be of benefit [82]. A decision to treat an underlying fixed stenosis in the face of acute infarct may therefore occur outside of this more hyperacute time frame. In this setting we are usually

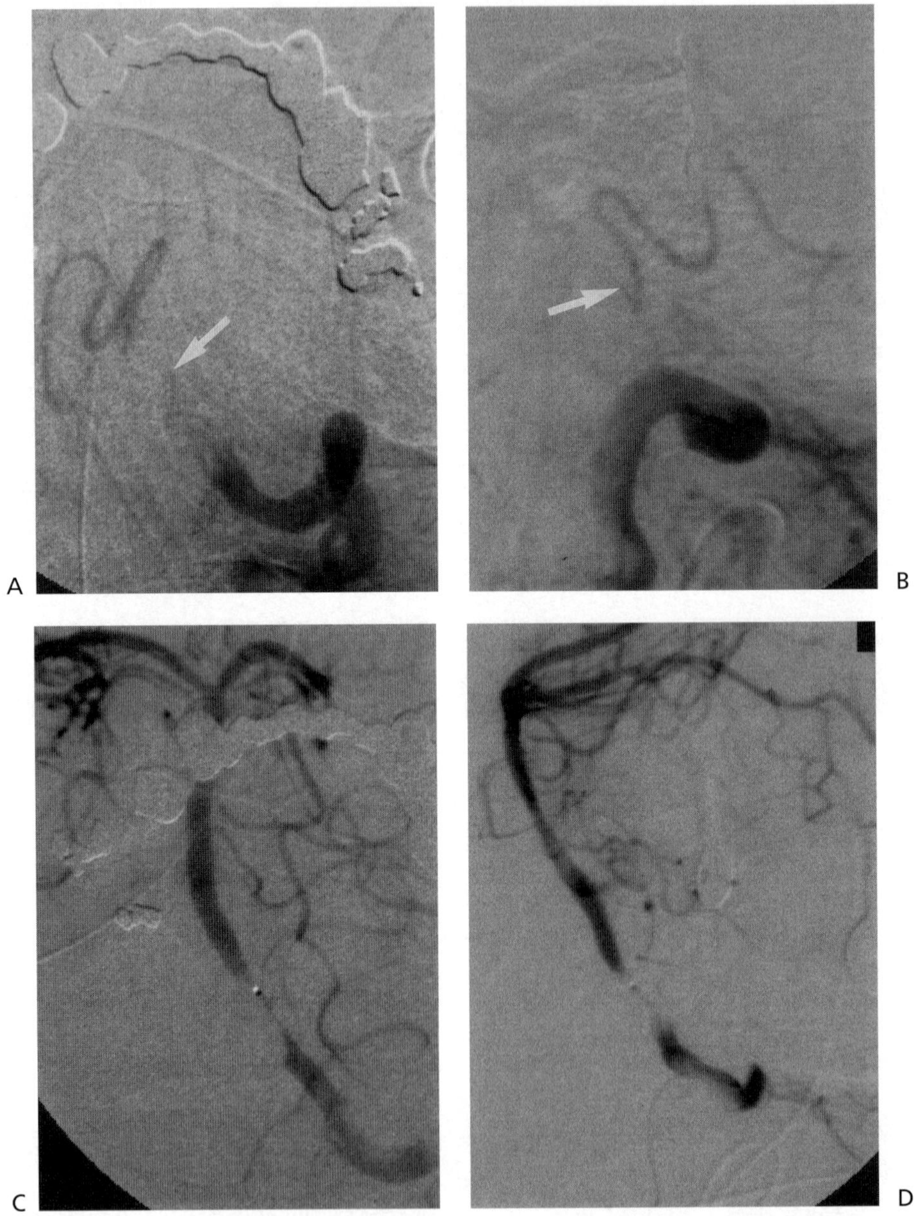

FIGURE 3-10. This 54-year-old male was seen approximately 2 hours into a coma. The CT workup was negative and angiography was performed. **A,B:** Anterior and lateral projections, respectively, from a left vertebral artery angiogram demonstrate complete occlusion of the left vertebral artery at the level of the PICA *(arrows),* without evidence of basilar artery filling. Injection of the right vertebral artery demonstrated that it ended in the PICA and with no communication to the basilar artery. **C,D:** Anterior and lateral views, respectively, from a selective angiogram through the microcatheter placed in the left vertebral artery just distal to the PICA. This demonstrates an approximately 1-cm area of severe luminal narrowing with normal flow seen distally in the basilar artery. *(Figure continues.)*

reluctant to perform angioplasty, unless there is an extreme situation where the patient is developing new progressive symptoms despite medical therapy. In general we prefer to wait at least 6 weeks following the acute stroke to perform angioplasty, because we feel that the risk of reperfusion bleeding in the ischemically injured capillary bed is too great. In the setting of acute stroke in which thrombolysis has been performed and an underlying stenosis has been shown to be present, there have been some limited case reports that have shown that angioplasty may be helpful to prevent rethrombosis [83–85]. Even in this setting we are reluctant to increase the perfusion pressure to the injured capillary bed distal to the stenosis by performing angioplasty. We therefore prefer to use anticoagulation and antiplatelet therapy, when possible, to maintain the lumen of the vessel and reperfuse the ischemic tissue. In addition, increasing perfusion with angioplasty may not alter outcome (Fig. 3-10). If further symptoms warrant considering angio-

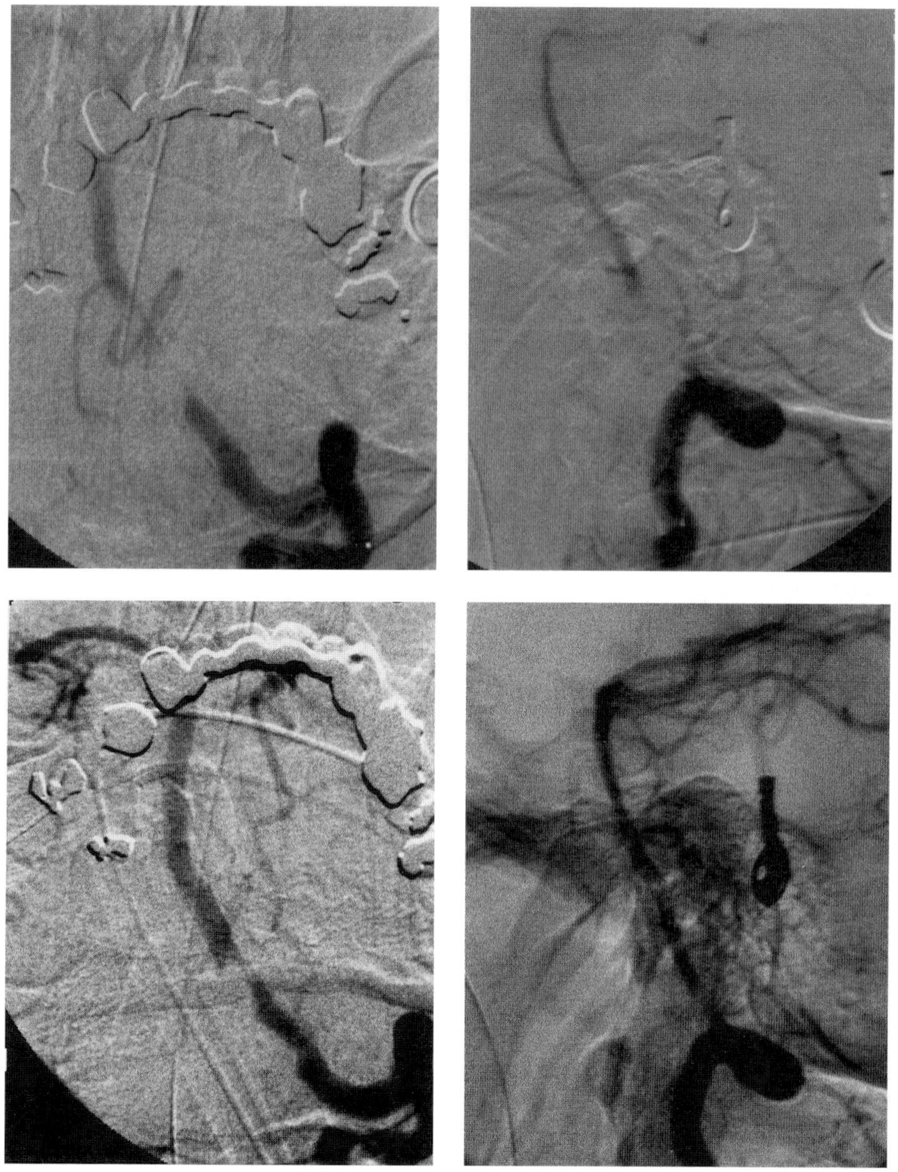

E F G H

FIGURE 3-10. *Continued.* **E,F:** Anterior and lateral views, respectively, from a left vertebral artery angiogram following intraarterial thrombolytic therapy. There is little improvement in the luminal diameter; however, antegrade flow is now reestablished through the left vertebral artery into the basilar circulation. **G,H:** Anterior and lateral views, respectively, from a left vertebral artery angiogram following angioplasty. Because the residual lumen was so severely stenosed it was decided to perform balloon angioplasty at the time of acute ischemic infarction. These angiographic views demonstrate the vessel following angioplasty, with mild reopening and improved distal flow through the area of stenosis. The patient was continued on anticoagulation. He succumbed to a large brainstem infarct, however, despite reestablishing antegrade flow and improving the flow with angioplasty.

plasty at a later point it can be considered. In the situation in which the underlying stenosis is quite severe and anticoagulation therapy has failed to maintain an open vessel, angioplasty may, however, be considered.

REFERENCES

1. Sacco RL, Kargman DE, Qiong G, et al. Race-ethnicity and determinants of intracranial atherosclerotic cerebral infarction. *Stroke* 1995;26:14–20.
2. Wityk RJ, Lehman D, Klag M, et al. Race and sex differences in the distribution of cerebral atherosclerosis. *Stroke* 1996;27: 1974–1980.
3. Feldmann E, Daneault N, Kwan E, et al. Chinese-white differences in the distribution of occlusive cerebrovascular disease. *Neurology* 1990;40:1541–1545.
4. Benesch CG, Chimowitz MI. Best treatment for intracranial arterial stenosis? 50 years of uncertainty. *Neurology* 2000;55: 465–466.
5. Hass WK, Fields WS, North RR, et al. Joint study of extracranial arterial occlusion II: arteriography, techniques, sites and complications. *JAMA* 1968;203:961–968.
6. Samuel KC. Atherosclerosis and occlusion of the internal carotid artery. *J Pathol Bacteriol* 1956;71:391–401.
7. Gorelick PB, Caplan LR, Langenberg P, et al. Clinical and angiographic comparison of asymptomatic occlusive disease. *Neurology* 1988;38:852–858.
8. Gorelick PB, Caplan LR, Hier DB, et al. Racial differences in the distribution of posterior circulation occlusive disease. *Stroke* 1985;16:785–790.
9. Caplan L, Babikian V, Helgason C, et al. Occlusive disease of the middle cerebral artery. *Neurology* 1985;35:975–982.
10. Yoo KM, Shin HK, Chang HM, et al. Middle cerebral artery occlusive disease. *J Stroke Cerebrovasc Dis* 1998;7:344–351.
11. Fisher CM, Gore I, Okabe N, et al. Atherosclerosis of the carotid and vertebral arteries—extracranial and intracranial. *J Neuropathol Exp Neurol* 1965;24:455–476.
12. Gorelick PB, Caplan LR, Hier DB, et al. Racial differences in the distribution of anterior circulation occlusive disease. *Neurology* 1984;34:54–59.
13. Nishimaru K, McHenry LC, Toole JF. Cerebral angiographic and clinical differences in carotid system transient ischemic attacks between American Caucasian and Japanese patients. *Stroke* 1984;15:56–59.
14. Bogousslavsky J, Barnett HJM, Fox AJ, et al. Atherosclerotic disease of the middle cerebral artery. *Stroke* 1986;17:1112–1120.
15. Marzewski DJ, Furlan AJ, St.Louis P, et al. Intracranial internal carotid artery stenosis: longterm prognosis. *Stroke* 1982;13: 821–824.
16. Hinton RC, Mohr JP, Ackerman RH, et al. Symptomatic middle cerebral artery stenosis. *Ann Neurol* 1979;5:152–157.
17. Bogousslavsky J, Regli F. Anterior cerebral artery territory infarction in the Lausanne Stroke Registry. *Arch Neurol* 1990;47: 144–150.
18. Muller-Kuppers M, Graf KJ, Pessin MS, et al. Intracranial vertebral artery disease in the New England Medical Center Posterior Circulation Registry. *Eur Neurol* 1997;37:146–156.
19. Shin HK, Yoo KM, Chang HM, et al. Bilateral intracranial vertebral artery disease in the New England Medical Center Posterior Circulation Registry. *Arch Neurol* 1999;56:1353–1358.
20. Pessin MS, Gorelick PB, Kwan ES, et al. Basilar artery stenosis: middle and distal segments. *Neurology* 1987;37: 1742–1746.
21. EC/IC Bypass Study Group. Failure of extracranial-intracranial arterial bypass to reduce the risk of ischemic stroke. *N Engl J Med* 1985;313:1191–1200.
22. Craig DR, Megura K, Watridge C, et al. Intracranial internal carotid artery stenosis. *Stroke* 1982;13:825–828.
23. Borozan PG, Schuler JJ, LaRosa MP, et al. The natural history of isolated carotid siphon stenosis. *J Vasc Surg* 1984;1:744–749.
24. Wechsler LR, Kistler JP, Davis KR, et al. The prognosis of carotid siphon stenosis. *Stroke* 1986;17:714–718.
25. Kappelle LJ, Elizsziw M, Fox AJ, et al. Importance of intracranial atherosclerotic disease in patients with symptomatic stenosis of the internal carotid artery. *Stroke* 1999;30:282–286.
26. Moulin DE, Lo R, Chiang J, et al. Prognosis in middle cerebral artery occlusion. *Stroke* 1985;16:282–284.
27. Moufarrij NA, Little JR, Furlan AJ, et al. Basilar and distal vertebral artery stenosis; long-term follow-up. *Stroke* 1986;178: 938–942.
28. WASID Study Group. Prognosis of patients with symptomatic vertebral or basilar artery stenosis. *Stroke* 1998;29: 1389–1392.
29. NASCET. Beneficial effect of carotid endarterectomy in symptomatic patients with high-grade carotid stenosis. *N Engl J Med* 1991;325:445–507.
30. Executive Committee for the Asymptomatic Carotid Atherosclerosis Study. Endarterectomy for asymptomatic carotid artery stenosis. *JAMA* 1995;273:1421–1428.
31. Barnett HJM. The Canadian Cooperative Study: a randomized trial of aspirin and sulfinpyrazone in threatened stroke. *N Engl J Med* 1978;299:23–59.
32. Antiplatelet Trialists' Collaboration. Secondary prevention of vascular disease by prolonged antiplatelet treatment. *BMJ* 1988; 296:320–331.
33. UK-TIA Study Group. The UK-TIA Aspirin Trial: the interim results. *BMJ* 1988;296:316–320.
34. The SALT Collaborative Group. Swedish Aspirin Low-Dose Trial (SALT) of 75 mg aspirin as secondary prophylaxis after cerebrovascular ischemic events. *Lancet* 1991;338:1345–1349.
35. The Dutch TIA Trial Study Group. A comparison of two doses of aspirin (30 mg vs. 283 mg a day) in patients after a transient ischemic attack or minor stroke. *N Engl J Med* 1991;325: 1261–1266.
36. Haas WK, Easton JD, Adams HP, et al. A randomized trial comparing ticlopidine hydrochloride with aspirin for the prevention of stroke in high-risk patients. *N Engl J Med* 1989;321: 501–507.
37. Gent M, Easton JD, Hachinski V, et al. The Canadian American Ticlopidine Study (CATS) in thromboembolic stroke. *Lancet* 1989;1:1215–1220.
38. CAPRIE Steering Committee. A randomized blinded trial of clopidogrel versus aspirin in patients at risk of ischaemic events. *Lancet* 1996;348:1329–1339.
39. Albers G. Atrial fibrillation and stroke. Three new studies, three remaining questions. *Arch Intern Med* 1994;154:1443–1448.
40. Chimowitz MI, Kokkinos J, Strong J, et al. The Warfarin-Aspirin Symptomatic Intracranial Disease Study. *Neurology* 1995;45: 1488–1493.
41. Caplan LR. *Caplan's stroke: a clinical approach.* Boston: Butterworth-Heinemann, 2000.

42. Major ongoing stroke trials. Warfarin versus aspirin for intracranial disease. *Stroke* 1999;30:2256–2261.
43. Thijs VN, Albers GW. Symptomatic intracranial atherosclerosis: outcome of patients who fail antithrombotic therapy. *Neurology* 2000;55:490–498.
44. Przybylski GJ, Yonas H, Smith HA. Reduced stroke risk in patients with compromised cerebral blood flow reactivity treated with artery bypass surgery. *J Stroke Cerebrovasc Dis* 1998;7:302–309.
45. Sundt TM, Smith HC, Campbell JK, et al. Transluminal angioplasty for basilar artery stenosis. *Mayo Clin Proc* 1980;55:673–680.
46. Higashida RT, Hieshima GB, Tsai FY, et al. Transluminal angioplasty of the vertebral and basilar artery. *AJNR Am J Neuroradiol* 1987;9:745–749.
47. Purdy PD, Devous MD Sr, Unwin DH, et al. Angioplasty of an atherosclerotic middle cerebral artery associated with improvement in regional cerebral blood flow. *AJNR Am J Neuroradiol* 1990;11:878–880.
48. Ahuja A, Guterman LR, Hopkins LN. Angioplasty for basilar artery atherosclerosis. Case report. *J Neurosurg* 1992;77:941–944.
49. Touho H, Ohnishi H, Karasawa J, et al. Percutaneous transluminal angioplasty for acute stroke due to stenosis of major cerebral vessels: report of two cases. *Surg Neurol* 1994;41:362–367.
50. Touho H, Takaoka M, Ohnishi H, et al. Percutaneous transluminal angioplasty for severe stenosis of the posterior cerebral artery: case report. *Surg Neurol* 1995;42:42–47.
51. Higashida RT, Tsai FY, Halbach VV, et al. Transluminal angioplasty for atherosclerotic disease of the vertebral and basilar arteries. *J Neurosurg* 1993;78:192–198.
52. Clark WM, Barnwell SL, Nesbit G, et al. Safety and efficacy of percutaneous transluminal angioplasty for intracranial atherosclerotic stenosis. *Stroke* 1995;26:1200–1204.
53. Terada T, Higashida RT, Halbach VV, et al. Transluminal angioplasty for arteriosclerotic disease of the distal vertebral and basilar arteries. *J Neurol Neurosurg Psychiatry* 1996;60:377–381.
54. McKenzie JD, Wallace RC, Dean BL, et al. Preliminary results of intracranial angioplasty for vascular stenosis caused by atherosclerosis and vasculitis. *AJNR Am J Neuroradiol* 1996;17:263–268.
55. Callahan AS, Berger BL. Balloon angioplasty of intracranial arteries for stroke prevention. *J Neuroimaging* 1997;7:232–235.
56. Takis C, Kwan ES, Pessin MS, et al. Intracranial angioplasty: experience and complications. *AJNR Am J Neuroradiol* 1997;18:1661–1668.
57. Touho H. Percutaneous transluminal angioplasty in the treatment of atherosclerotic disease of the anterior cerebral circulation and hemodynamic evaluation. *J Neurosurg* 1995;82:953–960.
58. Mori T, Fukuoka M, Kazita K, et al. Follow-up study after intracranial percutaneous transluminal cerebral balloon angioplasty. *AJNR Am J Neuroradiol* 1998;19:1525–1533.
59. Eckard DA, Zarnow DM, McPherson CM, et al. Intracranial internal carotid artery angioplasty: technique with clinical and radiographic results and follow-up. *AJNR Am J Neuroradiol* 1999;172:703–707.
60. Marks MP, Marcellus M, Norbash AM, et al. Outcome of angioplasty for atherosclerotic intracranial stenosis. *Stroke* 1999;30:1065–1069.
61. Connors JJ, Wojak JC. Percutaneous transluminal angioplasty for intracranial atherosclerotic lesions: evolution of technique and short-term results. *J Neurosurg* 1999;91:415–423.
62. Mori T, Kazita K, Mori K. Cerebral angioplasty and stenting for intracranial vertebral atherosclerotic stenosis. *AJNR Am J Neuroradiol* 1999;20:787–789.
63. Morris PP, Martin EM, Regan J, et al. Intracranial deployment of coronary stents for symptomatic atherosclerotic disease. *AJNR Am J Neuroradiol* 1999;20:1688–1694.
64. Malek AM, Higashida RT, Halbach VV, et al. Tandem intracranial stent deployment for treatment of an iatrogenic, flow-limiting, basilar artery dissection: technical case report. *Neurosurgery* 1999;45:919–924.
65. Horowitz MB, Pride GL, Graybeal DF, et al. Percutaneous transluminal angioplasty and stenting of midbasilar stenoses: three technical case reports and literature review. *Neurosurgery* 1999;45:925–931.
66. Gomez CR, Misra VK, Campbell MS, et al. Elective stenting of symptomatic middle cerebral artery stenosis. *AJNR Am J Neuroradiol* 2000;21:971–973.
67. Mori T, Kazita K, Chokyu K, et al. Short-term arteriographic and clinical outcome after cerebral angioplasty and stenting for intracranial vertebrobasilar and carotid atherosclerotic occlusive disease. *AJNR Am J Neuroradiol* 2000;21:249–254.
68. Rasmussen PA, Perl J, Barr JD, et al. Stent-assisted angioplasty of intracranial vertebrobasilar atherosclerosis: an initial experience. *J Neurosurg* 2000;92:771–778.
69. Gomez CR, Misra VK, Liu MW, et al. Elective stenting of symptomatic basilar artery stenosis. *Stroke* 2000;31:95–99.
70. Oelerich M, Lentscig MG, Zunker P, et al. Intracranial vascular stenosis and occlusion: comparison of 3D time-of-flight and 3D phase-contrast MR angiography. *Neuroradiology* 1998;40:567–573.
71. Furst G, Hofer M, Steinmetz H. Intracranial stenoocclusive disease: MR angiography with magnetization transfer and variable flip angle. *AJNR Am J Neuroradiol* 1996;17:1749–7557.
72. Jung HW, Chang KH, Choi DS, et al. Contrast-enhanced MR angiography for the diagnosis of intracranial vascular disease: optimum dose of gadopentetate dimeglumine. *AJR Am J Radiol* 1995;165:1251–1255.
73. Yano T, Kodama T, Suzuki Y, et al. Gadolinium-enhanced 3D time-of-flight MR angiography. *Acta Radiol* 1997;38:47–54.
74. Leclerc X, Gauvrit JY, Nicol L, et al. Contrast-enhanced MR angiography of the craniocervical vessels: a review. *Neuroradiology* 1999;41:867–874.
75. Katz DA, Marks MP, Napel SA, et al. Circle of Willis: evaluation with spiral CT angiography. MR angiography and conventional angiography. *Radiology* 1995;195:445–449.
76. Wong KS, Lam WW, Liang E, et al. Variability of magnetic resonance angiography and computed tomography in grading middle cerebral artery stenosis. *Stroke* 1996;27:1084–1087.
77. Wong KS, Liang EY, Lam WWM, et al. Spiral computed tomography angiography in the assessment of middle cerebral artery occlusive disease. *J Neurol Neurosurg Psychiatry* 1995;59:537–539.
78. Samuels OB, Joseph GJ, Lynn MJ, et al. A standardized method for measuring intracranial arterial stenosis. *AJNR Am J Neuroradiol* 2000;21:643–646.
79. Schueler BA, Rufenacht DA. Risk factors leading to cerebral arterial rupture by intravascular balloon. *AJNR Am J Neuroradiol* 1993;14:1085–1093.
80. Liu AY, Do HM, Albers GW, et al. Hyperfusion syndrome with hemorrhage after angioplasty for middle cerebral artery stenosis. *AJNR Am J Neuroradiol* 2001;22:1597–1601.
81. Wilenzt JR, Sanforn TA, Audenschild CC, et al. Platelet accumulation in experimental angioplasty: time course and relation to vascular injury. *Circulation* 1987;75:636–642.

82. Furlan A, Higashida R, Weschsler L, et al. Intra-arterial prourokinase for acute ischemic stroke. *JAMA* 1999;282:2003–2011.
83. Tsai FY, Berbrian B, Matovich V, et al. Percutaneous transluminal angioplasty adjunct to thrombolysis for acute middle cerebral artery rethrombosis. *AJNR Am J Neuroradiol* 1994;15:1823–1829.
84. Ueda T, Hatakeyama T, Kohno K, et al. Endovascular treatment for acute thrombotic occlusion of the middle cerebral artery: local intra-arterial thrombolysis combined with percutaneous transluminal angioplasty. *Neuroradiology* 1997;39:99–104.
85. Nakayama T, Tanaka K, Kaneko M, et al. Thrombolysis and angioplasty for acute occlusion of intracranial vertebrobasilar arteries. *J Neurosurg* 1998;88:919–922.

4

ENDOVASCULAR THERAPY FOR TREATMENT OF ACUTE ISCHEMIC STROKE

TODD A. KUETHER
GARY M. NESBIT
STANLEY L. BARNWELL

Treatment of acute ischemic stroke has received a great deal of recent attention. With the approval for the use of intravenous tissue plasminogen activator (t-PA) for the treatment of acute ischemic stroke and the completion of intraarterial thrombolysis trials of provrokinase, chemical thrombolysis has come to the fore [1]. Because provrokinase is unavailable at present, intraarterial t-PA has become a mainstay in cerebral thrombolysis.

Intravenous and intraarterial chemical thrombolysis does not come without a price, the risk of potentially lethal intracerebral hemorrhage (ICH). If technology could be developed that allowed the interventionist to remove the thrombus without exposing the patient to this serious risk of hemorrhage, it might expand the time window for treatment, complement chemical thrombolysis, or even obviate the need for chemical thrombolysis.

This chapter introduces more commonly used treatment regimens for acute ischemic stroke, such as intraarterial thrombolysis, and explores future modes of clot removal and other methods to treat acute ischemic stroke without the use of thrombolytic agents. It also provides information regarding our current techniques and approach to intraarterial thrombolysis.

BACKGROUND

Rationale for Intraarterial Thrombolysis

Stroke represents a major cause of death in the United States and a significant cause for long-term morbidity and loss of independence. Success demonstrated in the systemic fibrinolytic treatment of myocardial infarction raised the possibility of applying fibrinolysis in the treatment of acute ischemic stroke. This led to numerous intravenous thrombolysis trials including the recent positive randomized trial of intravenous t-PA, which demonstrated significant improvements in outcome within 3 hours of stroke onset [2]. Several randomized controlled trials have, however, shown no benefit to intravenous treatment 3 to 6 hours following the onset of ictus [3–8]. Due to the continued development of microcatheters over the past 15 years, these fibrinolytics may now be applied directly to the thrombus. The goal of direct fibrinolysis is the improvement of recanalization rates and extension of the treatment window for thrombolysis to beyond 3 hours after stroke onset.

Untreated acute stroke often has a poor outcome. The acute mortality rate for middle cerebral artery (MCA) strokes that are not treated is in the range of 12% to 28% [9–11]. More significantly these patients with untreated MCA strokes have an 80% risk of not returning to a favorable lifestyle. Those who do recover from a severe deficit do so early, suggesting that rapid spontaneous recanalization plays an important role in outcome [9]. The results in posterior circulation infarcts are even worse. Mortality rates of over 85% in vertebrobasilar occlusion have been reported for those given conservative, conventional treatment [12].

At present, thrombolysis for stroke in the United States is approved only in the form of recombinant t-PA (rt-PA) administered intravenously within 3 hours of symptom onset. This therapy was approved on the basis of a single randomized trial [13]. Other trials have failed to show a benefit for intravenous thrombolysis or demonstrated worse outcomes with these therapies [3–8]. Despite aggressive public education campaigns, the number of patients who seek treatment within the 3-hour window remains small, with less than 5% of all patients with stroke receiving intravenous t-PA [14–17]. Early recanalization is fundamental to clinical improvement. The recanalization rate for intravenous thrombolysis is low, ranging from 21% to 43%, although neither vascular occlusion nor recanalization was

T.A. Kuether: Dotter Interventional Institute, Oregon Health Sciences University, and Microneurosurgical Consultants, St. Vincent's/Providence, Portland, Oregon.

G.M. Nesbit: Dotter Interventional Institute, Oregon Health Sciences University, Portland, Oregon.

S.L. Barnwell: Department of Neurosurgery, Dotter Interventional Institute, Portland, Oregon.

documented in any of the recent major intravenous thrombolysis trials [18]. The Emergency Management of Stroke (EMS) Bridging Trial looked at the feasibility, efficacy, and safety of combined intravenous-intraarterial rt-PA for stroke within 3 hours of onset [19]. This small randomized study of 35 patients found that intravenous-intraarterial treatment provided better recanalization. However, this limited study did not show improvement in clinical outcomes and further study is required to determine its effectiveness. Anecdotal and case series evidence has shown the efficacy of intraarterial thrombolysis in recanalization with rates of 44% to 87% [9,11,12,18,20–26]. Most studies suffer from lack of internal controls and nonrandom patient selection but do suggest a trend toward improved outcome with intraarterial thrombolysis.

The best evidence for improved outcome comes from the two randomized control studies of intraarterial thrombolysis using prourokinase [11,26]. These studies demonstrated a relatively high recanalization rate (57.7% and 67% versus 14% and 17% for placebo). In one of the studies, the Prolyse in Acute Cerebral Thromboembolism II (PROACT II), patient enrollment was sufficient to show that the rate of recanalization was significantly higher for patients treated with a thrombolytic agent [11]. The primary end point for PROACT II was a modified Rankin score of no more than 2 after 90 days. This score (2 or less) indicates that a patient with stroke has slight or no disability and is able to live independently. The PROACT II trial demonstrated a 40% rate of favorable outcome (Rankin of 2 or lower) in the treatment group compared with 25% for the controls. This difference was statistically significant. The rate of symptomatic hemorrhage was 10.2% for the thrombolytic-treated group compared to 1.8% for the heparin-treated control group [11]. Despite this higher rate of symptomatic hemorrhage, clinical outcome was significantly improved using intraarterial thrombolysis.

The disadvantages of intraarterial delivery include its invasiveness, the inherent risks of angiography, the lack of facilities and personnel trained to perform the procedure, and the time required to initiate treatment (compared with intravenous thrombolysis). Indeed, intraarterial thrombolysis probably adds 30 to 60 minutes before beginning definitive treatment when compared with intravenous therapy. Rapid emergency room assessment and immediate transport from the radiology to the angiography department (after computed tomography [CT]) is imperative. Air transport may be used to deliver patients in a large geographic region within the time limits for treatment.

Thrombolytic Agents

Three main thrombolytic agents have been used for acute ischemic stroke treatment in various forms. They are streptokinase (STK), UK, and t-PA. None has proven clearly superior for intraarterial use. All work via a similar mechanism by activating the body's own fibrin-degrading enzyme, plasmin, but they do have significant differences. To lyse the clot, these activators must have available substrate (plasminogen), which is found within the clot and in circulating plasma.

STK shows no specific affinity for fibrin-bound plasminogen and therefore may have a greater systemic fibrinolytic effect than t-PA and a higher inherent risk for hemorrhage. Use of STK has largely been abandoned for acute stroke because several intravenous trials were halted after showing unacceptable rates of intracranial hemorrhage and early death [7].

UK, which has been unavailable for use due to a manufacturing issue, has been studied extensively. It does not show fibrin-bound plasminogen specificity and should have similar systemic effects to STK [27]. Doses for standard intraarterial UK range from 180,000 to 1.5 million units [9,20,22,23,25].

Prourokinase (Prolyse), a proenzyme similar to UK, shows fibrin-specific fibrinolysis and may have less systemic effect [28]. This drug has been most extensively studied in intraarterial stroke thrombolysis trials [11,26].

Due to the unavailability of UK, interventionists have turned to t-PA for thrombolysis in stroke. It is found in humans and is available derived from recombinant DNA in two forms in the United States, alteplase and reteplase. Its ability to activate plasminogen is greatly increased when the plasminogen is bound to fibrin rather than freely circulating [29]. This theoretically directs most of the anticoagulant activity toward the clot itself, rather than having a systemic effect, and accounts for its favored use in intravenous thrombolysis trials. The systemic half-life of t-PA is 5 minutes, but the thrombus-dissolving action by the bound t-PA lasts much longer. The two available forms differ in their affinity for and penetration of thrombus, although the advantages require further study in intraarterial stroke thrombolysis [30]. In case series comparing UK to t-PA for intraarterial thrombolysis, Zeumer et al. found no difference in recanalization rates between UK and t-PA for intracranial occlusion, but the type of occlusions included in the t-PA group were probably more difficult to treat [9]. One million units of UK are considered approximately equivalent to 10 mg t-PA, but direct human dose equivalents are not established, even for different preparations of t-PA [31,32]. Dose ranges are typically from 10 to 20 mg, although doses over 100 mg have been used intraarterially [9,33,34].

Other agents, both direct thrombolytics and agents that potentiate thrombolysis, are still undergoing study. Ancrod, which is derived from pit viper venom, lyses fibrinogen and promotes endogenous t-PA release [35]. Abciximab, a platelet glycoprotein IIb/IIIa inhibitor that decreases platelet aggregation, may play an adjunctive role in stroke treatment. Trials involving its use in acute myocardial infarction have shown it to be an effective adjunct [36]. In stroke thrombolysis, it is not currently recommended for routine use but should be considered for cases showing unusual resistance to thrombolysis or with recurrent occlusion after recanalization. Concerns about cerebral or systemic hemorrhage have been raised and are certainly a consideration when it is used in combination with heparin and t-PA, but the initial stroke data suggest that when it is used alone this risk may be low. A recent safety and efficacy study in 54 patients demonstrated that abciximab appeared to be safe when administered up to 24 hours after stroke onset and might improve functional outcome [37].

Mechanical Clot Disruption

Mechanical clot disruption includes any technique by which the interventionist mechanically disrupts the thrombus in the artery. In general, a thrombus that results in a significant neurologic deficit is usually sufficient in size to obstruct a cerebral artery more proximally than the very small distal branches. An embolus will lodge itself at the distal internal carotid artery (ICA) bifurcation or proximal M1 or M2 branch of the MCA, for example. The embolus is only a finite length, and the parent artery is in stasis but usually patent distal to the thrombus.

The goal of mechanical clot disruption is to rapidly establish blood flow and cerebral perfusion. As the thrombus is disrupted, the small emboli are carried into distal branches. If these emboli are small enough they will pass through the distal circulation. Otherwise, by disrupting the thrombus and reducing its size, the exposed surface area increases, which may facilitate clot dissolution by the body's intrinsic fibrinolytic system. Smaller emboli may also facilitate exogenous thrombolysis, resulting in some cortical rescue and neurologic improvement. The potential for distal embolization and worsening cortical perfusion exists and must be considered in each case. For example, if the internal carotid artery is occluded but the patient has good MCA flow through the circle of Willis or good leptomeningeal collaterals, reopening the carotid and exposing the patient to the risk of clot embolizing into the proximal or distal MCA must be considered.

Taking all of this into consideration, the potential advantages of mechanical thrombolysis are great. The first advantage is that it may significantly increase the time window for interventional stroke treatment [38]. With the use of thrombolytic agents, the window of opportunity is narrow, with a 3-hour window set for intravenous t-PA and typically a 6-hour window for intraarterial thrombolytic agents. These windows have been based partially on the risk of ICH associated with the use of thrombolytic agents. In the 3-hour window, symptomatic hemorrhage was approximately 10 times more likely to occur with t-PA (6.4% of patients) than with placebo (0.6%) [39]. For intravenous recombinant tissue-type plasminogen activator (alteplase) given up to 6 hours after onset, the overall risk of CT-detected ICH was 11.8% for the t-PA-treated patients compared with 3.1% for placebo patients [4]. Despite the increased incidence of symptomatic ICH, this did not lead to an increase in morbidity or mortality for the intravenous t-PA group in the 3-hour window [39,40]. On the basis of these results, intravenous t-PA was approved in the United States for use within 3 hours from onset of symptoms. For those treated within 6 hours of stroke onset with intraarterial recombinant prourokinase (r-proUK), the overall risk of symptomatic ICH within 24 hours was 15.4% compared with 7.1% for placebo [26]. In this study the heparin dose used did influence the hemorrhage frequency. These data support the rationale that by improving the efficacy of thrombolysis by using mechanical clot disruption, the dose of thrombolytic agents can be reduced, and this should in turn lower the risk of ICH.

Furthermore, one of the biggest problems associated with acute stroke treatment is getting patients to the hospital within these time limits. Mechanical clot disruption may eliminate the need for thrombolytic agents or significantly reduce the dose required, thereby extending the potential time frame for treatment. Perhaps of more importance, mechanical clot disruption may well speed the time to recanalization. The individual devices available now and those that may become available in the future are discussed in the latter part of the technique section of this chapter.

TECHNIQUE FOR INTRAARTERIAL THROMBOLYSIS

Patient Selection

Integral to the treatment algorithm for acute stroke is proper patient selection. We know some of the relative risk factors, but not their exact contribution or degree of risk. Not all patients will benefit from this treatment and many may be harmed. A symptomatic hemorrhage may convert a survivable event with some deficit into a life-threatening process. Evaluation of the current data for intravenous or intraarterial thrombolysis does not support stratification to treatment based on clinical factors, but certain trends in this analysis have suggested which patients do better with thrombolysis [41]. Patients with a National Institutes of Health Stroke Scale (NIHSS) score above 15 to 20 and with a hyperdense MCA sign or documented M1 occlusion tend not to do well with intravenous administration, and outcome may be improved with intraarterial thrombolysis.

Time is critical and medical evaluation must be swift and directed. A rapid assessment should be performed with a focused clinical history and neurologic evaluation using a stroke scale such as the NIHSS. Time of symptom onset, age, comorbid disease, history of hypertension, recent trauma, or TIA or stroke may increase the risk of hemorrhage with thrombolysis. A clinical evaluation of the patient should highlight these factors, and they should be considered in any decision to use thrombolytic agents in the patient with ischemic stroke.

Imaging also is used to help select the proper patient for treatment. After a rapid clinical assessment a noncontrast head CT is performed as quickly as possible. The purpose is to exclude hemorrhage. ICH, subdural hematoma, and subarachnoid hemorrhage are contraindications to thrombolysis. Other features of infarction may also be evaluated. Significant low attenuation in a large vascular territory implies a greater risk of postthrombolytic hemorrhage. One-third of patients treated with intravenous t-PA who had low attenuation of more than one-third of the MCA distribution went on to hemorrhage [42]. More recently, CT evaluation using the Alberta Stroke Programme Early CT Score (ASPECTS) found that patients with scores less than 7 were unlikely to make independent recovery despite intravenous thrombolytic therapy [43]. Findings such as loss of the insular ribbon or hypoattenuation in the basal ganglia are of uncertain risk but should be viewed with caution. More subtle findings, such as sulcal effacement, are more likely acceptable. Hyperdensity within the MCA is an inconstant, common finding with MCA occlusion and is not a contraindication to intraarterial thrombolysis. In time, other imaging modalities including xenon-enhanced CT, diffusion-perfusion MRI, magnetic resonance angiography (MRA), CT angiography (CTA), and single-photon emission computed tomography (SPECT) may play an increasingly important role in patient selection.

We generally use the following clinical and imaging criteria to select a patient for intraarterial therapy:

1. Neurologic deficit consistent with a large vessel territory vascular occlusion
2. Arrival time within 6 hours for anterior circulation, 12 hours for posterior circulation
3. CT findings
   a. No evidence of intracranial hemorrhage
   b. Less than one-third MCA territory hypodensity
   c. Less than 7 on the ASPECTS score (Fig. 4-1)
4. Vascular occlusion consistent with the neurologic deficit
5. Informed consent from family
6. Absent relative contraindications including: recent surgery, recent major trauma, and recent stroke
7. Controllable blood pressure below 185/110

Angiography

In advance of the procedure the National Institute of Neurological Disorders and Stroke (NINDS) recommends maintaining systolic blood pressure below 185 mm Hg and diastolic blood pressure below 110 mm Hg to reduce the risk of hemorrhage. Liberal conscious sedation should be used during the procedure. General anesthesia is not always required but can be advantageous when the patient is combative or aphasic. In our experience general anesthesia is rarely necessary and may slow initiation of treatment. Supplemental oxygen is given and a urinary catheter is placed. Suction is checked prior to initiation of the procedure. Medications, which may need to be ordered from the pharmacy,

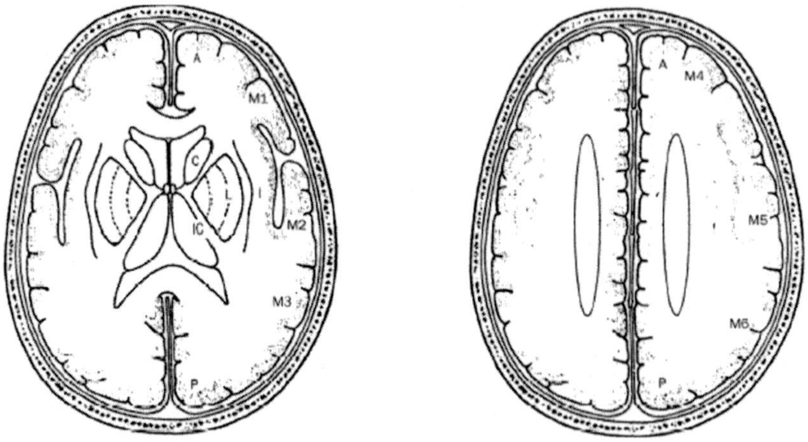

FIGURE 4-1. For the ASPECTS scoring system, the MCA is assigned 10 total points. A single point is subtracted in any area that shows early ischemic change, which is manifest as either focal swelling or hypoattenuation in the tissue for each of the regions. A normal CT, therefore, has 10 points, while 0 points indicates diffuse ischemic change in all of the regions of the MCA. A, anterior circulation; P, posterior circulation; C, caudate; L, lentiform; IC, internal capsule; I, insular ribbon; MCA, middle cerebral artery; M1, anterior MCA cortex; M2, MCA cortex lateral to insular ribbon; M3, posterior MCA cortex; M4, M5, and M6 are anterior, lateral, and posterior MCA territories immediately superior to M1, M2, and M3, rostral to basal ganglia. Subcortical structures are allotted 3 points (C, L, and IC). MCA cortex is allotted 7 points (insular cortex, M1, M2, M3, M4, M5, and M6). (From Barber PA, Demchuk AM, Zhang J, et al. Validity and reliability of a quantitative computed tomography score in predicting outcome of hyperacute stroke before thrombolytic therapy. ASPECTS Study Group. Alberta Stroke Programme Early CT Score. *Lancet* 2000;355: 1670–1674, with permission.)

will need to be obtained. A predefined plan coordinating the roles of the nurse, technologist, neurologist, and neurointerventionist is recommended.

The routine use of a femoral sheath is recommended. It allows easy exchange of guide catheters, takes only a minute to insert, and can greatly facilitate navigation with better torque control. It also allows for continuous accurate pressure monitoring. The sheath can be removed at the end of the procedure, and we are currently closing all arteriotomies with an endovascular suture device, which allows for the patient to remain anticoagulated if necessary.

Due to the importance of initiating treatment as quickly as possible, angiography should first evaluate the level of occlusion and the presence and adequacy of the circle of Willis, pial, and external carotid collaterals. We recommend assessing the involved vessel first. If enough information concerning the level of occlusion and degree of collateral flow can be obtained from this single injection, then thrombolysis can be immediately instituted. If the circle of Willis needs further evaluation, then other vessels are evaluated. For example, an M1 occlusion with good anterior cerebral artery filling needs no further evaluation. In contradistinction, a distal internal carotid occlusion may require evaluation of the contralateral carotid and possibly the vertebral artery to determine the most appropriate course.

For suspected basilar artery occlusion, the left subclavian artery is the initial vessel to evaluate to assess the origin of the vertebral artery. The vertebral artery is then catheterized and the posterior fossa studied in the lateral and anteroposterior projection. If only the proximal basilar artery fills, one or both common carotid arteries are studied to evaluate for posterior communicating artery supply. If the proximal or distal vertebral artery is occluded and there is no filling of the basilar artery, the right vertebral artery is studied.

The location of occlusion may help to determine the risk of hemorrhage with thrombolysis. Theron et al. have grouped patients into three categories based on carotid territory involved in order to predict therapeutic risk [44]. Group 1 has occlusion of the internal carotid artery with patency of the circle of Willis and lenticulostriate arteries. With sparing of the lenticulostriates, these patients present a relatively low risk for hemorrhage with treatment. Group 2 has occlusion of the cortical arteries but sparing of the lenticulostriates. These patients also have a relatively low risk of hemorrhage. Included in this group are branch, M2, or MCA bifurcation occlusion, although in bifurcation lesions some lenticulostriates may be involved. In group 3, the carotid terminus and the MCA are occluded, including the lenticulostriates. Within this category are those with occlusion of all the lenticulostriates, with or without an extensive internal carotid artery component, producing the densest ischemia and the highest risk for hemorrhage with thrombolytic agents. Patients with only partial lenticulostriate involvement have a moderate risk. Theron et al. also predict that the time available for safe treatment may be less than 6 hours with involvement of the lenticulostriates, or much longer if only cortical branches are occluded with good collaterals [44]. Hopefully, perfusion studies will give us better insight into this issue and help separate those who will benefit from those who may be harmed by thrombolysis.

Thrombolysis

Once the need for thrombolysis is confirmed, a blood sample for an activated clotting time (ACT) is drawn. This is normally below 140 seconds. Heparin is given at that time if the ACT is not markedly elevated. We follow the PROACT II guidelines of a 2,000 IU bolus and 500 IU/hr × 4 hours. Heparin usage and the dose have not been fully clarified and conflicting results persist. The PROACT trial demonstrated increases in both the recanalization and hemorrhage rates with higher heparin doses (100 IU/kg bolus followed by 1,000 IU/hr × 4 hours) compared with lower doses (2,000 IU bolus followed by 500 IU/hr × 4 hours). To minimize risk, the dose in the larger follow-up study (PROACT II) was reduced [26]. A tradeoff clearly exists between increased hemorrhage risk and prevention of rethrombosis.

We use t-PA for intraarterial thrombolysis, because it is readily available and we now have more extensive experience with this drug. Current recommendations for the use of t-PA included mixing the t-PA in a 1 mg to 1 ml ratio of t-PA to normal saline. The usual maximal dose is 20 mg, although higher doses have been used. It should not be mixed into a more dilute solution of less than 0.2 mg/ml, because this may disrupt the arginine-solubilizing agent in the product and could result in precipitation. A multicenter phase 2 study is about to begin in which a dose of up to 22 mg rt-PA will be given intraarterially over 2 hours. The t-PA is placed in a 1-ml syringe (1 mg), which is used for the bolus injections, followed by infusion of the remainder, most commonly by an infusion syringe pump. Although no direct equivalency is quoted, 1 mg of reteplase (Retavase) is approximately equal to 10 units of alteplase (Activase). A number of treatment methods have been proposed and outlined in the intraarterial stroke registry (Interventional Stroke Therapy Outcomes Registry [INSTOR]) (http://www.strokeregistry.org). It is our recommendation to become a site for this registry if you are involved in intraarterial stroke therapy.

Most favor embedding the microcatheter within the clot rather than just at the proximal face. A variation we favor involves traversing the clot, injecting a 1-ml bolus of t-PA distally, then lacing the thrombus with a second 1-ml aliquot as the microcatheter is slowly withdrawn in the thrombus, stopping in the proximal third.

Use of a guide catheter with an inner diameter of 0.05 inch or greater (5 Fr. or 6 Fr.) facilitates performance of "road mapping" via injection through the guide catheter around the microcatheter. We favor the use of a standard end-hole microcatheter because it allows more precise placement of the lytic agent into what is usually a short-segment (5-mm or less) occlusion.

Because the occluding thrombus will prevent adequate opacification of the artery, navigation is often blind. Knowledge of the arterial anatomy, particularly the location of the posterior communicating and anterior choroidal artery, the lenticulostriates, thalamostriates, and the vertebrobasilar branches, is essential to avoid puncture. Navigation of the microcatheter and microguidewire is slow and methodical and is usually straightforward without incident. Abnormal wire or catheter position, contrast extravasation, or a Cushing response (hypertension and bradycardia) may be signs of perforation. If a perforation is detected, the wire or microcatheter should not be withdrawn, because the device may be occluding the perforation. Vital signs are assessed, thrombolytic agents stopped, and heparin is reversed with protamine. If bleeding or deterioration continues, coils can be placed through the perforation. This may occlude the artery, but it is preferred to active hemorrhage.

An occlusion that does not resolve prompts reevaluation of the situation. An underlying stenosis may be present. The thrombus may be old and resistant to thrombolytic agents. The thrombus characteristics may alter the efficacy of thrombolysis. Clot, which is fresh, so-called *red thrombus,* responds much more rapidly to thrombolysis. Older clots, white thrombus, which is more typical of emboli, has more fibrin crosslinks, is relatively platelet rich and plasminogen poor, and may respond less well. Emboli may be calcified, mycotic, or composed of myxoma or plaque. The latter half of this section on technique addresses ways of mechanical clot removal, which may be useful for this group or in patients who cannot receive pharmaceutical thrombolytics.

Care after Thrombolysis

Postthrombolysis guidelines adapted from the intravenous National Institutes of Health (NIH) t-PA trial can be used, although no strict rules are published [13]. Close monitoring of the blood pressure is maintained, with the goal of maintaining the systolic blood pressure below 185 mm Hg. If good flow has been achieved and there is no hemodynamic stenosis, the blood pressure may be lowered even further. Heparin is usually discontinued and allowed to reverse spontaneously. A postthrombolysis CT is obtained to evaluate for hemorrhage. Large hematomas are generally the only type of hemorrhagic transformation that may alter the clinical course of ischemic stroke [45]. Repeated microcatheter injections can stain the infarcted basal ganglia with contrast, simulating hemorrhage (Fig. 4-2). We percutaneously close all arteriotomies to avoid hemorrhagic groin complications.

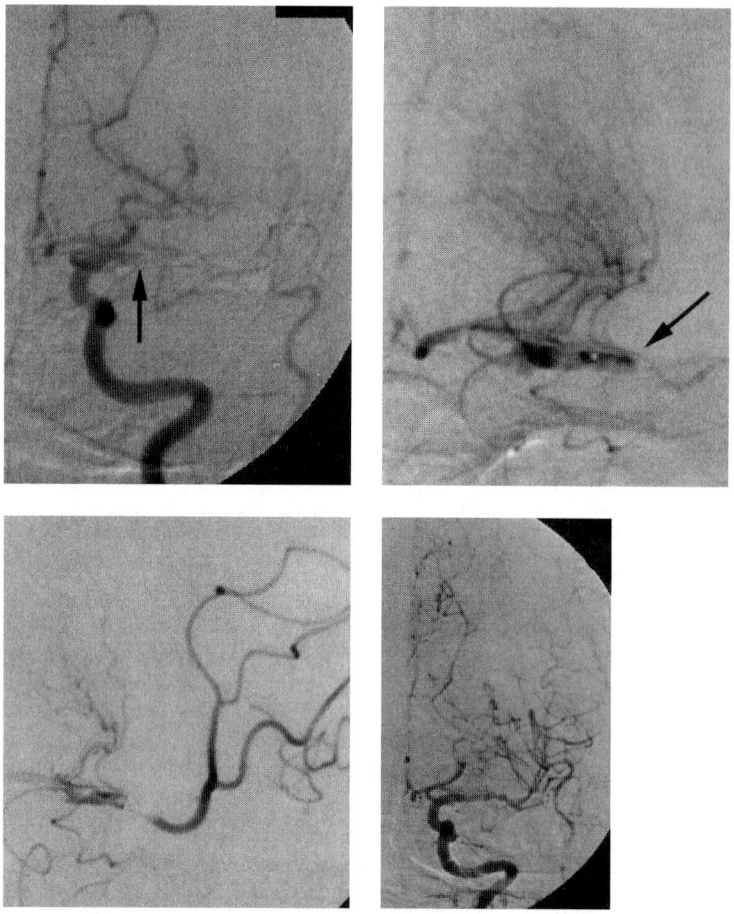

A,B

C,D

FIGURE 4-2. This 73-year-old woman developed acute onset of right hemiplegia and aphasia approximately 2 hours before coming to angiography. She was several days status post–thoracic aortic aneurysm repair. **A:** Anterior projection of a left carotid artery angiogram demonstrated an acute cutoff of the left MCA *(arrow).* The cervical portions of the carotid artery proximal to this were observed to be normal. **B:** Selective injection anterior projection with a microcatheter placed in the proximal M1 segment of the MCA demonstrates an acute cutoff of the vessel *(arrow).* Note the filling defects consistent with thrombus just proximal and distal to the catheter tip and the dense filling of the lenticulostriate arteries supplying the basal ganglia. **C:** Anterior projection selective left MCA M1 segment angiogram following approximately 5 mg of t-PA shows partial recanalization of the vessel with a continued filling defect representing a residual thrombus. **D:** Left internal carotid artery angiogram anterior projection following a total dose of 12.5 mg of t-PA shows recanalization of the left M1 segment and filling of the MCA opercular vessels. *(Figure continues.)*

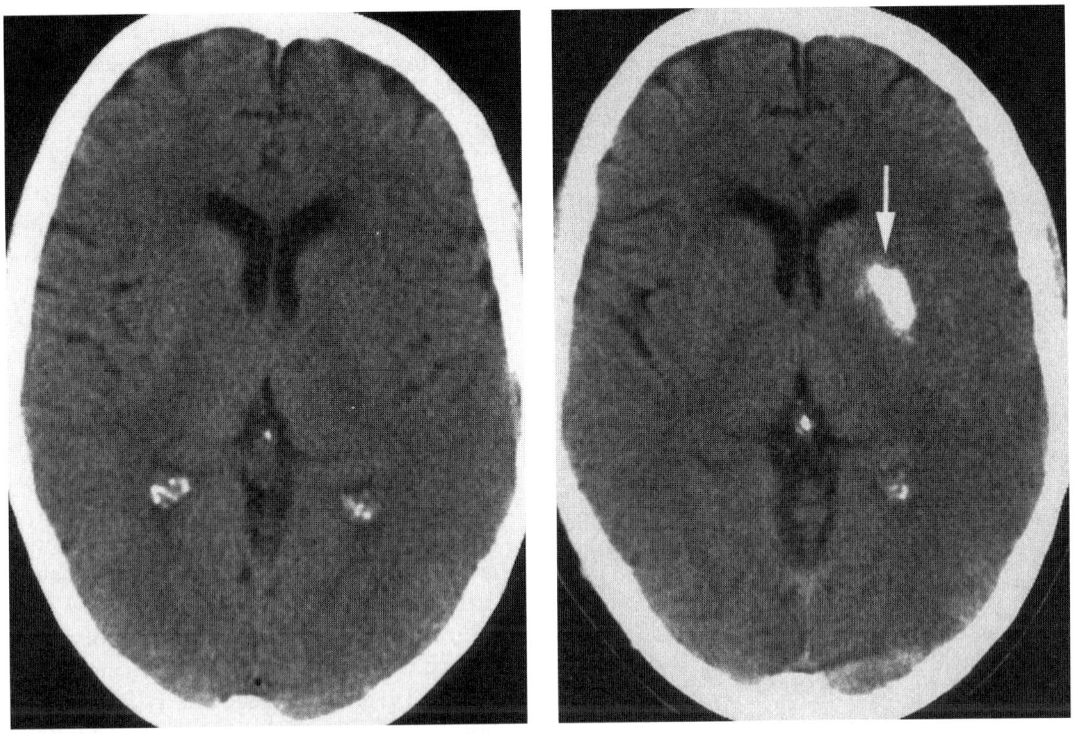

E F

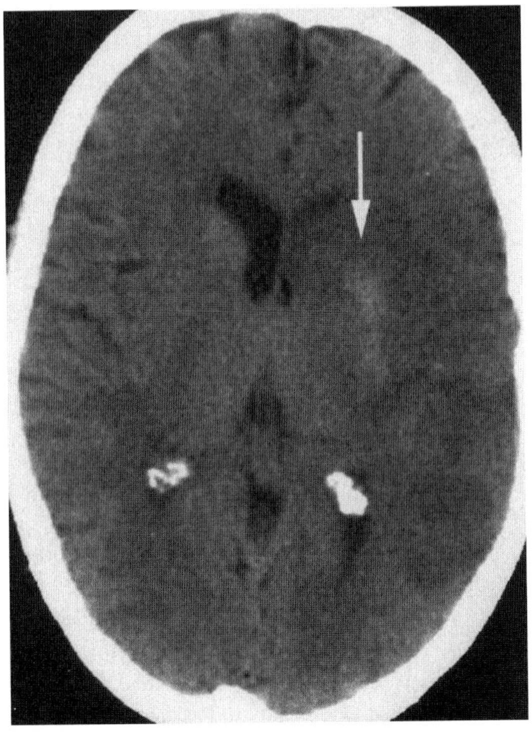

G

FIGURE 4-2. *Continued.* **E:** A single slice from a CT scan obtained immediately before angiography demonstrates some subtle loss of gray-white distinction in the posterior temporal lobe on the left side consistent with acute ischemic change. The study is otherwise unremarkable. **F:** CT scan immediately following thrombolysis demonstrates hyperdensity in the left basal ganglia, which is new since the initial CT scan *(arrow)*. The hypodensity and loss of gray-white distinction in the posterior temporal lobe is more pronounced than in the prior scan **(E)**. The area of hyperdensity may represent contrast stain or early hemorrhagic change. **G:** CT scan approximately 18 hours following the scan obtained in **(F)**. This shows edema accompanying ischemic change in a larger portion of the MCA territory. In addition, the area of hyperdensity has now cleared markedly since the prior scan with some minimal residual area of hyperdensity seen. This rapid clearing is much more consistent with contrast stain rather than a hematoma in this area. Following the procedure, the patient's right-sided weakness improved significantly and the aphasia also improved. At last follow-up the patient still had some residual aphasia and mild hemiparesis but was living independently. (From Michael P. Marks and Huy M. Do, unpublished material, with permission.)

Mechanical Clot Disruption—Current and Future Techniques

Guidewires

Perhaps the most primitive of devices for clot disruption is the simple microguidewire. As discussed previously in this chapter, during arterial thrombolysis, a microcatheter (usually an end-hole catheter) is navigated up to the proximal portion of the thrombus. Many times the microguidewire can be advanced easily through the thrombus into the distal vessel. Multiple passes through the clot is one form of mechanical disruption that may fragment the thrombus if it is not organized. In the case of thrombolysis, it is felt that this disruption aids in the process by increasing the surface area of the thrombus exposed to the lytic agent. This may be all that is required to promote thrombolysis of the clot [46].

Snares

These devices are essentially small lassos or baskets that have been designed to grasp objects from an endovascular approach (Fig. 4-3). They have been designed to retrieve endovascular devices, wires, and coils located inside the blood vessel. In the same context, one could potentially extract a dense fibrotic thrombus lodged inside a blood vessel. By passing the snare around the thrombus and cinching it, one may be able to pull it free from the intracranial circulation and remove it from the vasculature. The benefit and efficacy of this method have been anecdotally reported in a few cases to date. One such case is illustrated in Fig. 4-4. However, one must consider the potential loss of the thrombus into another vascular bed. This is one additional method that can be used to mechanically disrupt and potentially remove a thromboembolus, providing rapid recanalization. A number of new devices that incorporate this concept are currently under study.

Catheters

A number of experimental trials are underway with new microcatheters developed to assist in mechanical clot disruption and more thorough distribution of thrombolytic agents. These catheters are advanced into the thrombus, which they are designed to fragment as they are pulled back through the clot. These catheters must be agile enough to navigate to the site of the intracranial thrombus, yet rugged enough to effectively disrupt the organized thrombus. Mechanical catheter disruption may improve the efficacy of concomitant arterial thrombolysis so that the dose of lytic agent may be reduced to prevent bleeding complications.

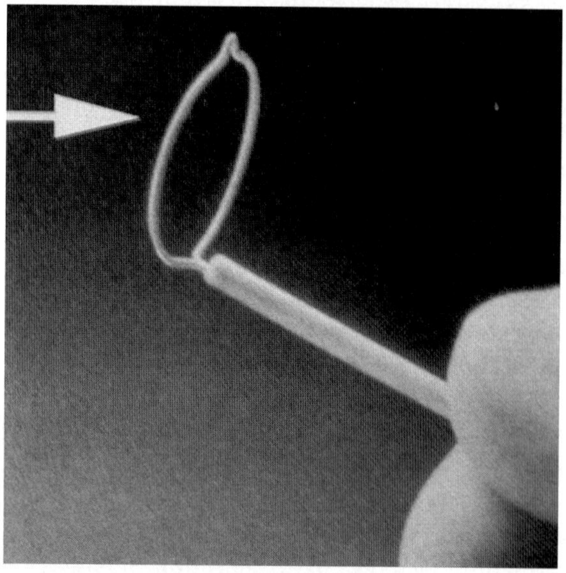

FIGURE 4-3. The 4-mm gooseneck snare (Microvena Corporation, White Bear Lake, MN). The snare *(arrow)* is seen prior to deployment and constriction of the snare loop around the thrombus.

Angioplasty

Percutaneous transluminal angioplasty (PTA) in acute stroke is used to treat atherosclerotic lesions, in both the extracranial and intracranial circulation, which are felt to be responsible for ischemic events. The balloon acts mechanically to dilate the vessel, resulting in a fracture of the intima, media, and atherosclerotic plaque. Complications that can be associated with this procedure include vessel spasm, dissection, occlusion, perforation, stroke, and death.

In the case of intracranial PTA, due to the risks associated with the procedure, it is used only in several situations. The first is in cases of intraarterial thrombolysis associated with an atheromatous lesion which reoccludes or does not sufficiently open after the initial thrombolytic treatment. Thrombolysis, when combined with PTA in patients whose symptoms reappear due to restenosis or reocclusion, can be an effective method of restoring patency and preventing reocclusion of the occluded artery [47]. The second indication for PTA is in those patients who are continuing to have clinically symptomatic stenotic lesions despite maximal medical therapy after the initial event. Under these circumstances PTA can be performed with a relatively low restenosis rate [48]. Finally, it can be used in patients who may be resistant to thrombolysis alone [49]. This type of rescue angioplasty (in patients who have not responded to thrombolytic therapy) may be of benefit to recanalize the still-thrombosed artery. These patients may have larger, older clots more resistant to thrombolysis alone (Fig. 4-5).

Unlike coronary angioplasty, primary intracranial angioplasty for acute stroke theoretically carries more risk. The occlusion in coronary vessels in acute myocardial infarction is almost always *in situ* thrombotic occlusion of an underlying stenosis. In the cerebral vasculature, it is usually embolic without a significant underlying lesion, and the amount of thrombus is greater. It is for this reason that recanalization may be more effective with thrombolysis in the cerebral vasculature versus primary angioplasty in the coronary vessels.

The use of extracranial angioplasty for acute stroke may involve high-grade stenotic lesions of the proximal internal carotid artery that lead to distal thromboemboli and carotid occlusion. It is felt that atherosclerotic disease at the bifurcation leads to clot formation. Before complete occlusion, this clot may embolize to the cerebral circulation, which corresponds to the onset of clinical symptoms. At any time thereafter, additional clot formation at the bifurcation may lead to an internal carotid occlusion. In this situation, PTA has been used successfully to recanalize the carotid artery and expedite intracranial thrombolysis [50]. However, the additional hemorrhage risk of hyperperfusion following proximal PTA must be considered.

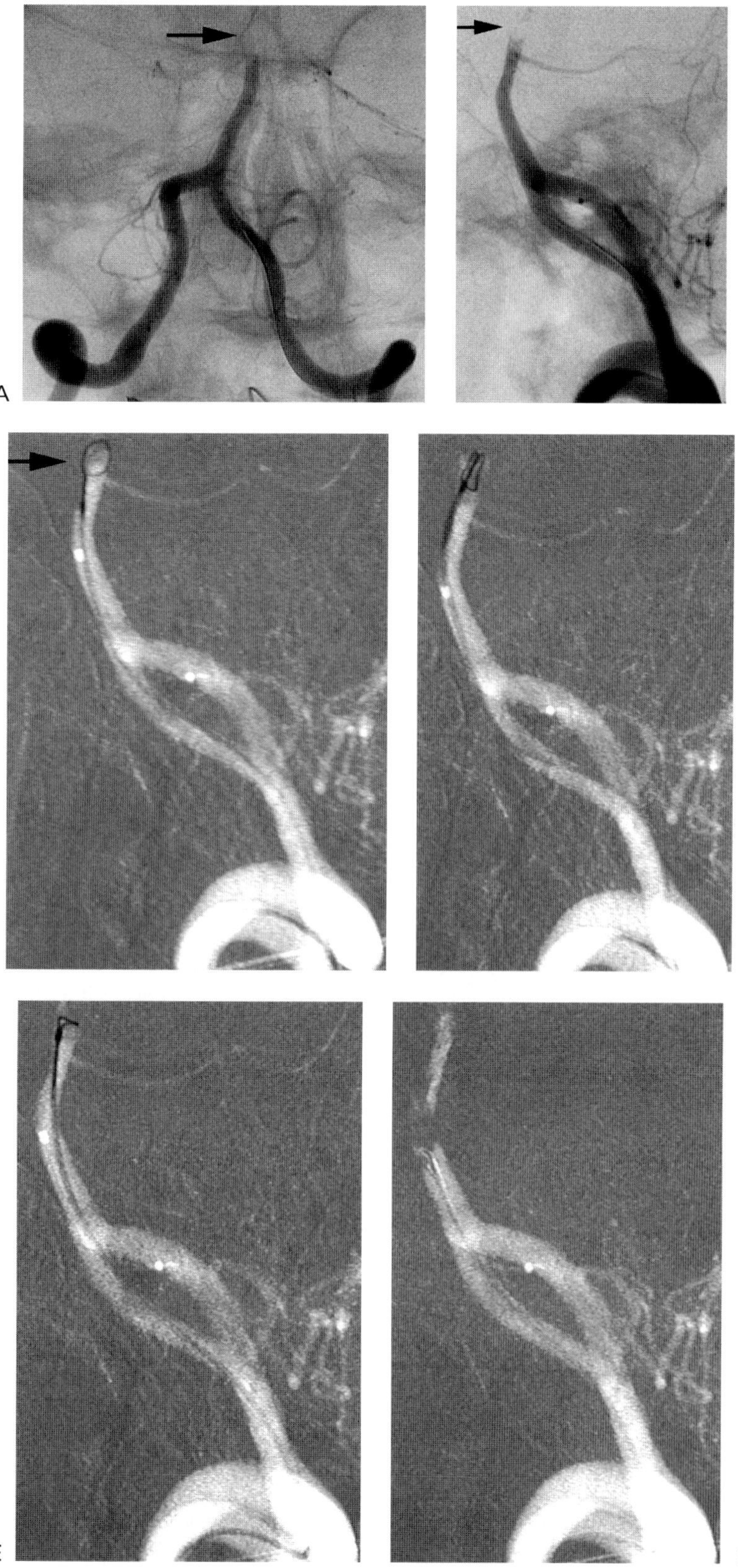

A B C D E F

FIGURE 4-4. This elderly patient deteriorated acutely after a coronary artery bypass surgery with aphasia, right-sided weakness, and progressive obtundation. Left vertebral artery angiography in the anterior **(A)** and lateral **(B)** projections demonstrates complete occlusion of the basilar tip by thrombus *(arrow),* with minimal filling of the superior cerebellar arteries. Due to the recent open heart surgery it was elected not to use thrombolytic agents. **C:** A snare *(arrow)* was brought just proximal to the thrombus. **D:** The snare was opened and pushed to the tip of the basilar artery and manipulated around the clot. The snare was tightened **(E)** and the thrombus was pulled down into a guide catheter **(F).** *(Figure continues.)*

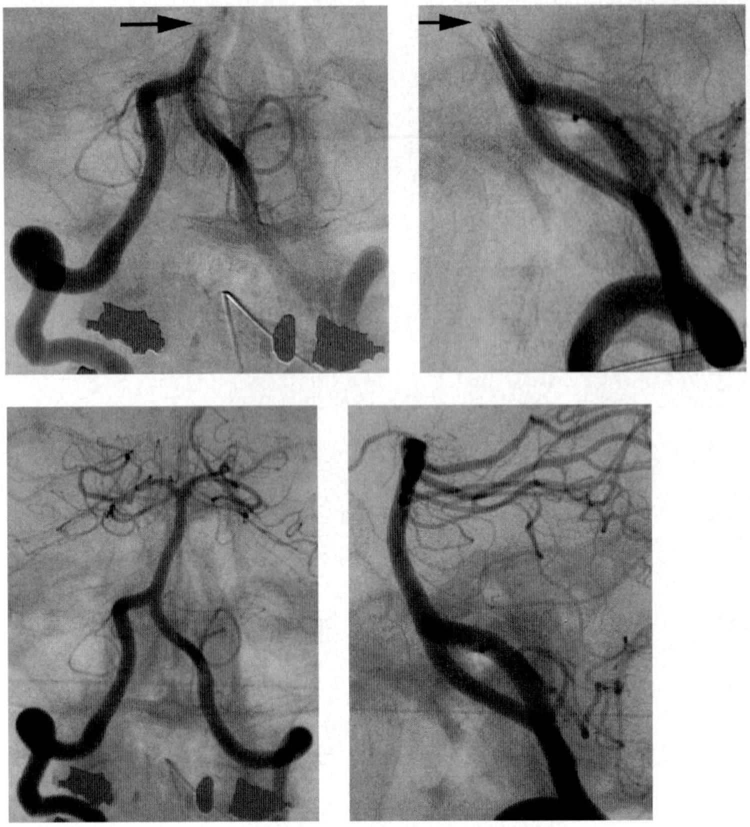

G,H

I,J

FIGURE 4-4. *Continued.* **G,H:** Angiograms demonstrate the thrombus *(arrow)* in the snare in the midbasilar artery. **I,J:** Following removal of the thrombus an angiogram was performed, showing complete resolution of the occlusion with normal patency of the basilar tip and its branches. Further study demonstrated an additional left M2 branch occlusion of the MCA.

Ultrasound

Trials are currently underway using a catheter (EKOS) that emits an ultrasonic frequency at the tip. The catheter (Fig. 4-6) is positioned within the thrombus and, when activated, produces an ultrasonic resonance meant to agitate the thrombus, allowing for the infused thrombolytic agent to better penetrate and lyse the clot. The goal is to improve the mechanical disruption of the thrombus and facilitate thrombolytic action with minimal vascular injury.

Lasers

This is another technology under aggressive investigation. A great deal of work has already been done characterizing the effects of laser angioplasty and endarterectomy. Most of the literature involves research done with argon ion and Nd:YAG (neodymium:yttrium aluminum garnet) lasers. Some studies have also been performed using a xenon chloride laser [51]. Both Nd:YAG and argon radiation have been shown to be capable of destroying atheromatous plaque. The major advantage of this technique is its ability to vaporize fresh thrombus and plaque without producing significant emboli. However, the problem *in vivo* is perforation of the artery wall, even in rather large, elastic arteries [52,53].

More recently, lasers have been applied to direct thrombectomy in acute stroke. Novel designs have included pulsed-dye or frequency-doubled Nd:YAG lasers tuned to the hemoglobin absorption peak. With very little energy absorbed into the blood vessel wall, this allows vaporization or photoacoustic mechanical disruption of the thrombus while minimizing the risk to the vessel wall. Prototypic microcatheter-mounted lasers, which can be navigated into a carotid or intracranial artery and used to disrupt the offending thrombus without requiring the use of thrombolytic agents, are being developed (Fig. 4-7). Preliminary clinical trials on several models using laser technology are currently underway.

Thrombectomy

This technique involves the extraction of the thrombus through the catheter, foregoing the risk of embolic complications seen with simple clot disruption. Once the thrombus is removed, flow is restored to the parent artery. Once again, the major obstacles which must be overcome are the flexibility required in these systems to navigate into the carotid arteries and even more tortuous intracranial arteries and safety issues related to vessel wall damage or perforation.

A simple approach to thrombectomy, which we have employed in cases of acute internal carotid artery occlusion,

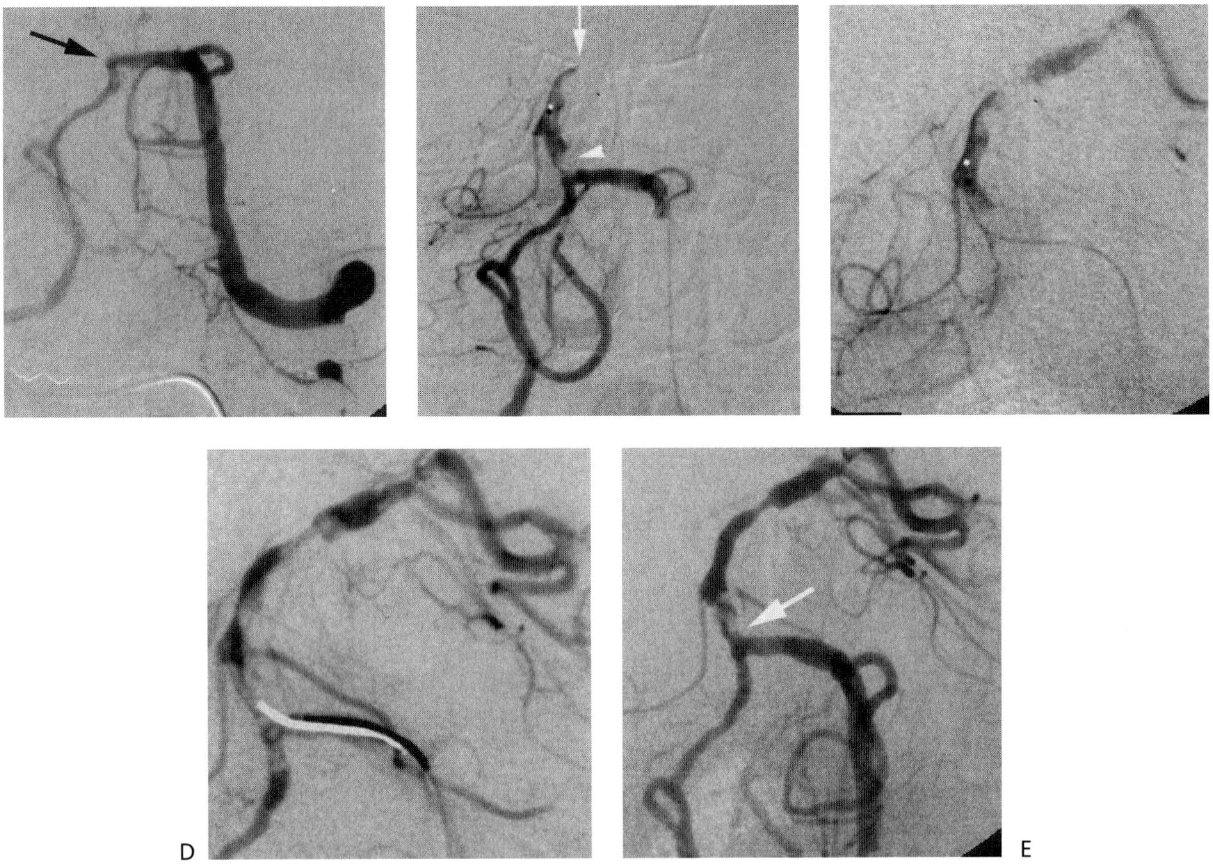

A,B C D E

FIGURE 4-5. This 59-year-old man with a known history of atherosclerotic disease involving the basilar artery became obtunded approximately 6 to7 hours prior to arriving at the angiography suite. At the time of arrival he was deeply comatose. **A:** Anterior view from an initial left vertebral artery injection demonstrates filling of the left vertebral artery up to the vertebral basilar junction *(arrow)* with reflux down the right vertebral artery. No filling of the basilar artery was noted. **B:** Selective injection with the microcatheter placed in the proximal basilar artery via the left vertebral artery. Complete cutoff of the basilar artery is again noted *(arrow).* In addition a filling defect, which may represent plaque or thrombus, is seen in the proximal basilar artery *(arrowhead).* **C:** Anterior projection from a selective injection was obtained after infusion of 10 mg of t-PA. Extensive thrombus of the proximal basilar artery is still noted, and there is poor antegrade filling of the distal basilar circulation. For this reason an angioplasty balloon was introduced into the basilar artery. This balloon was used to attempt to mechanically disrupt and fissure the clot to improve the response to thrombolysis. **D:** Anterior projection of a left vertebral artery angiogram obtained immediately after balloon dilatation of the thrombus-filled segments of the basilar artery shows some improved recanalization and flow in the basilar when compared to **(C)**. The patient then received additional thrombolysis to a total dose of 25 mg t-PA. **E:** Left vertebral artery angiogram shows recanalization of the vertebral basilar circulation following 25 mg of t-PA (total). Areas of residual stenoses are noted within the mid- and proximal basilar arteries (*proximal arrow* outlines the proximal stenoses). These were felt to represent atherosclerotic disease, clot resistant to thrombolysis, or both. Despite recanalization, the patient remained in coma and eventually succumbed to this ischemic episode due to the long period of complete basilar thrombosis. (From Michael P. Marks and Huy M. Do, unpublished material, with permission.)

involves simple suction thrombectomy to restore flow in the vessel. A large-bore guide catheter is navigated over a guidewire into the thrombus and a 60-ml syringe used to aspirate. The guide catheter is slowly withdrawn, allowing for more complete removal of the thrombus. This technique has been used in those cases of carotid occlusion in which the patient did not have enough collateral flow to perfuse the affected hemisphere. In general, patients with internal carotid artery occlusion seek treatment for either of two reasons. The first is when the internal carotid artery is occluded, with no middle or anterior cerebral artery occlusion. This type of patient becomes symptomatic when the circle of Willis is inadequate and internal carotid occlusion results in a significant reduction in flow to that hemisphere. By restoring flow in the internal carotid artery this flow deficit can be corrected. The second circumstance occurs when the

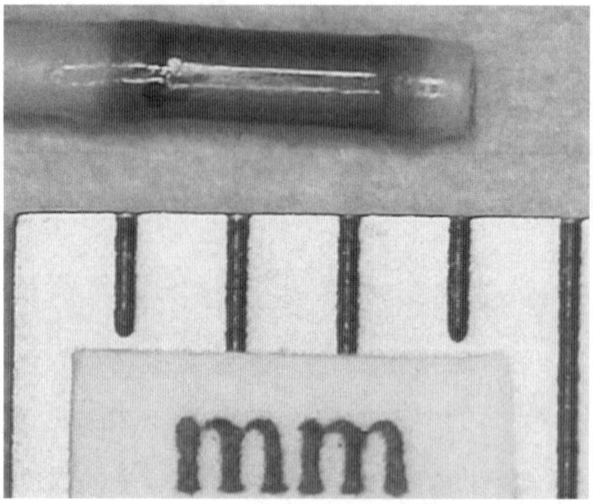

FIGURE 4-6. EKOS ultrasonographic catheter. The tip of the microcatheter is shown. A power setting in watts is selected and the catheter temperature is monitored during its use. Clinical trials are in progress.

internal carotid artery is occluded, and there has been distal embolic or thrombus propagation past the distal internal carotid artery bifurcation into the middle or anterior cerebral arteries. In this instance, recanalization of the distal occlusion should be performed, and then the need for recanalization of the internal carotid artery is assessed. Reopening of the internal carotid artery may not be necessary or may even be futile if the distal obstruction cannot be corrected.

The goal of suction thrombectomy is to remove as much thrombus as possible and minimize the amount of thrombolytic medication needed to achieve recanalization, or forego its use altogether. The assessment of collateral flow via the circle of Willis and leptomeninges is critical in selecting patients for such risky procedures. Figures 4-8 and 4-9 demonstrate two cases in which suction thrombectomy was used successfully. The first patient had no collaterals supplying the left hemisphere, and recanalization of the left carotid was necessary to reestablish flow. In the second case, there was a distal embolic occlusion but the patient had very marginal collateral vessels. By reestablishing flow in the internal carotid artery the collateral flow to the hemisphere was improved. This latter case also demonstrates when thrombolytic agents should be avoided due to the presence of infarct on the CT scan. We felt neither of these patients had good options other than attempting to reestablish flow in the internal carotid artery.

The AngioJet (Possis Medical, Minneapolis, MN) is an endovascular thrombectomy device that combines local vortex suction with mechanical disruption (Fig. 4-10). This catheter uses multiple retrograde high-pressure fluid jets directed into the primary evacuation lumen to create a hydrodynamic vortex that draws in, traps, and fragments adjacent thrombus. This debris is then simultaneously removed through the recovery lumen. This device has been tested in animal models and found to be safe with only mild injury to vessel walls [54]. It has been used in the peripheral circulation to treat extremity vessels, coronary arteries, and dialysis fistulae [55–60]. Most of the thrombus can be removed without significant particulate debris that is of major concern when considering carotid or intracranial thrombus removal.

Trials are underway in humans using the AngioJet in cases of acute carotid occlusion. A limited series has been reported using the thrombectomy device to open occluded internal carotid arteries in acute stroke [61]. In addition, a smaller version of this catheter is also undergoing clinical trials for intracranial thrombectomy. The AngioJet may be used to extract the thrombus in the artery and may have some advantages of suction thrombectomy discussed in the previous section. If this catheter technology is successful for intracranial use, thrombus could potentially be easily removed without requiring the use of lytics and without the concurrent risk of ICH.

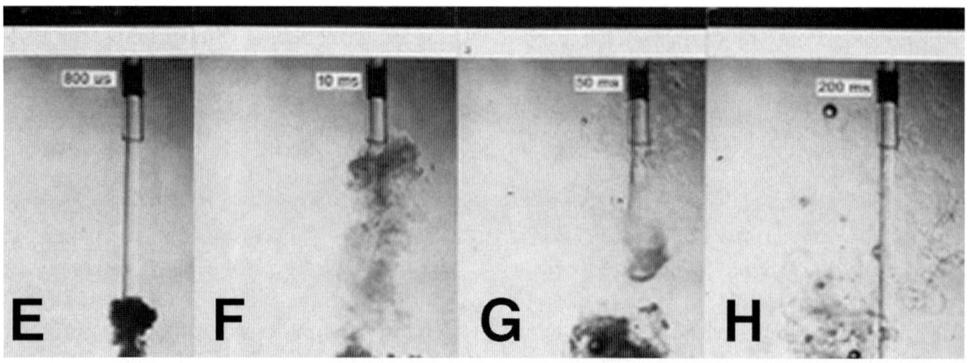

FIGURE 4-7. Laser catheter in development for use in stroke therapy. Tip of a microcatheter with column of flowing contrast material onto a surface thrombus. A single 2-μsec pulse had been given 50 μsec beforehand. A plume of disrupted thrombus is seen at 100 to 800 μsec **(E)** that disrupts the contrast column at 10 to 50 μsec **(F,G)** and that returns to normal at 200 μsec **(H).**

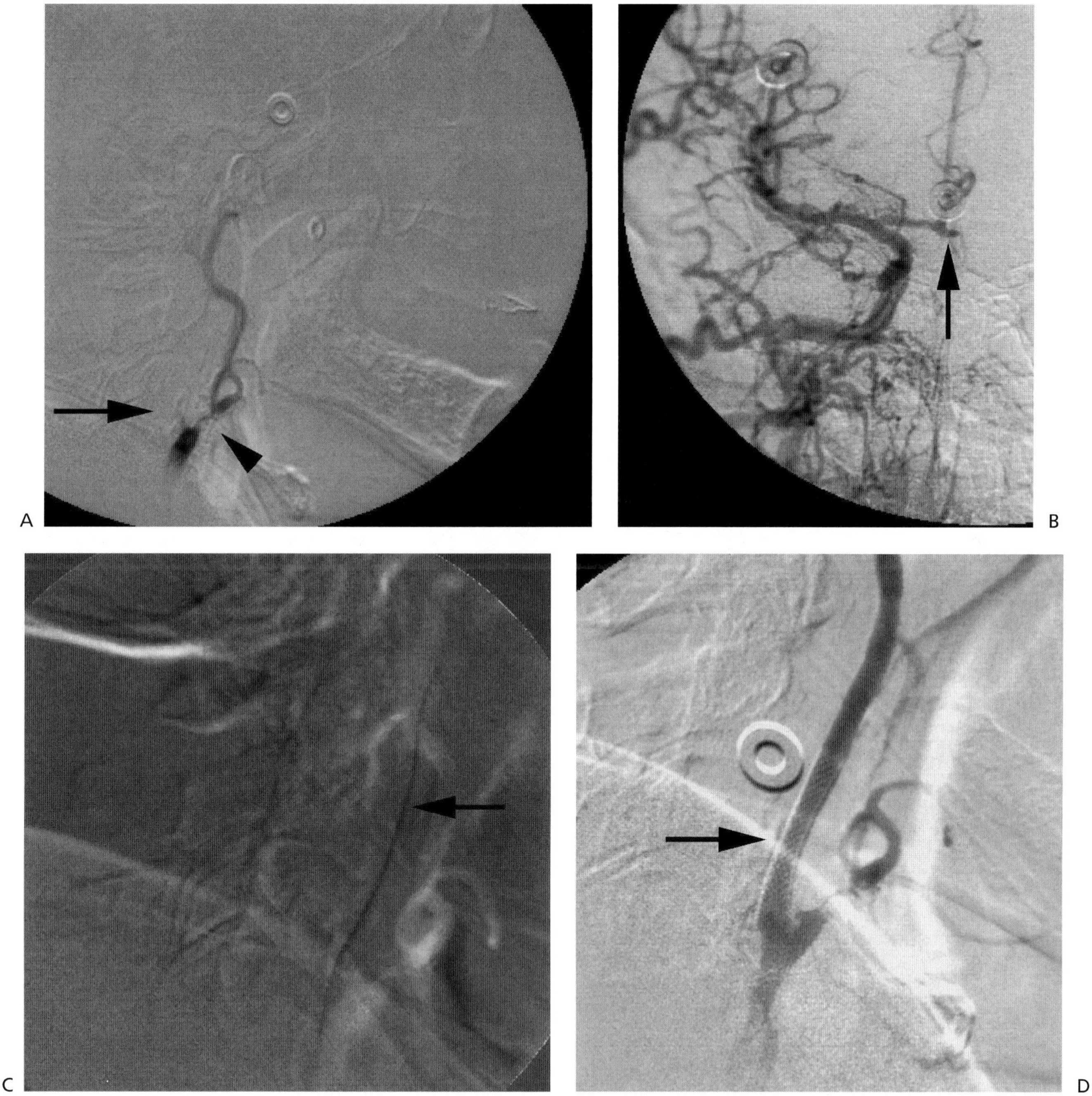

FIGURE 4-8. This 72-year-old right-handed man arrived 4 hours after onset of dense aphasia and right hemiplegia. Initial symptoms had begun 12 hours earlier, consisting of hesitancy of speech and mild facial weakness. **A:** The left common carotid artery (CCA) angiogram demonstrates complete occlusion of the cervical internal carotid artery (ICA) *(arrow),* with a calcified plaque at its origin and a significant external carotid artery (ECA) stenosis *(arrowhead).* **B:** The right CCA injection demonstrates no significant filling across the anterior communicating artery (ACoA) *(arrow)* to the left anterior cerebral artery (ACA) or left MCA. **C:** The patient was heparinized and a Glidewire *(arrow)* was navigated across the occlusion. A 6-Fr. guide catheter was advanced to the C2 level. Suction thrombectomy of the ICA was performed by applying suction to the guide catheter with a 60-ml syringe while slowly pulling back the guide catheter. Several 2- to 4-mm fragments of organized thrombus were removed. A contrast injection through this guide catheter demonstrated normal filling of the ICA beyond the stenosis and the left ACA and MCA, except for several small distal posterior left MCA branch occlusions. Due to the residual high-grade stenosis of the ICA at the carotid bifurcation, this was treated with angioplasty and stent placement with a 5-mm × 20-mm Wallstent (Schneider, Minneapolis, MN). Angiograms were obtained, which showed near-complete resolution of the cervical stenosis **(D),** with the stent in place *(arrow),* and filling of left ACA *(arrow)* and MCA *(arrowhead)* **(E)**. *(Figure continues.)*

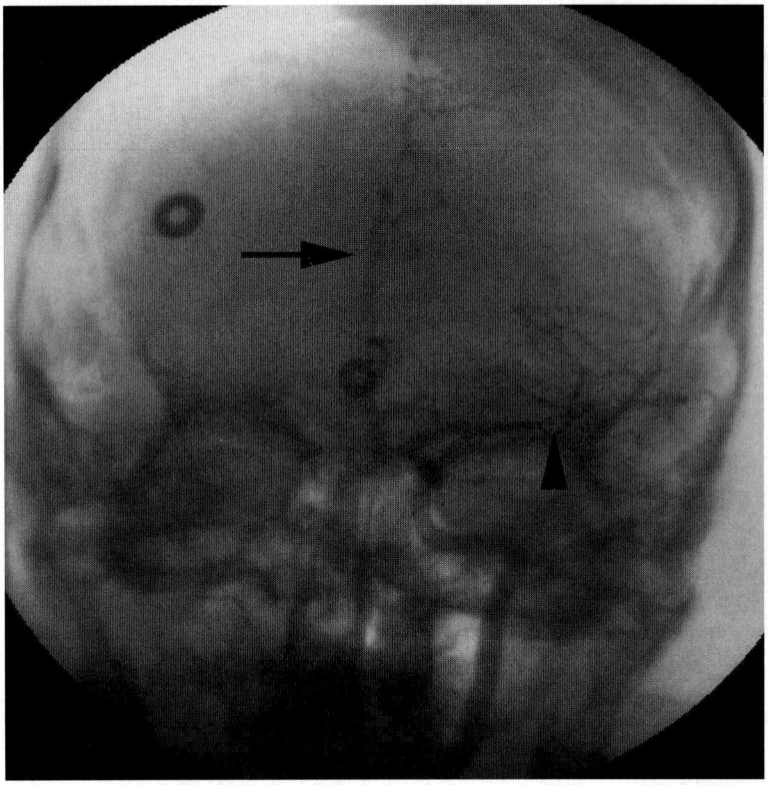

E

FIGURE 4-8. *Continued.* Flow was reestablished within 5 hours of stroke onset. Although flow was reestablished early in this patient's course, he made only a marginal recovery over the next 3 months and had persistent aphasia, right leg paresis, and arm plegia. This may have occurred because more than 12 hours had elapsed since the patient's first onset of speech difficulty and facial weakness, which prevented thrombolytic treatment of any intracranial branch occlusions.

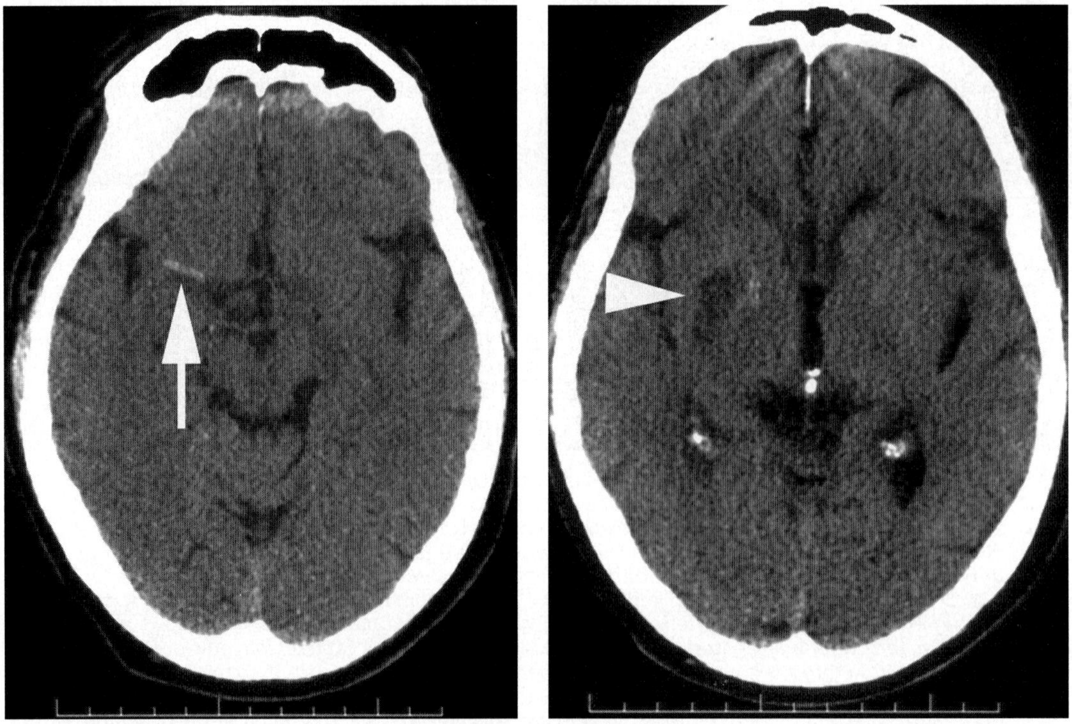

A B

FIGURE 4-9. This 67-year-old right-handed man had a sudden onset of left hemiplegia. The initial CT scan demonstrated a dense MCA sign. His symptoms largely resolved, except for some mild facial and arm weakness and a right Horner syndrome. He was placed on heparin. Overnight he had several episodes of transient hemiplegia, until the following morning when he developed a profound left hemiplegia. **A,B:** CT scanning was repeated in the morning and demonstrated the dense MCA sign *(arrow)* and a deep basal ganglia infarct *(arrowhead). (Figure continues.)*

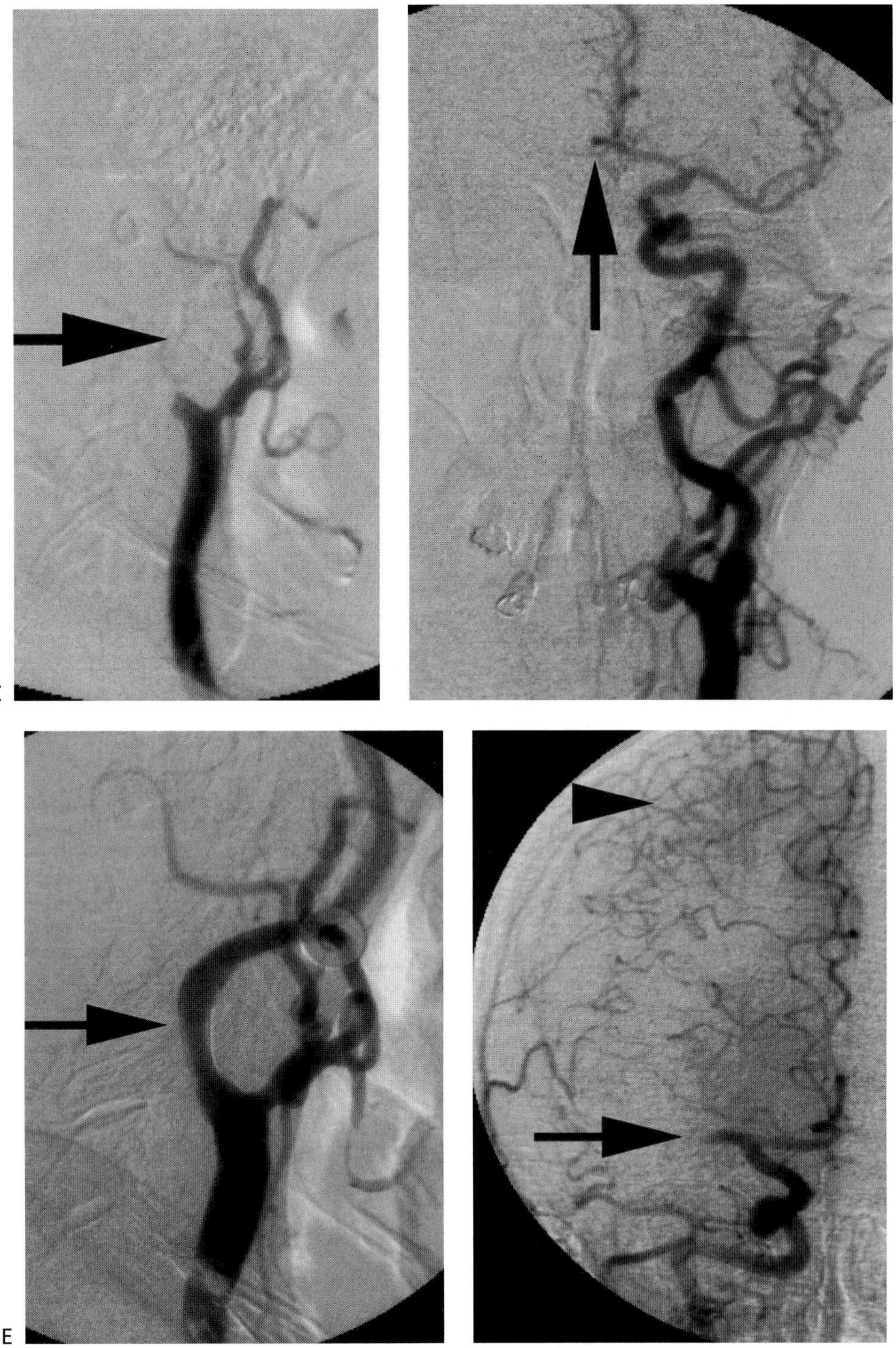

C D E F

FIGURE 4-9. *Continued.* **C:** The right CCA angiogram demonstrates complete occlusion of the cervical ICA, with a string of contrast proximally *(arrow).* Within the ICA was extensive thrombus, with no contrast filling the midcervical or intracranial ICA or its branches. **D:** The left CCA angiogram demonstrated minimal filling of the right ACA across the ACoA *(arrow)* but no flow into the right MCA. The left vertebral artery injection demonstrated no posterior communicating arteries (PCoA). Because there was a tight stenosis at the ICA origin, a Glidewire was used to cross the stenosis that was predilated with a 4-mm × 2-cm angioplasty balloon. The 9-Fr. guide catheter was navigated into the distal occluded right ICA and suction thrombectomy of the ICA was performed, with 5 cc of red and pink thrombus removed. Angioplasty and stent placement were performed using a 6-mm × 2-cm Wallstent. **E,F:** Right CCA angiograms showed near-complete resolution of the cervical stenosis *(arrow),* with filling of right ACA and a mid-M1 occlusion of the right MCA *(arrow).* The flow into the right ACA had significantly improved, with good filling of distal MCA branches via collaterals *(arrowhead)* from the ACA. Because of the presence of the right basal ganglia infarct this patient was not a candidate for thrombolysis. After the procedure, the patient continued to regain his strength. Within 4 days his only deficit was mild weakness of the left arm and a mild Horner syndrome. Six months later he was completely normal (no identifiable deficits) and had returned to work.

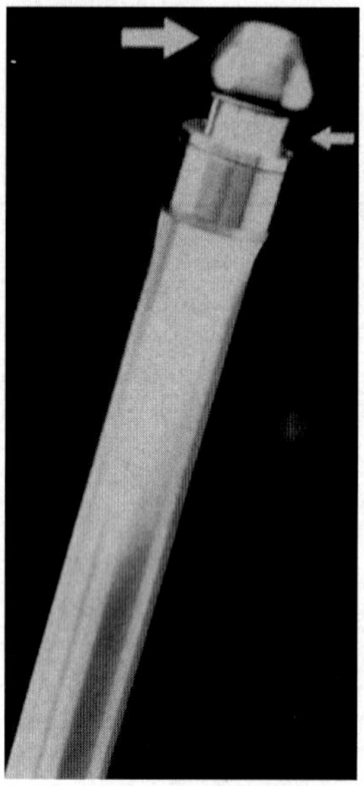

FIGURE 4-10. The AngioJet LF 140 Catheter (Possis Medical, Minneapolis, MN). High-pressure saline jets *(small arrow)* are directed into evacuation lumen from nozzles located in the catheter tip *(large arrow)*.

Cerebrovascular Stenting

This chapter would not be complete without mentioning the use of angioplasty and stents in the treatment of stroke. We have already briefly mentioned the use of angioplasty. In select cases, stents may also be deployed to maintain flow through vessels thought to be the cause of the stroke. For example, if a patient's underlying cause of stroke was a result of a highly stenotic lesion, then a stent may be deployed to maintain flow through the artery once the thrombus has been removed or lysed. Angioplasty may be necessary as an adjunct to stent placement to reopen the vessel lumen. The stent's purpose is to trap emboli during the angioplasty and to maintain luminal integrity. The risk of significant increases in perfusion to the involved brain and potential reperfusion hemorrhage must be weighed against the risk of rethrombosis. Another application for the use of stents is carotid dissection. Most carotid dissections can be treated effectively with anticoagulation. However, some patients may have embolic events despite heparin administration, due to the severity of the dissection and propensity for thrombus formation, or anticoagulant may be contraindicated (Fig. 4-11). If the dissection results in severe stenosis and a low-flow state, a stent may be necessary to maintain cerebral perfusion. In these cases, a stent may be used to tack intimal flaps and false lumens to the vessel wall and establish and maintain patency in the normal vessel lumen, thus preventing further emboli or hemodynamic compromise [62].

These same principles may be applied to the intracranial circulation. There have been anecdotal reports of the use of small stents in select cases of intracranial stenosis. Stents have been used in cases that have had problems of rethrombosis following thrombolytic recanalization. The underlying atheromatous stenosis causes a rapid rethrombosis even in the presence of systemic anticoagulation. As stent selection and technology improve, their use with angioplasty for intracranial lesions resulting in thrombosis and stroke may increase in the future.

Treatment of Proximal Occlusion

Until now we have discussed techniques that may be employed to restore flow through vessels after an acute stroke. However, it is always important to evaluate in each case the source of the stroke and the presence of collateral flow. A patient will become symptomatic only if the distal flow is occluded by thrombus or the collaterals are insufficient to maintain adequate perfusion. If the internal carotid artery is full of thrombus that may embolize distally, it may be in the patient's best interest to leave the carotid artery occluded. Thrombolysis may be performed through an occluded carotid by navigating the microcatheter through the proximal thrombus. Distal thrombolysis can then be carried out allowing reperfusion through collaterals. If the patient has an intact circle of Willis and distal thromboemboli, these collaterals will supply this distal branch once flow in the vessel has been restored.

One must carefully evaluate the need to restore flow in the internal carotid artery. Several cases have already been reviewed in which the carotid was the only supply to the hemisphere and recanalization was required to prevent massive infarction. However, in other cases proximal thrombus may serve as a source for recurring thromboemboli into distal vessels. If there is slow flow through a partially occluded carotid or vertebral artery, this may shower the intracranial circulation with emboli. In this situation a decision must be made to either remove or lyse the thrombus or permanently occlude the artery (Fig. 4-12). Once flow has been restored in the distal vasculature, it is equally important to consider whether treatment of the cause of the stroke is possible or necessary. In some instances permanent occlusion of the carotid artery may be the best alternative to prevent further ischemic events from thromboemboli.

Retrograde Transvenous Neuroperfusion

Although not mentioned above, this technique has been reported as a possible effective treatment for cerebral ischemia. Retrograde transvenous neuroperfusion (RTN), which is used extensively for cerebral protection during thoracic aortic surgery, has been applied to treating MCA occlusion in an animal model. A pump harvests arterial blood, which is pumped retrograde through the veins to reach the capillary bed. Pressures only moderately above venous pressures are necessary. The blood traverses the capillary bed to

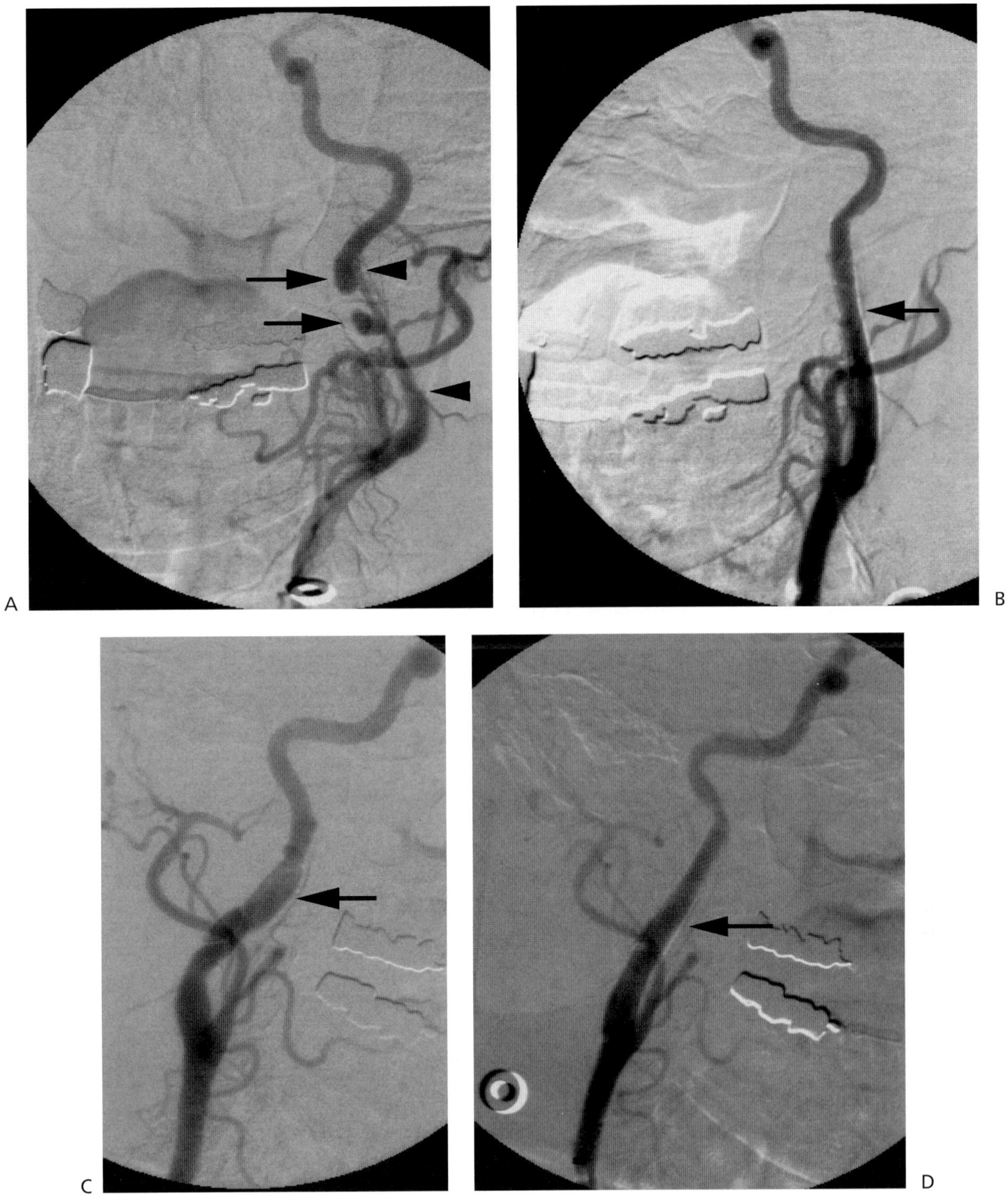

FIGURE 4-11. This patient is a 58-year-old woman who sustained bilateral ICA dissections after a motor vehicle accident. She suffered a left MCA-branch infarction. After anticoagulation therapy was stopped because of a retroperitoneal hematoma, she suffered a small area of infarction in the right hemisphere. The dissections were treated using carotid stenting to avoid systemic heparinization, which was contraindicated in her case. The dissections increased the degree of stenosis on the left and right sides over 2 weeks. **A:** The left CCA angiogram demonstrates marked irregularity and significant stenosis over an approximately 4-cm segment of the left cervical ICA *(arrowheads)* to approximately 1.5 cm below the petrous portion with two pseudoaneurysms *(arrows).* **B:** After Wallstent placement and gentle (less than 6 atmospheres) angioplasty to 6 mm, there was no significant residual stenosis *(arrow).* **C:** The right CCA angiogram demonstrates an irregular dissection of the cervical ICA *(arrow),* extending to approximately 1.5 cm proximal to the petrous portion. Although there is no specific stenosis, a series of spiral flaps can be seen which results in a significant decrease in flow through the region of dissection. **D:** After stenting and angioplasty of the right ICA in an identical fashion, there was excellent patency *(arrow)* and significant compression of the false lumen, which slowly filled, was in near stasis, and measured only 1 to 1.5 mm in diameter. The patient had no further ischemic events and was discharged to a rehabilitation center.

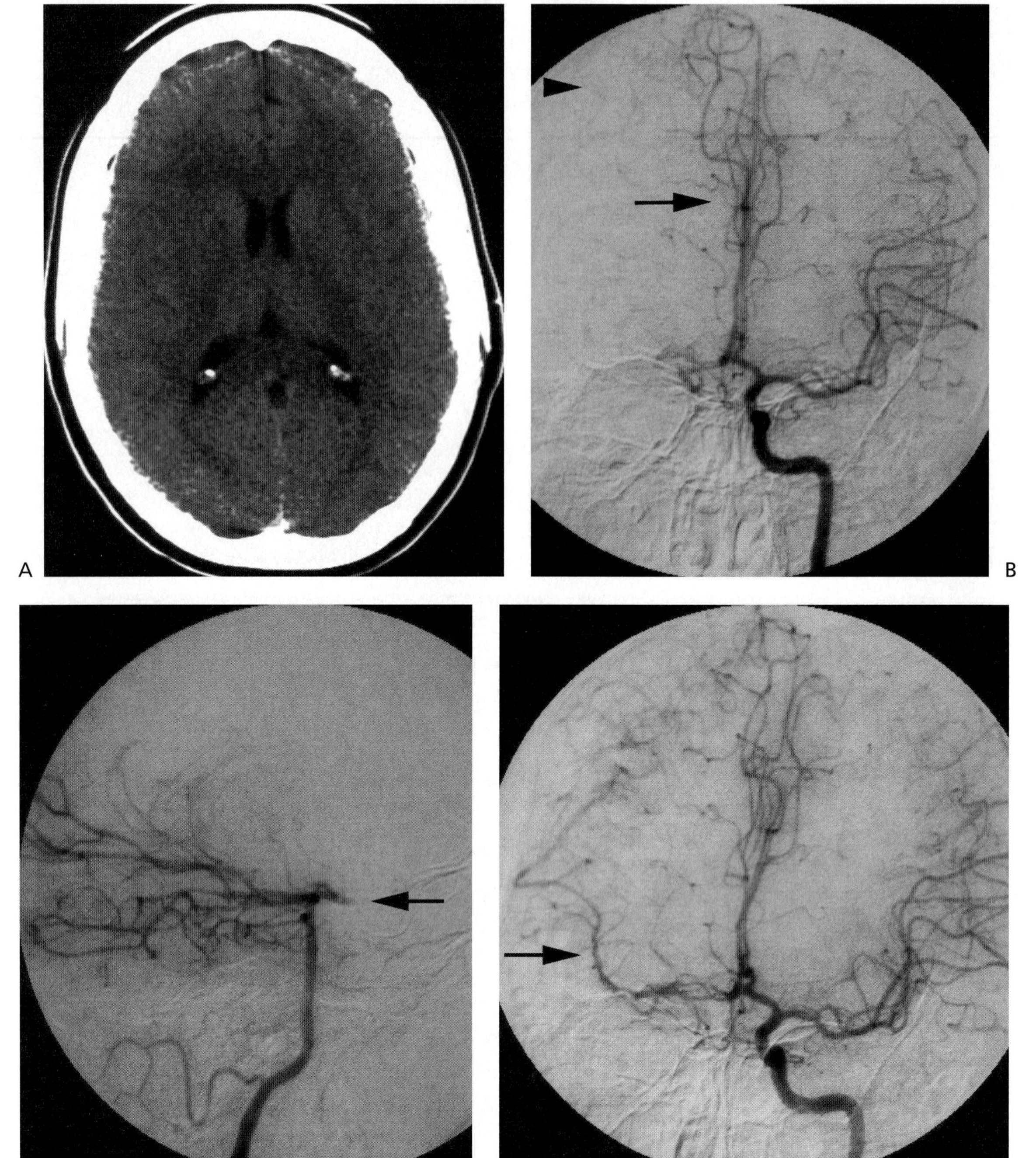

FIGURE 4-12. This 34-year-old right-handed woman sought treatment for an acute onset of left hemiparesis. **A:** The initial CT scan demonstrated no evidence of hemorrhage or infarct. The initial right CCA angiogram demonstrated complete occlusion of the ICA 1 cm distal to the bifurcation. **B:** The left ICA angiogram showed cross filling of the right ACA *(arrow)* but no filling of the right MCA, and moderate leptomeningeal collaterals are noted *(arrowhead)*. **C:** The left vertebral artery angiogram, lateral projection, demonstrates occlusion of the large right PCoA *(arrow)*. A microcatheter was navigated through the occluded right ICA and used to thrombolyse the right MCA. Following thrombolysis, the right MCA *(arrow)* filled from a combination of collateral flow from the left ICA via the ACoA **(D)** and the basilar artery via the right PCoA **(E)**. *(Figure continues.)*

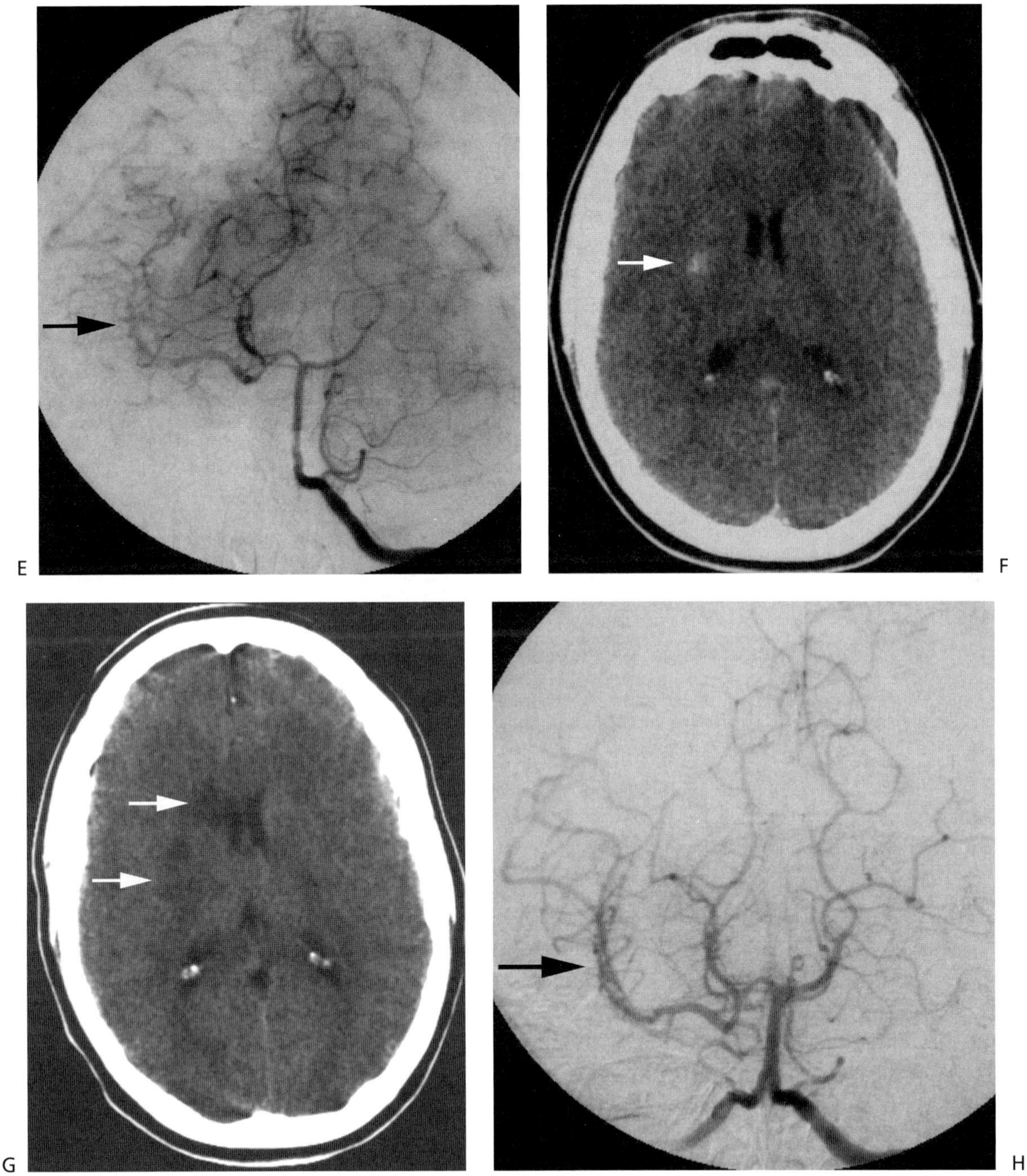

FIGURE 4-12. *Continued.* **F:** The patient's strength improved following the procedure and a repeat CT scan demonstrated no evidence of infarct, with high attenuation in the right basal ganglia *(arrow)* thought to be due to staining of contrast used during the preceding angiogram. The patient did well for 3 days until she had an acute worsening of her left hemiparesis. **G:** A repeat CT scan now showed evidence of infarct in the right caudate and basal ganglia *(arrows).* **H:** A vertebral angiogram demonstrated excellent flow in the right MCA *(arrow)* from the posterior circulation and the minimal residual thrombus in the distal M1 had cleared. *(Figure continues.)*

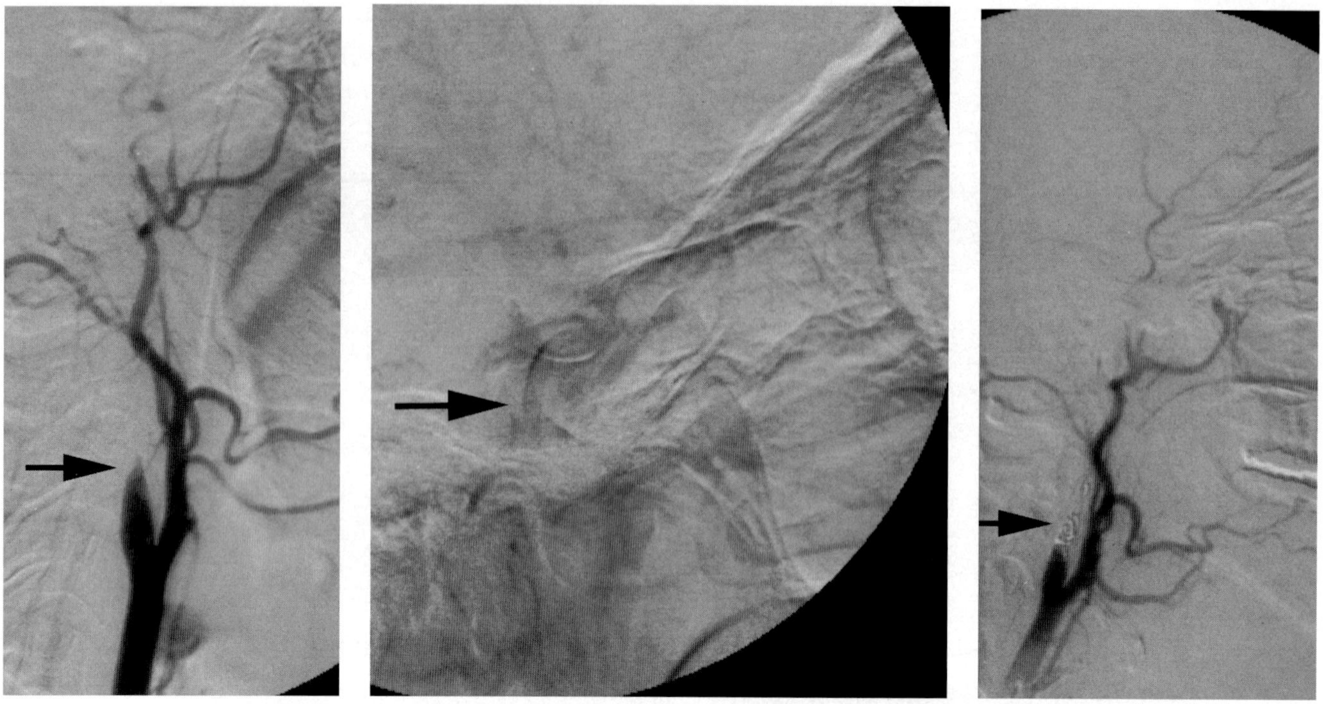

I,J K

FIGURE 4-12. *Continued.* **I:** The right CCA angiogram showed that the ICA appeared to be occluded *(arrow).* **J:** However, with close examination of the late arterial phase, extremely slow flow was identified through the upper cervical and petrous segment of the ICA *(arrow).* This type of flow through the nearly occluded ICA poses a significant risk for embolic phenomena, which were felt to be responsible for her recent neurologic deficit. **K:** Because she had excellent collateral flow from the posterior circulation, the ICA was occluded at its origin with multiple platinum coils *(arrow).*

exit through the redundant venous system. A study performed on ten baboons demonstrated a positive effect on somatosensory evoked potentials, stroke scores, and infarct size [63]. To maximize the benefit of RTN, it was instituted after 1 hour of ischemia. Future studies will address the ability of RTN to reduce or prevent stroke within several hours following ischemia. This may be one method which could be used to improve outcome and extend the time window during which thrombolytic agents or other therapies could be used to recanalize the occluded artery. However, most centers that would be able to perform RTN would also have access to intraarterial therapy (e.g., thrombolytic agents, mechanical thrombectomy), and a combined application might be more beneficial than arterial thrombolysis alone. In addition, the safety of RTN under conditions of thrombolysis has not yet been determined, because RTN is not a permanent treatment and arterial thrombolysis may still be necessary for definitive treatment.

CONCLUSION

The purpose of this chapter was to discuss the endovascular treatment strategies that can be used in the treatment of acute stroke. At the present time the mainstay of treatment is intraarterial or intravenous thrombolytic agents with t-PA. Much, however, is left to be refined. Techniques of delivery and dosing regimens are still under debate. In addition, improvements in imaging may help to better triage patients to intravenous or intraarterial treatment, and divert those with a poor response and high risk to some other treatment.

Other methods are also being developed to accomplish thrombus removal without the use of these agents, including mechanical clot disruption, laser thrombectomy, suction thrombectomy, and endovascular thrombectomy devices. In certain cases, a multimodality endovascular approach is required, which may involve other procedures, such as angioplasty, stenting, therapeutic occlusion, and retrograde transvenous perfusion.

With further technological advancements the safety and efficacy of these treatment options will only improve. We are getting closer to having catheter-based therapies which will allow for the rapid removal of thrombus from the intracranial circulation and the development of supportive therapies to maintain parent artery flow and prevent further embolic events.

REFERENCES

1. Brott T, Bogousslavsky J. Treatment of acute ischemic stroke. *N Engl J Med* 2000;343:710–722.

2. Anthony DC, Perry VH. Stroke: a double edged sword for cleaving clots? *Curr Biol* 1998;8:R274–R277.
3. Clark WM, Wissman S, Albers GW, et al. Recombinant tissue-type plasminogen activator (alteplase) for ischemic stroke 3 to 5 hours after symptom onset. The ATLANTIS Study: a randomized controlled trial. *JAMA* 1999;282:2019–2026.
4. ECASS II Investigators. Randomized double-blind placebo-controlled trial of thrombolytic therapy with intravenous alteplase in acute ischaemic stroke (ECASS II). *Lancet* 1998;352: 1245–1251.
5. Hacke W, Kaste M, Fieschi C, et al. Intravenous thrombolysis with recombinant tissue plasminogen activator for acute hemispheric stroke. *N Engl J Med* 1995;333:1581–1587.
6. Donnan GA, Davis SM, Chambers BR, et al. Streptokinase for acute ischemic stroke with relationship to time of administration. *JAMA* 1996;276:961–966.
7. The Multicenter Acute Stroke Europe Study Group. Thrombolytic therapy with streptokinase in acute ischemic stroke. *N Engl J Med* 1996;335:145–150.
8. The Multicenter Acute Stroke Trial—Italy (MAST-1) Group. Randomized controlled trial of streptokinase, aspirin and combination of both in treatment of acute ischemic stroke. *Lancet* 1995; 346:1509–1514.
9. Zeumer H, Freitag HJ, Zanella F, et al. Local intra-arterial fibrinolytic therapy in patients with stroke: urokinase versus recombinant tissue plasminogen activator (r-TPA). *Neuroradiology* 1993;35:159–162.
10. Chambers BR, Norris JW, Shurvell BL, et al. Prognosis of acute stroke. *Neurology* 1987;37:221–225.
11. Furlan AJ, Higashida R, Wechsler L, et al. PROACT II: Recombinant prourokinase (r-proUK) in acute cerebral thromboembolism: initial trial results—the PROACT II Investigators. Paper presented at: The 24th American Heart Association International Conference on Stroke and Cerebral Circulation; February 4, 1999; Nashville, TN.
12. Hacke W, Zeumer H, Ferbert A, et al. Intra-arterial thrombolytic therapy improves outcome in patients with acute vertebrobasilar occlusive disease. *Stroke* 1988;19:1216–1222.
13. National Institute of Neurological Disorders and Stroke—rt-PA Stroke Study Group. Tissue plasminogen activator for acute ischemic stroke. *N Engl J Med* 1995;333:1581–1587.
14. Chiu D, Krieger D, Vollar-Cordova C, et al. Intravenous tissue plasminogen activator for acute ischemic stroke—feasibility, safety, and efficacy in the first year of clinical practice. *Stroke* 1998;29:18–22.
15. Grond M, Stenzel C, Schmulling S, et al. Early intravenous thrombolysis for acute ischemic stroke in a community-based approach. *Stroke* 1998;29:1544–1549.
16. Zweifler RM, Brody D, Graves GC, et al. Intravenous t-PA for acute ischemic stroke: therapeutic yield of stroke code system. *Neurology* 1998;50:501–503.
17. Katzan IL, Furlan AJ, Lloyd LE, et al. Use of tissue-type plasminogen activator for acute ischemic stroke. The Cleveland area experience. *JAMA* 2000;283:1151–1158.
18. Sasaki O, Shigekazu T, Koike T, et al. Fibrinolytic therapy for acute embolic stroke: intravenous, intracarotid, and intra-arterial local approaches. *Neurosurgery* 1995;36:246–252.
19. Lewandowski CA, Frankel M, Tomsick TA, et al. EMS Bridging Trial investigators: combined intravenous and intra-arterial r-TPA versus intra-arterial therapy of acute ischemic stroke. *Stroke* 1999;30:2598–2605.
20. Mori E, Tabuchi M, Yoshida T, et al. Intracarotid urokinase with thromboembolic occlusion of the middle cerebral artery. *Stroke* 1988;19:802–812.
21. del Zoppo GJ, Ferbert A, Otis S, et al. Local intra-arterial fibrinolytic therapy in acute carotid territory stroke. A pilot study. *Stroke* 1988;19:307–313.
22. Barnwell SL, Nesbit GM, Clark WM. Local thrombolytic therapy for cerebrovascular disease: current Oregon Health Sciences University experience (July 1991 through April 1995). *J Vasc Interv Radiol* 1995;6:78S–82S.
23. Wijdicks EFM, Nichols DA, Thielen KR, et al. Intra-arterial thrombolysis in acute basilar artery thromboembolism: the initial Mayo Clinic experience. *Mayo Clin Proc* 1997;72:1005–1013.
24. Jansen O, von Kummer R, Forsting M, et al. Thrombolytic therapy in acute occlusion of the intracranial internal carotid artery bifurcation. *AJNR Am J Neuroradiol* 1995;16:1977–1986.
25. Casto L, Caverni L, Camerlingo M, et al. Intra-arterial thrombolysis in acute ischaemic stroke. Experience with a superselective catheter embedded in the clot. *J Neurol Neurosurg Psychiatry* 1996;60:667–670.
26. del Zoppo GJ, Higashida RT, Furlan AJ, et al. PROACT: a phase II randomized trial of recombinant pro-urokinase by direct arterial delivery in acute middle cerebral artery stroke. PROACT Investigators. Prolyse in acute cerebral thromboembolism. *Stroke* 1998;29:4–11.
27. Pessin MS, del Zoppo GL, Estol CG. Thrombolytic agent in the treatment of stroke. *Clin Neuropharmacol* 1990;13:271–289.
28. Pannell R, Burewich V. Prourokinase: a study of its stability in plasma and of a mechanism for its selective fibrinolytic effect. *Blood* 1986;67:1215–1223.
29. Hoylaerts M, Rigken DC, Lignen HR, et al. Kinetics of the activation of plasminogen by human plasminogen activator. Role of fibrin. *J Biol Chem* 1982;257:2912–2919.
30. Ouriel K, Katzen B, Mewissen M, et al. Reteplase in the treatment of peripheral arterial and venous occlusions: a pilot study. *J Vasc Interv Radiol* 2000;11:849–854.
31. Connors JJ, Wojak JC. Current directions in emergency stroke therapy. In: Connors JJ, Wojak JC, eds. *Interventional neuroradiology*. Philadelphia: WB Saunders, 1999.
32. Working Party on Thrombolysis in the Management of Limb Ischemia. Thrombolysis in the management of lower limb peripheral arterial occlusion—a consensus document. *Am J Cardiol* 1998;81:207–218.
33. Emergency Management of Stroke (EMS) Investigators. Combined intraarterial and intravenous t-PA for stroke. Paper presented at: The 22nd International Joint Conference on Stroke and Cerebral Circulation; February 8, 1997; Anaheim, CA.
34. Qureshi AI, Suri FK, Shatla AA, et al. Intraarterial recombinant tissue plasminogen activator for ischemia stroke: an accelerating dosing regimen. *Neurosurgery* 2000;47:473–479.
35. Atkinson RP. Ancrod in the treatment of acute ischaemic stroke. *Drugs* 1997;54:100–108.
36. Goklaney AK, Murphy JD, Hillegass WB. Abciximab therapy in percutaneous intervention: economic issues in the United States. *Eur Heart J* 1998;19:D52–58.
37. Abciximab in acute ischemic stroke: a randomized, double-blind, placebo-controlled, dose-escalation study. The Abciximab in Ischemic Stroke Investigators. *Stroke* 2000;31:601–609.
38. Barnwell S, Clark W, Nguyen T, et al. Safety and efficacy of delayed intraarterial urokinase therapy with mechanical clot disruption for thromboembolic stroke. *AJNR Am J Neuroradiol* 1994;15:1817–1822.
39. NINDS Investigators. Tissue plasminogen activator for acute ischemic stroke. The National Institute of Neurological Disorders and Stroke rt-PA Stroke Study Group. *N Engl J Med* 1995;333: 1581–1587.
40. NINDS t-PA Stroke Study Group. Intracerebral hemorrhage after intravenous t-PA therapy for ischemic stroke. *Stroke* 1997; 28:2109–2128.
41. National Institute of Neurological Disorders and Stroke. rt-PA Stroke Study Group. Generalized efficacy of t-PA for acute stroke subgroup analysis of the NINDS t-PA stroke trial. *Stroke* 1997; 26:2119–2125.

42. Hacke W, Kaste M, Fieschi C, et al. Intravenous thrombolysis with recombinant tissue plasminogen activator for acute hemispheric stroke, the European Cooperative Acute Stroke Study (ECASS). *JAMA* 1995;274:1017–1024.
43. Barber PA, Demchuk AM, Zhang J, et al. Validity and reliability of a quantitative computed tomography score in predicting outcome of hyperacute stroke before thrombolytic therapy. ASPECTS Study Group. Alberta Stroke Programme Early CT Score. *Lancet* 2000;355:1670–1674.
44. Theron J, Courtheoux P, Casasco A, et al. Local intraarterial fibrinolysis in the carotid territory. *AJNR Am J Neuroradiol* 1989; 10:753–765.
45. Fiorelli M, Bastianello S, von Kummer R, et al. Hemorrhagic transformation within 36 hours of a cerebral infarct: relationships with early clinical deterioration and 3-month outcome in the European Cooperative Acute Stroke Study I (ECASS I) cohort. *Stroke* 1999;30:2280–2284.
46. Nesbit G, Clark W, O'Neill O, et al. Intracranial intraarterial thrombolysis facilitated by microcatheter navigation through an occluded cervical internal carotid artery. *J Neurosurg* 1996;84: 387–392.
47. Ueda T, Hatakeyama T, Kohno K, et al. Endovascular treatment for acute thrombotic occlusion of the middle cerebral artery: local intra-arterial thrombolysis combined with percutaneous transluminal angioplasty. *Neuroradiology* 1997;39:99–104.
48. Higashida RT, Tsai FY, Halbach VV, et al. Interventional neurovascular techniques in the treatment of stroke—state-of-the-art therapy. *J Intern Med* 1995;237:105–115.
49. Ueda, T, Sakaki S, Ichiro N, et al. Angioplasty after intra-arterial thrombolysis for acute occlusion of intracranial arteries. *Stroke* 1998;29:2568–2574.
50. Spearman MP, Jungreis CA, Wechsler LR. Angioplasty of the occluded internal carotid artery. *AJNR Am J Neuroradiol* 1995; 16:1791–1796.
51. Grundfest W, Litvack F, Forrester J, et al. Laser ablation of human atherosclerotic plaque without adjacent tissue injury. *J Am Coll Cardiol* 1985;5:929–933.
52. Gillen G, Elliot A, Findlay I, et al. Recanalization of arteries by laser radiation. *J Med Eng Technol* 1984;8:215–217.
53. Lee G, Ikeda R, Theis J, et al. Acute and chronic complications of laser angioplasty: vascular wall damage and formation of aneurysms in the atherosclerotic rabbit. *Am J Cardiol* 1984;53: 290–293.
54. Sharafuddin M, Hicks M, Jenson M, et al. Rheolytic thrombectomy with use of the AngioJet-F105 catheter: preclinical evaluation of safety. *J Vasc Interv Radiol* 1997;8:939–945.
55. Silva JA, Ramee SR, Collins TJ, et al. Rheolytic thrombectomy in the treatment of acute limb-threatening ischemia: immediate results and six-month follow-up of multicenter AngioJet registry. Possis Peripheral AngioJet Study AngioJet Investigators. *Cathet Cardiovasc Diagn* 1998;45:386–393.
56. Nakagawa Y, Matsuo S, Yokoi H, et al. Stenting after thrombectomy with the AngioJet catheter for acute myocardial infarction. *Cathet Cardiovasc Diagn* 1998;43:327–330.
57. Dick A, Neuerburg J, Schmidt-Rode T, et al. Stenting after thrombectomy with the AngioJet catheter for acute myocardial infarction. *Cathet Cardiovasc Diagn* 1998;33:91–97.
58. Mathie AG, Bell SD, Saibil EA. Mechanical thromboembolectomy in acute embolic peripheral arterial occlusions with use of AngioJet Rapid Thrombectomy System. *J Vasc Interv Radiol* 1999;10:583–590.
59. Nakagawa Y, Matsuo S, Kimura T, et al. Thrombectomy with AngioJet catheter in native coronary arteries for patients with acute or recent myocardial infarction. *Am J Cardiol* 1999;83: 994–999.
60. Vesely TM, William D, Weiss M, et al. Comparison of the angiojet rheolytic catheter to surgical thrombectomy for the treatment of thrombosed hemodialysis grafter: Peripheral AngioJet Clinical Trial. *J Vasc Interv Radiol* 1999;10:1195–1205.
61. Bellon RJ, Putman CM, Budzik RF, et al. Rheolytic thrombectomy of the occluded internal carotid artery in the setting of acute ischemic stroke. *AJNR Am J Neuroradiol* 2001;22: 526–530.
62. Liu AY, Paulsen RD, Marcellus ML, et al. Long-term outcomes after carotid stent placement for treatment of carotid artery dissection (technique assessments). *Neurosurgery* 1999;45: 1368–1373.
63. Frazee JG, Luo X, Luan G, et al. Retrograde transvenous neuroperfusion: a back door treatment for stroke. *Stroke* 1998;29: 1912–1916.

Endovascular and Percutaneous Therapy of the Brain and Spine, edited by Michael P. Marks and Huy M. Do.
Lippincott Williams & Wilkins, Philadelphia © 2002.

5

INTRACRANIAL ANEURYSMS: OVERVIEW

MARCUS A. STOODLEY
BRYCE K.A. WEIR

An aneurysm is a dilation of any vascular structure, although arteries are far more commonly affected than veins. The term *aneurysm* is derived from the Greek *aneurysma,* meaning "a widening" [1]. Although aneurysms are relatively common in extracranial locations such as the aorta and splenic artery, those in the cerebral circulation are particularly sinister because they often affect young people and cause catastrophic loss of neurologic function. The large arteries at the base of the brain are predominantly affected, perhaps because of the unique morphology of arteries in this location, including a thinner wall, lack of external elastic lamina, and lack of surrounding supporting tissue. Aneurysms were initially thought to have a congenital etiology, but it is now recognized that the vast majority of cerebral aneurysms are a result of degenerative changes of the vessel wall.

Aneurysms of systemic arteries (often traumatic or syphilitic) were described from the time of Galen, but intracranial aneurysms were not recognized until the eighteenth century [2]. Direct surgical treatment of intracranial aneurysms was pioneered in 1933 by Dott, who applied strips of muscle to a ruptured aneurysm. The birth of modern aneurysm surgery occurred in 1937, when Dandy placed a silver clip across the neck of a posterior communicating artery aneurysm [2]. Aneurysm surgery was refined by the introduction of the operating microscope in the 1960s, careful microanatomical studies of the brain vasculature, and the development of reliable aneurysm clips. As a result of these efforts, the outcome after subarachnoid hemorrhage (SAH) is now determined largely by the severity of the initial hemorrhage and the patient's neurologic condition, rather than limitations of aneurysm obliteration techniques. Further refinement is occurring as endovascular therapy is being embraced as an additional technique, having already proved extremely useful in the treatment of difficult aneurysms. The refinement of biologically active detachable coils is likely to increase the use of endovascular techniques as a treatment for many aneurysms that were previously treated very successfully with surgical techniques.

M.A. Stoodley: Institute of Neurological Sciences, Prince of Wales Hospital, University of New South Wales, Randwick, New South Wales, Australia.
B.K.A. Weir: Departments of Surgery and Neurology, University of Chicago, Chicago, Illinois.

BACKGROUND

Epidemiology of Aneurysms and Subarachnoid Hemorrhage

Trauma is the most common cause of SAH, although the clinical picture is quite different from aneurysmal hemorrhage and the SAH tends to have a relatively minor influence on outcome. Aneurysmal rupture accounts for approximately 80% of nontraumatic SAH cases. Saccular aneurysms are by far the commonest type, although fusiform, dissecting, infectious, and traumatic aneurysms also cause SAH. Other causes of SAH include arteriovenous malformations (AVMs), arteritis, tumors, and cocaine use. Ruptured saccular aneurysms account for up to 15% of all strokes [3].

The reported annual incidence of SAH varies from 5 to 16 per 100,000 population, with the highest rates recorded in Japan and Finland [3–5]. In the United States each year there are approximately 25,000 cases of saccular aneurysmal SAH, which is less than 0.01% of the population. On average 18,000 of these patients die or remain disabled from the hemorrhage [6]. Autopsy, clinical, and angiographic studies have been used to estimate the prevalence of cerebral aneurysms, with reported rates varying from 0.3% to 9% of the population. A representative figure is approximately 2.4% [7,8]. It has been estimated that approximately one-half of the aneurysms will rupture at some stage.

There are gender, geographic, and racial variations in the prevalence and incidence of aneurysms and SAH. There is a female predominance of ruptured aneurysms, particularly with increasing age. Aneurysmal SAH occurs most frequently during the fifth and sixth decades of life, with the average age of onset approximately 51 years [9]. Higher rates of SAH are reported from Finland and Japan, while lower rates are reported from Africa, China, India, and the Middle East. It is not clear whether these lower rates are due to differences in health care, age distributions, or to true geographic differences. The roles of dietary and environmental factors are unknown. Compared with whites, blacks have approximately twice the risk of developing SAH [10]. There is no convincing evidence of seasonal or meteorologic influences on the incidence of SAH [9].

A familial tendency to form aneurysms is seen in a small proportion of patients. There is a particularly high incidence in Finland, where one study detected aneurysms in 12% of first-degree relatives of patients with SAH [11]. Patients with familial aneurysms tend to be younger, and the aneurysms are smaller when they rupture [12]. One-half of the familial aneurysms are on the middle cerebral artery. In most cases of familial aneurysms there appears to be a dominant pattern of inheritance. Multiple aneurysms are seen more commonly in patients with familial aneurysms [13].

Conditions Predisposing to Aneurysm Formation

Medical conditions associated with an increased risk of aneurysm formation include the general vascular risk factors hypertension, smoking, and a family history of stroke. Conditions with a proved or suspected increased risk of aneurysm formation include adult polycystic kidney disease, polycystic liver disease, sickle cell anemia, Marfan syndrome, pseudoxanthoma elasticum, fibromuscular dysplasia, moyamoya disease, Ehlers-Danlos syndrome type IV, tuberous sclerosis, hereditary hemorrhagic telangiectasia, Anderson-Fabry disease, and coarctation of the aorta [9,14, 15]. Up to 40% of patients with adult polycystic kidney disease harbor aneurysms, and as many as 10% will suffer an aneurysmal SAH during their lifetimes. These patients tend to have systemic hypertension, but it is believed that a genetically determined defect in the vascular wall accounts for aneurysm formation rather than hypertension being the underlying cause [16,17]. There is a male predominance, an increased frequency of middle cerebral artery aneurysms, and occurrence of SAH at a younger age when compared with other patients with aneurysms. The pathogenesis of aneurysms in patients with sickle cell disease is thought to be adhesion of abnormal erythrocytes to endothelial cells, with subsequent inflammation and injury to the vessel wall. Hemodynamic stress from the abnormal blood rheology could also be a factor. Appropriate fluid management in patients with sickle cell anemia is critical to avoid sludging [18]. An increased risk of SAH in patients with systemic lupus erythematosus has been reported. The inflammatory angiitis causes fibrinoid necrosis and destruction of elastic tissue, which predispose to vascular ectasia and occasionally saccular aneurysms. Aneurysms in patients with acute arteritis are usually not saccular and tend to be distally located and multiple [2].

Saccular aneurysms are present in up to 15% of patients with AVMs. These lesions are classified according to whether they arise from a feeding vessel, within the AVM nidus, or on unrelated arteries [19–21]. Intranidal aneurysms are associated with a higher risk of hemorrhage than AVMs without such an aneurysm. Patients with feeding-artery aneurysms suffer hemorrhage from the aneurysm approximately as frequently as with hemorrhage from the AVM. The formation of new aneurysms has been documented in patients with AVMs [22]. It is assumed that the high incidence of aneurysms in association with AVMs is related to hemodynamic stresses from high flow, although a common inherited vascular wall defect is another possibility.

The role of pregnancy as a risk factor for the formation and rupture of aneurysms is controversial. There is some evidence that the incidence of aneurysmal SAH is higher during pregnancy and the puerperium, with up to a fivefold increase being reported [23]. The hormonal and physiologic changes of pregnancy have been implicated in such cases.

Perhaps the most common condition associated with the development of cerebral aneurysms is congenital variation in the arrangement of the circle of Willis. For example, the majority of patients with anterior communicating artery aneurysms have asymmetric anterior cerebral arteries, and the aneurysm arises from the side of the larger artery in 95% of the cases [24].

CLASSIFICATION

Aneurysms are classified according to their size, location, and morphological and pathologic characteristics. These classifications are useful when assessing the natural history, appropriate treatment, and prognosis of each aneurysm type. Grading scales for assessing the clinical severity of hemorrhage have also been developed and these will be discussed below.

Classification by Size

Aneurysms are generally classified as small, large, or giant. Although this usually refers to saccular aneurysms, the same classification can be applied to other types. Most authors refer to small aneurysms as those with a maximal diameter of less than 10 mm; large, 10 to 25 mm; and giant, larger than 25 mm. Others have argued that the management of a 20-mm aneurysm does not differ from that of a 26-mm aneurysm and therefore include 20 mm aneurysms in the giant category.

Morphological and Etiologic Classification

Saccular Aneurysms

Saccular aneurysms (Fig. 5-1A) have the highest prevalence and incidence of all the morphological types. They form as

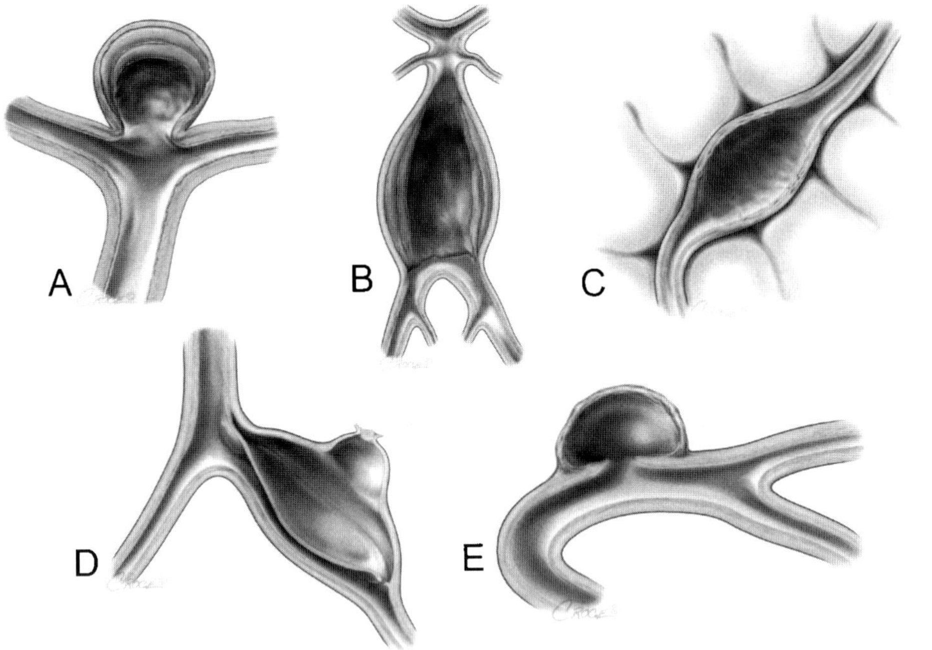

FIGURE 5-1. Schematic diagrams illustrating the morphologic classification of aneurysms: saccular **(A)**, fusiform **(B)**, infectious **(C)**, dissecting **(D)**, and false **(E)**.

outpouchings of the arterial wall, commonly at branching points, and their generally spherical shape has led to the synonym *berry* aneurysms. The wall of a saccular aneurysm is different from the wall of the parent artery. There is fragmentation and loss of the internal elastic lamina, loss of medial smooth muscle, and intimal proliferation [25]. The media becomes fibrosed, so that the histologic appearance of an aneurysmal wall is of intima and adventitia separated by a layer of fibrous tissue. The change from a normal arterial wall to the abnormal aneurysmal wall occurs abruptly at the aneurysmal neck, where on histologic study the internal elastic lamina can be seen to terminate. The parent vessels may show changes of atherosclerosis and even calcification, but in general the arterial wall adjacent to an aneurysm is relatively normal. Larger aneurysms develop intraluminal thrombosis and atherosclerotic changes and calcification in their walls, sometimes with neovascularization and organization of intraluminal hematoma. The neck of a saccular aneurysm usually remains a distinct outpouching from the parent artery. However, the neck in large and giant aneurysms sometimes encompasses the majority of the parent vessel, making the distinction between a saccular and fusiform aneurysm difficult.

Fusiform Aneurysms

In contrast to the outpouchings that characterize saccular aneurysms, fusiform aneurysms (see Fig. 5-1B) are dilations of an arterial segment, with circumferential involvement of the wall. The involved segment of artery can also be elongated. The term *dolichoectasia* has been used to describe tortuous and serpentine aneurysms of this type. Fusiform aneurysms are the most common aneurysms found in the general circulation, but they are less frequent than saccular aneurysms in the cerebral circulation. The vertebral and basilar arteries are the most common intracranial locations for these aneurysms. The usual underlying pathology is atherosclerotic change, with deposition of cholesterol, thickening of the media and intima, ulceration and hemorrhage, and intraluminal thrombosis. In some cases, the underlying pathology is weakening of the arterial wall by medial necrosis or degeneration of the internal elastic lamina, such as in Marfan syndrome. Thrombus commonly forms within the lumen of fusiform aneurysms. Perforating branches of the involved segments are often involved. Detection of a fusiform aneurysm in a patient under age 60 should raise suspicion about a nonatherosclerotic cause. Dissecting, infectious, and traumatic aneurysms can have a fusiform shape, but these aneurysms are classified separately.

Dissecting Aneurysms

Development of a tear in the intima allows blood under arterial pressure to force apart the layers of the arterial wall, forming a false lumen. Such dissections are usually located between layers of the media or between the media and the adventitia. The dissection may end blindly, rupture back into the lumen, or break through the adventitia into the subarachnoid space (see Fig. 5-1D). Although dissecting aneurysms may occur in previously normal arteries, there is often an underlying pathology such as Marfan syndrome, atherosclerosis, or fibromuscular dysplasia. Dissecting aneurysms affect extracranial and intracranial arteries.

Most extracranial dissecting aneurysms are of traumatic origin. The trauma can be relatively minor, such as from chiropractic manipulation. Other causes include atherosclerosis, fibromuscular dysplasia, and connective tissue disorders. Rupture of extracranial dissecting aneurysms is rare; the clinical picture is usually related to thromboembolic phenomena, or less often from hemodynamic consequences of stenosis or occlusion of the artery. Dissections of the extracranial carotid arteries usually do not extend beyond the skull base.

Intracranial dissections more commonly involve the posterior circulation than the anterior circulation. Collagen diseases are sometimes implicated, although hypertension and atherosclerosis are the most common causes [26]. Intracranial dissections are less commonly related to trauma [27]. Usually the pathology is similar to that of extracranial dissections, involving disruption of the intima with creation of a false lumen extending through the media and disruption of the adventitia in patients who have hemorrhage [28]. Occasionally a dissection originates as a spontaneous hemorrhage into an atherosclerotic plaque without disruption of the intima [26].

Infectious Aneurysms

The term *mycotic aneurysm* refers strictly to fungal infections and has been replaced by the more generic description *infectious,* because these aneurysms (see Fig. 5-1C) are usually the result of bacterial infection of the arterial wall. The most common organisms are *Staphylococcus* and *Streptococcus* species. Infection weakens the wall by destruction of the elastic lamina and media. Fusiform expansion of the arterial wall follows, although a saccular morphology is occasionally seen. Histologic study reveals acute or chronic inflammatory changes (or both) in the wall, with destruction of the intima and internal elastic lamina, necrosis of smooth muscle cells, and thrombosis. When the macroscopic appearances suggest a saccular anatomy, this is deceptive because there is usually no well-defined neck as there is with saccular aneurysms of degenerative etiology. Usually there is a systemic source of infection and bacterial emboli, such as bacterial endocarditis. Emboli tend to reach distal branches of the cerebral circulation and most commonly affect the middle cerebral artery branches, which receive the greatest proportion of the cerebral blood flow [29]. Approximately 5% of patients with endocarditis will develop infectious aneurysms. Intravenous drug abusers have an increasing risk of infectious aneurysms, and in these patients multiple organisms are often involved. Infectious aneurysms are commonly multiple. Fungal aneurysms are much less common and tend to involve the larger proximal arteries. They are commonly associated with thrombosis and cerebral ischemia. Direct invasion of arteries from intracranial infection, such as fungal meningitis, cavernous sinus thrombophlebitis, osteomyelitis, or empyema, is an uncommon source of infection for aneurysms.

False Aneurysms

A false aneurysm (see Fig. 5-1E) or pseudoaneurysm occurs when a vessel ruptures and the resulting hematoma and surrounding connective tissue form the wall of an "arterial expansion." The wall of such false aneurysms does not contain any normal elements of the arterial wall. Trauma (including iatrogenic vascular trauma) is the most common cause, and these aneurysms are sometimes referred to as traumatic aneurysms. Although a saccular appearance is common on angiography, there is generally no well-defined neck. These lesions are extremely friable and have a high risk of rupture. Vessel laceration can occur directly as a result of penetrating or missile injury and involve any of the intracranial arteries. Vessels particularly susceptible to disruption with closed head injury include the distal anterior cerebral artery from trauma against the free edge of the falx cerebri, the posterior cerebral artery injured against the free edge of the tentorium, the middle cerebral artery against the sphenoid ridge, and the internal carotid artery in or near the base of the skull related to a fracture.

Other Aneurysms

The angiographic appearance of a snakelike vascular channel through an aneurysm has been referred to as a *serpentine aneurysm.* These are usually originally saccular, although sometimes fusiform, aneurysms that have largely thrombosed, with a residual or recanalized lumen that gives the characteristic angiographic appearance.

Rare metastatic neoplastic aneurysms occur predominantly in peripheral internal carotid artery branches and result from infiltration of the vessel wall by hematogenously disseminated neoplastic cells. The internal elastic lamina and media are invaded, which leads to occlusion, aneurysm formation, and SAH. The lesions are often multiple and fusiform. Neoplasms associated with aneurysms include bronchogenic carcinoma, choriocarcinoma, and cardiac myxoma [30].

Fusiform aneurysms have been reported after radiation and intrathecal radioactive gold therapy. They tend to be midline, multiple, and have a high risk of enlargement and hemorrhage. Histopathologic examination reveals segmental necrosis and atherosclerotic changes, with fragmentation and loss of the internal elastic lamina.

Infundibula are small dilations at the origin of intracranial arteries, with the branch artery continuing from the dome. Approximately 7% of adults will have an infundibulum detectable on angiography [9]. Histologic examination reveals thinning or absence of the media and occasionally absence of the elastic lamina. They are most common at the origin of the posterior communicating artery. Although they rarely do, infundibula can rupture and can develop into aneurysms.

Classification by Location

The majority of saccular aneurysms are located at branching points of the large vessels of the circle of Willis. By convention, anatomical classifications of aneurysms refer to the branch of an artery where the aneurysm arises. An aneurysm arising from the internal carotid artery at the origin of the posterior communicating artery aneurysm is therefore referred to as a *posterior communicating artery aneurysm.* The rare aneurysms actually arising from the posterior communicating artery are called *true* posterior communicating artery aneurysms. When aneurysms are grouped together, they are referred to by the name of the parent artery. *Internal carotid artery aneurysms* therefore include all aneurysms of the internal carotid artery, regardless of the branch at which they arise. Aneurysms of the internal carotid, anterior cerebral, and middle cerebral artery and their branches are further grouped as *anterior circulation aneurysms,* whereas aneurysms of the vertebrobasilar system and its branches are referred to as *posterior circulation aneurysms.*

Aneurysms of the proximal intracranial internal carotid artery have been classified as *paraclinoid* aneurysms and subclassified as *carotid-ophthalmic, superior hypophyseal,* and *posterior carotid wall aneurysms.* Further important anatomical features of aneurysms include the direction of projection, the presence of loculations or blebs, and involvement of major branches in the aneurysmal neck.

Anatomical Distribution of Aneurysms

Over 90% of saccular aneurysms are on the vessels of the anterior circulation, distributed as follows: internal carotid artery, 26% to 30%; middle cerebral artery, 22% to 28%; and anterior cerebral artery, 40%. Up to 8% to 10% of saccular aneurysms involve arteries of the vertebrobasilar system [6,31]. Multiple aneurysms are detected in up to one-third of patients. Risk factors for multiplicity include hypertension, cigarette smoking, family history of cerebrovascular disease, female sex, and postmenopausal state [32].

There are differences in the distribution of aneurysms according to gender [2]. Of aneurysms arising from the internal carotid artery, two-thirds are in females and one-third are in males. In contrast, almost 60% of aneurysms of the anterior cerebral artery or anterior communicating artery occur in males and 40% occur in females. There is no difference between the sexes in the frequency of middle cerebral artery aneurysms.

PATHOPHYSIOLOGY

Saccular Aneurysm Formation and Rupture

Saccular aneurysms are no longer considered congenital in origin. Possible mechanisms of formation include oscillatory shear stress to the endothelium, enzymatic destruction of the arterial wall, immature collagen formation, or collagen deficiency [33]. There is good evidence that aneurysms form from hemodynamic stress, which is maximal at arterial bifurcations [33]. The pressure exerted at the apex of a bifurcation is much greater than on other parts of the wall. Study of the fluid dynamics and forces involved has proved difficult, partly because blood is a non-Newtonian fluid. However, blood flow in large and medium arteries is usually laminar, while turbulence occurs at bifurcations. The likelihood of flow within a tube being turbulent rather than laminar can be predicted by the Reynolds number. At arterial bifurcations there is a reduction in artery radius and blood flow velocity, and an increase in total cross-sectional area. This has the effect of lowering the Reynolds number from approximately 2,300 to 400, making turbulent flow more likely [33]. It has been postulated that the vibratory forces resulting from the hemodynamics and turbulence at arterial bifurcations cause large shear stresses against the endothelial surface and the underlying elastic lamina. Degeneration of the elastic lamina from these forces would weaken the wall at the point of the bifurcation [33]. This weakened part of the arterial wall is then subjected to the force of blood flowing in the direction of the parent artery. An outpouching then forms at the weak point to form an aneurysm, which usually projects in the direction of parent artery blood flow. Chronic arterial hypertension would exacerbate these changes. Atherosclerotic changes have also been invoked as a mechanism for the initial arterial wall weakening.

Expansion of the diameter of an aneurysm could be expected to increase the stress in the wall of the aneurysm. Application of the Laplace law would lead to the expectation of a linear increase in wall tension as the radius increases. However, the Laplace law assumes that the wall is linearly elastic, whereas the wall of an aneurysm is viscoelastic. As aneurysms enlarge, the relative contribution of elastic fibers in the wall decreases. An exponential increase in wall tension can therefore be expected as saccular aneurysms enlarge [33].

Flow within saccular aneurysms has been studied using various physical and computer models that have demonstrated entry of blood into the distal part of the aneurysmal opening, followed by circumferential flow in the aneurysm and reentry into the parent artery in the proximal portion of the aneurysmal opening (Fig. 5-2) [33]. Flow in the central part of the aneurysm is relatively stagnant, or contains vortices, which might predispose to thrombus formation.

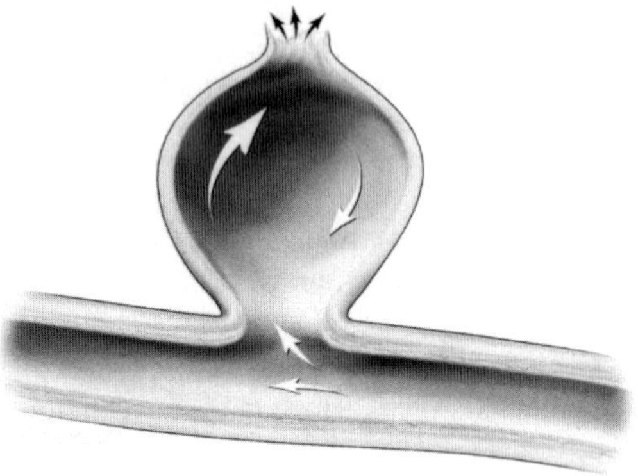

FIGURE 5-2. Flow within a saccular aneurysm. Blood enters the distal part of the neck, circulates around the circumference of the aneurysm, then reenters the parent artery at the proximal part of the neck. The most common point of rupture is at the apex of the dome. In large and giant aneurysms the center of the aneurysm has relatively stagnant or turbulent flow, which can predispose to thrombus formation.

Rupture of an aneurysm occurs most commonly at the apex of the fundus, less frequently at the sides, and rarely at the neck. Aneurysms rupture when the tension of the wall exceeds the force produced by the structural components [33]. Because the structural integrity of an aneurysmal wall is predominantly its collagen content, the force required to produce rupture is directly related to the elastic limit of collagen, which can be defined by the elastic modulus. The critical radius for rupture is determined by the elastic modulus, the wall thickness, and the intraaneurysmal pressure. For typical values of the elastic modulus, aneurysmal wall thickness (40 μm), and pressure (150 mm Hg), the critical radius for rupture has been calculated to be 4 mm [33]. It has been shown that vibration induces structural fatigue and this raises the possibility that vibration could play a role, not only in aneurysm formation, but also in rupture. It has been postulated that the resonant frequency between the pulsatile hemodynamic forces and the vibrational displacement of the aneurysmal wall plays a major role in degradation and rupture of the wall. The resonant frequency decreases as aneurysm size increases, which is consistent with the observation that rupture is more likely in larger aneurysms [33].

Fusiform Aneurysm Formation

As discussed above, fusiform aneurysms most often form in segments of artery affected by atherosclerosis. One potential mechanism of aneurysm formation is poststenotic dilation. Atherosclerotic plaques narrow the vessel diameter, which establishes abnormal hemodynamics, including turbulence, distal to the stenosis. The turbulent flow results in alternating high and low lateral pressure on the wall, with damage to the elastic lamina and intima. This process presumably reduces the tensile strength of the wall and leads to circumferential expansion in a similar fashion to fusiform aneurysms elsewhere in the body.

Aneurysmal Hemorrhage

The pathophysiologic responses to aneurysmal rupture depend largely on the volume of blood entering the subarachnoid space. Measurements of intracranial pressure during aneurysmal rebleeding reveal a rise of intracranial pressure to diastolic blood pressure levels [34]. There is therefore temporary circulatory arrest, with cerebral blood flow occurring only during systole [35]. Cessation of hemorrhage from the aneurysm is probably from platelet and thrombus occlusion of the rupture, aided by tamponade from the increased intracranial pressure.

Following SAH, there is a reduction in global cerebral blood flow and cerebral metabolic rate for oxygen [36]. In patients with vasospasm, there are further regional and sometimes multifocal reductions in cerebral blood flow [37]. Autoregulation to changes in blood pressure is also affected in patients with more severe SAH [38]. Loss of responsiveness to changes in arterial carbon dioxide levels occurs with even more severe brain damage.

Subarachnoid blood produces a meningeal inflammatory response, with evidence of polymorphs entering the subarachnoid space within hours of the ictus. These cells are followed by lymphocytes and monocytes. Although the precise mechanism of the inflammatory response is unknown, there could be contributions from potassium and hemoglobin released from red blood cells, and prostaglandins, bradykinin, and leukotrienes from platelets and white blood cells. The mechanism of the severe headache associated with SAH is also unknown; these inflammatory mediators may be involved by acting directly on nerve endings. Endothelial adhesion molecules are likely to be involved in the migration of leukocytes. The chronic inflammatory response is sometimes followed by fibrosis of the subarachnoid space, which can be seen as early as 10 days after the hemorrhage. Most erythrocytes are cleared from the subarachnoid space by hemolysis and phagocytosis; the evidence for some direct removal into the blood stream via the arachnoid villi is weaker [39,40].

At least some component of intraparenchymal hemorrhage occurs in up to 60% of patients. Aneurysms of the posterior circulation are less commonly complicated by intraparenchymal hemorrhage than anterior circulation lesions. Intraventricular hemorrhage occurs in approximately 25% of cases and is seen particularly with anterior communicating and basilar bifurcation aneurysms, which are close to the third ventricle. Intraparenchymal and intraventricular hemorrhages are associated with poorer outcome.

Acute subdural hematoma is an uncommon result of aneurysmal hemorrhage, occurring in less than 5% of cases. However, it is an important diagnosis to make so that appropriate angiography and treatment of the aneurysm is instituted. A ruptured aneurysm should be considered in any nontraumatic subdural hematoma, especially those located inferiorly over the convexity or subtemporally. When a subdural hematoma does result from an aneurysm, it is likely to have arisen from a posterior communicating artery or middle cerebral artery aneurysm that was adherent to the tentorium or sphenoid wing. Intraoperative rupture of these aneurysms is common, which mandates appropriate precautions for proximal artery control and blood volume replacement.

Cerebral edema commonly develops after SAH and is from a combination of vasogenic, cytotoxic, and hydrostatic mechanisms. Edema is exacerbated by hyponatremia from inappropriate antidiuretic hormone secretion or cerebral salt wasting.

Hydrocephalus

Hydrocephalus occurs in 10% to 40% of patients with SAH, and most of these patients will have symptoms or signs of increased intracranial pressure. The site of obstruction of cerebrospinal fluid is not always apparent; possible locations include the foramina of Monro, third ventricle, cerebral aqueduct, outlets of the fourth ventricle, the subarachnoid cisterns at the tentorial hiatus, and the arachnoid villi. Hydrocephalus can develop at various times after SAH. Hydrocephalus occurring within 3 days of the ictus is acute, between 3 days and 29 days is subacute, and after 29 days is chronic. Approximately 15% to 20% of patients with SAH develop acute hydrocephalus [41]. Hydrocephalus is more common in patients with more extensive SAH and especially in patients with ruptured anterior communicating artery aneurysms and intraventricular blood [42]. Increasing age, preexisting hypertension, use of antifibrinolytics, and hyponatremia all predict the development of hydrocephalus. Up to 15% of patients require permanent cerebrospinal fluid diversion by shunting. One-half of the patients who require external ventricular drainage require permanent shunting.

Vasospasm

Vasospasm is the delayed onset of focal or diffuse narrowing of intradural cerebral arteries after SAH. It commences after day 3 and reaches a peak after 7 to 10 days. Vasospasm can occur in association with subarachnoid blood of any cause, but the thickest subarachnoid clots occur after aneurysmal SAH and vasospasm is most common in this situation. Two-thirds of patients with SAH will have vasospasm detectable on angiography during the second week after the SAH, and approximately one-half of these patients will develop ischemic neurologic deficits. Mortality and permanent morbidity from vasospasm occur in up to 14% of patients with SAH [6,43] The risk of developing vasospasm is highest in patients with thick subarachnoid blood and occurs predominantly in arteries surrounded by thick clots, but any of the large- and medium-sized intracranial arteries can be involved [44,45] Although a higher volume of subarachnoid blood is also associated with a worse initial neurologic condition, higher intracranial pressure, and hydrocephalus, the subsequent development of vasospasm is an independent predictor of poor outcome. Aside from the effects of the original hemorrhage, vasospasm is the leading cause of poor outcome and accounts for up to 15% of patient deaths [6].

The initial process of vasospasm appears to be contraction of medial smooth muscle, followed by corrugation of the elastic lamina and longitudinal furrowing of the intima. There is thickening of all arterial wall layers. There is subendothelial proliferation, vacuolation, and necrosis of smooth muscle cells, medial fibrosis, smooth muscle and fibroblast proliferation, collagen deposition, and platelet aggregation [42]. The endothelial cells desquamate, and there is loss of tight junctions in the remaining endothelial cells [43]. The adventitia has an inflammatory cell infiltrate and there is degeneration of perivascular nerve terminals. On gross inspection, vasospastic arteries are pale and narrow. During the following 6 weeks there is resolution of the luminal diameter and intimal changes, but there can be persisting medial fibrosis.

It is accepted that subarachnoid blood clot causes vasospasm, but the precise mechanism remains unclear. Removal of clot from the subarachnoid space within 3 days prevents vasospasm, so irreversible processes are not established at the time of the hemorrhage [43,46] There is good evidence that hemoglobin and its breakdown products are responsible for vasospasm. However, a single agent responsible for prolonged vasospasm has not been identified. In addition to hemoglobin and its metabolites, possible contributors include free radicals, adenosine triphosphate, and an imbalance between physiologic constrictors, such as endothelins and prostaglandins, and physiologic vasodilators, such as nitric oxide or prostacyclin [47]. Some experimental studies have indicated that inflammation plays an important role but is not prominent after intracranial SAH [47].

NATURAL HISTORY

Subarachnoid Hemorrhage

The natural history of aneurysmal SAH is difficult to determine. Studies of outcome prior to the widespread adoption of early surgical treatment are not relevant to current standards of diagnosis and medical management. It is clear, however, that the overall prognosis of untreated SAH is poor. The major contributors to mortality are the effects of the initial hemorrhage, rebleeding, vasospasm, and surgical and medical complications. Approximately 10% to 15% of patients suffering an SAH die immediately and do not reach

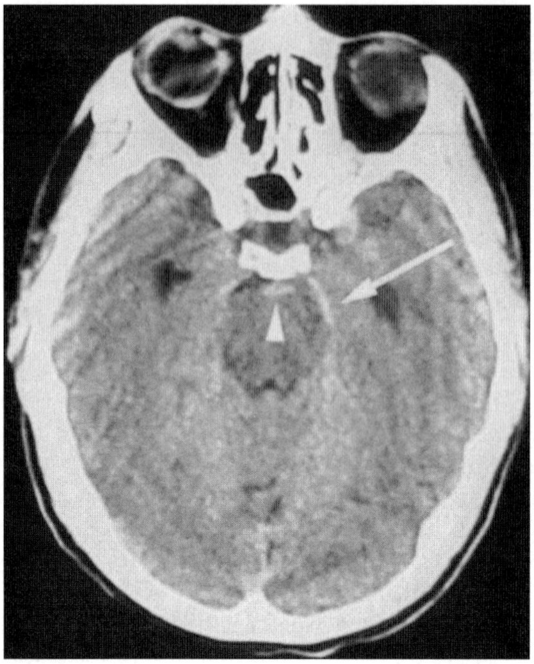

FIGURE 5-3. CT findings in a case of benign perimesencephalic hemorrhage. There is a thin layer of subarachnoid blood in the ambient cistern *(arrow)* and the interpeduncular cistern *(arrowhead).*

a hospital. Including these deaths, the total mortality rate 1 month after SAH is approximately 60% [48]. The risk of rebleeding is 50% within the first 6 months, decreases to 10% by 1 year postictus, and gradually reaches 3% per year. The highest risk of rebleeding is during the first 2 weeks, and especially the first 2 days [9]. Mortality from rebleeding is even higher than from the original hemorrhage and approaches 70% [49].

The prognosis for patients with normal angiographic results after SAH is considerably better than for patients with ruptured aneurysms. When the initial angiogram is normal, a follow-up angiogram should be performed to check for aneurysms that were thrombosed at the time of the original study, except for patients with a perimesencephalic type of hemorrhage (Fig. 5-3). The chance of demonstrating a lesion in a second angiogram in patients with this pattern of hemorrhage is so low that it is rarely justified. The cause of hemorrhage in these cases remains unknown, although venous rupture has been implicated. The symptoms are less severe than with aneurysmal SAH, are of slower onset, and vasospasm is unlikely. Magnetic resonance imaging (MRI) and magnetic resonance angiography (MRA) are helpful when initial angiographic results are negative.

Unruptured Aneurysms

Symptomatic unruptured aneurysms have a different natural history than incidentally discovered lesions. In the cooperative aneurysm study, 32 patients with symptomatic unruptured aneurysms had conservative management. The mortality from SAH was 25% at 3 years after diagnosis [50]. The risk of rupture after a warning headache has been reported to be 60%, while the risk for aneurysms with symptoms of focal compression is up to 6.5% per year [51,52].

The risk of rupture of asymptomatic aneurysms remains a controversial topic. Epidemiologic and clinical data have been used to calculate that if the prevalence of aneurysms is 0.5% and the annual incidence of SAH is 10 per 100,000 population, the rate of rupture is 2% per year [9]. There are numerous retrospective studies providing some guide to the risk of hemorrhage. In a study of 130 patients with 161 unruptured aneurysms, none of the lesions under 10 mm in maximal diameter ruptured during a mean follow-up of 8.3 years. The mean diameter of aneurysms that did rupture in this study was 21 mm. It was suggested that the discrepancy between this average size and the average size of all ruptured aneurysms (7.5 mm) was because aneurysms decreased in size after rupture. Yasui et al. followed 234 patients with unruptured aneurysms. Over 6 years, 34 patients bled, for an average annual rupture rate of 2.3%. The 5-year survival rate in a further study of 54 patients with 72 unruptured aneurysms was 56% and the annual bleeding rate was almost 2% [53]. In this group, the average size of ruptured aneurysms was 13 mm, but in 4 of the 11 patients with SAH, the ruptured aneurysm was 4 to 5 mm in diameter. In a long-term study of 142 patients with 181 unruptured aneurysms, there was a 1.4% annual rate of SAH [51]. Most of the unruptured aneurysms in this group were detected because the patient originally had a different aneurysm that ruptured. Aneurysm size was the only variable associated with rupture.

The most comprehensive natural history data currently available come from the International Study of Unruptured Intracranial Aneurysms (ISUIA), although these are still retrospective data [54]. This report provided evidence that there is a different natural history for patients with a history of SAH than for patients without such a history. Participating centers in North America and Europe enrolled 2,621 patients. A retrospective component consisting of 1,449 patients with 1,937 aneurysms was divided into two groups, those patients who had no history of a SAH (727 patients) and those who had a SAH from a different aneurysm (722 patients). Treatment mortality and morbidity were assessed in the prospective component of 1,172 patients. The results of this study indicated a very low (below 0.05%) annual risk of rupture for patients harboring small (less than 10 mm) aneurysms who had not previously had a SAH. Aneurysms of the same size in the group of patients who had previously suffered a SAH from a different aneurysm had a much higher risk of rupture (0.5% per year). The risk of aneurysms larger than 10 mm rupturing was approximately 1% per year in each group. Among patients with giant aneurysms, the rupture rate was 6% over the first year. Aneurysm location was also associated with rupture; posterior circulation and posterior communicating artery aneurysms were more prone to hemorrhage. The mortality from aneurysms that did rupture was 66%. The 5-year survival rate for the entire cohort was 89%. The findings of this study have been criticized on the basis that the retrospective cohort of patients with unruptured aneurysms was selected for no treatment and that this introduced a systematic bias into the patient selection [55]. Whether these results are representative of the risk faced by all patients with unruptured aneurysms remains to be determined.

The finding by the ISUIA that small aneurysms have a very low risk of rupture is difficult to reconcile with SAH being most frequently caused by aneurysms 7 to 10 mm in diameter [3]. This has led to a suggestion that this size range is critical for rupture, in contrast to the 10-mm size indicated by the ISUIA. Alternative explanations include a much higher prevalence of aneurysms 7 to 10 mm in diameter, a decrease in aneurysm size after rupture, or rupture of aneurysms soon after they form. The latter explanation, that aneurysms grow quickly and either stabilize or rupture, appears to be the most credible.

The Stroke Council of the American Heart Association has published recommendations for the management of patients with unruptured intracranial aneurysms [3]. According to this group, the available data (level IV and V evidence) support the following recommendations: (a) treatment of small incidental intracavernous aneurysms is generally not indicated, (b) symptomatic intradural aneurysms of all sizes should be considered for treatment, (c) unruptured aneurysms in patients with an acute SAH from another aneurysm warrant consideration for treatment, (d) small incidental aneurysms in patients without a history of acute SAH should not generally be treated (exceptions could include young patients, aneurysms approaching 10 mm in size, aneurysms with daughter sacs, patients with a positive family history of aneurysms, and changes in aneurysm size or configuration on follow-up imaging), and (e) asymptomatic aneurysms larger than 10 mm in diameter warrant strong consideration for treatment [3].

Decisions regarding the management of unruptured aneurysms must also take into account the results of surgical treatment for these cases. In a series of 202 cases, an excellent or good outcome was achieved in all the patients with aneurysms under 10 mm and in 95% of patients with aneurysms measuring 11 to 25 mm. Excellent or good outcomes were achieved in 79% of patients with giant aneurysms [56]. In the prospective component of the ISUIA, the combined morbidity and mortality rate was approximately 15% 1 year after surgery. The only independent predictor of outcome was patient age.

CLINICAL FEATURES

Subarachnoid and Intracerebral Hemorrhage

Warning symptoms prior to the hemorrhage have been documented in up to 50% of patients with SAH. Sentinel headaches are thought to represent minor hemorrhages; occasionally there are chronic headaches [2]. Meningism and photophobia are generally not present. The interval between a warning headache and a subsequent SAH varies. One-half occur within 1 week and 90% occur within 6 weeks. Up to 50% of the patients who subsequently have SAH come to medical attention at the time of the warning headache [57].

The hallmark of intracranial hemorrhage of any type is the sudden onset of severe headache. SAH causes meningeal irritation. Therefore nuchal rigidity, fever, photophobia, and reduced level of consciousness are prominent clinical features. Focal neurologic deficits and seizures are not common unless there is associated intraparenchymal hemorrhage. Of patients arriving at the hospital, 10% will be unconscious and a further 45% will have had a brief loss of consciousness [2].

Intracerebral hematoma is most likely with distal anterior cerebral artery, anterior communicating artery, and middle cerebral bifurcation aneurysms. Approximately two-thirds of patients with ruptured aneurysms in these locations will have intracerebral hemorrhage. The size and location of intracerebral clots correlates with outcome.

Assessment of Subarachnoid Hemorrhage Severity

Grading scales have been developed to assess the severity of the clinical picture. These are used to compare outcomes and to estimate the prognosis of patients with SAH. The most commonly used scales are the Hunt and Hess grade (Table 5-1) and the World Federation of Neurosurgical So-

TABLE 5-1. MODIFIED HUNT AND HESS GRADING SCALE FOR ASSESSING CLINICAL SEVERITY OF SUBARACHNOID HEMORRHAGE

Grade	Description
0	Unruptured aneurysm[a]
I	Asymptomatic, or mild headache and slight nuchal rigidity
II	Moderate to severe headache, nuchal rigidity, no neurologic deficit except cranial nerve palsy
III	Mild focal deficit, drowsiness, or confusion
IV	Stupor, moderate to severe hemiparesis, possible early decerebrate rigidity, vegetative disturbances
V	Deep coma, decerebrate rigidity, moribund

[a]Grade 0 was not included in the original scale.
From Hunt WE, Hess RM. Surgical risk as related to time of intervention in the repair of intracranial aneurysms. *J Neurosurg* 1968;28:14–20, with permission.

TABLE 5-2. WORLD FEDERATION OF NEUROSURGICAL SOCIETIES SCALE FOR GRADING CLINICAL SEVERITY OF SUBARACHNOID HEMORRHAGE

Grade	Glasgow Coma Scale Score	Motor Deficit
1	15	No
2	13–14	No
3	13–14	Yes
4	7–12	Yes or no
5	3–6	Yes or no

From Teasdale GM, Drake CG, Hunt W, et al. A universal subarachnoid hemorrhage scale: report of a committee of the World Federation of Neurosurgical Societies. *J Neurol Neurosurg Psychiatry* 1988;51:1457, with permission.

cieties (WFNS) Scale (Table 5-2), which takes into account the Glasgow Coma Scale score and is probably a more accurate predictor of outcome. In practice, few patients score Hunt and Hess grade II and the scale is therefore not as discriminatory as the WFNS scale.

The amount of subarachnoid blood is a predicting factor for the development of vasospasm and for outcome. Fisher published a scale of SAH severity based on the thickness and location of blood seen on computed tomography (CT) scan (Table 5-3) [44]. The highest incidence of spasm is in patients with Fisher grade 3.

Other Signs and Symptoms of Saccular Aneurysms

Other signs and symptoms of aneurysms include mass effect, seizures, embolic phenomena, and bruit. Mass effect is unusual in nongiant aneurysms except for paraclinoidal and posterior communicating artery aneurysms. Neurologic deficits from giant aneurysms are usually of gradual onset. Cranial nerve palsies from small and large aneurysms can have a sudden onset, presumably due to rapid expansion or thrombosis of the aneurysm. The third cranial nerve is most commonly affected, usually from a posterior communicating artery or superior cerebellar artery aneurysm. Retroorbital pain is a prominent feature of aneurysm-related third cranial nerve palsies. Visual loss from optic nerve compression by an ophthalmic artery aneurysm is relatively common. An alternative, and uncommon, mechanism of visual loss is from optic chiasm compression by an inferiorly projecting anterior communicating artery aneurysm. These lesions are usually painless. The sixth cranial nerve is occasionally compressed by a midbasilar artery or intracavernous carotid aneurysm. Intracavernous carotid aneurysms can cause a cavernous sinus syndrome, with palsies of the third, fourth, fifth, and sixth cranial nerves. Rupture of an intracavernous aneurysm produces proptosis and chemosis. Erosion of the sphenoid sinus by an intracavernous or intrapetrous aneurysm and subsequent rupture can lead to epistaxis. Any sudden-onset, painful cranial nerve palsy should be regarded as caused by an aneurysm until proved otherwise, and treated as an emergency. Sudden enlargement of the aneurysm is probably responsible for such symptoms, and rupture of the aneurysm should be considered imminent. Although the relatively common oculomotor neuropathy associated with diabetes is generally painless and spares the pupil, even these cases should be investigated for a possible aneurysm.

TABLE 5-3. FISHER GRADE OF THE SEVERITY OF SUBARACHNOID HEMORRHAGE DETERMINED BY THE THICKNESS OF BLOOD DEMONSTRATED ON COMPUTED TOMOGRAPHY

Grade	Subarachnoid Blood on Computed Tomography
1	No subarachnoid blood
2	Diffuse subarachnoid hemorrhage or vertical layers <1 mm thick
3	Localized subarachnoid clot or layers of hemorrhage ≥1 mm thick
4	Intracerebral or intraventricular clot with diffuse or no subarachnoid blood

From Fisher CM, Kistler JP, Davis JM. Relation of cerebral vasospasm to subarachnoid hemorrhage visualized by computerized tomographic scanning. *Neurosurgery* 1980;6:1–9, with permission.

Symptoms from mass effect of aneurysms on the brain are uncommon. Giant dominant hemisphere middle cerebral artery aneurysms can cause dysphasia or even hemiparesis. Aneurysms of the basilar artery or its branches can compress the brainstem, with corresponding neurologic deficits (Fig. 5-4). Thalamic syndrome from a small internal carotid artery bifurcation aneurysm has been reported [58].

Rupture of an intracavernous carotid aneurysm will create a carotid-cavernous fistula, with cranial neuropathies, pain, bruit, chemosis, and proptosis. Patients with this problem are at very low risk of intradural hemorrhage, and the main concern is preservation of vision and elimination of the bruit. Bruits can also be the only complaint associated with large or giant unruptured intradural aneurysms.

Epilepsy is an unusual symptom of unruptured aneurysms. Compression of the cerebral cortex and calcification of the aneurysm are predisposing factors. The most common location is the middle cerebral artery, and the aneurysm causes complex partial seizures. Ischemic symptoms related to embolism or thrombosis occur with up to 25% of symptomatic unruptured aneurysms and are most common with giant lesions of the internal carotid and middle cerebral arteries. Detection of completely asymptomatic aneurysms is becoming more frequent with improvements in noninvasive imaging techniques.

Features of Nonsaccular Aneurysms

Extracranial arterial dissections are often asymptomatic, although they can cause pain and Horner syndrome from

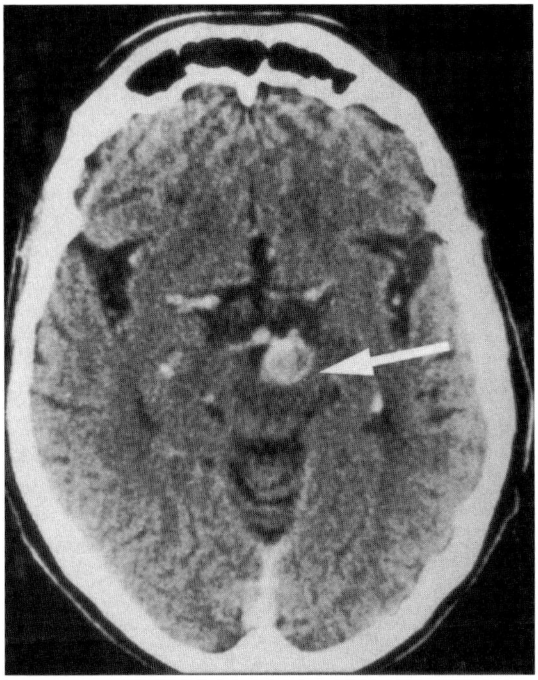

FIGURE 5-4. CT demonstrates an unruptured posterior cerebral artery aneurysm compressing the cerebral peduncle. This patient had ipsilateral oculomotor nerve paresis and contralateral hemiparesis, which resolved after the aneurysm was clipped.

disruption of sympathetic fibers in the arterial wall, thromboembolic phenomena, or hemodynamic insufficiency from stenosis or occlusion. Intracranial fusiform aneurysms cause mass effect more commonly than hemorrhage. The posterior circulation is usually involved, so the clinical picture includes brainstem signs, cranial neuropathy, and hydrocephalus. The less common anterior circulation fusiform aneurysms are associated with seizures, visual loss, or hemispheric signs and symptoms.

Infectious aneurysms become apparent most commonly with SAH without any premonitory neurologic symptoms or signs. Focal neurologic deficit related to thrombosis of the parent artery is often seen in addition to SAH. Traumatic (false) aneurysms usually are associated with delayed hemorrhage after a head injury, but early rupture is occasionally seen. The risk of rebleeding is high.

DIAGNOSIS

Subarachnoid Hemorrhage

CT is a highly sensitive method for detecting acute intracranial blood clots. Scans performed within 48 hours of a SAH will be positive in over 95% of cases. The consequences of missing the diagnosis of SAH are so grave that there should be a low threshold for performing lumbar puncture when there is clinical suspicion of a hemorrhage that is not confirmed by CT. Unfortunately, a warning hemorrhage may not be detectable by CT or lumbar puncture. MRI can be used instead of lumbar puncture to look for intracranial hemorrhage in patients who are evaluated more than 24 to 48 hours after the ictus. Acute blood is not well demonstrated on routine MRI or MRA, but these studies may show an aneurysm or other vascular lesion and may demonstrate an acutely thrombosed aneurysm missed with angiography.

Computed Tomography

In addition to confirming the diagnosis of SAH, CT findings can provide evidence of the location and pathology of the underlying lesion (Fig. 5-5) [44]. In most situations, angiography is performed to provide detailed information, so contrast is not usually given with the CT scan. However, in some acute situations, in which an intracranial hematoma requires urgent evacuation without time for angiography, a rapid CT scan with contrast can provide useful information about the location and size of the aneurysm.

Magnetic Resonance Imaging

MRI provides exquisite anatomical detail in multiple planes. The anatomical information provided by MRI is particularly useful for giant aneurysms. MRI is less sensitive for detecting acute bleeding than CT but is more useful in detecting early ischemic changes. The contents of aneurysm are better demonstrated with MRI than with CT. MRI will often demonstrate intramural blood of varying ages from dissecting aneurysms.

MRA can detect aneurysms as small as 3 mm, but the anatomy is not as well defined as on digital subtraction angiography. In addition, functional information about dominant parent arteries and collateral flow provided by digital subtraction angiography is not available with MRA. MRA is a useful tool for screening patients at risk of harboring an unruptured aneurysm.

Digital Subtraction Angiography

Intraarterial contrast angiography (Fig. 5-6) remains the standard method for delineating the anatomical details of an aneurysm and the related arteries. Adequate angiographic examination to localize and determine the anatomy of an aneurysm and the cerebral circulation requires bilateral carotid and vertebral injections. Valuable information about the anatomy of an aneurysm, and in particular its neck, can often be obtained with oblique views. Compression of a carotid artery during contralateral carotid injection or vertebral injection (Allcock test) can provide additional anatomical and functional information about the anterior and posterior communicating arteries. Rotational angiography and angiography with three-dimensional reconstruction provide excellent visualization of the anatomical arrangements. Mul-

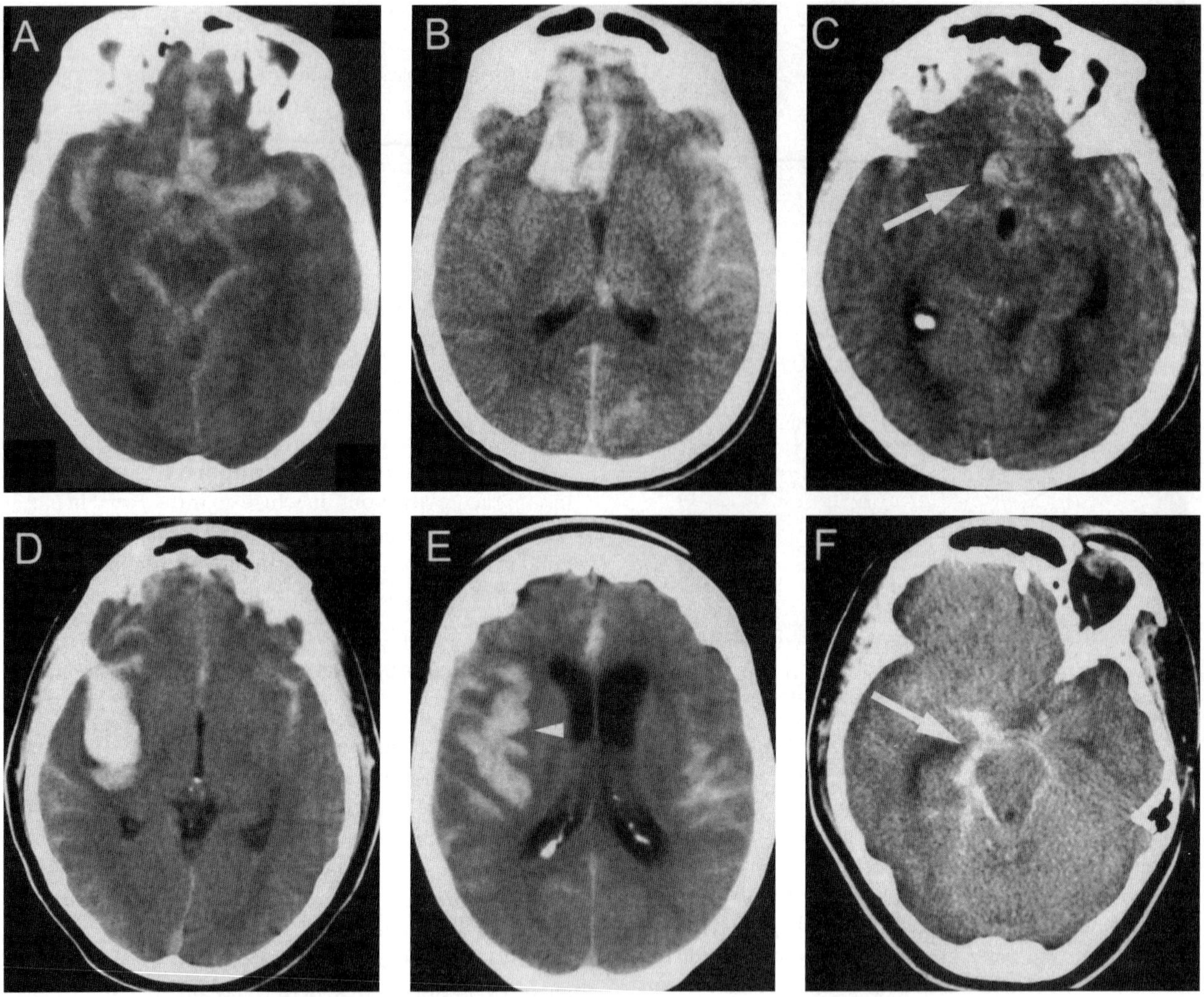

FIGURE 5-5. CT findings in SAH. **A:** Diffuse SAH. There is thick clot in the anterior interhemispheric fissure, but the hemorrhage is so widespread that there is little localizing value. **B:** Diffuse SAH with a large hematoma within the gyrus rectus. This pattern is virtually pathognomonic of an anterior communicating artery aneurysm arising from the junction of the anterior cerebral artery and the anterior communicating artery on the side contralateral to the hematoma. **C:** Diffuse SAH with a small hematoma in the gyrus rectus. This has the same diagnostic value as **(B)**. **D:** Temporal lobe hematoma in conjunction with SAH that is highly suggestive of a middle cerebral artery aneurysm. **E:** Thick clot within the sylvian fissure is also highly suggestive of a ruptured middle cerebral artery aneurysm. The insular cortex is seen as a corrugated border *(arrowhead)* medial to the hematoma, which helps to differentiate such a hemorrhage from a hypertensive hemorrhage. **F:** Thick subarachnoid blood in the ambient cistern *(arrow)* was from a ruptured posterior cerebral artery aneurysm.

tiple aneurysms are sufficiently frequent to warrant a complete investigation, even if a single injection demonstrates the offending aneurysm. An exception might be the elderly patient in whom carotid angiography demonstrates an aneurysm of the anterior circulation and a vertebral injection is unlikely to demonstrate an aneurysm that will be treated electively.

Angiographic findings of dissecting aneurysms include stenosis, the pearl-and-string sign (a series of dilations alternating with narrowing, a beaded luminal appearance), a true double lumen, or complete occlusion. Fusiform aneurysms can appear as dilated segments of artery, but usually also have irregular stenosis and double or false lumens. False aneurysms have an irregular contour and delayed filling and emptying. These aneurysms do not usually occur at branch points and there is not a well-defined neck. Infectious aneurysms usually are demonstrated as fusiform dilations on peripheral branches.

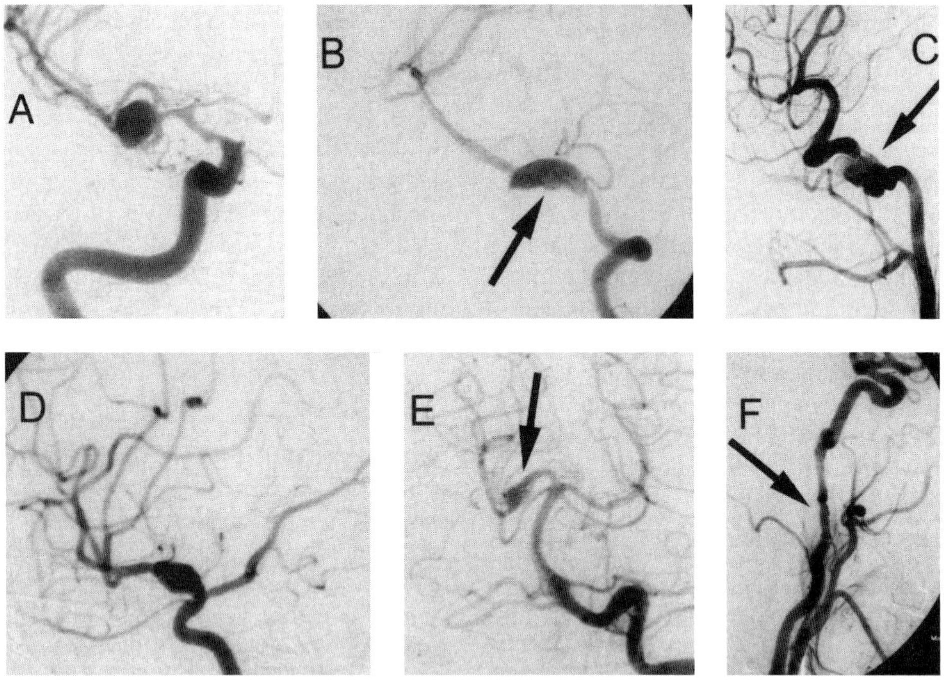

FIGURE 5-6. Digital subtraction angiograms demonstrate various types of aneurysm. **A:** Saccular aneurysm arises from the bifurcation of the middle cerebral artery. The apparently narrow neck seen on the angiogram can be misleading; the neck often involves the major branches also. **B:** Fusiform aneurysm of the left vertebral artery. There was extensive intraluminal thrombus, which gives part of the aneurysm an irregular appearance *(arrow).* **C:** Posttraumatic false aneurysm of the petrous and intracavernous internal carotid artery. The true lumen of the internal carotid artery was stenosed by the aneurysm *(arrow).* **D:** Fungal infectious aneurysm. Most bacterial aneurysms involve distal branches, but fungal aneurysms are usually proximal and fusiform. **E:** Intracranial dissecting aneurysm of the posterior cerebral artery *(arrow).* **F:** Extracranial dissecting aneurysm of the internal carotid artery, which was also affected by fibromuscular dysplasia *(arrow).* The acute dissection in this case was demonstrated on MRI, which revealed blood products within the arterial wall.

Cerebral Blood Flow Studies

The role of routine cerebral blood flow studies for SAH is limited. Patients with vasospasm will have reduced blood flow and increased oxygen extraction fraction in the regions supplied by the narrowed arteries, but the diagnosis of vasospasm is generally made by other means. Jugular venous oxygen saturation monitoring is a useful guide to the global oxygen extraction and can be used to assist with management of increased intracranial pressure. Blood flow studies (often during temporary occlusion) are desirable if proximal occlusion, trapping, or revascularization surgery is being considered.

TREATMENT

Nonoperative Management of Subarachnoid Hemorrhage

Patients with SAH should be managed in an intensive care or high-dependency unit. Care is taken to provide an environment that minimizes stimuli, so that the patient can rest quietly. Laxatives are generally prescribed so that constipation and straining at stool are avoided. Particular attention is paid to blood pressure, fluid, and electrolyte management. Nutritional support should be commenced early after SAH, in the same manner that patients with head injuries are treated. Unconscious patients managed with intubation and mechanical ventilation should have their intracranial pressure monitored. Usually these patients have a ventricular catheter, which provides ideal measurements with a fluid-filled or coaxial transducer and has the huge advantage of permitting drainage to control intracranial pressure. When a ventricular catheter has not been placed, intracranial pressure can be monitored with an intraparenchymal transducer.

Steroids have been used for their neuroprotective effects and possible benefits in reduction of cerebral edema, prevention of vasospasm, and the prevention of hydrocephalus. None of these effects has been proved in patients with SAH and steroid use is not recommended. Steroids have numerous side effects, including peptic ulceration and hemorrhage, hyperglycemia, infection, and psychosis. Sucralfate or histamine receptor antagonists are often used for ulcer prophylaxis when steroids are being used. Long-term prophylactic use of anticonvulsant medication has not been demonstrated to reduce the risk of developing epilepsy after trauma or SAH. Although seizures occur in 10% to 30% of patients with SAH, the majority happen in patients with poor neurologic grade, and those with cortical and subcortical hematomas, ruptured middle cerebral artery aneurysms, and infarcts from vasospasm. We reserve the use of anticonvulsants for these high-risk patients [59]. Although effective in reducing rebleeding, antifibrinolytic agents were found to have a negative effect on overall outcome because of a higher incidence of vasospasm and hydrocephalus. A recent interesting report has suggested that administering tranexamic acid immediately after SAH reduces very early rebleed rates during the period before clipping or coil placement is possible [60].

Management of Medical Complications

Electrolyte Abnormalities

Electrolyte abnormalities are common after SAH, especially hyponatremia and hypothalamic dysfunction associated with a ruptured anterior communicating artery aneurysm. Hyponatremia affects up to one-third of patients and is most likely to occur between the second and tenth days after a SAH. Cerebral edema, seizures, and reduced level of consciousness are exacerbated by a low serum sodium content. Loss of plasma volume in the presence of a normal serum sodium level can occur due to secretion of atrial natriuretic factor. The differentiation between hypervolemia from the syndrome of inappropriate antidiuretic hormone (which is rare) and hypovolemia from natriuresis (which is relatively common) can be difficult, but it is important. Restriction of fluid intake in the latter condition can be extremely detrimental, especially in patients who also have vasospasm. Daily monitoring of serum electrolytes in the early stages after a SAH is essential.

Hyperglycemia

Hyperglycemia in association with SAH is presumably a stress response to the hemorrhage. Use of glucocorticoids further elevates the serum glucose. Particular attention should be paid to elderly or overweight patients who may have undiagnosed diabetes mellitus. Hyperglycemia can contribute to a reduced level of consciousness and can be primarily responsible for focal or generalized seizures. The use of insulin to treat hyperglycemia is controversial because of concerns that it will exacerbate cerebral edema.

Thromboembolic Complications

Patients with SAH are at risk of developing thromboembolic complications, which occur in approximately 2% of cases. The risk of deep venous thrombosis is higher if there is a neurologic deficit, especially if there is lower limb paresis. Some authors have advocated the use of subcutaneous heparin in addition to stockings in the immediate posthemorrhagic or postsurgical period. Heparinization is contraindicated when there is an unsecured ruptured aneurysm. Anticoagulation within 10 days of surgery for a ruptured aneurysm should be avoided, and an inferior vena cava filter is recommended for patients with extensive deep venous thrombosis or pulmonary embolus during this period, or where the ruptured aneurysm cannot be secured [42].

Hypertension

Severe hypertension should be treated immediately because it increases the risk of aneurysmal rebleeding. However, it should be remembered that an elevated blood pressure can be a homeostatic response to increased intracranial pressure, and lowering the blood pressure excessively carries a risk of cerebral ischemia. Pain, hypoxia, and agitation can further elevate the blood pressure and these should be avoided or treated. Systemic hypertension increases the transmural pressure and therefore the risk of rebleeding. The transmural pressure will be particularly high if increased intracranial pressure is treated without concomitant treatment of systolic hypertension. Sedation and analgesia are often sufficient to control the blood pressure.

Cardiac and Pulmonary Complications

Electrocardiography often reveals arrhythmias in patients after a SAH [61]. It is likely that they contribute to the loss of consciousness and sudden death that can occur after aneurysmal rupture. Arrhythmias are most common early after the hemorrhage. Although usually benign, ventricular tachycardia, flutter, and fibrillation can occur. The precise mechanism of cardiac arrhythmias in these patients is not known, but sympathetic outflow changes from hypothalamic damage are possibly responsible. Treatment of cardiac arrhythmias after a SAH should be no different than the treatment of arrhythmias in other patients.

Pneumonia is the most common pulmonary complication after a SAH. It is a significant contributor to mortality, but this is generally in patients who are in poor neurologic condition. Adult respiratory distress syndrome is seen occasionally. The use of inhaled nitric oxide has been reported to improve oxygenation in these patients [62].

Gastrointestinal Ulceration and Bleeding

Gastroduodenal ulcerations that occur in association with intracranial disease are called *Cushing ulcers.* Hemorrhage from these ulcers has been reported in up to 4% of patients after an aneurysmal SAH [63]. Antacids and histamine receptor blockers are commonly used for prophylaxis, although no convincing evidence for their efficacy exists.

Hemorrhagic complications from peptic ulcer disease are not reported commonly in contemporary series of patients with SAH.

Management of Vasospasm

The clinical effects of vasospasm generally include a reduction in level of consciousness and the development of focal neurologic deficit, depending on the arteries involved. Signs that should heighten suspicion of impending neurologic deficit from vasospasm include worsening headache, fever, increasing meningismus, and hyponatremia. These findings may precede the sudden onset of neurologic deficit.

The diagnosis of vasospasm can be made with certainty only with cerebral angiography. Transcranial Doppler ultrasonographic measurements of blood flow velocities greater than 120 cm/sec in the middle cerebral artery are suggestive of vasospasm, and values over 200 cm/sec are usually associated with ischemic neurologic deficits. Measurements of velocity in the middle cerebral artery are the most reliable, with a reported sensitivity of approximately 60% and specificity of 100% [64]. Greater sensitivity can be obtained with serial recordings that demonstrate a rapid rise (more than 50 cm/sec per day) in velocity [40].

Hypotension, hypovolemia, hyponatremia, and increased intracranial pressure either exacerbate vasospasm or contribute to its ischemic effects. Fluid management is therefore crucial in the prevention and treatment of symptomatic vasospasm. Maintenance of normal intravascular volume with crystalloids, colloids, and blood, if necessary, and increasing blood pressure and cardiac output (in the event of late ischemia) have been used to treat the effects of vasospasm. There are cardiac, pulmonary, and hematologic complications associated with deliberate fluid overload, including heart failure and myocardial ischemia, pulmonary edema, hyponatremia, coagulopathy, and complications related to invasive monitoring catheters. In asymptomatic low-risk patients the key to successful prophylaxis is the avoidance of hypotension and anemia. Central venous pressure should be kept within the normal range. A Swan-Ganz catheter should be considered in patients in whom inotropic agents are being used to elevate blood pressure, but we do not favor routine placement.

The calcium-channel antagonist nimodipine has been used widely in the management of patients with SAH. It was originally introduced for its putative cerebroselective smooth muscle relaxation properties. Although improved outcomes and a reduction in symptomatic vasospasm have been demonstrated [65], it appears that this is more likely from its neuronal protective effects, which are probably mediated by preventing the influx of calcium ions. Other possible effects include dilating small collateral vessels, and the induction of hypotension that resulted in administration of more fluids [40]. Several large randomized trials were performed over the last decade to examine the efficacy of tirilazad mesylate in improving outcome from SAH. Despite early encouraging results, no significant differences were detected in the treatment and placebo groups and tirilazad has not been approved for use in SAH by the Food and Drug Administration. Metaanalyses of these trials have suggested that there might be a reduction in the incidence of clinical vasospasm in poor-grade patients, especially in males [40,66]. Early reports of the efficacy of intravenous and intracisternal nitrovasodilators are encouraging [40].

Endovascular methods for treating vasospasm include intraarterial injection of papaverine and mechanical angioplasty with balloon dilation. Angiographic and clinical results can be dramatic, with improvement in up to 75% of patients. Papaverine has the advantage that catheterization of distal branches is not always necessary, but selective administration to severely affected vessels can be difficult, because flow goes preferentially into unaffected arteries. Papaverine can cause acute increases in intracranial pressure and its effects tend to be temporary [40]. Balloon dilation has a longer-lasting effect but cannot be used for distal small arteries. There is a risk of arterial dissection, occlusion, or rupture with this technique, in addition to the risks of reperfusion injury and hemorrhagic transformation of infarcted brain. Case selection for these treatments remains controversial. Many patients who develop ischemic neurologic deficits can be managed successfully with medical treatment and these patients should not be subjected to the risks of procedures. However, the effectiveness of endovascular procedures is greatest when used early, and a delay while determining whether medical management is effective could result in irreversible cerebral infarction. The role and timing of angioplasty remain unresolved.

Surgical Management of Aneurysms

The era of microsurgical techniques has seen significant advances in the surgical management of intracranial aneurysms, and most aneurysms are now approachable surgically. Outcome is determined predominantly by the severity of the original hemorrhage. Good neurosurgical and anesthetic techniques involve the avoidance of arterial hypertension or hypotension, excessive retractor pressure, and perforation of arteries and veins. Advances in perioperative management and prevention of aneurysmal rupture are likely to improve the outlook of patients with cerebral aneurysms.

Indications for Surgery

It is accepted that occlusion of a ruptured aneurysm is generally indicated to eliminate the risk of rebleeding. In an individual patient, factors such as advanced age, poor clinical grade, and associated medical conditions may influence the treatment recommendations. Whether advanced age is an independent predictor of poor outcome remains unclear, and many authors advocate managing patients on the basis of clinical grade rather than age [67]. Coexisting medical problems can increase the risk of poor outcome in patients with SAH. However, except in the most unstable patients, the risk of rebleeding is generally higher than the risk of intervening.

The appropriate management strategy for poor-grade patients is controversial. Approaches include no treatment, treatment of young patients only, delayed treatment if neurologic improvement occurs, and aggressive treatment regardless of neurologic grade. Clearly many patients have such severe neurologic injury that good recovery is not possible. However, it is often difficult to predict which patients are capable of making a good recovery, and a pessimistic approach probably denies many patients the opportunity to recover. The mortality of grade 5 patients who are untreated is over 90%. With selective delayed treatment, up to 20% of patients will make a favorable recovery. A favorable outcome has been reported in up to 50% of poor-grade patients who were treated aggressively [67]. A major concern with an aggressive approach is the possibility that more patients will survive in a severely disabled state; however, a similar number of vegetative and severely disabled survivors has been reported with aggressive and pessimistic approaches [67]. It is therefore reasonable to treat all but the most severely affected patients with early aggressive treatment to provide every opportunity for recovery. Control of respiration and ventricular cerebrospinal fluid drainage are essential adjuncts in poor-grade cases. Clearly therapy should not be continued in the absence of neurologic recovery within a reasonable timeframe.

Indications for Treatment of Unruptured Aneurysms

Symptomatic unruptured aneurysms should be regarded as highly dangerous lesions that require urgent management. A patient with an acute oculomotor nerve palsy should be regarded with particular concern; the risk of rupture is high and these aneurysms should be treated as soon as possible after diagnosis.

The management of asymptomatic unruptured aneurysms remains controversial. There are no level I, II, or III studies of the natural history and management risks of unruptured aneurysms to guide decision making [3]. The risk of rupture of these aneurysms is discussed in the section on natural history, along with a summary of the recently published guidelines from the Stroke Council of the American Heart Association. The lifetime risk of rupture of an unruptured aneurysm detected at age 60 has been estimated at less than 5% [68,69]. Prophylactic obliteration of asymptomatic aneurysms in elderly patients should probably be restricted to patients with large aneurysms who are otherwise healthy.

Patients with unruptured aneurysms in association with AVMs present a special problem. Aneurysms that are distal on feeding arteries have a high rate of spontaneous resolution after treatment of the AVM, but proximal aneurysms usually persist [20]. There is a risk of hemorrhage from such aneurysms after sudden obliteration of the AVM, perhaps because the aneurysm is exposed to a higher transmural pressure when the low-resistance shunt is removed. Although opinions vary, it is generally recommended that aneurysms associated with AVMs be treated before treatment of the AVM [22].

Patients with polycystic kidney disease have a high incidence of SAH, but the natural history of unruptured aneurysms in these patients is unknown. Until more precise natural history data are obtained, it is recommended that accessible aneurysms in otherwise healthy patients with polycystic kidney disease be treated [16].

Unruptured aneurysms are more likely to rupture subsequently if they progressively enlarge, develop loculations, attain large size, have a midline location, are associated with a previously ruptured aneurysm, and if the patients harboring them are young, smokers, or have certain medical conditions [70].

Timing of Surgery

A strong argument has been made for early surgery to address the high rates of rebleeding and attendant mortality that patients are exposed to within the first few days after an aneurysmal SAH. Additional benefits from securing an aneurysm soon after SAH include an improved ability to treat vasospasm if it occurs, and a shorter (and less expensive) hospital stay. Others have recommended that surgery be delayed to achieve optimal operating conditions without brain swelling. Advocates of delayed surgery cite better surgical results in these patients, but there is good evidence that early surgery has a beneficial effect on overall management outcome [6,31,71–75]. In the International Cooperative Study on the Timing of Aneurysm Surgery, 78% of good-grade patients who had early surgery had a favorable outcome, compared with 69% of patients who had surgery more than 14 days after the event [6,71]. This was a nonrandomized study; however, there was a statistically significant better outcome after early surgery in the subgroup of patients treated in North American centers [71]. The appropriate timing for poor-grade patients is less clear. In a prospective study of poor-grade patients (including Hunt and Hess grade III), there was a management mortality of 38% in patients who underwent surgery within 3 days of the event, compared with 70% when surgery was performed between 4 and 6 days, and over 80% when surgery was delayed for 7 days or more [76].

A patient who delays seeking medical help after SAH presents a difficult management problem, especially when there is established vasospasm. Physical manipulation of arteries during surgery is thought to exacerbate vasospasm, but there is some experimental evidence to refute this [77]. The mechanism of spasm seen at the time of surgery is almost certainly different from the mechanism of delayed vasospasm, and mechanical spasm appears to respond well to topical application of papaverine. In addition, provided appropriate fluid management is administered prior to surgery, delayed surgery does not appear to increase the risk of vasospasm or ischemic deficit [78]. Prompt occlusion of the aneurysm in this situation has the additional advantage of allowing safer hypertensive and endovascular therapy for spasm [79].

General Principles of Surgery for Saccular Aneurysms

The essential goal of surgical or endovascular treatment of an aneurysm is to exclude it from the circulation without damaging adjacent vascular or neural structures. This can be achieved in the majority of cases with appropriate anesthesia, intraoperative monitoring, and neuroprotective agents. Adequate brain relaxation is crucial for safe exposure of aneurysms after a SAH. A lumbar drain or ventricular catheter is inserted prior to surgery or at the beginning of surgery in the majority of cases. The need for cerebrospinal fluid drainage is less compelling when the aneurysm is unruptured. Insertion of a ventricular catheter to manage hydrocephalus does carry a risk of aneurysmal rebleeding [80], so if a ventricular catheter is inserted preoperatively it is kept at approximately 20 cm H_2O to minimize the effect on the transmural pressure gradient. Further brain relaxation during surgery is achieved with the routine use of hyperventilation, mannitol, and furosemide. The role of intraoperative neuroprotective agents is controversial. Agents used for this purpose have included etomidate, propofol, and thiopental.

Intracerebral hematomas with significant mass effect should be evacuated and the aneurysm clipped at the same time. Partial evacuation of the hematoma to allow brain relaxation and exposure and clipping of the aneurysm is probably a safer approach than complete hematoma removal before clipping the aneurysm. Experimental and clinical studies support the surgical or fibrinolytic removal of subarachnoid clot within 3 days after SAH to prevent vasospasm [40,46]. The benefit of surgical clot removal in humans has not been proved, perhaps related to the extensive dissection required around an injured brain and the risk of damaging cortex or perforating arteries during the process.

Early proximal arterial control is essential for the safe exposure and dissection of any intracranial aneurysm. Generally this is achieved by early exposure of the internal carotid or vertebral artery. When the aneurysm involves the proximal intracranial internal carotid artery, exposure of the artery proximal to the aneurysm can often be achieved with removal of the anterior clinoid process. With large and very proximal aneurysms, it is of significant benefit to expose the cervical carotid artery, not just for proximal control, but also for suction decompression as an adjunct to clip placement [81].

The use of temporary clips to reduce intraaneurysmal pressure during critical periods of dissection is preferred to systemic hypotension [82]. Application of a temporary clip with slight elevation of the blood pressure achieves softening of the aneurysm so that neck dissection and clip placement are safer, while allowing reasonable collateral flow. Intraoperative neurophysiologic monitoring is a useful guide to the safe duration of temporary clipping. Provided there are no neurophysiologic changes in the region supplied by the temporarily occluded artery, a temporary clip can be maintained for 15 minutes or more.

Direct occlusion of the aneurysmal neck is the preferred surgical treatment. In some cases it is impossible or too dangerous to clip the aneurysmal neck. Surgical options in these cases include proximal ligation, trapping, and wrapping. Cervical common or internal carotid ligation was used in the premicrosurgery era in the treatment of anterior circulation aneurysms. This reduced the risk of rebleeding within the first 6 months but did not alter the long-term rehemorrhage rate [49]. There is also some evidence that wrapping provides some protection against rebleeding. In one series of 60 cases followed for 10 years, the rebleeding rate within the first 6 months was 8.6% and then 1.5% per year [83]. Surgical revascularization of branches distal to a trapped aneurysm is a useful adjunct to the management of difficult aneurysms. Intraoperative methods used to confirm aneurysmal occlusion and preserve the parent artery and major branches include microvascular Doppler ultrasonography and intraoperative angiography.

Surgical Approaches

It is beyond the scope of this chapter to provide a detailed description of the various surgical approaches to intracranial aneurysms; however, a brief description of some of the principles will be given.

The patient is positioned so that the head is above the level of the heart and extended so that gravity will assist with retraction. Approaches to the circle of Willis make extensive use of bone removal at the skull base to minimize the brain retraction required. Most anterior circulation aneurysms are approached from a pterional, or transsylvian, route. With this approach it is important that the anterior fossa floor and sphenoid wing are drilled flat, so that frontal lobe retraction is minimized. In most cases the first intracranial maneuver is to achieve proximal control by preparing the internal carotid artery for possible temporary clipping. Dissection can then proceed along the internal carotid artery and its branches until the aneurysm is reached. The arachnoid dissection involved frees up the frontal and temporal lobes for retraction. Splitting the sylvian fissure facilitates frontal and temporal lobe retraction and is required to some degree for the exposure of most anterior circulation aneurysms. Anterior cerebral artery aneurysms distal to the anterior communicating artery are approached from an interhemispheric direction.

The approach to posterior circulation aneurysms is more complex. Many aneurysms in the region of the basilar apex can also be approached from a pterional direction. The sylvian fissure is split widely and the corridor of approach is between the internal carotid artery and third cranial nerve, or between the optic nerve and internal carotid artery. A low angle of approach for high basilar bifurcation aneurysms is achieved by removing the orbital rim and the zygomatic arch. Alternatives for basilar apex region aneurysms include the subtemporal approach or modifications of it. These provide a more direct route to the aneurysm but can make visualization of the contralateral branches difficult. For more low-lying posterior circulation aneurysms, middle fossa, transpetrous, retrosigmoid, transcondylar, and suboccipital approaches are used.

Endovascular Management of Aneurysms

Surgical obliteration of a ruptured aneurysm remains the procedure of choice, provided it is technically feasible and there are no medical conditions that would contraindicate surgery. However, treatment decisions are preferably made by a neurovascular team that includes the interventional neuroradiologist, neurovascular surgeon, and stereotactic radiosurgeon. (The radiosurgeon will not have input for aneurysm management but is an integral member of the team for management of AVMs and other conditions.)

Early clinical and angiographic results indicate that the treatment-related complications of endovascular therapy for aneurysms compare favorably to surgery [3]. The long-term efficacy remains unproved and there have been some concerns about the rebleeding rate for treated aneurysms [3]. A metaanalysis of 1,383 patients revealed a complication rate of only 3.7% but an incomplete obliteration rate of 46% [84]. The long-term rebleeding rate of incompletely obliterated aneurysms treated with coils remains unclear. Although coils can result in complete obliteration of aneurysms as determined angiographically, there is concern about long-term recanalization because the internal surface does not reendothelialize after the coil is placed (Fig. 5-7). It is likely that advances in the technology of coil materials will solve this problem in the near future.

In general, coil placement is reserved for patients who are considered high surgical risks, who are medically unsuitable for surgery, or who refuse open surgery. However, the location of some aneurysms, such as the intracavernous carotid artery and basilar apex, dictates that endovascular treatment is preferable if possible.

Other endovascular treatments for aneurysms include proximal occlusion (usually with a preceding test occlusion) and proximal occlusion or trapping in combination with revascularization surgery. Endovascular management of vasospasm has been discussed above.

Treatment of Nonsaccular Aneurysms

Dissecting Aneurysms

Neurologic deficits from extracranial dissecting aneurysms are generally related to thromboembolism. Extracranial dis-

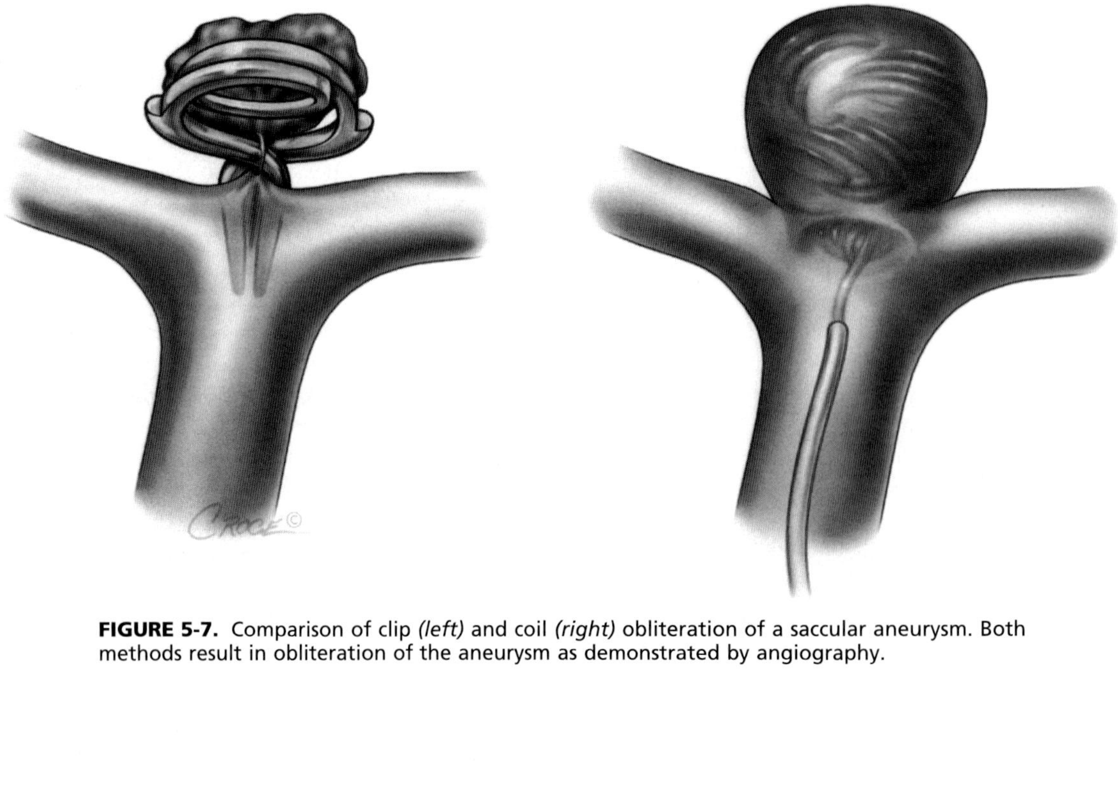

FIGURE 5-7. Comparison of clip *(left)* and coil *(right)* obliteration of a saccular aneurysm. Both methods result in obliteration of the aneurysm as demonstrated by angiography.

sections tend to heal well spontaneously, so the aim of treatment in most cases is to prevent thromboembolic events while the intima heals [85]. Anticoagulation or antiplatelet therapy for an empirical period of 3 months and follow-up angiography is commonly advised, although there are no clear therapeutic guidelines [86]. Revascularization surgery with bypass grafts or excision and replacement of the affected segment is reserved for the unusual case with symptomatic hemodynamic insufficiency that is confirmed on blood flow studies. Asymptomatic dissections may be treated with anticoagulation to prevent embolic events, but there is no conclusive evidence to support this. Endovascular treatment with angioplasty and stents has been reported [85,87].

Dissection of intracranial arteries is much less common and more problematic to treat. Rupture with SAH is a much more common result of intracranial dissections than of extracranial lesions, so anticoagulation is usually contraindicated. Thrombolytic therapy has been used in selected unruptured cases [88]. The prognosis in children is surprisingly dismal [2]. Trapping or resection of the dissected segment combined with revascularization using external carotid or saphenous vein bypass grafts is recommended for patients with transient ischemic symptoms or SAH when it is technically feasible to do so. Proximal occlusion (surgical or endovascular), wrapping, or stenting can be considered, particularly for posterior circulation aneurysms with hemorrhage [27].

Fusiform Aneurysms

Treatment of fusiform aneurysms is formidable, whether surgically or endovascularly. Symptomatic progression despite anticoagulant therapy can justify wrapping, resection, occlusion, reconstruction with clips, grafting, or decompression by thrombectomy. Surgery is technically difficult and carries a high risk. Reconstruction of fusiform aneurysms carries a high risk of injury to perforating branches involved in the aneurysm, and pathologic walls tend to rebulge. Current endovascular therapies are also limited, although stenting may become a useful method for reinforcing the walls of these lesions.

Infectious Aneurysms

Prolonged antibiotic therapy is mandatory for patients with infectious aneurysms, regardless of other treatment. Unruptured aneurysms can be treated with antibiotics alone, but these patients should have serial angiography (every 2 to 4 weeks) to ensure resolution occurs. Obliteration of the aneurysm is indicated when a SAH occurs. Surgical management usually requires trapping and excision of the aneurysm, with revascularization when eloquent brain is at ischemic risk. Location and excision of these aneurysms is often difficult, because they often reside deep in sulci. Infectious aneurysms are friable and rupture easily. Recently, endovascular occlusion of the parent artery proximal to the aneurysm has produced favorable results and this may be a preferable treatment, except when eloquent brain is supplied by the artery [29].

The mortality from ruptured infectious aneurysms treated only with antibiotics is up to 80%. Modern multimodality treatment can yield good results in 80% of cases [29]. Survival from intracranial fungal aneurysms is distinctly unusual and would require aggressive surgery with *en bloc* resection.

False Aneurysms

The risk of rebleeding from traumatic false or pseudoaneurysms is high. Once detected, these lesions should be resected or trapped. Revascularization is indicated to preserve flow to eloquent regions of brain. Endovascular occlusion or stenting is likely to play an increasing role with proximal lesions.

Aneurysms in Children

Up to 4% of aneurysms are detected in patients younger than 18. An underlying disorder predisposing to aneurysm formation can be identified in up to one-half of the patients. SAH is the most common reason for seeking treatment, although mass effect is more common than in adults [89]. The clinical features of SAH in very young patients are less characteristic than in adults and include irritability, vomiting, and a reduced level of consciousness. Seizures occur in 25% of pediatric patients with SAH. Aneurysms are distinctly unusual in patients less than 5 years of age. In contrast to the epidemiology of aneurysms in the adult population, there is a male predominance, perhaps because disorders associated with aneurysms are more common in males [90]. Saccular aneurysms are the most common type, but traumatic and infectious aneurysms appear to be more common than in adults. The most common site for saccular aneurysms in children is the internal carotid artery bifurcation, followed by the anterior cerebral artery [2,91]. Some series have suggested that posterior circulation and giant aneurysms are relatively more common in children [90,92]. Giant aneurysms in children are associated with mass effect rather than hemorrhage, except in infants when SAH is the usual problem. In children under 5 years of age, the most common locations are the middle cerebral artery and basilar bifurcation [89]. Proximal middle cerebral artery aneurysms are as common in this group as aneurysms of the middle cerebral artery bifurcation [91]. Multiple aneurysms are less common in children than in adults. The distribution of clinical grades and outcomes is similar to adults with a SAH [91]. Treatment of patients with aneurysms in this age group is similar to that of adults. The greater potential for neurologic recovery in children should be considered when treating patients who are in poor condition. The rate of angiographic vasospasm is similar in children to that in adults, but the risk of developing delayed ischemic deficits appears to be less. The risk of ischemia is also less in children treated with proximal ligation. The value of nimodipine has not been established in children.

Giant Aneurysms

Approximately 5% of cerebral aneurysms will reach 2.5 cm or more in diameter and these lesions pose significant management problems. The most common problem with these giant aneurysms is still rupture, but compared with small and large aneurysms they more commonly cause mass effect, transient ischemic attacks, and seizures. Giant carotid-ophthalmic aneurysms are more common in women than men. The natural history of these aneurysms is extremely poor—the 5-year survival rate after diagnosis in untreated patients is less than 20%. Surgical occlusion of giant aneurysms remains the preferred treatment in most cases. These aneurysms often contain intraluminal thrombus, have large necks, and involve the origins of major branches—all factors that make endovascular therapy less attractive. To achieve effective surgical reconstruction, attention must be paid to adequate exposure of the aneurysm and all related branches, control of all related arteries, and decompression of the aneurysm prior to clip application [93]. Giant aneurysms of the posterior circulation are particularly difficult lesions to treat surgically. The confined space, and involvement of main branches and critical perforating arteries makes adequate exposure and reconstruction difficult.

Alternative treatments to clipping of the neck should be considered. These include proximal occlusion and trapping, with or without distal revascularization. Proximal occlusion of anterior and posterior circulation aneurysms has been relatively successful in reducing the risk of hemorrhage and in many cases is a far preferable treatment to the high risk of direct surgery [94].

Outcome

Only one-third of patients suffering a SAH make a full recovery. Adverse prognostic factors for good outcome include advanced age, poor neurologic condition, loss of consciousness, and comorbid atherosclerotic illnesses [6]. Elderly patients have a higher incidence of hypertension and tend to be in poorer neurologic condition than younger patients. Aneurysm location in the posterior circulation, especially the basilar artery, is also associated with a worse outcome. Thick subarachnoid clots, intraparenchymal hemorrhage, and intraventricular hemorrhage are all associated with worse outcome.

Patients with a good physical recovery can suffer neuropsychologic deficits that may be detected only with detailed examinations [95,96]. There is some evidence that the cognitive outcome is slightly better after aneurysm coil placement than after clipping [97]. However, the most important factor in neuropsychologic outcome is the severity of the original hemorrhage [97,98]. Patients with a left-sided middle cerebral artery aneurysm suffer greater impairments of social contact, communication, and cognition than patients with other aneurysms [98].

REFERENCES

1. Haubrich WS. *Medical meanings. a glossary of word origins.* San Diego: Harcourt Brace Jovanovich, 1984.
2. Weir B. *Aneurysms affecting the nervous system.* Baltimore: Williams and Wilkins, 1987.
3. Bederson JB, Awad IA, Wiebers DO, et al. Recommendations for the management of patients with unruptured intracranial aneurysms. A statement for healthcare professionals from the Stroke Council of the American Heart Association. *Stroke* 2000;31: 2742–2750.
4. Kiyohara Y, Ueda K, Hasuo Y, et al. Incidence and prognosis of subarachnoid hemorrhage in a Japanese rural community. *Stroke* 1989;20:1150–1155.
5. Sarti C, Tuomilehto J, Salomaa V, et al. Epidemiology of subarachnoid hemorrhage in Finland from 1983 to 1985. *Stroke* 1991;22:848–853.
6. Kassell NF, Torner JC, Haley EC, et al. The International Cooperative Study on the Timing of Aneurysm Surgery. Part 1: overall management results. *J Neurosurg* 1990;73:18–36.
7. Stehbens WE. The pathology of intracranial arterial aneurysms and their complications. In: Fox JL, ed. *Intracranial aneurysms.* New York: Springer-Verlag, 1983:272–357.
8. Atkinson JL, Sundt TM, Houser OW, et al. Angiographic frequency of anterior circulation intracranial aneurysms. *J Neurosurg* 1989;70:551–555.
9. Weir B. *Subarachnoid hemorrhage: causes and cures.* New York: Oxford University Press, 1998.
10. Broderick JP, Brott T, Tomsick T, et al. The risk of subarachnoid and intracerebral hemorrhages in blacks as compared with whites. *N Engl J Med* 1992;327:568.
11. Ronkainen A, Hernesniemi J, Ryynanen M. Familial subarachnoid hemorrhage in east Finland, 1977–1990. *Neurosurgery* 1993;33:796–797.
12. Ronkainen A, Hernesniemi J, Tromp G. Special features of familial intracranial aneurysms: report of 215 familial aneurysms. *Neurosurgery* 1995;35:43–46.
13. Lozano AM, Leblanc R. Familial intracranial aneurysms. *J Neurosurg* 1987;66:522–528.
14. Alberts MJ. Subarachnoid hemorrhage and intracranial aneurysms. In: Alberts MJ, ed. *Genetics of cerebrovascular disease.* Armonk, NY: Futura Publishing, 1999.
15. Geevarghese SK, Powers T, Marsh JW, et al. Screening for cerebral aneurysm in patients with polycystic liver disease. *South Med J* 1999;92:1167–1170.
16. Lozano AM, Leblanc R. Cerebral aneurysms and polycystic kidney disease: a critical review. *Can J Neurol Sci* 1992;19:222–227.
17. Belz MM, Hughes RL, Kaehny WD, et al. Familial clustering of ruptured intracranial aneurysms in autosomal dominant polycystic kidney disease. *Am J Kidney Dis* 2001;38:770–776.
18. Preul MC, Cendes F, Just N, et al. Intracranial aneurysms and sickle cell anemia: multiplicity and propensity for the vertebrobasilar territory. *Neurosurgery* 1998;42:971–977.
19. Meisel HJ, Mansmann U, Alvarez H, et al. Cerebral arteriovenous malformations and associated aneurysms: analysis of 305 cases from a series of 662 patients. *J Neurosurg* 2000;46:793–800.

20. Redekop G, TerBrugge K, Montanera W, et al. Arterial aneurysms associated with cerebral arteriovenous malformations: classification, incidence, and risk of hemorrhage. *J Neurosurg* 1998; 89:539–546.
21. Westphal M, Grzyska U. Clinical significance of pedicle aneurysms on feeding vessels, especially those located in infratentorial arteriovenous malformations. *J Neurosurg* 2000;92:995–1001.
22. Thompson RC, Steinberg GK, Levy RP, et al. The management of patients with arteriovenous malformations and associated intracranial aneurysms. *Neurosurgery* 1998;43:202–211.
23. Wong MC, Giuliani MJ, Haley E. Cerebrovascular disease and stroke in women. *Cardiology* 1990;77[Suppl 2]:80–90.
24. Yaşargil MG. *Microneurosurgery. Vol II: clinical considerations, surgery of the intracranial aneurysms and results.* Stuttgart: Georg Thieme Verlag, 1984.
25. Stehbens WE. Aneurysms. In: Stehbens WE, Lie JT, eds. *Vascular pathology.* New York: Chapman and Hall Medical, 1995: 377–414.
26. Sakata N, Takebayashi S, Kojima M, et al. Different roles of arteriosclerosis in the rupture of intracranial dissecting aneurysms. *Histopathology* 2001;38:325–327.
27. Malek AM, Halbach VV, Phatouros CC, et al. Endovascular treatment of a ruptured intracranial dissecting vertebral aneurysm in a kickboxer. *J Trauma* 2000;48:143–145.
28. Mizutani T, Kojima H, Asamoto S, et al. Pathological mechanism and three-dimensional structure of cerebral dissecting aneurysms. *J Neurosurg* 2001;94:712–717.
29. Chun JY, Smith W, Halbach VV, et al. Current multimodality management of infectious intracranial aneurysms. *Neurosurgery* 2001;48:1203–1213.
30. Seigle JM, Caputy AJ, Manz HJ, et al. Multiple oncotic intracranial aneurysms and cardiac metastasis from choriocarcinoma: case report and review of the literature. *Neurosurgery* 1987;20:39–42.
31. Miyaoka M, Sato K, Ishii S. A clinical study of the relationship of timing to outcome of surgery for ruptured cerebral aneurysms. A retrospective analysis of 1622 cases. *J Neurosurg* 1993;79: 373–378.
32. Ellamushi HE, Grieve JP, Jager HR, et al. Risk factors for the formation of multiple intracranial aneurysms. *J Neurosurg* 2001; 94:728–732.
33. Hademenos GJ, Massoud TF. The physics of cerebrovascular disease. In: Greenbaum E, ed. *Biological physics series.* New York: Springer-Verlag, 1998.
34. Nornes H. The role of intracranial pressure in the arrest of hemorrhage in patients with ruptured intracranial aneurysm. *J Neurosurg* 1973;39:226–234.
35. Hassler W, Steinmetz H, Pirschel J. Transcranial Doppler study of intracranial circulatory arrest. *J Neurosurg* 1989;71:195–201.
36. Grubb RL, Raichle ME, Eichling JO, et al. Effects of subarachnoid hemorrhage on cerebral blood volume, blood flow, and oxygen utilization in humans. *J Neurosurg* 1977;46:446–453.
37. Meyer CH, Lowe D, Meyer M, et al. Progressive change in cerebral blood flow during the first three weeks after subarachnoid hemorrhage. *Neurosurgery* 1983;12:58–76.
38. Voldby B, Enevoldsen EM, Jensen FT. Cerebrovascular reactivity in patients with ruptured intracranial aneurysms. *J Neurosurg* 1985;62:59–67.
39. Griebel RW, Black PM, Pile-Spellman J, et al. The importance of "accessory" outflow pathways in hydrocephalus after experimental subarachnoid hemorrhage. *Neurosurgery* 1989;24: 187–192.
40. Macdonald RL, Weir B. *Cerebral vasospasm.* San Diego: Academic Press, 2001.
41. Graff-Radford NR, Torner J, Adams HP, et al. Factors associated with hydrocephalus after subarachnoid hemorrhage. A report of the Cooperative Aneurysm Study. *Arch Neurol* 1989;46: 744–752.
42. Chicoine MR, Dacey RG. Clinical aspects of subarachnoid hemorrhage. In: Welch KMA, Caplan LR, Reis DJ, et al., eds. *Primer on cerebrovascular diseases.* San Diego: Academic Press, 1997: 425–432.
43. Macdonald RL. Cerebral vasospasm. *Neurosurg Q* 1995;5:73–97.
44. Fisher CM, Kistler JP, Davis JM. Relation of cerebral vasospasm to subarachnoid hemorrhage visualized by computerized tomographic scanning. *Neurosurgery* 1980;6:1–9.
45. Kistler JP, Crowell RM, Davis KR, et al. The relation of cerebral vasospasm to the extent and location of subarachnoid blood visualized by CT scan: a prospective study. *Neurology* 1983;33: 424–436.
46. Findlay JM, Kassell NF, Weir BKA, et al. A randomized trial of intraoperative, intracisternal tissue plasminogen activator for the prevention of vasospasm. *Neurosurgery* 1995;37:168–178.
47. Weir B, Macdonald RL, Stoodley M. Etiology of cerebral vasospasm. *Acta Neurochir Suppl* 1999;72:27–46.
48. Pakarinen S. Incidence, aetiology, and prognosis of primary subarachnoid haemorrhage. A study based on 589 cases diagnosed in a defined urban population during a defined period. *Acta Neurol Scand* 1967;43[Suppl]29:1–28.
49. Jane JA, Winn HR, Richardson AE. The natural history of intracranial aneurysms: rebleeding rates during the acute and long term period and implication for surgical management. *Clin Neurosurg* 1977;24:176–184.
50. Locksley HB. Natural history of subarachnoid hemorrhage, intracranial aneurysms and arteriovenous malformations. *J Neurosurg* 1966;25:321–368.
51. Wiebers DO, Whisnant JP, Sundt T, et al. The significance of unruptured intracranial saccular aneurysms. *J Neurosurg* 1987; 66:23–29.
52. Juvela S, Porras M, Heiskanen O. Natural history of unruptured intracranial aneurysms: a long-term follow-up study. *J Neurosurg* 1993;79:174–182.
53. Yasui N, Suzuki A, Nishimura H, et al. Long-term follow-up study of unruptured intracranial aneurysms. *Neurosurgery* 1997; 40:1155–1159.
54. The ISUIA Investigators. Unruptured intracranial aneurysms: risks of rupture and risks of surgical intervention. *N Engl J Med* 1998;339:1725–1733.
55. Ausman JI. The New England Journal of Medicine report on unruptured aneurysms: a critique. *Surg Neurol* 1999;51: 227–229.
56. Solomon RA, Fink ME, Pile-Spellman J. Surgical management of unruptured intracranial aneurysms. *J Neurosurg* 1994;80: 440–446.
57. Hauerberg J, Andersen BB, Eskesen V, et al. Importance of the recognition of a warning leak as a sign of a ruptured intracranial aneurysm. *Acta Neurol Scand* 1991;83:61–64.
58. Stoodley MA, Warren JD, Oatey PE. Thalamic syndrome caused by unruptured cerebral aneurysm. Case report. *J Neurosurg* 1995; 82:291–293.
59. Stoodley MA, Macdonald RL, Weir BK. Surgical treatment of middle cerebral artery aneurysms. *Neurosurg Clin N Am* 1998; 9:823–834.
60. Fridriksson S, Hillman J, Saveland H, et al. Immediate short-term antifibrinolytic treatment with tranexamic acid in SAH to prevent very early rebleeds—a prospective multicenter study. Paper presented at: World Federation of Neurosurgical Societies 12th World Congress of Neurosurgery; 2001; Sydney, Australia.
61. Andreoli A, di Pasquale G, Pinelli G, et al. Subarachnoid hemorrhage: frequency and severity of cardiac arrhythmias. A survey of 70 cases studied in the acute phase. *Stroke* 1987;18:558–564.
62. Grady RE, Strickland RA, Fabi AY, et al. Intraoperative use of

nitric oxide during intracranial aneurysm clipping in a patient with acute respiratory distress syndrome. *J Neurosurg Anesthesiol* 1999;11:124–126.
63. Kassell NF, Boarini DJ. Perioperative care of the aneurysm patient. *Contemp Neurosurg* 1984;6:1–6.
64. Sloan MA, Haley EC, Kassell NF, et al. Sensitivity and specificity of transcranial Doppler ultrasonography in the diagnosis of vasospasm following subarachnoid hemorrhage. *Neurology* 1989;39:1514–1518.
65. Tettenborn D, Dycka J. Prevention and treatment of delayed ischemic dysfunction in patients with aneurysmal subarachnoid hemorrhage. *Stroke* 1990;21[Suppl 12]:85–89.
66. Haley EC, Kassell NF, Apperson-Hansen C, et al. A randomized, double-blind, vehicle-controlled trial of tirilazad mesylate in patients with aneurysmal subarachnoid hemorrhage: a cooperative study in North America. *J Neurosurg* 1997;86:467–474.
67. Le Roux PD, Elliott JP, Newell DW, et al. Predicting outcome in poor-grade patients with subarachnoid hemorrhage: a retrospective review of 159 aggressively managed cases. *J Neurosurg* 1996;85:39–49.
68. Inagawa T, Hada H, Katoh Y. Unruptured intracranial aneurysms in elderly patients. *Surg Neurol* 1992;38:364–370.
69. Dell S. Asymptomatic cerebral aneurysm: assessment of its risk of rupture. *Neurosurgery* 1982;10:162–166.
70. Weir B. Unruptured intracranial aneurysms—a review. *J Neurosurg* 2002;96:3–42.
71. Kassell NF, Torner JC, Jane JA, et al. The International Cooperative Study on the Timing of Aneurysm Surgery. Part 2: surgical results. *J Neurosurg* 1990;73:37–47.
72. Disney L, Weir B, Petruk K. Effect on management mortality of a deliberate policy of early operation on supratentorial aneurysms. *Neurosurgery* 1987;20:695–701.
73. Chyatte D, Fode NC, Sundt TM. Early versus late intracranial aneurysm surgery in subarachnoid hemorrhage. *J Neurosurg* 1988;69:326–331.
74. Hernesniemi J, Vapalahti M, Niskanen M, et al. One-year outcome in early aneurysm surgery: a 14 years experience. *Acta Neurochir (Wien)* 1993;122:1–10.
75. Milhorat TH, Krautheim M. Results of early and delayed operations for ruptured intracranial aneurysms in two series of 100 consecutive patients. *Surg Neurol* 1986;26:123–128.
76. Disney L, Weir B, Grace M. Factors influencing the outcome of aneurysm rupture in poor grade patients: a prospective series. *Neurosurgery* 1988;23:1–9.
77. Findlay JM, Macdonald RL, Weir BK, et al. Surgical manipulation of primate cerebral arteries in established vasospasm. *J Neurosurg* 1991;75:425–432.
78. Solomon RA, Onesti ST, Klebanoff L. Relationship between the timing of aneurysm surgery and the development of delayed cerebral ischemia. *J Neurosurg* 1991;75:56–61.
79. Le Roux PD, Newell DW, Eskridge J, et al. Severe symptomatic vasospasm: the role of immediate postoperative angioplasty. *J Neurosurg* 1994;80:224–229.
80. Pare L, Delfino R, Leblanc R. The relationship of ventricular drainage to aneurysmal rebleeding. *J Neurosurg* 1992;76:422–427.
81. Batjer HH, Samson DS. Retrograde suction decompression of giant paraclinoid aneurysms: technical note. *J Neurosurg* 1990;73:305–306.
82. Chang HS, Hongo K, Nakagawa H. Adverse effects of limited hypotensive anesthesia on the outcome of patients with subarachnoid hemorrhage. *J Neurosurg* 2000;92:971–975.
83. Todd NV, Tocher JL, Jones PA, et al. Outcome following aneurysm wrapping: a 10-year follow-up review of clipped and wrapped aneurysms. *J Neurosurg* 1989;70:841–846.
84. Brilstra EH, Rinkel GJ, van der Graaf Y, et al. Treatment of intracranial aneurysms by embolization with coils: a systematic review. *Stroke* 1999;30:470–476.
85. Schievink WI. The treatment of spontaneous carotid and vertebral artery dissections. *Curr Opin Cardiol* 2000;15:316–321.
86. Engelter ST, Lyrer PA, Kirsch EC, et al. Long-term follow-up after extracranial internal carotid artery dissection. *Eur Neurol* 2000;44:199–204.
87. Redekop G, Marotta T, Weill A. Treatment of traumatic aneurysms and arteriovenous fistulas of the skull base by using endovascular stents. *J Neurosurg* 2001;95:412–419.
88. Leistner S, Hartmann A, Marx P, et al. Successful thrombolytic treatment of intracranial carotid occlusion due to dissection. *Eur Neurol* 2001;45:284–285.
89. Ferrante L, Fortuna A, Celli P, et al. Intracranial arterial aneurysms in early childhood. *Surg Neurol* 1988;29:39–56.
90. Meyer FB, Sundt TM, Fode NC, et al. Cerebral aneurysms in childhood and adolescence. *J Neurosurg* 1989;70:420–425.
91. Proust F, Toussaint P, Garnieri J, et al. Pediatric cerebral aneurysms. *J Neurosurg* 2001;94:733–739.
92. Roach ES, Riela AR. *Pediatric cerebrovascular disorders.* Armonk, NY: Futura Publishing, 1995.
93. Kopitnik T, Samson D. Surgical management of the patient with a giant cerebral aneurysm. In: Welch KMA, Caplan LR, Reis DJ, et al., eds. *Primer on cerebrovascular diseases.* San Diego: Academic Press, 1997:475–480.
94. Drake CG, Peerless SJ, Ferguson GG. Hunterian proximal arterial occlusion for giant aneurysms of the carotid circulation. *J Neurosurg* 1994;81:656–665.
95. Ogden JA, Utley T, Mee EW. Neurological and psychosocial outcome 4 to 7 years after subarachnoid hemorrhage. *Neurosurgery* 1997;41:25–34.
96. Ogden JA, Mee EW, Henning M. A prospective study of impairment of cognition and memory and recovery after subarachnoid hemorrhage. *Neurosurgery* 1993;33:572–586.
97. Hadjivassiliou M, Tooth CL, Romanowski CA, et al. Aneurysmal SAH: cognitive outcome and structural damage after clipping or coiling. *Neurology* 2001;56:1672–1677.
98. Hutter BO, Kreitschmann-Andermahr I, Gilsbach JM. Health-related quality of life after aneurysmal SAH: impacts of bleeding severity, computerized tomography findings, surgery, vasospasm, and neurological grade. *J Neurosurg* 2001;94:241–251.

Endovascular and Percutaneous Therapy of the Brain and Spine, edited by Michael P. Marks and Huy M. Do.
Lippincott Williams & Wilkins, Philadelphia © 2002.

6

INTRAANEURYSMAL ENDOVASCULAR THERAPY

YUICHI MURAYAMA
FERNANDO VIÑUELA

Microsurgical clipping of intracranial aneurysms has been the therapeutic gold standard for treatment of intracranial aneurysms [1]. This surgical technique achieves complete aneurysmal occlusion with preservation of the parent artery and important arterial perforators in a vast number of patients. However, its procedural morbidity and mortality rates are increased by specific risk factors, such as aneurysm location (deep versus superficial), size (small, large, or giant), patient age, and medical conditions. Therefore, patients with these relatively high risk factors would benefit from therapeutic alternatives to exclude the aneurysm from the circulation, thus preventing aneurysmal growth, rupture, or rerupture. Since the early 1970s, endovascular treatment of selected cases of intracranial aneurysms has become a therapeutic alternative to direct surgical clipping. This chapter will discuss the history, present techniques, and future developments in intraaneurysmal endovascular treatment for aneurysms. Chapter 7 covers the technique of parent vessel occlusion.

BACKGROUND

Intracranial aneurysms are the main cause of nontraumatic subarachnoid hemorrhage (SAH) [2]. Autopsy studies estimate that up to 5% of the general population may harbor intracranial aneurysms [3]. However, the true prevalence of intracranial aneurysms and the risk of rupture remain difficult to ascertain [4].

With few exceptions, these lesions make their presence known after a rupture produces SAH. The rate of morbidity and mortality related to aneurysmal rupture remains high (45% overall during the first year) [3]. At least 15% of patients are found dead after the initial hemorrhage. The mortality rate during the first 2 weeks is 20% to 30% for patients surviving the initial hemorrhage. Rebleeding is a major cause of death and disability in the untreated patient.

The risk of rebleeding during the 2 weeks after the first hemorrhage is approximately 20% and increases to 33% 1 month and 50% 6 months afterward [5]. The mortality rate from this second hemorrhage is 40% to 50%. The risk of rebleeding gradually diminishes but does not reach zero. Approximately 5% to 6% of long-term survivors can be expected to rebleed annually, depending on the aneurysm size, location, and the patient's clinical picture [6]. Aside from the risk of fatality, there is significant patient disability.

In more than 50% of survivors of SAH, the disability is serious, and approximately 64% of patients discharged home after aneurysmal occlusion never achieve the quality of life they enjoyed before aneurysmal rupture [7].

Accordingly, both ruptured and unruptured intracranial aneurysms constitute a significant public health problem. The estimated lifetime cost (including hospitalization, treatment, morbidity, and mortality) for patients hospitalized with unruptured intracranial aneurysms in the United States is $522.5 million annually, and $1.76 billion for patients with aneurysmal SAH [8]. A more complete discussion of epidemiology and natural history for intracranial aneurysms is covered in Chapter 5.

Endovascular Treatment Using Balloons

Serbinenko [9], Debrun et al. [10], and Kerber [11] succeeded in overcoming the natural obstacle of the circle of Willis using microcatheters and balloons and, for the first time, navigated inside intracranial arteries. Their technical success launched the genesis of modern interventional neuroradiology [12–17].

The first significant contribution of modern interventional neuroradiology in the treatment of intracranial aneurysms was the proximal balloon occlusion of the parent artery in large and giant aneurysms. It required the use of preembolization temporary arterial occlusion with concomitant electroencephalographic (EEG) and clinical assessment

Y. Murayama and F. Viñuela: Division of Interventional Neuroradiology, UCLA School of Medicine and Medical Center, Los Angeles, California.

of brain functions [18]. If the patient tolerated the temporary balloon occlusion for 30 minutes or more, the parent artery was then permanently occluded with detachable balloons or coils. If the patient failed this functional test, an external carotid-internal carotid (EC-IC) bypass preceded the permanent arterial occlusion. The overall procedural morbidity and mortality rate of this technique is approximately 4% to 5%.

The development of smaller catheters and balloons launched the technique of balloon occlusion of the aneurysm while preserving the parent artery [19]. The main drawback of this technique was that the fragile wall of the aneurysm underwent stress while adapting to the shape of the balloon, thus carrying the risk of aneurysmal rupture. This procedural complication increased in ruptured aneurysms. In addition, due to the frequent mismatch between the shapes of the aneurysm and the balloon, a potentially dangerous residual neck often remained after aneurysmal occlusion. For these reasons and also because of the secondary balloon deflation, it became clear that it was unlikely that this technique would one day replace microsurgical clipping of intracranial aneurysms.

Microcoil Therapy

In the late 1980s, the endovascular occlusion of aneurysms included "pushable" microcoils [20]. These coils were softer than balloons, although they could not be retrieved after being deployed into the sac of the aneurysm. This technical limitation increased the possibility of untoward coil migration into the parent artery. In 1991, Guglielmi et al. reported the use of electrolytically detachable platinum coils (GDCs) [21,22]. This platinum coil, approved by the U.S. Food and Drug Administration (FDA) in 1995, is soft, adapts to different sizes and shapes of aneurysms, can be retrieved and repositioned as many times as needed, and is detached from a stainless steel guidewire using a small electric current. Today, more than 70 types of GDCs allow physicians to select the best coil for each type of intracranial aneurysm (Fig. 6-1). The addition of #10 and #18, soft and regular, two- (2-D) and three-dimensional (3-D) GDCs has also improved immediate and long-term anatomical and clinical outcomes.

The development of a new generation of coated microcatheters and microguidewires facilitated intracranial navigation well beyond the circle of Willis, and peripheral aneurysms can now be occluded using endovascular techniques.

Currently, a controlled detachment coil system is the gold standard for endovascular occlusion of incidental or ruptured intracranial aneurysms [23–28]. It does not require brain manipulation. The incidence of delayed cerebral arterial vasospasm is similar to that associated with surgical clipping [29], and its procedural morbidity and mortality rate in experienced hands is approximately 5%.

In January 2000, the FDA made available a second controlled-release coil system in the United States for intraaneurysmal therapy. This system is known as the ACT (anatomically compliant 3-D) microcoil system (Micrus Corporation). The system is similar to the GDC in that it is a soft, compliant, platinum coil system. The system differs from the GDC in that it has a heat-resistant detachment mechanism that fractures a fiber and thereby effects release between the coil pusher and the coil. This attachment mechanism produces a rapid (less than 5-second) release time. The ACT is available in a 3-D spherical shape as well as the more conventional helical shape.

Long-term cerebral angiographic follow-up has shown that the overall recanalization rate of aneurysms embolized with the GDC system varies between 20% to 25%. It oscillates between 5% and 10% in small aneurysms with small necks to 45% to 50% in large and giant aneurysms [23, 28].

Aneurysm recanalization is related to coil remodeling at the level of the aneurysmal inflow zone produced by the water hammer effect of the arterial flow. In aneurysms with a wide neck (4 mm or more) it is difficult to achieve a dense coil packing at the level of the neck inflow zone without increasing the risk of untoward coil migration into the parent artery or intracranially. The addition of 3-D GDC [30] and the balloon-assisted technique [31–34], and the incorporation of intracranial microstents [35–40] may well improve long-term anatomical outcomes.

The 3-D GDCs permit a stronger anchoring of the microcoil within the aneurysm and allow denser aneurysm packing than regular microcoils. This coil is used as a first coil to form a basket-like shape. Additional helical GDCs can be deposited in the basket area. Aneurysm recanalization rates using 3-D GDC seem lower than those with standard GDC alone, although no series have been published to document this.

The balloon-assisted technique may require a temporary blocking of the neck of the aneurysm with a nondetachable balloon while deploying the GDC. This technique requires a bifemoral approach and the handling of intracranial balloons, even though it improves the anchoring of the microcatheter within the aneurysm. This better catheter anchoring increases the density of the coil packing of the neck of the aneurysm and in particular of the aneurysmal inflow zone. Preliminary data on long-term angiographic follow-up performed in aneurysms treated with the balloon-assisted technology suggest a decreased percentage of aneurysm recanalization. Its procedural morbidity and mortality rate has been reported to be similar to that of the standard GDC technique [32].

Microstents and Liquid Embolic Agents

The deployment of intracranial microstents across the neck of a wide-necked aneurysm and in a limited number of fusiform aneurysms has also improved the anatomical and

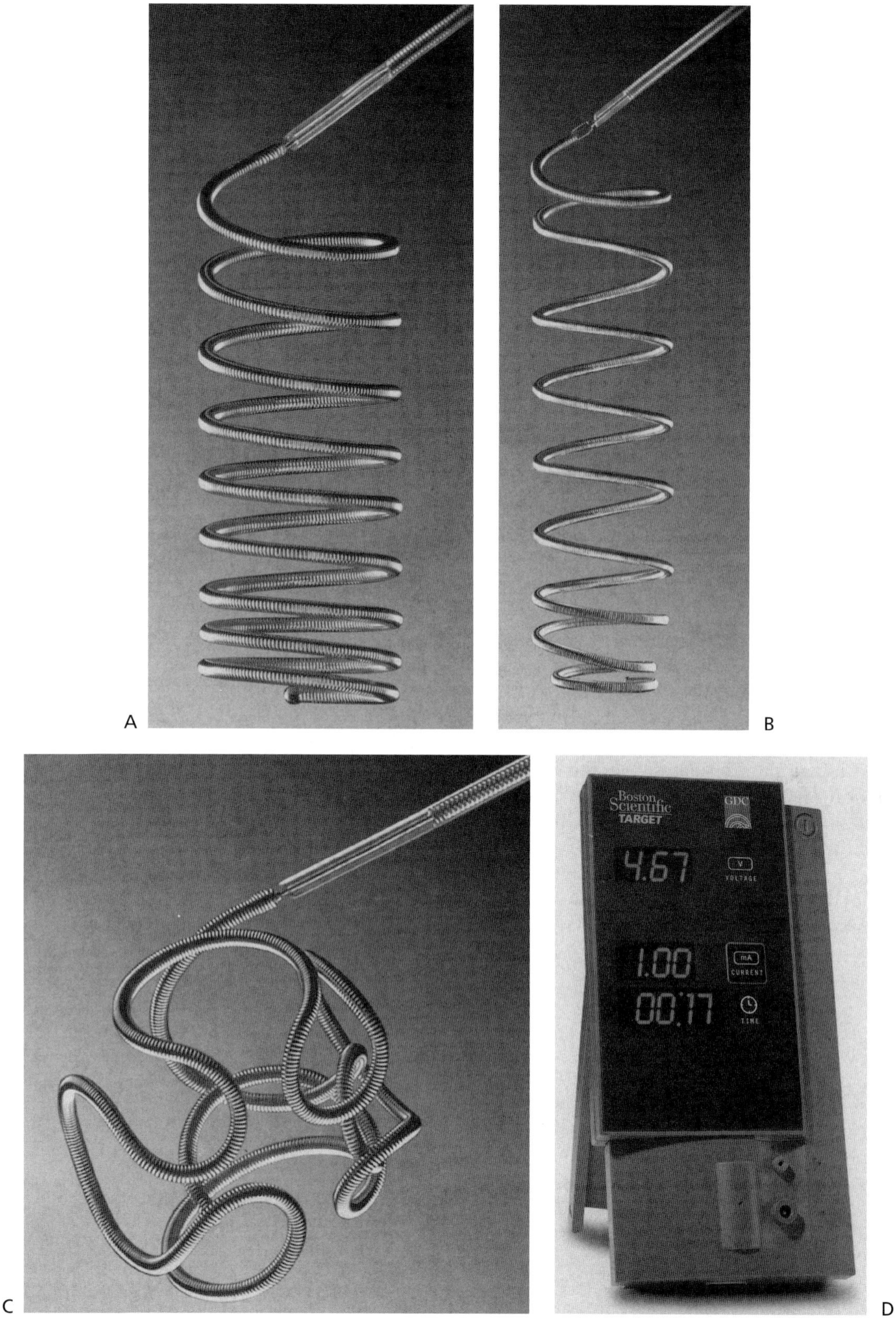

FIGURE 6-1. The Guglielmi Detachable Coil (GDC) system. **A:** Standard GDC. **B:** Two-dimensional GDC. **C:** Three-dimensional GDC. **(D):** SynerG detachment power supply unit.

clinical outcomes. Most microstents used today in neurointerventional procedures have been inherited from the cardiovascular experience in coronary artery stenting. They may need to be specifically modified in their tractability and thrombogenicity to overcome the winding curves of the brain circulation as well as the smaller caliber of intracranial arteries. Nonetheless, an increasing number of articles in the neurosurgical and neurointerventional literature report anatomical and clinical successes in cases that could not be treated several years ago [35–40].

Debrun et al. reported the use of acrylics for embolization of aneurysms in the animal laboratory in 1984 [41]. In 1992, Kinugasa and Mandai et al. reported the use of cellulose acetate polymer (CAP) as an embolic material used for the endovascular occlusion of aneurysms [42,43]. They emphasized the importance of gravity as an important factor in keeping the liquid embolic agent within the aneurysm and used proximal temporary occlusion (either balloon or manual hand compression) of the parent artery during CAP injection [42–48]. Taki et al. used ethylene-vinyl alcohol copolymer (EVAL) as a liquid embolic agent to occlude intracranial aneurysms [49]. This liquid agent was originally developed for the embolization of brain arteriovenous malformations.

More recently, another formula of ethylene-vinyl copolymer (Onyx) has developed. We have done an experimental study using Onyx in combination with protective agents such as GDCs, temporary balloon occlusion of the parent artery, temporary balloon occlusion of the neck of the aneurysm, and microstents [50]. The findings of this study suggest these devices do allow for more filling of the aneurysms but do not necessarily totally preclude migration of Onyx into the parent artery. Preliminary clinical experience using the technique of Onyx delivery with concomitant temporary balloon occlusion of the aneurysmal neck in patients harboring large and giant aneurysms has begun to be collected.

Single-center Experience for Intraaneurysmal Embolization of Intracranial Aneurysms

In an effort to describe the current use of intraaneurysmal coil therapy we report our experience at the University of California, Los Angeles (UCLA) with GDC embolization of 728 patients with 824 aneurysms. Table 6-1 shows the clinical features of our patient population. Of 359 patients with acute SAH (49.3%), 67 had nonacute SAH (9.2%) (treatments were performed 15 days after the hemorrhagic episode), 209 patients had incidental aneurysms (28.7%), 70 had intracranial mass effect (9.6%), and 23 patients (3.2%) had other presenting symptoms.

Five hundred eighty-five aneurysms were located in the anterior circulation (71%) and 239 were in the posterior circulation (29%). The distribution of the aneurysms is detailed in Table 6-2.

In the early phase of our experience we had a dominant referral pattern of posterior circulation aneurysms. This type of referral expressed the higher surgical morbidity and mor-

TABLE 6-1. CLINICAL FEATURES

Clinical Features	Patients	
	No.	%
SAH, acute	359	49.3
SAH, nonacute	67	9.2
Incidental	209	28.7
Mass effect	70	9.6
Others	23	3.2
Total	728	100

SAH, subarachnoid hemorrhage.

TABLE 6-2. DISTRIBUTION OF ANEURYSMS

Location	Aneurysms	
	No.	%
Anterior Circulation		
Anterior communicating	130	15.8
Posterior communicating	114	13.8
Carotid-ophthalmic	103	12.5
Carotid-paraclinoid	85	10.2
MCA	68	8.3
Intracavernous/petrous	27	3.3
ICA bifurcation	24	2.9
Anterior choroidal	14	1.7
Anterior cerebral	12	1.5
Others	8	1.0
Total	585	71.0
Posterior Circulation		
Basilar tip	117	14.2
Basilar trunk	48	5.8
Vertebral artery	30	3.6
Posterior cerebral	22	2.7
PICA	21	2.5
Others	1	0.1
Total	239	29.0

MCA, middle cerebral artery; ICA, internal carotid artery; PICA, posterior inferior cerebellar artery.

TABLE 6-3. ANATOMICAL RESULTS

Anatomical Result	Aneurysms	
	No.	%
Complete	481	66.1
Neck remnant	276	37.9
Incomplete	26	3.6
Attempts	41	5.6
Total	824	113.2

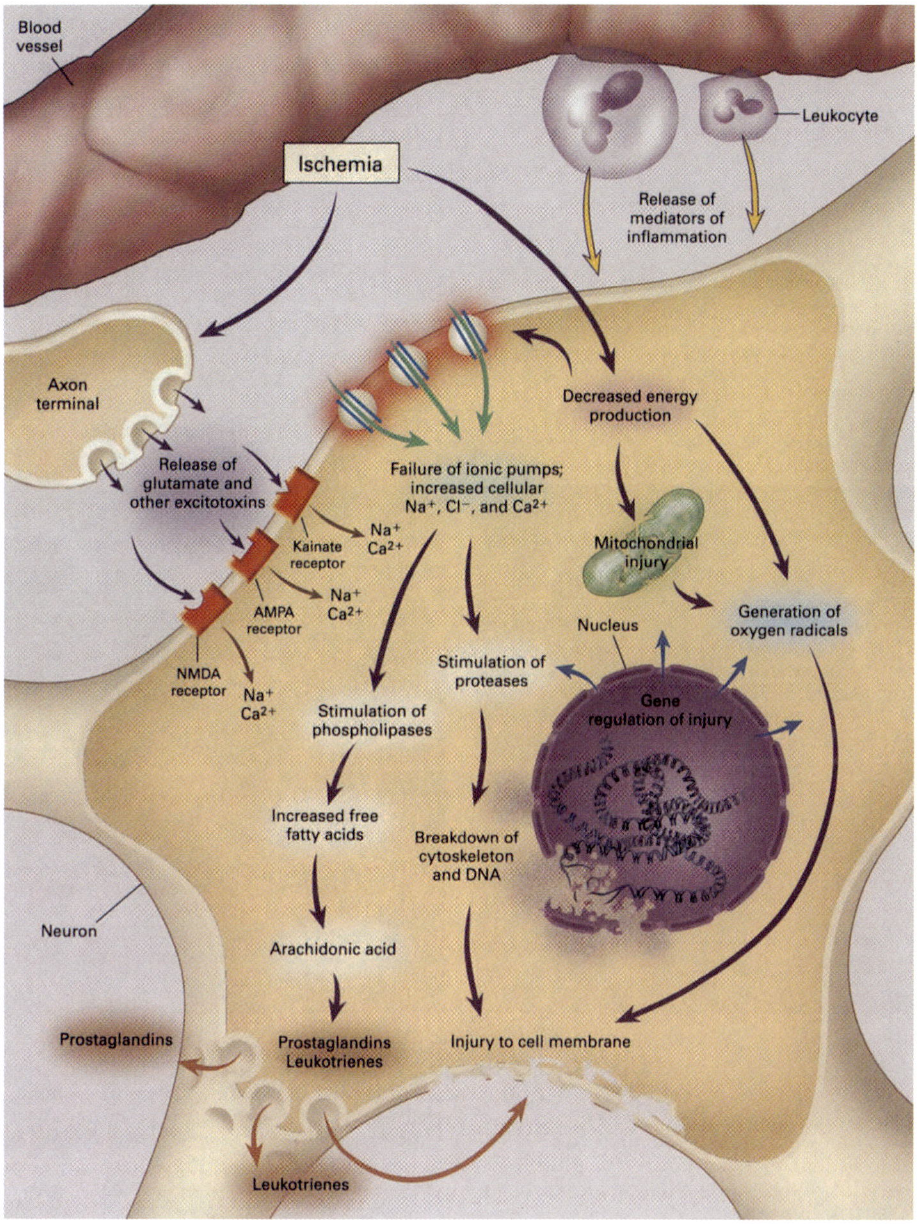

COLOR FIGURE 1-1. The ischemic cascade. (From Brott T, Bogousslavsky J. Treatment of acute ischemic stroke. *N Engl J Med* 2000;343:710–722, with permission.)

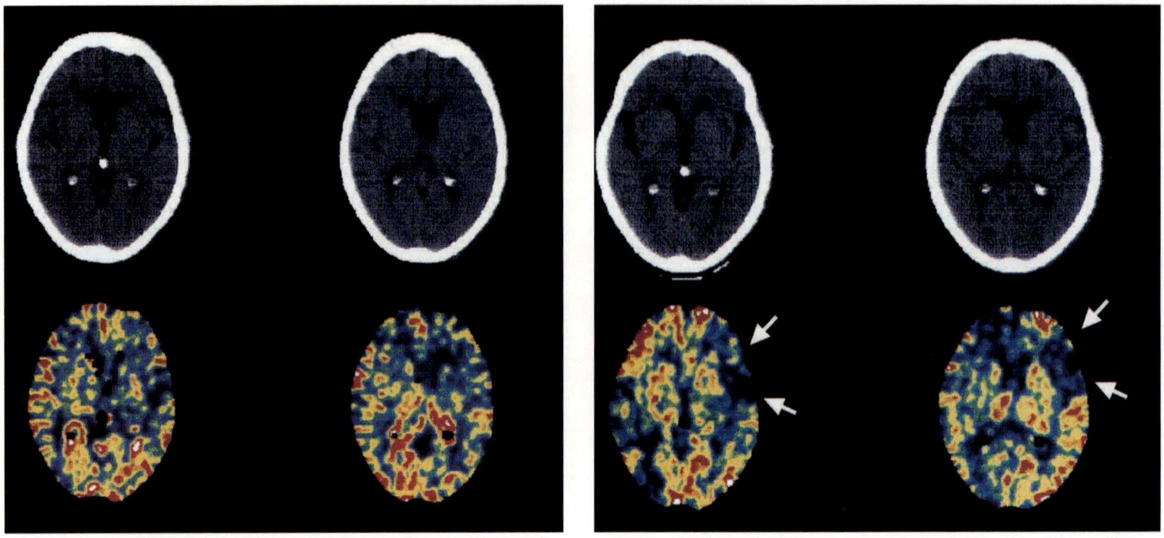

C D

COLOR FIGURE 3-9. This 81-year-old woman developed left hemispheric TIAs despite therapeutic levels of anticoagulation with warfarin. These were manifest as periods of dysphasia. **C,D:** Xenon-CT with axial CT and blood-flow map images are shown on two contiguous slices before **(C)** and after **(D)** acetazolamide challenge 1 day prior to balloon angioplasty. Loss of cerebrovascular autoregulation is most notable in the left frontal lobe as demonstrated by paradoxically low cerebral blood flow after acetazolamide administration. Note *arrows* between areas on the postacetazolamide scans. The color-coding scale is defined in units of ml/100 g tissue per minute. (From Liu AY, Do HM, Alpers GW, et al. Hyperperfusion syndrome with hemorrhage after angioplasty for middle cerebral artery stenosis. *AJNR Am J Neuroradiol* 2001;22:1597–1601, with permission.)

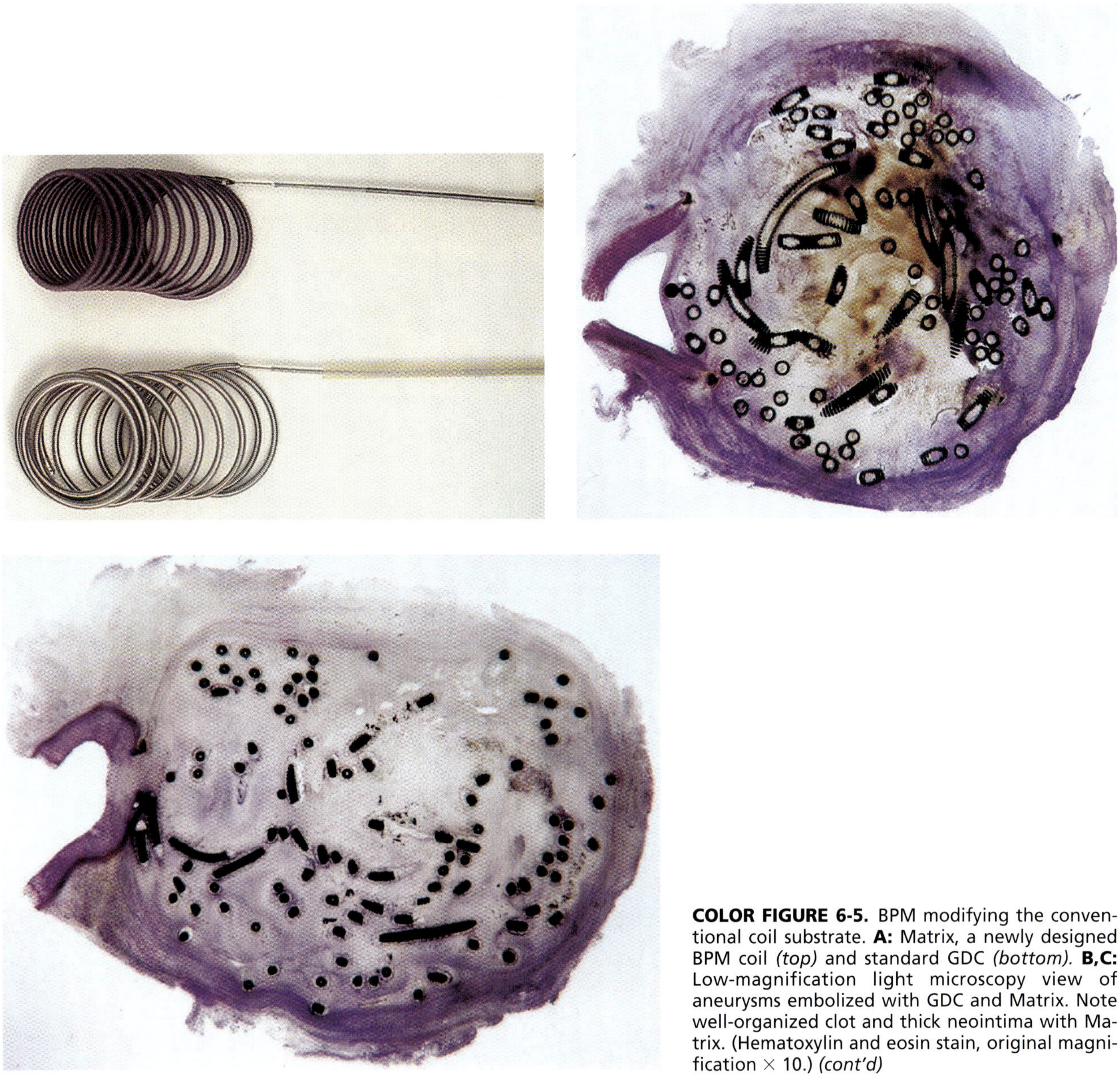

A B C

COLOR FIGURE 6-5. BPM modifying the conventional coil substrate. **A:** Matrix, a newly designed BPM coil *(top)* and standard GDC *(bottom).* **B,C:** Low-magnification light microscopy view of aneurysms embolized with GDC and Matrix. Note well-organized clot and thick neointima with Matrix. (Hematoxylin and eosin stain, original magnification × 10.) *(cont'd)*

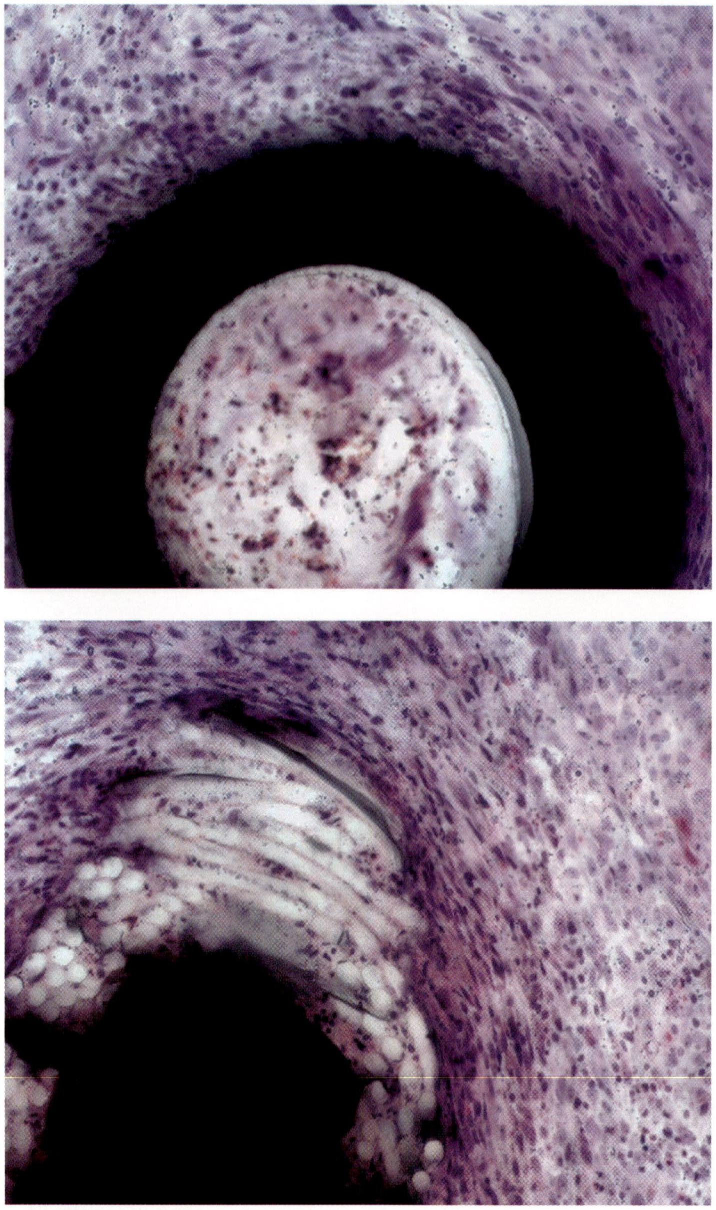

D

E

COLOR FIGURE 6-5. *(Continued)* **D,E:** High-magnification light microscopy view of aneurysms treated with GDC and Matrix. BPM outer layer is seen around the inner platinum core. Moderate inflammatory reaction is present, with foreign body giant cell reactions. (Hematoxylin and eosin stain, original magnification × 25.)

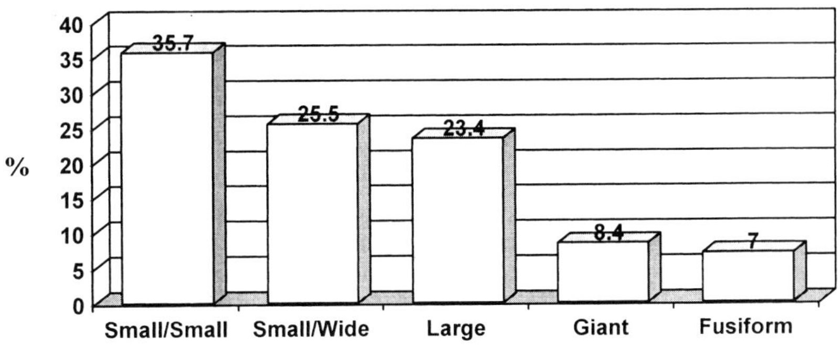

FIGURE 6-2. Graph of size and distribution of aneurysm cases.

TABLE 6-4. ANATOMICAL RESULT AND ANEURYSM SIZE

Aneurysm	No.	Complete	Neck Remnant	Incomplete
SS	316	245 (77.5%)	60 (19%)	3 (0.9%)
SW	214	95 (44.4%)	99 (46.3%)	2 (0.9%)
Large	179	84 (46.9%)	71 (39.7%)	12 (6.7%)
Giant	62	13 (21%)	42 (67.7%)	5 (8.1%)

SS, small aneurysm, small neck; SW, small aneurysm, wide neck.

tality rate not infrequently related to this kind of aneurysm. After the FDA approval of the GDC technique in 1995, our referral pattern became similar to that of a standard neurosurgical practice, although there is still a higher incidence of posterior circulation aneurysms. The most common location was the carotid ophthalmic-paraclinoid segment (22.8%), followed by anterior communicating artery (15.8%), and basilar tip (14.2%). Figure 6-2 shows the size distribution of our aneurysm cases.

The immediate and long-term anatomical results of the GDC technique are influenced by multiple factors. In our opinion, the most important are (a) anatomical characteristics of the aneurysm, (b) hemodynamic control of the aneurysmal inflow zone, and (c) the biologic response elicited by the GDC technique when deposited in an aneurysm. Tables 6-3 and 6-4 summarize our anatomical results with intraaneurysmal coil placement.

A complete GDC occlusion was achieved in 77.5% of small aneurysms with a small neck, in 44.4% of small aneurysms with a wide neck, in 46.9% of large aneurysms, and in 21% of giant aneurysms. A neck remnant was observed in 19% of small aneurysms with a small neck, in 46.3% of small aneurysms with a wide neck, in 39.7% of large aneurysms, and in 67.7% of giant aneurysms.

In wide-necked or large-to-giant aneurysms, it is more difficult to obtain a dense aneurysm packing without increasing the risk of coil herniation across the neck of the aneurysm. An aneurysm can be successfully and permanently occluded with the GDC system when a compact mesh of coils has been deposited in the body and particularly across the neck of the aneurysm. This is the main reason why the best anatomical results of our series are identified in small aneurysms with a small neck. Our percentage of complete aneurysmal occlusion dramatically dropped in small aneurysms with a wide neck and in large and giant aneurysms. When further treatment of these neck remnants was performed, 25% of aneurysms developed progressive thrombosis, 25% were unchanged, and 50% developed aneurysm recanalization (23).

The overall immediate morbidity rate of the 728 patients treated at UCLA (Tables 6-5 and 6-6) was 6.8%, and the perioperative mortality rate was 2.2%. In the anterior circu-

TABLE 6-5. IMMEDIATE CLINICAL OUTCOME

	Anterior	Posterior	Total
Total patients	508	220	728
Morbidity	36 (4.9%)	14 (1.9%)	50 (6.8%)
Mortality	8 (1.1%)	8 (1.1%)	16 (2.2%)

TABLE 6-6. DETAILED IMMEDIATE CLINICAL OUTCOME

Immediate Clinical Outcome	Patients	
	No.	%
Improved	3	0.4
Unchanged/intact	656	90.1
New neurologic deficit	50	6.8
Death	16	2.2
N/A	3	0.4
Total	728	100

N/A, not available.

TABLE 6-7. IMMEDIATE MORBIDITY AND MORTALITY AND CLINICAL PICTURE

	No. Patients	Morbidity		Mortality	
		No.	%	No.	%
SAH acute	359	30	8.4	14	3.9
SAH nonacute	67	5	7.5	0	0
Incidental	209	10	4.8	1	0.05
Mass effect	70	5	7.1	0	0
Others	23	0	0	0	0
Total	728	50	6.8	15	2.0

SAH, subarachnoid hemorrhage.

lation (508 patients with 585 aneurysms), we observed a 4.9% morbidity rate and a 1.1% mortality rate. In the posterior circulation (220 patients with 239 aneurysms), a 1.9% morbidity rate and a 1.1% mortality rate were recorded.

Table 6-7 outlines the immediate morbidity and mortality as a function of initial clinical features. Patients with acute SAH (359 patients) had an 8.4% morbidity rate and a 3.9% mortality rate. The incidence of symptomatic arterial vasospasm was approximately 20% to 30%. There was a linear correlation between the severity of Hunt and Hess grading and the increased incidence of vasospasm [29]. Cases of nonacute SAH (67 patients) had a 7.5% morbidity rate and a mortality rate of zero. The higher morbidity rate observed in patients with acute SAH is related to the severity of the primary disease plus an increased incidence of aneurysm perforation. Patients with incidental aneurysms (209 patients) showed a 4.8% morbidity rate and a 0.5% mortality rate, and patients who had mass effect (70 patients) had a 7.1% morbidity rate and a mortality rate of zero.

Table 6-8 outlines the immediate morbidity and mortality rates as a function of anatomical location. In contrast to the neurosurgical experience, aneurysm location plays a minor role in the incidence of morbidity associated with the GDC technology. Most intracranial aneurysms can be safely catheterized with the present generation of microcatheters and guidewires. Extreme vascular tortuosity in brachiocephalic arteries and post-SAH arterial vasospasm may increase the technical difficulty. The anatomical characteristics of the aneurysm remain the most important factor when considering anatomical outcome and morbidity and mortal-

TABLE 6-8. IMMEDIATE MORBIDITY AND MORTALITY AND ANEURYSM LOCATION

Location	No. Aneurysms	Morbidity		Mortality	
		No.	%	No.	%
Anterior Circulation					
Anterior communicating	130	8	6.2	4	3.1
Posterior communicating	114	7	6.1	0	0
Carotid-ophthalmic	103	7	6.8	0	0
Carotid-paraclinoid	85	1	1.2	1	1.2
MCA	68	4	5.9	1	1.5
Intracavernous/petrous	27	1	3.7	0	0
ICA bifurcation	24	2	8.3	2	8.3
Anterior choroidal	14	1	7.1	0	0
Anterior cerebral	12	2	16.7	0	0
Others	8	0	0	0	0
Total	585	33	5.6	8	1.4
Posterior Circulation					
Basilar tip	117	6	5.1	3	2.6
Basilar trunk	48	4	8.3	2	4.2
Vertebral artery	30	2	6.7	2	6.7
Posterior cerebral	22	3	13.6	0	0
PICA	21	2	9.5	1	4.8
Others	1	0	0	0	0
Total	239	17	7.1	8	3.3

MCA, middle cerebral artery; ICA, internal carotid artery; PICA, posterior inferior cerebellar artery.

TABLE 6-9. LONG-TERM CLINICAL OUTCOME AFTER EMBOLIZATION

Long-term Clinical Outcome	Patients No.	Patients %
Improved	113	15.5
Unchanged/intact	518	71.2
New neurologic deficit	28	3.8
Death	39	5.4
N/A	30	4.1
Total	728	100

N/A, not available.

TABLE 6-10. PROCEDURAL COMPLICATIONS

Procedural Complication	Patients No.	Patients %*
Cerebral embolization	17	2.3
Aneurysm perforation	17	2.3
Parent artery occlusion	16	2.2
Coil migration	3	0.4
Parent vessel narrowing	3	0.4
Coil rupture	3	0.4
Arterial dissection	3	0.4
New mass effect	1	0.1
Total	63	8.5

* % of total patients (728).

ity rates. In our experience, wide-necked anterior communicating aneurysms pointing upward and backward are the most difficult to treat with GDCs. The microcatheter tends to have an unstable position and the coil migrates downward into the anterior communicating artery. The balloon-assisted technique is difficult to use due to the small size of the anterior cerebral artery complex.

The presence of cerebral vasospasm does not preclude the catheterization of a distally located aneurysm. In a limited number of cases, it is necessary to perform angioplasty of the spastic artery in order to enter the ruptured aneurysm. This maneuver does not appear to increase the rate of aneurysmal rerupture.

Table 6-9 shows the long-term clinical outcome in patients followed for 6 months to 8 years after embolization. We were not able to obtain telephone or direct contact with 30 of the patients (4.1%). Four hundred thirty-four (59.6%) were neurologically intact, and 84 (11.5%) remained neurologically unchanged when compared with their clinical pictures after the procedure. Twenty-eight (3.8%) had neurologic deterioration, and 39 died (5.4%). Twelve deaths were related to GDC procedural complications (30.7%), 16 were associated with the severity of the SAH, and 14 patients died of unrelated causes (e.g., bacterial endocarditis, acquired immunodeficiency syndrome [AIDS], ventriculitis).

Ten patients with acute SAH had a postembolization delayed aneurysmal rerupture (10 of 359 patients; 2.8%). All cases showed a significant coil remodeling at the aneurysmal inflow zone and exposure of the body of the aneurysm to the blood flow. In our experience, no cases of rerupture were observed in aneurysms showing a stable neck remnant in long-term angiographic follow-ups. The significance of a small-neck remnant after incomplete GDC coil placement is unknown. Thorough long-term angiographic and clinical follow-up is needed to learn their natural history in order to be able to make therapeutic decisions. The use of microstents, with GDCs, may be one solution to a limited number of giant, saccular, or fusiform intracranial aneurysms. The involvement of large or perforating arteries in the body of these aneurysms remains unsolved by the endovascular technique.

Figure 6-3 shows the relationship between aneurysm size and recanalization. Aneurysm recanalization was frequently seen with large and giant aneurysms. Because of the variety of coils available, such as soft coil and 3-D coils, and the new balloon-assisted technique, the risk of recanalization of small-to-wide aneurysms may be significantly improved.

Table 6-10 summarizes procedural complications, which included aneurysm perforation (2.3%), parent artery occlusion (2.2%), cerebral embolization (2.3%), and arterial dissection of brachycephalic arteries (0.4%). Aneurysm perforation is more rarely seen today due to the marked mechanical improvement of delivery systems and GDCs. It is more often observed in acutely ruptured aneurysms and seldom seen in incidental aneurysms. This complication can

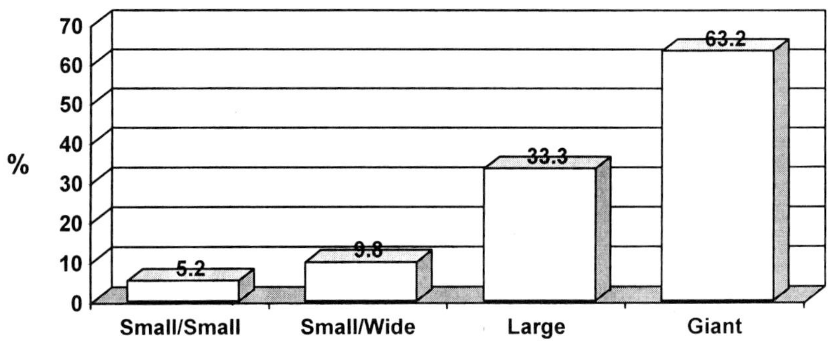

FIGURE 6-3. Graph showing relationship between aneurysm size and recanalization.

be fatal if it happens in the early phase of embolization. If it occurs when most of the aneurysm has been filled with GDCs, it may produce only mild-to-moderate temporary neurologic deterioration.

A parent artery occlusion is usually caused by herniation of GDCs into the parent artery. This complication may be reduced if an appropriate vascular mapping of the aneurysm is achieved (biplane standard angiography, 3-D computed tomographic angiography [CTA], 3-D digital angiography). Three-dimensional imaging is particularly useful in middle cerebral and anterior communicating aneurysms, as well as in large fusiform aneurysms. In giant fusiform aneurysms, it best shows the relationship between the body of the aneurysm and the ostia of normal arteries. After identifying these normal arteries, arterial bypass may be required before surgical or endovascular aneurysm trapping is done.

Cerebral embolization has been the most frequent procedural complication. It has substantially decreased in frequency with the use of pre- and postembolization systemic anticoagulation, followed by a regimen of aspirin and ticlopidine for at least 3 months. This therapeutic regimen is useful in wide-necked aneurysm or in cases showing GDC coil protrusion into the parent artery. This is particularly risky in anterior communicating and middle cerebral artery aneurysms.

Limitations of Microcoil Therapy

Critical analysis of long-term anatomical results of aneurysms treated with GDCs shows three important limitations. First, GDC compaction and aneurysm recanalization may occur [59,60]. It is more often seen in small aneurysms with a wide neck (5 mm or more) and in large or giant aneurysms (Fig. 6-4). Second, tight and complete GDC packing in large or giant aneurysms may increase the aneurysmal mass effect on adjacent brain parenchyma or in cranial nerves [43].

The third limitation arises because the standard platinum GDC coil is biologically inert and elicits a delayed mild clot organization and maturation in an aneurysm [61–63]. Guglielmi et al. first reported mild-to-moderate thrombus organization and development of a neoendothelium across the aneurysmal neck in experimental aneurysms in swine embolized with GDCs [21]. Spetzger et al. and Reul et al., using experimental bifurcation aneurysms in rabbits, reported open spaces, absence of organized thrombus, and lack of neoendothelial formation even at 3 and 6 months after embolization with GDCs [64,65]. However, the same authors reported in a later article the presence of endothelial-like tissue in the same rabbit aneurysm treated with GDCs.

Mawad et al. showed the formation of neointima covering the aneurysmal neck in over 60% of aneurysms in a canine sidewall aneurysm model [61]. Tenjin et al. reported similar histologic findings in a primate aneurysm model [63]. Tamatani et al. reported *in vitro* results [62].

In humans, the histopathologic changes in aneurysms treated with GDCs have seldom been documented [66–71]. Molyneux et al. reported postmortem histologic results of two intracranial wide-necked aneurysms that had been incompletely occluded with GDCs 2 and 6 months before death [70]. The coils were embedded in a largely nonorganized thrombus and no neoendothelial coverage of the neck of the aneurysm was observed.

Mizoi et al. [69] reported histologic findings from a patient with an anterior communicating aneurysm previously treated with GDCs. This aneurysm recanalized 6 months later and was surgically clipped. Histology of the resected

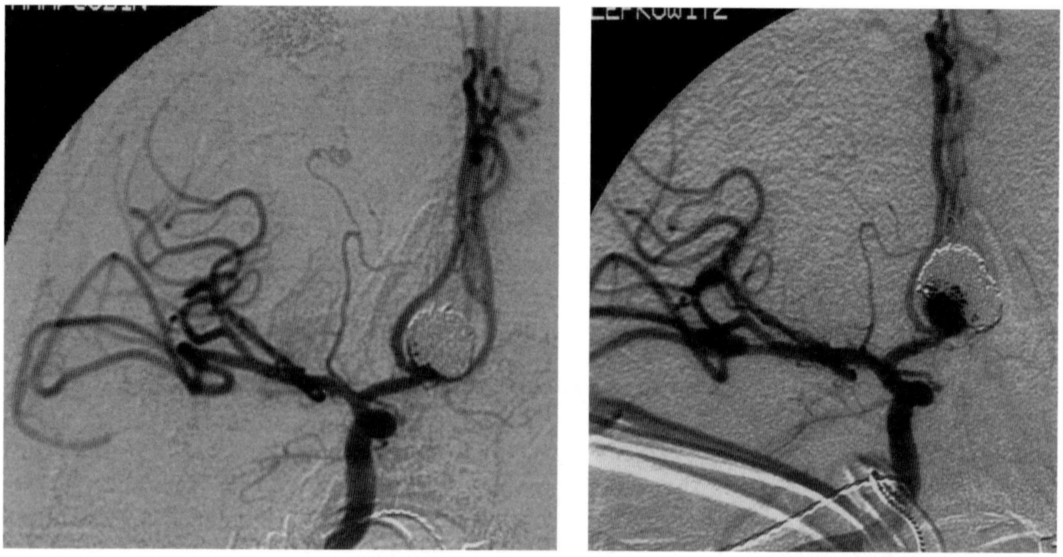
A B

FIGURE 6-4. Coil compaction and aneurysm remodeling. **A:** Large anterior communicating aneurysm was embolized with GDCs. Small neck remnant was seen. **B:** Three-month postembolization angiogram demonstrates aneurysm recanalization and coil remodeling.

aneurysm revealed the presence of a nonorganized intraaneurysmal thrombus that was directly exposed to the blood circulation. No neointimal coverage of the neck of the aneurysm was observed.

Horowitz et al. [67] examined a basilar artery aneurysm with electron microscopy 4 weeks after GDC embolization. They reported cellular proliferation at the edges of the neck of the aneurysm, and they concluded that these cells were either endothelial or fibroblastic in nature.

Koizumi et al. [68], in another electron microscopy study, documented a complete lining of endothelial-like cells across the orifice of a posterior communicating aneurysm in a patient who died 4 weeks after treatment with interlocking detachable platinum coils.

Shimizu et al. reported the postmortem histologic results in wide-necked aneurysms treated with GDCs 6 weeks prior to death [71]. They described some inflammatory response in the aneurysmal wall but no intraluminal clot organization or neoendothelial coverage of the neck of the aneurysms.

However, Castro et al. [72] reported abundant fibrous connective tissue in carotid ophthalmic and middle cerebral aneurysms in a 33-year-old patient treated with GDCs 33 months before death. The GDCs were firmly attached to the walls of the aneurysms, and in one aneurysm a thick, dense layer of collagenous tissue completely covered the neck. A single neoendothelial layer totally covered the collagenous tissue bridging the neck of the aneurysm.

Stiver et al. [73] reported a postmortem histology of an anterior communicating aneurysm treated 36 hours prior to death. They reported a discrete membrane composed mainly of fibrin covering the neck of the aneurysm and excluding it from the parent artery.

Bavinzski et al. reported that of 16 aneurysms studied from 3 to 40 days after GDC embolization, six aneurysms were completely occluded with formation of a thin membrane over the neck of the aneurysm, and five aneurysms showed a thin incomplete membrane covering the aneurysmal neck [66]. This important article also showed a probable evolution of aneurysmal healing, with GDCs embedded in nonorganized thrombus 1 week after embolization. An incomplete replacement of intraluminal clot by fibrous tissue was reported. Of note, one giant wide-necked aneurysm examined 54 months after embolization showed partial aneurysmal occlusion.

FUTURE IMPROVEMENTS TO MICROCOIL THERAPY

A series of articles recently published in the neurointerventional literature emphasizes the need to bring biomolecular and tissue-engineering resources to the forefront of microcoil development for the treatment of aneurysms. It is known that the platinum coil elicits mild and delayed biologic response when deployed into an aneurysm. Tamatani et al. reported no endothelial proliferation on the platinum coil surface in an *in vitro* study [62]. Surface modifications of GDCs using a bioactive material may induce acceleration of clot maturation and remodeling in an aneurysm. This biologic modification may anchor the coil and decrease coil compaction and aneurysm recanalization.

Previous attempts to increase coil thrombogenicity have been centered on increasing their surface area with fabric stands such as Dacron [74] and polyester [75] and by placing coils into a thrombin solution prior to their use [76].

Recently, some investigators have modified the surface of GDCs by coating them with extracellular matrix proteins such as collagen or polyurethane [77,78]. However, protein coating on a platinum surface is usually weak and it may be easily removed during coil delivery through microcatheters. Polyurethane coating, in particular, has the problem of increasing coil rigidity and decreasing memory of shape. Murayama et al. used a high-energy ion implantation in combination with a protein coating to modify the surface of GDCs [79–81]. They used aneurysms manufactured in swine. Ion implantation is a physicochemical modification process that uses the impingement of a high-energy ion beam onto the surface of protein-coated GDCs. After ion implantation, the coated protein is embedded into the platinum structure, resulting in a homogeneous, biologically active coil surface. Murayama et al. reported that these biologically modified GDCs elicited stronger clot maturation and remodeling when they were compared to standard GDCs, in aneurysms manufactured in swine. Kallmes et al. evaluated modified GDC using growth factors or genetically modified cells [82, 83].

Tissue engineering is a scientific field that encompasses tissue repair and replacement using bioactive materials [84–91]. It is an emerging interdisciplinary field that includes implantation of cell-containing or cell-free devices that induce regeneration of functional human tissue. This approach relies on the purification and large-scale production of "signal" to molecules like growth factors and cytokines, to assist in biomaterial-guided tissue regeneration.

Bioabsorbable polymeric materials (BPM) are being used in 3-D scaffolds to which cells attach and grow to reconstitute tissues. These techniques are currently used to regenerate tissues such as skin, bone, cartilage, ureters, and vessels. Cerebral aneurysms may be considered defects of normal arterial tissue and they can be repaired using such tissue-engineering technology.

Basic science and clinical research on the medical use of BPM have increased during the past decade. The ideal BPM to be used in aneurysms requires special design criteria. (a) The surface should permit cellular adhesion and growth, (b) neither the polymer nor its degradation products should provoke excessive inflammation, or local or systemic toxicity, (c) the material should be processed into 3-D structures, and (d) the polymer should be absorbed once it has served its purpose of providing a template for tissue regeneration.

Because foreign materials carry a potential risk of causing chronic inflammation, the scaffold degradation rate should be adjustable to match the rate of tissue regeneration by the cell type of interest. Synthetic polymers such as polylactide (PLA), polyglycolic acid (PGA), and polyglycolic–poly-L-lactic acid (PLGA) copolymer meet all these criteria [84].

Endovascular embolic implants made from bioabsorbable polymers could be used to create an intraaneurysmal scaffold that could generate a permanent, mature connective tissue retraction of this aneurysmal "scar" and could also decrease the mass effect observed with large or giant aneurysms. As a general rule, polymers with a faster bioabsorption time elicit a stronger inflammatory reaction. Modifying the copolymer ratio may change this inflammatory reaction and bioabsorption rate.

Recently, a newly designed hybrid platinum BPM coil (Matrix) was developed at UCLA Medical Center (Fig. 6-5). A 90:10 ratio of polyglycolic–to–poly-L-lactic acid copolymers were used as BPM. The inner platinum core provided memory and radiopacity, and it preserved the core platinum coil for its mechanical properties. The histologic reaction of this new Matrix coil prototype was compared with the standard GDC coil in 24 aneurysms created in 12 swine [92]. This preliminary study showed that the Matrix coil accelerated aneurysmal fibrosis and intensified neointima coverage of the aneurysmal neck when compared with standard GDCs. No parent artery stenosis or occlusion was noted. There was also evidence of aneurysmal retraction as documented by a 3-month angiographic follow-up.

Future developments of biologically active embolic

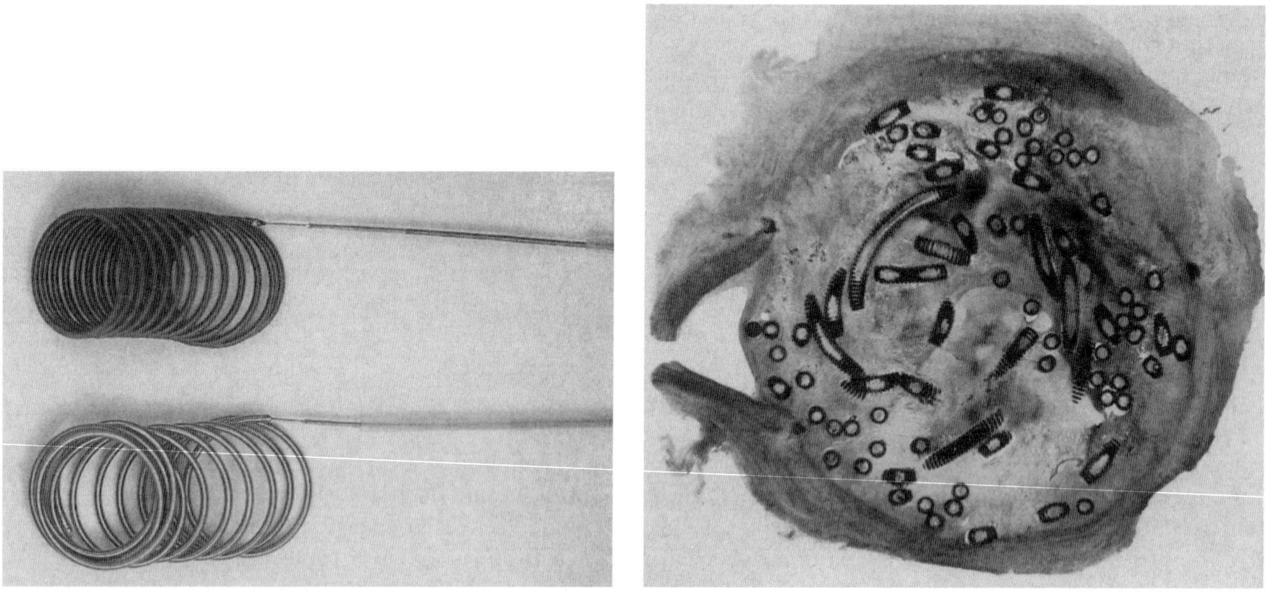

A B

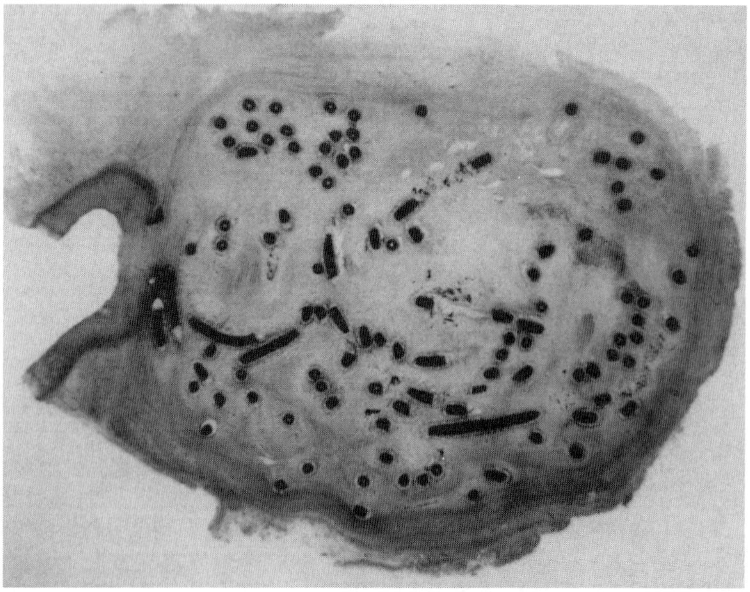

C

FIGURE 6-5. BPM modifying the conventional coil substrate. **A:** Matrix, a newly designed BPM coil *(top)* and standard GDC *(bottom).* **B,C:** Low-magnification light microscopy view of aneurysms embolized with GDC and Matrix. Note well-organized clot and thick neointima with Matrix. (Hematoxylin and eosin stain, original magnification × 10). *(Figure continues.)*

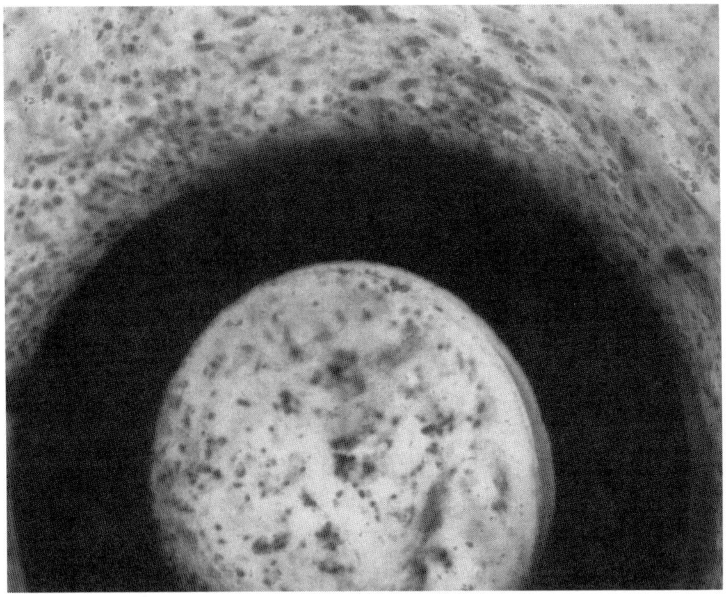

D

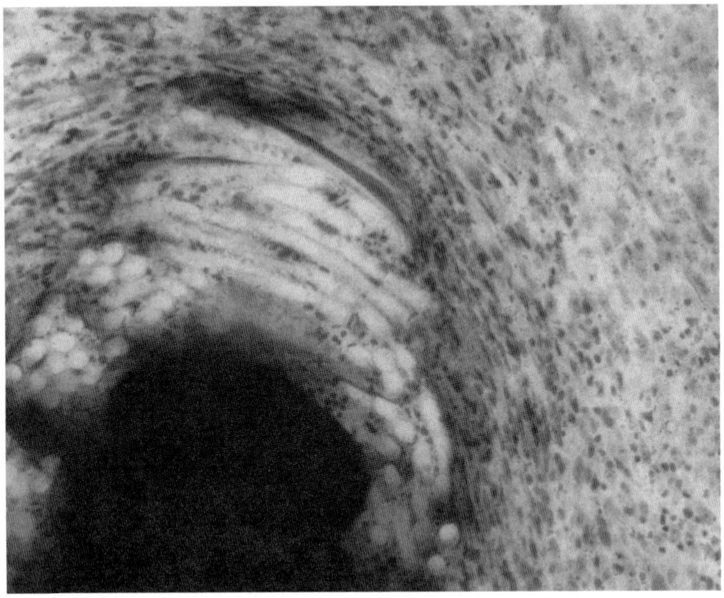

E

FIGURE 6-5. *Continued.* **D,E:** High-magnification light microscopy view of aneurysms treated with GDC and Matrix. BPM outer layer is seen around the inner platinum core. Moderate inflammatory reaction is present, with foreign body giant cell reactions. (Hematoxylin and eosin stain, original magnification × 25.) (See Color Figure 6-5.)

agents should have a very positive impact on the anatomical and clinical outcomes of aneurysms treated via the endovascular route. Present histologic results in animal models show that the molecular and histologic responses elicited by these materials accelerate clot remodeling, reinforce coil anchoring, and may induce aneurysmal retraction due to collagen transformation. A faster and thicker neointima and neoendothelial coverage of the neck of experimental aneurysms in swine has also been noted.

TECHNIQUE FOR INTRAANEURYSMAL EMBOLIZATION USING MICROCOILS

In the early phases of GDC clinical use, this therapy was mainly used in surgically difficult or unclippable aneurysms or in patients in poor neurologic or medical condition. After 1995, the most important factors modifying its use have been aneurysm morphology and the patients' clinical and neurologic status. Any patient harboring a saccular aneurysm may be a potential candidate for endovascular GDC occlusion. Small, wide-necked and large and giant aneurysms represent a technical challenge. Recent incorporation of 3-D coils, balloon-assisted technique and microstent deployment have enabled the endovascular therapist to treat more of these aneurysms.

The therapeutic plan needs to be discussed between the vascular neurosurgeon and the interventional neuroradiologist. The patient's clinical condition, the aneurysm location and size, and the therapist's personal experience need to be factored into any therapeutic decision. In the future it is hoped that a prospective, double-blind, randomized trial comparing anatomical and clinical outcomes of surgery and endovascular techniques will improve our ability to objectively offer these therapeutic alternatives.

Patient Evaluation

Patients with acute SAH are admitted to a neurologic intensive care unit. A thorough neurologic evaluation is performed, including the Hunt and Hess classification (see Chapter 5). A cerebral CT scan is obtained to evaluate blood distribution in the subarachnoid space (Fisher classification), status of brain parenchyma, and size of the ventricles. In patients harboring wide-necked or complex-shaped aneurysms, 3-D CTA [51–54] and 3-D digital angiography [55, 56] provide important anatomical information for endovascular and neurosurgical therapeutic planning. This 3-D anatomical information is often critical for aneurysms located in the middle cerebral and anterior communicating as well as basilar tip arteries (Fig. 6-6).

The biplane digital subtraction angiographic (DSA) system with roadmap guidance is essential for modern endovascular procedures to avoid image-related complications. More recently, the 3-D DSA system provides better anatomical information for interventional procedures.

A complete angiographic exploration of the aneurysm precedes the endovascular procedure. It is essential to find the appropriate radiographic position that separates the neck of the aneurysm from normal arterial branching and perforating arteries (lenticulostriate and posterior thalamoperforate arteries). This is an extremely important element of GDC embolization (Fig. 6-7). This same angiographic position will be used to evaluate immediate and long-term anatomical results.

A 6- or 7-French (Fr.) sheath is positioned in the femoral artery. A complete angiographic evaluation of the anterior and posterior fossa arterial circulation is done. Particular attention is paid to a ruptured aneurysm, additional unruptured aneurysms, and local or generalized arterial vasospasm.

Once a decision has been made to perform endovascular treatment, the patient should undergo general anesthesia. This provides better control of the vital hemodynamic parameters and avoids untoward complications, such as aneurysm perforation or dissection of the vessel due to the patient's unexpected movements. It is also allows the therapist to obtain good quality roadmap imaging.

Systemic heparinization decreases the chance of thromboembolic complications from the guiding catheters or untoward clot formation on protruding coils through wide-necked aneurysms. In hyperacute aneurysms, systemic heparinization may be used after the aneurysm has been partially embolized and its ruptured site has been excluded from circulation.

It is important to evaluate the aneurysm projection before embolization. Appropriate head positioning provides better angiographic imaging. For example, if the basilar tip

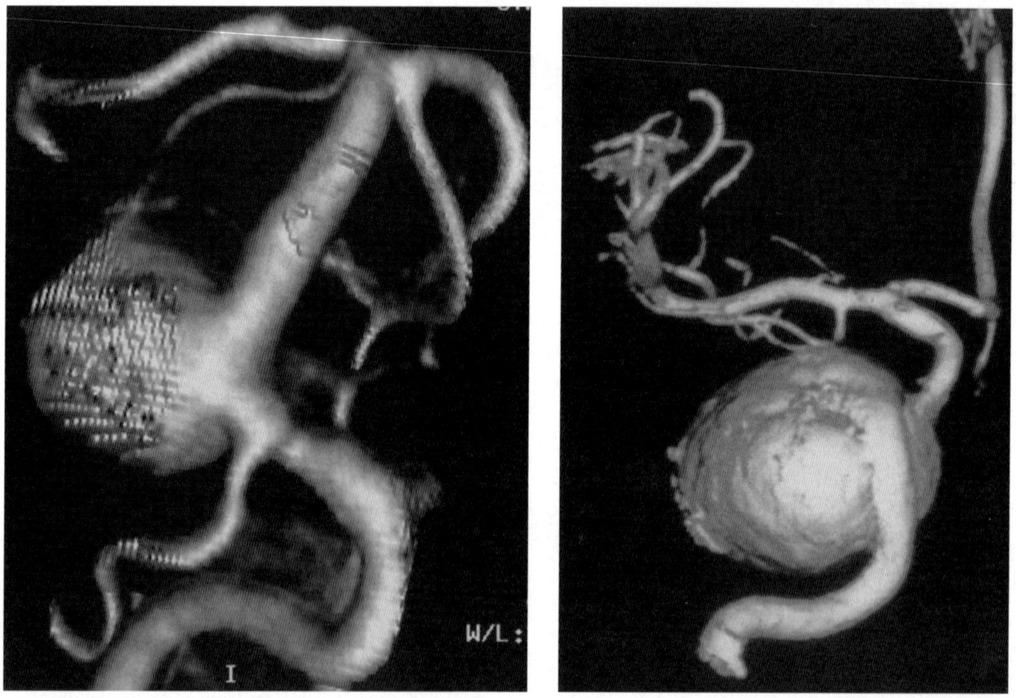

A B

FIGURE 6-6. Three-dimensional anatomical depiction of aneurysms. **A:** Three-dimensional CT angiogram of basilar trunk aneurysm. **B:** Large ICA angiogram, 3-D DSA angiogram. (**B:** From Philips Medical Systems, with permission.)

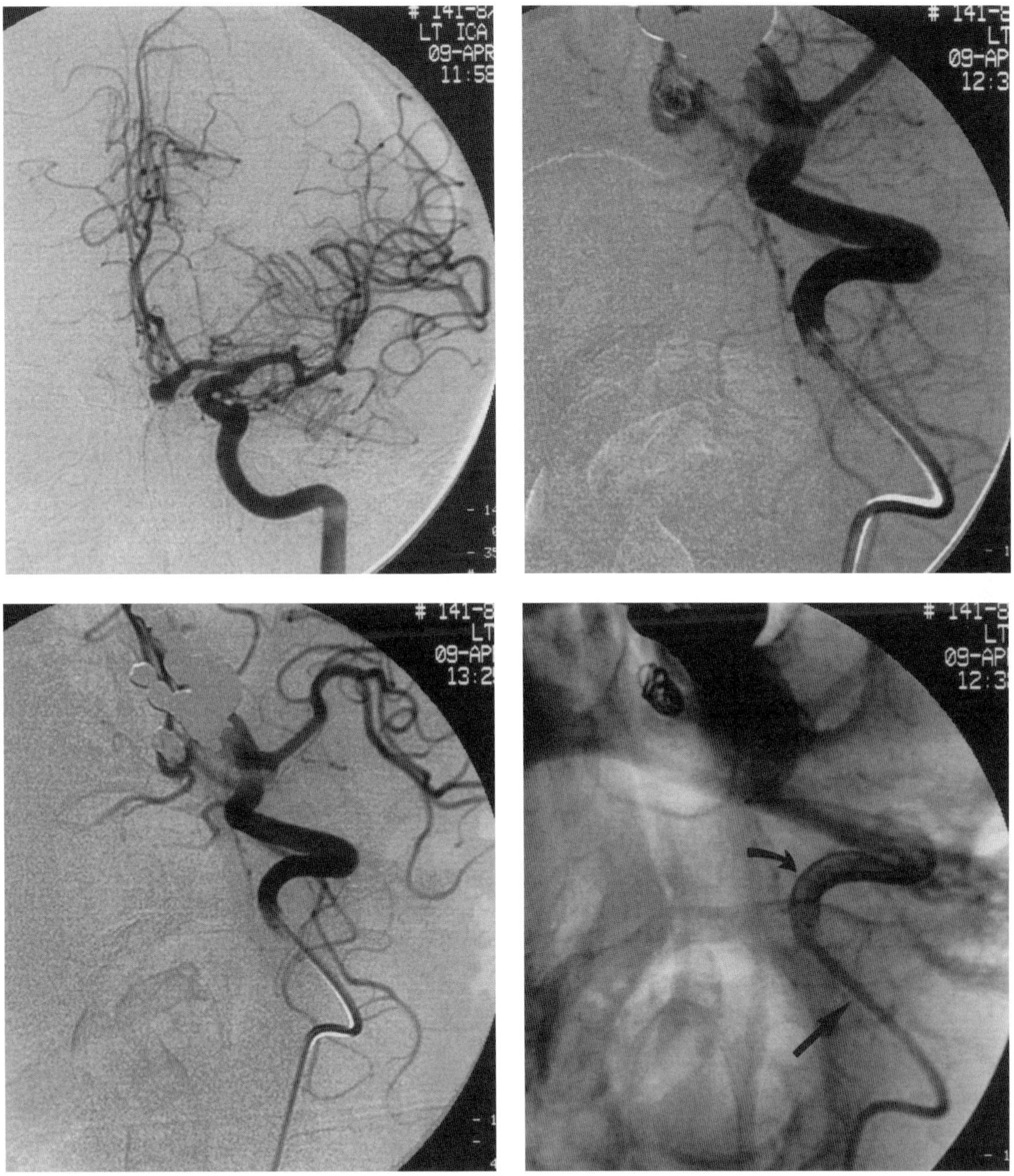

FIGURE 6-7. Anterior communicating artery aneurysm. **A:** Left carotid angiogram demonstrates the anterior communicating aneurysm; however, the true aneurysmal neck is indistinct. **B:** Extreme Waters view demonstrates the relationship between parent arteries and aneurysmal neck. The first GDC was successfully placed in the sac of the aneurysm. **C:** Postembolization angiogram shows complete packing of the aneurysm. **D:** Nonsubtraction view of the anterior communicating aneurysm shows triaxial system. Note Tracker 38 catheter *(curved arrow)* in the internal carotid artery and coaxial Tracker 10 microcatheter *(straight arrow).*

aneurysm is pointing forward, the patient's head should be vertex up to obtain the best DSA projection without extreme image intensifier tube angle. This is similar to surgical head positioning used to obtain better surgical view.

A 6- or 7-Fr. guiding catheter is positioned in the internal carotid or vertebral artery and roadmapping of the aneurysm is performed. In patients with tortuous arteries it may be necessary to use a triaxial catheter system. A triaxial system is useful for embolization when patients with tortuous brachiocephalic arteries produce unstable anchoring of the microcatheter in an aneurysm. It comprises a 7-Fr. guiding catheter placed in the common carotid or subclavian artery and a soft 5-Fr. catheter, such as the Tracker 38, located as distal as possible into the internal carotid or vertebral artery (Fig. 6-7). This double guiding system provides a strong support to the microcatheter deployed through the Tracker 38 catheter. The Tracker 38 catheter can be placed into the intracranial internal carotid artery (ICA) or vertebral arteries. This system decreases the friction of the microcatheter while negotiating tortuous arteries in the neck, because it is supported by the Tracker 38 catheter. The triaxial system has proven useful in the embolization of anterior communicating aneurysms in the elderly population and of vertebrobasilar circulation aneurysms when the ostium of the vertebral artery is tortuous or stenosed.

A new generation of braided microcatheters is now available in 0.010-, 0.014-, and 0.018-inch sizes. The 0.014-inch is the most popular because it can deliver either size 10 or 18 (0.010- or 0.018-inch) microcoils. This type of microcatheter has better trackability, and more resistance and strength than regular microcatheters. Braided catheters are also less likely to kink when making steep vascular turns, such as in intracavernous internal carotid or distal vertebral arteries. Braided microcatheters are more difficult to shape with steam than standard microcatheters, and they tend to jump forward if given excessive tension. This natural sudden forward movement needs to be controlled when the microcatheter is positioned in an aneurysm and, in particular in a small aneurysm, due to the risk of perforation.

In aneurysms that form an acute angle with the parent artery, such as superior hypophyseal, anterior choroidal, and sometimes anterior communicating aneurysms, the catheterization may be improved by shaping the angle of the tip of the catheter to match the anatomical angle to be negotiated. An unbraided microcatheter, such as the FasTracker, may be a better choice in these circumstances because it keeps its shape longer than the braided microcatheters.

Today numerous excellent 0.010- and 0.014-inch microguidewires are available from a variety of manufacturers to guide the microcatheter into an intracranial aneurysm. There has been a significant improvement in their strength, tip control, trackability, and durability of hydrophilic coating. They can be safely maneuvered distal to the circle of Willis into cortical arteries that are 2 and 3 mm in diameter. These guidewires need to be withdrawn slowly from the microcatheter situated in an aneurysm to minimize the possibility of untoward forward jumping of the microcatheter and possible aneurysm perforation. This is particularly true in cases with difficult anatomy due to tortuous arteries in the neck. The microcatheter should be permanently flushed with saline to decrease internal friction of the GDC coil produced by blood aspirated into the catheter tip.

The goal of GDC embolization of an aneurysm is to obtain complete and tight packing of the aneurysm. This anatomical outcome is more likely to produce a complete and permanent aneurysmal occlusion. A spectrum of more than 70 types of microcoils, including standard 0.010- and 0.018-inch, and 2-D and 3-D, soft, stretch resistant, and ultrasoft coils are available.

A special effort should be made to obtain a tight packing of the neck inflow zone. This inflow zone is defined as the area of the aneurysmal neck that receives the largest amount of the blood flow entering the aneurysm. It is in this particular area of the neck of the aneurysm where aneurysm recanalization develops.

The initial coil size is chosen to approximate the maximal aneurysm diameter. In general, a shorter and softer coil is preferred for a ruptured aneurysm or for placement in a very torturous vessel. For example, one might choose a 10-mm–long coil rather than 20-mm–long coil because it imparts less friction. If possible, the first coil should cross the neck of the aneurysm as many times as possible, to obtain an immediate change of blood flow pattern, decreasing pressure in the aneurysmal rupture site. When a GDC 3-D coil is used as the first coil, one may see a typical rotational movement of the coil while it is deployed. The coil may leave the aneurysm and reenter, searching for a strong 3-D anchoring (Fig. 6-8).

If the rupture site of the aneurysm is identified, we endeavor not to touch it either with the microcatheter or with the microcoils. In most cases, the change of flow produced by the coils delivered around the "bleb" is sufficient to elicit thrombosis in this area. The coil delivery needs to continue until the aneurysm bleb no longer fills with contrast material.

After endovascular coil occlusion of an aneurysm, systemic heparinization is reversed in most cases, with the exception of patients harboring wide-necked aneurysms. In those aneurysms, there is a large coil surface in contact with blood flow, increasing the chances of untoward thrombosis *in situ* and distal embolic complications. Systemic heparinization may be prolonged for 24 hours and then followed with aspirin for 6 months and clopidigrel for 3 months. This therapeutic regimen has decreased postembolization thromboembolic complications.

Special Technical Issues

Several modifications to our techniques have been used to improve the treatment of wide-necked aneurysms. Balloon-assisted technology (BAT) was first reported by Guglielmi et al. in 1992 and popularized and perfected by Moret et al. [33] as an important technical adjunct in wide-necked aneurysm. BAT requires the inflation of a balloon across the neck of the aneurysm while deploying GDCs (Fig. 6-9). The inflated balloon blocks the parent artery and stabilizes the microcatheter and microcoil in the aneurysm, allowing the deployment of a denser mesh of GDCs. The inflated balloon decreases the chances of untoward migration of the GDC coil into the parent artery or intracranially. This technique is very useful in wide-necked carotid ophthalmic, superior hypophyseal, and midtrunk basilar aneurysms. In experienced hands, the BAT carries a procedural morbidity and mortality rate similar to that of the standard GDC tech-

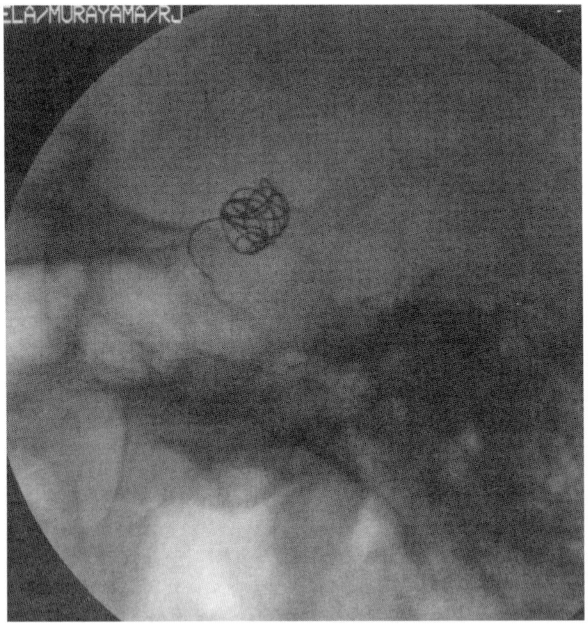

A

FIGURE 6-8. Use of 3-D GDC in coil placement. **A:** Unsubtracted view demonstrates configuration of 3-D GDC at the time of placement in the sac of unruptured superior hypophyseal artery aneurysm. **B:** Subtraction angiogram showing the shape of 3-D GDC in the aneurysmal sac. **C:** Postembolization angiogram shows small protrusion of 3-D GDC loop.

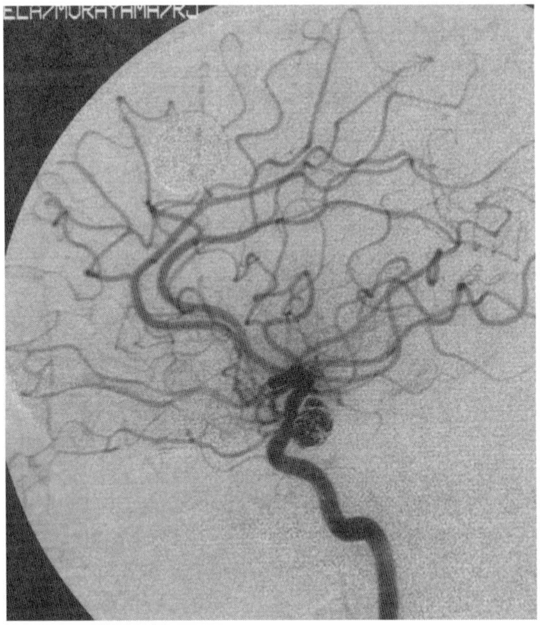

B

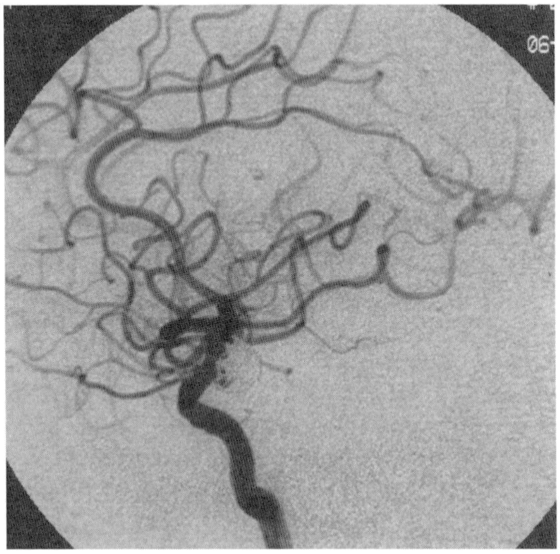

C

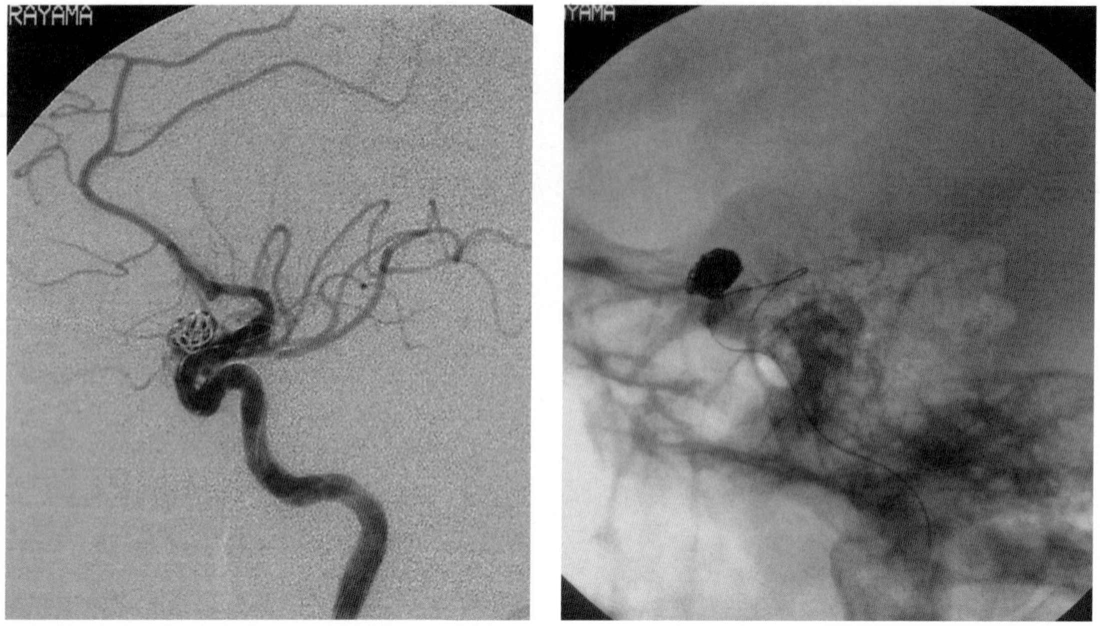

A B

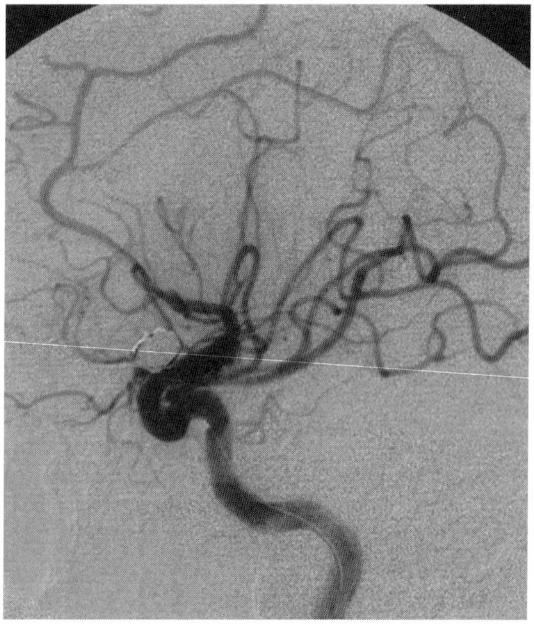

C

FIGURE 6-9. Demonstration of the balloon assist technique. **A:** Unruptured wide-necked carotid ophthalmic aneurysm. Three-dimensional GDC was used as first coil. **B:** The aneurysm was tightly packed with GDC using the balloon remodeling technique. **C:** Postembolization angiogram showed near-complete occlusion of the aneurysm.

nique. Several microballoon products are now available on the market. To avoid intraaneurysmal high pressure, the microballoon should not be inflated at the distal portion of the aneurysmal neck (stump effect). Another alternative to treating the wide-necked aneurysm may be a technique that combines clipping followed by coil treatment (Fig. 6-10).

The GDC Trispan coil has been recently developed to be used in wide-necked aneurysms [57]. It consists of a trifoliate coil ("tulip" coil) that is positioned in the neck of the aneurysm while deploying the standard GDCs through a second microcatheter (Fig. 6-11). The Trispan is then detached at the end of the procedure. Preliminary clinical experience suggests it is useful in terminal aneurysms such as basilar tip aneurysms or internal carotid bifurcation aneurysms. This system appears to have serious limitations in lateral wall aneurysms.

An increasing number of papers reported in the neurosurgical and neurointerventional literature emphasize the deployment of microstents associated with GDCs for the endovascular occlusion of large wide-necked and fusiform aneurysms (Fig. 6-12) [37–40].

The present generation of microstents inherited from the cardiovascular experience has achieved sufficient suppleness to negotiate arteries at the skull base and beyond. Most

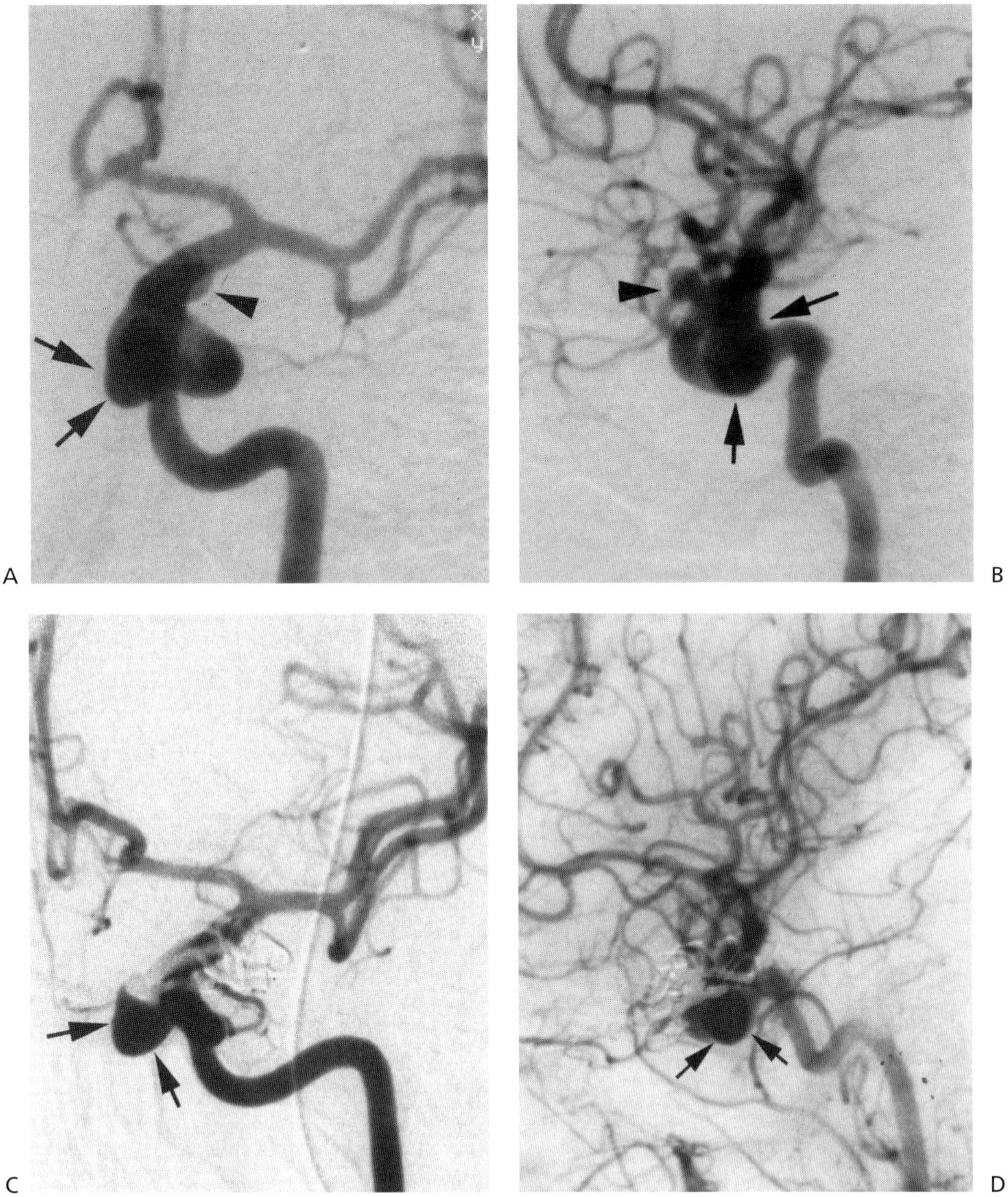

FIGURE 6-10. Use of combined clipping and coil placement for an aneurysm. This 56-year-old woman with multiple aneurysms had two noted in the left internal carotid artery circulation. **A,B:** Left internal carotid artery angiogram, anterior and lateral views, respectively. This demonstrates two aneurysms, a smaller ophthalmic artery aneurysm *(arrowhead)* and a larger broad-based paraclinoid-cavernous aneurysm *(arrows)*. The broad-based paraclinoid-cavernous aneurysm was not considered a good morphology for coil placement (due to the large neck), and because the aneurysm extended into the cavernous sinus it was not considered amenable to surgery alone. For this reason, combined clipping and coil placement was performed. During surgery the ophthalmic aneurysm was clipped. The anterior clinoid process was removed and the dural ring was opened to expose the clinoidal segment of the internal carotid artery. The upper portion of the aneurysm was successfully clipped to narrow the neck in advance of coil placement. **C,D:** Left internal carotid artery angiogram, anterior and lateral projections, respectively, following surgery. This demonstrated the continued filling of the cavernous segment of the aneurysm with narrowing of the neck following clipping *(arrows)*. *(Figure continues.)*

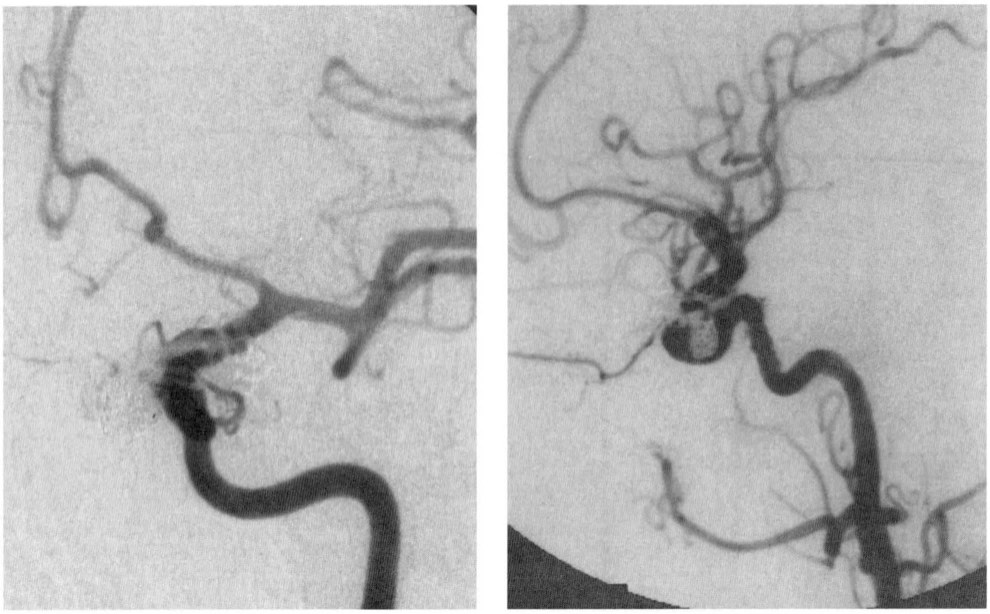

E F

FIGURE 6-10. *Continued.* **E,F:** Left internal carotid artery angiogram, anterior and lateral projections following coil placement. A series of GDCs were used to obliterate the remaining portion of the aneurysm. (From Michael P. Marks and Huy M. Do, unpublished material, with permission.)

clinical cases are confined to large aneurysms at the skull base, such as carotid ophthalmic, posterior communicating, and fusiform vertebral and basilar trunk aneurysms. The deployment of the microstent(s) across the neck of the aneurysm is followed by catheterization of the aneurysm with a microcatheter across the struts of the stents, followed by GDC packing of the aneurysm. The microstent keeps the GDCs inside the aneurysm while sparing the lumen of the parent artery. The preliminary anatomical and clinical outcomes are encouraging. Intracranial microstents have seldom been deployed in smaller arteries such as middle cerebral and posterior cerebral arteries. Further improvements in microstents' mechanical and biologic properties need to be achieved before tackling arteries smaller than 3.5 mm in diameter.

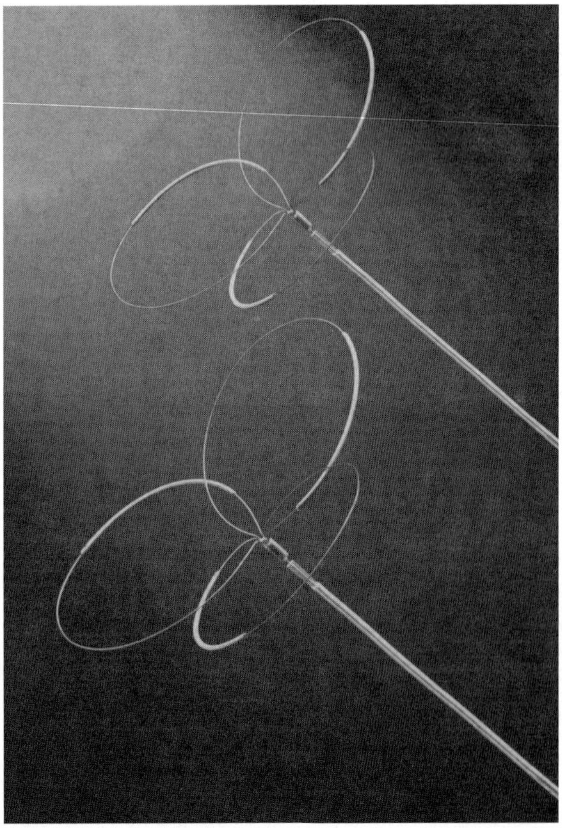

FIGURE 6-11. Trispan GDC.

Liquid embolic agents are potential alternatives for the treatment of the cerebral aneurysm (Fig. 6-13). Onyx (Micro Therapeutics, Irvine, CA) is a biocompatible polymer (ethylene-vinyl alcohol copolymer, EVOH), dissolved in its organic solvent, dimethyl sulfoxide (DMSO). The EVOH is composed of a random mixture of two subunits, ethylene (hydrophobic) and vinyl alcohol (hydrophilic). Micronized tantalum powder is added to the polymer–solvent mixture to obtain appropriate radiopacity. When this mixture contacts a liquid agent such as blood, DMSO rapidly diffuses away from the mixture causing *in situ* precipitation and solidification of the polymer. The liquid agent becomes spongy and occlusive without adhering to the vascular wall. A multicenter study using the liquid embolic agent Onyx is being conducted by the manufacturer in Europe and the United States. A neck protection balloon with or without

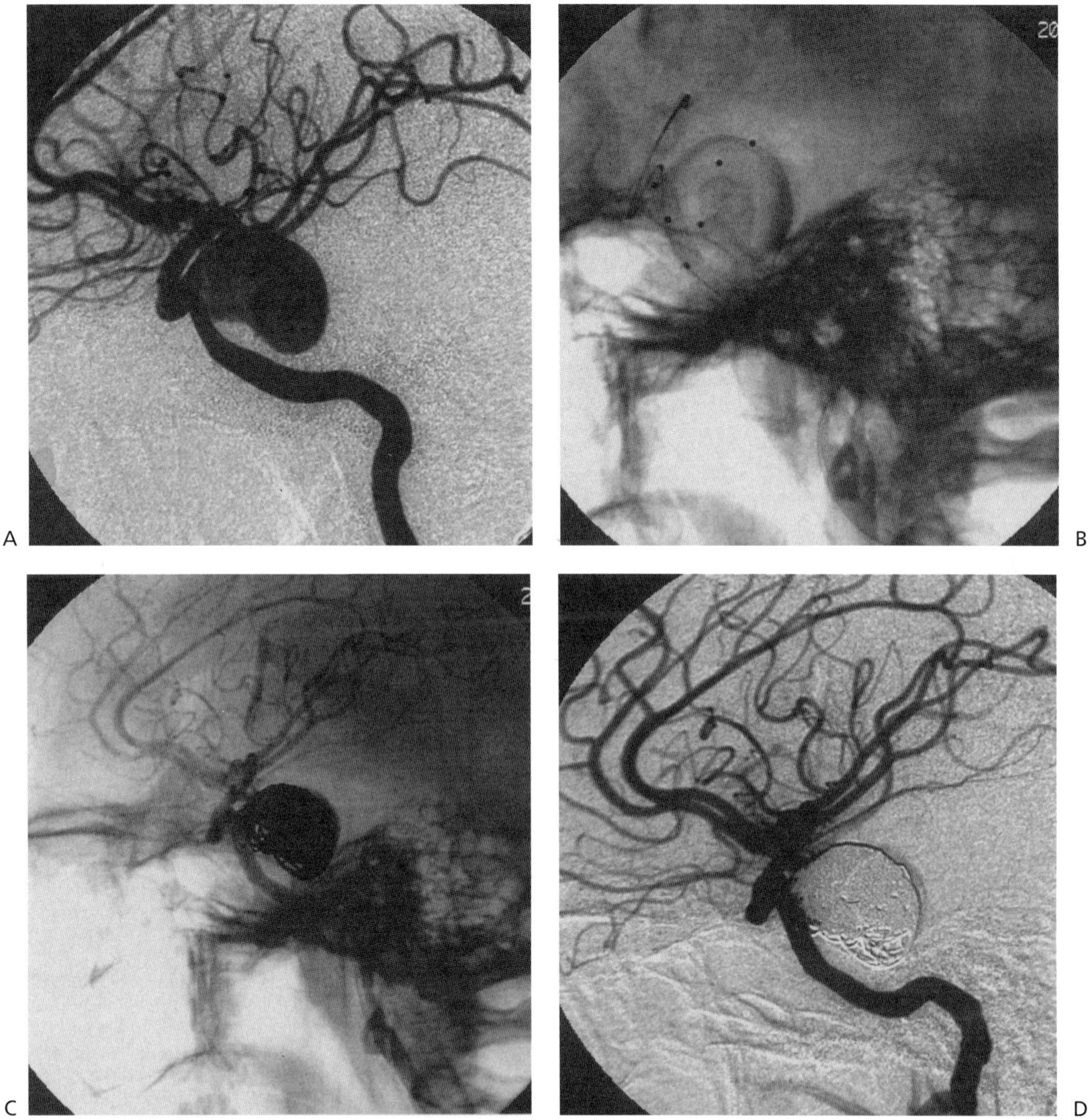

FIGURE 6-12. Coil placement following microstent placement. **A:** Large cavernous ICA aneurysm. **B:** A GFX microstent (4 mm × 12 mm) deployed across the neck of the aneurysm. **C:** Microcoils were delivered through stent struts. **D:** Successful stenting and coil embolization resulted in near-complete occlusion of the aneurysm.

microstent placement across the neck of the aneurysm is required to prevent liquid migration into the parent artery. Because of the high viscosity of the material, a specially designed high-pressure resistant microcatheter system is necessary.

The presence of a post-SAH arterial vasospasm does not preclude the GDC embolization of a ruptured aneurysm [29,58]. The interventional neuroradiologist may navigate through spastic arteries, occlude the ruptured aneurysm, and then perform angioplasty in the circle of Willis.

In most cases, it is not necessary to dilate the artery first with angioplasty in order to reach the ruptured aneurysm. However, balloon or chemical angioplasty may precede the GDC occlusion of an aneurysm, if necessary. The current clinical experience among interventional neuroradiologists indicates that it does not appear to increase the rate of aneurysmal rerupture.

The endovascular manipulation of symptomatic arterial vasospasm may need to be performed in those patients failing triple H therapy. A patient at risk for ischemic injury

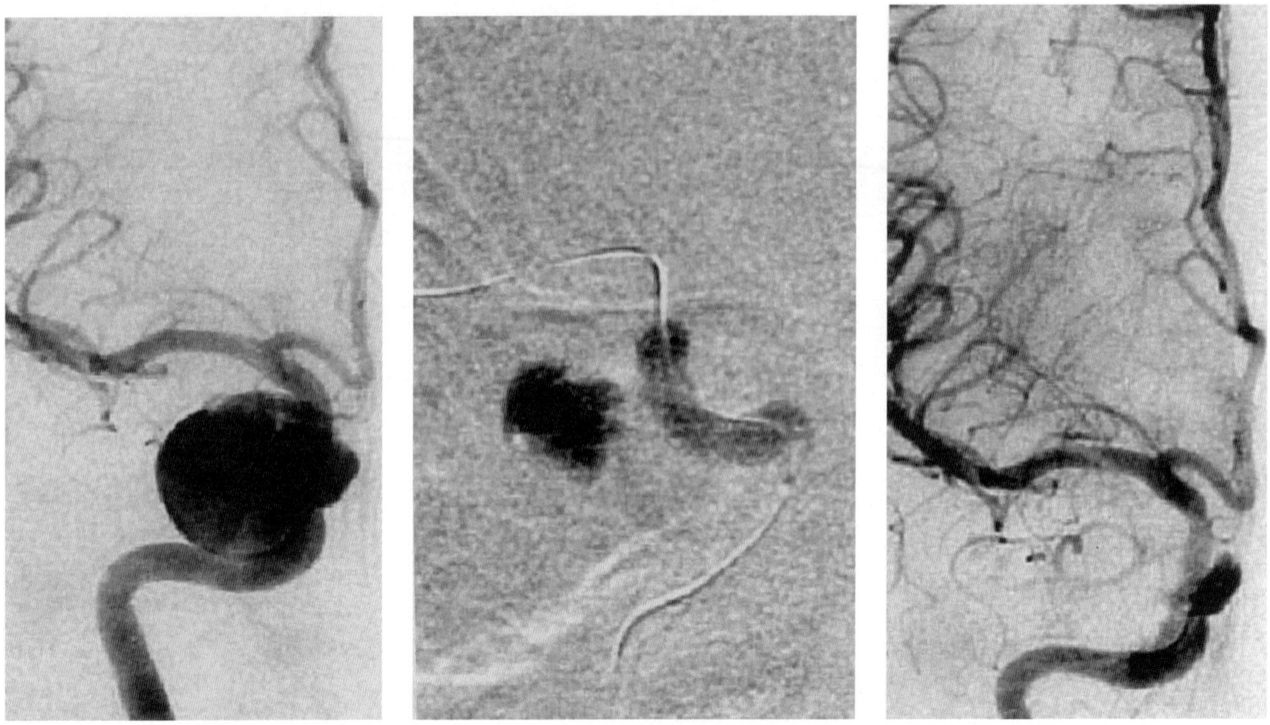

A,B C

FIGURE 6-13. Clinical use of Onyx for treatment of giant ICA aneurysm. **A:** Giant cavernous carotid aneurysm with wide neck. **B:** Roadmap image showing delivery of Onyx behind inflated blocking balloon. **C:** Control DSA following embolization. (From M. Mawad, unpublished material, with permission.)

often requires a complete cerebral angiogram and immediate mechanical or chemical angioplasty, or both, of the symptomatic arterial territory. These endovascular maneuvers are more fully discussed in Chapter 8.

ACKNOWLEDGEMENT

We gratefully acknowledge Dr. Yih-Lin Nien for assistance in the preparation of this manuscript.

REFERENCES

1. Zabramski JM, Spetzler RF. Surgery of intracranial aneurysms. In: *Stroke: pathophysiology, diagnosis, and management.* New York: Churchill Livingstone, 1992:1055–1092.
2. Kassell NF, Torner JC. Aneurysmal rebleeding: a preliminary report from the Cooperative Aneurysm Study. *Neurosurgery* 1983;13:479–481.
3. Weir B. *Aneurysms affecting the nervous system.* Baltimore: Williams & Wilkins, 1987.
4. Unruptured intracranial aneurysms—risk of rupture and risks of surgical intervention. International Study of Unruptured Intracranial Aneurysms Investigators. *N Engl J Med* 1998;339: 1725–1733.
5. Sahs A. *Intracranial aneurysms and subarachnoid hemorrhage: a cooperative study.* Philadelphia: JB Lippincott Co, 1969.
6. Nishioka H, Torner JC, Graf CJ, et al. Cooperative study of intracranial aneurysms and subarachnoid hemorrhage: a long-term prognostic study. II. Ruptured intracranial aneurysms managed conservatively. *Arch Neurol* 1984;41:1142–1146.
7. Ropper AH, Zervas NT. Outcome 1 year after SAH from cerebral aneurysm. Management morbidity, mortality, and functional status in 112 consecutive good-risk patients. *J Neurosurg* 1984;60: 909–915.
8. Weibers DO, Torner JC, Meissner I. Impact of unruptured intracranial aneurysms on public health in the United States. *Stroke* 1992;23:1416–1419.
9. Serbinenko FA. Balloon catheterization and occlusion of major cerebral vessels. *J Neurosurg* 1974;41:125–145.
10. Debrun G, Lacour P, Caron JP, et al. Detachable balloon and calibrated-leak balloon techniques in the treatment of cerebral vascular lesions. *J Neurosurg* 1978;49:635–649.
11. Kerber C. Balloon catheter with a calibrated leak: a new system for superselective angiotherapy and occlusive catheter therapy. *Radiology* 1976;120:547–549.
12. Taki W, Handa H, Yamagata S, et al. Balloon embolization of a giant aneurysm using a newly developed catheter. *Surg Neurol* 1979;12:363–365.
13. Fox AJ, Viñuela F, Pelz DM, et al. Use of detachable balloons for proximal artery occlusion in the treatment of unclippable cerebral aneurysms. *J Neurosurg* 1987;66:40–46.
14. Higashida RT, Halbach VV, Dormandy B, et al. Endovascular treatment of intracranial aneurysms with a new silicone microballoon device: technical considerations and indications for therapy. *Radiology* 1990;174:687–691.
15. Higashida RT, Halbach VV, Dowd CF, et al. Intracranial aneurysms: interventional neurovascular treatment with detachable balloons—results in 215 cases. *Radiology* 1991;178:663–670.
16. Fox AJ, Drake CG. Detachable balloon embolization for intracranial aneurysms. *J Neurosurg* 1990;73:157–159.

17. Higashida RT, Halbach VV, Dowd CF, et al. Interventional neurovascular treatment of a giant intracranial aneurysm using platinum microcoils. *Surg Neurol* 1991;35:64–68.
18. Morioka T, Matsushima T, Fujii K, et al. Balloon test occlusion of the internal carotid artery with monitoring of compressed spectral arrays (CSAs) of electroencephalogram. *Acta Neurochir (Wien)* 1989;101:29–34.
19. Higashida RT, Halbach VV, Barnwell SL, et al. Treatment of intracranial aneurysms with preservation of the parent vessel: results of percutaneous balloon embolization in 84 patients. *AJNR Am J Neuroradiol* 1990;11:633–640.
20. Casasco AE, Aymard A, Gobin YP, et al. Selective endovascular treatment of 71 intracranial aneurysms with platinum coils. *J Neurosurg* 1993;79:3–10.
21. Guglielmi G, Viñuela F, Dion J, et al. Electrothrombosis of saccular aneurysms via endovascular approach. Part 2: preliminary clinical experience. *J Neurosurg* 1991;75:8–14.
22. Guglielmi G, Viñuela F, Sepetka I, et al. Electrothrombosis of saccular aneurysms via endovascular approach. Part 1: electrochemical basis, technique, and experimental results. *J Neurosurg* 1991;75:1–7.
23. Viñuela F, Duckwiler G, Mawad M. Guglielmi detachable coil embolization of acute intracranial aneurysm: perioperative anatomical and clinical outcome in 403 patients. *J Neurosurg* 1997; 86:475–482.
24. Tateshima S, Murayama Y, Gobin YP, et al. Endovascular treatment of basilar tip aneurysms using Guglielmi detachable coils: anatomic and clinical outcomes in 73 patients from a single institution. *Neurosurgery* 2000;47:1332–1342.
25. Murayama Y, Viñuela F, Duckwiler GR, et al. Embolization of incidental cerebral aneurysms by using the Guglielmi detachable coil system. *J Neurosurg* 1999;90:207–214.
26. Solander S, Ulhoa A, Viñuela F, et al. Endovascular treatment of multiple intracranial aneurysms by using Guglielmi detachable coils. *J Neurosurg* 1999;90:857–864.
27. Malisch TW, Guglielmi G, Viñuela F, et al. Intracranial aneurysms treated with the Guglielmi detachable coil: midterm clinical results in a consecutive series of 100 patients. *J Neurosurg* 1997;87:176–183.
28. Byrne JV, Sohn MJ, Molyneux AJ, Chir B. Five-year experience in using coil embolization for ruptured intracranial aneurysms: outcomes and incidence of late rebleeding. *J Neurosurg* 1999;90: 656–663.
29. Murayama Y, Malisch T, Guglielmi G, et al. Incidence of cerebral vasospasm after endovascular treatment of acutely ruptured aneurysms: report on 69 cases. *J Neurosurg* 1997;87:830–835.
30. Cloft HJ, Joseph GJ, Tong FC, et al. Use of three-dimensional Guglielmi detachable coils in the treatment of wide-necked cerebral aneurysms. *AJNR Am J Neuroradiol* 2000;21:1312–1314.
31. Cottier JP, Pasco A, Gallas S, et al. Utility of balloon-assisted Guglielmi detachable coiling in the treatment of 49 cerebral aneurysms: a retrospective, multicenter study. *AJNR Am J Neuroradiol* 2001;22:345–351.
32. Lefkowitz MA, Gobin YP, Akiba Y, et al. Balloon-assisted Guglielmi detachable coiling of wide-necked aneurysma: part II—clinical results. *Neurosurgery* 1999;45:531–538.
33. Moret J, Cognard C, Weill A, et al. Reconstruction technic in the treatment of wide-neck intracranial aneurysms. Long-term angiographic and clinical results. Apropos of 56 cases. *J Neuroradiol* 1997;24:30–44.
34. Levy DI, Ku A. Balloon-assisted coil placement in wide-necked aneurysms. Technical note. *J Neurosurg* 1997;86:724–727.
35. Fessler RD, Ringer AJ, Qureshi AI, et al. Intracranial stent placement to trap an extruded coil during endovascular aneurysm treatment: technical note. *Neurosurgery* 2000;46:248–253.
36. Higashida RT, Smith W, Gress D, et al. Intravascular stent and endovascular coil placement for a ruptured fusiform aneurysm of the basilar artery. Case report and review of the literature. *J Neurosurg* 1997;87:944–949.
37. Horowitz MB, Miller G III, Meyer Y, et al. Use of intravascular stents in the treatment of internal carotid and extracranial vertebral artery pseudoaneurysms. *AJNR Am J Neuroradiol* 1996;17: 693–696.
38. Lanzino G, Wakhloo AK, Fessler RD, et al. Efficacy and current limitations of intravascular stents for intracranial internal carotid, vertebral, and basilar artery aneurysms. *J Neurosurg* 1999;91: 538–546.
39. Lylyk P, Ceratto R, Hurvitz D, et al. Treatment of a vertebral dissecting aneurysm with stents and coils: technical case report. *Neurosurgery* 1998;43:385–388.
40. Mericle RA, Lanzino G, Wakhloo AK, et al. Stenting and secondary coiling of intracranial internal carotid artery aneurysm: technical case report. *Neurosurgery* 1998;43:1229–1234.
41. Debrun GM, Varsos V, Liszczak TM, et al. Obliteration of experimental aneurysms in dogs with isobutyl-cyanoacrylate. *J Neurosurg* 1984;61:37–43.
42. Kinugasa K, Mandai S, Terai Y, et al. Direct thrombosis of aneurysms with cellulose acetate polymer. Part II: preliminary clinical experience. *J Neurosurg* 1992;77:501–507.
43. Mandai S, Kinugasa K, Ohmoto T. Direct thrombosis of aneurysms with cellulose acetate polymer. Part I: results of thrombosis in experimental aneurysms. *J Neurosurg* 1992;77:497–500.
44. Kinugasa K, Mandai S, Tsuchida S, et al. Direct thrombosis of a pseudoaneurysm after obliteration of a carotid-cavernous fistula with cellulose acetate polymer: technical case report. *Neurosurgery* 1994;35:755–760.
45. Kinugasa K, Mandai S, Tsuchida S, et al. Cellulose acetate polymer thrombosis for the emergency treatment of aneurysms: angiographic findings, clinical experience, and histopathological study. *Neurosurgery* 1994;34:694–701.
46. Kinugasa K, Kamata I, Hirotsune N, et al. Early treatment of subarachnoid hemorrhage after preventing rerupture of an aneurysm. *J Neurosurg* 1995;83:34–41.
47. Kinugasa K, Mandai S, Kamata I, et al. Prophylactic thrombosis to prevent new bleeding and to delay aneurysm surgery. *Neurosurgery* 1995;36:661–667.
48. Sugiu K, Kinugasa K, Mandai S, et al. Direct thrombosis of experimental aneurysms with cellulose acetate polymer (CAP): technical aspects, angiographic follow up, and histological study. *J Neurosurg* 1995;83:531–538.
49. Taki W, Nishi S, Yamashita K, et al. Selection and combination of various endovascular techniques in the treatment of giant aneurysms. *J Neurosurg* 1992;77:37–42.
50. Murayama Y, Viñuela F, Tateshima S, et al. Endovascular treatment of experimental aneurysms by use of a combination of liquid embolic agents and protective devices. *AJNR Am J Neuroradiol* 2000;21:1726–1735.
51. Kato Y, Sano H, Katada K, et al. Application of three-dimensional CT angiography (3D-CTA) to cerebral aneurysms. *Surg Neurol* 1999;52:113–122.
52. Korogi Y, Takahashi M, Katada K, et al. Intracranial aneurysms: detection with three-dimensional CT angiography with volume rendering—comparison with conventional angiographic and surgical findings. *Radiology* 1999;211:497–506.
53. Rieger J, Hosten N, Neumann K, et al. Initial clinical experience with spiral CT and 3D arterial reconstruction in intracranial aneurysms and arteriovenous malformations. *Neuroradiology* 1996;38:245–251.
54. Villablanca JP, Martin N, Jahan R, et al. Volume-rendered helical computerized tomography angiography in the detection and characterization of intracranial aneurysms. *J Neurosurg* 2000;93: 254–264.
55. Anxionnat R, Bracard S, Macho J, et al. 3D angiography. Clinical

interest. First applications in interventional neuroradiology. *J Neuroradiol* 1998;25:251–262.
56. Anxionnat R, Bracard S, Ducrocq X, et al. Intracranial aneurysms: clinical value of 3d digital subtraction angiography in the therapeutic decision and endovascular treatment. *Radiology* 2001; 218:799–808.
57. Turk AS, Rappe AH, Villar F, et al. Evaluation of the TriSpan neck bridge device for the treatment of wide-necked aneurysms: an experimental study in canines. *Stroke* 2001;32:492–497.
58. Murayama Y, Uda K, Gobin YP, et al. Combined GDC embolization and angioplasty for ruptured aneurysm associated with symptomatic vasospasm. *J Neurosurg* 2000(abst).
59. Fernandez Zubillaga A, Guglielmi G, Viñuela F, et al. Endovascular occlusion of intracranial aneurysms with electrically detachable coils: correlation of aneurysm neck size and treatment results. *AJNR Am J Neuroradiol* 1994;15:815–820.
60. Hayakawa M, Murayama Y, Duckwiler GR, et al. Natural history of the neck remnant of a cerebral aneurysm treated with the Guglielmi detachable coil system. *J Neurosurg* 2000;93:561–568.
61. Mawad ME, Mawad JK, Cartwright J Jr, et al. Long-term histopathologic changes in canine aneurysms embolized with Guglielmi detachable coils. *AJNR Am J Neuroradiol* 1995;16:7–13.
62. Tamatani S, Ozawa T, Minakawa T, et al. Histological interaction of cultured endothelial cells and endovascular embolic materials coated with extracellular matrix. *J Neurosurg* 1997;86: 109–112.
63. Tenjin H, Fushiki S, Nakahara Y, et al. Effect of Guglielmi detachable coils on experimental carotid artery aneurysms in primates. *Stroke* 1995;26:2075–2080.
64. Reul J, Spetzger U, Weis J, et al. Endovascular occlusion of experimental aneurysms with detachable coils: influence of packing density and perioperative anticoagulation. *Neurosurgery* 1997;41: 1160–1168.
65. Spetzger U, Reul J, Weis J, et al. Microsurgically produced bifurcation aneurysms in a rabbit model for endovascular coil embolization. *J Neurosurg* 1996;85:488–495.
66. Bavinzski G, Talazoglu V, Killer M, et al. Gross and microscopic histopathological findings in aneurysms of the human brain treated with Guglielmi detachable coils. *J Neurosurg* 1999;91: 284–293.
67. Horowitz MB, Purdy PD, Burns D, et al. Scanning electron microscopic findings in a basilar tip aneurysm embolized with Guglielmi detachable coils. *AJNR Am J Neuroradiol* 1997;18: 688–690.
68. Koizumi T, Kawano T, Kazekawa K, et al. Histological findings in aneurysm treated with IDC: scanning electron microscopical study [in Japanese]. *No Shinkei Geka* 1997;25:1027–1031.
69. Mizoi K, Yoshimoto T, Takahashi A, et al. A pitfall in the surgery of a recurrent aneurysm after coil embolization and its histological observation: technical case report. *Neurosurgery* 1996;39: 165–169.
70. Molyneux AJ, Ellison DW, Morris J, et al. Histological findings in giant aneurysms treated with Guglielmi detachable coils. Report of two cases with autopsy correlation. *J Neurosurg* 1995;83: 129–132.
71. Shimizu S, Kurata A, Takano M, et al. Tissue response of a small saccular aneurysm after incomplete occlusion with a Guglielmi detachable coil. *AJNR Am J Neuroradiol* 1999;20:546–548.
72. Castro E, Fortea F, Villoria F, et al. Long-term histopathologic findings in two cerebral aneurysms embolized with Guglielmi detachable coils. *AJNR Am J Neuroradiol* 1999;20:549–552.
73. Stiver SI, Porter PJ, Willinsky RA, et al. Acute human histopathology of an intracranial aneurysm treated using Guglielmi detachable coils: case report and review of the literature. *Neurosurgery* 1998;43:1203–1208.
74. Knuckey NW, Haas R, Jenkins R, et al. Thrombosis of difficult intracranial aneurysms by the endovascular placement of platinum-Dacron microcoils. *J Neurosurg* 1992;77:43–50.
75. Ahuja AA, Hergenrother RW, Strother CM, et al. Platinum coil coatings to increase thrombogenicity: a preliminary study in rabbits. *AJNR Am J Neuroradiol* 1993;14:794–798.
76. McLean GK, Stein EJ, Burke DR, et al. Steel occlusion coils: pretreatment with thrombin. *Radiology* 1986;158:549–550.
77. Szikora I, Wakhloo AK, Guterman LR, et al. Initial experience with collagen-filled Guglielmi detachable coils for endovascular treatment of experimental aneurysms. *AJNR Am J Neuroradiol* 1997;18:667–672.
78. Dawson RC III, Shengelaia GG, Krisht AF, et al. Histologic effects of collagen-filled interlocking detachable coils in the ablation of experimental aneurysms in swine. *AJNR Am J Neuroradiol* 1996;17:853–858.
79. Murayama Y, Viñuela F, Suzuki Y, et al. Ion implantation and protein coating of detachable coils for endovascular treatment of cerebral aneurysms: concepts and preliminary results in swine models. *Neurosurgery* 1997;40:1233–1244.
80. Murayama Y, Suzuki Y, Viñuela F, et al. Development of a biologically active Guglielmi detachable coil for the treatment of cerebral aneurysms. Part I: in vitro study. *AJNR Am J Neuroradiol* 1999;20:1986–1991.
81. Murayama Y, Viñuela F, Suzuki Y, et al. Development of the biologically active Guglielmi detachable coil for the treatment of cerebral aneurysms. Part II: an experimental study in a swine aneurysm model. *AJNR Am J Neuroradiol* 1999;20:1992–1999.
82. Kallmes DF, Williams AD, Cloft HJ, et al. Platinum coil-mediated implantation of growth factor-secreting endovascular tissue grafts: an in vivo study. *Radiology* 1998;207:519–523.
83. Kallmes DF, Borland MK, Cloft HJ, et al. In vitro proliferation and adhesion of basic fibroblast growth factor-producing fibroblasts on platinum coils. *Radiology* 1998;206:237–243.
84. Freed LE, Vunjak-Novakovic G, Biron RJ, et al. Biodegradable polymer scaffolds for tissue engineering. *Biotechnology (N Y)* 1994;12:689–693.
85. Langer R. New methods of drug delivery. *Science* 1990;249: 1527–1533.
86. Langer R. Angiogenesis—biomedical technology. *EXS* 1992;61: 23–25.
87. Langer R, Vacanti JP. Tissue engineering. *Science* 1993;260: 920–926.
88. Langer R. Drug delivery and targeting. *Nature* 1998;392:5–10.
89. Langer R. Biomaterials in drug delivery and tissue engineering: one laboratory's experience. *Acc Chem Res* 2000;33:94–101.
90. Langer R. Tissue engineering. *Mol Ther* 2000;1:12–15.
91. Lendlein A, Schmidt AM, Langer R. AB-polymer networks based on oligo(varepsilon-caprolactone) segments showing shape-memory properties. *Proc Natl Acad Sci U S A* 2001;98:842–847.
92. Murayama Y, Viñuela F, Tateshima S, et al. Bioabsorbable polymeric material coils for embolization of intracranial aneurysms: a preliminary experimental study. *J Neurosurg* 2001;94:454–463.

7

PARENT VESSEL OCCLUSION FOR CEREBRAL ANEURYSMS AND PSEUDOANEURYSMS

HARRY J. CLOFT

In 1784, John Hunter performed the first treatment of an aneurysm by proximal arterial ligation [1]. Hunter ligated the feeding artery to a popliteal artery aneurysm, which reduced the flow to the aneurysm while allowing the distal circulation to be supplied by collateral arteries. In recognition of this pioneering operation, the treatment of aneurysms by proximal occlusion of the feeding artery has come to be known as *Hunterian occlusion.* Keen [2] reported the first proximal ligation of the carotid artery for the treatment of an intracranial aneurysm in 1890. After Dandy described the clipping of an intracranial aneurysmal neck, it soon became clear that such clipping, when possible, was more effective than proximal ligation [3]. However, because clipping of the aneurysmal neck is not always feasible, surgical ligation of an artery remains a viable therapy for cerebral aneurysms.

Beginning in the 1970s, surgical ligation for the treatment of cerebral aneurysms was gradually replaced by endovascular techniques. Endovascular arterial sacrifice for intracranial aneurysms began in the early 1970s with the pioneering work of Serbinenko, who used detachable latex balloons for parent artery sacrifice [4,5]. In the 1980s, the treatment of aneurysms by endovascular arterial sacrifice using latex balloons was reported at multiple North American medical centers [6–8]. Also in the 1980s, Hieshima et al. and Higashida et al. developed a silicone balloon to be used for endovascular arterial sacrifice [9,10]. Silicone balloons were eventually approved by the U.S. Food and Drug Administration (FDA) for endovascular arterial sacrifice in 1998.

Since the Guglielmi detachable coil (GDC; Target Therapeutics, Boston Scientific Corporation, Natick, MA) was approved by the FDA for cerebral aneurysm therapy in September of 1995, embolization with retrievable coils has become the primary endovascular technique for the treatment of intracranial saccular aneurysm. The use of this technique is discussed in Chapter 6. Patients are currently treated with parent vessel sacrifice when it is not possible or safe to treat them with a technique that will preserve flow through the parent vessel (i.e., surgical clipping or endovascular coil embolization). Endovascular arterial sacrifice remains a viable therapy for a subset of patients with cerebral aneurysms, and it is quite safe and effective in appropriately selected patients.

BACKGROUND

Carotid Artery Circulation

Aneurysms located in the subarachnoid space are treated to prevent subarachnoid hemorrhage, which can be life-threatening. Smaller aneurysms (<10 mm) in the subarachnoid space can generally be treated with surgical clipping or endosaccular coil embolization. Aneurysms treated by parent artery endovascular sacrifice tend to be large (≥10 mm) or giant (≥25 mm). Aneurysms equal to and greater than 10 mm in diameter have been shown to have an increased risk of subarachnoid hemorrhage relative to smaller aneurysms [11]. Giant aneurysms in the subarachnoid space have a particularly dangerous natural history. Within 5 years of diagnosis, approximately 80% of patients with untreated giant aneurysms are severely disabled or dead secondary to cerebral infarction, brainstem compression, or subarachnoid hemorrhage [12].

Cavernous carotid artery aneurysms are not generally life-threatening because they rarely cause subarachnoid hemorrhage [13–15]. Unlike the treatment of subarachnoid aneurysms, which is aimed at the prevention of hemorrhage, the treatment of cavernous carotid aneurysms is aimed at the alleviation of symptoms [15]. Patients with cavernous carotid artery aneurysms may have cranial nerve deficits due to mass effect, carotid-cavernous fistula, decreased visual

H. J. Cloft: Departments of Radiology and Neurosurgery, Mayo Clinic, Rochester, Minnesota.

acuity, or headache (especially retroorbital) [15,16]. Rarely, cavernous carotid artery aneurysms can extend into the sphenoid sinus and cause life-threatening epistaxis [17].

Most cavernous carotid aneurysms are large or giant at the time of diagnosis, and they usually require carotid sacrifice for cure. Cavernous carotid aneurysms with a definable neck can be treated with GDC embolization and parent vessel preservation [18]. Small, asymptomatic cavernous aneurysms can usually be observed conservatively, because they pose no immediate threat that would justify exposing the patient to the risks of therapy [19].

When planning carotid occlusion as a treatment for supraclinoid aneurysms, consideration must be given to the possibility of continued blood flow to the aneurysm through the ophthalmic artery or through the circle of Willis (Fig. 7-1). With large or giant ophthalmic segment aneurysms, it is sometimes effective to place GDCs in the aneurysm, allowing them to extend into and occlude the parent carotid artery as well, followed by balloon occlusion of the cervical carotid artery. Not all aneurysms are amenable to this kind of coil sacrifice, however.

Aneurysms treated by carotid occlusion have been shown to involute, thus reducing mass effect [19–21]. Cranial neuropathies caused by giant cavernous aneurysms will usually improve following carotid occlusion [16,20,21], but long-standing neuropathies are less likely to improve. Visual symptoms from anterior visual pathway compression will improve in a minority of cases following endovascular carotid sacrifice [19].

New advances in endovascular and surgical techniques will likely continue to reduce the need for carotid sacrifice for cerebral aneurysm. Stents [22,23] and surgery under circulatory arrest are examples.

Pseudoaneurysms and ruptures of the carotid artery can be caused by malignancy, infection, or trauma. These pseudoaneurysms sometimes require endovascular carotid sacrifice for effective treatment (Fig. 7-2). Advanced head and neck squamous cell carcinoma can invade adjacent arteries and cause a clinical entity known as *carotid blowout syndrome* [24–27]. Carotid blowout syndrome is caused by the invasion of the carcinoma into the artery wall, which leads to life-threatening hemorrhage, either externally through a cutaneous fistula or into the pharynx. The bleeding can be due to invasion of an external carotid artery branch, the internal carotid artery, or common carotid artery. Bleeding from an external carotid artery branch is usually easily treated by coil embolization of the bleeding branch. Bleeding from the internal carotid or common carotid artery generally requires endovascular carotid sacrifice. Any attempt to preserve the common or internal carotid artery exposes the patient to recurrent blowout, because invasion of the artery by carcinoma will continue. The arterial blowout site must be considered an infected wound because it communicates with the skin surface or the pharynx. It is probably wise to minimize the amount of foreign material used to occlude the carotid artery, because the foreign material may serve as a nidus of continued infection. Simple balloon occlusion with the balloons located at a distance above and below the blowout site may be the best way to minimize such infection.

If the patient does not tolerate test balloon occlusion, extracranial-intracranial (EC-IC) bypass surgery is generally not practical because of the patient's poor condition secondary to the malignancy. In this circumstance, it may be possible to spare the carotid artery by embolizing only the pseudoaneurysm [26]. Embolizing only the pseudoaneurysm will likely only temporarily prevent bleeding, however, because of the presence of carcinoma and an absence of normal tissue healing in the region of the blowout.

Stents have been suggested as a therapeutic alternative to carotid sacrifice in patients with carotid blowout syndrome [76]. Stents can be nidi for infection and, if not covered by a membrane that is impermeable to blood, the stent will very probably not stop the bleeding. Even if they survive their hemorrhages, patients with carotid blowout secondary to carcinomatous invasion have a dismal prognosis because of their advanced malignancies. Treating active hemorrhage with endovascular therapy may add only weeks or months to the patients' overall survival. The goal is to stop the bleeding, because hemorrhage through a cutaneous fistula or into the pharynx is an objectionable way to die. It is important to remember that these patients do not have long to live, and stopping the hemorrhage by causing a stroke because of an inadequate circle of Willis is not in their best interest. The physician, patient, and family should reach an understanding regarding realistic expectations about the procedure and the ultimate prognosis. The physician must be very sensitive to the wishes of the patient and family when considering the treatment options under these dire circumstances.

Sometimes endovascular carotid sacrifice is required for traumatic [28–30] or iatrogenic [31–34] injury to the carotid artery. Pseudoaneurysms of the internal carotid artery resulting from dissection rarely result in embolization or arterial rupture and can usually be medically treated with antiplatelet agents after early anticoagulation [35]. Should symptoms of a pseudoaneurysm of the cervical internal carotid artery warrant more aggressive therapy, they can often be treated with a carotid-sparing procedure, using stent placement followed by coil embolization of the pseudoaneurysm [36–38] rather than endovascular arterial sacrifice. Because pseudoaneurysms resulting from dissection are much less likely to recur than cancerous pseudoaneurysms, carotid-sparing procedures are more feasible with pseudoaneurysms resulting from dissection.

Carotid-cavernous fistula is another manifestation of traumatic rupture of the internal carotid artery. Occasionally, carotid-cavernous fistula cannot be occluded at the site of fistula and sacrifice of the internal carotid artery becomes necessary [39].

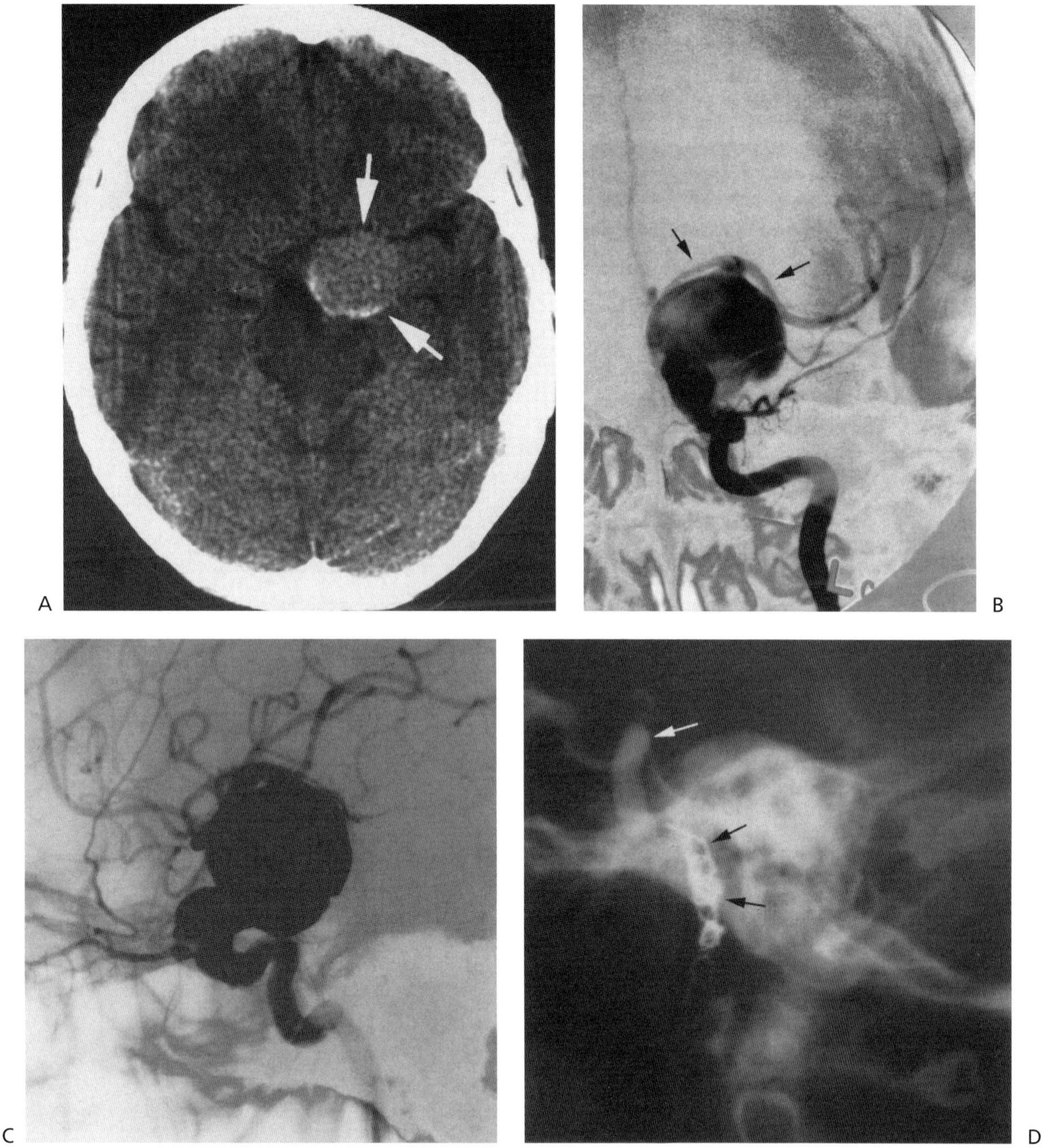

FIGURE 7-1. This 18-year-old woman was admitted to the hospital with severe retroorbital pain and markedly decreased visual acuity in the left eye. She had a giant left supraclinoid carotid artery aneurysm. In addition, the patient was at the end of the second trimester of a normal pregnancy. Her workup with a lumbar puncture confirmed that she had sustained a subarachnoid hemorrhage. **A:** Axial CT scan demonstrates a slightly hyperdense giant aneurysm in the left supraclinoid region *(arrows)*. **B,C:** Left carotid angiograms, anterior and lateral projections, respectively, demonstrate a giant fusiform aneurysm involving the entire supraclinoid carotid artery. The dilation of the carotid extends from the infraclinoid region and up to the bifurcation. The aneurysm is seen to supply the anterior and middle cerebral arteries *(arrows)*. It was recommended that the patient continue the pregnancy for approximately 6 more weeks to improve fetal lung maturity. Endovascular trapping of the aneurysm was not judged to be possible because the entire supraclinoid carotid artery was involved. Coiling of the entire segment of the aneurysm was also judged to be relatively higher risk because of the giant size of the lesion. For this reason, test occlusion was performed, followed by carotid sacrifice at the level of the cavernous carotid artery, recognizing that a portion of the aneurysmal segment would continue to fill via ophthalmic and posterior communicating artery collateral vessels. **D:** Left lateral plain film after carotid artery sacrifice demonstrates a balloon in the petrous and proximal cavernous artery segment *(white arrow)* with coil packing proximal *(black arrows)*. *(Figure continues.)*

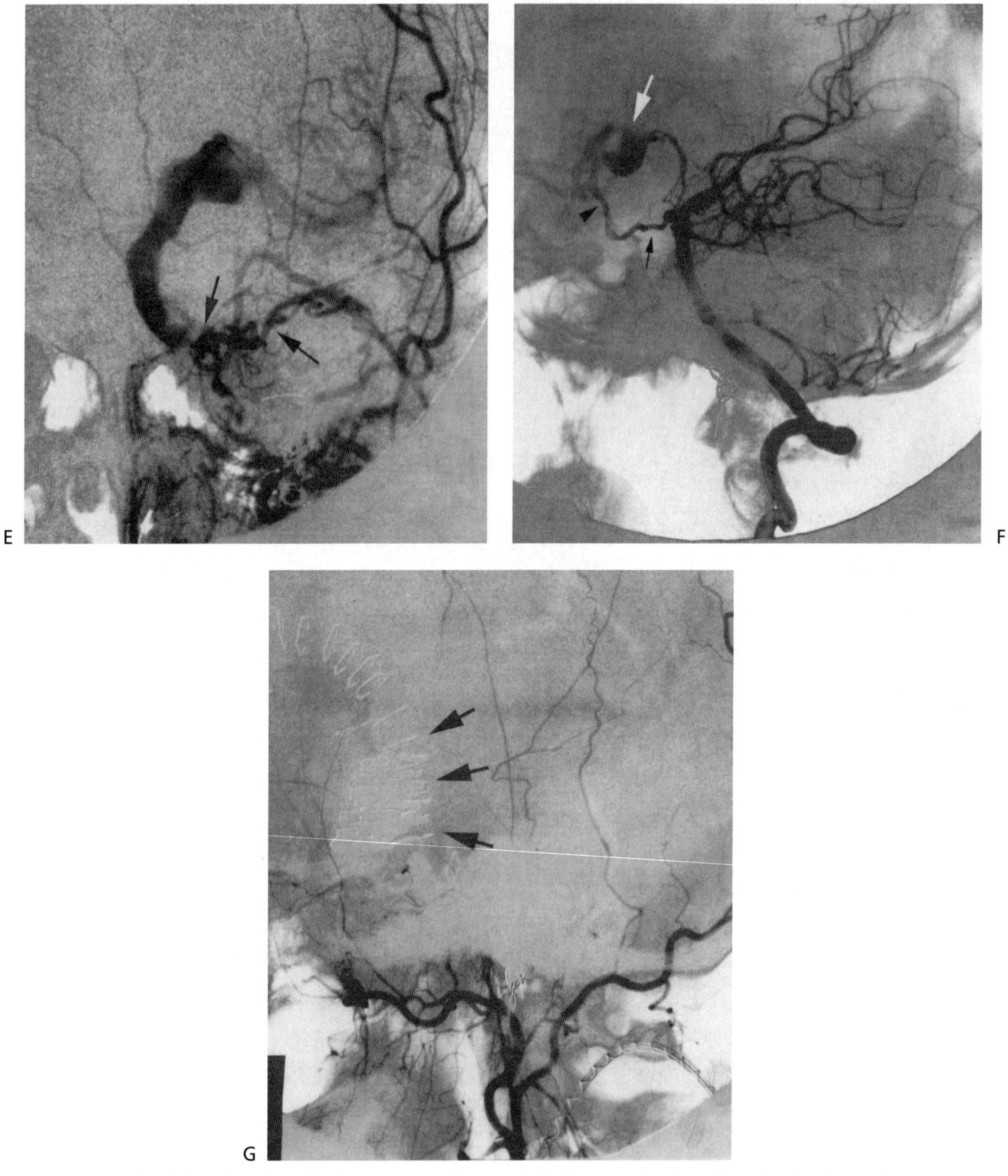

FIGURE 7-1. *Continued.* **E:** Common carotid artery injection, anterior view, 6 weeks after internal carotid artery sacrifice. This demonstrates continued filling of the aneurysmal segment with marked thrombosis and shrinkage of the aneurysm. This filling is noted to come from ophthalmic artery collateral vessels *(arrows).* **F:** Left vertebral artery angiogram, lateral projection, also 6 weeks after deliberate carotid artery sacrifice. This demonstrates filling of the supraclinoid artery segment *(arrowhead)* via the posterior communicating arteries *(black arrow),* with subsequent filling of the aneurysm *(white arrow).* The patient had an uncomplicated cesarean section and delivery after this angiogram was made. Because there was continued filling of the aneurysm, carotid sacrifice below the level of the bifurcation was performed surgically with a series of clips. **G:** Left external carotid artery control angiogram after surgery. A series of clips have been placed along the length of the aneurysm *(arrows)* and no filling of the aneurysm is observed. Preoperatively, she had had decreased visual acuity in the left eye, and this continued postoperatively. One year after her procedures, she was otherwise neurologically intact. (From Michael P. Marks and Huy M. Do, unpublished material, with permission.)

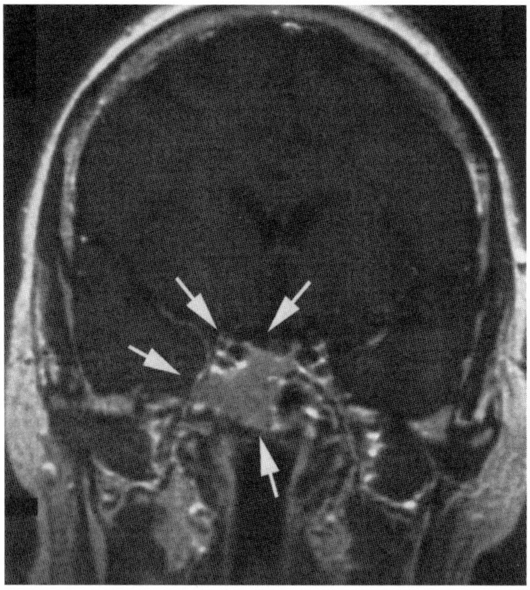
A

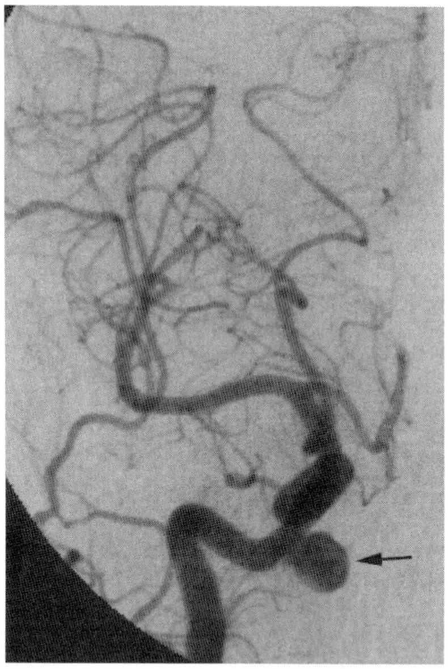
B

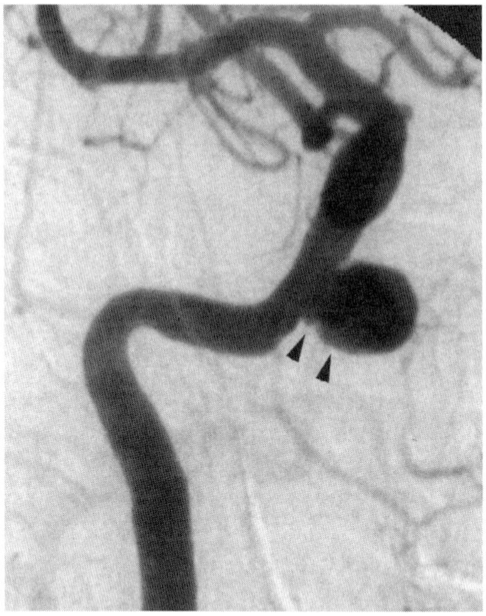
C

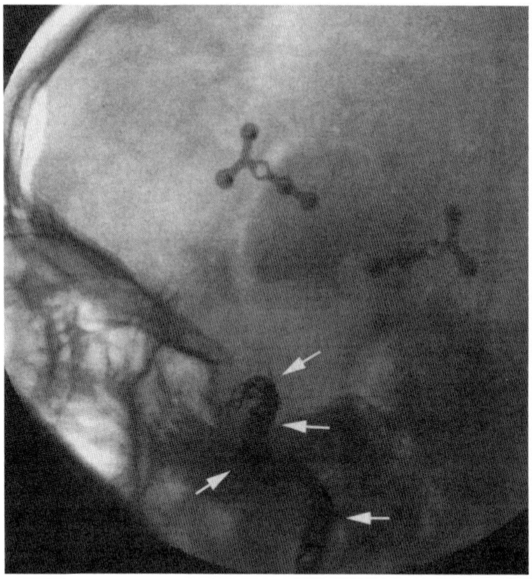
D

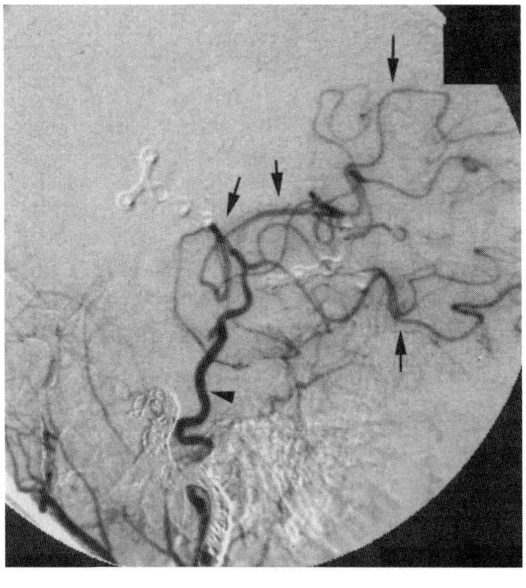
E

FIGURE 7-2. This 73-year-old woman developed a pseudoaneurysm in the right internal carotid artery following a transphenoidal biopsy of a skull base tumor. **A:** Coronal T1-weighted post–gadolinium MRI demonstrates a tumor mass in the sphenoid sinus region extending into the right cavernous sinus *(arrows)*. The patient underwent transphenoidal biopsy and at that time had profuse bleeding through the operative site, which required extensive packing. **B,C:** Right carotid artery angiograms, anterior projection, demonstrate a pseudoaneurysm of the petrous segment of the carotid artery (*arrow,* **B**). On the more magnified view, the irregularities of this aneurysm can be seen (*arrowheads,* **C**). The patient underwent an EC-IC bypass because she did not tolerate test occlusion. After this, carotid sacrifice was performed. **D:** Lateral plain film. Coils were placed across the perforated area of the carotid artery, effectively trapping the aneurysm *(arrows)*. **E:** Right external carotid artery control angiogram, lateral projection, after carotid sacrifice. Brisk filling of the middle cerebral artery circulation *(arrows)* is occurring via the superficial temporal artery graft *(arrowhead)*. No filling of the aneurysm was seen. (From Michael P. Marks and Huy M. Do, unpublished material, with permission.)

Most of the delayed strokes occurring following carotid sacrifice are probably due to thromboembolism. Mathis et al. [40] summarized the data from five reports [7,16,23–25] of endovascular carotid sacrifice after passing a test balloon occlusion with clinical neurologic examination alone, finding 9 (4.7%) permanent strokes in 192 patients. Surgical sacrifice of the carotid artery has a higher stroke risk than endovascular sacrifice [6,16,20,41]. The higher risk associated with surgical occlusion may be due to surgical sacrifice being performed without anticoagulation to prevent emboli and a tendency for a longer stump distal to the point of occlusion that will accumulate more thrombus. It is unlikely that any test will ever predict the risk of embolic stroke with carotid or vertebral artery sacrifice. The embolic stroke risk will probably be best managed with pharmacologic prophylaxis. This pharmacologic prophylaxis has traditionally been anticoagulation with heparin, but antiplatelet agents may play an important role in the future.

Balloon failure can occur immediately or in a delayed manner [34,42–44]. If a balloon fails and deflates partially or completely, it will embolize distally and may cause ischemic injury. It is sometimes possible to deflate the balloon percutaneously, thereby decreasing the size and clinical significance of the embolized balloon [43]. If percutaneous balloon deflation fails, surgical embolectomy may be necessary [42,44].

Cavernous cranial nerve deficits [6,7,45] and severe retroorbital pain [6] occur when cavernous aneurysms thrombose. These symptoms probably result from inflammation and swelling secondary to thrombosis and usually respond quickly to nonsteroidal antiinflammatory drugs.

Because sacrifice of the carotid artery results in increased flow through the contralateral carotid artery and the circle of Willis, induction of aneurysm formation is a theoretical risk [20,46–49]. New aneurysms formed during the long term, following carotid ligation in 3 of 27 patients reported by Fujiwara et al. [46] and in 1 of 58 patients reported by Larson et al. [20]. Tomsick et al. [50] performed a metaanalysis of 11 reported series of patients with aneurysm who were treated with carotid occlusion. The incidence of subarachnoid hemorrhage in the 510 patients in this series was found to be 0.4 per 100 patient-years of follow-up [50]. The aneurysms causing subarachnoid hemorrhage following carotid occlusion are usually located on the anterior communicating artery, which receives a markedly increased flow following the procedure. The incidence of subarachnoid hemorrhage in patients treated with carotid occlusion is 40 times higher than in the general population and 5 times higher than in patients with previous subarachnoid hemorrhage not treated with carotid occlusion [51].

Vertebral Artery Circulation

Large saccular and fusiform vertebrobasilar aneurysms sometimes require treatment with unilateral or bilateral endovascular vertebral artery sacrifice [7,52–55]. Treatment of distal vertebral artery aneurysms with unilateral vertebral artery endovascular sacrifice [7,12,52,55,56] is rather straightforward and carries a low risk if the contralateral vertebral artery is large enough to provide adequate blood supply to the basilar artery. Elimination of flow to the aneurysm with preservation of flow to the posterior inferior cerebellar artery is usually possible (Fig. 7-3). If the aneurysm is located on the vertebral artery distal to the origin of the posterior inferior cerebellar artery (PICA), the aneurysmal lumen and parent vessel can be completely filled with coils. If the aneurysm is located proximal to the origin of the PICA, the vertebral artery can be occluded proximal to the PICA, resulting in collateral supply from the contralateral vertebral artery to the distal vertebral artery and PICA. In rare cases it may not be possible to maintain direct flow to the PICA (Fig. 7-4).

Treatment of basilar artery aneurysms with parent artery occlusion is problematic because critical blood supply to the brainstem must be preserved in order for the patient to survive. Unilateral vertebral artery endovascular sacrifice will sometimes alter flow sufficiently to lead to basilar aneurysm thrombosis [12,53]. Bilateral vertebral artery endovascular sacrifice has been used occasionally to treat basilar artery aneurysms [7,52–54]. Bilateral vertebral artery sacrifice carries a higher risk than unilateral sacrifice, because the success of the procedure depends upon collateral flow to the basilar artery from the anterior circulation through the posterior communicating arteries. Rarely, endovascular sacrifice of the basilar artery has been used to treat aneurysms [12,54,55]. This procedure carries a high risk and cannot be tolerated by many patients, but it has been used successfully on occasion to treat difficult basilar artery aneurysms.

Even if collateral blood supply is sufficient to allow a patient to tolerate bilateral vertebral artery sacrifice or basilar artery sacrifice, devastating stroke from thrombosis of perforating arteries remains a risk. Indeed, some patients with basilar artery fusiform aneurysm have ischemic symptoms secondary to thrombosis [57], and these symptoms might be exacerbated by thrombosis precipitated by endovascular arterial sacrifice. Perforating arteries providing blood supply to the brainstem have been demonstrated on autopsy to arise from fusiform basilar trunk aneurysms [58,59]. Controlled anticoagulation with heparin may be critical to prevent catastrophic basilar thrombosis following endovascular arterial sacrifice [59].

Vertebral artery dissecting aneurysms are an infrequent cause of subarachnoid hemorrhage. Histologically, there is fragmentation of the internal elastic lamina, intramural hemorrhage, and extension of the dissection plane through the adventitia [61,62]. The angiographic findings include a combination of luminal narrowing and dilation, and perhaps a double lumen [62]. Vertebral artery dissecting aneurysms are particularly dangerous, because the rerupture rate

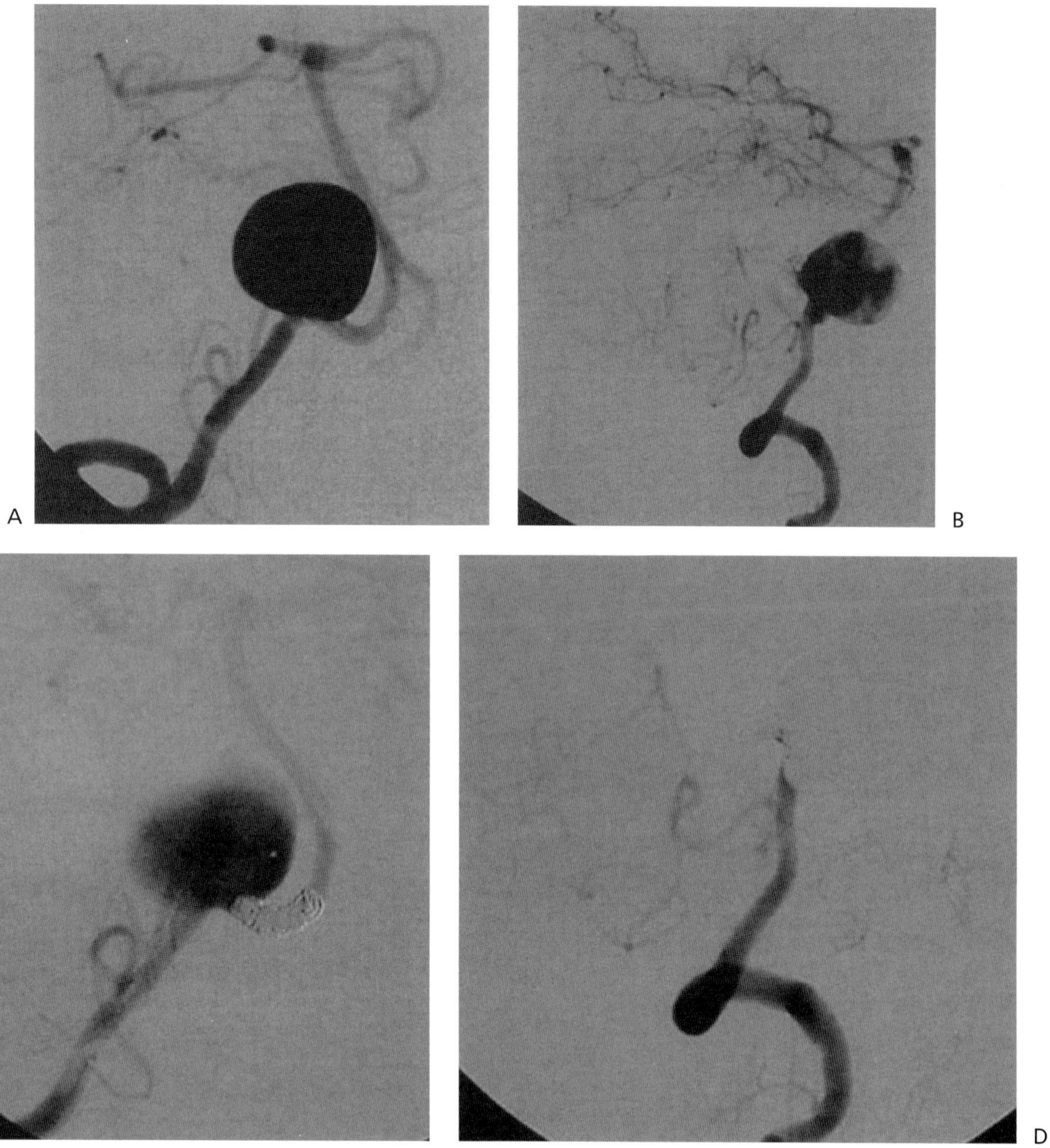

FIGURE 7-3. Giant vertebral artery aneurysm distal to posterior inferior cerebellar artery in a 48-year-old woman. **A,B:** A detachable silicone balloon could not be navigated distal to the aneurysm, so coil embolization was performed. The vertebral artery distal to the aneurysm was embolized with GDCs **(C)**, followed by coil embolization of the aneurysm **(D)**.

is very high, approximately 50% within the 24 hours following the initial hemorrhage [60,63,64]. The entire intradural dissected segment should be sacrificed to prevent rehemorrhage [63,65,66]. Occlusion of the vertebral artery proximal to the dissected segment does not always prevent rehemorrhage [63,67]. Coils rather than balloons should be used to embolize the diseased arterial segment, because the radial force exerted by a balloon could cause arterial rupture. GDCs are softer than pushable coils and therefore probably are safer for this application. The PICA can usually be spared. If PICA sacrifice is necessary to treat the entire dissected segment, a surgical revascularization procedure using the occipital artery may be needed to prevent infarction. Sometimes bilateral vertebral artery dissecting aneurysms occur, which might require sacrifice of both vertebral arteries if this can be tolerated by the patient [68,69].

Infrequently, intracranial vertebral artery dissections cause an ischemic stroke rather than subarachnoid hemorrhage. There is little risk of hemorrhage in patients who have an ischemic stroke, so endovascular sacrifice of the vertebral artery is not usually indicated [70].

Stents have been proposed for treatment of dissecting

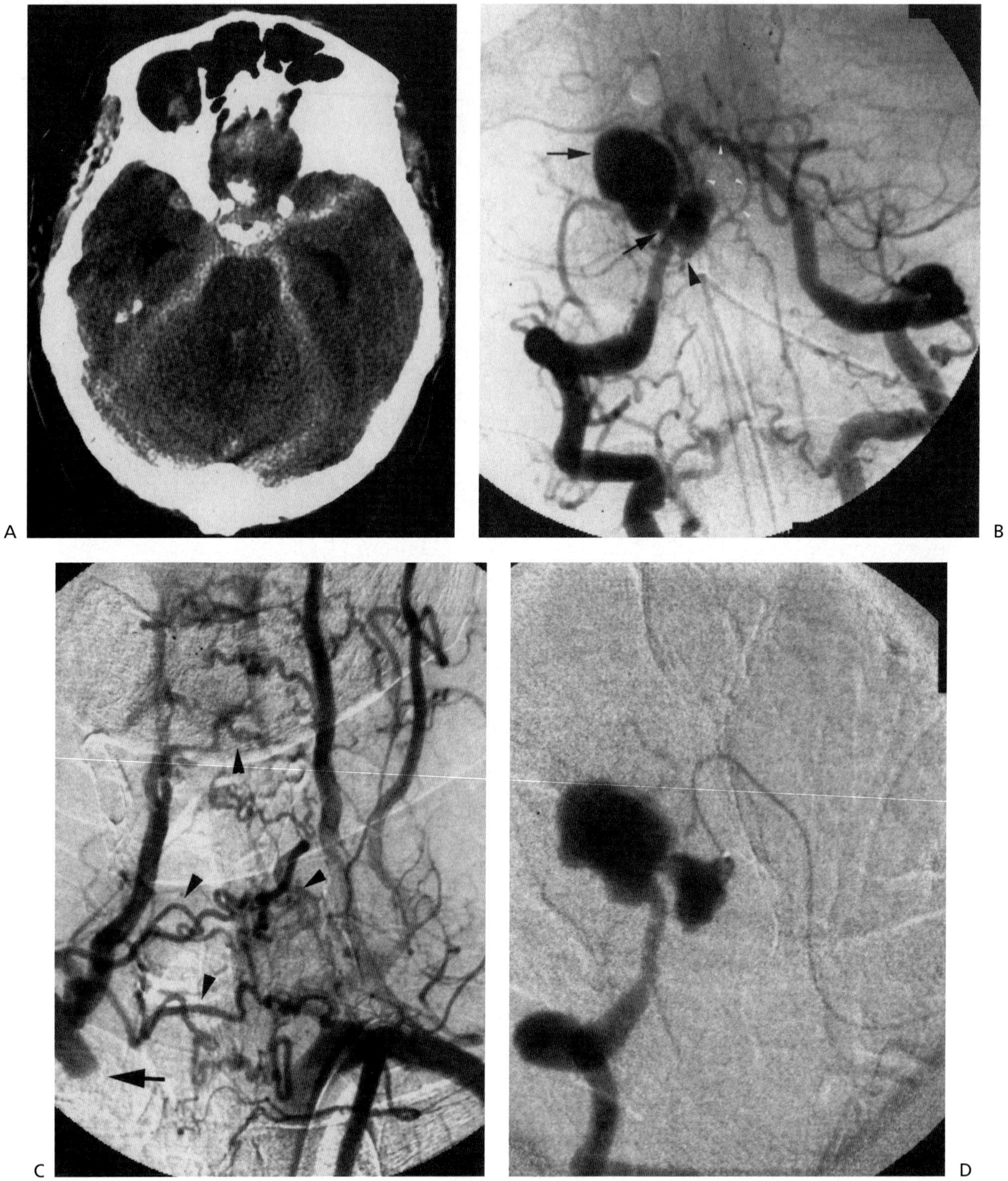

FIGURE 7-4A–D.

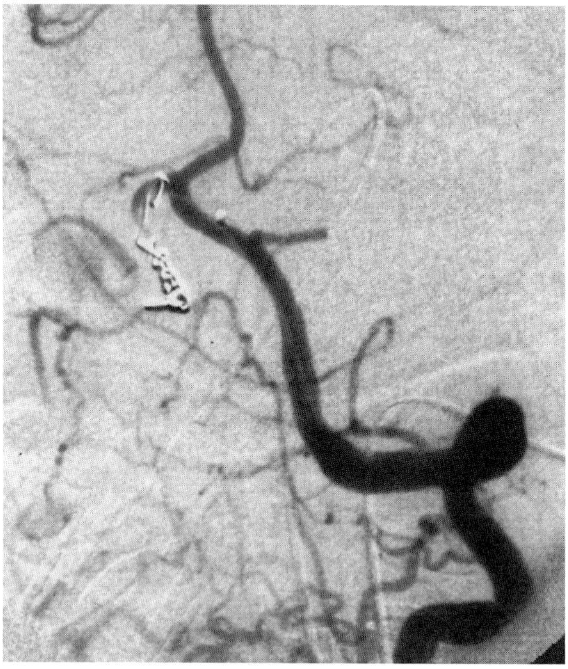

E

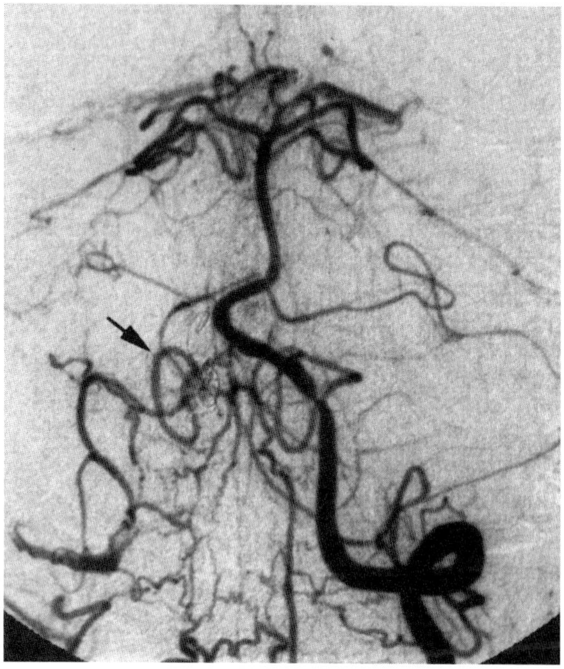

F

FIGURE 7-4. This 62-year-old woman was admitted in a coma following a subarachnoid hemorrhage (Hunt and Hess grade IV). **A:** Axial CT scan demonstrates extensive subarachnoid hemorrhage, which was most prominent in the posterior fossa. **B:** Left vertebral artery angiogram, anterior projection. Injection of the left vertebral artery demonstrated reflux across the vertebrobasilar junction into the right vertebral artery with filling into the cervical segment of the vertebral artery, suggesting a proximal occlusion or severe stenosis in the right vertebral artery circulation. A dysplastic segment of the right vertebral artery just proximal to the takeoff of the PICA *(black arrowhead)* was seen. In addition, a second area of dilation appeared more saccular in nature *(arrows)*. The right PICA was observed to fill from the proximal margin of this dilated region *(white arrowheads)*. **C:** Left subclavian artery angiogram, anterior projection, cervical view. Injection of the left subclavian artery demonstrated that there was an occlusion of the right subclavian at its point of origin *(arrow)*. In addition to the flow that traveled retrograde down the vertebral artery from the vertebrobasilar junction as noted on **(B)**, extensive cervical collaterals were revascularizing the vertebral and subclavian systems on the right side *(arrowheads)*. **D:** Anterior projection of a superselective distal right vertebral artery angiogram. The microcatheter has been placed at the distal end of the dysplastic segment in the right vertebral artery, demonstrating the anatomy of the two aneurysms more clearly. Because there was a proximal occlusion with retrograde flow into the aneurysms and an extensive collateral system was present, it was decided to occlude the inflow from the distal portion of the right vertebral artery with coils. They were placed in the normal segment of the right vertebral artery in an effort to occlude and thrombose the aneurysm. **E:** Left vertebral artery angiogram anterior projection following coil occlusion of the distal right vertebral artery demonstrates occlusion of retrograde flow into the aneurysmal complex. **F:** Anterior projection of a left vertebral artery angiogram made about 6 months after endovascular treatment demonstrates an extensive collateral network with revascularization of the right PICA *(arrow)* and nonfilling of the aneurysm. After an extensive stay in a rehabilitation facility (6 months) the patient had returned home, was living independently, and had no neurologic deficits. (From Michael P. Marks and Huy M. Do, unpublished material, with permission.)

aneurysm of the vertebral artery by Lylyk et al. [71,72]. It remains unproved that porous stents will prevent future subarachnoid hemorrhage in these patients. In addition there may be an excessively high complication rate due to intraprocedural rupture caused by application of radial force using a relatively sharp, rigid metal device in a fragile, ruptured artery. Covering stents with a membrane that is impermeable to blood and improving the flexibility of stents may allow safer treatment of dissecting aneurysms of the vertebral artery in the future. Stent technology will be most useful in patients who have inadequate collateral flow from the anterior circulation or contralateral vertebral artery and therefore cannot tolerate endovascular vertebral artery sacrifice without bypass surgery.

PICA dissections can also occur and can cause subarachnoid hemorrhage [67,73,74]. Surgical or endovascular occlusion of the dissected segment is usually well tolerated, but a surgical bypass from the occipital artery to the PICA can be performed if there is concern about inadequate collateral supply [73].

Distal Aneurysms

Small distal aneurysms can be treated by sacrifice of the involved distal arterial segment. These aneurysms are often mycotic. Unruptured mycotic aneurysms may be treated with antibiotics alone, but ruptured mycotic aneurysms are usually treated by sacrifice of the involved arterial segment [75]. The traditional surgical therapy of mycotic aneurysm consists of parent artery occlusion and aneurysm resection [75]. Endovascular parent artery occlusion is an acceptable alternative therapy for mycotic aneurysms. The parent vessel is inflamed and probably quite fragile, so all endovascular maneuvers should be performed very gently to prevent rebleeding.

Endovascular therapy of mycotic aneurysms has been reported in three cases by Khayata et al. [76], in one case by Frizzell et al. [77], and in two cases by Cloft et al. [78]. Khayata et al. used N-butyl cyanoacrylate in one case, autologous clot in another, and platinum coils in the third. Frizzell et al. and Cloft et al. used platinum coils in their cases. Chaloupka et al. [79] reported two cases of small distal superior cerebellar artery aneurysms treated with parent artery occlusion using platinum microcoils. Treatment was successful in all of these cases.

Detachable balloons used for permanent occlusion of the internal carotid and vertebral arteries to treat aneurysms are too large for use in distal small arteries. Parent vessel occlusion adjacent to a mycotic aneurysm can be accomplished using short coils, which allow for controlled, accurate occlusion at a very distal location. The advantage of retrievable versus nonretrievable coils were recently pointed out in a letter by Debrun [80], responding to the report of two cases of distal superior cerebellar artery aneurysms by Chaloupka et al. [79]. The controlled detachability of the short GDCs allows them to be carefully positioned and repositioned, and even retrieved, prior to detachment. This is a significant advantage over coils placed with a coil pusher, in which coils cannot be repositioned or retrieved once they are deployed. Injecting coils with fluid is uncontrolled, and could result in a higher incidence of aneurysmal rupture because of the rapid burst of increased pressure that would occur when the coil is injected.

TEST BALLOON OCCLUSION

When arterial sacrifice is being considered as a therapy for cerebral aneurysm, test balloon occlusion is used to determine if the patient can hemodynamically tolerate arterial sacrifice. Abrupt internal carotid artery occlusion without test balloon occlusion results in a 26% stroke rate and a 12% mortality rate [81]. Test balloon occlusion evaluates the adequacy of collateral flow, primarily through the circle of Willis. It is meant to test whether or not occlusion of a carotid or vertebral artery will result in inadequate blood flow to the brain, thereby allowing physicians to avoid the complication of ischemic stroke. Matas [82] was the first to describe a test of tolerance to carotid artery occlusion, using digital compression to achieve temporary occlusion. The development of balloons for endovascular use [4,5] made temporary testing of arteries with balloon catheters possible. Such testing is clinically useful, because patients who fail test balloon occlusion are thought to be at extremely high risk of stroke with internal carotid sacrifice or prolonged temporary occlusion [41].

A false-negative test balloon occlusion (stroke with endovascular arterial sacrifice despite passed test balloon occlusion test) can occur if the patient's hemodynamic parameters during the test balloon occlusion are different from the parameters following permanent occlusion (e.g., hypertension during test balloon occlusion, or hypotension following permanent occlusion). Unrecognized balloon inflation failure, placement of the test balloon proximal to an important collateral artery that will be lost with permanent sacrifice, and thromboembolism occurring following arterial sacrifice can also lead to a false-negative test balloon occlusion. False positive tests may occur if too much saline is infused through the balloon catheter lumen [83] or if the patient is dehydrated or otherwise abnormally hypotensive.

If a patient develops a neurologic deficit or has signs of diminished perfusion on an adjunctive test during test balloon occlusion, extracranial-intracranial bypass surgery can be performed to improve circulation prior to permanent carotid occlusion [84–90]. In two clinical series of endovascular carotid sacrifice, however, extracranial-intracranial arterial bypass did not appear to protect against postocclusion cerebral ischemia [86,88].

Vertebral artery test balloon occlusion is not frequently required and has not been investigated as much as has carotid artery test balloon occlusion. Vertebral artery test occlusion has been reported only in small series [52,53]. As with carotid test balloon occlusion, it is important to evaluate collateral circulation with angiography, with particular attention given to the other vertebral artery and the posterior communicating arteries. Patients with a contralateral large vertebral artery essentially always pass the test balloon occlusion, whereas those without a sizable vertebral artery almost always fail (although they may pass if they have large posterior communicating arteries). Attention should be paid to the presence of a vertebral artery origin of the anterior spinal artery, because occlusion of the origin of the anterior spinal artery could cause a devastating spinal cord infarction. Occasionally it is necessary to perform test balloon occlusion of both vertebral arteries simultaneously or test balloon occlusion of the basilar artery. The use of adjunctive tests for vertebral artery test occlusion has not been reported.

Complications do occasionally occur with test balloon occlusion. Although the complications of test balloon occlusion are similar to those of cerebral angiography, there is some added risk resulting from potential injury to the artery by the radial force of the balloon and the added procedural duration resulting from the test occlusion period. Mathis et al. reported the results of 500 test balloon occlusion procedures [40]. They reported a 1.6% neurologic complication rate (1.2% transient and 0.4% permanent). Transient cranial nerve deficits have been reported to occur during balloon inflation in the cavernous carotid artery, but they resolve shortly following balloon deflation [91].

Adjunctive Testing

A number of adjunctive tests have been used to try to predict the adequacy of collateral flow after permanent arterial occlusion and thereby reduce the number of false-negative results from balloon occlusions that occur when using the clinical neurologic examination alone. Unfortunately, no adjunctive test has been validated in controlled clinical trials. It has not been proven that any adjunctive test is better than any other, nor has it been proven that any adjunctive test makes carotid sacrifice safer than clinical testing alone. The complication rate of endovascular carotid and vertebral artery sacrifice is relatively low, regardless of which adjunctive test is used, and most complications are probably thromboembolic stroke not predicted by any adjunctive test. Therefore, a large number of patients would be required in a study that attempted to show that a particular adjunctive test is a better predictor of the ischemic stroke risk than test balloon occlusion using the clinical neurologic examination alone.

The theoretical premise of adding an adjunctive test to test balloon occlusion is that there is likely a subgroup of patients who pass the clinical test without neurologic deficit yet have sufficiently altered blood flow to put them at a significant risk of delayed ischemic stroke. Abrupt internal carotid artery occlusion without test balloon occlusion results in a 26% stroke rate and a 12% mortality rate [81]. Clinical testing alone with test balloon occlusion identifies the majority of patients at risk for ischemic stroke following carotid sacrifice. McIvor et al. [41] summarized the data from five reports [7,16,92–94] of internal carotid sacrifice after clinical passage of a test balloon occlusion, finding 9 (4.7%) permanent strokes in 192 patients. Because the overall risk of carotid sacrifice following passage of test balloon occlusion using clinical neurologic examination alone is fairly low, and this risk is probably largely due to embolic strokes which cannot be predicted by test balloon occlusion, it is difficult to definitively show an added benefit of any adjunctive test. Another impediment to demonstrating the predictive value of an adjunctive test is that most investigators consider it unethical to perform permanent carotid occlusion on patients who demonstrate an abnormality on an adjunctive test. Patients who fall below thresholds for passing an adjunctive test are almost never treated with endovascular sacrifice, which makes it impossible ever to measure the predictive value of the adjunctive test.

Positron emission tomography (PET) [95,96], single-photon emission computed tomography (SPECT) [97–105], and stable xenon-enhanced computed tomography (xenon CT) [81,106–110] have all been used as adjunctive tests to evaluate regional perfusion during test balloon occlusion. All three techniques offer similar perfusion information, and the decision to use one of these techniques depends largely on convenience and equipment availability. Perfusion imaging sometimes demonstrates a decrease in perfusion in the absence of clinical symptoms during balloon test occlusion. This decreased perfusion suggests that permanent carotid sacrifice is more likely to result in a delayed neurologic deficit. At some institutions, local decreased perfusion is an indication for extracranial-intracranial bypass surgery prior to carotid sacrifice [85]. If normal perfusion is demonstrated on an adjunctive test during carotid test balloon occlusion, a delayed ischemic deficit may still occur [81,101], perhaps most often as a result of embolic stroke.

Additionally, patients who pass adjunctive test criteria currently used do not seem to have any significantly lower risk of carotid occlusion than patients who have been tested by clinical neurologic examination alone. Stable xenon CT as an adjunctive test was studied by Linskey et al. [81], who reported a permanent stroke risk of 10% in 31 patients who underwent endovascular carotid sacrifice after passing a test balloon occlusion using stable xenon CT as an adjunctive test. This stroke rate is not an improvement over the risk of stoke with clinical neurologic testing alone.

The value of PET imaging during test balloon occlusion for predicting the risk of stroke with permanent carotid sacrifice has been studied in one small series [95]. Neurologic sequelae developed in none of the eight patients undergoing permanent internal carotid artery occlusion, when during the test balloon occlusion they had no clinical symptoms and a cerebral blood flow decrease of less than 10 ml/100 g per minute on PET imaging. Cerebral infarction developed following carotid sacrifice in one of five patients (20%) who, during the test balloon occlusion, had no clinical symptomatology and cerebral blood flow fell to 25 to 35 ml/100 g per minute on the occluded side. This study is too small to make statistically valid conclusions.

Stable xenon CT and PET give a quantitative assessment of cerebral blood flow that can be used to determine if a patient is an appropriate candidate for endovascular carotid sacrifice. Normal cerebral blood flow is 50 ml/100 g per minute [81]. Cerebral blood flow below 40 ml/100 g per minute results in cessation of protein synthesis [111]. Spontaneous electrical activity, as measured by electroencephalography (EEG), has been shown to stop when cerebral blood flow reaches 20 ml/100 g per minute [112]. The threshold for abnormal perfusion during test balloon occlusion was chosen to be 30 ml/100 g per minute for stable xenon CT [81] and 25 to 35 ml/100 g per minute for PET [95].

The value of SPECT imaging during test balloon occlusion for predicting the risk of stroke with permanent carotid sacrifice is not known. SPECT can give qualitative information about regional cerebral blood flow but does not offer the quantitative blood flow information obtained with stable xenon CT and PET. Patients with asymmetric perfusion on SPECT imaging during balloon test occlusion are simply assumed to be at high risk for stroke with carotid sacrifice at centers that use this adjunctive test, yet this assumption has never been, and may never be, scientifically validated. SPECT enables a "memory of blood flow" during temporary ischemia to determine the character of quick diffusion and slow washout, which cannot be performed by other methods of cerebral blood flow measurement.

A new, simple adjunctive test is to angiographically evaluate asymmetry of cerebral perfusion during test balloon occlusion [21]. While the balloon is inflated to occlude the carotid artery, the contralateral carotid artery is injected with contrast material while digital subtraction imaging is performed in the anteroposterior projection. Patients with asymmetric filling of the cortical veins are assumed to be at high risk of cerebral infarction if carotid sacrifice is performed.

Indirect Adjunctive Testing

Indirect measurements of cerebral perfusion such as carotid stump pressure measurements [21,109,113,114], transcranial Doppler evaluation of middle cerebral artery velocity [115–118], and cerebral oximetry [119] have been proposed as adjunctive tests during carotid test occlusion, but these techniques remain speculative and have not been widely accepted.

EEG has been used at some centers as an adjunctive measurement of cerebral function during carotid test balloon occlusion [94,120–124]. Whether or not EEG changes during test balloon occlusion are predictive of ischemic stroke following permanent occlusion remains unclear.

Hypotensive challenge has been suggested as a means of increasing the predictive value of test balloon occlusion [98, 103,125,126]. If test occlusion under normotension has been tolerated, the patient's blood pressure is lowered to two-thirds mean systemic blood pressure [125] or to 50 to 70 mm Hg [84] with intravenous nitroprusside. Alternatively, Polin et al. [127] contend that patients should be hemodynamically optimized and monitored with an arterial line and Swan-Ganz catheter before and after permanent balloon occlusion. Although opinions may differ regarding what are the best hemodynamic conditions under which to perform test balloon occlusion, it is clearly important that physicians consider the hemodynamic conditions that a patient would be likely to experience in the foreseeable future when interpreting test balloon occlusion results. It is important for patients to be well hydrated and at their baseline blood pressure when performing test occlusion to avoid a false-positive test, and it is probably equally important that they not be at a blood pressure significantly above their baseline so as to avoid a false-negative test. It is essential for all physicians involved in the planning of the patient's care to understand that the results of the test balloon occlusion can be considered valid only for the hemodynamic conditions under which the test was performed. Assumptions cannot be made about the patient's ability to tolerate arterial occlusion under hemodynamic conditions different from those during the test balloon occlusion.

TECHNIQUE FOR PARENT VESSEL OCCLUSION

Test Balloon Occlusion

When getting consent for the procedure from the patient, the patient should be informed of the entire plan for therapy. It is important for both the patient and the physician performing the test to understand what the treatment plan is following either a "failed" or a "passed" test balloon occlusion.

A complete cerebral angiogram to evaluate the circle of Willis is performed prior to test balloon occlusion. It may be clear from an angiogram alone that a patient will not tolerate endovascular arterial sacrifice; for example, carotid sacrifice will not be tolerated in a patient with aplasia of the ipsilateral anterior cerebral artery A1 segment and the ipsilateral posterior communicating artery. Compression of the carotid artery on the side of potential arterial sacrifice while injecting the contralateral carotid artery can aid assessment of blood flow across the anterior communicating artery. Similarly, compression of the carotid artery on the side of potential arterial sacrifice while injecting the dominant vertebral artery will aid in the assessment of blood flow across the posterior communicating artery to the anterior circulation. It is often important to examine angiographically the cervical portion of the carotid and vertebral arteries to evaluate for occlusive disease which might affect the patient's ability to tolerate carotid sacrifice. The presence of aneurysms other than the one being treated by the arterial sacrifice needs to be addressed at the outset of treatment, because the endovascular arterial sacrifice could affect the treatment options and natural history of these other aneurysms. External carotid angiography should be performed if an extracranial-intracranial bypass graft is being considered.

All patients must have a complete neurologic examination by the interventional neuroradiologist performing the procedure. This is to establish the patient's baseline neurologic status immediately prior to test balloon occlusion. Repeated, detailed clinical neurologic examinations are then performed by the same person who performed the baseline examination at 5-minute intervals during balloon occlusion. The balloon occlusion test is carried out for 15 to 30 minutes [7,41,84,85,125] or until a new neurologic deficit develops. A new neurologic deficit during test balloon occlusion referable to the vascular territory being tested constitutes a test failure, indicating that permanent arterial sacrifice will likely result in a permanent neurologic deficit. Sedation should be avoided, if possible, because it can alter nonspecifically the neurologic status of the patient. In patients who are substantially neurologically compromised at the time of test occlusion, such as those who have suffered a severe subarachnoid hemorrhage, it will not be possible to perform a meaningful test with clinical examination alone.

Consideration must also be given to the patient's potential to develop vasospasm when subarachnoid hemorrhage has occurred. A patient with subarachnoid hemorrhage may tolerate endovascular arterial sacrifice initially but subsequently decompensate due to vasospasm. It may be wise in such cases to defer endovascular arterial sacrifice until after the period of potential vasospasm.

A 6-French (Fr.) femoral artery sheath is needed if only a test balloon occlusion is to be performed. If a permanent balloon occlusion using detachable balloons is likely to be performed immediately following a passed test balloon occlusion, a 7- or 8-Fr. femoral sheath will be required. Full anticoagulation with intravenous heparin (activated clotting time greater than 300 seconds) prior to balloon inflation is necessary to prevent thromboembolic complications.

The characteristics of the balloon chosen for test balloon occlusion are important.

A compliant balloon is necessary to minimize risk of arterial wall injury with inflation. Noncompliant angioplasty balloons are not appropriate for test balloon occlusion, because they are more likely to injure the artery. The non-detachable silicone balloon (Target, Boston Scientific; Natick, MA) and latex occlusion balloon (Medi-tech, Boston Scientific; Natick, MA) are currently the most common balloons used for test balloon occlusion.

The latex occlusion balloon may be used safely in patients without bifurcation stenosis and with straight segments of the internal carotid artery. It is generally placed in the artery to be tested using a catheter exchange technique. Heparinized saline is infused through the central lumen. If saline is infused too fast, a false-positive test occlusion can occur due to dilution of blood perfusing the brain.

The non-detachable silicone balloons for test occlusions require more operator experience but carry the advantage of being highly atraumatic because they are extremely compliant. Because they are mounted on a microcatheter, they can be maneuvered through a stenosis of the carotid bifurcation and can be placed distally within the internal carotid artery system, including intracranial segments. The disadvantages of the silicone balloon are that it is more expensive and requires a guide catheter. Less experienced operators will find the silicone balloon more difficult to use.

Test occlusion is performed with the inflated balloon as close to the level of expected permanent occlusion as is technically feasible. While observing with fluoroscopy, the balloon is carefully inflated to achieve the minimal inflation necessary to provide complete vessel occlusion. A digital "roadmap" can be used to gauge the appropriate size of the artery. Complete occlusion can be confirmed by injection of radiographic contrast material through the central lumen of the balloon catheter or through the guiding catheter. Our test occlusions are generally conducted with neurologic testing performed every 5 minutes for 30 minutes, or until a new neurologic deficit appears. A new neurologic deficit should resolve almost instantaneously following deflation of the balloon. Whatever adjunctive tests are to be used need to be integrated into the test balloon occlusion and should be part of the plan from the beginning.

Permanent Balloon Occlusion

The patient must tolerate test balloon occlusion prior to undergoing permanent endovascular arterial sacrifice. It is usually most convenient to perform endovascular arterial sacrifice immediately following balloon occlusion, provided that the patient tolerates the test balloon occlusion.

The procedure is performed from a transfemoral arterial approach. Detachable silicone balloons with maximal volumes up to 0.9 ml require a 7-Fr. guide catheter. For detachable balloons with maximal volumes greater than 0.9 ml, an 8-Fr. guiding catheter is required.

Silicone balloons (Fig. 7-5) must be filled with isoosmolar solution, because the silicone is a permeable membrane and the volume of the balloon can change as a result of osmotic shifts of fluid. Visipaque 270 (Nycomed Amersham; Princeton, NJ) is a suitable contrast agent to use to inflate the balloon, because it is isoosmolar. All balloons are test inflated to check for leaks in the valve. The balloon is then mounted onto the microcatheter.

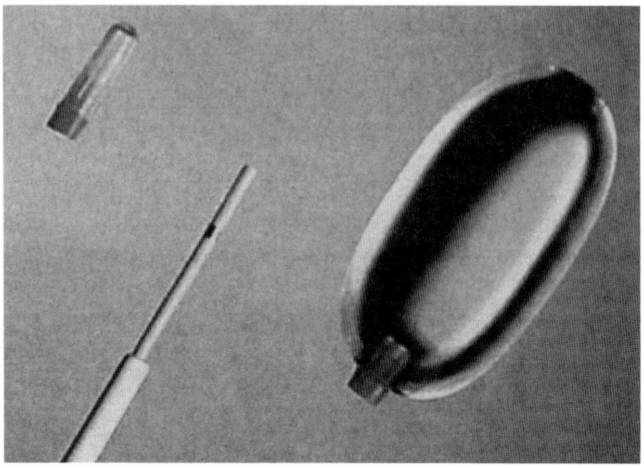

FIGURE 7-5. Detachable silicone balloon before *(left)* and after *(right)* inflation. The microcatheter to deliver the balloon is shown at center.

A 0.010-inch diameter guidewire can be placed inside the lumen of the microcatheter to improve "pushability," but this partially obstructs the microcatheter lumen and thereby increases the time needed for balloon inflation and deflation. The operator must be careful to not push the detachable balloon off of the microcatheter with the microguidewire.

Before detaching a balloon, a second balloon should be already prepared for deployment. This is important if the first balloon malfunctions and deflates; it will be necessary to rapidly insert and deploy the second balloon to reduce flow behind the first balloon that embolized. A second, nondetachable balloon can be used as a safety balloon, solely for the purpose of stabilizing the placement of the first balloon and eliminating blood flow at the time of detachment [128]. When the balloon is positioned at the desired point of detachment, continuous gradual tension is applied to the microcatheter until detachment occurs (Fig. 7-6).

Because balloon failures are not rare, it is wise to perform endovascular arterial sacrifice with at least two detachable balloons to assure permanent occlusion and reduce the risk of distal balloon embolism. The first balloon should be positioned as distally as possible, to minimize the carotid stump in which thrombus will form distal to the balloon. Aneurysm trapping may reduce the risk of postocclusion embolic events after endovascular carotid sacrifice [86]. Trapping of the aneurysm also likely provides better protection from hemorrhage. Proximal occlusion alone can sometimes lead to recurrent hemorrhage [56,129]. It is not always feasible, however, to trap the aneurysm without compromising important branches distal to the aneurysm. It can also be technically difficult to advance a balloon distal to a large aneurysm, and efforts to do so can dislodge intraluminal thrombus. A balloon should not be placed at the carotid bulb, because a baroreceptor response resulting in systemic hypotension can occur because of the pressure exerted by the balloon.

The silicone balloons are more slippery than latex balloons, so they are more prone to slip backward during detachment. Therefore, they may need more inflation to generate enough radial force to maintain their position. Small balloons tend to slip along the walls of the artery more because there is less friction.

Microcoils have been found to be a safe and effective alternative to detachable balloons for carotid occlusion [130–132]. Temporary flow arrest during coil occlusion has been recommended to prevent distal embolization of thrombus forming on the coils before flow is completely arrested [132,133]. Temporary flow arrest may not be necessary, however, if aggressive anticoagulation with heparin is used [130]. Another alternative is the use of a covered stent sewed close at the distal end to create a windsock-like device that causes instant flow arrest [134].

At some hospitals, the patient is transferred to the intensive care unit for placement of a Swan-Ganz catheter and arterial line if endovascular arterial sacrifice is anticipated [127]. These devices assist in optimizing the patient's hemodynamic status before, during, and after the procedure. The patient is well hydrated and the central venous pressure and wedge pressure are kept high. This is particularly important during the first days after permanent occlusion, because focal ischemic symptoms often resolve with aggressive hemodynamic therapy (i.e., optimal hydration and blood pressure).

After endovascular arterial sacrifice, the patient should be sent to the intensive care unit overnight with heparinization (partial thromboplastin time at 2. to 2.5-times normal). Bed rest should be maintained in the intensive care unit for 24 hours. The patient should also take oral aspirin (325 mg/day). Patients should avoid strenuous activity for 2 weeks after endovascular arterial sacrifice.

Prophylactic anticoagulation with heparin during and after endovascular arterial sacrifice may reduce the frequency of postocclusion embolic events after endovascular carotid sacrifice [86]. Antiplatelet agents may provide additional protection from embolic complications, but this remains to be proved [86]. Careful attention to postoperative anticoagulation, hydration, and blood pressure management is essential to minimizing delayed ischemia following carotid or vertebral artery endovascular sacrifice.

Intraoperative Temporary Balloon Occlusion and Suction Decompression

Intraoperative temporary balloon occlusion and suction decompression is sometimes useful in assisting surgical clipping of large internal carotid artery aneurysms, which are difficult to control proximally [135–138]. The patient must be placed on a radiolucent operating table and the head must be positioned in a radiolucent frame. A double-lumen balloon catheter is placed in the carotid artery by a transfemoral route. After surgical placement of a temporary clip distal to the aneurysm, the balloon is inflated proximal to the aneurysm, and blood is aspirated through the balloon catheter in an effort to collapse the aneurysm. The decompression of the aneurysm allows the surgeon to manipulate a "slack" rather than "tight" aneurysmal sac. This maneuver provides for easier dissection of the aneurysm and accurate clip placement. The balloon also gives proximal control to prevent or control bleeding in case of intraoperative aneurysmal rupture. After clip placement, the balloon is deflated and angiography is performed to assure precise clip placement.

The surgery must take place with the patient on a radiolucent table and the head positioned in a radiolucent head holder. A 6-Fr. sheath is placed in the common femoral artery prior to the craniotomy. The 6-Fr. sheath lumen will allow reinfusion of blood around the 5-Fr. occlusion balloon catheter. A 5-Fr. occlusion balloon catheter with a central lumen is used to allow blood aspiration. The occlusion balloon catheter is placed in the internal carotid artery ipsi-

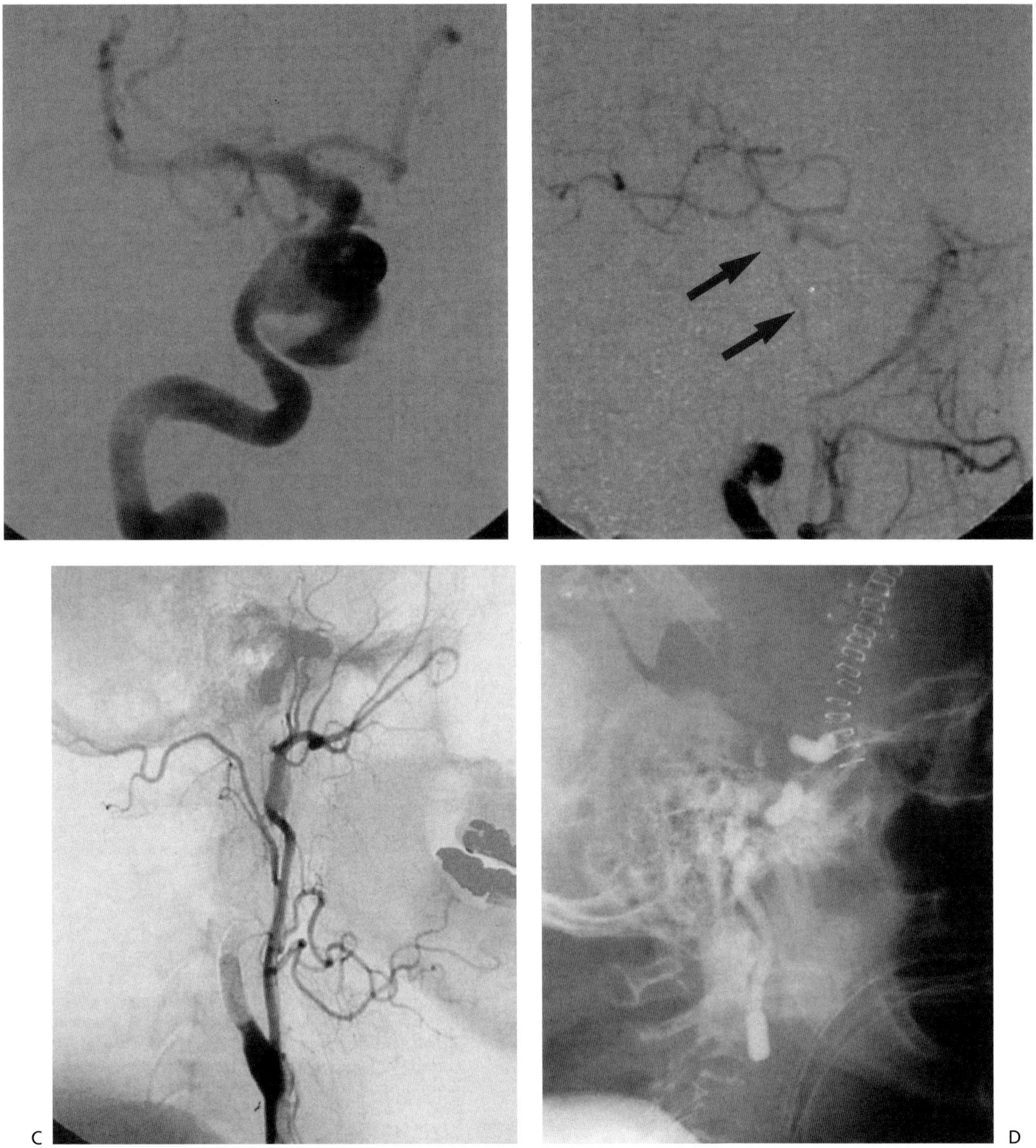

FIGURE 7-6. **A:** Giant cavernous carotid aneurysm in a 43-year-old woman who did not tolerate test balloon occlusion. A bypass was performed from the superficial temporal artery *(arrows)* to the middle cerebral artery **(B),** followed immediately by endovascular sacrifice of the internal carotid artery with three detachable silicone balloons **(C,D).**

lateral to the aneurysm after the patient's head is restrained in the head holder to avoid movement of head and neck while the catheter is in place. The internal carotid artery is catheterized with a diagnostic angiography catheter and then the balloon catheter is inserted into the internal carotid artery using an exchange technique. It is generally safest to place the balloon in a straight segment of the cervical internal carotid artery. While observing with fluoroscopy, the balloon is inflated with radiographic contrast material to determine the inflation volume necessary for internal carotid artery occlusion. The balloon is then left deflated until it is needed. The balloon catheter central lumen is continuously infused with heparinized saline. When the operating neurosurgeon wants the balloon inflated for suction decompression to facilitate clip placement, the balloon will be inflated with the predetermined volume of radiographic contrast material (fluoroscopy is usually not available at this time because the operating neurosurgeon will be in the midst of clipping the aneurysm). When the balloon is inflated to facilitate clipping, blood is aspirated through the catheter lumen with syringes and put back into the patient through the sheath side port. The balloon is then deflated when the operating neurosurgeon has clipped the aneurysm. An angiogram can be performed by injecting radiographic contrast material through the central lumen of the balloon catheter to assess the adequacy of aneurysm treatment. If the aneurysm ruptures intraoperatively, quick inflation of the balloon will help to control the bleeding.

REFERENCES

1. Hunter J. *The works of James F. Palmer,* vol 3. London: Longmans, Rees, Orme, Brown, Green, and Longmans, 1837: 594–612.
2. Keen WW. Intracranial lesions. *Med News (N Y)* 1890;57:443.
3. Dandy WE. Intracranial aneurysm of the internal carotid artery: cured by operation. *Ann Surg* 1938;107:654–659.
4. Serbinenko FA. Balloon catheterization and occlusion of major cerebral vessels. *J Neurosurg* 1974;41:125–145.
5. Serbinenko FA. Balloon occlusion of saccular aneurysms of the cerebral arteries. *Vopr Neirokhir* 1974;7:8–15.
6. Debrun G, Fox A, Drake C, et al. Giant unclippable aneurysms: treatment with detachable balloons. *AJNR Am J Neuroradiol* 1981;2:167–173.
7. Fox AJ, Viñuela F, Pelz DM, et al. Use of detachable balloons for proximal artery occlusion in the treatment of unclippable cerebral aneurysms. *J Neurosurg* 1987;66:40–46.
8. Berenstein A, Ransohoff J, Kupersmith M, et al. Transvascular treatment of giant aneurysms of the cavernous carotid and vertebral arteries. Functional investigation and embolization. *Surg Neurol* 1984;21:3–12.
9. Hieshima GB, Grinnell VS, Mehringer CM. A detachable balloon for therapeutic transcatheter occlusions. *Radiology* 1981; 138:227–228.
10. Higashida RT, Hieshima GB, Halbach VV, et al. Intravascular detachable balloon embolization of intracranial aneurysms. Indications and techniques. *Acta Radiol Suppl* 1986;369:594–596.
11. Unruptured intracranial aneurysms—risk of rupture and risks of surgical intervention. International Study of Unruptured Intracranial Aneurysms Investigators. *N Engl J Med* 1998;339: 1725–1733.
12. Steinberg GK, Drake CG, Peerless SJ. Deliberate basilar or vertebral artery occlusion in the treatment of intracranial aneurysms. Immediate results and long-term outcome in 201 patients. *J Neurosurg* 1993;79:161–173.
13. Horowitz M, Fichtel F, Samson D, et al. Intracavernous carotid artery aneurysms: the possible importance of angiographic dural waisting. A case report. *Surg Neurol* 1996;46:549–552.
14. Lee AG, Mawad ME, Baskin DS. Fatal subarachnoid hemorrhage from the rupture of a totally intracavernous carotid artery aneurysm: case report. *Neurosurgery* 1996;38:596–599.
15. Kupersmith MJ, Hurst R, Berenstein A, et al. The benign course of cavernous carotid artery aneurysms. *J Neurosurg* 1992;77: 690–693.
16. Vazquez Anon V, Aymard A, Gobin YP, et al. Balloon occlusion of the internal carotid artery in 40 cases of giant intracavernous aneurysm: technical aspects, cerebral monitoring, and results. *Neuroradiology* 1992;34:245–251.
17. Sudhoff H, Stark T, Knorz S, et al. Massive epistaxis after rupture of intracavernous carotid artery aneurysm. Case report. *Ann Otol Rhinol Laryngol* 2000;109:776–778.
18. Halbach VV, Higashida RT, Dowd CF, et al. Cavernous internal carotid artery aneurysms treated with electrolytically detachable coils. *J Neuroophthalmol* 1997;17:231–239.
19. Vargas ME, Kupersmith MJ, Setton A, et al. Endovascular treatment of giant aneurysms which cause visual loss. *Ophthalmology* 1994;101:1091–1098.
20. Larson JJ, Tew JM Jr, Tomsick TA, et al. Treatment of aneurysms of the internal carotid artery by intravascular balloon occlusion: long-term follow-up of 58 patients. *Neurosurgery* 1995;36:26–30.
21. van Rooij WJ, Sluzewski M, Metz NH, et al. Carotid balloon occlusion for large and giant aneurysms: evaluation of a new test occlusion protocol. *Neurosurgery* 2000;47:116–122.
22. Mericle RA, Lanzino G, Wakhloo AK, et al. Stenting and secondary coiling of intracranial internal carotid artery aneurysm: technical case report. *Neurosurgery* 1998;43:1229–1234.
23. Phatouros CC, Sasaki TY, Higashida RT, et al. Stent-supported coil embolization: the treatment of fusiform and wide-neck aneurysms and pseudoaneurysms. *Neurosurgery* 2000;47: 107–113.
24. Citardi MJ, Chaloupka JC, Son YH, et al. Management of carotid artery rupture by monitored endovascular therapeutic occlusion (1988–1994). *Laryngoscope* 1995;105:1086–1092.
25. Chaloupka JC, Putman CM, Citardi MJ, et al. Endovascular therapy for the carotid blowout syndrome in head and neck surgical patients: diagnostic and managerial considerations. *AJNR Am J Neuroradiol* 1996;17:843–852.
26. Chaloupka JC, Roth TC, Putman CM, et al. Recurrent carotid blowout syndrome: diagnostic and therapeutic challenges in a newly recognized subgroup of patients. *AJNR Am J Neuroradiol* 1999;20:1069–1077.
27. Macdonald S, Gan J, McKay AJ, et al. Endovascular treatment of acute carotid blow-out syndrome. *J Vasc Interv Radiol* 2000; 11:1184–1188.
28. Higashida RT, Halbach VV, Tsai FY, et al. Interventional neurovascular treatment of traumatic carotid and vertebral artery lesions: results in 234 cases. *AJR Am J Roentgenol* 1989;153: 577–582.
29. Han MH, Sung MW, Chang KH, et al. Traumatic pseudoaneurysm of the intracavernous ICA presenting with massive epistaxis: imaging diagnosis and endovascular treatment. *Laryngoscope* 1994;104:370–377.
30. Ramadan F, Rutledge R, Oller D, et al. Carotid artery trauma:

a review of contemporary trauma center experiences. *J Vasc Surg* 1995;21:46–55.

31. Hudgins PA, Browning DG, Gallups J, et al. Endoscopic paranasal sinus surgery: radiographic evaluation of severe complications. *AJNR Am J Neuroradiol* 1992;13:1161–1167.
32. Raymond J, Hardy J, Czepko R, et al. Arterial injuries in transsphenoidal surgery for pituitary adenoma; the role of angiography and endovascular treatment. *AJNR Am J Neuroradiol* 1997; 18:655–665.
33. Britt RH, Silverberg GD, Prolo DJ, et al. Balloon catheter occlusion for cavernous carotid artery injury during transsphenoidal hypophysectomy. Case report. *J Neurosurg* 1981;55:450–452.
34. Tranmer BI, Humphreys RP, Chuang SH. Microsurgical recovery of a migrated balloon from the internal carotid artery of a child. *Neurosurgery* 1985;16:381–386.
35. Guillon B, Brunereau L, Biousse V, et al. Long-term follow-up of aneurysms developed during extracranial internal carotid artery dissection. *Neurology* 1999;53:117–122.
36. Bush RL, Lin PH, Dodson TF, et al. Endoluminal stent placement and coil embolization for the management of carotid artery pseudoaneurysms. *J Endovasc Ther* 2001;8:53–61.
37. Liu AY, Paulsen RD, Marcellus ML, et al. Long-term outcomes after carotid stent placement treatment of carotid artery dissection. *Neurosurgery* 1999;45:1368–1373.
38. Marks MP, Dake MD, Steinberg GK, et al. Stent placement for arterial and venous cerebrovascular disease: preliminary experience. *Radiology* 1994;191:441–446.
39. Lewis AI, Tomsick TA, Tew JM Jr. Management of 100 consecutive direct carotid-cavernous fistulas: results of treatment with detachable balloons. *Neurosurgery* 1995;36:239–245.
40. Mathis JM, Barr JD, Jungreis CA, et al. Temporary balloon test occlusion of the internal carotid artery: experience in 500 cases. *AJNR Am J Neuroradiol* 1995;16:749–754.
41. McIvor NP, Willinsky RA, TerBrugge KG, et al. Validity of test occlusion studies prior to internal carotid artery sacrifice. *Head Neck* 1994;16:11–16.
42. Swann KW, Heros RC, Debrun G, et al. Inadvertent middle cerebral artery embolism by a detachable balloon: management by embolectomy. Case report. *J Neurosurg* 1986;64:309–312.
43. Kallmes DF, Cloft HJ, Chadduck JB, et al. Percutaneous deflation of a vertebral artery occlusion balloon that migrated to the axillary artery. *J Vasc Interv Radiol* 1997;8:809–812.
44. Linskey ME, Sekhar LN, Hecht ST. Emergency embolectomy for embolic occlusion of the middle cerebral artery after internal carotid artery balloon test occlusion. Case report. *J Neurosurg* 1992;77:134–138.
45. Eskridge JM, Harris AB, Finch L, et al. Carotid sinus syndrome and embolization procedures. *AJNR Am J Neuroradiol* 1993; 14:818–820.
46. Fujiwara S, Fujii K, Fukui M. De novo aneurysm formation and aneurysm growth following therapeutic carotid occlusion for intracranial internal carotid artery (ICA) aneurysms. *Acta Neurochir (Wien)* 1993;120:20–25.
47. Timperman PE, Tomsick TA, Tew JM Jr, et al. Aneurysm formation after carotid occlusion. *AJNR Am J Neuroradiol* 1995; 16:329–331.
48. Dyste GN, Beck DW. De novo aneurysm formation following carotid ligation: case report and review of the literature. *Neurosurgery* 1989;24:88–92.
49. Clark WC, Ray MW. Contralateral intracranial aneurysm formation as a late complication of carotid ligation. *Surg Neurol* 1982;18:458–462.
50. Tomsick TA, Van Loevern H, Tew JM, et al. Delayed complications of balloon occlusion of the internal carotid artery for unclippable aneurysm. *J Neurovasc Dis* 1997 March/April:64–67.
51. Miller CA, Hill SA, Hunt WE. "De novo" aneurysms. A clinical review. *Surg Neurol* 1985;24:173–180.
52. Sluzewski M, Brilstra EH, van Rooij WJ, et al. Bilateral vertebral artery balloon occlusion for giant vertebrobasilar aneurysms. *Neuroradiology* 2001;43:336–341.
53. Aymard A, Gobin YP, Hodes JE, et al. Endovascular occlusion of vertebral arteries in the treatment of unclippable vertebrobasilar aneurysms. *J Neurosurg* 1991;74:393–398.
54. Pelz DM, Viñuela F, Fox AJ, et al. Vertebrobasilar occlusion therapy of giant aneurysms. Significance of angiographic morphology of the posterior communicating arteries. *J Neurosurg* 1984;60:560–565.
55. Higashida RT, Halbach VV, Cahan LD, et al. Detachable balloon embolization therapy of posterior circulation intracranial aneurysms. *J Neurosurg* 1989;71:512–519.
56. Chang SD, Marks MP, Steinberg GK. Recanalization and rupture of a giant vertebral artery aneurysm after hunterian ligation: case report. *Neurosurgery* 1999;44:1117–1121.
57. Flemming KD, Josephs K, Wijdicks EF. Enlarging vertebrobasilar dolichoectasia with subarachnoid hemorrhage heralded by recurrent ischemia. Case illustration. *J Neurosurg* 2000;92:504.
58. Forsting M, Resch KM, von Kummer R, et al. Balloon occlusion of a giant lower basilar aneurysm: death due to thrombosis of the aneurysm. *AJNR Am J Neuroradiol* 1991;12:1063–1066.
59. Ling F, Zhank H, Wand D, et al. The role of controlled anticoagulation in balloon occluding vertebral arteries to treat giant fusiform aneurysms of the basilar artery. *Interventional Neuroradiology* 1999;5:145–150.
60. Nakatomi H, Nagata K, Kawamoto S, et al. Ruptured dissecting aneurysm as a cause of subarachnoid hemorrhage of unverified etiology. *Stroke* 1997;28:1278–1282.
61. Friedman AH, Drake CG. Subarachnoid hemorrhage from intracranial dissecting aneurysm. *J Neurosurg* 1984;60:325–334.
62. Pozzati E, Andreoli A, Limoni P, et al. Dissecting aneurysms of the vertebrobasilar system: study of 16 cases. *Surg Neurol* 1994;41:119–124.
63. Kurata A, Ohmomo T, Miyasaka Y, et al. Coil embolization for the treatment of ruptured dissecting vertebral aneurysms. *AJNR Am J Neuroradiol* 2001;22:11–18.
64. Tsukahara T, Wada H, Satake K, et al. Proximal balloon occlusion for dissecting vertebral aneurysms accompanied by subarachnoid hemorrhage. *Neurosurgery* 1995;36:914–920.
65. Halbach VV, Higashida RT, Dowd CF, et al. Endovascular treatment of vertebral artery dissections and pseudoaneurysms. *J Neurosurg* 1993;79:183–191.
66. Yamaura I, Tani E, Yokota M, et al. Endovascular treatment of ruptured dissecting aneurysms aimed at occlusion of the dissected site by using Guglielmi detachable coils. *J Neurosurg* 1999;90:853–856.
67. Nakatomi H, Nagata K, Kawamoto S. Persistent patent pseudolumen of ruptured dissecting aneurysm involving the posterior inferior cerebellar artery after proximal clipping. *Acta Neurochir (Wien)* 1999;141:533–536.
68. Kubo Y, Miura K, Suzuki M, et al. Development of a dissecting aneurysm on the vertebral artery immediately after occlusion of the contralateral vertebral artery: a case report. *Neurosurg Rev* 1998;21:177–180.
69. Redekop G, TerBrugge K, Willinsky R. Subarachnoid hemorrhage from vertebrobasilar dissecting aneurysm treated with staged bilateral vertebral artery occlusion: the importance of early follow-up angiography: technical case report. *Neurosurgery* 1999;45:1258–1262.
70. Yoshimoto Y, Wakai S. Unruptured intracranial vertebral artery dissection. Clinical course and serial radiographic imagings. *Stroke* 1997;28:370–374.
71. Lylyk P, Ceratto R, Hurvitz D, et al. Treatment of a vertebral

dissecting aneurysm with stents and coils: technical case report. *Neurosurgery* 1998;43:385–388.
72. Lylyk P, Cohen JE, Ceratto R, et al. Combined endovascular treatment of dissecting vertebral artery aneurysms by using stents and coils. *J Neurosurg* 2001;94:427–432.
73. Dinichert A, Rufenacht DA, Tribolet N. Dissecting aneurysms of the posterior inferior cerebellar artery: report of four cases and review of the literature. *J Clin Neurosci* 2000;7:515–520.
74. Lefkowitz MA, Teitelbaum GP, Giannotta SL. Endovascular treatment of a dissecting posteroinferior cerebellar artery aneurysm: case report. *Neurosurgery* 1996;39:1036–1039.
75. Clare CE, Barrow DL. Infectious intracranial aneurysms. *Neurosurg Clin N Am* 1992;3:551–566.
76. Khayata MH, Aymard A, Casasco A, et al. Selective endovascular techniques in the treatment of cerebral mycotic aneurysms. Report of three cases. *J Neurosurg* 1993;78:661–665.
77. Frizzell RT, Vitek JJ, Hill DL, et al. Treatment of a bacterial (mycotic) intracranial aneurysm using an endovascular approach. *Neurosurgery* 1993;32:852–854.
78. Cloft HJ, Kallmes DF, Jensen ME, et al. Endovascular treatment of ruptured, peripheral cerebral aneurysms: parent artery occlusion with short Guglielmi detachable coils. *AJNR Am J Neuroradiol* 1999;20:308–310.
79. Chaloupka JC, Putman CM, Awad IA. Endovascular therapeutic approach to peripheral aneurysms of the superior cerebellar artery. *AJNR Am J Neuroradiol* 1996;17:1338–1342.
80. Debrun G. Retrievable versus nonretrievable coils. *AJNR Am J Neuroradiol* 1997;18:1389–1390.
81. Linskey ME, Jungreis CA, Yonas H, et al. Stroke risk after abrupt internal carotid artery sacrifice: accuracy of preoperative assessment with balloon test occlusion and stable xenon-enhanced CT. *AJNR Am J Neuroradiol* 1994;15:829–843.
82. Matas R. Testing the efficiency of the collateral circulation as a preliminary to the occlusion of the great surgical arteries. *Arch Surg* 1911;53:1–43.
83. Russell EJ, Goldberg K, Oskin J, et al. Ocular ischemic syndrome during carotid balloon occlusion testing. *AJNR Am J Neuroradiol* 1994;15:258–262.
84. Hacein-Bey L, Connolly ES Jr, Duong H, et al. Treatment of inoperable carotid aneurysms with endovascular carotid occlusion after extracranial-intracranial bypass surgery. *Neurosurgery* 1997;41:1225–1234.
85. Barnett DW, Barrow DL, Joseph GJ. Combined extracranial-intracranial bypass and intraoperative balloon occlusion for the treatment of intracavernous and proximal carotid artery aneurysms. *Neurosurgery* 1994;35:92–98.
86. Abruzzo T, Joseph GJ, Owens DS, et al. Prevention of complications resulting from endovascular carotid sacrifice: a retrospective assessment. *Neurosurgery* 2000;46:910–917.
87. Hacein-Bey L, Connolly ES Jr, Mayer SA, et al. Complex intracranial aneurysms: combined operative and endovascular approaches. *Neurosurgery* 1998;43:1304–1313.
88. Hawkins TD. Extracranial/intracranial anastomosis in therapeutic balloon occlusion of the internal carotid artery. *Acta Radiol Suppl* 1986;369:73–76.
89. Yonas H, Kaufmann A. Combined extracranial-intracranial bypass and intraoperative balloon occlusion for the treatment of intracavernous and proximal carotid artery aneurysms. *Neurosurgery* 1995;36:1234.
90. Peerless SJ, Ferguson GG, Drake CG. Extracranial-intracranial (EC/IC) bypass in the treatment of giant intracranial aneurysms. *Neurosurg Rev* 1982;5:77–81.
91. Lopes DK, Mericle RA, Wakhloo AK, et al. Cavernous sinus syndrome during balloon test occlusion of the cervical internal carotid artery. Report of two cases. *J Neurosurg* 1998;89:667–670.
92. Higashida RT, Halbach VV, Dowd C, et al. Endovascular detachable balloon embolization therapy of cavernous carotid artery aneurysms: results in 87 cases. *J Neurosurg* 1990;72:857–863.
93. Weil SM, van Loveren HR, Tomsick TA, et al. Management of inoperable cerebral aneurysms by the navigational balloon technique. *Neurosurgery* 1987;21:296–302.
94. Andrews JC, Valavanis A, Fisch U. Management of the internal carotid artery in surgery of the skull base. *Laryngoscope* 1989;99:1224–1229.
95. Brunberg JA, Frey KA, Horton JA, et al. [^{15}O]H_2O positron emission tomography determination of cerebral blood flow during balloon test occlusion of the internal carotid artery. *AJNR Am J Neuroradiol* 1994;15:725–732.
96. Katano H, Nagai H, Mase M, et al. Measurement of regional cerebral blood flow with H2(15)O positron emission tomography during Matas test. Report of three cases. *Acta Neurochir (Wien)* 1995;135:70–77.
97. Monsein LH, Jeffery PJ, van Heerden BB, et al. Assessing adequacy of collateral circulation during balloon test occlusion of the internal carotid artery with ^{99m}Tc-HMPAO SPECT. *AJNR Am J Neuroradiol* 1991;12:1045–1051.
98. Komiyama M, Khosla VK, Tamura K, et al. A provocative internal carotid artery balloon occlusion test with ^{99m}Tc-HMPAO CBF mapping: report of three cases. *Neurol Med Chir (Tokyo)* 1992;32:747–752.
99. Peterman SB, Taylor A Jr, Hoffman JC Jr. Improved detection of cerebral hypoperfusion with internal carotid balloon test occlusion and ^{99m}Tc-HMPAO cerebral perfusion SPECT imaging. *AJNR Am J Neuroradiol* 1991;12:1035–1041.
100. Furuhata S, Kubo A, Kawase T, et al. A simple technique to measure regional cerebral blood flow during intravascular balloon clamping. *Radioisotopes* 1988;37:336–338.
101. Lorberboym M, Pandit N, Machac J, et al. Brain perfusion imaging during preoperative temporary balloon occlusion of the internal carotid artery. *J Nucl Med* 1996;37:415–419.
102. Walker BS, Mathews D, Batjer H, et al. Detection of cerebral hypoperfusion during trial carotid occlusion with reversal following extracranial-intracranial bypass prior to permanent occlusion. *Clin Nucl Med* 1994;19:499–503.
103. Tanaka F, Nishizawa S, Yonekura Y, et al. Changes in cerebral blood flow induced by balloon test occlusion of the internal carotid artery under hypotension. *Eur J Nucl Med* 1995;22:1268–1273.
104. Mathews D, Walker BS, Purdy PD, et al. Brain blood flow SPECT in temporary balloon occlusion of carotid and intracerebral arteries. *J Nucl Med* 1993;34:1239–1243.
105. Moody EB, Dawson RC III, Sandler MP. ^{99m}Tc-HMPAO SPECT imaging in interventional neuroradiology: validation of balloon test occlusion. *AJNR Am J Neuroradiol* 1991;12:1043–1044.
106. de Vries EJ, Sekhar LN, Horton JA, et al. A new method to predict safe resection of the internal carotid artery. *Laryngoscope* 1990;100:85–88.
107. Erba SM, Horton JA, Latchaw RE, et al. Balloon test occlusion of the internal carotid artery with stable xenon/CT cerebral blood flow imaging. *AJNR Am J Neuroradiol* 1988;9:533–538.
108. Tan WS, Jafar JJ, Abejo R, et al. Regional cerebral blood flow assessment prior to balloon detachment in the treatment of intracranial giant aneurysms. *Acta Radiol Suppl* 1986;369:116–119.
109. Okudaira Y, Arai H, Sato K. Cerebral blood flow alteration by acetazolamide during carotid balloon occlusion: parameters reflecting cerebral perfusion pressure in the acetazolamide test. *Stroke* 1996;27:617–621.
110. Witt JP, Yonas H, Jungreis C. Cerebral blood flow response

pattern during balloon test occlusion of the internal carotid artery. *AJNR Am J Neuroradiol* 1994;15:847–856.

111. Xie Y, Mies G, Hossmann KA. Ischemic threshold of brain protein synthesis after unilateral carotid artery occlusion in gerbils. *Stroke* 1989;20:620–626.
112. Sharbrough FW, Messick JM Jr, Sundt TM Jr. Correlation of continuous electroencephalograms with cerebral blood flow measurements during carotid endarterectomy. *Stroke* 1973;4: 674–683.
113. Kurata A, Miyasaka Y, Tanaka C, et al. Stump pressure as a guide to the safety of permanent occlusion of the internal carotid artery. *Acta Neurochir (Wien)* 1996;138:549–554.
114. Morishima H, Kurata A, Miyasaka Y, et al. Efficacy of the stump pressure ratio as a guide to the safety of permanent occlusion of the internal carotid artery. *Neurol Res* 1998;20:732–736.
115. Giller CA, Mathews D, Walker B, et al. Prediction of tolerance to carotid artery occlusion using transcranial Doppler ultrasound. *J Neurosurg* 1994;81:15–19.
116. Sorteberg A, Sorteberg W, Bakke SJ, et al. Cerebral haemodynamics in internal carotid artery trial occlusion. *Acta Neurochir (Wien)* 1997;139:1066–1073.
117. Hetzel A, von Reutern G, Wernz MG, et al. The carotid compression test for therapeutic occlusion of the internal carotid artery. Comparison of angiography with transcranial Doppler sonography. *Cerebrovasc Dis* 2000;10:194–199.
118. Schneweis S, Urbach H, Solymosi L, et al. Preoperative risk assessment for carotid occlusion by transcranial Doppler ultrasound. *J Neurol Neurosurg Psychiatry* 1997;62:485–489.
119. Takeda N, Fujita K, Katayama S, et al. Cerebral oximetry for the detection of cerebral ischemia during temporary carotid artery occlusion. *Neurol Med Chir (Tokyo)* 2000;40:557–563.
120. Sazonova OB, Serbinenko FA, Smirnov NA, et al. Electroencephalography in aneurysms of the internal carotid artery during endovascular operations. *Zh Vopr Neirokhir Im N N Burdenko* 1987:30–39.
121. Morioka T, Matsushima T, Fujii K, et al. Balloon test occlusion of the internal carotid artery with monitoring of compressed spectral arrays (CSAs) of electroencephalogram. *Acta Neurochir (Wien)* 1989;101:29–34.
122. Cloughesy TF, Nuwer MR, Hoch D, et al. Monitoring carotid test occlusions with continuous EEG and clinical examination. *J Clin Neurophysiol* 1993;10:363–369.
123. Hacke W, Zeumer H, Ringelstein EB. EEG controlled occlusion of the internal carotid artery during angiography. *Neuroradiology* 1981;22:19–22.
124. Herkes GK, Morgan M, Grinnell V, et al. EEG monitoring during angiographic balloon test carotid occlusion: experience in sixteen cases. *Clin Exp Neurol* 1993;30:98–103.
125. Standard SC, Ahuja A, Guterman LR, et al. Balloon test occlusion of the internal carotid artery with hypotensive challenge. *AJNR Am J Neuroradiol* 1995;16:1453–1458.
126. Dare AO, Chaloupka JC, Putman CM, et al. Failure of the hypotensive provocative test during temporary balloon test occlusion of the internal carotid artery to predict delayed hemodynamic ischemia after therapeutic carotid occlusion. *Surg Neurol* 1998;50:147–156.
127. Polin RS, Shaffrey ME, Jensen ME, et al. Medical management in the endovascular treatment of carotid-cavernous aneurysms. *J Neurosurg* 1996;84:755–761.
128. Masaryk TJ, Perl J II, Wallace RC, et al. Detachable balloon embolization: concomitant use of a second safety balloon. *AJNR Am J Neuroradiol* 1999;20:1103–1106.
129. Gurian JH, Viñuela F, Gobin YP, et al. Aneurysm rupture after parent vessel sacrifice: treatment with Guglielmi detachable coil embolization via retrograde catheterization: case report. *Neurosurgery* 1995;37:1216–1220.
130. Barr JD, Lemley TJ. Endovascular arterial occlusion accomplished using microcoils deployed with and without proximal flow arrest: results in 19 patients. *AJNR Am J Neuroradiol* 1999; 20:1452–1456.
131. Braun IF, Hoffman JC Jr, Casarella WJ, et al. Use of coils for transcatheter carotid occlusion. *AJNR Am J Neuroradiol* 1985; 6:953–956.
132. Graves VB, Perl J II, Strother CM, et al. Endovascular occlusion of the carotid or vertebral artery with temporary proximal flow arrest and microcoils: clinical results. *AJNR Am J Neuroradiol* 1997;18:1201–1206.
133. Connors JJ III, Wojak JC. Permanent carotid artery occlusion should not be performed using fibered coils without proximal flow arrest. *J Vasc Interv Radiol* 1996;7:947–948.
134. Singer RJ, Dake MD, Norbash A, et al. Covered stent placement for neurovascular disease. *AJNR Am J Neuroradiol* 1997;18: 507–509.
135. Fahlbusch R, Nimsky C, Huk W. Open surgery of giant paraclinoid aneurysms improved by intraoperative angiography and endovascular retrograde suction decompression. *Acta Neurochir (Wien)* 1997;139:1026–1032.
136. Shucart WA, Kwan ES, Heilman CB. Temporary balloon occlusion of a proximal vessel as an aid to clipping aneurysms of the basilar and paraclinoid internal carotid arteries: technical note. *Neurosurgery* 1990;27:116–119.
137. Mizoi K, Takahashi A, Yoshimoto T, et al. Combined endovascular and neurosurgical approach for paraclinoid internal carotid artery aneurysms. *Neurosurgery* 1993;33:986–992.
138. Ng PY, Huddle D, Gunel M, et al. Intraoperative endovascular treatment as an adjunct to microsurgical clipping of paraclinoid aneurysms. *J Neurosurg* 2000;93:554–560.

Endovascular and Percutaneous Therapy of the Brain and Spine, edited by Michael P. Marks and Huy M. Do.
Lippincott Williams & Wilkins, Philadelphia © 2002.

8

ENDOVASCULAR THERAPY FOR VASOSPASM

HUY M. DO
MICHAEL P. MARKS

Subarachnoid hemorrhage (SAH)–induced cerebral vasospasm is a well-recognized complication of aneurysmal rupture. Each year in North America, some 40,000 individuals experience SAH from ruptured intracranial aneurysms [1, 2]. Aneurysmal rupture has a high rate of morbidity and mortality, resulting in death in approximately one-third of patients and permanent severe neurologic deficits in another one-third [3–5]. Ischemic injury to the brain due to cerebral vasospasm is a major cause of the morbidity and mortality of this disease.

Aneurysmal rerupture was previously the major cause of morbidity and mortality in patients who survived the initial hemorrhagic event, with a case-fatality rate of approximately 70% for persons who rebled [2,6]. A shift to earlier surgical and endovascular treatment during the last several decades due to improved diagnosis of SAH, rapid referral to specialized centers, and results of the International Cooperative Study on the Timing of Aneurysm Surgery [3,4,7] has reduced the frequency of this potentially life-threatening complication. The overall trial results from this cooperative study that included 3,521 patients worldwide found no difference between early and delayed surgery. In contrast, the subgroup of patients treated in North American centers, where surgery was planned between days 0 and 3 after SAH, showed improved outcome after early surgery [7]. Seven hundred seventy-two (21.9% of the total study population) patients admitted from days 0 to 3 after SAH were accrued in North American centers. Overall mortality for patients treated surgically on days 0 to 3 was similar to that of patients who had surgery on days 11 to 32. However, the patients who had early surgery had a significantly higher rate of good recovery (70.9% versus 61.7%, $p < 0.01$). Patients undergoing operations during days 7 to 10 had nearly twice the mortality of patients in either the early or later intervals.

Because of this greater stress on early surgery, ischemic injury due to cerebral vasospasm has emerged as the leading cause of poor outcome and death after SAH, affecting nearly one-third of patients [4,8–10]. In this chapter, we will review the natural history, pathophysiology, diagnosis, and basis for practical medical and endovascular management of vasospasm. We will then discuss the use of neuroendovascular techniques of intracranial percutaneous transluminal balloon angioplasty (PTA) and intraarterial papaverine infusion.

BACKGROUND

Cerebral vasospasm may be defined as delayed focal or diffuse narrowing of arteries following SAH. Although the most common cause of vasospasm is aneurysmal SAH, it may be seen following hemorrhage from arteriovenous malformations, tumors, trauma, and perimesencephalic hemorrhage [11–14]. There are two definitions for cerebral vasospasm, angiographic vasospasm and clinical vasospasm.

Angiographic vasospasm follows a relatively consistent temporal course and may be entirely asymptomatic. The narrowing is time dependent and is rarely present before the third day after hemorrhage, with peak incidence 6 or 7 days after ictus [4,7,11,15–17]. Forty to seventy percent of patients have been found to have angiographic evidence of vasospasm when studied from 4 to 17 days after the initial bleed. Repeat cerebral angiography usually demonstrates a gradual resolution of angiographic vasospasm, with a return to normal vessel diameter within 2 to 3 weeks following hemorrhage.

Clinical vasospasm is the syndrome of ischemic sequelae produced by the progressive narrowing of large and small cerebral arteries. It occurs in about one-third of patients. It is manifest by a delayed ischemic neurologic deficits syndrome (DINDS) that may resolve or progress to permanent cere-

H.M. Do: Departments of Radiology and Neurosurgery, Stanford University School of Medicine, Stanford, California.
M.P. Marks: Departments of Radiology and Neurosurgery, Stanford University Medical Center, Stanford, California.

bral infarction [17]. Ultimately the patient may become increasingly less responsive and progress to coma and death. Cerebral infarction occurs in approximately 50% of symptomatic cases. The time course of clinical vasospasm parallels that of angiographic vasospasm. The incidence of clinical vasospasm is clearly lower than that of angiographic vasospasm. The Cooperative Aneurysm Study found an incidence of angiographic vasospasm in over 50% and clinical vasospasm in 32% of patients [8].

Subarachnoid Hemorrhage and Cerebral Blood Flow

Aneurysmal SAH results in a myriad of systemic and intracranial alterations [6,18]. Among these is increased intracranial pressure, reduced cerebral blood flow (CBF), decreased tissue oxygen supply, impaired autoregulation of carbon dioxide reactivity, and intravascular volume and electrolyte derangements. Understanding of the pathophysiology of delayed cerebral vasospasm from ruptured aneurysms came about in the last half-century. In 1949, Robertson [19] analyzed the postmortem findings of a series of patients with ruptured aneurysms and found frequent cerebral infarction in the territory of the cerebral arteries that were surrounded by dense subarachnoid blood. In 1951, Ecker and Reimenschneider [20] first reported angiographic cerebral vasospasm following aneurysmal SAH in humans. They hypothesized that arterial spasm played an important role following spontaneous rupture of intracranial aneurysms, and stated that excessive spasm may produce unfavorable effects by impairing the circulation of the brain. Other investigators further defined the clinical and angiographic characteristics of cerebral vasospasm, demonstrated the prognostic significance, and established the characteristic time course [8,10, 16,21–24]. The true significance of DINDS and stroke from vasospasm was also confirmed by CBF studies [25–29].

A wide range of CBF is compatible with normal neurologic function. In healthy individuals, regional CBF averages between 50 and 70 ml/100 g of brain per minute. Symptoms of cerebral ischemia and electrical dysfunction occur when CBF is reduced to less than 20 ml/100 g of brain per minute. Cellular structural damage and death occur when CBF falls below 15 ml/100 g of brain per minute [17,30]. These thresholds help explain the discordance in the incidences of angiographic and clinical vasospasm. A patient with angiographic evidence of cerebral vasospasm may have marginally sufficient CBF and still be neurologically normal.

Following SAH, CBF is reduced to 30% to 40% of normal values [18]. CBF appears to recover in patients with good Hunt and Hess grades but not in poor-grade patients [31,32]. In a study correlating the CBF, somatosensory evoked potentials, CT scan grade, and neurologic grade in patients with aneurysmal SAH, Fazl et al. [31] observed that CBF averaged 49 ml/100 g of brain per minute in Hunt and Hess grade I patients and 37 ml/100 g of brain per minute in grade V patients. Regional CBF depends on not only the distribution and severity of the arterial spasm, but also on the presence of large (communicating arterial segments) and leptomeningeal collateral blood supply, and other factors such as cerebral perfusion pressure, blood volume, and hematocrit.

Etiology of Vasospasm

It is generally accepted that the breakdown and release of blood products in the subarachnoid space are responsible for SAH-induced vasospasm, but the exact pathophysiologic mechanism is still the subject of intense research. Numerous experimental animal preparations and methods have been used to study the effects of SAH on the cerebrovascular circulation [33,34]. Experimental models include dog, cat, rat, rabbit, goat, monkey, cow, isolated vessels, and cell culture of cerebrovascular cells. Experimental methods to induce and simulate SAH include single or double cisternal injection of autologous blood, direct cerebral vessel puncture, and injection of blood products, lysate, clots, hemoglobin, or cerebrospinal fluid (CSF). These models and methods have been used to study cerebral autoregulation, endothelium-dependent mechanisms, smooth muscle cell mechanisms, gene activation, cerebral microcirculation, and gene therapy.

The most common experimental approach is to induce SAH by intracisternal injection of blood into canine subjects and subsequently study the effects of SAH and their underlying molecular mechanisms on the brain. On the basis of its ability to accurately predict human SAH events the primate model, in which clot is surgically placed around the larger arteries at the skull base, appears to be the best model [34]. Recently, more reductionist approaches using isolated macro- and microvessels and cell cultures from smaller animals, such as rats or rabbits, are now more commonly used for such studies. These methods have the advantage of studying molecular mechanisms relevant to SAH under simplified conditions, and the information gathered can be used in the interpretation of data obtained from whole-brain studies [33].

Suggested theories for the relationship between blood products and vasospasm revolve around the concept of release of vasoactive substances such as prostaglandin, oxyhemoglobin, histamines, angiotensin, serotonin, bilirubin, and thromboxane [17]. The presence of oxyhemoglobin has been found to be an important factor in the initiation of vasospasm. Red blood cells (RBCs) break down and release oxyhemoglobin starting at day 2 and peaking at day 7 after SAH [35]. Investigators have found that with time, incubated RBCs become more contractile [35,36]. Following SAH in the clinical setting, RBCs are trapped in the CSF and disappear by hemolysis, similar to *in vitro* studies. Furthermore, the time course of vasospasm parallels the increasing levels of oxyhemoglobin that are seen. Oxyhemoglobin has been found to decrease the levels of vasodilators such as prostacyclin and increase the levels of vasoconstrictors, such as prostaglandins and thromboxane, from blood vessels [17,35,36]. The hemoglobin moiety has been implicated in the release of oxygen free radicals (oxygen and hydroxyl). Oxyhemoglobin undergoes autooxidation to methemoglobin, thus releasing the superoxide-anion free radical O_2 [37]. Iron compounds released during RBC lysis are also known to be potent catalysts in the generation of reactive free radicals such as the hydroxyl radical [38]. These free radicals then initiate a cascade of lipid peroxidation and prostaglandin production that are thought to contribute to development of cerebral vasospasm. Despite successes of compounds designed to inhibit the effects of these vasoconstrictors in animal studies [39,40], transferring these positive results to the clinical arena has been disappointing. One such compound is the 21-aminosteroid, tirilazad. Although it has been shown in the laboratory that tirilazad is highly effective at inhibiting iron-dependent lipid peroxidation and significantly diminishing vasospasm in animal models, this drug was found not to be of significant benefit in the management of vasospasm in a clinical trial [41].

Through a variety of molecular mechanisms such as ion channel activation and inhibition, SAH causes smooth muscle cell depolarization and contraction and subsequent vasospasm [17]. With prolonged vasoconstriction, vascular smooth muscles cells may become fixed into their shortened configuration by deposition or rearrangement, or both, of extracellular collagen matrix. Compression of this extracellular connective tissue matrix may explain why intraarterial balloon angioplasty appears to relieve vasospasm permanently [42,43]. Morphological changes in the blood vessel wall with subendothelial fibrosis, migration, and proliferation of smooth muscle cells, and infiltration of lymphocytes, plasma cells, and macrophages are secondary, nonspecific histologic changes that may also contribute to delayed vasospasm [17].

Clinical studies have shown that greater amounts of blood, as seen on computed tomography (CT), following aneurysm rupture can be an important predictor of clinically symptomatic vasospasm. Fisher et al. [24] published a classic article that correlated CT findings and clinical course of 47 patients with acutely ruptured aneurysms (Table 8-1). They found out that when blood was undetectable (grade 1) or mildly diffusely distributed (grade 2), the incidence of symptomatic vasospasm was rare, occurring in only 2 of 18 cases. However when CT demonstrated subarachnoid clots larger than 5 mm × 3 mm or layers of blood 1-mm thick or greater in the cerebral fissures and basal cisterns (grade 3), symptomatic vasospasm almost always followed, occurring in 23 of 24 patients. Qureshi et al. [44] prospectively collected data from a placebo-treated group in a multicenter trial of tirilazad mesylate to develop a scheme for early identification of patients at risk for clinical vasospasm after aneurysmal SAH. These authors found that the thickness of clot seen on noncontrast head CT scans is one of four independent predictors of symptomatic vasospasm. The other three predictors were early rise in transcranial Doppler (TCD) velocity of the middle cerebral artery (MCA), Glasgow coma scale score below 14, and rupture of anterior cerebral artery (ACA) or internal carotid artery (ICA) aneurysms. Intraventricular or intraparenchymal hemorrhage was part of the initial Fisher classification; however, it was not found to be a risk factor of development of symptomatic vasospasm by the Cooperative Aneurysm Study [8]. Certainly patients with small amounts of blood (low-grade scores by either the Fisher or modified Fisher classification) can develop symptomatic vasospasm [45], so the amount of clot noted on CT alone is not an absolute predictor of clinical vasospasm.

TABLE 8-1. FISHER GRADE OF SUBARACHNOID HEMORRHAGE DETERMINED BY COMPUTED TOMOGRAPHY

Grade	CT Findings
1	No subarachnoid blood
2	Diffuse subarachnoid hemorrhage or vertical layers <1 mm thick
3	Localized subarachnoid clot or layers of hemorrhage ≥1 mm thick
4	Intracerebral or intraventricular clot with diffuse or no subarachnoid blood

From Fisher CM, Kistler JP, Davis JM. Relation of cerebral vasospasm to subarachnoid hemorrhage visualized by computerized tomographic scanning. *Neurosurgery* 1980;6:1–9, with permission.

Zabramski et al. [46] used a canine model to demonstrate a direct correlation between the volume and timing of hemorrhage and the severity of vasospasm. Increasing the volume of blood in this animal model, from 9 to 15 ml of blood delivered over 24 hours, produced more severe arterial spasm. Delay of the final injection of blood to 96 hours in the 15-ml hemorrhage group resulted in even more intense spasm. Serial angiographic evaluation demonstrated this vasospasm resolved over about 3 weeks. Finally, small, late rebleeding episodes resulted in the rapid onset of intense spasm. Their results support the clinical impression that, in general, the severity of spasm is related to the volume of hemorrhage and, in addition, suggest that the time course of hemorrhage may play a significant role in determining the overall severity of chronic cerebral vasospasm.

DIAGNOSTIC STUDIES

CT is still the diagnostic imaging study of choice for detection of SAH. Chakeres and Bryan in 1986 performed an *in vitro* comparison of the magnetic resonance (MR) T1-

and T2-weighted signal intensities and CT attenuation values of simulated SAH [47]. They concluded that MR was better at distinguishing varying blood and CSF mixtures on the basis of relaxation times when compared with CT attenuation change. However, CT attenuation change was better at distinguishing the density of clot from normal brain when compared with MR signal intensity. Acute SAH appeared isointense to brain on these conventional sequences. Recently, fluid-attenuated inversion recovery (FLAIR) MR imaging sequences have been shown by *in vivo* experiments and small clinical series to have better sensitivity than CT for the detection of SAH [48–50]. Logistical problems are often associated with obtaining emergent MR scans in acutely ill patients, and a prospective comparison of the two imaging modalities needs to be performed for MR to become the study of choice to evaluate patients with acute SAH.

Transcranial Doppler Ultrasonography

TCD ultrasonography has greatly helped in the diagnosis of vasospasm. This modality uses range-gated pulsed Doppler insonation through the thinner part of the skull to determine blood velocity in the larger arteries in the region of the circle of Willis. TCD often fails to detect vasospasm in arteries beyond the circle of Willis [51]. It is a noninvasive test performed at the bedside. Elevated cerebral arterial blood velocity is highly correlated with angiographic vasospasm in SAH. Normative values for major cerebral arteries have been established [52]. Blood flow velocity in the middle cerebral artery (MCA) has been most highly correlated with angiographic vasospasm. The normal blood flow velocity range for the proximal MCA is 30 to 80 cm/sec with an average of 62 cm/sec. Mild to moderate arterial spasm of the MCA correlates to a TCD velocity of greater than 120 cm/sec, and a velocity greater than 200 cm/sec indicates severe vasospasm. To differentiate generalized increased CBF due to a hyperdynamic state from vasospasm, the ratio of the MCA-to-ICA velocity (the Lindegaard ratio) can be calculated, with a ratio greater than 3 indicative of vasospasm [53]. The sensitivity and specificity of TCD in the detection of MCA vasospasm is approximately 85% to 95% [30]. Specific TCD velocity levels that correspond to the degree of vasospasm have not been firmly established for the posterior circulation. However increasing blood flow velocity in the basilar and distal vertebral arteries on serial examinations suggests vasospasm of the posterior circulation. Clearly the TCD findings must be interpreted in the context of neurologic examination. High TCD velocity does not necessarily indicate cerebral ischemia, because patients with vasospasm may be asymptomatic.

Cerebral Blood Flow Studies

Noninvasive modalities to assess regional CBF, including xenon CT, single-photon emission computed tomography (SPECT), positron emission tomography (PET), and MR perfusion imaging, may also be helpful in guiding therapy for vasospasm [30,54]. Yonas et al. [55] used xenon CT to document depressed CBF specific to the distribution of cerebral arteries with vasospasm. A CBF below 15 ml/100 g of brain per minute resulted in eight of nine patients developing infarction, whereas no patient with CBF greater than 18 ml/100 g of brain per minute developed infarction. Preliminary studies have shown the clinical promise and feasibility of advanced neuroimaging techniques such as CT perfusion imaging, MR diffusion-weighted imaging (DWI), MR contrast dynamic perfusion-weighted imaging (PWI), and MR spectroscopy in the evaluation of post-SAH patients at risk for vasospasm [56–59]. In a small clinical series, Condette-Auliac et al. [58] found DWI abnormalities in all patients with both asymptomatic and symptomatic vasospasm defined by TCD-determined MCA average blood velocity rates above 120 cm/sec. No DWI lesions were seen in the group of patients without vasospasm. Bracard et al. [56] reported a case in which MCA angioplasty resulted in reversal of DWI changes, PWI evidence of oligemia, and regression of clinical deficits.

Cerebral Angiography

Digital subtraction angiography is the definitive method to diagnose cerebral vasospasm. MR angiography and CT angiography have been used to evaluate the anatomy and morphology of intracranial aneurysms, but they have not played a role in the diagnosis or management of delayed ischemic deficit. A three- or four-vessel cerebral angiogram is routinely obtained during the admission period and initial evaluation of patients with SAH to search for a ruptured intracranial aneurysm. This baseline study is usually available for comparison when angiography is requested to confirm suspected symptomatic vasospasm. Angiographic evidence of cerebral vasospasm should correspond to a location that explains a neurologic deficit. Angiography used to confirm vasospasm has an acceptable risk. The risk of permanent neurologic deficit associated with angiography in patients with vasospasm has been reported to be lower than the risk of new permanent neurologic deficit in patients undergoing workup for transient ischemic attack or ischemic stroke (1.8% versus 3.7%, $p = 0.001$) [60]. The postoperative angiogram can also be used to identify other abnormalities related to the aneurysm clipping. In one large retrospective series these included aneurysmal remnants from incomplete clipping (5.7% of aneurysms), new aneurysms (2.9% of patients), and vessel occlusion (5.7% of patients) [61].

MEDICAL THERAPY

A number of strategies have been developed to manage cerebral vasospasm. Preventive measures include preoperative management in the form of early surgery and the use of calcium-channel antagonists. Postoperative or postendovascular therapy management includes hypertensive, hypervolemic, and hemodilution therapy, often called *triple H therapy*.

Calcium-channel blockers, particularly oral nimodipine, have been shown to reduce delayed ischemic deficits related to vasospasm [62]. Pickard et al. [10] conducted a randomized prospective double-blinded study on 199 patients in which oral nimodipine was given in a dosage of 60 mg every 4 hours, started within 4 days of SAH, and continued in survivors for 21 days. This trial demonstrated a 34% reduction in cerebral infarction and 40% reduction in poor outcome. The placebo group had a 36% rate of death or severe disability compared with 17% in the treatment group. In addition, 83% of the nimodipine group had a good recovery or moderate disability compared with 64% in the placebo group. These differences were statistically significant. The mechanism of action of calcium-channel blockers does not appear to be vessel dilation but rather improvement of leptomeningeal collateral flow, microcirculation enhancement, or a direct protective effect of neuronal cells [10,63]. However nimodipine should be discontinued if severe hypotension is present to avoid further decrease in cerebral perfusion pressure [30].

The rationale for triple H therapy is based upon the observation that the reduction of CBF results when vasospasm is accompanied by imbalances of cerebral autoregulation [17,30,64]. As arterial narrowing increases, cerebral vascular resistance shifts from the penetrating arterioles to the major branches of the circle of Willis and the proximal conducting vessels. Once this shift occurs, the brain that is fed by these narrowed branches loses its capacity for autoregulation. Blood flow through the narrowed proximal branches then becomes the factor limiting CBF, and cerebral perfusion varies directly with blood pressure.

$$\left[Q = \frac{\pi r^4 P}{8\ Ln}\right]$$

Poiseuille's Law (above) describes the relationship of blood flow (Q) with blood pressure (P), vessel radius (r), vessel length (L), and blood viscosity (n). Simplistically speaking, blood flow increases with higher pressure, large-vessel radius, and decreasing blood viscosity. Therefore, when resistance is fixed by proximal vessel narrowing, the only options available for increasing flow are to decrease fluid viscosity or to increase perfusion pressure. Colloid (5% albumin) and crystalloid fluids are administered to achieve volume expansion and raise the central venous pressure by approximately 10 mm Hg, or to achieve a central pulmonary venous pressure of approximately 50 mm Hg. This also lowers the patient's hematocrit (blood viscosity), resulting in a further increase in blood flow. The oxygen-carrying capacity of blood is not affected unless the hematocrit is reduced below 30%. If the systemic blood velocity does not rise sufficiently with volume expansion, vasopressor therapy with dopamine, dobutamine, and phenylephrine may be required.

Although triple H therapy has become the standard of care in most medical centers managing SAH, data from prospective randomized controlled trials are sparse and inconclusive [65–67]. Multiple reports have, however, shown that DINDS can be reversed by hypervolemia and induced hypertension. Kassell et al. [64] reported that hypervolemic, hypertensive therapy successfully reversed the neurologic deterioration from angiographically proven arterial spasm in 47 of 58 patients. The improvement was permanent in 43 patients and transient in 4. The most advantageous time to institute triple H therapy is soon after the onset of symptomatic vasospasm, when deficits are mild. If the patient becomes symptomatic while under maximal medical therapy, it is unlikely that the deficit will reverse with time unless more aggressive techniques are used.

ENDOVASCULAR THERAPY

When maximal medical therapy fails and the CT scan does not show a large infarction, endovascular treatment with balloon angioplasty has been clinically beneficial. Numerous reports have described profound improvement in neurologic deficits for patients with vasospasm refractory to other modes of therapy who are treated with transluminal angioplasty [68–75]. In selected patient populations, such as those with vasospasm of the smaller arteries beyond the first order segment, intraarterial papaverine infusions have also been used successfully to treat symptomatic vasospasm [30, 76–78].

Percutaneous Transluminal Angioplasty

The effects of angioplasty are summarized as follows: significant clinical improvement occurs in 60% to 80% of patients, often within minutes of the angioplasty; normal angiographic caliber is achieved in nearly all cases which persist without recurrent vasospasm; and evidence of improved CBF by TCD ultrasonography or SPECT correlates with clinical improvement. The efficacy of angioplasty in restoring persistent luminal arterial caliber supports the concept of passive maintenance of arterial narrowing in established vasospasm (Fig. 8-1).

Zubkov et al. [68,69] introduced the concept of using endovascular balloon angioplasty to dilate severely vasospastic large arteries in the region of the circle of Willis in carefully selected patients. They reported balloon dilations in 52 patients with symptomatic vasospasm, resulting in improvement in CBF and ischemic deficits in 87% of patients [69]. Higashida et al. [70] performed angioplasty in 99 vascular territories in 28 patients. In 17 patients (61%) angioplasty resulted in clinical improvement. Two patients (7%)

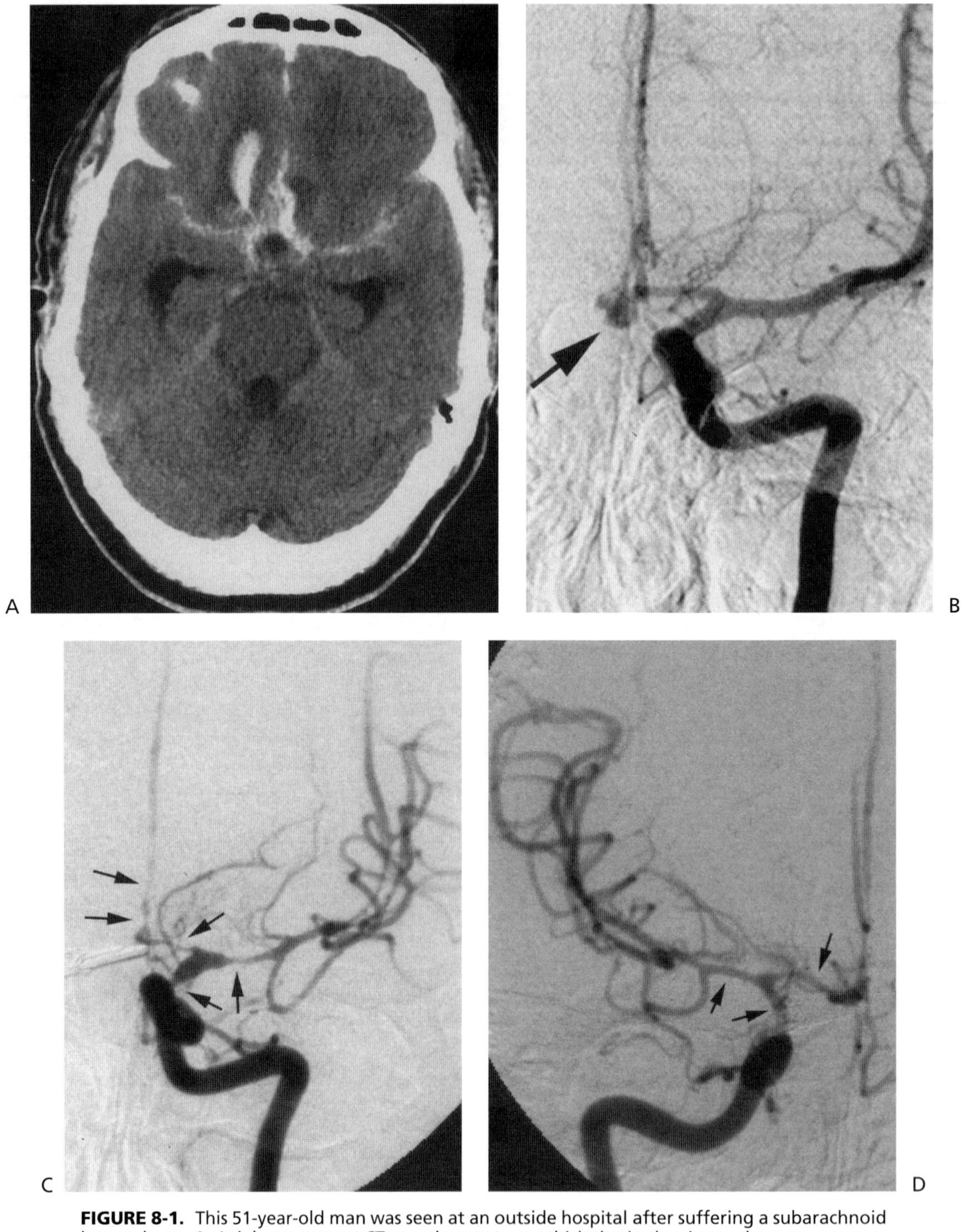

FIGURE 8-1. This 51-year-old man was seen at an outside hospital after suffering a subarachnoid hemorrhage. **A:** Axial noncontrast CT scan demonstrates thick clot in the cisternal spaces, a parenchymal hemorrhage in the right frontal lobe (Fisher grade 4), and evidence of hydrocephalus. **B:** Left internal carotid artery angiogram anterior projection demonstrates an anterior communicating artery aneurysm *(arrow).* After this angiogram and CT scan were made, the patient was taken to the operating room and the anterior communicating artery aneurysm was clipped. Seven days later, he began experiencing a decreased level of consciousness and was transferred to our institution. **C,D:** Left internal carotid artery and right internal carotid artery angiograms anterior projection done 8 days after subarachnoid hemorrhage. These demonstrate severe vasospasm in the left internal carotid artery circulation *(arrows)* **(C),** and moderate vasospasm in the right internal carotid artery circulation *(arrows)* **(D).** Because there was evidence of vasospasm involving the anterior cerebral artery circulation and more distal portions of the middle cerebral artery circulation bilaterally, 240 mg of papaverine was infused in each carotid circulation. Following this a guidewire-directed silicone balloon was used to perform angioplasty in the supraclinoid carotid and middle cerebral artery M1 segment in both the right and left circulations. *(Figure continues.)*

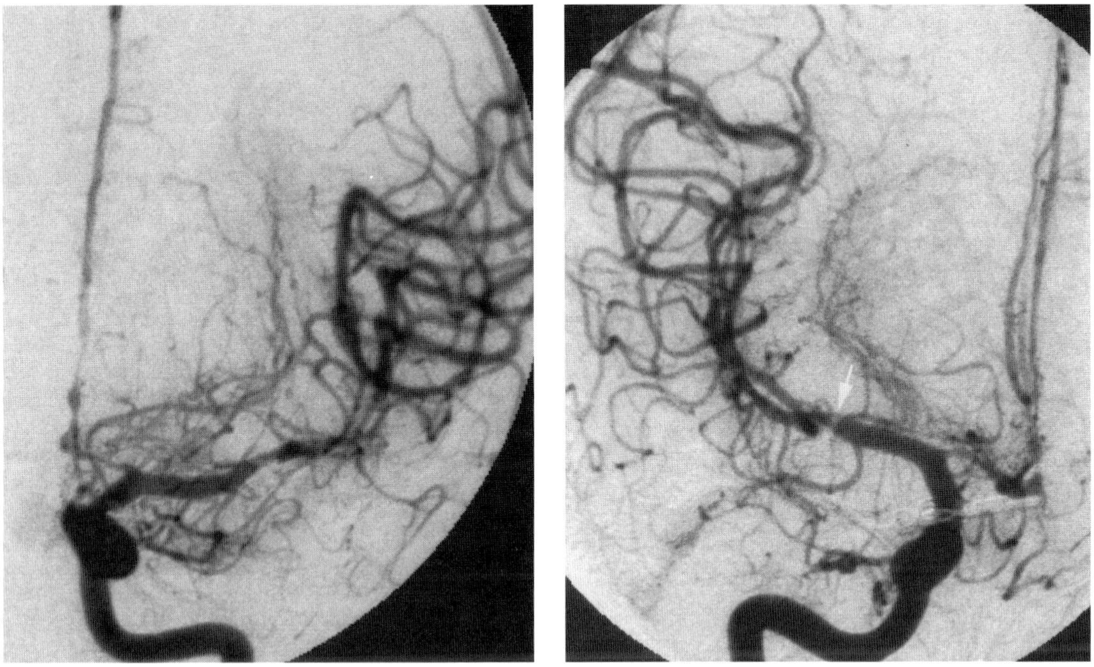

E F

FIGURE 8-1. *Continued.* **E,F:** Left internal carotid artery and right internal carotid artery anterior projections, respectively, following balloon angioplasty demonstrating dilation of these segments and augmented perfusion to the cerebral circulation bilaterally. There is a small area of residual stenosis at the middle cerebral artery bifurcation in the right circulation *(arrow)* **(F)**, which was not dilated. Over the next 24 hours, the patient's mental status improved. He was able to leave the hospital and return to work.

remained in poor condition, and nine patients (32%) died despite treatment.

Eskridge et al. [71] reported a retrospective uncontrolled study of 50 cases treated with angioplasty after failure of maximal medical therapy of postaneurysmal SAH vasospasm. Ninety-four percent of the patients were treated within 2 weeks of SAH, 64% treated within 12 hours of symptom onset, and 92% within 18 hours. Sixty-one percent showed significant neurologic improvement within 72 hours, 4% died immediately following the procedure, and 2% deteriorated. Significant neurologic improvement was defined as a two-level increase in motor strength or Glasgow coma scale within 48 to 72 hours of angioplasty. Thirty-three percent did not improve. It was found that the longer the duration of vasospasm, the more difficult it was to perform balloon angioplasty. These investigators also demonstrated improved TCD velocities and improvement in brain perfusion following angioplasty. Long-term results from this group are also promising, although there may be selection biases in such follow-up reports. Song et al. [30] followed more than 20 patients with TCD studies 3 to 7 years after angioplasty procedures and all have been normal. Three patients had normal-appearing angiograms 18 months after angioplasty.

Bejjani et al. [73] retrospectively reviewed their results with angioplasty for 31 patients with vasospasm. They found greater clinical improvement in the 21 patients (68%) who were treated early (within 24 hours of clinical deterioration). In spite of delayed angioplasty being used in a significant number of the study patients, 25 of 27 patients (92%) available for follow-up were found to have good outcome (Glasgow outcome scale score = 1).

Rosenwasser et al. [75] attempted to determine the optimal time window for angioplasty relative to symptom onset. Ninety-three patients in this report underwent endovascular treatment for medically refractory clinical vasospasm. Seventy-three patients (60%) had Hunt and Hess grades of III or IV. The Glasgow outcome scale was determined after 6 to 31 months and was available in 84 patients. Fifty-one patients underwent endovascular treatment within 2 hours of symptom onset, while 33 were treated more than 2 hours after the development of clinical vasospasm. Both groups had similar angiographic improvement (90%) after treatment. However, the group treated within 2 hours of symptom onset showed a 70% sustained clinical improvement, compared with only 40% for the group treated beyond 2 hours ($p < 0.01$).

These reports stress the importance of timing to make endovascular therapy effective. Clinical vasospasm must be quickly and reliably recognized and the patient must be treated early in the disease process to prevent cerebral infarction. Intracranial balloon angioplasty requires a high level of neuroradiologic expertise and is often available only at major referral medical centers [79]. Angioplasty is limited primarily to the large proximal intracranial arteries due to the risk of vessel rupture if the balloon is advanced beyond a first-order vessel.

Earlier treatment is usually associated with better patient survival and outcome. Based upon basic research indicating that balloon angioplasty prior to development of vasospasm can prevent its development [42], a small pilot study by Muizelaar et al. has shown the feasibility of prophylactic balloon angioplasty in patients with Fisher grade 3 SAH [80]. Prophylactic angioplasty was performed in the distal internal carotid artery, A1, M1, and P1 segments bilaterally in 13 patients. Despite a low incidence of subsequent clinical vasospasm and DINDS, the mortality rate of angioplasty was 7.7%. This increased risk in comparison to results of series of angioplasty of patients with developed vasospasm may be because prophylactic angioplasty involves dilation of arteries of normal diameter that can result in exceeding the maximal diameter of these arteries and rupturing them. A randomized trial based upon this study is currently underway.

Intraarterial Papaverine Infusion

Papaverine hydrochloride is a member of the benzylisoquinoline group of alkaloids. It was originally prepared as a crude alkaloid derivative of opium but is now manufactured synthetically. It has no narcotic properties and is capable of producing diffuse dilation of arteries and arterioles. Its mechanism of action is not definitively known. The average half-life is about 1 hour [81].

Papaverine has been used in the treatment of clinical and experimental cerebral vasospasm by intravenous, intrathecal, and intraarterial administrations. In a rabbit model of vasospasm due to SAH, papaverine will reverse angiographic spasm in the first 3 days after its appearance; however, vasospasm becomes refractory to papaverine treatment after 5 to 9 days [82]. The initial arterial narrowing after SAH is thought to be due to vasoactive substances released near and adjacent to the involved arterial wall. Subsequent changes in vessel wall compliance and distensibility are late phenomena associated with tissue damage and permanent structural change [82]. Despite encouraging results in early reports of a small series of patients, the overall clinical results of recent studies of intraarterial papaverine for the treatment of vasospasm have been less enthusiastic [78,83–85].

Patients treated with papaverine infusion have not shown a statistically significant improvement in the 3-month Glasgow outcome scale when compared with those given medical therapy alone [84]. Intraarterial papaverine has also not been shown to be effective in permanently reversing cerebral hypoperfusion. Vajkoczy et al. have reported on the effects of intraarterial papaverine on regional CBF and hemodynamically relevant cerebral vasospasm [85]. In this prospective study, eight patients with cerebral vasospasm after SAH were entered into the study. Before papaverine infusion, thermal diffusion microprobes were implanted into the white matter of each affected vascular territory for regional CBF monitoring. During and after papaverine infusion, mean arterial blood pressure, intracranial pressure, cerebral perfusion pressure, thermal diffusion regional CBF, and cerebral vascular resistance were recorded continuously. The authors found that papaverine infusion significantly increased regional CBF from 7.13 ± 1.6 to 37.9 ± 6.6 ml/100 g of brain per minute, indicating reversal of cerebral hypoperfusion. This regional CBF response was dependent upon the degree of vasospasm and reduced perfusion within the vascular territory. However, long-term analysis of regional CBF demonstrated that this beneficial effect of papaverine on cerebral hyperperfusion was only transient, disappearing within 3 hours of treatment. Regional CBF and cerebral vascular resistance returned to baseline values after this time. There was a lack of correlation between TCD ultrasonography and thermal diffusion regional CBF measurement, suggesting that TCD is not suited for CBF base neurologic monitoring after intraarterial papaverine infusion. The authors concluded that intraarterial papaverine infusion is not effective in permanently reversing cerebral hyperperfusion in patients with post-SAH cerebral vasospasm.

Intraarterial injections of papaverine can elicit rapid improvement in vasoconstriction as shown on immediate control angiography, but its vasodilatory effect persists for only a short time and there is no strong evidence of sustained clinical improvement in patients treated only with intraarterial papaverine for symptomatic vasospasm [86]. In this instance, papaverine infusion may need to be infused repeatedly, with the associated risk of continued and repeat angiography [86,87]. Papaverine infusion has also been implicated in increased intracranial pressure and seizures [88, 89].

TECHNIQUE FOR ENDOVASCULAR THERAPY

Patient Evaluation

Balloon angioplasty of symptomatic cerebral vasospasm is considered the primary endovascular treatment for vasospasm, because it directly addresses the anatomic basis of the disease. Post-SAH patients with clinical evidence of new neurologic deficits, in whom other possible causes have been excluded and who have angiographically documented vasospasm in the vascular territory responsible for their symptoms, should be treated aggressively with angioplasty. Because the best results are seen when patients are treated early after the onset of symptoms, care and effort must be taken to treat these patients in an emergent or semi-emergent manner. Balloon angioplasty for treatment of cerebral vasospasm in the presence of cerebral infarction is controversial and varies from institution to institution. Reluctance to perform angioplasty in the presence of CT evidence of infarction is due to the fear of reperfusion hemorrhage.

Proper treatment requires careful evaluation of the patient in advance of treatment. Determination of which patient to treat requires communication between the clinical neuroscience subspecialties involved, taking into account the patients' overall clinical state and available neuroimaging data. The risk and benefit to the patient must be weighed prior to embarking on this procedure.

The clinical features of cerebral vasospasm can be quite diverse because they depend on several variables, including the severity and location of arterial narrowing, the age and clinical condition of the patient, complicating factors such as elevated intracranial pressure or systemic hypotension, and the extent of collateral circulation to the ischemic brain. Approximately 50% of patients with angiographic vasospasm remain asymptomatic. The development of DINDS occurs only when the limits of compensatory mechanisms (cerebrovascular autoregulation and maximization of tissue oxygen extraction ratio) have been surpassed.

Post-SAH DINDS from delayed vasospasm should be considered when the patient develops new neurologic deficits that are not explained by other causes [54,90]. DINDS associated with symptomatic vasospasm generally occurs shortly after the onset of angiographic vasospasm. In the anterior or carotid circulation, signs and symptoms include hemiparesis, hemisensory deficits, apathy, visual disturbances, dysphasia, and changes in the level of consciousness. In the posterior or vertebrobasilar circulation, manifestations may be subtle and include brainstem signs such as dysarthria, diplopia, vertigo, ataxia, decreased gag reflex, respiratory difficulty, and altered sensorium. The onset of neurologic signs may be preceded by fever, increased meningismus, and nonspecific lightheadedness. Symptoms and signs may progress steadily in severity or fluctuate, and are often associated with change in intravascular volume status or blood pressure. Progression to a permanent cerebral infarction occurs in about one-half of untreated symptomatic patients [90].

The diagnosis of cerebral vasospasm is based largely on careful sequential clinical neurologic examination. A high index of suspicion, with awareness of risk factors and the temporal course of the disease, is needed to make the diagnosis. Changes in neurologic condition of the patient should alert the physician to exclude other causes of deterioration such as hydrocephalus, seizures, cerebral edema, electrolyte disturbances, sepsis, drug reactions, respiratory insufficiency, and recurrent or new intracranial hemorrhage. Cerebral ischemia from other causes such as embolic disease from the aneurysm should also be considered. Head CT, serum electrolyte and blood gas determinations, and monitoring of intracranial pressure are appropriate studies performed at this stage. If these alternative causes are excluded, then delayed neurologic deterioration is most likely due to the ischemic consequences of vasospasm. Appropriate diagnostic tests such as TCD, previously discussed, will aid greatly in the evaluation.

Angioplasty

Methods for balloon angioplasty have been well described in the literature [30,69–75]. However, the basic technique remains the same. Because the patient is neurologically impaired, every effort must be made to obtain informed consent from a legal guardian. The potential risk of stroke or death that is related to balloon angioplasty must be explained in detail. Although the risk associated with balloon angioplasty is not yet clearly defined, it is likely to be 1% to 3% [69–75]. Using the Seldinger technique, a 6-French vascular sheath is placed in the common femoral artery. Diagnostic angiography may either be performed through a diagnostic catheter or through the larger-bore guiding catheter. The potential benefit of using the larger guiding catheter is to save time so that one may then embark on angioplasty earlier. Prior to introduction of the catheter, systemic anticoagulation is initiated with a bolus of 3,000 to 5,000 units of intravenous heparin followed by an additional 1,000 units each hour. Adequate anticoagulation should be confirmed with serial measurements of an activated coagulation time to achieve a time 2- to 2.5-times greater than normal.

The suspected cerebrovascular territory in jeopardy should be interrogated first. Although early reports of angioplasty with less compliant balloon catheter systems had good safety profiles, newer balloon designs made with highly compliant silicone are now used predominantly. The silicone balloons will elongate and conform to the lumina of the arteries, therefore decreasing the risk of vessel perforation or rupture. Two basic silicone balloon catheter designs are available. A 3-mm nondetachable low-pressure balloon attached to the end of a microcatheter, or a similar size balloon in an over-the-wire system, can be used to perform angioplasty. We generally prefer an over-the-wire system because it allows for better placement and control of the angioplasty balloon in the intracranial circulation. Balloon inflation is performed with a solution of 1:1 contrast-to-saline ratio. Care must be taken to purge the balloon and catheter dead space of air prior to introduction of the system into the intracranial circulation. For the nondetachable silicone balloon, introduction of a soft 0.001-inch guidewire to near the distal tip of the microcatheter will give the system some added stiffness and pushability, and will assist in introducing the system into the guiding catheter. The guidewire can be removed prior to balloon inflation. Balloon angioplasty of a vasospastic segment can be performed only from proximal to distal if a nondetachable balloon is used. With the over-the-wire system, angioplasty may be performed either from proximal to distal or from distal to proximal. It is of the utmost importance to perform inflation lightly and cautiously. This is to prevent catastrophic vessel rupture. In contradistinction to techniques of peripheral and coronary vascular angioplasty in which the balloon is inflated to near its maximal volume with high pressures to

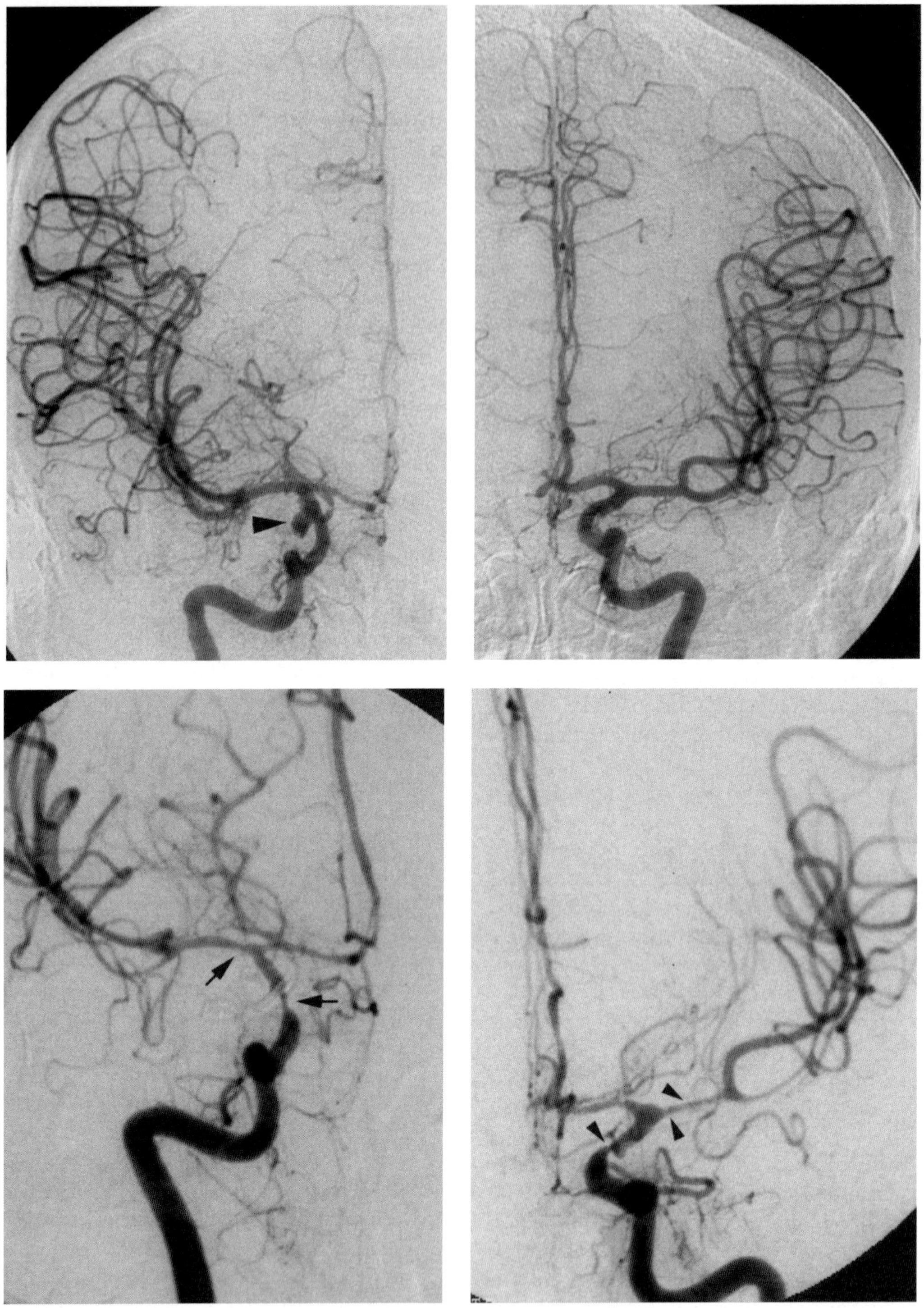
A B C D

FIGURE 8-2. This 44-year-old woman was seen at an outside hospital with a severe headache and evidence of a subarachnoid blood on CT scan. She had reported having headaches and double vision starting about 2 weeks before this. **A,B:** Right internal carotid artery and left internal carotid artery angiograms anterior projections, respectively, done on the day of the patient's subarachnoid hemorrhage demonstrate a right posterior communicating artery aneurysm *(arrowhead).* This was clipped. On postoperative day 6, the patient was confused and agitated, and a cerebral angiogram at the outside hospital showed evidence of vasospasm. After this, she was transferred. **C,D:** Right internal carotid artery and left internal carotid artery angiograms, respectively, in the anterior projection demonstrate moderate-to-severe vasospasm bilaterally. This is seen in the supraclinoid carotid segment and middle cerebral artery segment of the right internal carotid artery *(arrows)* and similarly seen in the left internal carotid artery circulation *(arrowheads).* The patient underwent balloon angioplasty of these segments using a 3-mm guidewire-directed silicone balloon. *(Figure continues.)*

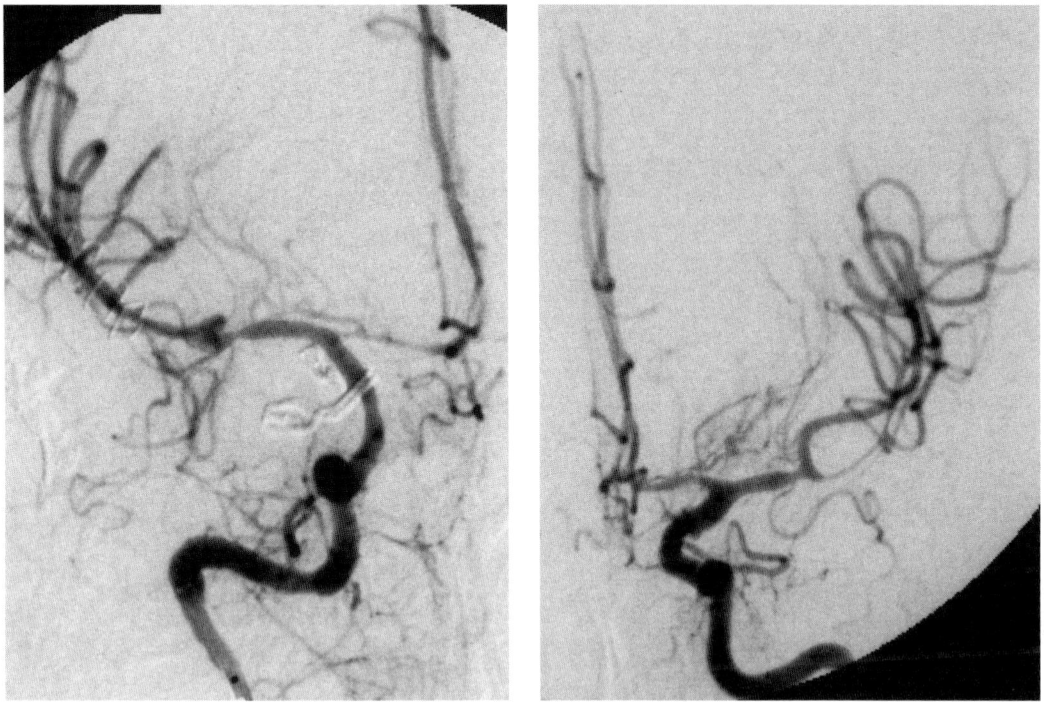

E F

FIGURE 8-2. *Continued.* **E,F:** Right internal carotid artery and left internal carotid artery angiograms, respectively, in the anterior projection following balloon angioplasty. Because the posterior communicating artery segment of the internal carotid artery had recently undergone clipping, this right internal carotid artery segment was dilated more gingerly, still allowing increased blood flow into the right carotid circulation, but it was not dilated as maximally as on the left side (compare **[E]** and **[F]**).

stretch the vessel segment, and to create fissures within the atherosclerotic intima, intracranial angioplasty should be performed gently with low pressures (approximately 0.5 atmosphere). Frequent roadmap refreshments or controlled angiograms should be performed to monitor the results and effects of angioplasty.

In the anterior circulation, angioplasty is generally performed in the supraclinoid carotid and M1 segment of the MCA (see Fig. 8-1). In general, angioplasty of the A1 segment of the anterior cerebral artery is more difficult. This is especially true with the nondetachable balloon but also applies to an over-the-wire balloon system. In the posterior circulation, angioplasty can be performed from the distal intradural portion of the vertebral artery to the P1 segment. Care must be taken to study the anatomy of the circle of Willis to assess whether the P1 segments are truly vasospastic or merely represent hypoplastic segments due to prominent posterior communicating arteries. Advancement of the balloon and inflation beyond the proximal M2, A1, and P1 segments carries a higher risk of vessel rupture due to the small size of these vascular segments and the discrepancy between the vessel diameter and balloon size, and therefore should be discouraged. Because of the limit of resolution of digital subtraction angiography, it may sometimes be quite difficult to discern changes in balloon size or see the contrast medium within the balloon lumen when one is inflating the balloon. Balloon angioplasty in more proximal segments may also result in vessel rupture, formation of thrombus with resultant thromboembolic ischemia, intracerebral hemorrhage from rupture or from reperfusion hemorrhage associated with an infarction in the territory of the repaired vessel, and vascular dissection leading to hemorrhagic or ischemic problems. Care must be taken when performing angioplasty across a recently ruptured aneurysm (Fig. 8-2). When the ruptured aneurysm is unprotected, endovascular coiling should be considered, particularly if the spasm is proximal in the circulation and treatment will result in higher perfusion pressures to the aneurysm (Fig. 8-3).

It is prudent to have tissue plasminogen activator (t-PA) and protamine sulfate in the neuroangiography suite readily available for use in the event of ischemic or hemorrhagic complications. When there is an acutely ruptured aneurysm or recently coiled ruptured aneurysm, t-PA should be used judiciously and may well be contraindicated. No matter what the circumstance, t-PA use requires close monitoring of the patient's neurologic status during the infusion.

Intraarterial Papaverine

Although papaverine has failed to supplant angioplasty as the primary endovascular treatment of cerebral vasospasm, it may be a useful adjunct to situations in which angioplasty

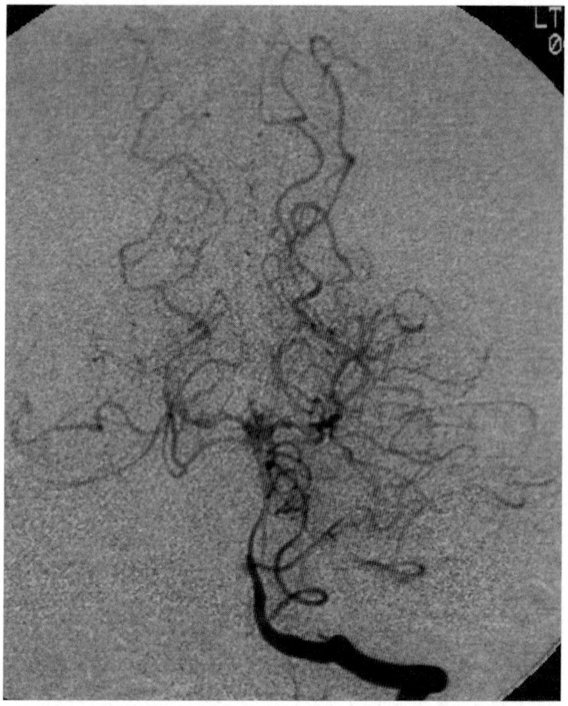

A

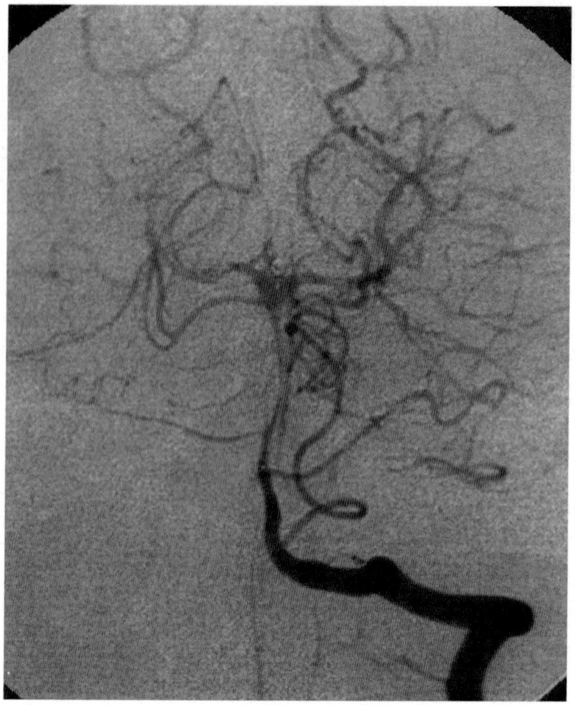

B

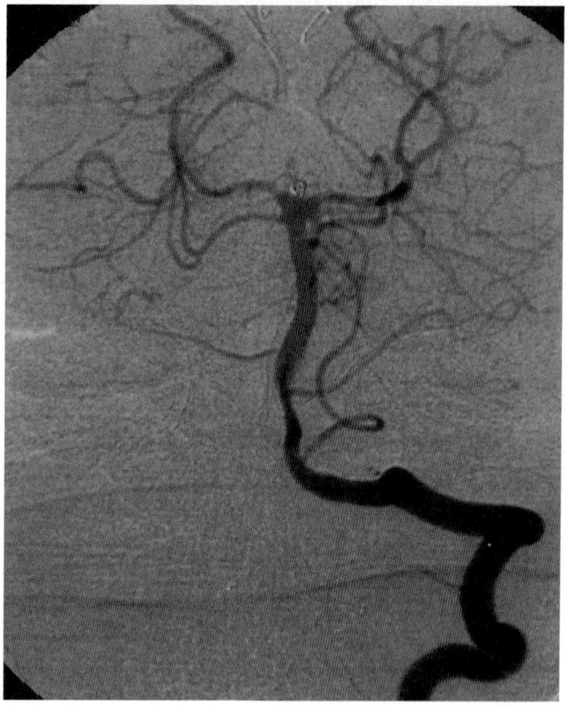

C

FIGURE 8-3. This patient suffered subarachnoid hemorrhage due to a small basilar tip aneurysm and had severe basilar trunk vasospasm. **A:** Left vertebral artery angiogram anterior projection demonstrates a 2-mm basilar apex aneurysm with severe vasospasm of the basilar artery. A microcatheter was directed into the aneurysm and the aneurysm was occluded with a GDC coil. **B:** Left vertebral artery angiogram anterior projection following coil occlusion of the basilar apex aneurysm demonstrates continued vasospasm. After coil embolization, balloon angioplasty of the basilar artery was performed. **C:** Left vertebral artery angiogram anterior projection demonstrates dilation of the basilar artery segment with improved flow noted throughout the posterior circulation. The coiled aneurysm remains occluded. (From Y. Murayama and F. Viñuela, unpublished material, with permission.)

is found to be difficult due to severely stenotic or fibrotic blood vessels. In this instance, papaverine infusion may be performed to dilate the spastic proximal arterial segments to facilitate angioplasty balloon navigation and inflation. It also may provide some short-term benefit in harder-to-reach proximal arteries, such as the A1 segment (Fig. 8-4), or in more distal arteries beyond the safe reach of angioplasty balloon therapy.

Papaverine hydrochloride is supplied as a 3% concentration, 30 mg/ml, in an acidic mixture of pH 3.3. The preparation also contains the preservative chlorobutanol. Papaverine is unstable in neutral or basic solutions. In addition, pH dependency on papaverine solution stability concentration has also been found to affect solution stability. Papaverine may form crystal precipitates, with crystal size up to 100 μm, when mixed with human serum at 3% or 0.3%

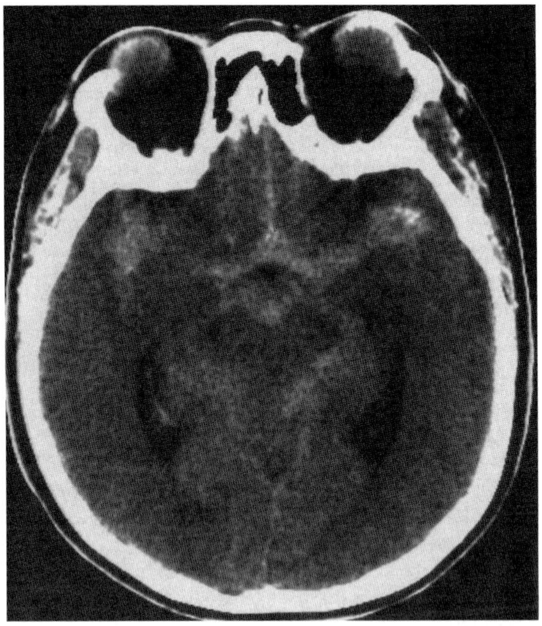

A

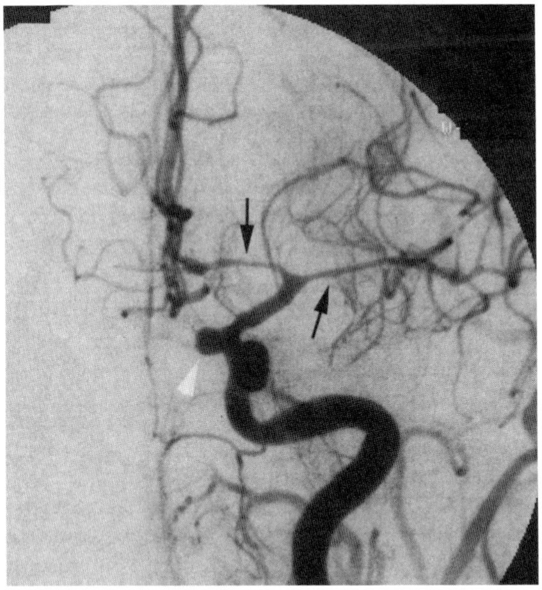

B

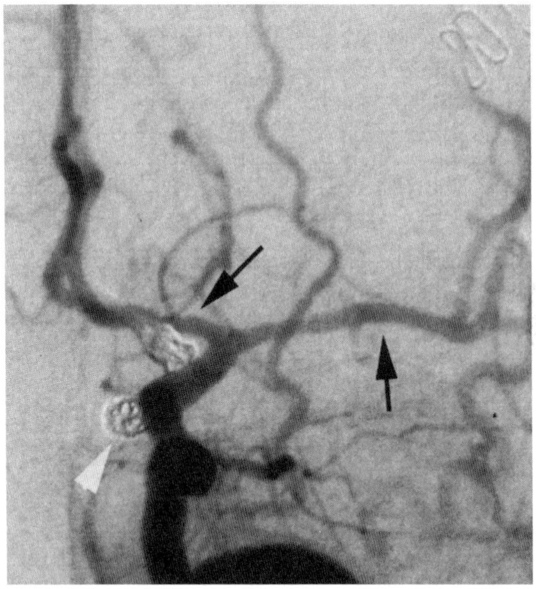

C

FIGURE 8-4. This 49-year-old woman was taken to an outside hospital after being found unconscious. **A:** A CT scan at the outside hospital demonstrated diffuse subarachnoid hemorrhage with thick clots (Fisher grade 3). An angiogram done at this time demonstrated an anterior communicating artery aneurysm and a left paraclinoid artery aneurysm. The anterior communicating artery aneurysm underwent clipping. Following surgery the patient was alert and following commands. Approximately 5 days after this, she became obtunded and experienced right-sided weakness. Repeat CT scan demonstrated a question of new subarachnoid blood, and an angiogram showed vasospasm in the left internal carotid artery circulation. She was transferred to our institution. **B:** Left internal carotid artery angiogram at the time of transfer demonstrates the left paraclinoid artery aneurysm *(white arrowhead)* and marked vasospasm in the anterior and middle cerebral artery circulations *(arrows)*. Because there was a question of repeat bleeding and concurrent vasospasm, the aneurysm was coil occluded. Papaverine was then administered to dilate both the middle and anterior cerebral artery circulation. **C:** Left internal carotid artery anterior projection following endovascular coiling and papaverine administration demonstrates occlusion of the aneurysm *(white arrowhead)* and dilation of the A1 and M1 segments of the internal carotid circulation.

concentrations. The lower of these concentrations can be resuspended with agitation or turbulence of the human serum. Also, a precipitate has been seen when a 3% papaverine solution was mixed with heparinized saline in concentrations of 2,000 to 10,000 units of heparin per liter. Precipitate formation has also been reported with ionic contrast media in multiple clinical situations [81,91]. The typical papaverine concentration infused is 0.3%, produced by diluting 300 mg of papaverine in 100 ml of normal saline. The entire 300-mg dose is administered into the affected vascular territory over 20 to 30 minutes, either using incremental manual injection or by continuous machine injection. It is important to ensure that the microcatheter is not in a wedged position or catheterizing a small branch, such as a perforating branch or ophthalmic artery. If more than one vascular territory is involved, additional infusions of 300 mg of papaverine can be given. Care must be taken to monitor the systemic blood pressure as well as the intracranial pressure to prevent systemic hypotension and increased intracranial pressure [30,88]. The microcatheter tip is typically placed beyond the origin of the ophthalmic artery in the supraclinoid ICA. Further superselective catheterization of the MCA or ACA is up to the discretion of the operator. In the posterior circulation, the catheter is typically placed below the region affected by the vasospasm. Papaverine infusion can be given in smaller aliquots, with frequent control angiograms to monitor the changes of vasodilatory effects of the agent and also for microcatheter repositioning.

Side effects reported with the use of intraarterial papaverine have included transient neurologic events such as pupillary dilation, transient hemiparesis, and respiratory arrest [81, 92,93].

Mydriasis is a common phenomenon with papaverine infusion, particularly when the catheter is proximal to the ophthalmic artery. Hendrix et al. [93] reported five cases of ipsilateral pupillary dilation that developed during local intraarterial infusion of papaverine. All patients were being treated for symptomatic vasospasm secondary to SAH. In each case, the tip of the infusion catheter was positioned in the internal carotid artery in close proximity to the origin of the ophthalmic artery. The effect on the pupil is transient and resolves quickly with discontinuation of papaverine infusion. Infusions into the posterior circulation have been associated with respiratory arrest and also carry the potential for cardiac dysfunction. The risk is increased with infusion into the distal vertebral artery or proximal basilar trunk below the origin of the anterior inferior cerebellar artery and likely due to transient depression of medullary respiratory and cardiovascular nuclei [81]. Systemic hypertension has not been reported as a side effect when infused at the rates described above but has been reported with faster infusion of papaverine, particularly when infusion of multiple vascular territories were required [81]. If systemic hypotension is observed, the infusion should be terminated. The etiology of transient neurologic events seen with papaverine infusion is not completely understood but may be related to the formation of papaverine microcrystals demonstrated by *in vitro* experiments [81,91].

REFERENCES

1. Ljunggren B, Saveland H, Brandt L, et al. Early operation and overall outcome in aneurysmal subarachnoid hemorrhage. *J Neurosurg* 1985;62:547–551.
2. Mayberg MR, Batjer HH, Dacey R, et al. Special report: a statement for healthcare professionals from a special writing group of the stroke council, American Heart Association. *Circulation* 1994;90:2592–2605.
3. Kassell NF, Torner JC, Haley EC Jr, et al. The international cooperative study on the timing of aneurysm surgery. Part 1. Overall management results. *J Neurosurg* 1990;73:18–36.
4. Kassell NF, Torner JC, Haley EC Jr, et al. The international cooperative study on the timing of aneurysm surgery. Part 2. Surgical results. *J Neurosurg* 1990;73:37–47.
5. Ropper AH, Zervas NT. Outcome 1 year after SAH from cerebral aneurysms: management morbidity, mortality, and functional status in 112 consecutive good-risk patients. *J Neurosurg* 1994; 60:909–915.
6. Solenski NJ, Haley EC Jr, Kassell NF, et al. Medical complications of aneurysmal subarachnoid hemorrhage: a report of the multicenter, cooperative aneurysm study. *Crit Care Med* 1995; 23:1007–1017.
7. Haley EC Jr, Kassell NF, Torner JC. International cooperative study on the timing of aneurysm surgery: the North American experience. *Stroke* 1992;23:205–214.
8. Adams HP Jr., Kassell NF, Torner JC, et al. Predicting cerebral ischemia after aneurysmal subarachnoid hemorrhage: influences of clinical condition, CT results, and antifibrinolytic therapy. *Neurology* 1987;37:1586–1591.
9. Petruk KC, West M, Mohr F, et al. Nimodipine treatment in poor-grade aneurysm patients: results of multicenter double-blind placebo-controlled trial. *J Neurosurg* 1988;68:505–517.
10. Pickard JG, Murray GD, Illingworth R, et al. Effect of oral nimodipine on cerebral infarction and outcome after subarachnoid hemorrhage: British aneurysm nimodipine trial. *BMJ* 1989;298: 636–642.
11. Mayberg MR, Batjer HH, Dacey R, et al. Guidelines for the management of aneurysmal subarachnoid hemorrhage. *Stroke* 1994;25:2315–2328.
12. Le Roux P, Haglund M, Mayberg MR, et al. Symptomatic cerebral vasospasm following tumor resection. *Surg Neurol* 1991;36: 25–31.
13. Martin NA, Doberstein C, Zane C, et al. Posttraumatic cerebral arterial spasm: transcranial Doppler ultrasound, cerebral blood flow, and angiographic findings. *J Neurosurg* 1992;77:575–583.
14. Schievink WI, Wijdicks EF, Spetzler RF. Diffuse vasospasm after pretruncal nonaneurysmal subarachnoid hemorrhage. *AJNR Am J Neuroradiol* 2000;21:521–523.
15. Weir, B, Disney L, Grace M. Daily trends in white blood cell count and temperature after subarachnoid hemorrhage from aneurysm. *Neurosurgery* 1989;25:161–167.
16. Kwak R, Niizuma H, Ohi T, et al. Angiographic study of cerebral vasospasm following rupture of intracranial aneurysms. Part 1. Time of appearance. *Surg Neurol* 1979;11:257–262.
17. Zabramski JM, Hamilton MG. Cerebral vasospasm. In: Carter LP, Spetzler RF, eds. *Neurovascular surgery.* New York: McGraw-Hill, 1995:583–601.
18. McKhann GM, Le Roux PD. Perioperative and intensive unit care of patients with aneurysmal subarachnoid hemorrhage. *Neurosurg Clin N Am* 1998;9:595–613.
19. Robertson EG. Cerebral lesions due to intracranial aneurysms. *Brain* 1949;72:150–185.
20. Ecker A, Reimenschneider PA. Arteriographic demonstration of spasm of the intracranial arteries. *J Neurosurg* 1951;8:660–667.
21. Pool JL. Cerebral vasospasm. *N Engl J Med* 1958;259: 1259–1264.
22. Stornelli SA, French JD. Subarachnoid hemorrhage: factors in prognosis and management. *J Neurosurg* 1964;21:769–780.
23. Allcock JM, Drake CG. Ruptured intracranial aneurysms: the role of arterial spasm. *J Neurosurg* 1965;22:21–29.
24. Fisher CM, Kistler JP, Davis JM. Relation of cerebral vasospasm to subarachnoid hemorrhage visualized by computerized tomographic scanning. *Neurosurgery* 1980;6:1–9.
25. Geraud G, Trmoulet M, Guell A, et al. The prognostic value of noninvasive CBF measurement in subarachnoid hemorrhage. *Stroke* 1984;15:301–305.
26. Symon L. Disordered cerebrovascular physiology in aneurysmal subarachnoid hemorrhage. *Acta Neurochir (Wien)* 1978;41:7–22.
27. Heilbrun MP, Olesen J, Lassen NA. Regional cerebral blood flow studies in subarachnoid hemorrhage. *J Neurosurg* 1972;37: 36–44.
28. Martin NA, Carter LP, Spetzler RF. Measurement of regional cerebral blood flow in aneurysm surgery. *Clin Neurosurg* 1985; 32:79–104.
29. Powers WJ, Grubb RL Jr, Baker RP, et al. Regional cerebral blood flow and metabolism in reversible ischemia due to vasospasm: determination by positron emission tomography. *J Neurosurg* 1985;62:539–546.
30. Song JK, Elliott JP, Eskridge JM. Neuroradiologic diagnosis and treatment of vasospasm. *Neuroimaging Clin N Am* 1997;7: 819–835.
31. Fazl M, Houlden DA, Weaver K. Correlation between cerebral blood flow, somatosensory evoked potentials, CT scan grade and

neurological grade in patients with subarachnoid hemorrhage. *Can J Neurol Sci* 1991;18:453–457.
32. Origitano TC, Wascher TM, Reichman OH, et al. Sustained increased cerebral blood flow with prophylactic hypertensive hypervolemic hemodilution (triple H therapy) after subarachnoid hemorrhage. *Neurosurgery* 1990;27:729–740.
33. Dietrich HH, Dacey RG Jr. Molecular keys to the problems of cerebral vasospasm. *Neurosurgery* 2000;46:517–530.
34. Megyesi JF, Vollrath B, Cook DA, et al. *In vivo* animal models of cerebral vasospasm: a review. *Neurosurgery* 2000;46:448–461.
35. Macdonald RL, Weir BKA. A review of hemoglobin and the pathogenesis of cerebral vasospasm. *Stroke* 1991;22:971–982.
36. Osaka K. Prolonged vasospasm produced by the breakdown products of erythrocytes. *J Neurosurg* 1977;47:403–411.
37. Ikeda Y, Long DM. The molecular basis of brain injury and brain edema: the role of oxygen free radicals. *Neurosurgery* 1990; 27:1–11.
38. Sasaki T, Tanishima T, Asano T, et al. Significance of lipid peroxidation in the genesis of chronic vasospasm following rupture of an intracranial aneurysm. *Acta Neurochir Suppl* 1979;28: 536.
39. Hall ED, McCall JM, Chase RL, et al. Nonglucocorticoid steroid analog of methylprednisolone duplicates its high-dose pharmacology in models of central nervous system trauma and neuronal membrane damage. *J Pharmacol Exp Ther* 1987;242:137–142.
40. Vollmer DG, Kassell NF, Hongo K, et al. Effect of the nonglucocorticoid 21-aminosteroid U74006F on experimental cerebral vasospasm. *Surg Neurol* 1989;31:190–194.
41. Haley EC Jr, Kassell NF, Apperson-Hansen C, et al. A randomized, double-blind, vehicle-controlled trial of tirilazad mesylate in patients with aneurysmal subarachnoid hemorrhage. *J Neurosurg* 1997;86:467–474.
42. Megyesi JF, Findlay JM, Vollrath B, et al. *In vivo* angioplasty prevents the development of vasospasm in canine carotid arteries: pharmacological and morphological analyses. *Stroke* 1997;28: 1216–1224.
43. Honma Y, Fujiwara T, Irie K, et al. Morphological changes in human cerebral arteries after percutaneous transluminal angioplasty for vasospasm caused by subarachnoid hemorrhage. *Neurosurgery* 1995;36:1073–1081.
44. Qureshi AI, Sung GY, Razumovsky AY, et al. Early identification of patients at risk for symptomatic vasospasm after aneurysmal subarachnoid hemorrhage. *Crit Care Med* 2000;28:984–990.
45. Schaller C, Rohde V, Meyer B, et al. Amount of subarachnoid blood and vasospasm: current aspects—a transcranial Doppler study. *Acta Neurochir (Wein)* 1995;136:67–71.
46. Zabramski JM, Spetzler RF, Bonstelle C. Chronic cerebral vasospasm: effect of volume and timing of hemorrhage in a canine model. *Neurosurgery* 1986;18:1–6.
47. Chakeres DW, Bryan RN. Acute subarachnoid hemorrhage: *in vitro* comparison of magnetic resonance imaging and computed tomography. *AJNR Am J Neuroradiol* 1986;7:223–228.
48. Woodcock RJ Jr, Short J, Do HM, et al. Imaging of acute subarachnoid hemorrhage with a fluid-attenuated inversion recovery sequence in an animal model: comparison with non-contrast enhanced CT. *AJNR Am J Neuroradiol* 2001;22:1698–1703.
49. Perl J II, Tkach JA, Porras-Jimenez M, et al. Hemorrhage detected using MR imaging in the setting of acute stroke: an in vivo model. *AJNR Am J Neuroradiol* 1999;20:1863–1870.
50. Noguchi K, Ogawa A, Inugami A, et al. Acute subarachnoid hemorrhage: MR imaging with fluid-attenuated inversion recovery pulse sequences. *Radiology* 1995;196:773–777.
51. Newell DW, Grady MS, Eskridge JM, et al. Distribution of angiographic vasospasm after subarachnoid hemorrhage: implications for diagnosis by transcranial Doppler ultrasonography. *Neurosurgery* 1990;27:574–577.
52. Aaslid R, Markwalder TM, Nornes H. Noninvasive transcranial Doppler ultrasound recording of flow velocity in basal cerebral arteries. *J Neurosurg* 1982;57:769–774.
53. Lindegaard KF, Nornes H, Bakke SJ, et al. A noninvasive Doppler ultrasound method for the evaluation of patients with subarachnoid hemorrhage. *Acta Radiol Diagn (Stockh)* 1986;369: 96–98.
54. Newell DW, Elliott JP, Eskridge JM, et al. Endovascular therapy for aneurysmal vasospasm. *Crit Care Clin* 1999;15:685–699.
55. Yonas H, Sekhar L, Johnson SW, et al. Determination of irreversible ischemia by xenon-enhanced computed tomographic monitoring of cerebral blood flow in patients with symptomatic vasospasm. *Neurosurgery* 1989;24:368–372.
56. Bracard S, Anxionnat R, Auliac S, et al. Relevance of diffusion and perfusion weighted MRI for endovascular treatment of vasospasm in subarachnoid hemorrhage. *J Neuroradiol* 2001;28: 27–32.
57. Rowe J, Blamire AM, Domingo Z, et al. Discrepancies between cerebral perfusion and metabolism after subarachnoid hemorrhage: a magnetic resonance approach. *J Neurol Neurosurg Psychiatry* 1998;64:98–103.
58. Condette-Auliac S, Bracard S, Anxionnat R, et al. Vasospasm after subarachnoid hemorrhage: interest in diffusion-weighted MR imaging. *Stroke* 2001;32:1818–1824.
59. Rordorf G, Koroshetz WJ, Copen WA, et al. Diffusion and perfusion-weighted imaging in vasospasm after subarachnoid hemorrhage. *Stroke* 1999;30:599–605.
60. Cloft HJ, Joseph GJ, Dion JE. Risk of cerebral angiography in patients with subarachnoid hemorrhage, cerebral aneurysm, and arteriovenous malformation: a meta-analysis. *Stroke* 1999;30: 317–320.
61. Le Roux PD, Elliott JP, Eskridge JM, et al. Risks and benefits of diagnostic angiography after aneurysm surgery: a retrospective analysis of 597 studies. *Neurosurgery* 1998;42:1248–1254.
62. Feigin VL, Rinkel GJE, Algra A. Calcium antagonists for aneurysmal subarachnoid hemorrhage. *Cochrane Database Syst Rev* 2001; 2.
63. Meyer FB. Calcium antagonists and vasospasm. *Neurosurg Clin N Am* 1990;1:367–376.
64. Kassell NF, Peerless SJ, Durwald QJ, et al. Treatment of cerebral vasospasm with intravascular volume expansion and induced arterial hypertension. *Neurosurgery* 1982;11:337–343.
65. Feigin VL, Rinkel GJE, Algra A, et al. Circulatory volume expansion for aneurysmal subarachnoid hemorrhage. *Cochrane Database Syst Rev* 2001;2.
66. Rosenwasser RH, Delgago TE, Buchheit WA, et al. Control of hypertension and prophylaxis against vasospasm in cases of subarachnoid hemorrhage. *Neurosurgery* 1983;12:658–661.
67. Lennihan L, Solomon RA, Mayer SA, et al. Effect of volume therapy on cerebral blood flow after subarachnoid hemorrhage. *Neurology* 1994;44[Suppl]:862.
68. Zubkov YN, Nikiforov BM, Shustin VA. Balloon catheter technique for dilatation of constricted cerebral arteries after aneurysmal SAH. *Acta Neurochir* 1984;70:65–79.
69. Zubkov YN, Alexander LF, Smith RR, et al. Angioplasty of vasospasm: is it reasonable? *Neurol Res* 1994;16:9–11.
70. Higashida RT, Halbach VV, Dowd CF, et al. Intravascular balloon dilatation therapy for intracranial arterial vasospasm: patient selection, technique, and clinical results. *Neurosurg Rev* 1992;15: 89–95.
71. Eskridge JM, McAuliffe W, Song JK, et al. Balloon angioplasty for the treatment of vasospasm: results of first 50 cases. *Neurosurgery* 1998;42:510–517.
72. Coyne TJ, Montanera WJ, Macdonald RL, et al. Percutaneous transluminal angioplasty for cerebral vasospasm after subarachnoid hemorrhage. *Can J Surg* 1994;37:391–396.

73. Bejjani GK, Bank WO, Olan WJ, et al. The efficacy and safety of angioplasty for cerebral vasospasm after subarachnoid hemorrhage. *Neurosurgery* 1998;42:979–986.
74. Firlik AD, Kaufmann AM, Jungreis CA, et al. Effect of transluminal angioplasty on cerebral blood flow in the management of symptomatic vasospasm following aneurysmal subarachnoid hemorrhage. *J Neurosurg* 1997;86:830–839.
75. Rosenwasser RH, Armonda RA, Thomas JE, et al. Therapeutic modalities for the management of cerebral vasospasm: timing of endovascular options. *Neurosurgery* 1999;44:975–979.
76. Clouston JE, Numaguchi Y, Zoarski GH, et al. Intraarterial papaverine infusion for cerebral vasospasm after subarachnoid hemorrhage. *AJNR Am J Neuroradiol* 1995;16:27–38.
77. Marks MP, Steinberg GK, Lane B. Intraarterial papaverine for the treatment of vasospasm. *AJNR Am J Neuroradiol* 1993;14: 822–826.
78. Kaku Y, Yonekawa Y, Tsukahara T, et al. Superselective intraarterial infusion of papaverine for the treatment of cerebral vasospasm after subarachnoid hemorrhage. *J Neurosurg* 1992;77:842–847.
79. Chaturvedi S, St Pierre ME, Bertasio B. Cerebral angioplasty practice at major medical centers in the United States. *Neuroradiology* 2000;42:218–220.
80. Muizelaar JP, Zwienenberg M, Rudisill NA, et al. The prophylactic use of transluminal balloon angioplasty in patients with Fisher grade 3 subarachnoid hemorrhage: a pilot study. *J Neurosurg* 1999;91:51–58.
81. Mathis JM, Jensen ME, Dion JE. Technical considerations on intraarterial papaverine hydrochloride for cerebral vasospasm. *Neuroradiology* 1997;39:90–98.
82. Vorkapic P, Bevan RD, Benan JA. Pharmacologic irreversible narrowing in chronic cerebral vasospasm in rabbits is associated with functional damage. *Stroke* 1990;21:1478–1484.
83. Kassell NF, Helm G, Simmons N, et al. Treatment of cerebral vasospasm with intra-arterial papaverine. *J Neurosurg* 1992;77: 848–852.
84. Polin RS, Hansen CA, German P, et al. Intra-arterially administered papaverine for the treatment of symptomatic cerebral vasospasm. *Neurosurgery* 1998;42:1256–1267.
85. Vajkoczy P, Horn P, Bauhuf C, et al. Effect of intra-arterial papaverine on regional cerebral blood flow in hemodynamically relevant cerebral vasospasm. *Stroke* 2001;32:498–505.
86. Numaguchi Y, Zoarski GH, Clouston JE, et al. Repeat intra-arterial papaverine for recurrent cerebral vasospasm after subarachnoid hemorrhage. *Neuroradiology* 1997;39:751–759.
87. Elliott JP, Newell DW, Lam DJ, et al. Comparison of balloon angioplasty and papaverine infusion for the treatment of vasospasm following aneurysmal subarachnoid hemorrhage. *J Neurosurg* 1998;88:277–284.
88. McAuliffe W, Townsend M, Eskridge JM, et al. Intracranial pressure changes induced during papaverine infusion for treatment of vasospasm. *J Neurosurg* 1995;83:430–434.
89. Carhuapoma JR, Qureshi AI, Tamargo RJ, et al. Intra-arterial papaverine-induced seizures: case report and review of the literature. *Surg Neurol* 2001;56:159–163.
90. Mayberg MR. Cerebral vasospasm. *Neurosurg Clin N Am* 1998; 9:615–627.
91. Mathis JM, DeNardo A, Thibault L, et al. In vitro evaluation of papaverine hydrochloride incompatibilities: a simulation of intraarterial infusion for cerebral vasospasm. *AJNR Am J Neuroradiol* 1994;15:1665–1670.
92. Mathis JM, DeNardo A, Jensen ME. Transient neurological events associated with intra-arterial papaverine infusion for subarachnoid hemorrhage induced vasospasm. *AJNR Am J Neuroradiol* 1994;15:1671–1674.
93. Hendrix LE, Dion JE, Jensen ME, et al. Papaverine-induced mydriasis. *AJNR Am J Neuroradiol* 1994;15:716–718.

Endovascular and Percutaneous Therapy of the Brain and Spine, edited by Michael P. Marks and Huy M. Do.
Lippincott Williams & Wilkins, Philadelphia © 2002.

9

ARTERIOVENOUS MALFORMATIONS: OVERVIEW

IAN G. FLEETWOOD
GARY K. STEINBERG

Arteriovenous malformations (AVMs) are pathologic networks of arteriovenous shunts. They usually take the form of a compact nidus fed by one or more arteries and emptying into one or more veins. These lesions of the central nervous system can affect children and adults. Their clinical features and natural history can be quite variable. In this chapter we explore the various facets of high-flow AVMs, focusing on their clinical features, hemorrhage risk, treatment indications, and the role of microsurgical and radiosurgical management. Endovascular treatment, which forms a significant tool in the armamentarium used in treating these lesions, is covered in detail in the following chapter (Chapter 10). In this chapter we do not cover other vascular malformations of the central nervous system, such as dural arteriovenous fisutulas, vein of Galen malformations, capillary telangiectasias, developmental venous anomalies, or cavernous malformations. Dural arteriovenous fistulas are discussed separately (Chapter 11), as are carotid-cavernous fistulas (Chapter 12). Spinal AVMs are also the subject of another chapter in this volume (Chapter 16). Readers are directed to several contemporary reviews of AVM management [1, 2], as well as the American Heart Association guidelines for management of patients with AVMs [3].

DEFINITION

Most readers of this volume are familiar with the nature of AVMs. They are generally thought to be congenital lesions of the cerebral vasculature consisting of variably sized nidi. The AVM nidus is a tangle of arteriovenous shunts that is fed by one or more arteries. There is no intervening capillary network and therefore the arterial blood is shunted directly into the venous system, which is represented by one or multiple veins. These veins travel either superficially or deeply but eventually drain into the cerebral venous sinuses. There can be intervening brain parenchyma within an AVM nidus, however it is thought to be nonfunctional. Anatomically, AVMs can be located anywhere in the central nervous system, including the cerebral hemispheres, basal ganglia and thalamus, cerebellum, brainstem, and within the ventricular system.

EPIDEMIOLOGY AND DEMOGRAPHICS

The actual incidence and prevalence of AVMs is not well defined. For decades, estimates have been quoted in the literature based on early clinical and autopsy studies. However, few (if any) comprehensive studies of AVM incidence and prevalence have been conducted in a nonbiased population-based fashion. Based on data presented in the Cooperative Study of Intracranial Aneurysms and Subarachnoid Hemorrhage, Michelsen estimated the prevalence to be 0.14% (or 140 per 100,000) [4]. However, this was strictly an extrapolation and its derivation has been criticized in more recent work [5]. The often-cited autopsy series of McCormick estimates the prevalence to be 521 per 100,000 [6], but this data was accumulated from two centers over a period of 19 years and has certain limitations as well. In the pediatric population the prevalence is thought to be lower because only 10% to 20% of AVMs are diagnosed in children. Garza-Mercado et al. estimated the prevalence in pediatric populations to be 0.014% to 0.028%, but this figure was derived using Michelsen's original estimate and the estimated proportion of pediatric AVMs [7]. According to the work of Brown et al., in the general population the prevalence of hemorrhage from vascular malformations is 7.5 per 100,000 people [8]. In a recent reanalysis of previous publications to clarify the incidence and prevalence of cerebral AVMs as accurately as possible, Berman et al. concluded that it is not currently feasible to definitively establish the prevalence of AVMs in the population [5]. However, they estimated the prevalence of active (at-risk) disease to be less

I.G. Fleetwood: Department of Neurosurgery and Stanford Stroke Center, Stanford University School of Medicine, Stanford, California.
G.K. Steinberg: Department of Neurosurgery and Stanford Stroke Center, Stanford University, Stanford, California.

than 10.3 per 100,000 (or approximately 0.01% of the population), noting that once disease is detected in this cohort, patients will often be treated and therefore no longer at risk. This figure is remarkably lower than previous estimates derived from the Cooperative Study (0.14%) [4] and large autopsy series (0.52%) [6], and Berman et al. systematically explain the reasons that previous prevalence figures should be considered unfounded and overestimates. Most recently, Hillman reported a population-based study in which 135 *de novo* AVMs were diagnosed in a captive population of 986,000 persons over an 11-year period, yielding an annual incidence rate of 1.24 per 100,000 population [9], similar to the rate of 1.11 per 100,000 described by Brown et al. [10]. Many patients will remain asymptomatic, and therefore accurate incidence and prevalence statistics may not be attainable even through prospective research.

Most AVMs occur in patients aged 20 to 40 years [11–13]. This has been borne out in numerous retrospective and prospective studies of patients with AVMs [11,14]. In the largest and most recent study directed specifically at determining the demographic characteristics of patients with AVMs, the average age at diagnosis was 31.2 years [15]. However, approximately 8% to 20% of AVMs occur in children [7,11,16–20]. The tendency for delayed diagnosis has been attributed to both increasing tortuosity and progressive changes in the abnormal vessels as well as to actual growth of the AVM. In large reported series of patients with AVMs, the sex distribution was essentially equal with a slight male preponderance. In the 453 patients with AVMs evaluated in the Cooperative Study in 1966, 52% were male [11]. Of the 662 patients managed endovascularly by Mansmann et al. and reported in 2000, 57% were male [14]. Of the 1,289 patients studied by several groups worldwide and reported in 2000, 55% were male [15], and of 1,479 patients described by Karlsson et al., 51% were male [21].

EMBRYOLOGY

The cause of AVMs is unknown [22]. AVMs are considered congenital lesions [23,24,30]. Pfeifer originally suggested that AVMs form through persistence of one (or multiple) arteriovenous fistula that is normally present, but this theory has largely been rejected [25,26]. Most clinicians adopt Yasargil's theory regarding the nature of AVMs [27]. It is proposed that the lesions develop due to maldevelopment during Streeter's 2 to 5 stage. These lesions are thought to develop from a proliferative capillaropathy. Citing Evans' work demonstrating that the primitive cerebral vasculature exists as a capillary network, he implicates maldevelopment of the stages of vessel maturation into the normal arterial and venous structures adjacent to the capillaries. He also refers to the studies by Dandy suggesting the persistence of primordial arteriovenous connections [28], as well as that of Olivecrona and Ladenheim [29] hypothesizing agenesis of the capillary system of the mesoderm during embryogenesis. A third possibility includes secondary destruction of the capillary network, creating direct arteriovenous connections. Suggesting that there is a middle ground between these theories, Yasargil proposed that there was not complete agenesis or secondary destruction, but rather abnormal development of the capillaries that he referred to as *proliferative capillaropathy.* These vessels would then undergo metamorphic angiodysplasia into the abnormal vessels seen in AVMs.

However, two interesting theories or modifications to previous theories regarding the development of AVMs have been published over the past several years. Mullan et al. recently reviewed the embryology of the cerebral vascular system [30]. It was mentioned that although cerebral AVMs are considered to be congenital lesions, they are often impossible to identify in utero or with perinatal ultrasonography. This suggests either that the lesions are too small to detect in these early stages or that they actually develop after birth. It is further suggested that the absence of a middle cerebral vein may predict the later formation of an AVM. The authors remind us that most AVMs do not drain into the tentorial sinus, indicating that the timing of AVM formation is possibly near the 80-mm stage. The multitude and lack of functional architecture is thought to indicate that "dedicated" AVM vessels represent a primitive vessel type. Their observations led the authors to speculate that AVMs form during a stage of absorption of the multiple pial-dural subarachnoid veins (40- to 80-mm stage), with potential for growth thereafter.

The congenital nature of AVMs is considered implicit by many. Although seldom diagnosed in childhood, these lesions are assumed to be congenital even when diagnosed in adulthood. This notion is challenged in a review paper by Lasjaunias [22]. He indicates that AVMs are the result of biologic dysfunction of the remodeling process at the capillovenous junction [22]. Noting that intracranial blood vessels are influenced by an ongoing process of genetically controlled maintenance and homeostasis, he suggests that abnormalities such as AVMs could be a result of this renewal process, rather than a result of the original construction of the vascular tree. In discussion of the embryology of AVMs, he concludes that large ones should be formed by a mutation early in embryogenesis and smaller ones should be formed by a causative event later. According to this theory, AVMs should not grow, and he speculates that growth as reported in the literature may be due to a secondary angiopathy or angiogenesis following ischemia or hemorrhage. He notes that in genetic syndromes associated with AVMs, such as hemorrhagic hereditary telangiectasia (HHT, also known as Rendu-Osler-Weber syndrome), there may be an abnormality in the postcapillary venule, resulting in venous remodeling failure. Finally, he comments on the role of vascular remodeling, as originally described by Gibbons and Dzau [31], in AVM biology and postulates that a cerebral AVM is ultimately the result of a congenital event. This initial event may or may not be morphologically apparent at birth but may change as the result of vascular remodeling. The target of remodeling is thought to be the venous side of the capillovenous junction. The subsequent generation of an AVM is said to be the result of secondary triggers including mechanical, hormonal, pharmaceutical, hemodynamic, thermal, radiation, viral, infective, and metabolic factors that lead to the eventual phenotype of the AVM.

Interestingly, Stapf and Mohr have pointed out in a recent review article that there are no reports documenting the diagnosis of cerebral AVMs in utero; however, this diagnosis can be made sonographically or by magnetic resonance imaging (MRI) during the prenatal period for infants born with vein of Galen malformations [32]. This would appear to contradict theories that suggest the embryonic nature of AVMs, but the basis for this speculation is only from case reports.

CLINICAL FEATURES AND NATURAL HISTORY

Patients with intracranial AVMs generally tend to experience intracranial hemorrhage, seizures or epilepsy, headaches, or focal neurologic deficit. Although not generally a primary symptom, many patients are found to suffer from cognitive difficulties or developmental delay. Depending on location of the AVM nidus, hydrocephalus can also contribute to the symptom complex. In addition to the above, several unusual clinical features have been described, representing peculiar manifestations of focal deficits. Many patients have multiple simultaneous difficulties from the AVM.

In an early study, Waltimo compared a group of patients who sought treatment for seizures alone to a group that suffered only from hemorrhages [33]. It was determined that the group with seizures had AVMs of smaller volumes than the group that had hemorrhages, confirming an earlier observation of MacKenzie [34]. Much effort has been directed to determining what leads to the various clinical features in patients with AVM and, despite numerous studies, certain factors in the clinical picture of AVMs remain controversial. Additionally, various studies have attempted to elaborate on the natural history of AVMs as a function of their original clinical picture. Nonetheless, in the upcoming sections we will summarize what is known about the clinical features and natural history in patients following diagnosis of AVM.

Hemorrhage

Natural History

Intracranial hemorrhage is potentially the most devastating consequence of intracranial AVM. The majority of studies dealing with the natural history of AVMs have examined the propensity of these lesions to cause hemorrhage and, although this has been well studied over the past two decades, there is still some uncertainty regarding the likelihood of a patient with an AVM to suffer hemorrhage. Because many of the early studies estimating hemorrhage risk were retrospective, many of the data presented are based on patients whose AVMs were diagnosed due to nonhemorrhagic clinical pictures, with epilepsy, focal neurologic deficit, or headache, and then followed clinically thereafter. However, more often the data are derived from cohorts of patients who were managed nonoperatively because the anatomical location of their AVM was not favorable for surgery [1]. In such instances, a selection bias limits conclusions about the true natural history of AVMs. Although the natural history has been reviewed in several forums [4,35–38], we will summarize these data again here, including recent advances.

One of the earliest attempts to determine the natural history of AVMs included not only those patients selected for nonsurgical management, but also those who had undergone nondefinitive surgical procedures [39]. Svien and McRae followed 68 patients for intervals up to 30 years and 11 died of causes attributable to their AVMs (16%). The method of reporting does not allow specific determination of annual risk.

Later, Troupp et al. first described their cohort of 137 patients selected for nonsurgical management [40]. With a mean follow-up of greater than 4.5 years, 24% of patients were disabled and 10% were dead from factors attributable to their AVMs. They also noted that patients with parietal, central, and infratentorial AVMs had a much higher hemorrhage rate. This cohort formed the foundation of what would later be considered a definitive study of the natural history of AVMs [41]. In 1972, Forster et al. reported the long-term follow-up of a cohort managed between 1935 and 1965. Among the 35 patients managed conservatively there was a mean follow-up duration of 12 years, and 29% of patients had suffered new hemorrhage and 17% had died as a result of hemorrhage [42]. This is comparable to the mortality rate of 16% derived in the review by Pool of 523 patients [43]. Another sizable cohort of conservatively managed patients was described by Guidetti and Delitala in 1980 [12]. They observed 50 patients whose AVMs were deemed unfavorable for surgical resection or who refused to undergo surgery. During an unspecified long-term follow-up period, the mortality rate was 20%, and 17 patients suffered an intracranial hemorrhage.

Although these earlier studies began to delineate roughly the natural history of AVMs, it was not until two decades ago that we truly began to develop a better understanding of the hemorrhage risks associated with AVMs. These studies are summarized in Table 9-1. Graf et al. studied 57 patients who had nonruptured AVMs for a mean duration of 4.8 years and found an annual hemorrhage rate of 2% to 3% over as long as 20 years of follow-up [44]. In those whose lesions had ruptured, the mean follow-up was 2 years and the hemorrhage rate was 6% per year during the first year, returning to a baseline rate of 2% per year for the following 20 years. Fults and Kelly found that the rebleeding

TABLE 9-1. NATURAL HISTORY OF HEMORRHAGE FROM AN AVM

Author, Year	Overall Rate[a]	Previous Hemorrhage[a]	No Prior Hemorrhage[a]	Morbidity	Mortality
Graf, 1983	—	6% in year 1 2% for 20 yr	2–3% 2–3% in those with seizures	—	12.7% *per hemorrhage* (17/134 bleeds)
Fults, 1984	—	2.0–3.0%	—	—	40.5% *per hemorrhage* (17/42 bleeds)
Crawford, 1986	2.1–3.0%	2.5–3.6%	1.65–1.70% 1.5%–2.2% in those with seizures	—	1.6–1.8% per yr in those who bled 1.4–2.0% per yr in those who did not bleed
Brown, 1988	—	—	2.25% (18.5% of patients bled over 8.2 yr) 1.3% after 1 yr 2.2% after 15 yr	—	29% (9/31 patients who hemorrhaged, died)
Itoyama, 1989	—	6.9% in first yr 1.91% after 5 yr 0.92% after 15 yr	4.8% in first yr 1.9% after 5 yr 1.3% after 10 yr	—	—
Ondra, 1990	4.0%	3.9%	4.3% in those with seizures 3.9% in those without seizure or hemorrhage	1.7% per year	1% per yr
Brown, 1996	—	—	—	—	17.6% *30-day mortality* from first AVM hemorrhage
Mast, 1997	—	32.9% in first yr 11.3% thereafter (17.8% overall)	2.2% in all patients without hemorrhage	—	—

AVM, arteriovenous malformation.
[a]All rates annualized (i.e., % per year).

rate fell from 3% per year after 5 years to 2% per year after 10 years [45].

Since then, Crawford et al. reported the natural history of 217 patients managed conservatively for a mean duration of 10.4 years without any surgical procedures or radiation [46]. Using life survival analyses, they determined that 20 years after diagnosis there was a 42% risk of hemorrhage (2% per annum). The average hemorrhage risk over 20 years was higher in those patients who had originally suffered a hemorrhage, roughly 2.5% per year in those who had bled versus 1.65% per year in those who had not bled. Patients with epilepsy had a smaller risk of bleeding, while those with a neurologic deficit had an even lesser risk. None of their patients with incidentally diagnosed AVMs suffered hemorrhage during the follow-up period.

Brown et al. performed retrospective analysis of 166 patients diagnosed with AVM. The significant difference between this group and other groups of patients with AVMs was that none of these patients had previously suffered a clinically documented hemorrhage. The authors were able to obtain a mean follow-up of 8.2 years and found the mean hemorrhage risk was 2.2% per year [47]. They also noted the percentage of survivors who had not suffered an intracranial hemorrhage was greatly decreased by 10 years after the diagnosis of AVM was made and that the hemorrhage risk remained significant for 20 years following original diagnosis. Itoyama et al. studied 50 patients who were selected for nonsurgical management, some of whom had previously ruptured AVMs [13]. They found that in those who had had a rupture, the risk of rehemorrhage during the initial year was 6.9%, but after 15 years the average annual rate was 0.92%. In those patients who had not bled previously, the annual rate of hemorrhage was 4.8% during the first year but fell to 1.3% after 10 years.

The work of Ondra et al. is generally considered a definitive study of the natural history of AVMs because of the impressive follow-up period of up to 24 years, yet these patients were also subject to a selection bias when conservative management was selected [40,41]. In this cohort, the yearly hemorrhage rate in those with prior hemorrhage was 3.9%, compared to a rate of 4.3% in those with seizures and 3.9% in those with other features such as headache and asymptomatic bruits. There were no statistically significant differences between these groups with respect to hemorrhage risk.

Using these previously derived estimates of the annual risk of hemorrhage in conjunction with actuarial survival data, Kondziolka et al. determined the approximate lifetime risk of hemorrhage for a patient as a function of age when diagnosed [48]. These data are presented in Table 9-2. Simplifying this information further, Brown commented that a similar estimate of lifetime hemorrhage risk could be achieved by subtracting the patient's age (in years) from 105 [49]. Thus, a patient who is diagnosed with an AVM at age 35 would be predicted to have a lifetime hemorrhage risk of 70%.

TABLE 9-2. SIMPLE RISK PREDICTIONS FOR HEMORRHAGE FROM AN AVM AS A FUNCTION OF AGE

Age	Life Expectancy Following Hemorrhage	Risk of Hemorrhage During Patient's Lifetime[a]		
		2% Per Yr	3% Per Yr	4% Per Yr
0	76	79	90	96
15	62	71	85	92
25	52	65	80	88
35	43	58	73	83
45	34	50	65	75
55	25	40	53	64
65	18	31	42	52
75	11	20	29	36
85	6	11	17	22

AVM, arteriovenous malformation.
[a]Risk of hemorrhage during remainder of life assuming various annual risks for bleeding.

A different approach to this problem was taken by Karlsson et al. [21]. Using the reliable hemorrhage data from 1,479 of their 2,262 patients with AVMs, they derived a mathematical formula that predicted the annual hemorrhage risk for a patient at a given age. They found that hemorrhage risk increases with age and that the annual risks for first hemorrhage for patients aged 10, 25, 50, and 70 were 2%, 5%, 7%, and 10%, respectively (Fig. 9-1). This expectation is different from prior natural history studies that predicted a constant rate of hemorrhage over time. However, given the large clinical experience and sound mathematics, this new concept certainly deserves significant consideration and future study.

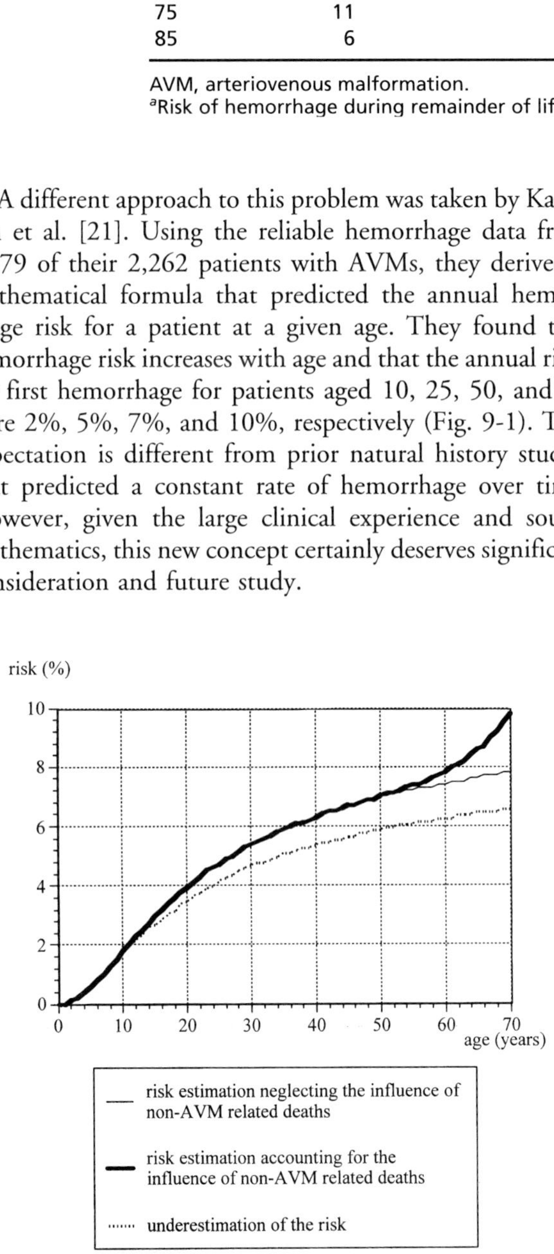

FIGURE 9-1. Annual risk of hemorrhage from an AVM as a function of age of the patient. (From Karlsson B, Lindquist C, Johansson A, et al. Annual risk for the first hemorrhage from untreated cerebral arteriovenous malformations. *Minim Invasive Neurosurg* 1997;40:40–46, with permission.)

Most recently, Mast et al. published what is probably the only prospective determination of hemorrhage risk from an AVM [50]. Consistent with previous authors, they found that for patients who had not suffered prior hemorrhage, the annual hemorrhage risk is 2.2%. However, in the group that had originally experienced hemorrhage their findings were strikingly divergent from previous estimates, with the risk being 32.9% during the first year and 11.3% annually thereafter.

Finally, as we will discuss below, deep location and deep venous drainage are thought to predispose to hemorrhage. Our experience with 96 patients with AVMs of the basal ganglia and thalamus has revealed that the natural history of hemorrhage following original diagnosis is substantially greater than the risk described in these previous reports. We found that the risk of hemorrhage from an AVM in this location is 9.8% per patient-year [51].

In summary, despite numerous attempts to quantify the natural history of hemorrhage for a patient with AVM, there is still no absolutely definitive data. Most would agree that the annual risk is probably 2% to 4% and higher for those with deep AVMs. Recent prospective work challenges this notion, suggesting that the rate may be even higher, and there is controversy regarding how this projects to the patient's lifetime risk of hemorrhage.

Clinical Features, and Morbidity and Mortality from Hemorrhage

Despite the relatively low annual risk of hemorrhage, the majority of symptomatic patients with AVMs will have intracranial hemorrhage. In the above-mentioned natural history studies, the proportion of patients who were originally diagnosed with hemorrhage ranged from 51% to 72% [8, 13,39–42,44,46,50]. Two recent large clinical studies described initial hemorrhage in 53% to 68% of a combined total of over 3,500 patients with AVMs [15,21]. In Hillman's recent population-based study, 69.6% of patients ex-

FIGURE 9-2. This 22-year-old left-handed male telecommunications specialist with long-standing migraine headaches sought treatment for a sudden headache. **A:** A noncontrast CT scan demonstrated a small focal hemorrhage in the right sylvian fissure region *(arrow),* and **(B,C)** subsequent MRI confirmed the presence of an underlying 2-cm AVM *(arrows).* **D,E:** Initial diagnostic angiography demonstrated the AVM nidus *(black arrows)* and feeding arteries primarily from the middle cerebral artery with superficial venous drainage *(open arrow).* We considered this a Spetzler-Martin grade II AVM because of the location adjacent to the inferior motor area and corona radiata. Given his young age and presence of hemorrhage, we recommended treatment for this patient. *(Figure continues.)*

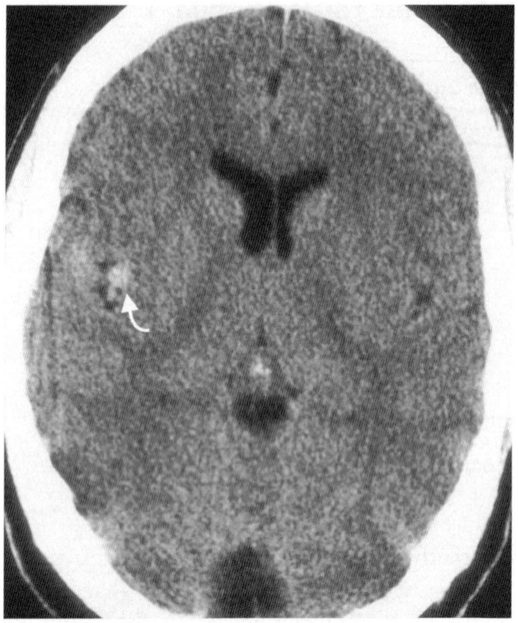
A

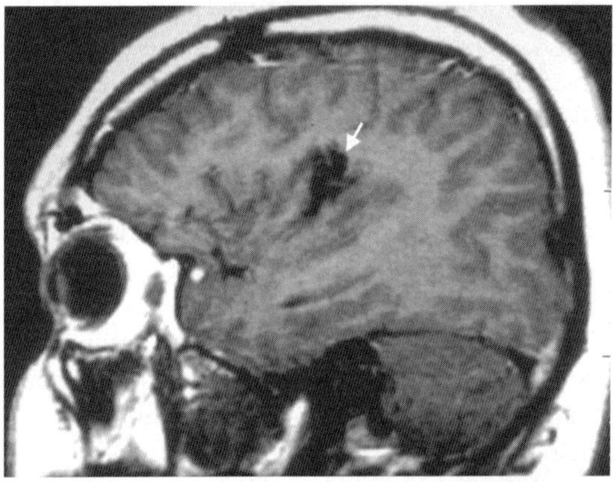
B

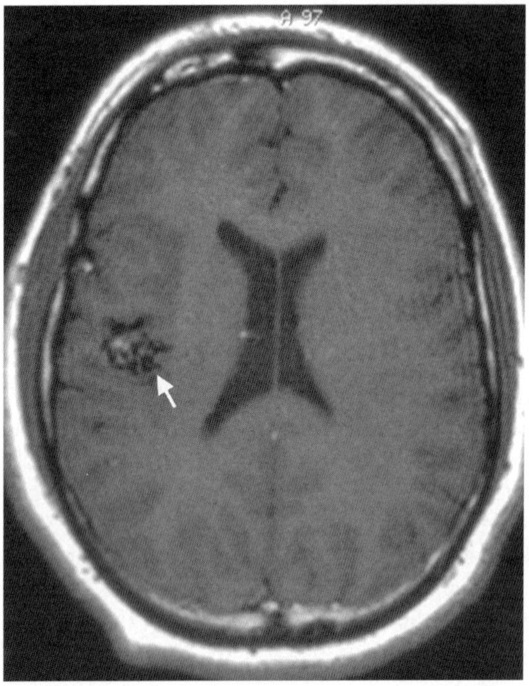
C

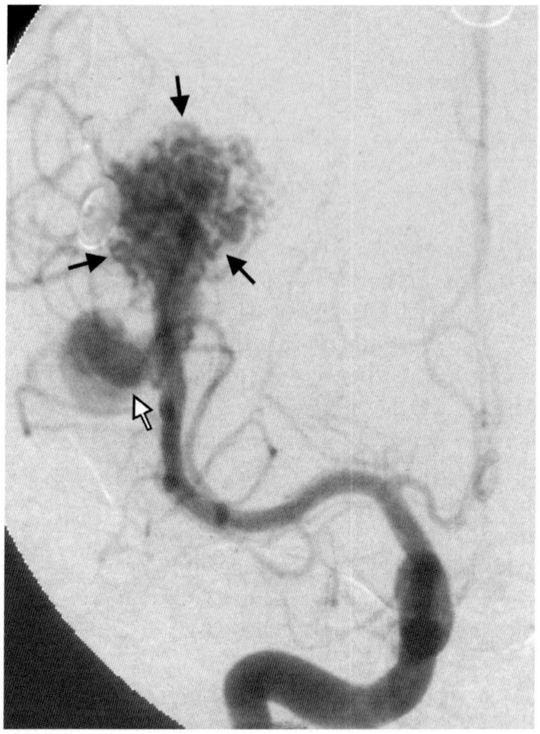
D

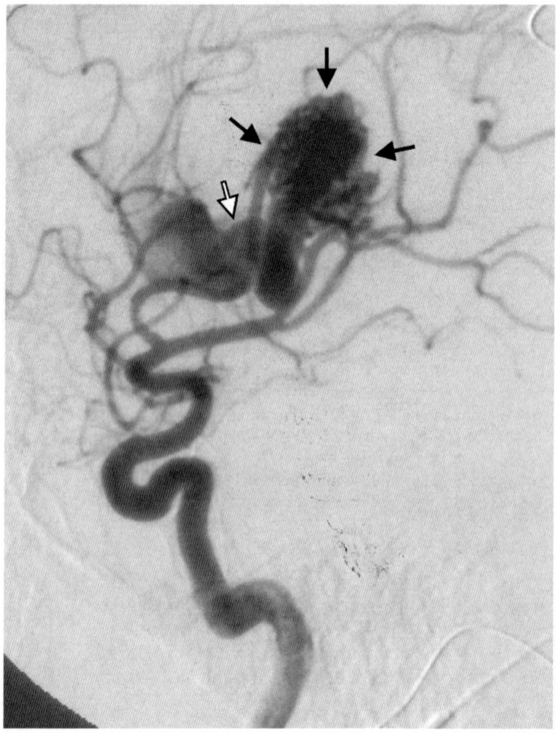
E

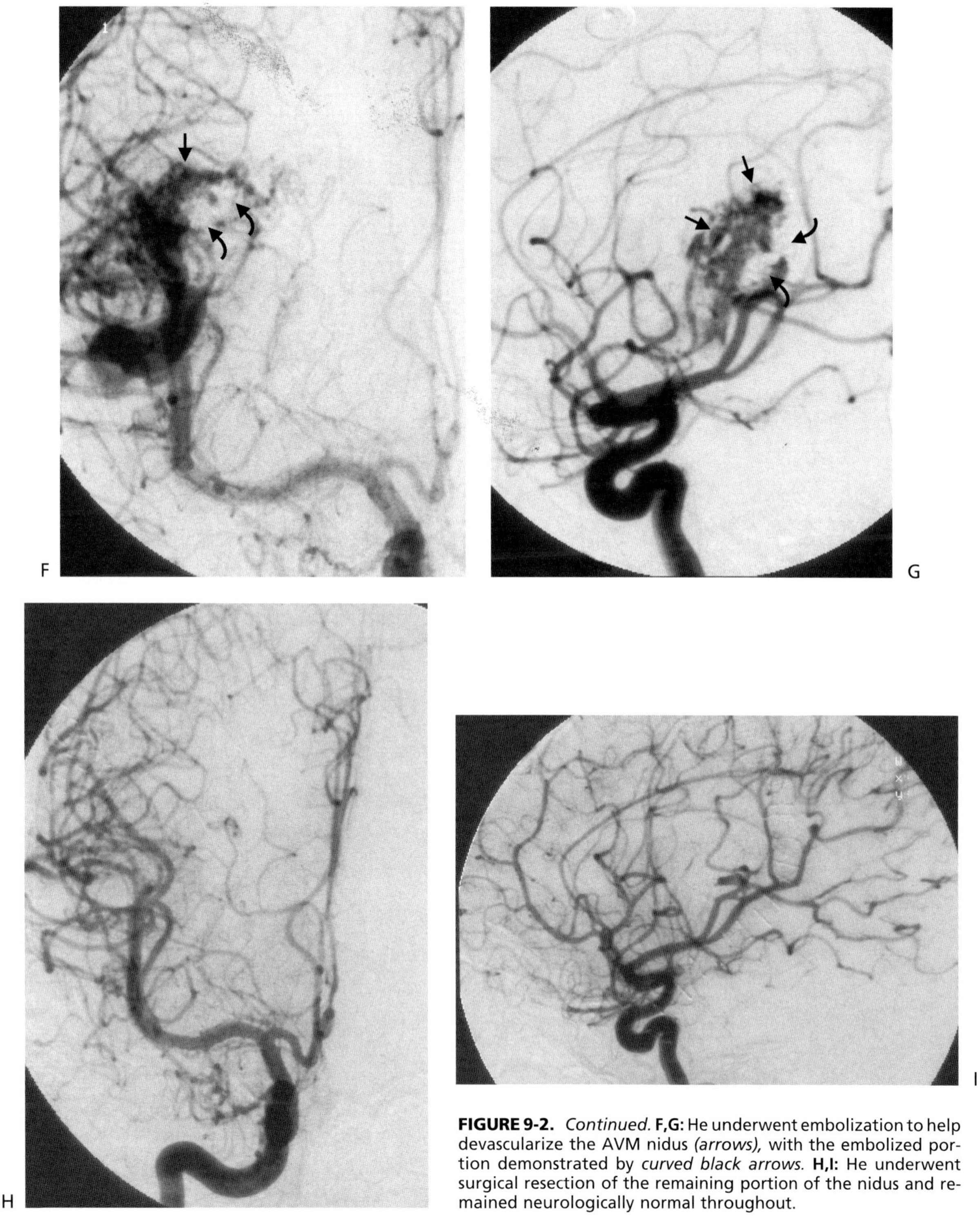

FIGURE 9-2. *Continued.* **F,G:** He underwent embolization to help devascularize the AVM nidus *(arrows),* with the embolized portion demonstrated by *curved black arrows.* **H,I:** He underwent surgical resection of the remaining portion of the nidus and remained neurologically normal throughout.

perienced hemorrhage from their AVMs [9]. Data from the Cooperative Study of Intracranial Aneurysms and Subarachnoid Hemorrhage showed that approximately 68% of patients had a hemorrhage prior to admission to the study, and the peak period for bleeding was between ages 15 and 20 years [11]. Seventy-two percent of AVMs had bled by the time the patients reached 40 years of age [11]. Thus, from these numerous studies it can be seen that between one-half and three-fourths of patients with AVMs will come to clinical attention with an intracranial hemorrhage (Figs. 9-2 and 9-3).

The effects of intracranial hemorrhage from an AVM

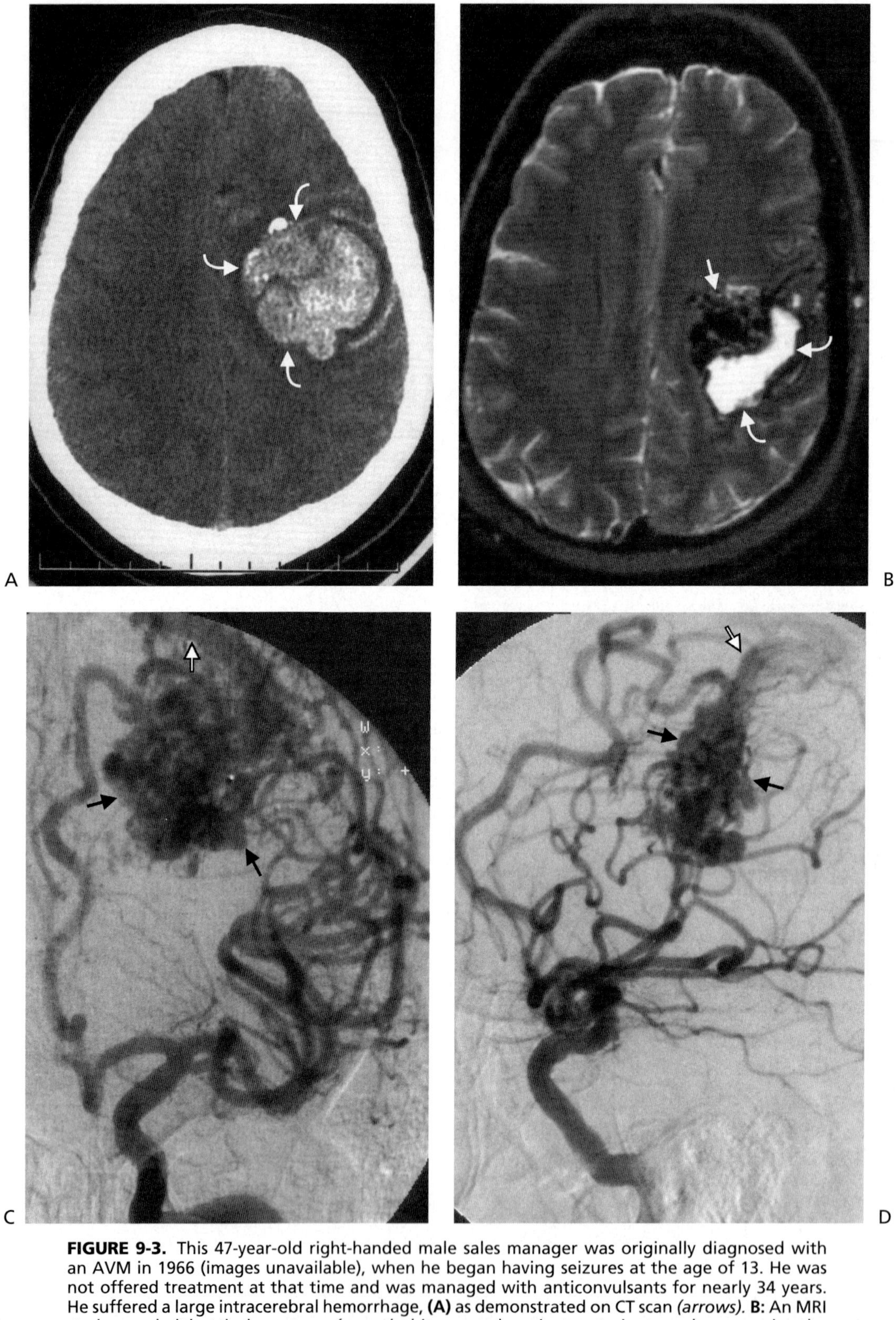

FIGURE 9-3. This 47-year-old right-handed male sales manager was originally diagnosed with an AVM in 1966 (images unavailable), when he began having seizures at the age of 13. He was not offered treatment at that time and was managed with anticonvulsants for nearly 34 years. He suffered a large intracerebral hemorrhage, **(A)** as demonstrated on CT scan *(arrows).* **B:** An MRI study revealed that the hematoma *(curved white arrows)* was just posterior to and compressing the AVM nidus *(small white arrows).* **C,D:** Angiography demonstrated a 4-cm AVM *(black arrows)* in the left frontoparietal region with superficial drainage *(open arrows)*—a Spetzler-Martin grade III AVM. The hematoma was managed conservatively, and he was left with a dense right hemiparesis and significant expressive dysphasia from which he made an incomplete recovery. *(Figure continues.)*

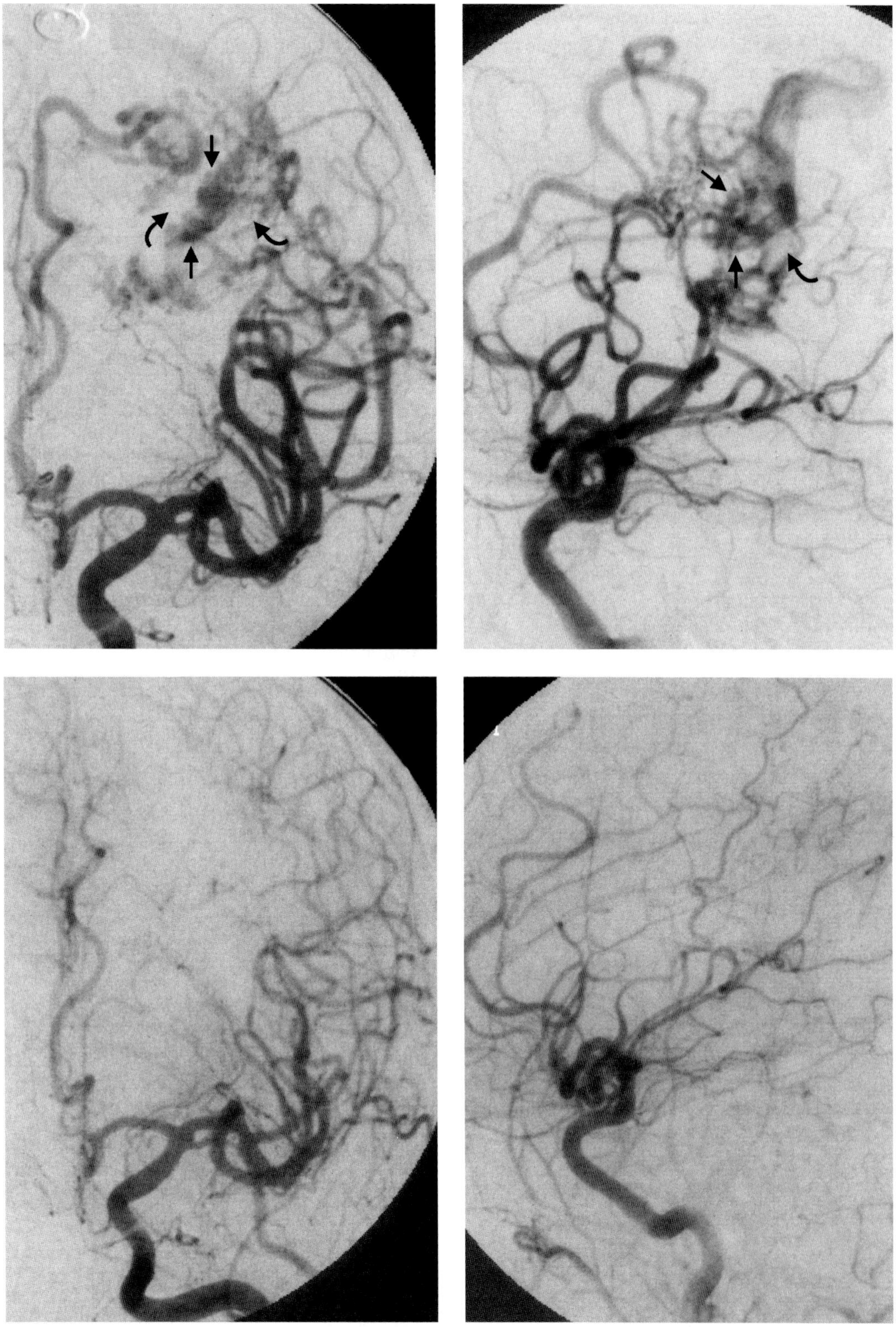

FIGURE 9-3. *Continued.* Twelve weeks post hemorrhage, to allow further clinical recovery and resolution of the hematoma, he underwent two sessions of embolization, resulting in a substantial decrease in the size of the AVM nidus *(straight arrows)* **(E,F),** with the embolized area demonstrated by *curved arrows.* The remainder of the nidus was resected microsurgcially using image guidance, somatosensory evoked potential monitoring, mild intraoperative hypothermia, and relative hypotension to minimize surgical risks. **G,H:** Postoperative angiography showed cure of the AVM, and the patient incurred no new neurologic deficits related to treatment but had persistent weakness and dysphasia related to his original hemorrhage.

will be unique in each patient and are largely dependent on the anatomical location of the AVM. While some hemorrhages will result in headaches or seizures, others can produce focal neurologic deficits (see Fig. 9-3). The morbidity following hemorrhage from an AVM is generally less significant than that from an aneurysm. However, morbidity is clearly the most important concern for those surviving the initial hemorrhage. In the Cooperative Study data, as many as 58% of patients suffered a neurologic deficit as a result of the original hemorrhage, and the hemorrhage rate was 74% (207 of 280) of a large series from Mayo Clinic [52]. The early work of Graf et al. demonstrated that 81.3% of 134 patients developed a neurologic deficit immediately following an intracranial hemorrhage, and deficit was much more common (90.2%) and more severe in the presence of an intracerebral hematoma [44]. Crawford et al. found a lower rate of permanent disability following hemorrhage, with only 6% suffering major deficit and 25% developing a minor handicap by the time of hospital discharge [53]. Brown et al. found significant disability in 23% of those who had survived the hemorrhage from an AVM. This was much higher than the rate of permanent disability in those patients not suffering hemorrhage (7%) [47]. More recently, 50% of patients from a prospective database were found to have hemorrhaged at the time of their diagnosis [54]. Of the patients who had the hemorrhage confirmed by imaging studies, 84% were either deficit free or completely independent in their activities of daily living. Only 3% incurred severe disability (Rankin score 4 to 5) and 13% were moderately disabled (Rankin score 2 to 3). These authors found that parenchymal hemorrhage was more likely to be associated with a focal deficit (52%). The authors cite their low morbidity rate following hemorrhage as a reason to reassess current treatment regimens for AVMs, given that their findings are lower than previously reported rates. They contrast these rates to their own reported rates of 8% morbidity and mortality during the multidisciplinary management of patients with AVM using surgery, embolization, and radiosurgery [55]. However, they acknowledge the attenuating effect of a referral bias on observed morbidity as well as their likely underestimation of mortality rates for the same reasons.

The majority of AVM hemorrhages are not fatal. Several authors have quantified the mortality rate after an AVM bleed. Early work showed the initial mortality rate to be roughly 6% following hemorrhage [39], while others found this rate to be higher (10.8% to 12.7%) [44,46]. The mortality rate from a second hemorrhage in the series of Svien and McRae was 13% [39]. Brown et al. found that the risk of death following rupture of an AVM was 29%, with most patients succumbing within 24 hours of the hemorrhage [47]. More recently, Ondra et al. have estimated the mortality rate in a different way. They did not discuss the initial death rate in their series, but they determined that following diagnosis there was an annual mortality rate of approximately 1% from AVM hemorrhage, regardless of initial symptomatology [41]. Twenty-three percent of their population ultimately died from an AVM hemorrhage, similar to the 20% mortality described by Abad et al. after conservative management of unruptured AVMs [56].

Risk Factors for Hemorrhage

Although hemorrhage is clearly the dominant mode of discovery for patients with AVM, of more specific interest to such patients is the likelihood they will suffer a hemorrhage or rehemorrhage following diagnosis. This topic has been most commonly addressed in retrospective studies that correlate clinical and angioarchitectural features with hemorrhage. Although these studies provide valuable data, it is impossible to know if these results can be extrapolated to predict a risk of subsequent hemorrhage. This is being addressed currently in prospective trials. Several factors consistently have been found to put patients at higher risk for hemorrhage from an AVM (Table 9-3). One of the most widely reported is small size (generally smaller than 2.0 to 3.0 cm) [44] [12,57–60]. In the series of Crawford et al., patients with small AVMs were more likely to have had hemorrhage as the major initial symptom [46]. However, this was not statistically significant. This relationship had previously been described by Graf et al., who found that patients with small AVMs had a 52% risk of rehemorrhage within 5 years after diagnosis, while those with large AVMs had only a 10% risk [44]. Hemorrhage was more likely in those with small (<3 cm) AVMs [52]. Small size as a risk factor for hemorrhage was most recently corroborated by Stiver and Ogilvy, who reported on a series of 12 patients, all with AVM nidus diameter <1 cm, and all of whom had suffered intracranial hemorrhage [61].

Deep, central, or periventricular location has also been described by several authors as a risk factor for hemorrhage [40] (Fig. 9-4). In some reports deep location is reported in association with deep venous drainage, but in others deep venous drainage is considered an independent risk factor [59,60,62–65].

High hemodynamic resistance or shunt resistance was reported as a risk factor for hemorrhage by Parkinson and Bachers [57]. This has also been studied by Spetzler et al., who found that small AVMs with high feeding artery pressures, and therefore small differences between feeding artery pressure and mean arterial pressure, are more likely to experience hemorrhage [58]. Duong et al. found that mean feeding artery pressure as measured during superselective angiography was a risk factor for hemorrhage in multivariate analysis [65], confirming earlier work by the same group [59]. Although Norris et al. prospectively studied numerous AVM angioarchitectural features previously shown to create hemorrhage risk, the only factor in their study to increase the risk of hemorrhage was slow arterial filling with contrast material [66]. This probably correlates with high feeding

TABLE 9-3. FACTORS INFLUENCING THE RISK OF HEMORRHAGE FROM AN AVM

Risk Factor	Influence	Reference
Venous stenosis	Increases	Willinsky et al., 1988 [67]
	Increases (except for cortical AVMs)	Nataf et al., 1997 [64]
		Mansmann et al., 2000 [14]
Deep venous drainage	Increases	Marks et al., 1990 [62]
		Crawford et al., 1986 [46]
		Kader et al., 1994 [59]
		Nataf et al., 1997 [64]
Small nidus (independent)	Increases (2×)	Crawford et al., 1986 [46]
		Spetzler et al., 1992 [58]
		Mansmann et al., 2000 [14]
Small nidus in a deep location	Increases	Kader et al., 1994 [59]
Deep location	Increases	Marks et al., 1990 [62]
Hemodynamic factors	Increases	Kader et al., 1994 [59]
Associated aneurysm (any)	Increases	Willinsky et al., 1988 [67]
	Increases	Marks et al., 1990 [62], 1992 [206]
	No effect	Mansmann et al., 2000 [14]
Original clinical picture with hemorrhage	Increases likelihood of future hemorrhage	Mast et al., 1997 [50]
Slow arterial filling with contrast material	Increases risk	Norris et al., 1999 [66]
High feeding artery pressure	Increases risk	Spetzler et al., 1992 [58]
	Increases risk (independent of nidus size)	Kader et al., 1994 [59]
Angiomatous change	Decreases	Marks et al., 1990 [62,95]

AVM, arteriovenous malformation.

artery pressure, consistent with the findings of other authors.

In addition to the above, venous stenosis has also been found unfavorable for patients with AVMs and is correlated with hemorrhage [67]. Most recently this was confirmed by Nataf et al. in a study of 160 patients [64]. Pollock et al. also identified a single draining vein as a risk factor for hemorrhage [68]. Interestingly, Stapf et al. recently reported that arterial supply by more than one major circle of Willis vessel was protective against hemorrhage [69]. They defined these lesions as being in arterial "border zones." It may be that feeding the malformation from multiple sources serves to reduce feeding artery pressure, although this was not specifically addressed in that report. Similarly, the presence of angiomatous change (arterial supply to an AVM from a vascular distribution not normally supplying that territory) may protect against hemorrhage [62,95].

The issue of which factors determine the risk of hemorrhage from an AVM has recently been addressed in two complementary fashions. Mansmann et al. retrospectively evaluated 662 patients with AVM and determined the angioarchitectural features that were associated with hemorrhage in 348 of these patients [14]. This study involved only patients undergoing endovascular therapy for their AVMs and therefore incurred a selection bias. They determined that venous stenosis was the greatest predictor of hemorrhage in a multivariate analysis and also indicated that AVM-associated aneurysms were not a significant risk factor for hemorrhage, which was also the finding of the others [60,65]. The issue of AVM-associated aneurysms is controversial and others have found these to increase the risk of hemorrhage [62,63,67,70,71].

Location in a deep or periventricular area has been associated with a higher risk of hemorrhage at the time of initial evaluation as described by prior studies [62,63]. As mentioned above, we recently reviewed the series of 96 patients seen at Stanford University with basal ganglia and thalamus AVMs and found that following diagnosis with or without hemorrhage, the annual risk of subsequent hemorrhage was 9.8% per patient [51]. This is much higher than the natural history of AVMs in general and seems to corroborate the concept that deep venous drainage and deep location indicate a higher risk for hemorrhage.

All of the aforementioned studies are retrospective in nature. Perhaps the only report to address this dilemma using a prospective database was performed by the group at Columbia University, who confirmed that deep venous drainage is an independent risk factor for hemorrhage [50]. Clinical factors associated with hemorrhage have been studied less extensively than angiographic factors, but several authors have described parameters that might increase the risk of hemorrhage from an AVM. These include a prior bleed [68], a history of hypertension [60], and male gender [50,67].

Seizures

AVMs may induce neuronal degeneration of parenchymal tissues adjacent to the AVM nidus in the form of deafferentation. Regardless, it is generally thought that the seizure

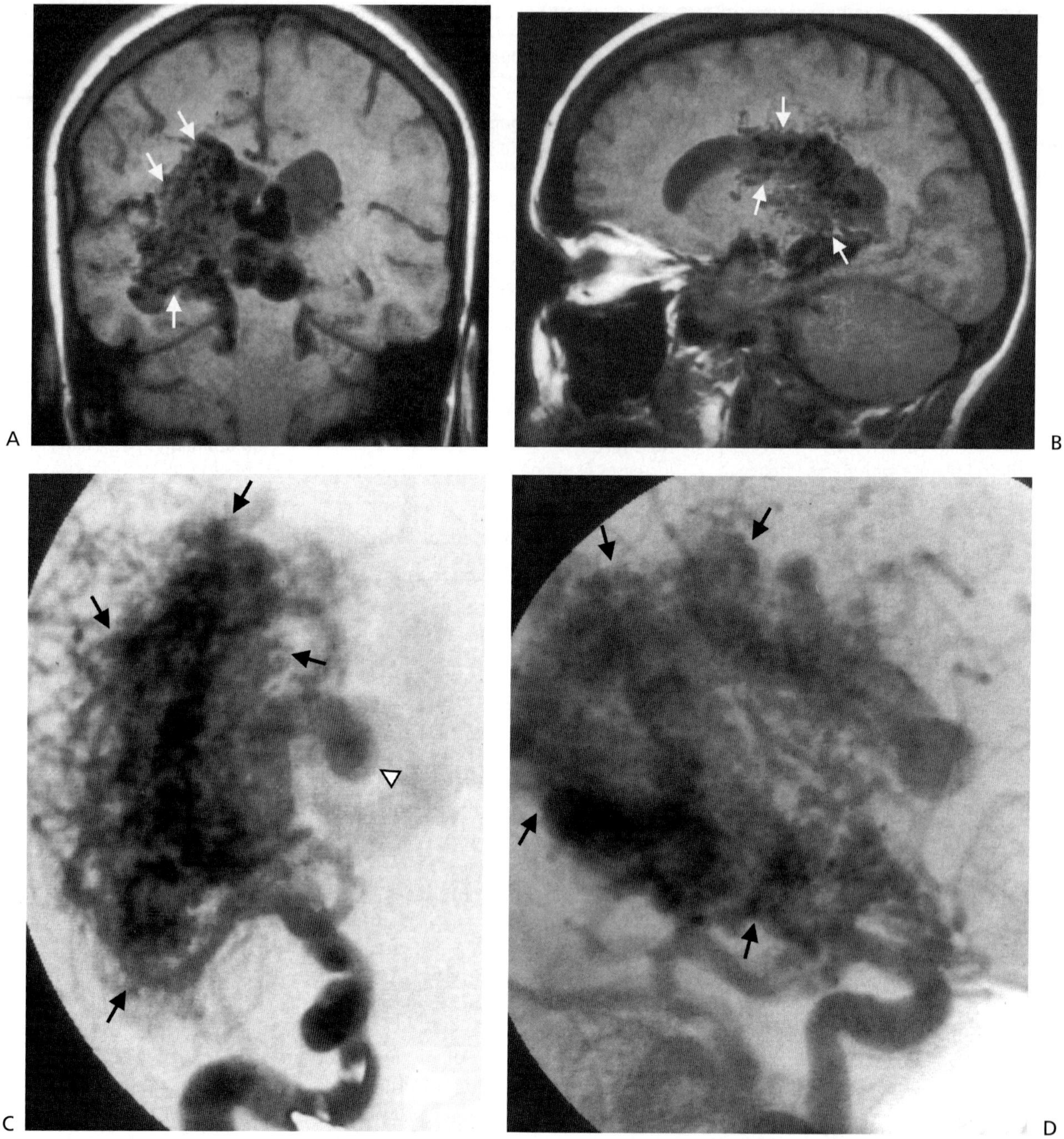

FIGURE 9-4. This 30-year-old woman originally sought treatment following intraparenchymal and intraventricular hemorrhage from a large AVM in the right basal ganglia and thalamus, fed by both the anterior and posterior circulations. She was originally treated with helium ion radiosurgery in 1987 (20 GyE to a volume of 3,500 mm^3). She had residual hemiparesis and ataxia from the original bleed; however, this was progressive in nature. **A,B:** She had significant residual volume demonstrated on an MRI in 1989 *(arrows),* and **(C,D)** angiography demonstrated the limited response to her prior radiation treatment *(black arrows).* This was considered a Spetzler-Martin grade IV AVM. *(Figure continues.)*

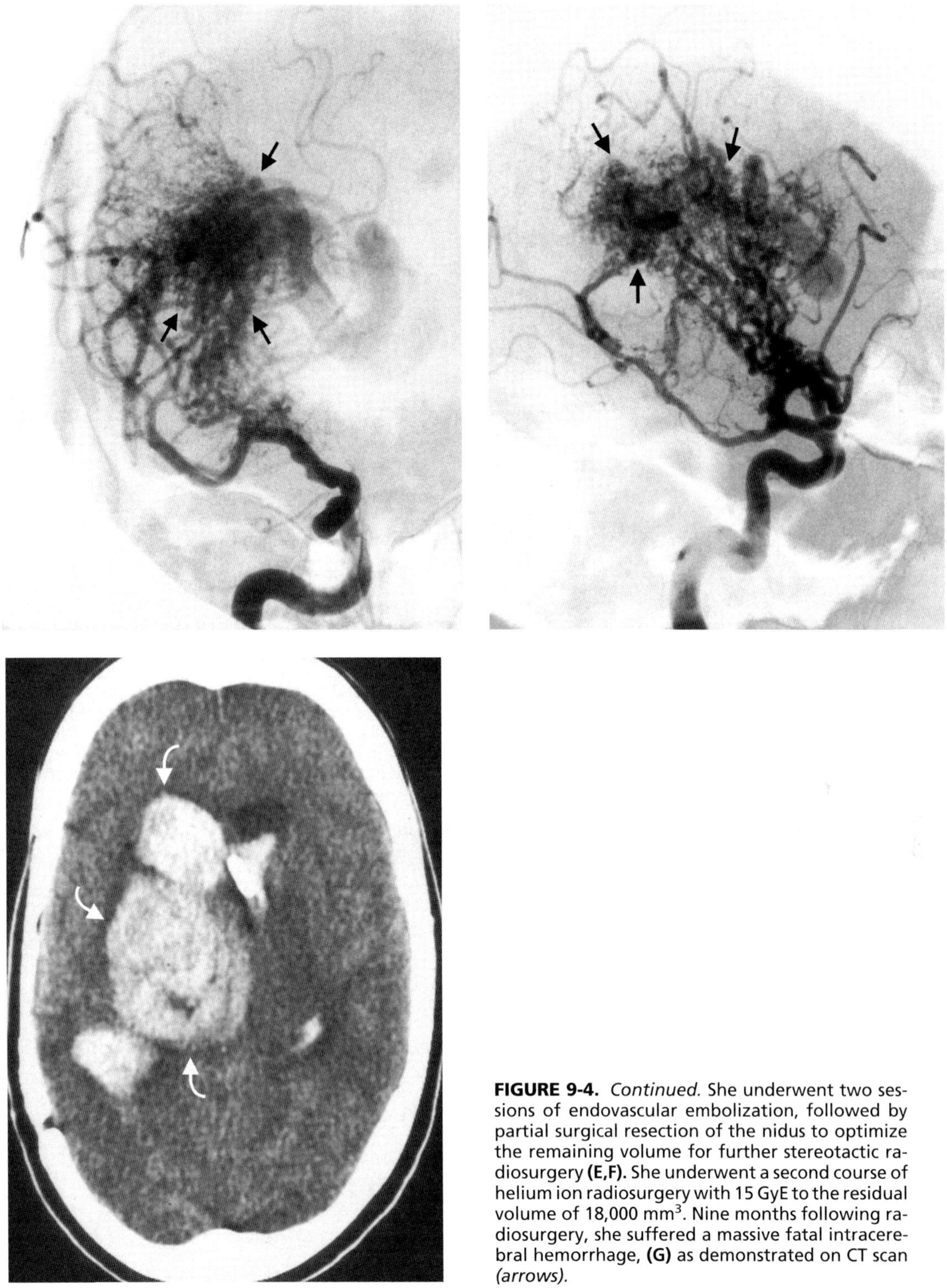

FIGURE 9-4. *Continued.* She underwent two sessions of endovascular embolization, followed by partial surgical resection of the nidus to optimize the remaining volume for further stereotactic radiosurgery **(E,F).** She underwent a second course of helium ion radiosurgery with 15 GyE to the residual volume of 18,000 mm^3. Nine months following radiosurgery, she suffered a massive fatal intracerebral hemorrhage, **(G)** as demonstrated on CT scan *(arrows).*

focus is in the parenchyma surrounding the AVM nidus and not the nidus itself. Possible mechanisms include gliosis, hemorrhage, or ischemia secondary to the "steal" phenomenon [4,72]. Secondary epileptogenesis resulting from hemosiderin deposition at the site of previous subclinical hemorrhage has also been postulated by Yeh et al. [73].

Clinical Picture with Seizures and Natural History of Epilepsy

Seizures are second to intracranial hemorrhage in frequency among patients with AVMs. They were the initial feature in 28% of patients in the Cooperative Study [11] and 36%

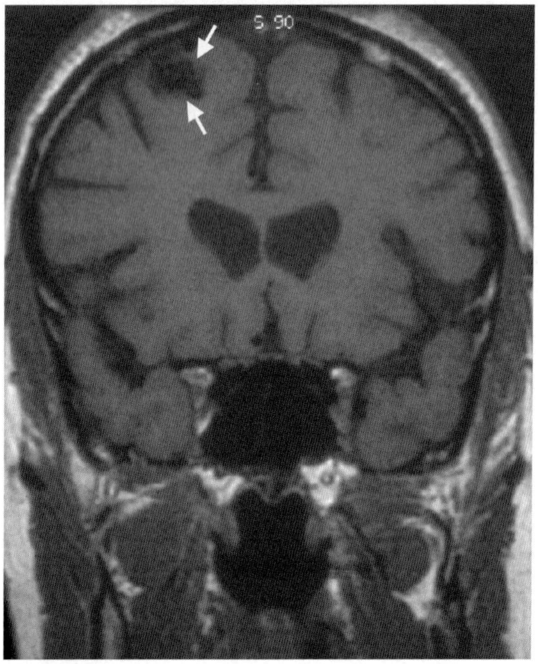

A

FIGURE 9-5. This 62-year-old right-handed male physician experienced an episode of left jaw numbness, **(A)** prompting an MRI scan, which demonstrated a small right frontal AVM *(white arrows).* In retrospect, he had also experienced a prior focal motor seizure of his left hand. **B,C:** Angiography confirmed a small (1.5-cm) AVM *(black arrows)* with superficial venous drainage *(open arrows)* (Spetzler-Martin grade I). He desired treatment and we recommended surgical excision alone. Following surgery he was completely neurologically intact and returned to work on the third postoperative day. *(Figure continues.)*

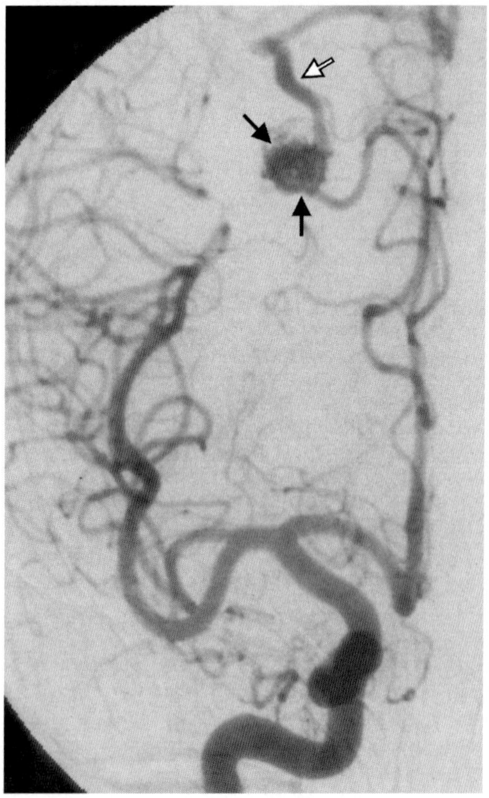

B

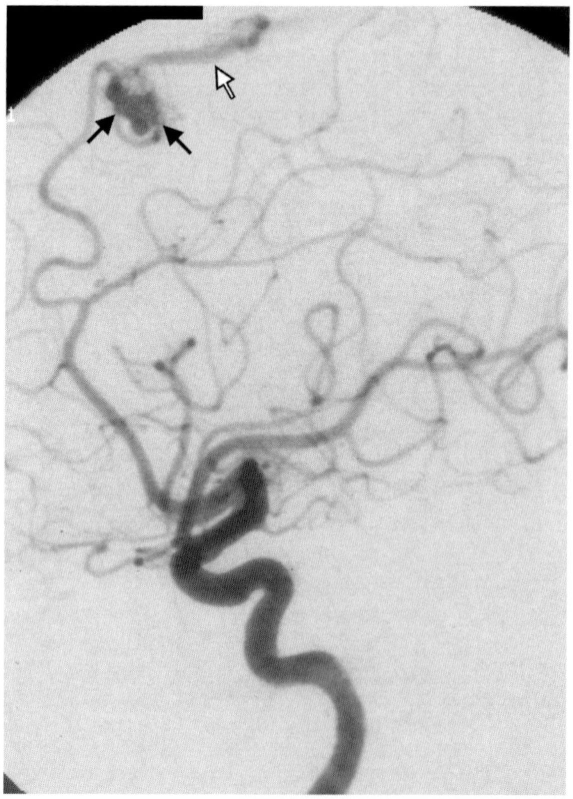

C

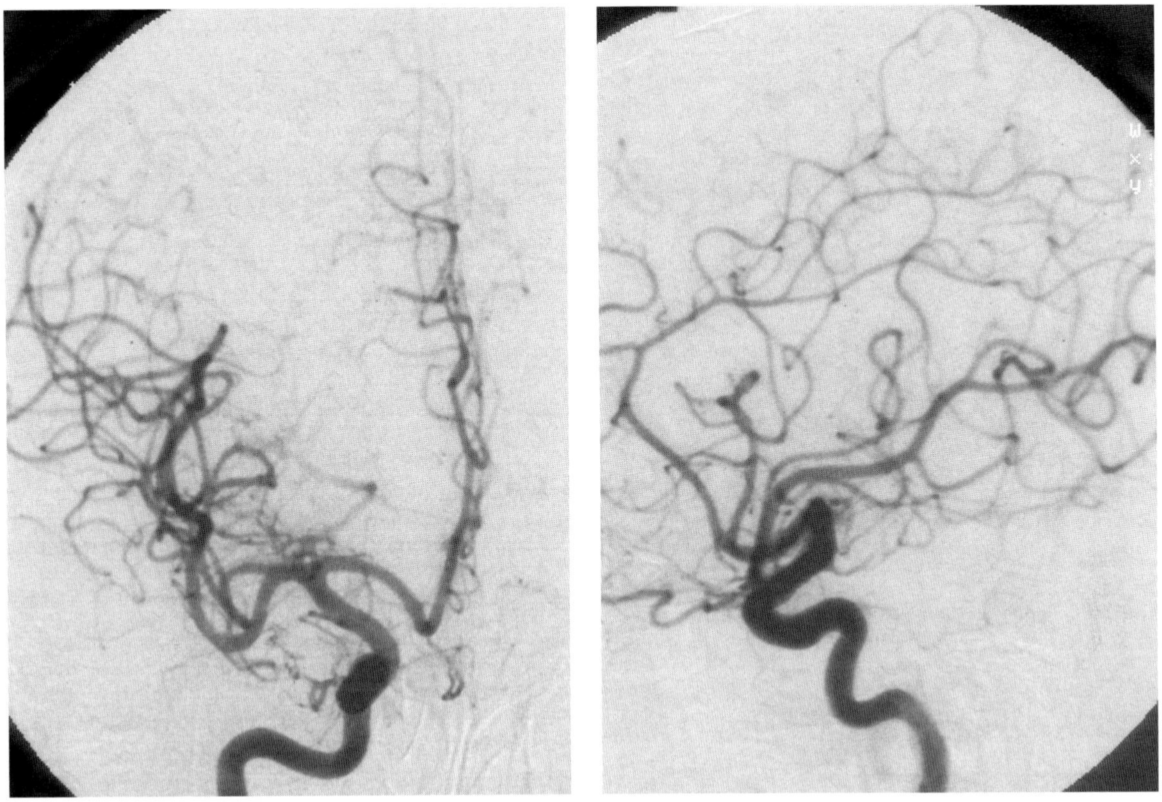

D E

FIGURE 9-5. *Continued.* **D,E:** Postoperative angiography demonstrated complete obliteration of the arteriovenous shunting.

of patients studied by Leblanc et al. [74]. As could be expected, all seizure types are seen in patients with AVMs, including simple partial, complex partial, partial seizures with secondary generalization, and generalized tonic-clonic seizures. AVMs producing seizures include cortical lesions, subcortical lesions, and even those affecting the deep structures.

In the AVM natural history studies, seizures were present at the time of diagnosis in 23.8% to 57.7% of patients [13,39–42,47,50]. In a natural history series that excluded patients with hemorrhage, Brown et al. found seizures in 57.7% of their patients [47]. In the natural history study by Graf et al., 21.1% of patients with unruptured AVMs had seizures alone, but an additional 52.6% had seizures with some other manifestation of the AVM such as focal deficit [44]. In the study by Crawford et al., these patients constituted 23% of the group [46]. In Graf's patients with ruptured AVMs, 32.1% had seizures, but the seizure preceded the bleed in only 10.4% of these patients. In Crawford's series, this group accounted for only 8%.

In clinical reports describing the management of patients with AVMs, the range of patients with seizures is wider. Among patients eventually treated surgically, 8% to 50% originally had seizures [34,43,52,56,75–78], while the rate of epilepsy is higher in those with AVMs of the temporal lobe or sylvian fissure [79,80]. Of patients eventually treated with radiosurgery, 13.3% to 47% originally had convulsions [42,53,72,78,81–87]. Seizures were more likely (statistically significant) to be the initial symptom in patients with large AVMs (45% of 49 patients) or medium-sized AVMs (25% of 153 patients) than they were in patients with small AVMs (25% of 106 patients) [52], a relationship that has been described by others. The seizure type varied and was more common (statistically significant) in patients with AVMs larger than 25 mm. Seizures were more common in patients with frontal lobe AVMs (73%) [87].

In a larger clinical series, the recently reported worldwide experience of Hofmeister et al. found that the incidence of generalized focal seizures in 1,289 patients was 30% [15]. In the large cohort of 2,262 patients reported by Karlsson et al., only 16% had epilepsy at the time of diagnosis [21]. Most recently, Hillman reported that in a large population-based study, 20% of patients had sought treatment for seizures, leading to the diagnosis of their AVMs [9]. In summary, there is a wide range reported for the occurrence of seizures at the time of AVM discovery, likely a function of the selection biases present in the individual studies. Although most report that approximately 20% to 30% of patients arrive with seizures, the range is from 8% to 58% (Figs. 9-5 to 9-8; see Fig. 9-3).

The natural history of epilepsy associated with AVMs has been studied less extensively than the risk of hemor-

text continued on p. 222

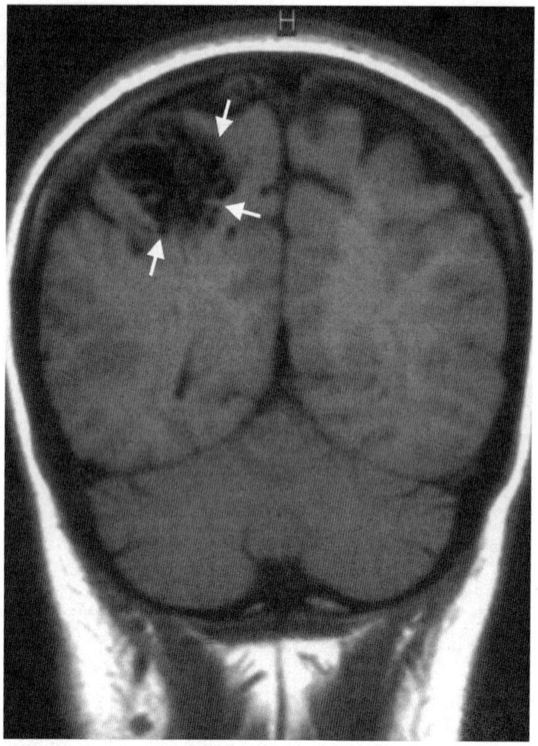

A

FIGURE 9-6. This 44-year-old female nurse was diagnosed with an AVM following the onset of sensory seizures involving the left face and arm. **A:** Her MRI shows a 3.5-cm AVM *(arrows)* in an eloquent location (right parietal region). The AVM nidus was demonstrated on angiography (RICA—**[B,C]** LICA—**[D,E]** *black arrows*) and venous drainage was superficial *(open arrow)* in **(C)**, making this a Spetzler-Martin grade III AVM. **B,C:** Her AVM showed independent filling from the right middle cerebral artery *(black arrows)*. *(Figure continues.)*

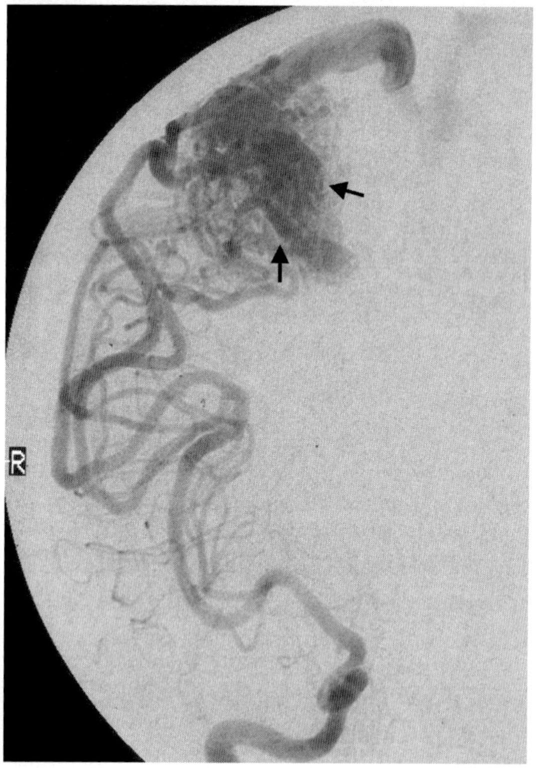

B

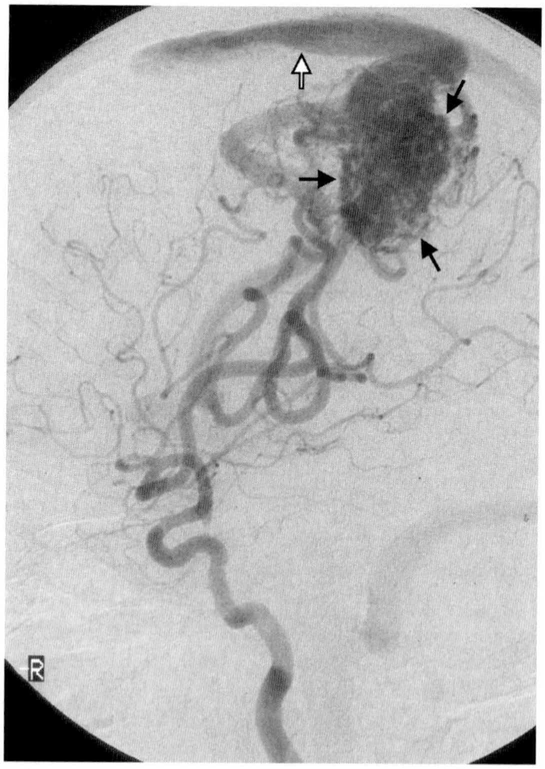

C

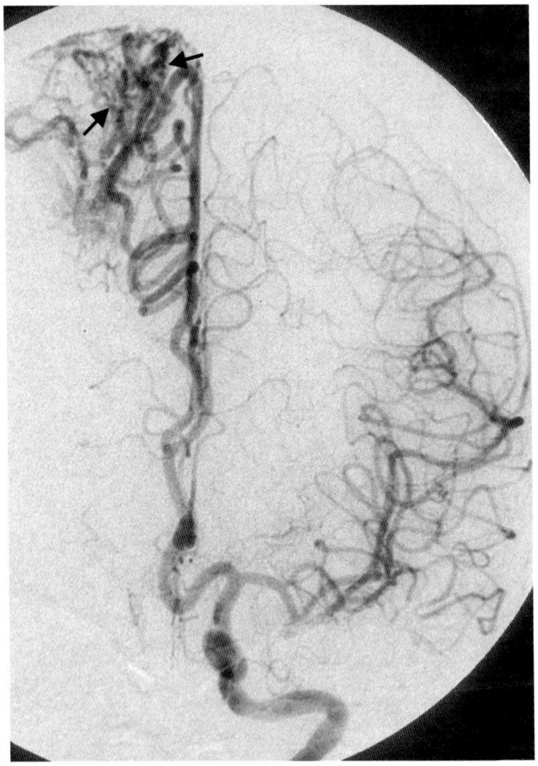

D

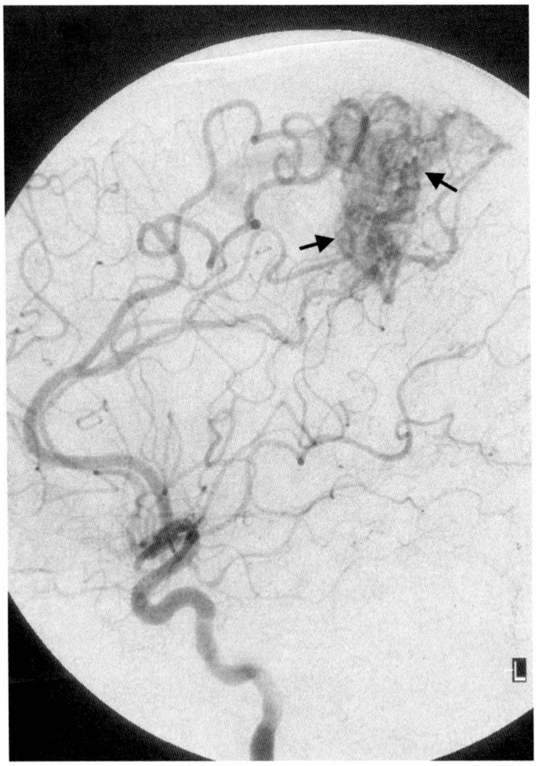

E

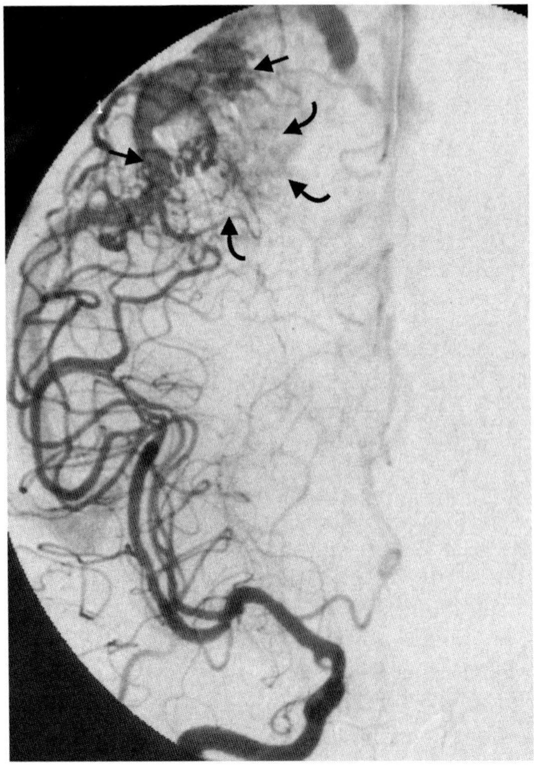

F

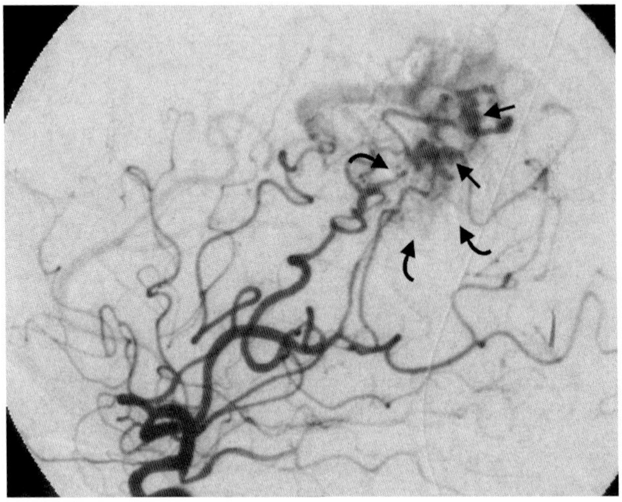

G

FIGURE 9-6. *Continued.* **(D,E)** and the left anterior cerebral artery (via the anterior communicating artery) *(arrows).* She underwent two embolization procedures of the left-sided arterial supply to the AVM, resulting in partial devascularization of that portion of the nidus (RICA—**[F,G]** LICA—**[H,I]** *straight black arrows,* with the embolized portion surrounded by *curved black arrows*). *(Figure continues.)*

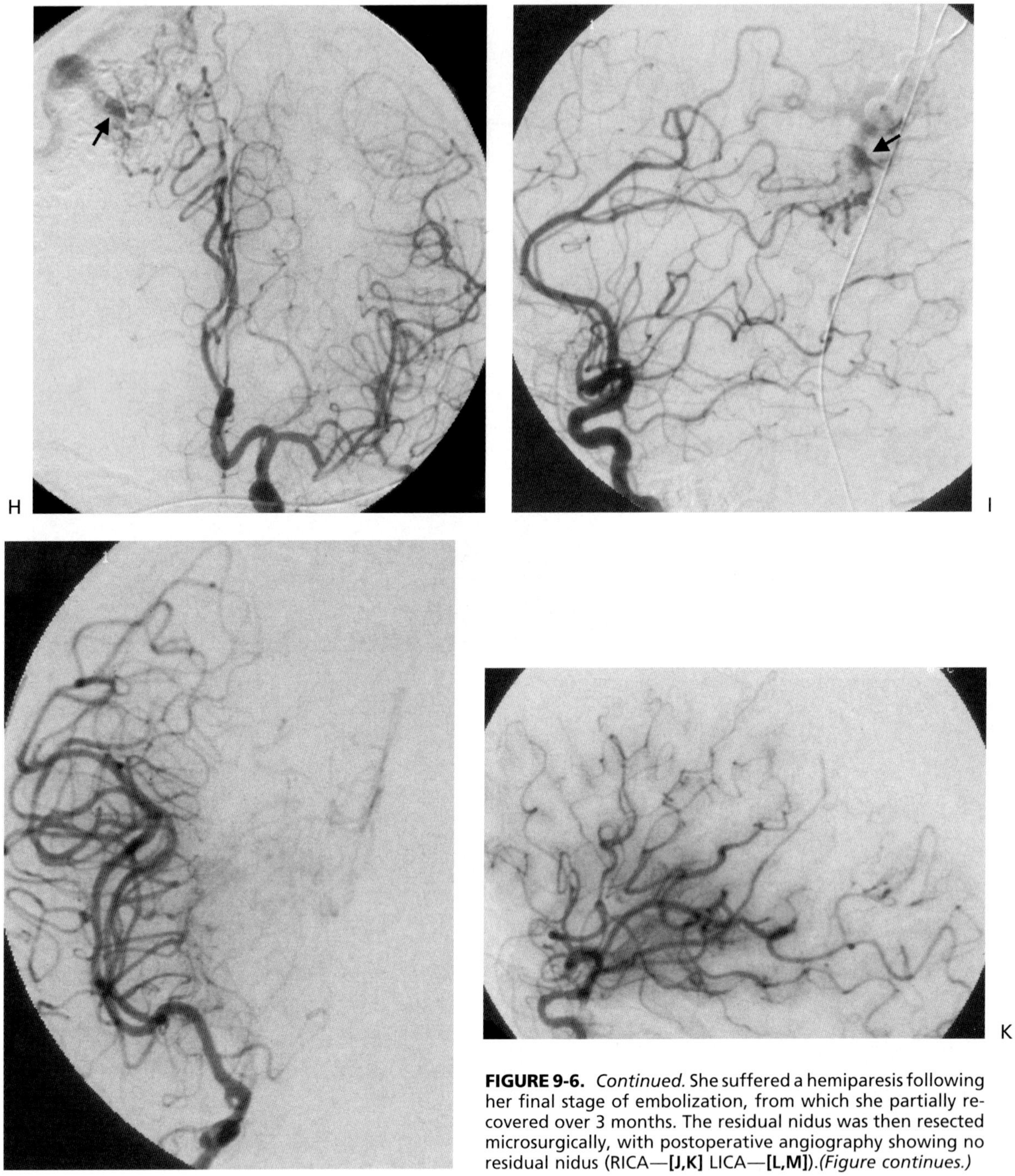

FIGURE 9-6. *Continued.* She suffered a hemiparesis following her final stage of embolization, from which she partially recovered over 3 months. The residual nidus was then resected microsurgically, with postoperative angiography showing no residual nidus (RICA—**[J,K]** LICA—**[L,M]**).*(Figure continues.)*

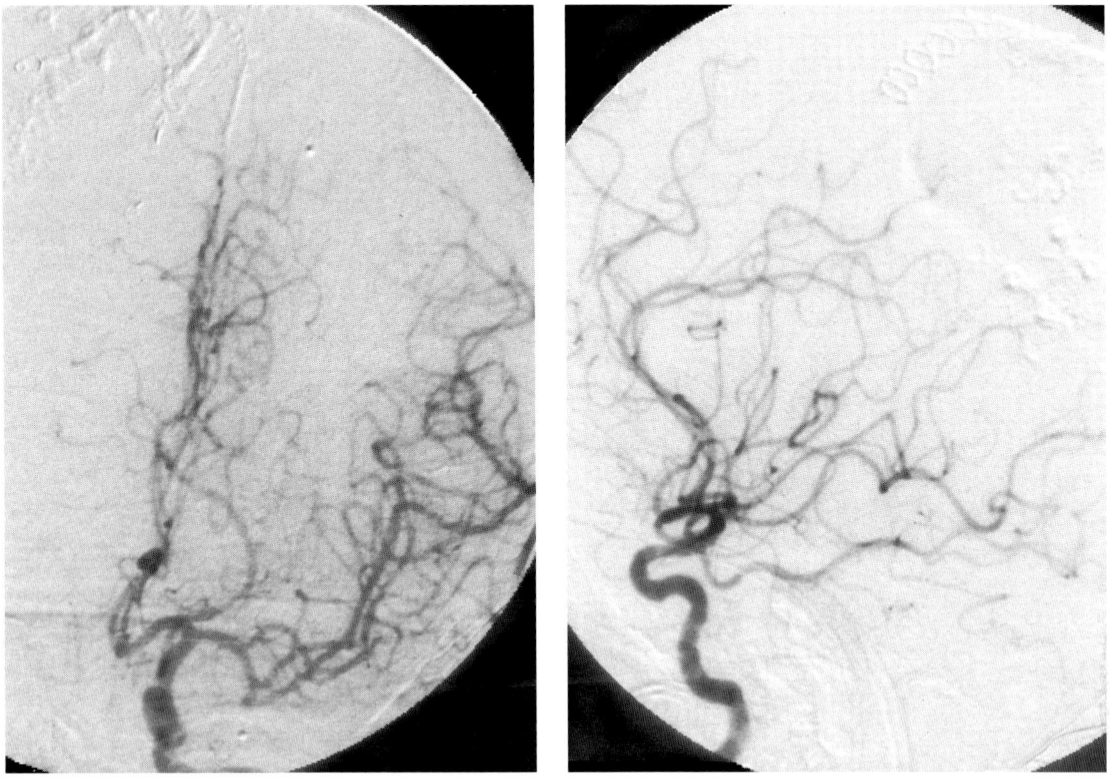
L M

FIGURE 9-6. *Continued.* She had a transient worsening of her hemiparesis after surgery but returned to baseline. With physical therapy she then recovered almost completely.

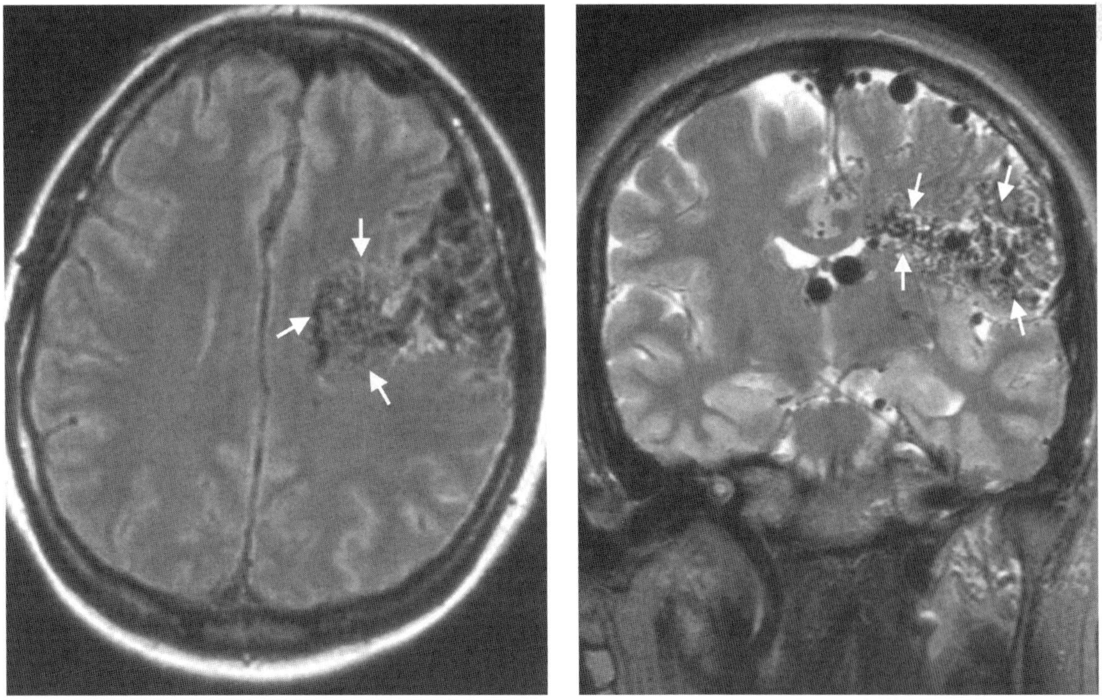
A B

FIGURE 9-7. This 43-year-old right-handed woman with a long-standing history of migraine headaches experienced simple partial seizures and mild right-sided weakness. **A,B:** Investigations included an MRI showing her AVM involving the left inferior frontal and superior temporal regions extending to the ventricular surface *(small white arrows). (Figure continues.)*

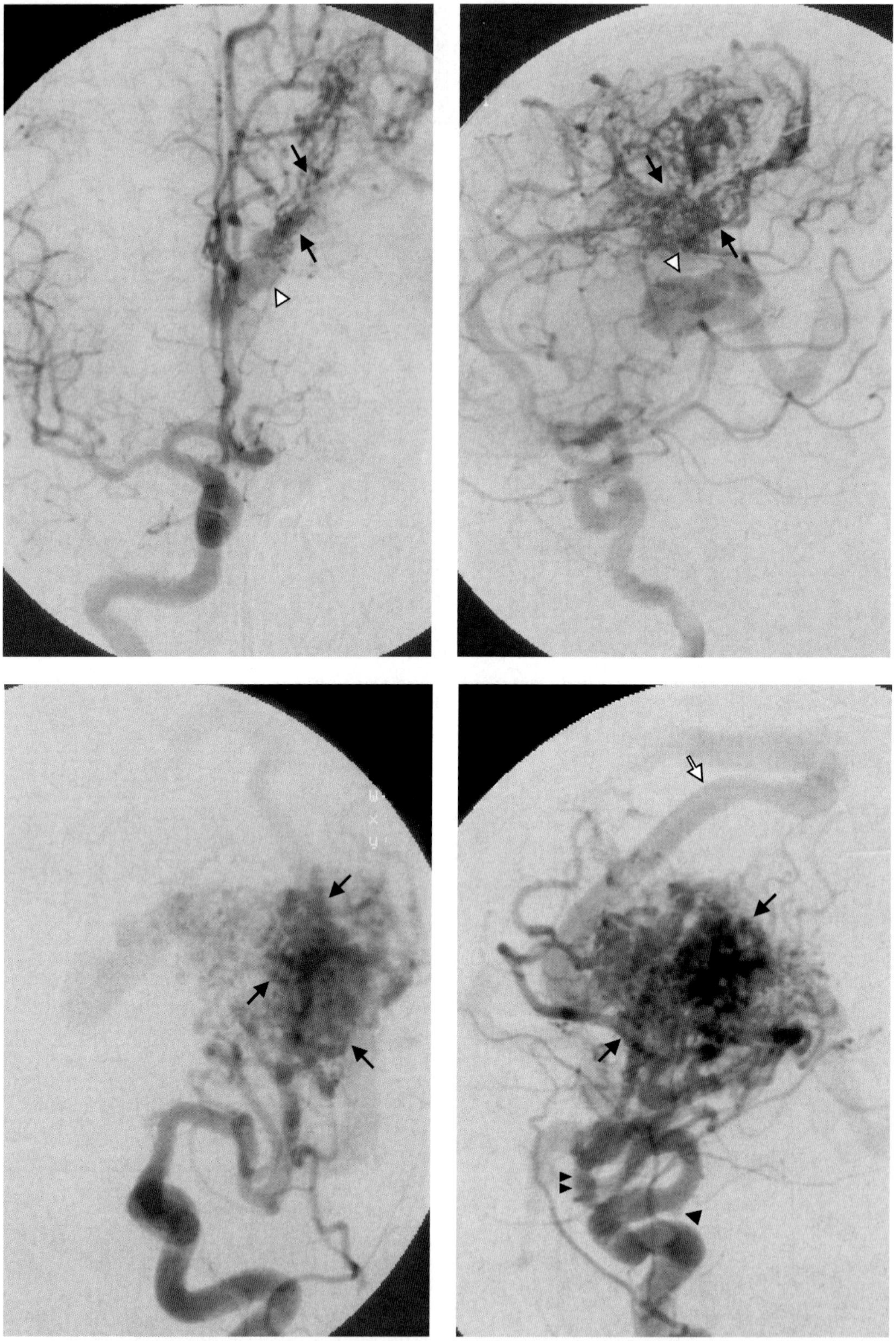

C D E F

FIGURE 9-7. *Continued.* **C–F:** On angiography, the AVM nidus measured 6 cm, was eloquent, demonstrated deep venous drainage *(open arrowheads)* **(C,D)** and was Spetzler-Martin grade V. **C,D:** A portion of the AVM filled from the right internal carotid circulation via the anterior communicating artery *(black arrows)* with primarily deep venous drainage *(open arrowheads).* **E,F:** The majority of the AVM filled through branches of the left anterior and middle cerebral arteries *(black arrows)* and had superficial venous drainage *(open arrow).* Because of the patient's young age, treatment of the AVM was advised. *(Figure continues.)*

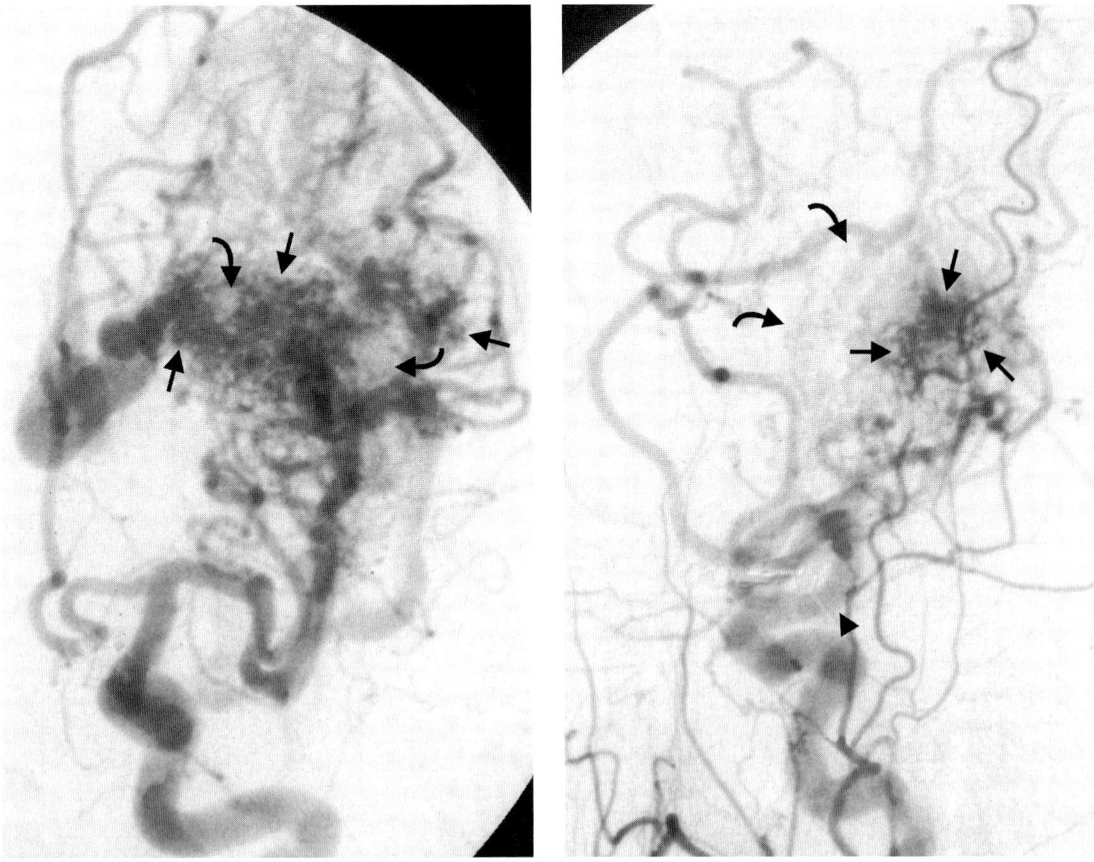

G H

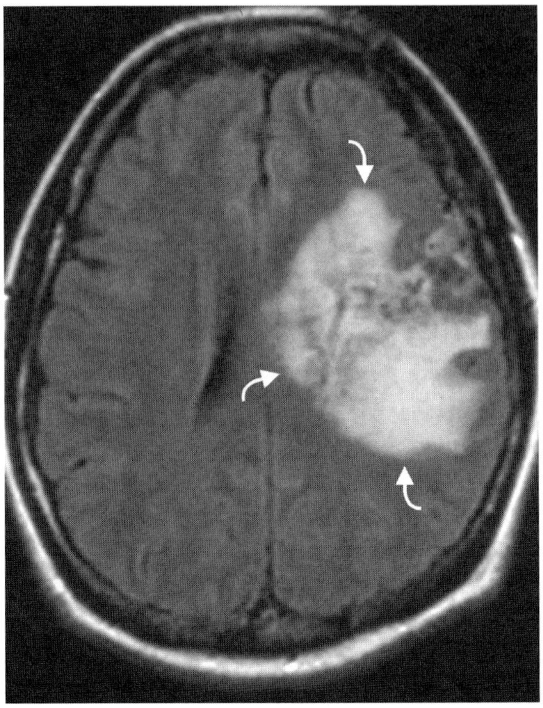

I

FIGURE 9-7. *Continued.* However, we first recommended obliteration of her type II flow-related aneurysms arising from the left posterior communicating *(single arrowhead)* **(F)** and anterior communicating arteries *(double arrowhead)* **(F)** to prevent hemorrhage from these aneurysms during treatment of the AVM nidus. After surgical clipping of the aneurysms *(arrowhead)* **(H)**, and *(double arrowhead)* **(K)**, she underwent three embolization procedures (LICA—**[G,H]**) with a reduction in the nidus size *(straight black arrows)*, with the embolized portion surrounded by *curved black arrows*. Because of the anatomical location of the AVM and the size of the residual nidus, she was treated with proton beam radiosurgery (25 GyE to a volume of 31.4 cm^3). Within 6 months of radiosurgery, she began to develop fluctuating expressive dysphasia and headaches related to significant radiation-induced white matter edema *(arrows)* **(I)**. *(Figure continues.)*

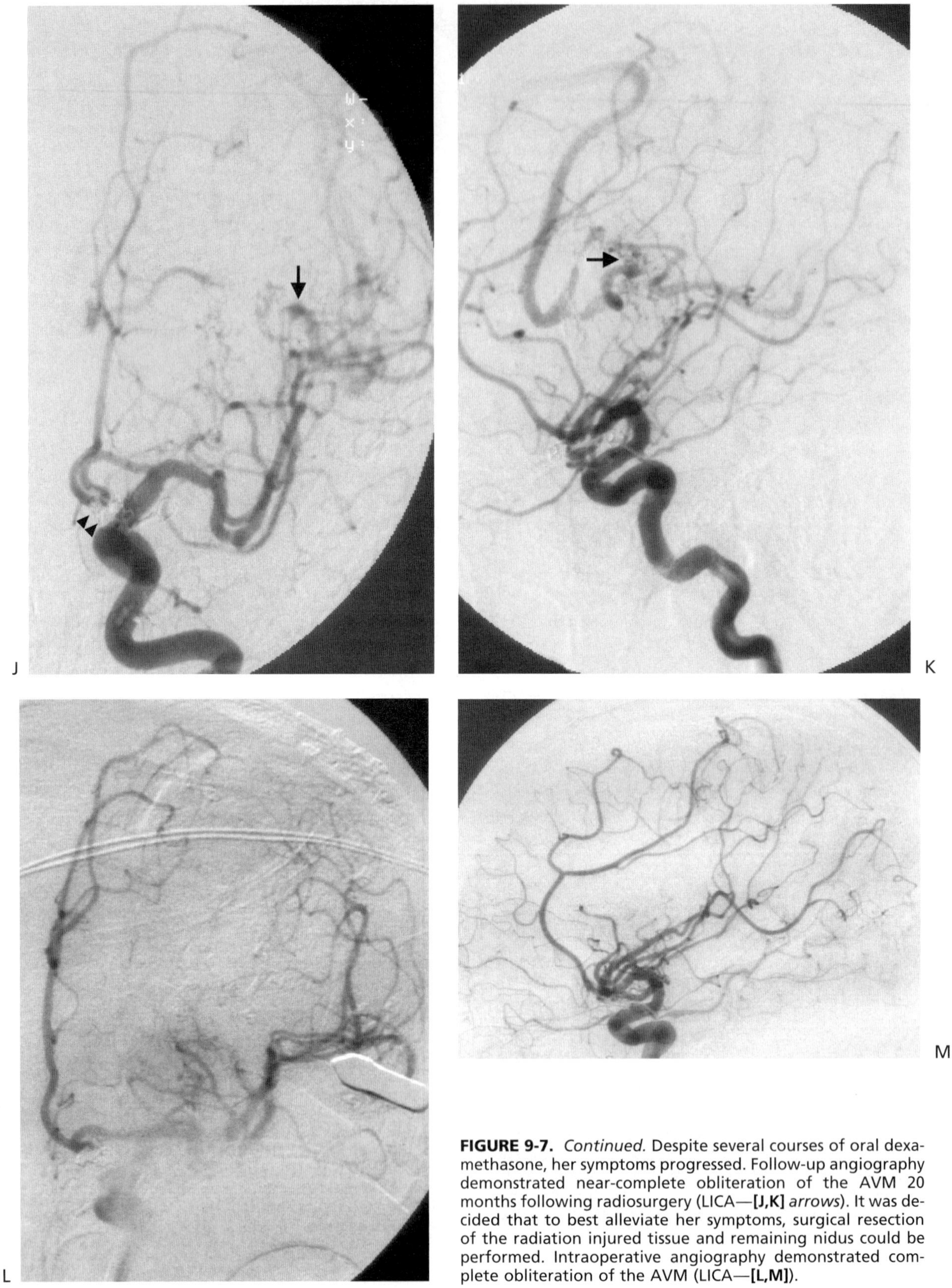

FIGURE 9-7. *Continued.* Despite several courses of oral dexamethasone, her symptoms progressed. Follow-up angiography demonstrated near-complete obliteration of the AVM 20 months following radiosurgery (LICA—**[J,K]** *arrows*). It was decided that to best alleviate her symptoms, surgical resection of the radiation injured tissue and remaining nidus could be performed. Intraoperative angiography demonstrated complete obliteration of the AVM (LICA—**[L,M]**).

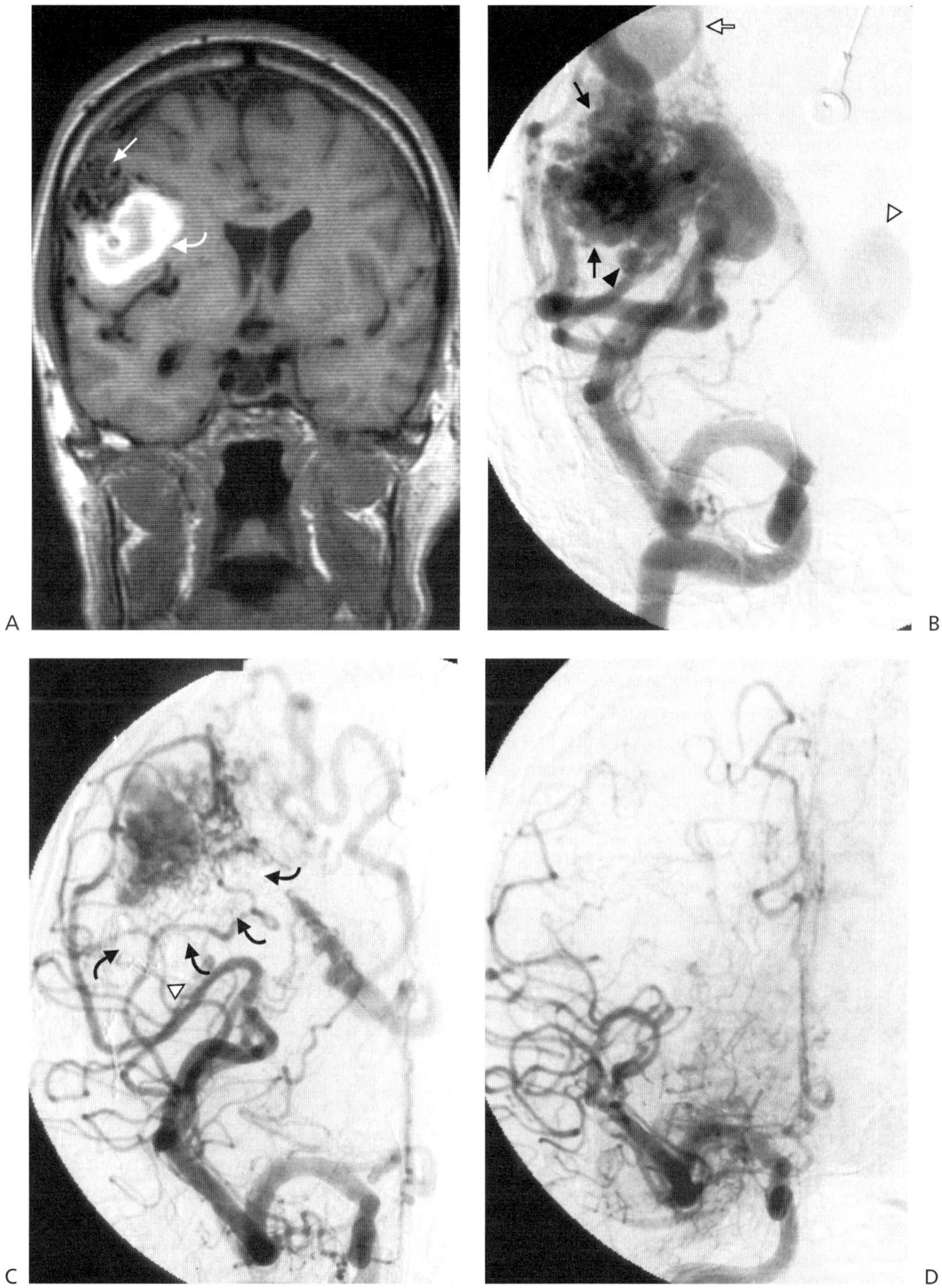

FIGURE 9-8. This 42-year-old right-handed man had originally had onset of seizures a decade earlier. Although surgical resection was recommended at that time, he decided to pursue medical treatment only (anticonvulsant therapy). He then sought treatment after 10 years for a right scotoma and left homonymous hemianopia, left arm paraesthesia, and left leg weakness. **A:** MRI scan demonstrated a subacute hemorrhage *(curved arrow)* adjacent to the AVM nidus *(straight arrow).* **B:** The diagnostic angiogram revealed that MCA vessels were the dominant feeding arteries and the venous drainage was both deep *(open arrowhead)* and superficial *(open arrow).* The AVM nidus *(black arrows)* measured 3.5 cm, making this a Spetzler-Martin grade IV AVM. The angiogram also showed a type III distal flow-related aneurysm *(black arrowhead)* arising from one of the MCA branches. **C:** Therefore, he underwent image-guided surgical clipping of the aneurysm, followed by two sessions of embolization that resulted in significant reduction in size of the AVM nidus. Note embolization material in the thrombosed AVM *(curved arrows)* and surgical clip on obliterated aneurysm *(open arrowhead).* He then underwent resection of the remaining AVM nidus using image guidance. The patient suffered mild left hand weakness following surgery, but this returned to normal within 6 weeks. **D:** His postoperative angiogram demonstrated complete obliteration of the AVM.

rhage, likely because of the more immediate contribution to morbidity presented by a hemorrhage. The risk of developing epilepsy following the diagnosis of an AVM is not well documented. Crawford et al. found that the risk of developing seizures during 20-year follow-up was 18%, with a greater risk in those patients who had originally had a hemorrhage (22%) [46]. As one might expect, the risk was higher for patients with temporal lobe AVMs. Seizure control with anticonvulsants has not been the specific focus of many reports. However, several series do comment that medical control of epilepsy is relatively easy to accomplish [47,57,76,77,88].

Risk of Hemorrhage in Patients with Seizures

Of the natural history studies discussed in the preceding sections, few addressed the risk of hemorrhage following diagnosis of an AVM in patients with seizures but without hemorrhage [42,44,46] (see Fig. 9-3). In the conservatively managed cohort of their study, Forster et al. found that for those with epilepsy who had never bled, there was a 25% chance of suffering hemorrhage over the ensuing 15 years [42]. That same risk (25%) was realized over merely 4 years in those who had previously bled once and over only 1 year in those who had bled twice, suggesting that the risk of hemorrhage is lower in those who have seizures. Fults and Kelly reported on 26 patients who originally came in with seizures and were followed for a mean duration of 11 years [45]. In this group the hemorrhage rate was 26.9%, and mortality attributable to the AVM was 7.7%. In two early natural history studies, the risk of hemorrhage was roughly 1.5% to 3.0% per year, very similar to the rates in patients without seizures [44,46].

Headache

As many as 24% of patients with AVMs will have headache as the initial or primary manifestation [34], although in larger series aimed at identifying demographic characteristics of a large number of patients, the proportion with headaches was only 14% [15] (Fig. 9-9). In studying a series of 70 patients with occipital AVMs, Kupersmith et al. found headache to be as common a symptom as visual field deficits, and more common than hemorrhage or epilepsy [89]. They noted that the symptoms associated with occipital AVMs can closely mimic those of migraine headache (including unilateral pain, throbbing nature, and visual symptomatology), and this can sometimes lead to a delay in diagnosis of the underlying vascular malformation. Kupersmith et al. discovered that patients with AVMs in this location were more likely to have dural vessels supplying the AVM [89]. Interestingly, patients with AVMs in this location who had headaches had a significantly lower risk of subsequent AVM rupture [89]. Two recent case reports also discuss this phenomenon. In the first patient, migraines with visual aura resolved completely after the AVM was treated with radiosurgery and went on to complete obliteration [90]. In the second, daily migraines with visual aura were described in a patient with an occipital AVM [91]. Headache severity and aura frequency were improved with partial obliteration of the AVM nidus after two gamma knife radiosurgery treatments. One series reported improvement or cure of headaches in 68% of patients treated with stereotactic radiosurgery [92].

Neurologic Deficit

Because AVMs represent mass lesions and can affect the blood flow to surrounding and distant parenchymal regions, patients commonly have focal neurologic deficits that are a function of the anatomical area and physiologic disturbance created by the AVM. Early descriptions of the steal phenomenon were made by Pool and Norlen [43,93]. Focal neurologic deficit is a less common clinical manifestation in a patient with an AVM than is hemorrhage or seizures. In a large recent study the incidence of focal deficit was only 7% [15]. As in the Cooperative Study, 72% of patients in Batjer and Samson's series experienced hemorrhage, while the other 28% had progressive deficits related to steal phenomenon from the AVM [94]. Because this is a less common clinical picture for the patient with AVM, attempts to correlate morphological characteristics with progressive neurologic deficit have been more limited. However, large AVM size and the presence of angiomatous feeding vessels have been found to correlate with progressive neurologic deficit [95].

In a large series of 70 patients with occipital AVMs, visual symptoms were present in 56% at the time of diagnosis and were more common in patients with AVMs affecting the medial aspect of the occipital lobe than those involving the lateral aspect or anterior portion [89]. Prior hemorrhage was associated with a significantly higher risk of visual field loss, and these patients also had more severe visual symptoms [89]. These results compared favorably with an earlier reported series describing a smaller number of patients with medial occipital lobe AVMs, in which homonymous visual field deficits were present in 67% of patients whose AVMs had hemorrhaged [96]. Symptoms included scintillating scotomas, jagged flickering fortification images, transient and permanent homonymous hemianopia, blurred vision, hemifield spots, tunnel vision, and diplopia [89]. Finally, it was also noted by these authors that one-half of patients with normal visual fields who were treated in a multidisciplinary fashion went on to develop a field deficit, while only 30% of patients who had a field deficit prior to treatment experienced improvement in the deficit [89]. A more unusual focal feature is that of pathologic laughter, which has been described with AVMs in the region of the midbrain as well as with other lesions in the hypothalamus [97].

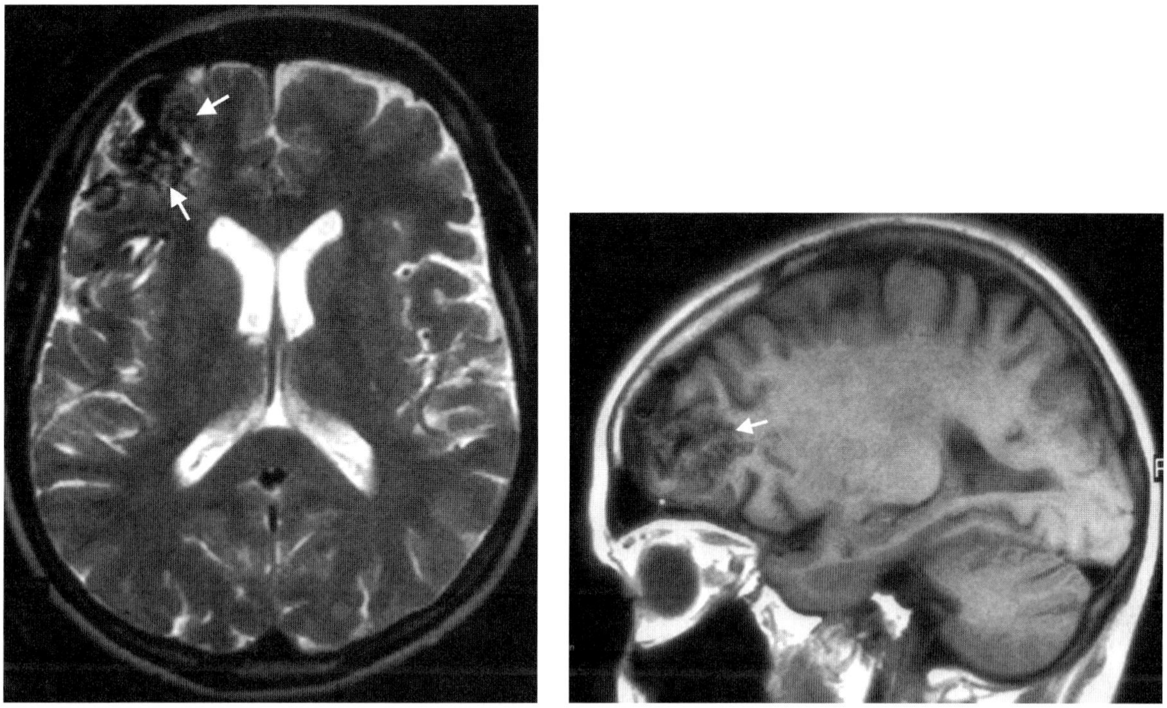

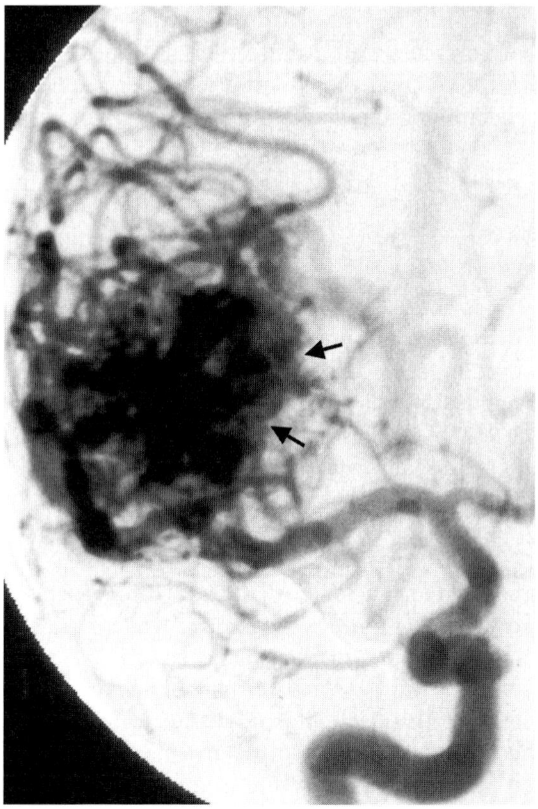

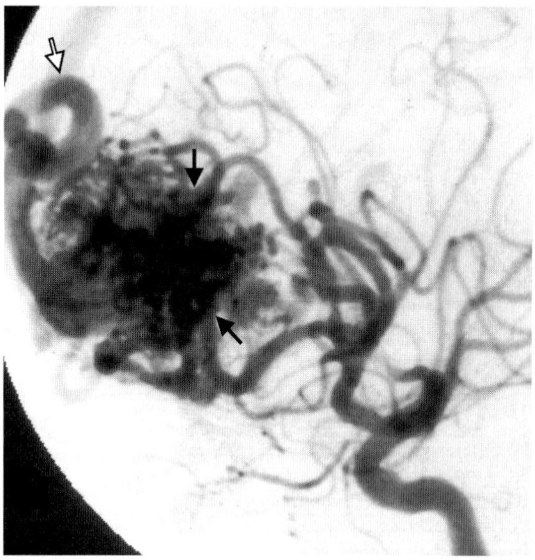

FIGURE 9-9. This 68-year-old right-handed retired school principal presented with a vague history of headaches that did not appear related to her incidentally discovered AVM. **A,B:** MRIs demonstrated a 3-cm right frontal AVM *(arrows)*. **C,D:** Subsequent angiography revealed the nidus *(arrows)* being fed from branches of the right middle cerebral artery. The venous drainage was entirely into the superior sagittal sinus. With no involvement of eloquent parenchyma, this was a Spetzler-Martin grade II AVM. Because of her age and lack of symptoms, we did not recommend treatment.

Cognitive Impairment

Most clinical studies of patients with AVM are retrospective analyses and therefore do not assess routinely for developmental delay or cognitive difficulties in this population, and certainly some of the cognitive deficits described below could actually be considered focal deficits. However, when these factors are specifically studied, as many as 66% of patients are found to have had difficulty during school years with at least one skill (reading problems, impulsivity, disorganization, drawing problems, mathematical problems, writing disorders, attention deficit, listening problems, speech problems) [98]. This was significantly different from an age- and education-matched control population in a retrospective analysis of 44 adult patients with AVMs, and there was no difference attributable to AVM hemorrhage or AVM size [98]. These rates were also higher than national rates for learning disorders and, additionally, there were nonsignificant trends toward need for tutoring or summer school and delays in developmental milestones.

Several studies have evaluated certain cognitive functions more specifically. Lazar et al. evaluated transfer of language function in three patients with left frontal AVMs. They found evidence on Wada-type testing and functional MRI studies that expressive language function had relocalized to areas in the right hemisphere analogous to the Broca area in the left hemisphere, while receptive language function remained in the left temporoparietal region and was affected by the Wada test [99]. In a similar study performed by the same group, there was anterior relocation of language function in patients with left temporoparietal AVMs in the region of the Wernicke area, such that Wada testing of the left prefrontal region led to Wernicke aphasia [100].

Arteriovenous Malformations Associated with Syndromes

Hereditary Hemorrhagic Telangiectasia

HHT, or Rendu-Osler-Weber syndrome, is an autosomal dominant disorder with an incidence of approximately 1: 10,000 with a reported range of 1:2,351 to 1:39,216 [101]. The defect has been mapped to chromosomes 9q and 12q [102–104]. Clinical manifestations include mucocutaneous telangiectasias and AVMs affecting multiple organ systems including the lung and brain. Cerebral manifestations are predominantly from infection or ischemia. The risk of having an AVM in this population is higher than the risk in the general population. In a study by Willemse et al. [105], 12% (24 of 196) of patients with HHT had cerebral AVMs. They calculated the annual hemorrhage risk to be 0.36% to 0.56%, which is much lower than in the general AVM population. Another recent paper relating to AVMs in patients with HHT suggests again that the risk is actually quite low. In a study of 321 patients with HHT, only 10 had AVMs (3.1%), with only seven of these patients having ruptured AVMs (2.1%) [106]. In fact, in this population, the risk of developing neurologic consequences of a pulmonary arteriovenous fistula (cerebral ischemia or abscess) was higher than the risk of hemorrhage from an AVM, prompting the authors to recommend against screening for cerebral AVMs [106]. Conversely, patients with HHT make up an extremely small portion of the population of patients with AVMs. In a retrospective study of 638 patients with AVMs, only 14 (2%) had an associated diagnosis of HHT [107]. In this population, all of the AVMs were 3 cm or less in diameter, over 96% were asymptomatic, and all were cortically based. Patients with HHT who have at least one AVM have a marked propensity for multiple AVMs.

Wyburn-Mason Syndrome

Encephaloretinofacial angiomatosis, or Wyburn-Mason syndrome, is a rare condition involving unilateral vascular malformations of the diencephalon or mesencephalon, ipsilateral retina, and face, with or without cognitive changes [108–111]. Subarachnoid and intracerebral hemorrhages have been reported, and the rare clinical features related to an AVM depend on the anatomical location of the malformation. These vascular malformations tend to follow the optic tracts and radiations [112] and, due to the deep-seated nature of these AVMs, treatment is complicated and frequently multimodal in nature.

Pediatric Arteriovenous Malformations

AVMs are the most common anomalies affecting the cerebral vasculature in children [12,113] and are roughly 10 times more frequent than pediatric aneurysms [7,114], therefore deserving special consideration. However, the overall prevalence of symptomatic AVMs in the pediatric population is low and, as previously mentioned, pediatric AVMs account for only 8% to 20% of all AVMs [7,11, 16–20]. Children with AVMs can obviously experience hemorrhage, seizures, headaches, or focal deficits like adult patients do. However, in the pediatric population AVMs can produce enough arteriovenous shunting to cause high-output congestive heart failure. Hydrocephalus and macrocrania are also relatively unique manifestations of AVMs in childhood and, in particular, infancy.

Although the natural history of hemorrhage and seizures has been studied to some degree in adults, there is little complementary data in pediatric populations. Hemorrhage is the most common clinical feature, as it is in adults [16, 113]. Numerous authors have noted that the hemorrhage rate in children is higher than in adults [16,17,19,115]. As many as 75% to 80% of children with AVMs will have intracerebral hemorrhage [116], and AVMs represent the most common cause of pediatric hemorrhagic stroke [24, 117]. This was recently confirmed in a study of nontraumatic intraparenchymal hemorrhages in children, in which one-third of hemorrhages were due to an AVM or fistula [118]. In a small uncontrolled study, Celli et al. found that within their series of pediatric patients with AVMs, the hemorrhage rate after 10 years of conservative management was greater in those who were diagnosed prior to age 15 years [17]. Additionally, they performed a metaanalysis demonstrating that the risk of hemorrhage after symptom onset was statistically significantly higher in children than in adults, and this relationship was more pronounced in those who originally were diagnosed without hemorrhage. As previously discussed, small size is an independent risk factor for AVM hemorrhage and D'Aliberti et al. found that pediatric AVMs were generally smaller than adult AVMs, possibly leading to their increased rate of symptomatic hemorrhage [18]. Alternatively, Di Rocco et al. indicate that a disproportionate occurrence of deep AVMs in the basal ganglia thalamus might account for the greater hemorrhage rate in children [116]. However, in most series there is no higher frequency of such angioarchitectural features that might explain the higher hemorrhage risk compared to adults. On the other hand, some think angioarchitecture in pediatric AVMs tends to be simpler [18]. They tend to be fed by fewer vessels and some reports indicate that they affect deep structures less frequently. This is in keeping with the theory that AVMs are progressive lesions with the tendency to grow.

The mortality risk in children following initial hemorrhage is also thought to be higher than that in the adult population. Humphreys et al. found that 24% of children died following AVM hemorrhage either before or after treatment [114], which is higher than the more widely quoted 10% for adults. There are no reliable natural history data for AVMs specifically in children; however, two series calculate the short-term risk of subsequent hemorrhage. In a literature review, it was noted that for children with AVMs who did not undergo treatment, the average 10-year mortality was 23% [17]. The 5-year risk of rehemorrhage from an AVM in a child has been reported to be 25% [113]. Some authors feel that symptomatic AVMs in juveniles should always be considered for surgical excision [7]. Approximations of risk such as these, coupled with the protracted life expectancy of pediatric patients, are often cited as indication to pursue treatment. Others have noted that children tend to make a better recovery than adults and therefore should be treated earlier. Gerszten et al. surmised that early treatment of pediatric AVMs is almost always warranted because of the high cumulative risk of hemorrhage or rehemorrhage over their lifetimes [72]. Gerosa et al. also described the high mortality rate following conservative treatment and recommended surgical therapy for children with AVMs [16].

Although AVMs represent the most common cause of pediatric brain hemorrhage, they are an uncommon cause for pediatric epilepsy. In a community-based study of 613 children with newly diagnosed epilepsy, 488 underwent imaging studies and only one was found to have an AVM [119]. Among series of children with AVMs, the rate of seizures, or epilepsy, is 11.5% to 30% [7,16,17,120,121].

TREATMENT

Grading Systems

Many grading systems have been designed for AVMs in order to clarify treatment risk and outcome. Among these, the scale proposed in 1986 by Spetzler and Martin has become most widely adopted [122]. Additionally, it has been validated in a prospective fashion [123]. Before presenting this scale in detail, we will review its predecessors and other scales that have not become as widely adopted.

In 1977, Luessenhop and Gennarelli developed an early grading scale that was based on the number of angiographically identifiable feeding arteries [124]. The highest grade was IV, based on the premise at the time that lesions with more than four major feeding arteries could be treated only by hemispherectomy. Using their classification scheme, there was no morbidity or mortality in grade I AVMs, 6% morbidity and no mortality in grade II AVMs, and 30% morbidity and 20% mortality in grade III AVMs. They did not treat any patients with grade IV lesions and concluded that for grade III AVMs, location and clinical status of the patient were more important than anatomical grade.

Subsequently, Parkinson and Bachers proposed a classification scheme in 1980 based on angioarchitecture [57]. This was based on anatomical and physiologic characteristics of the AVM and attempted to draw comparisons to possible embryologic origins of AVMs. This also did not come into general use as a grading scale.

Pasqualin et al. evaluated AVM nidus volume, location, anatomy of feeding arteries and venous drainage, and transcranial Doppler (TCD) ultrasonographic measurements of flow velocity [125]. Using these factors they could predict morbidity and mortality and, in certain instances, postoperative hematoma. However, this classification scheme involved many variables, some of which are not typically measured in patients with AVM (TCD velocity), and also was not widely used.

Pertuiset et al. studied the predictability of outcome in patients with supratentorial AVMs according to anatomical, hemodynamic, and clinical factors [126]. However, this scale was complex and devised to predict operability and surgical strategy, with a minimal score of 3 and a maximum of 69, and varying management recommendations for patients with scores over 30 (surgery not advised), 21 to 30 (several-stage operations recommended), 11 to 20 (two-stage operation), and less than 11 (single-stage operation for radical excision). It has not been used by subsequent authors in a widespread fashion.

The Spetzler-Martin classification scheme is accepted as the standard for assessing the surgical risk associated with

TABLE 9-4. SPETLZER-MARTIN GRADING[a] OF SURGICAL RISKS ASSOCIATED WITH AVM RESECTION

AVM Factor	Points
Nidus Size	
<3 cm	1
3–6 cm	2
>6 cm	3
Deep Venous Drainage	
Absent	0
Present	1
Location	
Noneloquent	0
Eloquent	1

AVM, arteriovenous malformation.
[a]Grade is determined by adding total points.

a patient's AVM. This scale stratifies AVMs according to the size of the nidus, the eloquence of the surrounding brain, and the presence or absence of venous drainage (Table 9-4). In prospective follow-up, it was determined that AVMs graded I, II, or III were safely treated by surgical excision alone, with low morbidity and little mortality. On the other hand, patients with lesions graded IV and V incurred significant morbidity and mortality with surgical treatment. Subsequent work by groups at other centers, including Deruty et al. [127] and Heros et al., has also validated this work [76]. Heros et al. studied 153 patients who underwent surgical resection of AVMs and found a high correlation between Spetzler-Martin grade and outcome. Grading according to the Spetzler-Martin scale is applied in all clinical examples (see Figs. 9-2 to 9-9).

However, not all published series have been in agreement with this grading scale. Hartmann et al. recently found that in their 124 patients there was not a universally low complication rate in grade I to III AVMs, and there was not a progressive increase in complication rates from grades I to V [128]. Although the assessment of deep venous drainage and AVM nidus size leaves little room for variability among those rating them, recent work has suggested that eloquence of AVM location is interpreted differently at various institutions [15].

Indications for Treatment

The general principle surrounding AVM treatment, regardless of modality, must be to eliminate the threat of intracranial hemorrhage while at the same time preserving neurologic function and avoiding complications [129]. Several authors have explored the question of whether or not unruptured AVMs should be treated and the issue has been approached in several fashions. Initially, Aminoff reviewed the literature surrounding operative and nonoperative management of AVMs and incorporated an assessment of natural history. He concluded that there was no clear advantage to the surgical management of unruptured AVMs [130].

Fisher used the technique of decision analysis in his assessment and, in doing so, noted the complexity of the factors contributing to the ultimate decision, such as patient's age, efficacy and risks of treatment, and natural history of AVMs [131]. This model estimated that open surgery was the best treatment option for a young (38-year-old) patient with a Spetzler-Martin grade III AVM who lacked significant concurrent disease (American Society of Anesthesiologists 1 to 2). However, if there was significant disease, the model predicted that radiosurgery was a better option. Additionally, radiosurgery was favored for larger AVMs (Spetzler-Martin grade IV or V). The natural history of the lesion never supported the conservative treatment path for these patients. This analysis assumed that embolization procedures preceding radiosurgery led to a 25% increase in cure rates. In a similar decision analysis paper, the authors also recommended treatment, in the form of elective surgical resection, for young patients with unruptured AVMs demonstrating favorable angioarchitectural features [132]. Interestingly, the results of these recent decision analyses were contrary to an earlier decision analysis study performed on unruptured AVMs published prior to the advent of multidisciplinary AVM treatment with embolization and radiosurgery and more definitive studies documenting natural history of these lesions. In the earlier study, it was determined that conservative therapy was the preferred method of managing an unruptured AVM [133]. Although useful in prompting the clinician to consider all potential outcomes for a given patient, we feel that these methods oversimplify the complexity of any given patient's lesion. Nonetheless, these serial decision analyses demonstrate that the development of radiosurgery and embolization, allowing multidisciplinary treatment of AVMs, has resulted in a positive impact on patient outcome with treatment and argue against conservative management in most cases.

Based on his assessment of natural history studies of patients whose AVMs had and had not previously ruptured, Flamm concluded that the long-term risks were similar and advocated treatment for patients following the diagnosis of an AVM [134]. In an earlier report, Pool and Potts found that 56% of the patients they managed conservatively went on to die or develop severe disability [135]. Similarly, Luessenhop demonstrated that in an untreated cohort of AVM patients, 20% died and another 30% developed severe disability within 10 years of diagnosis [136].

In weighing the natural history against the risks of treatment, Mattle et al. also advocated treatment of all AVMs [1]. They recommended surgical treatment for grade I to III AVMs and multimodal treatment for grades IV and V AVMs, with a more conservative approach taken with older patients harboring high-grade AVMs. Patients with Spetzler-Martin grade IV and V AVMs require careful consideration before being enrolled in a treatment protocol. Some advocate treatment of these lesions only when there is progressive symptomatology as a result of repeated hemorrhage [137].

In considering all of the above, one must undertake treatment of AVMs with the primary goal being complete obliteration of the AVM nidus and disappearance of arteriovenous shunting. It has long been thought that incomplete AVM resection does not confer protection against future hemorrhagic events [130]. Davis and Symon have demonstrated that following incomplete resection, the annual risk of hemorrhage is 2.6% [138]. Abad et al. obtained incomplete resections of the AVM nidus in 13 patients, and 46% of them either died or suffered hemorrhage from the residual nidus [56]. In the series of Amacher et al., 6 of 16 patients (37.5%) with incomplete AVM resections suffered rehemorrhage [75]. The risk of recurrent hemorrhage from a residual nidus was echoed in a more recent case report as well [139].

In some patients, the daunting anatomical location or size of the AVM may lead neurosurgeons or interventional neuroradiologists to deem an AVM "incurable." In these situations, consideration might be given to partial treatment of the AVM in order to reduce arteriovenous shunting and alleviate a patient's symptoms, or at least slow their progression. We have employed this philosophy to treat several incurable AVMs, believing that palliative treatment may help relieve symptoms such as headache, seizures, or progressive neurologic deficit. However, a recent study indicates that such palliative treatment may not confer any advantage to the patient and might instead be more threatening than the natural history of the AVM [140]. Miyamoto et al. reported on 43 patients, 24 of whom were treated in an intentionally palliative fashion, using partial embolization, radiosurgery, or subtotal resection. They found the annual rate of hemorrhage in this subset of patients following such treatment was 17%. The major morbidity rate was 23% and the mortality rate was nearly 10%, with 75% of mortality being directly attributable to the treatment. They recommended a conservative approach to patients with incurable AVMs. With improved treatment strategies involving multimodal therapy and improved knowledge of the natural history, the indications for treatment of patients with AVMs are becoming broader. We treat most patients with the exception of the elderly, medically infirm, or some patients who are minimally symptomatic (see Fig. 9-9).

Children have the longest life expectancy of any cohort with AVMs and therefore inherently have the highest lifetime risk of hemorrhage (see Fig. 9-3). Obviously, if age and hemorrhage risk become the primary considerations in decision making, then the presence of an AVM alone might be considered an indication for treatment. Several authors have reported series of pediatric patients with AVMs both treated and observed. Based on his early experience treating 36 children with AVMs, in which 10 of 14 patients who had originally had seizures alone went on to hemorrhage within 7 years, So recommended that all AVMs in children should be obliterated [113]. Gerosa et al. also described the high mortality rate following conservative treatment and recommended surgical therapy for children with AVMs [16].

The treatment of epilepsy associated with an AVM is a controversial topic. Although seizures can be managed medically (see Figs. 9-3 and 9-6), there is a cohort of patients who will become refractory to pharmacological treatment and may benefit from obliteration of their AVMs. Patients whose seizures are controlled with anticonvulsants and are otherwise asymptomatic represent a difficult group. Although treatment might not be indicated based on their seizure control, the issue of long-term hemorrhage risk and the patient's age again become important.

The psychologic dilemma that harboring an AVM creates for a patient is worthy of mention [1,141]. The patient who has seen the angiogram or been told of the potential for AVM hemorrhage, albeit small, may be compelled to pursue treatment despite any recommendations by the neurologist or neurosurgeon. We certainly do not commonly invoke this factor as an indication for surgery and it should never be used as the sole indication to proceed. However, in a small subset of patients it becomes a real issue and a legitimate indication for consideration of treatment.

When it is determined that treatment is indeed indicated, the next dilemma revolves around what treatment modality is best for a given patient. In general, endovascular embolization is used as an adjunctive treatment. It can be used strategically to remodel an AVM prior to microsurgical or radiosurgical treatment and will rarely be used in isolation to achieve cure of an AVM. Occasionally, a very small AVM can be obliterated completely using embolization alone. The debate that currently rages loudest however, is whether to treat patients initially with surgery or radiosurgery. In the absence of randomized clinical trials, there is no correct answer.

This issue was addressed by several groups [142–145], who indicated that the primary differences between the treatments are their short- and long-term outcomes. Surgery offers an immediate chance of curing the AVM with removal of the nidus and elimination of arteriovenous shunting, but the effects of radiosurgery are not achieved completely for several years. On the other hand, the risks of surgery are fractionally higher than the risks of radiosurgery, as elaborated upon in the following sections of this chapter. The following represents a composite list of the advantages of surgical management as recently described by several experienced neurosurgeons [142,143,145]:

1. Surgery results in higher cure rates than radiosurgery.
2. Surgery provides immediate protection from future hemorrhage.

3. Surgery is associated with fewer posttreatment hemorrhages than radiosurgery.
4. Symptomatic recurrence of an angiographically obliterated AVM following surgery is exquisitely rare.
5. AVM obliteration is not a certain consequence of radiosurgery.
6. Hemorrhage during the latent period following radiosurgery is not a benign event.
7. Microsurgical resection of AVMs is increasingly safe and postoperative deficits tend to improve over time.

On the other hand, the same authors elaborate the following points that argue in favor of pursuing radiosurgical treatment:

1. Some AVM patients are unable to undergo surgical resection without an unacceptable risk.
2. Smaller AVMs (less than or equal to 3 cm) respond better than larger ones to radiosurgery, both in terms of lesion obliteration and radiation complications.
3. For most small AVMs, both radiosurgery and microsurgery have high rates of success.
4. Surgical therapy is invasive.
5. Perioperative hemorrhage can occur as a result of residual AVM, hyperemia, or venous infarction.
6. Surgical results are surgeon specific.

Pikus et al. compared radiosurgery to microsurgery and found that patients treated by microsurgery were more likely to enjoy obliteration of their AVMs, and less likely to suffer posttreatment hemorrhage, die, or develop a new neurologic deficit [146]. Regardless of all the prior published series, the treatment decision for a given patient will incorporate not only published data, but also the biases and tendencies of the treating team, the resources of the medical facility, and the preferences of the patient. In the absence of a randomized trial comparing radiosurgery to microsurgery, the latter elements have the potential to weigh more heavily in the decision than they probably should.

Because it is usually performed as an outpatient procedure, it is commonly believed that radiosurgery is performed more economically than microsurgery. However, the only published series that describe a cost-benefit analysis of the two modalities both favor surgical resection of the AVM. In the study of Nussbaum et al., primary surgical management resulted in extended quality-adjusted life expectancy and an overall cost savings to society of over $7,500 per patient [147]. In an analysis by Porter et al., surgery provided 0.98 years of additional quality-adjusted life years and was also more cost effective over the long term [148].

Endovascular Embolization

Endovascular embolization of AVMs is covered in detail in Chapter 10 and therefore not dealt with in this chapter. We defer detailed discussion of this technique to experts in the field. Suffice to say that the advantages of superselective angiography and advanced endovascular techniques in diagnosing and treating AVMs include improved understanding of the hemodynamics, physiology, and functional localization of an AVM, better visualization of components of an AVM fed from different vessels, and improved diagnosis and treatment of associated conditions such as arterial flow-related aneurysms and segments of venous stenosis. Although its use without adjunctive surgery or radiosurgery is only likely to result in a cure of 6% to 20% of AVMs, embolization can generally be performed with low risk of morbidity or mortality [1].

Microsurgery

Microsurgical resection remains the proven gold standard treatment for accessible AVMs that can be removed with minimal surgical risk [72]. Batjer reminds us that surgical treatment of an AVM is seldom undertaken with the goal of improving the patient's actual neurologic status [143]. In most instances, the stated goal of treatment is to eliminate the risk of future hemorrhage and neurologic deterioration. Because no immediate gain is offered to the patient, surgical morbidity and mortality rates must be kept to a minimum in order to make surgical management worthwhile. Other treatment modalities such as embolization or radiosurgery do not always result in complete obliteration of the AVM nidus but can be used in concert with surgery to obliterate it.

Surgical Results, Morbidity, and Mortality

With these principles in mind, several of the significant surgical series will be reviewed, concentrating on the rate of nidus obliteration and the procedural complications. Microsurgery, with or without adjunctive embolization, is considered first-line therapy for grade I and II AVMs [137] (see Fig. 9-5). These AVMs tend to be small (<3 cm), with or without deep venous drainage, and not necessarily involving eloquent cortex. Although some of these patients may benefit from embolization in order to control deep feeding arteries, the surgical risk is relatively low and offers immediate elimination of hemorrhage risk without the 24- to 36-month latency period associated with radiosurgery. Larger and more challenging AVMs generally require a multidisciplinary approach, as described in more detail below.

During the last decade, several institutional series have been published that demonstrate the efficiency with which patients with AVMs can be treated microsurgically. Heros et al. provided long-term follow-up (mean 3.8 years) on 153 patients [76]. Although 24.2% had significant morbidity during the immediate postoperative period, only 7.8% had permanent deficits, indicating that many of the neurologic deficits seen soon after AVM surgery tend to resolve with time. Mortality related to the AVM was 1.3% and all lesions were completely obliterated angiographically. These results also demonstrated reliably favorable results in patients with grades I to III AVMs and less favorable results in those with higher grade lesions.

Sisti et al. surgically resected 67 small (<3 cm) AVMs, 45% of which were located in deep eloquent areas [149]. They cured 94% of their patients and only one patient (1.5%) developed permanent significant morbidity related to surgery. There were no operative deaths. As part of their analysis of their surgical series, Piepgras et al. determined that the life expectancy of their 280 patients who underwent surgery for AVM resection was no different than that of an appropriate control population [52]. Although this series focused on surgical treatment of epilepsy, there were five acute and five delayed deaths attributable to the AVM, for a mortality rate of approximately 3.6%.

In a series from Germany of 62 patients, small AVMs (<3 cm) deemed amenable to radiosurgery or endovascular treatment were surgically excised [150]. More than 98% of these patients were cured following surgery and permanent deficits were seen after surgery in only 3.2%, with no mortality. More recently, this same group confirmed the findings of Heros et al. [76,151]. The early postoperative morbidity rate was 39.3%, but only 10.6% of patients suffered permanent deficits, of which only 7.3% were major deficits [151].

Several authors have addressed the surgical management of AVMs in specific anatomical areas of the brain [79,80, 94,152–156]. To review these series in detail is beyond the scope of this chapter. However, in many instances these specialized series represent technically challenging anatomical locations, and the authors were able to obtain excellent obliteration rates (88.9% to 100%) with minimal new morbidity (0% to 22.2%) or mortality (0% to 17%).

With growing experience with surgical management of AVMs, there are more reports that specifically examine the factors contributing to a negative outcome following microsurgical AVM resection. The onset of delayed neurologic deterioration following surgical resection of AVMs was studied retrospectively by Morgan et al. [157], who found that the Spetzler-Martin scale accurately predicted immediate deficits but not those occurring later. They emphasize that vigilance must be maintained during the postoperative period in order to prevent physiologic and hemodynamic complications that may cause delayed deterioration following an otherwise successful operation for extirpation of an AVM. In analyzing their series of 200 AVMs that were surgically resected, these authors elaborated several factors that increase the risk of postoperative deterioration. Their 30-day operative mortality was only 0.5%, but they studied factors leading to postoperative morbidity. Specifically, they found that postoperative hypertension led to hemorrhage in four patients who had undergone resection of large AVMs. Another four patients developed vasospasm, and this was more common in patients who had undergone dissection near the more proximal segments of the major intracranial arteries. Two patients developed delayed progressive symptoms from venous stasis or thrombosis. The authors emphasize the need to manage patients' blood pressure very tightly following the removal of the arteriovenous shunt in those with large AVMs, and suggest the selective use of nimodipine in patients for whom extensive dissection near major intracranial vessels is necessary.

In another recent analysis of outcome following surgery for cerebral AVMs, Hartmann et al. studied 124 patients who underwent surgical resection of an AVM in the modern era (1990 to 1998) at a tertiary care facility experienced in the surgical management of AVMs [128]. In long-term follow-up averaging 12 months, 38% of these patients incurred surgery-related neurologic deficits. However, less than one-sixth of these deficits were disabling (6%), representing a better outcome than has been recently reported from pooled data published by the same authors [55]. In this recent study, significant associations were drawn between (any) postoperative neurologic deficit and increasing Spetzler-Martin grade, female gender, AVM size, and the presence of deep venous drainage (independently) [128]. The use of preoperative endovascular embolization did not have any impact on the rate of postoperative neurologic deficit. These authors did not make specific recommendations to reduce procedural morbidity, but speculated that current grading systems might be too insensitive to accurately predict risk, and suggested that other parameters be studied more closely. Schaller et al. also recently found a relationship between surgical morbidity and the Spetzler-Martin scale, but stated that the predictive value of this scale could be increased by subdividing the eloquence of an AVM into less eloquent (visual cortex) and highly eloquent (brainstem, basal ganglia and motor cortex) [151]. Although intuitive to a certain extent, continued assessment and reassessment of surgical results will improve not only the ability to predict which patients will incur neurologic morbidity but perhaps also the ability to select patients for alternative forms of therapy.

Finally, Barrow makes the noteworthy point that most surgical series focus on transient and permanent neurologic sequelae of surgery and by their retrospective nature do not report "minor" complications of surgery such as pulmonary infections, deep venous thrombosis, pulmonary emboli, and urinary tract infections [144,145]. Although these other complications are generally not reported, they do have the potential to slow neurologic recovery and thus should be reported.

Seizure Control Following Surgery

There is a question whether or not medically controlled seizures constitute an indication for surgery. One way to assess this issue is to evaluate the ability of AVM treatment to control or cure seizures. Outcome with respect to epilepsy and seizures has been the primary focus of relatively few reports to date [52,73,158] but has been reported in several general AVM series [42,57,76,159].

Many authors have reported good results controlling epilepsy following AVM nidus removal, although there are conflicting results in the literature. Trumpy and Eldevik abolished seizures in 50% of the patients they operated on [77]. Guidetti and Delitala cured 53% of their patients with epilepsy by resecting the AVM [12]. As many as 70% of patients in the series of Leblanc et al. were seizure free or nearly seizure free following AVM nidus resection and resection of surrounding epileptogenic tissue [74]. A similarly positive result was obtained in 75% of patients who had resection of the AVM nidus and epileptogenic focus by Yeh et al. [158]. In the report by Heros et al., more than one-half of all patients with preoperative seizures were cured or their seizure activity declined significantly [76]. However, Forster et al. reported that 22% of their patients developed new seizures, 14% of which were permanent, patients who were seizure free preoperatively [42]. In their series, only 4% of those who underwent surgery had seizures that could be controlled completely with anticonvulsants, and another 14% derived some reduction in seizure frequency [42].

In a report looking specifically at seizure outcome, Piepgras et al. showed that 83% of their 102 patients with preoperative seizures were seizure free postoperatively, with a minimal follow-up duration of 2 years [52]. They also reported that only 6% of patients who were seizure free preoperatively went on to develop postoperative seizures. Interestingly, these authors reported that they did not treat patients primarily for seizures but rather to eliminate the risk of future hemorrhage. Inasmuch, they did not pursue extranidal resection of potentially epileptogenic parenchyma. Despite this, their results with respect to seizure control were more favorable than those of others who resected surrounding epileptogenic tissue [74]. Of course, depending on the eloquence of the lesion, resection of such perinidal tissue may not always be an option.

In a second recent paper looking specifically at seizure outcome, Yeh et al. studied 54 patients following surgical excision of AVMs causing seizures and found that postoperative seizure control was best predicted by age at seizure onset (<30 years), short duration of preoperative seizures (<1 year), and AVM location in noneloquent areas that did not limit resection of epileptogenic foci [73]. They advocate cortical resection for optimal seizure control, particularly in patients with early-onset or long-standing seizures. Other series have also reported less encouraging results with seizure control following surgery, but these results tend to come from older literature. These included Parkinson and Bachers, who comment that postoperative seizures are just as likely as preoperative seizures [57], and Drake, who suggested that resection of the AVM nidus alone is ineffective in control of seizures [159]. Murphy found no difference in the number of seizure-free patients managed surgically than those managed medically [88].

Results of Surgery for Pediatric Arteriovenous Malformations

Numerous series have described the results of microsurgical resection of AVMs in children [18,24,114,116,120,121,160], and fewer have described multimodal management of pediatric AVMs [20,116]. Review of this literature suggests that pediatric AVMs can be resected with high obliteration rates in most series, causing minimal procedural morbidity and mortality.

Malik et al. reported on 46 children with AVMs (excluding vein of Galen malformations and dural arteriovenous fistulas) managed over a 48-year period [24]. They analyzed a group of seven younger children separately and found that all AVMs diagnosed before age 5 were >5 cm in longest diameter, and these patients commonly had congestive heart failure, hydrocephalus, and cranial bruit. Only one of these patients had suffered hemorrhage. Due to the size of these malformations, they were generally considered inoperable. Although surgery was performed on three patients, two died. Two other pediatric patients eventually died of factors related to the AVM. In children aged 3 to 18 years, 28 of 39 (71.8%) suffered hemorrhage, while the other 11 (28.2%) had seizures. Despite an overall mortality of 7% (both were children <2 years of age), they achieved excellent or good outcomes in 85% of 27 patients who underwent surgery and concluded that surgical excision is the best treatment for pediatric AVMs. They commented that 70% of children who were not treated for the AVM after an initial hemorrhage went on to suffer a repeat hemorrhage. Their mortality rate was somewhat higher than reported in other pediatric series [17], however the obvious limitation in their study was the extended interval during which patients were treated, spanning a long period of neurosurgical advancement. In their review, Celli et al. found an operative mortality of 8.5% in 1,027 adult patients undergoing surgery for an AVM, but only 2.6% in 133 children [17].

In a large experience managing 101 pediatric patients with cerebral AVMs over 32 years, Humphreys et al. operated on 78 children [114]. They were able to completely obliterate 73.1% of the AVMs, with six children needing additional resections to obtain cure. Following surgery, 76.9% of patients were neurologically intact or had a nonlimiting deficit and the operative mortality rate was 8%. This series was updated in 1992, with 132 patients managed over 40 years [121]. At that time the complete obliteration rate had been obtained in 70 of 104 patients who underwent surgery. Death following hemorrhage from an AVM was significantly more likely for patients with cerebellar lesions. Following surgery, 67% of children were neurologically normal.

In their series of children with vascular malformations,

Caldarelli et al. described 26 patients with AVMs, 19 of which were supratentorial [120]. They were able to resect 19 of these lesions with no mortality, and 58% of their patients returned to normal. They cite a better chance of recovery in children than in adults as a reason to pursue treatment in children whose AVMs have not ruptured. However, they advised against microsurgical treatment of brainstem AVMs and recommend radiosurgery as the primary treatment for these patients. A few authors have indirectly compared pediatric and adult AVMs. D'Aliberti et al. reported a 15-year experience during which they treated 19 children with AVMs [18]. This group was compared with a group of 120 adults with AVMs managed over the same period. They determined that children tend to have more severe clinical symptoms but at the same time tend to have a better clinical outcome. Eighty-nine percent of the children they treated made a good recovery while 11% had a moderate disability.

Recently, Di Rocco et al. described their experience managing 37 pediatric patients with AVMs over a 17-year period. In their experience, the best predictors of patient outcome were the occurrence of hemorrhage prior to treatment as well as the neurologic status of the patient at the time of diagnosis [116]. In their series, most patients (62%) were managed by surgery alone. No patients were treated exclusively with endovascular therapy while 8% were treated with radiation alone. A combination of treatments was used to treat 23% of patients and 11% were not treated. The four patients in their series who died following treatment were all in extremely poor neurologic condition beforehand. With a mean follow-up duration of nearly 5.5 years, they report 68% of their patients led a normal life. Menovsky and van Overbeeke reviewed the microsurgical management of AVMs in children and concluded that surgical resection provided the best protection against hemorrhage and therefore should be the treatment modality of choice whenever possible. In their analysis they included 21 series published as early as the 1970s, in the pre-CT (i.e., before computed tomography) era. In the majority of the reports, the mortality rate was generally less than 10% and in most series the surgical morbidity was less than 20%, with 85% of children having a good or excellent neurologic outcome [160].

Reoperation

Repeated surgery for AVMs has not been widely described and, apart from intentional staging of a procedure, is generally reserved for patients who develop recurrent AVMs or those who have residual AVM following treatment. Batjer and Samson addressed this in patients undergoing reoperation after incomplete surgical resection or embolization [161]. They commented that, although the principles of resection are generally similar to a native operation, the devascularizing effects of microsurgery are more long-standing. In their experience, patients who have residual AVMs following incomplete embolization tend to recruit more leptomeningeal, perforating, and dural feeders, possibly due to recruitment by the remaining nidus. Our group has described the experience with surgical resection of residual AVMs following radiosurgery [162,163]. The interval following irradiation varied from 1 to 11 years in 33 patients whose AVMs were not cured by radiosurgery. In the majority of these patients (84.8%) complete obliteration was achieved, while only 12% worsened clinically following surgery. Interestingly, intraoperative findings were that these AVMs were less vascular and technically more easy to resect, likely due to partial thrombosis, endothelial proliferation, and hyalinization of vessel walls.

Stereotactic Radiosurgery

Stereotactic radiosurgery offers an essential component in the modern treatment of AVMs. Although radiosurgery is an established treatment for AVMs, continuous improvements in technique promise better results. Radiation can be delivered stereotactically through one of three systems: gamma knife, linear accelerator, or heavy charged particle (proton beam or helium ion). The first two, using photons, are more common and will be the focus of this discussion. Radiosurgery can be employed as the primary individual therapy for a given AVM, and it can be used following subtotal microsurgical resection of an AVM or following incomplete endovascular obliteration of an AVM. As radiosurgery has become more widespread, additional information has become available regarding treatment planning, prediction of successful outcome, and prediction of risks.

At present it is difficult to draw direct efficacy comparisons between published series of patients treated surgically and those treated with radiosurgery. Decisions to proceed with one form of treatment or the other depend on the preference of the patient, preference of the physician or surgeon, size and complexity of the AVM, institutional resources, and local referral patterns.

We generally reserve radiosurgery for treatment of more difficult AVMs or treatment of AVMs in patients who are medically infirm (see Figs. 9-4 and 9-7). It is seldom used for small, easily accessible, noneloquent AVMs such as Spetzler-Martin grade I and II lesions. In fact, some authors indicate that the residual hemorrhage risk and incomplete response to radiosurgery preclude its use in surgically accessible AVMs [137]. Deep AVMs and those located in critical structures are often not amenable to surgical extirpation without unfavorable risk of morbidity. In this regard, radiosurgery should not be viewed as an alternative to surgery, but rather as an adjunctive treatment that can be used to treat AVMs or portions of those that are not surgically accessible. The treating physician must be certain to present treatment options in a responsible, logical, and scientific fashion. Situations will arise in which the patient with a low-grade and easily accessible AVM is attracted to the minimally invasive nature of radiosurgery, although the AVM might be best treated by microsurgical excision to eliminate the hemorrhage risk immediately.

Results of Radiosurgery

The efficacy of radiosurgery in curing patients with lesions <3 cm in maximal diameter or 10 cm^3 in volume has been well established over the last decade [92,164–169]. These patients will experience angiographic cure 65% to 85% of the time, while those with larger AVMs treated by radiosurgery are at higher risk for treatment failure [170–172]. Several studies have shown that AVMs with volumes >10 cm^3 have a higher rate of treatment failure [92,170,173]. Consistent with this, increasing Spetzler-Martin grade has been shown to be a risk factor for treatment failure [170]. The latent interval between treatment and obliteration is usually 2 to 3 years.

In order to obtain these results, several observations have been made at centers with experienced clinicians. The marginal dose was of paramount importance in the series of 838 patients treated by gamma knife, reported by Karlsson et al., regardless of AVM volume [174]. Miyawaki et al., in a multicenter report, also demonstrated the importance of the minimal peripheral dose. In their series, no patients treated with a minimal dose <1,400 cGy had obliterated AVMs [171]. Other studies have also found reduced obliteration rates when the minimal dose falls below 1,400 to 1,500 cGy [92,170]. Several factors have been shown to negatively impact AVM obliteration rates and contribute to treatment failure. In patients treated after intracerebral hemorrhage, changes in AVM nidus morphology following hematoma resolution can have a negative effect [172]. Patients failing radiosurgical treatment after prior embolization may have incomplete obliteration due to recanalization of embolized portions of the nidus [169,171,172,175]. However, many of these reports rely on embolization with particulate material (specifically polyvinyl alcohol), which has been found to have high recanalization rates (see Chapter 10). Technical errors in treatment planning are also commonly cited reasons for incomplete obliteration [170,172, 173], but in some cases deliberately inadequate doses must be given due to the proximity to eloquent brain [172]. Finally, some AVM treatment failures have been attributed to "radiobiologic resistance" [176], although at the present time this is poorly understood. Interestingly, Bhatnagar et al.[207] recently reported that risk factors for cardiovascular disease, that might be expected to increase AVM obliteration, had no discernible effect on AVM obliteration.

Predicting Complications of Radiosurgery

As experience with radiosurgery has grown and patient selection has improved, several authors have attempted to define factors that might lead to complications of radiosurgery. In a large study that combined data from several centers, 102 of 1,255 patients (8%) developed neurologic deficits following AVM radiosurgery [177]. Fatal complications in this series were rare (0.2%) and parenchymal injuries were the most common complication (6.4%). Worsened seizures were rare (0.8%), as were cranial nerve injuries (1%). Kihlstrom et al. documented delayed imaging findings in a small group of patients 8 to 23 years after radiosurgical AVM treatment [178]. All 18 patients were asymptomatic but showed cyst formation on MRI (28%), contrast enhancement (61%), or T2-weighted hyperintensity (17%). Changes were independent of radiation dose and unrelated to AVM recanalization. Others have documented cyst formation in case reports of three patients who developed symptoms such as focal neurologic deficits or seizures [179, 180,180]. Recently, Pollock and Brown described their patients with cyst formation and reviewed the literature to arrive at recommendations for management of these cysts [181]. They concluded that for most patients with symptomatic cysts, a cystoperitoneal catheter could be used to shunt the cyst, but patients failing this technique might require excision of the cyst. The factors leading to radiation injury in general have been studied by the Pittsburgh group [182]. In 38 of 85 patients who developed problems after gamma knife radiosurgery it was found that the "12-Gy volume" (the total volume of tissue, including the target lesion, receiving a dose of 12 Gy or more) was significantly associated with permanent postradiosurgical sequelae [182]. They developed the significant postradiosurgery injury expression (SPIE) score, a measure of radiosurgical risk related to AVM location.

Hemorrhage Risk Following Radiosurgery

The known latency between radiosurgery and AVM obliteration leaves a period of 24 to 36 months during which the patient's AVM still has flow. Several recent studies have demonstrated clearly that during this period there is a persistent risk of hemorrhage between 1.8% and 7.4% per year. This is essentially no different from the natural history of AVM hemorrhage following diagnosis [92,166,183–186]. In a sizable retrospective analysis, Karlsson et al. identified 56 patients from a cohort of 1,593 who suffered AVM hemorrhage during the 2-year latency period following gamma knife radiosurgery for an AVM (1.8% per year) [186]. Posttreatment hemorrhage was related to patient's age, AVM volume, minimal dose, and average dose. Using their data, they developed a complicated model for prediction of hemorrhage in this situation that predicts a higher hemorrhage risk after treatment for patients with large AVMs and older individuals, and lower risk for those who are treated with higher radiation doses. Large AVM size was also determined to be a risk factor for posttreatment hemorrhage in earlier work by Friedman et al. [184], while Pollock et al. found that an unsecured proximal aneurysm was a risk factor for hemorrhage following radiosurgical AVM treatment in their patients [185].

Seizure Control Following AVM Radiosurgery

Many authors have reported seizures occurring in the immediate period following radiosurgery (<24 hours), but these events are generally discounted from long-term postradiosurgery follow-up studies [81,86,164]. The exact mechanism is unknown, however there is no apparent impact on long-term seizure control. In our practice, we administer a single dose of phenytoin 500 mg immediately following radiosurgery to prevent seizures and have not had a patient seize in more than 5 years.

For the treatment of epilepsy related to AVMs, stereotactic radiosurgery has had varying results. In the series of patients from Leningrad treated with proton beam radiosurgery, deep AVMs (75%) and parietal AVMs (60%) had the best results with respect to seizure control [84]. The effect of irradiation on seizures was also greater in smaller AVMs (<6 cm^3) [84]. Over 55% (16 of 29) of patients became seizure free. Patients with simple partial seizures had the poorest results. Interestingly, seizure control was not necessarily related to degree of nidus obliteration demonstrated on follow-up angiography. Some patients had complete AVM obliteration but no change in their seizure frequency. Others had seizure control without complete AVM nidus obliteration. The authors speculate that there may have been an effect of the radiation itself on the surrounding parenchymal tissue. Heavy particle helium ion radiosurgery was reported to improve seizure control in 63% of patients [92].

In another series of patients treated with linear accelerator (LINAC) radiosurgery at the University of Florida, 59% were seizure free and 19% had reduction of seizure frequency of more than 75% compared with their pretreatment seizure frequency [87]. Effect on epilepsy was similar in patients with large and small AVMs. The majority of patients who became seizure free after radiosurgery did so during the first 3 months. This group also found that there was reduction in seizure frequency even in those patients who did not achieve AVM thrombosis, suggesting a direct effect on epileptogenic neurons.

Kurita et al. studied a cohort of 35 patients who had seizures, whose AVMs had never ruptured, and who were treated with gamma knife radiosurgery [81]. Twenty-eight of 35 (80%) were seizure free at mean follow-up duration of 43 months (some of whom remained on anticonvulsant medications). They found a statistically significant correlation between persistence of seizures, number (>5) or frequency (>1 per month) of pretreatment seizures, and pretreatment duration (>6 months) of seizures. They also observed that resolution of seizures began to occur within months following irradiation, much sooner than the expected course for involution of the AVM.

Others have reported seizure control (seizure free or significant improvement) in 51% to 94% of patients treated with radiosurgery [83,164,165]. Although Sutcliffe et al. cured 38% of patients of seizures and improved seizures in 22% of 49 patients, they found a positive relationship between degree of AVM nidus obliteration and seizure control [86]. This has not been the finding of many authors since then. Colombo et al. [187] reported that seizures were no better in their patients following radiosurgery, while Seifert et al. reported worsening of seizures in more than 10% of their patients [188]. Gerszten et al. observed that 3% of 72 children developed new seizures following gamma knife radiosurgery [72]. The discordance between AVM obliteration rate and latency to seizure control described in most studies is not entirely understood. Explanations for the efficacy of radiosurgery in treating seizures include reduction of ischemia from decreased arteriovenous shunting [12,189, 190] and direct effect of radiation on abnormal neurons.

Management of Associated Aneurysms

Aneurysms associated with AVMs represent an important concurrent diagnosis that has a significant impact on the course of therapy for a given patient [70,191,192]. With an incidence of 7.5% to 17% and as high as 58% on superselective angiographic studies [193], these aneurysms occur with greater frequency than aneurysms in the general population and are probably related to the hemodynamic stress imposed by increased flow through the AVM. Aneurysms can be located within the AVM nidus (intranidal, type IV), or on vessels that supply the AVM (proximal flow-related, type II; or distal flow-related, type III) (see Figs. 9-7 and 9-8). Aneurysms located in remote locations are not flow related (type I). As described above, intranidal aneurysms increase the risk of hemorrhage from an AVM and we advocate treating these lesions endovascularly at the time of initial embolization of the AVM nidus. Distal flow-related aneurysms arise from vessels that are at higher risk for hypertensive changes following partial or complete obliteration of the AVM nidus, and we therefore also treat these aneurysms microsurgically or endovascularly prior to commencing staged treatment of the AVM nidus. In one study, these aneurysms were noted to regress following complete nidus treatment [71], but this was based on study of only five patients and is not a uniform finding in our experience. Other authors have recently described the disappearance of these distal aneurysms when they were included in the radiation field for gamma knife radiosurgery [194]. Radiosurgery is certainly not a conventional treatment for aneurysms and for this reason we do not employ this approach. In theory, the most significant increase in feeding artery pressure should occur in the distal branches of arteries feeding an AVM [195] and, therefore, aneurysms in this location may be at higher risk for rupture immediately following obliteration of an AVM if left unprotected. For these reasons, we advocate treatment of distal flow-related aneurysms prior to embarking on treatment of the AVM nidus. Finally, proximal flow-related aneurysms arising from the circle of Willis represent the last type of aneurysm that requires special attention during the treatment of an AVM. These aneurysms are less likely to regress with treatment of the AVM nidus [71] and may hemorrhage before, during, or after treatment of the AVM nidus [70]. Again, we tend to treat these lesions microsurgically or endovascularly before commencing AVM treatment (see Figs. 9-7 and 9-8).

Role of Multimodal Treatment of Arteriovenous Malformations

We have developed a multidisciplinary approach to AVMs, which is summarized in Table 9-5 [142]. We intentionally tend to incorporate several staged treatment sessions into the therapeutic approach to our patients, particularly if there are coexisting flow-related aneurysms (see Figs. 9-7 and 9-8). For patients with AVMs more than 3.0 cm in diameter, we almost always recommend one or more sessions of staged endovascular embolization, with the goal of reducing the nidus size or eliminating deep feeding arteries to facilitate subsequent treatment by microsurgery or radiosurgery (see Figs. 9-3, 9-4, 9-6, and 9-7). Decisions following embolization incorporate the clinical and neurologic status of the patient, the anatomical location of the remaining portion of the AVM nidus, and the accessibility to feeding arteries and draining veins. On one hand, we may recommend radiosurgery for a superficial AVM nidus that is partially embolized and easily accessible surgically in a young patient who is neurologically intact and has not suffered previous hemorrhage. Alternatively, we may recommend surgical resection of a small AVM that is deeply located if the patient is debilitated by a previous hemorrhage, even though the same nidus in a different patient might be treated by radiosurgery.

Based on our experience with AVM-associated aneurysms, we tend to manage such aneurysms primarily. Aneurysms can sometimes be obliterated via an endovascular approach and this technique is particularly useful when the aneurysm is intranidal. For proximal and distal flow-related aneurysms we often advocate surgical clipping of the aneurysm prior to initial management with staged endovascular embolization procedures, unless our interventional colleagues are confident that the aneurysm can be obliterated endovascularly. Depending on the morphology and accessibility of the AVM nidus, patients typically receive between two and nine embolization sessions prior to definitive treatment of the AVM nidus by microsurgical resection or radiosurgery. We usually offer radiosurgery to patients with deep or inaccessible AVMs remaining after embolization. Additionally, we avoid microsurgical approaches to lesions in eloquent areas unless the patient has been left with a significant deficit from a hemorrhage prior to treatment. The method of radiosurgery employed is generally a function of the size of AVM nidus remaining after embolization. If the residual nidus is small, we treat the patient at our own institution using linear accelerator–based radiosurgery (either frame-based or frameless cyberknife). Alternatively, for a large residual AVM nidus that is not amenable to microsurgical resection following embolization, we enroll the patient in our heavy-particle (proton beam) radiosurgery program in conjunction with Loma Linda University Medical Center (see Figs. 9-4 and 9-7). Following radiosurgery, we follow the patient with MRI studies every 6 months in order to monitor for radiation-induced edema (see Fig. 9-7), as well as to follow the loss of flow voids suggesting progressive nidus obliteration. In most instances, we do not obtain control angiography until 3 years following radiation administration. In some situations, patients will require repeat radiosurgery for particularly large AVMs (see Fig. 9-4). However, sometimes following incomplete or failed radiosurgical treatment of an AVM, the residual nidus may have been altered such that it is now amenable to treatment by either microsurgical resection, embolization followed by microsurgery or even, rarely, embolization alone.

Microsurgical resection of AVMs provides the best opportunity to obtain a complete angiographic obliteration and thus cure an AVM and eliminate the risk of future hemorrhage. As such, we tend to resect the remaining AVM nidus following embolization when the nidus is in a safely accessible location (see Figs. 9-2, 9-3, 9-6, and 9-8). We perform all these operations using stereotactic image guidance in order to assist with planning of the craniotomy and

TABLE 9-5. FACTORS AFFECTING THE APPROACH TO AVMS AND RECOMMENDED TREATMENT OPTIONS

AVM Size	Noncritical Location	Critical Location
Small (≤3.0 cm)	1. Microsurgical resection 2. Stereotactic radiosurgery, if poor surgical risk 3. Occasionally, embolization aimed at complete thrombosis	1. Stereotactic radiosurgery 2. Occasionally, microsurgical resection or embolization if multiple hemorrhages
Large (>3.0 cm)	1. Embolization followed by microsurgical resection 2. Embolization followed by stereotactic radiosurgery, if poor surgical risk	1. Embolization followed by stereotactic radiosurgery 2. Stereotactic radiosurgery alone if poor embolization candidate (proton beam XRT for AVMs >3.5 cm)

AVM, arteriovenous malformation; XRT, stereotactic radiosurgery.

intraoperative decision making. This is particularly useful in the latter stages of AVM resection when the deepest portion of the AVM is approached. The deeper structures are less likely to shift, and therefore the accuracy of their registration remains reliable throughout the operation. It is at this final stage of AVM resection when the dissection is most tedious that the added information from image guidance is most useful. We undertake all these operations with various forms of intraoperative neuroprotection. Intraoperative hypothermia is routinely employed, with the goal core temperature being 33° C. Neurophysiologic monitoring is also a routine adjunctive measure used to minimize risk of neurologic injury. Somatosensory evoked potentials are monitored in all cases, and brainstem auditory evoked responses are monitored for infratentorial and thalamic AVMs. In certain instances intraoperative electroencephalography is performed, and intraoperative cortical mapping is used in appropriate patients. As the dissection proceeds, the anesthesiologist induces intraoperative hypotension to a mean arterial pressure of about 60 to 65 mm Hg to minimize the risk of hemorrhage from the AVM. The numerous small and large feeding arteries are coagulated using bipolar electrocautery. In the relatively common instance that an artery or arteriole is refractory to bipolar electrocautery, we advocate the use of Sundt titanium micro-AVM clips (Codman) to assure hemostasis. As has been well described, the venous drainage from the AVM, whether it be deep or superficial, is left intact until the arterial inflow has been completely obliterated, again to avoid intraoperative hemorrhage. On the rare occasion that there is excessive bleeding from the parenchymal wall abutting the dissected surface of an AVM, residual nidus should be suspected. This can be interrogated intraoperatively either by exploration or angiography. Intraoperative angiography is considered essential in these patients and when performed using the radiolucent head frame and state-of-the-art image intensification equipment, image quality rivals that which can be obtained in the angiography suite. The added time at the end of the resection is minimal and allows important decisions to be made immediately in the case of an unexpected residual AVM component. If there is any doubt regarding the quality of the intraoperative image, a formal postoperative angiogram is performed. The time involved in obtaining the intraoperative angiogram allows the patient to begin rewarming such that core temperature is normal upon arrival in the intensive care unit. There the patient is observed for at least 24 hours, with strict pharmacological control of the mean arterial pressure at approximately 65 to 75 mm Hg.

As referred to above, the morphology and anatomy of a particular AVM determine which course of treatment will be used preferentially. There is an argument for entertaining a multidisciplinary approach for all AVMs. However, the adjunctive use of preoperative embolization of a Spetzler-Martin grade I or II AVM offers relatively less overall benefit and potentially more combined risk than a staged multidisciplinary approach to a deep-seated eloquently positioned AVM. Patients with these more difficult lesions require thoughtful consideration of the potential role of microsurgery, endovascular embolization, and stereotactic radiosurgery, considering the benefits and risks of all the procedures together. For example, a patient with a large, dominant hemisphere, perirolandic AVM might benefit from staged embolization followed by microsurgical resection with cortical mapping. On the other hand, another patient with a deep thalamic AVM might receive more benefit from a single embolization session followed by stereotactic radiosurgery. In any case, the treatment of these more difficult AVMs by a team of neurosurgeons, neuroradiologists, and radiation oncologists skilled in the management of these patients is essential.

Menovsky and van Overbeeke recently reviewed multimodal treatment of pediatric AVMs [160]. While commenting that such multidisciplinary reports came from highly specialized institutions, they noted that mortality rates were generally less than 10%, with no mortality in the majority of series. Multimodal treatment of pediatric AVMs was recently described by Hoh et al., who presented the first large series of 40 patients managed in this fashion [20]. Using various combinations of surgery, embolization, and radiosurgery, 95% had a good or excellent clinical outcome (Glasgow outcome scale score of 4 or 5), while their mortality rate was only 2.5%. Complete obliteration was achieved in 92.9%.

Recurrent Arteriovenous Malformations

Finally, the concept of recurrent AVMs has been a topic of recent interest in the literature. Although the overwhelming majority of patients will not develop recurrent AVM after angiographic obliteration, there have been numerous reports over the past decade of recurrence causing either hemorrhage or seizures after previous angiographically proven obliteration [121,196–201]. Although the majority of these patients were children at the time of their original treatment [121,196,198], a few recent reports describe this phenomenon in adults as well [197,199,200,202]. We have experience with only one such patient and, interestingly, she suffered an intracranial hemorrhage 10 years following the angiographically documented obliteration of her AVM after helium ion radiosurgery. Serial MRI studies failed to show any evidence of a recurrent lesion, and an angiogram 1 year after the hemorrhage also failed to demonstrate a nidus. We postulate that the lesion must have recanalized and then was obliterated by the mass effect from the hemorrhage. This was recently described in a population of adults with AVMs treated by gamma knife radiosurgery [203]. Various theories have been invoked to explain this phenomenon. The most common explanation relates back to the Yasargil's theory of a proliferative capillaropathy acting on an immature cerebral vasculature [27]. The role of vascular endothelial growth factor has also been proposed but definitive proof is lacking [204]. A recent case report describes the development of a second distinct AVM in a child following successful treatment of the first AVM with gamma knife radiosurgery, also suggesting a proliferative process in the immature vasculature [205]. These few case reports and small series remind us that although there have been significant advances in the management of cerebral AVMs over the past several decades, we still do not fully understand the mechanisms that cause them. Further knowledge of AVM formation and growth may improve the efficacy and safety of our treatment strategies in the future.

ACKNOWLEDGEMENT

We thank Beth Hoyte for assistance with preparation of the figures. This work was supported by funding from Bernard and Ronni Lacroute, the William Randolph Hearst Foundation, and John and Dodie Rosekrans.

REFERENCES

1. Mattle HP, Schroth G, Seiler RW. Dilemmas in the management of patients with arteriovenous malformations. *J Neurol* 2000;247:917–928.
2. Fleetwood IG, Steinberg GK. Arteriovenous malformations. *Lancet* 2002;359:863–873.
3. Ogilvy CS, Stieg PE, Awad I, et al. Recommendations for the management of intracranial arteriovenous malformations: a statement for healthcare professionals from a special writing group of the Stroke Council, American Stroke Association. *Circulation* 2001;103:2644–2657.
4. Michelsen WJ. Natural history and pathophysiology of arteriovenous malformations. *Clin Neurosurg* 1979;26:307–313.
5. Berman MF, Sciacca RR, Pile-Spellman J, et al. The epidemiology of brain arteriovenous malformations. *Neurosurgery* 2000; 47:389–396.
6. McCormick WF. Pathology of vascular malformations of the brain. In: Wilson CB, Stein BM, eds. *Intracranial arteriovenous malformations.* Baltimore: Williams & Wilkins, 1984:44–63.
7. Garza-Mercado R, Cavazos E, Tamez-Montes D. Cerebral arteriovenous malformations in children and adolescents. *Surg Neurol* 1987;27:131–140.
8. Brown RDJ, Wiebers DO, Torner JC, et al. Frequency of intracranial hemorrhage as a presenting symptom and subtype analysis: a population-based study of intracranial vascular malformations in Olmsted County, Minnesota. *J Neurosurg* 1996;85: 29–32.
9. Hillman J. Population-based analysis of arteriovenous malformation treatment. *J Neurosurg* 2001;95:633–637.
10. Brown RDJ, Wiebers DO, Torner JC, et al. Incidence and prevalence of intracranial vascular malformations in Olmsted County, Minnesota, 1965 to 1992. *Neurology* 1996;46: 949–952.
11. Perret G, Nishioka H. Report on the cooperative study of intracranial aneurysms and subarachnoid hemorrhage. Section VI. Arteriovenous malformations. An analysis of 545 cases of craniocerebral arteriovenous malformations and fistulae reported to the cooperative study. *J Neurosurg* 1966;25:467–490.
12. Guidetti B, Delitala A. Intracranial arteriovenous malformations. Conservative and surgical treatment. *J Neurosurg* 1980; 53:149–152.
13. Itoyama Y, Uemura S, Ushio Y, et al. Natural course of unoperated intracranial arteriovenous malformations: study of 50 cases. *J Neurosurg* 1989;71:805–809.
14. Mansmann U, Meisel J, Brock M, et al. Factors associated with intracranial hemorrhage in cases of cerebral arteriovenous malformation. *Neurosurgery* 2000;46:272–281.
15. Hofmeister C, Stapf C, Hartmann A, et al. Demographic, morphological, and clinical characteristics of 1289 patients with brain arteriovenous malformation. *Stroke* 2000;31:1307–1310.
16. Gerosa MA, Cappellotto P, Licata C, et al. Cerebral arteriovenous malformations in children (56 cases). *Childs Brain* 1981; 8:356–371.
17. Celli P, Ferrante L, Palma L, et al. Cerebral arteriovenous malformations in children. Clinical features and outcome of treatment in children and in adults. *Surg Neurol* 1984;22:43–49.
18. D'Aliberti G, Talamonti G, Versari PP, et al. Comparison of pediatric and adult cerebral arteriovenous malformations. *J Neurosurg Sci* 1997;41:331–336.
19. Sheikh BY, Hassounah M, Al Moutare K, et al. Childhood intracranial arteriovenous malformation in Saudi Arabia. *Childs Nerv Syst* 1999;15:262–266.
20. Hoh BL, Ogilvy CS, Butler WE, et al. Multimodality treatment of nongalenic arteriovenous malformations in pediatric patients. *Neurosurgery* 2000;47:346–358.
21. Karlsson B, Lindquist C, Johansson A, et al. Annual risk for the first hemorrhage from untreated cerebral arteriovenous malformations. *Minim Invasive Neurosurg* 1997;40:40–46.
22. Lasjaunias P. A revised concept of the congenital nature of cerebral arteriovenous malformations. *Interv Neuroradiol* 1997;3: 275–281.
23. Takashima S, Becker LE. Neuropathology of cerebral arteriovenous malformations in children. *J Neurol Neurosurg Psychiatry* 1980;43:380–385.
24. Malik GM, Sadasivan B, Knighton RS, et al. The management of arteriovenous malformations in children. *Childs Nerv Syst* 1991;7:43–47.
25. Campbell ACP. The vascular architecture of the cat's brain: a study by vital injection. *Res Nerv Ment Dis* 1938;18:69–93.
26. Scharrer E. Arteries and veins in the mammalian brain. *Anat Rec* 1940;78:173–196.
27. Yasargil MG. Pathological considerations. In: Yasargil MG, ed. *Microneurosurgery IIIA.* New York: Thieme, 1987:49–58.
28. Dandy WE. Arteriovenous aneurysm of the brain. *Arch Surg* 1928;17:190–243.
29. Olivecrona H, Ladenheim J. *Congenital arteriovenous aneurysms of the carotid and vertebral arterial systems,* 1st ed. Berlin: Springer, 1957.
30. Mullan S, Mojtahedi S, Johnson DL, et al. Embryological basis of some aspects of cerebral vascular fistulas and malformations. *J Neurosurg* 1996;85:1–8.
31. Gibbons GH, Dzau VJ. The emerging concept of vascular remodeling. *N Engl J Med* 1994;330:1431–1438.
32. Stapf C, Mohr JP. New concepts in adult brain arteriovenous malformations. *Curr Opin Neurol* 2000;13:63–67.
33. Waltimo O. The relationship of size, density and localization of intracranial arteriovenous malformations to the type of initial symptom. *J Neurol Sci* 1973;19:13–19.
34. MacKenzie I. The clinical presentation of cerebral angioma. A review of 50 cases. *Brain* 1953;76:184–214.
35. Luessenhop AJ. Natural history of cerebral arteriovenous malformations. In: Wilson CB, Stein BM, eds. *Intracranial arterio-*

venous malformations. Baltimore: Williams & Wilkins, 1984: 12–23.
36. Wilkins RH. Natural history of intracranial vascular malformations: a review. *Neurosurgery* 1985;16:421–430.
37. Jane JA, Kassell NF, Torner JC, et al. The natural history of aneurysms and arteriovenous malformations. *J Neurosurg* 1985; 62:321–323.
38. Wilkins RH. Natural history of arteriovenous malformations of the brain. In: Barrow DL, ed. *Intracranial arteriovenous malformations.* Park Ridge: American Association of Neurological Surgeons, 1990:31–44.
39. Svien HJ, McRae JA. Arteriovenous anomalies of the brain: fate of patients not having definitive surgery. *J Neurosurg* 1965;23: 23–28.
40. Troupp H, Marttila I, Halonen V. Arteriovenous malformations of the brain. Prognosis without operation. *Acta Neurochir (Wien)* 1970;22:125–128.
41. Ondra SL, Troupp H, George ED, et al. The natural history of symptomatic arteriovenous malformations of the brain: a 24-year follow-up assessment. *J Neurosurg* 1990;73:387–391.
42. Forster DM, Steiner L, Hakanson S. Arteriovenous malformations of the brain. A long-term clinical study. *J Neurosurg* 1972; 37:562–570.
43. Pool JL. Treatment of arteriovenous malformations of the cerebral hemispheres. *J Neurosurg* 1962;19:136–141.
44. Graf CJ, Perret GE, Torner JC. Bleeding from cerebral arteriovenous malformations as part of their natural history. *J Neurosurg* 1983;58:331–337.
45. Fults D, Kelly DLJ. Natural history of arteriovenous malformations of the brain: a clinical study. *Neurosurgery* 1984;15: 658–662.
46. Crawford PM, West CR, Chadwick DW, et al. Arteriovenous malformations of the brain: natural history in unoperated patients. *J Neurol Neurosurg Psychiatry* 1986;49:1–10.
47. Brown RDJ, Wiebers DO, Forbes G, et al. The natural history of unruptured intracranial arteriovenous malformations. *J Neurosurg* 1988;68:352–357.
48. Kondziolka D, McLaughlin MR, Kestle JRW. Simple risk predictions for arteriovenous malformation hemorrhage. *Neurosurgery* 1995;37:851–855.
49. Brown RDJ. Simple risk predictions for arteriovenous malformation hemorrhage [Letter]. *Neurosurgery* 2000;46:1024.
50. Mast H, Young WL, Koennecke HC, et al. Risk of spontaneous haemorrhage after diagnosis of cerebral arteriovenous malformation. *Lancet* 1997;350:1065–1068.
51. Fleetwood IG, Marcellus ML, Levy RP, et al. Deep arteriovenous malformations of the basal ganglia and thalamus: natural history. *J Neurosurg* (submitted).
52. Piepgras DG, Sundt TMJ, Ragoowansi AT, et al. Seizure outcome in patients with surgically treated cerebral arteriovenous malformations. *J Neurosurg* 1993;78:5–11.
53. Crawford PM, West CR, Shaw MD, et al. Cerebral arteriovenous malformations and epilepsy: factors in the development of epilepsy. *Epilepsia* 1986;27:270–275.
54. Hartmann A, Mast H, Mohr JP, et al. Morbidity of intracranial hemorrhage in patients with cerebral arteriovenous malformation. *Stroke* 1998;29:931–934.
55. Mast H, Koennecke HC, Meisel J, et al. Therapy of cerebral arteriovenous malformations. *Nervenarzt* 1998;69:287–295.
56. Abad JM, Alvarez F, Manrique M, et al. Cerebral arteriovenous malformations. Comparative results of surgical vs conservative treatment in 112 cases. *J Neurosurg Sci* 1983;27:203–210.
57. Parkinson D, Bachers G. Arteriovenous malformations. Summary of 100 consecutive supratentorial cases. *J Neurosurg* 1980; 53:285–299.
58. Spetzler RF, Hargraves RW, McCormick PW, et al. Relationship of perfusion pressure and size to risk of hemorrhage from arteriovenous malformations. *J Neurosurg* 1992;76:918–923.
59. Kader A, Young WL, Pile-Spellman J, et al. The influence of hemodynamic and anatomic factors on hemorrhage from cerebral arteriovenous malformations. *Neurosurgery* 1994;34: 801–808.
60. Langer DJ, Lasner TM, Hurst RW, et al. Hypertension, small size, and deep venous drainage are associated with risk of hemorrhagic presentation of cerebral arteriovenous malformations. *Neurosurgery* 1998;42:481–489.
61. Stiver SI, Ogilvy CS. Micro-arteriovenous malformations: significant hemorrhage from small arteriovenous shunts. *Neurosurgery* 2000;46:811–818.
62. Marks MP, Lane B, Steinberg GK, et al. Hemorrhage in intracerebral arteriovenous malformations: angiographic determinants. *Radiology* 1990;176:807–813.
63. Turjman F, Massoud TF, Viñuela F, et al. Correlation of the angioarchitectural features of cerebral arteriovenous malformations with clinical presentation of hemorrhage. *Neurosurgery* 1995;37:856–862.
64. Nataf F, Meder JF, Roux FX, et al. Angioarchitecture associated with haemorrhage in cerebral arteriovenous malformations: a prognostic statistical model. *Neuroradiology* 1997;39:52–58.
65. Duong DH, Young WL, Vang MC, et al. Feeding artery pressure and venous drainage pattern are primary determinants of hemorrhage from cerebral arteriovenous malformations. *Stroke* 1998;29:1167–1176.
66. Norris JS, Valiante TA, Wallace MC, et al. A simple relationship between radiological arteriovenous malformation hemodynamics and clinical presentation: a prospective, blinded analysis of 31 cases. *J Neurosurg* 1999;90:673–679.
67. Willinsky R, Lasjaunias P, TerBrugge K, et al. Brain arteriovenous malformations: analysis of the angio-architecture in relationship to hemorrhage (based on 152 patients explored and/or treated at the hospital de Bicetre between 1981 and 1986). *J Neuroradiol* 1988;15:225–237.
68. Pollock B, Flickinger JC, Lunsford LD, et al. Factors that predict the bleeding risk of cerebral arteriovenous malformations. *Stroke* 1996;27:1–6.
69. Stapf C, Mohr JP, Sciacca RR, et al. Incident hemorrhage risk of brain arteriovenous malformations located in the arterial borderzones. *Stroke* 2000;31:2365–2368.
70. Thompson RC, Steinberg GK, Levy RP, et al. The management of patients with arteriovenous malformations and associated intracranial aneurysms. *Neurosurgery* 1998;43:202–212.
71. Redekop G, TerBrugge K, Montanera W, et al. Arterial aneurysms associated with cerebral arteriovenous malformations: classification, incidence, and risk of hemorrhage. *J Neurosurg* 1998;89:539–546.
72. Gerszten PC, Adelson PD, Kondziolka D, et al. Seizure outcome in children treated for arteriovenous malformations using gamma knife radiosurgery. *Pediatr Neurosurg* 1996;24: 139–144.
73. Yeh HS, Tew JM Jr., Gartner M. Seizure control after surgery on cerebral arteriovenous malformations. *J Neurosurg* 1993;78: 12–18.
74. Leblanc R, Feindel W, Ethier R. Epilepsy from cerebral arteriovenous malformations. *Can J Neurol Sci* 1983;10:91–95.
75. Amacher AL, Allcock JM, Drake CG. Cerebral angiomas: the sequelae of surgical treatment. *J Neurosurg* 1972;37:571–575.
76. Heros RC, Korosue K, Diebold PM. Surgical excision of cerebral arteriovenous malformations: late results. *Neurosurgery* 1990;26:570–578.
77. Trumpy JH, Eldevik P. Intracranial arteriovenous malforma-

tions: conservative or surgical treatment? *Surg Neurol* 1977;8: 171–175.

78. Moody RA, Poppen JL. Arteriovenous malformations. *J Neurosurg* 1970;32:503–511.
79. Malik GM, Seyfried DM, Morgan JK. Temporal lobe arteriovenous malformations: surgical management and outcome. *Surg Neurol* 1996;46:106–115.
80. Zimmerman G, Lewis AI, Tew JM Jr. Pure sylvian fissure arteriovenous malformations. *J Neurosurg* 2000;92:39–44.
81. Kurita H, Kawamoto S, Suzuki I, et al. Control of epilepsy associated with cerebral arteriovenous malformations after radiosurgery. *J Neurol Neurosurg Psychiatry* 1998;65:648–655.
82. Hosobuchi Y, Fabricant J, Lyman J. Stereotactic heavy-particle irradiation of intracranial arteriovenous malformations. *Appl Neurophysiol* 1987;50:248–252.
83. Falkson CB, Chakrabarti KB, Doughty D, et al. Stereotactic multiple arc radiotherapy. III—influence of treatment of arteriovenous malformations on associated epilepsy. *Br J Neurosurg* 1997;11:12–15.
84. Heikkinen ER, Konnov B, Melnikov L, et al. Relief of epilepsy by radiosurgery of cerebral arteriovenous malformations. *Stereotact Funct Neurosurg* 1989;53:157–166.
85. Kjellberg RN, Hanamura T, Davis KR, et al. Bragg-peak proton-beam therapy for arteriovenous malformations of the brain. *N Engl J Med* 1983;309:269–274.
86. Sutcliffe JC, Forster DM, Walton L, et al. Untoward clinical effects after stereotactic radiosurgery for intracranial arteriovenous malformations. *Br J Neurosurg* 1992;6:177–185.
87. Eisenschenk S, Gilmore RL, Friedman WA, et al. The effect of LINAC stereotactic radiosurgery on epilepsy associated with arteriovenous malformations. *Stereotact Funct Neurosurg* 1998; 71:51–61.
88. Murphy MJ. Long-term follow-up of seizures associated with cerebral arteriovenous malformations. Results of therapy. *Arch Neurol* 1985;42:477–479.
89. Kupersmith MJ, Vargas ME, Yashar A, et al. Occipital arteriovenous malformations: visual disturbances and presentation. *Neurology* 1996;46:953–957.
90. Kurita H, Shin M, Kirino T. Resolution of migraine with aura caused by an occipital arteriovenous malformation. *Arch Neurol* 2000;57:1219–1220.
91. Spierings EL. Daily migraine with visual aura associated with an occipital arteriovenous malformation. *Headache* 2001;41: 193–197.
92. Steinberg GK, Fabrikant JI, Marks MP, et al. Stereotactic heavy-charged-particle Bragg-peak radiation for intracranial arteriovenous malformations. *N Engl J Med* 1990;323:96–101.
93. Norlen G. Arteriovenous aneurysms of the brain. Report of ten cases of total removal of the lesion. *J Neurosurg* 1949;6: 475–494.
94. Batjer H, Samson D. Arteriovenous malformations of the posterior fossa. Clinical presentation, diagnostic evaluation, and surgical treatment. *J Neurosurg* 1986;64:849–856.
95. Marks MP, Lane B, Steinberg G, et al. Vascular characteristics of intracerebral arteriovenous malformations in patients with clinical steal. *AJNR Am J Neuroradiol* 1991;12:489–496.
96. Martin NA, Wilson CB. Medial occipital arteriovenous malformations. Surgical treatment. *J Neurosurg* 1982;56:798–802.
97. Alusi SH, Colquhoun I, Sensky T, et al. Pathologic laughter resulting from a large midbrain arteriovenous malformation. *Mov Disord* 1999;14:185–189.
98. Lazar RM, Connaire K, Marshall RS, et al. Developmental deficits in adult patients with arteriovenous malformations. *Arch Neurol* 1999;56:103–106.
99. Lazar RM, Marshall RS, Pile-Spellman J, et al. Interhemispheric transfer of language in patients with left frontal cerebral arteriovenous malformation. *Neuropsychologia* 2000;38:1325–1332.
100. Lazar RM, Marshall RS, Pile S, et al. Anterior translocation of language in patients with left cerebral arteriovenous malformation. *Neurology* 1997;49:802–808.
101. Guttmacher AE, Marchuk DA, White RI. Hereditary hemorrhagic telangiectasia. *N Engl J Med* 1995;333:918–924.
102. Shovlin CL, Hughes JM, Tuddenham EG, et al. A gene for hereditary haemorrhagic telangiectasia maps to chromosome 9q3. *Nat Genet* 1994;6:205–209.
103. McDonald MT, Papenberg KA, Ghosh S, et al. A disease locus for hereditary haemorrhagic telangiectasia maps to chromosome 9q33-34. *Nat Genet* 1994;6:197–204.
104. Johnson DW, Berg JN, Gallione CJ, et al. A second locus for hereditary hemorrhagic telangiectasia maps to chromosome 12. *Genome Res* 1995;5:21–28.
105. Willemse RB, Mager JJ, Westerman CJ, et al. Bleeding risk of cerebrovascular malformations an hereditary hemorrhagic telangiectasia. *J Neurosurg* 2000;92:779–784.
106. Maher CO, Piepgras DG, Brown RDJ, et al. Cerebrovascular manifestations in 321 cases of hereditary hemorrhagic telangiectasia. *Stroke* 2001;32:877–882.
107. Matsubara S, Manzia JL, TerBrugge KG, et al. Angiographic and clinical characteristics of patients with cerebral arteriovenous malformations associated with hereditary hemorrhagic telangiectasia. *AJNR Am J Neuroradiol* 2000;21:1016–1020.
108. Theron J, Newton TH, Hoyt WF. Unilateral retinocephalic vascular malformations. *Neuroradiology* 1974;7:185–196.
109. Roman G, Fisher M, Perl DP, et al. Neurological manifestations of hereditary hemorrhagic telangiectasia (Rendu-Osler-Weber disease): report of 2 cases and review of the literature. *Ann Neurol* 1978;4:130–144.
110. Kikuchi K, Kowada M, Sakamoto T, et al. Wyburn-Mason syndrome: report of a rare case with computed tomography and angiographic evaluations. *J Comput Tomogr* 1988;12:111–115.
111. Patel U, Gupta SC. Wyburn-Mason syndrome. A case report and review of the literature. *Neuroradiology* 1990;31:544–546.
112. Willinsky RA, Lasjaunias P, TerBrugge K, et al. Multiple cerebral arteriovenous malformations (AVMs). Review of our experience from 203 patients with cerebral vascular lesions. *Neuroradiology* 1990;32:207–210.
113. So SC. Cerebral arteriovenous malformations in children. *Childs Brain* 1978;4:242–250.
114. Humphreys RP, Hendrick EB, Hoffman HJ. Arteriovenous malformations of the brain. *Concepts Pediatr Neurosurg* 1988; 8:146–164.
115. Mori K, Murata T, Hashimoto N, et al. Clinical analysis of arteriovenous malformations in children. *Childs Brain* 1980;6: 13–25.
116. Di Rocco C, Tamburrini G, Rollo M. Cerebral arteriovenous malformations in children. *Acta Neurochir (Wien)* 2000;142: 145–148.
117. Hladky JP, Lejeune JP, Blond S, et al. Cerebral arteriovenous malformations in children: report on 62 cases. *Childs Nerv Syst* 1994;10:328–333.
118. Al-Jarallah A, Al-Rifai MT, Riela AR, et al. Nontraumatic brain hemorrhage in children: etiology and presentation. *J Child Neurol* 2000;15:284–289.
119. Berg AT, Testa FM, Levy SR, et al. Neuroimaging in children with newly diagnosed epilepsy: a community-based study. *Pediatrics* 2000;106:527–532.
120. Caldarelli M, Di Rocco C, Iannelli A, et al. Combined manage-

ment of intracranial vascular malformations in children. *J Neurosurg Sci* 1997;41:315–324.
121. Kondziolka D, Humphreys RP, Hoffman HJ, et al. Arteriovenous malformations of the brain in children: a forty year experience. *Can J Neurol Sci* 1992;19:40–45.
122. Spetzler RF, Martin NA. A proposed grading system for arteriovenous malformations. *J Neurosurg* 1986;65:476–483.
123. Hamilton MG, Spetzler RF. The prospective application of a grading system for arteriovenous malformations. *Neurosurgery* 1994;34:2–7.
124. Luessenhop AJ, Gennarelli TA. Anatomical grading of supratentorial arteriovenous malformations for determining operability. *Neurosurgery* 1977;1:30–35.
125. Pasqualin A, Barone G, Cioffi F, et al. The relevance of anatomic and hemodynamic factors to a classification of cerebral arteriovenous malformations. *Neurosurgery* 1991;28:370–379.
126. Pertuiset B, Ancri D, Kinuta Y, et al. Classification of supratentorial arteriovenous malformations. A score system for evaluation of operability and surgical strategy based on an analysis of 66 cases. *Acta Neurochir (Wien)* 1991;110:6–16.
127. Deruty R, Pelissou-Guyotat I, Mottolese C. Prognostic value of Spetzler's grading system in a series of cerebral AVMs treated by combined management. *Acta Neurochir (Wien)* 1994;131:169–175.
128. Hartmann A, Stapf C, Hofmeister C, et al. Determinants of neurological outcome after surgery for brain arteriovenous malformation. *Stroke* 2000;31:2361–2364.
129. Nanda A. Controversies in neurosurgery: microsurgery versus radiosurgery for arteriovenous malformations—introduction. *Clin Neurosurg* 1999;45:11–12.
130. Aminoff MJ. Treatment of unruptured cerebral arteriovenous malformations. *Neurology* 1987;37:815–819.
131. Fisher WS. Therapy of AVMs: a decision analysis. *Clin Neurosurg* 1995;42:294–312.
132. Auger RG, Wiebers DO. Management of unruptured intracranial arteriovenous malformations: a decision analysis. *Neurosurgery* 1992;30:561–569.
133. Iansek R, Elstein AS, Balla JI. Application of decision analysis to management of cerebral arteriovenous malformation. *Lancet* 1983;1:1132–1135.
134. Flamm ES. Clinical decision making on the management of intracranial vascular malformations. In: Barrow DL, ed. *Intracranial arteriovenous malformations.* Park Ridge: American Association of Neurological Surgeons, 1990:227–233.
135. Pool JL, Potts DG. Arteriovenous malformations and other vascular anomalies. In: Pool JL, Potts DG, eds. *Aneurysms and arteriovenous anomalies of the brain: diagnosis and treatment.* New York: Harper & Row, 1965:326–373.
136. Luessenhop AJ. Operative treatment of arteriovenous malformations. In: Morley TP, ed. *Current controversies in neurosurgery.* Philadelphia: WB Saunders, 1976:203–209.
137. Pascual-Castroviejo I, Pascual-Pascual JI, Blazquez MG, et al. Spontaneous occlusion of an intracranial arteriovenous malformation. *Childs Brain* 1977;3:169–179.
138. Davis C, Symon L. The management of cerebral arteriovenous malformations. *Acta Neurochir (Wien)* 1985;74:4–11.
139. Guo WY, Karlsson B, Ericson K, et al. Even the smallest remnant of an AVM constitutes a risk of further bleeding. Case report. *Acta Neurochir (Wien)* 1993;121:212–215.
140. Miyamoto S, Hashimoto N, Nagata I, et al. Posttreatment sequelae of palliatively treated cerebral arteriovenous malformations. *Neurosurgery* 2000;46:589–594.
141. Heros RC, Tu YK. Is surgical therapy needed for unruptured arteriovenous malformations? *Neurology* 1987;37:279–286.
142. Steinberg GK, Marks MP. Intracranial arteriovenous malformation: therapeutic options. In: Batjer H, ed. *Cerebrovascular disease.* Philadelphia: Lippincott–Raven Publishers, 1997:727–742.
143. Batjer HH. Treatment decisions in brain AVMs: the case for and against surgery. *Clin Neurosurg* 2000;46:319–325.
144. Barrow DL. Controversies in neurosurgery: microsurgery versus radiosurgery for arteriovenous malformations—the case for microsurgery. *Clin Neurosurg* 1999;45:13–17.
145. Barrow DL. Controversies in neurosurgery: microsurgery versus radiosurgery for arteriovenous malformations—the case for microsurgery. *Clin Neurosurg* 2000;46:285–294.
146. Pikus HJ, Beach ML, Harbaugh RE. Microsurgical treatment of arteriovenous malformations: analysis and comparison with stereotactic radiosurgery. *J Neurosurg* 1998;88:641–646.
147. Nussbaum ES, Heros RC, Camarata PJ. Surgical treatment of intracranial arteriovenous malformations with an analysis of cost-effectiveness. *Clin Neurosurg* 1995;42:348–369.
148. Porter PJ, Shin AY, Detsky AS, et al. Surgery versus stereotactic radiosurgery for small, operable cerebral arteriovenous malformations: a clinical and cost comparison. *Neurosurgery* 1997;41:757–764.
149. Sisti MB, Kader A, Stein BM. Microsurgery for 67 intracranial arteriovenous malformations less than 3 cm in diameter. *J Neurosurg* 1993;79:653–660.
150. Schaller C, Schramm J. Microsurgical results for small arteriovenous malformations accessible for radiosurgical or embolization treatment. *Neurosurgery* 1997;40:664–672.
151. Schaller C, Schramm J, Haun D. Significance of factors contributing to surgical complications and to late outcome after elective surgery of cerebral arteriovenous malformations. *J Neurol Neurosurg Psychiatry* 1998;65:547–554.
152. Yamada S. Arteriovenous malformations in the functional area: surgical treatment and regional cerebral blood flow. *Neurol Res* 1982;4:283–322.
153. Waga S. Surgical treatment of arteriovenous malformations in the lateral ventricle. *Neurol Res* 1986;8:18–24.
154. Solomon RA, Stein BM. Management of arteriovenous malformations of the brainstem. *J Neurosurg* 1986;64:857–864.
155. Yamada S, Brauer FS, Knierim DS. Direct approach to arteriovenous malformations in functional areas of the cerebral hemisphere. *J Neurosurg* 1990;72:418–425.
156. Nagata S, Matsushima T, Fujii K, et al. Lateral ventricular arteriovenous malformations: natural history and surgical indications. *Acta Neurochir (Wien)* 1991;112:37–46.
157. Morgan MK, Sekhon LH, Finfer S, et al. Delayed neurological deterioration following resection of arteriovenous malformations of the brain. *J Neurosurg* 1999;90:695–701.
158. Yeh HS, Kashiwagi S, Tew JM Jr., et al. Surgical management of epilepsy associated with cerebral arteriovenous malformations. *J Neurosurg* 1990;72:216–223.
159. Drake CG. Cerebral arteriovenous malformations: considerations for and experience with surgical treatment in 166 cases. *Clin Neurosurg* 1979;26:145–208.
160. Menovsky T, van Overbeeke JJ. Cerebral arteriovenous malformations in childhood: state of the art with special reference to treatment. *Eur J Pediatr* 1997;156:741–746.
161. Batjer HH, Samson DS. Reoperation for aneurysms and vascular malformations. *Clin Neurosurg* 1992;39:140–171.
162. Steinberg GK, Chang SD, Levy RP, et al. Surgical resection of large incompletely treated intracranial arteriovenous malformations following stereotactic radiosurgery. *J Neurosurg* 1996;84:920–928.
163. Chang SD, Steinberg GK, Levy RP, et al. Microsurgical resection of incompletely obliterated intracranial arteriovenous mal-

formations following stereotactic radiosurgery. *Neurol Med Chir (Tokyo)* 1998;38[Suppl]:200–207.
164. Lunsford LD, Kondziolka D, Flickinger JC, et al. Stereotactic radiosurgery for arteriovenous malformations of the brain. *J Neurosurg* 1991;75:512–524.
165. Steiner L, Lindquist C, Adler JR, et al. Clinical outcome of radiosurgery for cerebral arteriovenous malformations. *J Neurosurg* 1992;77:1–8.
166. Colombo F, Pozza F, Chierego G, et al. Linear accelerator radiosurgery of cerebral arteriovenous malformations: an update. *Neurosurgery* 1994;34:14–20.
167. Friedman WA, Bova FJ, Mendenhall WM. Linear accelerator radiosurgery for arteriovenous malformations: the relationship of size to outcome. *J Neurosurg* 1995;82:180–189.
168. Yamamoto Y, Coffey RJ, Nichols DA, et al. Interim report on the radiosurgical treatment of cerebral arteriovenous malformations. The influence of size, dose, time, and technical factors on obliteration rate. *J Neurosurg* 1995;83:832–837.
169. Schlienger M, Atlan D, Lefkopoulos D, et al. Linac radiosurgery for cerebral arteriovenous malformations: results in 169 patients. *Int J Radiat Oncol Biol Phys* 2000;46:1135–1142.
170. Ellis TL, Friedman WA, Bova FJ, et al. Analysis of treatment failure after radiosurgery for arteriovenous malformations. *J Neurosurg* 1998;89:104–110.
171. Miyawaki L, Dowd C, Wara W, et al. Five year results of LINAC radiosurgery for arteriovenous malformations: outcome for large AVMS. *Int J Radiat Oncol Biol Phys* 1999;44:1089–1106.
172. Kwon Y, Jeon SR, Kim JH, et al. Analysis of the causes of treatment failure in gamma knife radiosurgery for intracranial arteriovenous malformations. *J Neurosurg* 2000;93[Suppl 3]:104–106.
173. Gallina P, Merienne L, Meder JF, et al. Failure in radiosurgery treatment of cerebral arteriovenous malformations. *Neurosurgery* 1998;42:996–1002.
174. Karlsson B, Lax I, Soderman M. Can the probability for obliteration after radiosurgery for arteriovenous malformations be accurately predicted? *Int J Radiat Oncol Biol Phys* 1999;43:313–319.
175. Pollock BE, Flickinger JC, Lunsford LD, et al. Factors associated with successful arteriovenous malformation radiosurgery. *Neurosurgery* 1998;42:1239–1244.
176. Pollock BE, Kondziolka D, Lunsford LD, et al. Repeat stereotactic radiosurgery of arteriovenous malformations: factors associated with incomplete obliteration. *Neurosurgery* 1996;38:318–324.
177. Flickinger JC, Kondziolka D, Lunsford LD, et al. A multi-institutional analysis of complication outcomes after arteriovenous malformation radiosurgery. *Int J Radiat Oncol Biol Phys* 1999;44:67–74.
178. Kihlstrom L, Guo WY, Karlsson B, et al. Magnetic resonance imaging of obliterated arteriovenous malformations up to 23 years after radiosurgery. *J Neurosurg* 1997;86:589–593.
179. Kim MS, Lee SI, Sim JH. A case of very large cyst formation with gamma knife radiosurgery for an arteriovenous malformation. *Stereotact Funct Neurosurg* 1999;72[Suppl 1]:168–174.
180. Hara M, Nakamura M, Shiokawa Y, et al. Delayed cyst formation after radiosurgery for cerebral arteriovenous malformation: two case reports. *Minim Invasive Neurosurg* 1998;41:40–45.
181. Pollock BE, Brown RD. Management of cysts arising after radiosurgery to treat intracranial arteriovenous malformations. *Neurosurgery* 2001;49:259–264.
182. Flickinger JC, Kondziolka D, Lunsford LD, et al. Development of a model to predict permanent symptomatic postradiosurgery injury for arteriovenous malformation patients. Arteriovenous Malformation Radiosurgery Study Group. *Int J Radiat Oncol Biol Phys* 2000;46:1143–1148.
183. Pollock BE, Lunsford LD, Kondziolka D, et al. Patient outcomes after stereotactic radiosurgery for "operable" arteriovenous malformations. *Neurosurgery* 1994;35:1–7.
184. Friedman WA, Blatt DL, Bova FJ, et al. The risk of hemorrhage after radiosurgery for arteriovenous malformations. *J Neurosurg* 1996;84:912–919.
185. Pollock BE, Flickinger JC, Lunsford LD, et al. Hemorrhage risk after stereotactic radiosurgery of cerebral arteriovenous malformations. *Neurosurgery* 1996;38:652–661.
186. Karlsson B, Lax I, Soderman M. Risk for hemorrhage during the 2-year latency period following gamma knife radiosurgery for arteriovenous malformations. *Int J Radiat Oncol Biol Phys* 2001;49:1045–1051.
187. Colombo F, Benedetti A, Pozza F, et al. Linear accelerator radiosurgery of cerebral arteriovenous malformations. *Neurosurgery* 1989;24:833–840.
188. Seifert V, Stolke D, Mehdorn HM, et al. Clinical and radiological evaluation of long-term results of stereotactic proton beam radiosurgery in patients with cerebral arteriovenous malformations. *J Neurosurg* 1994;81:683–689.
189. Spetzler RF, Selman WR. Pathophysiology of cerebral ischemia accompanying arteriovenous malformations. In: Wilson CB, Stein BM, eds. *Intracranial arteriovenous malformations.* Baltimore: Williams & Wilkins, 1984:24–31.
190. Leblanc R, Little JR. Hemodynamics of arteriovenous malformations. *Clin Neurosurg* 1990;36:299–317.
191. Cockroft KM, Thompson RC, Steinberg GK. Aneurysms and arteriovenous malformations. *Neurosurg Clin N Am* 1998;9:565–576.
192. Fleetwood IG, Steinberg GK. The management of aneurysms associated with arteriovenous malformations. In: Winn HR, LeRoux PD, eds. *Management of cerebral aneurysms.* Baltimore: WB Saunders, 2002 *(in press).*
193. Turjman F, Massoud TF, Viñuela F, et al. Aneurysms related to cerebral arteriovenous malformations: superselective angiographic assessment in 58 patients. *AJNR Am J Neuroradiol* 1994;15:1601–1605.
194. Vymazal J, Liscak R, Novotny JJ, et al. The role of gamma knife radiosurgery in arteriovenous malformation with aneurysms. *Stereotact Funct Neurosurg* 1999;72[Suppl 1]:175–184.
195. Gao E, Young WL, Pile-Spellman J, et al. Cerebral arteriovenous malformation feeding artery aneurysms: a theoretical model of intravascular pressure changes after treatment. *Neurosurgery* 1997;41:1345–1348.
196. Kader A, Goodrich JT, Sonstein WJ, et al. Recurrent cerebral arteriovenous malformations after negative postoperative angiograms. *J Neurosurg* 1996;85:14–18.
197. Gabriel EM, Sampson JH, Wilkins RH. Recurrence of a cerebral arteriovenous malformation after surgical excision. Case report. *J Neurosurg* 1996;84:879–882.
198. Sathi S, Mascott CR, Liu SS, et al. Recurrence of arteriovenous malformation in children. *J Neurosurg* 1996;84:364a(abst).
199. Lanzino G, Fergus A, Jensen ME, et al. Recurrence of arteriovenous malformations [Letter]. *J Neurosurg* 1996;85:1196–1197.
200. Hino A, Fujimoto M, Iwamoto Y, et al. An adult case of recurrent arteriovenous malformation after complete surgical excision: a case report. *Surg Neurol* 1999;52:156–159.
201. Fraudenstein D, Duffner F, Ernemann U, et al. Recurrence of a cerebral arteriovenous malformation after surgical excision. *Cerebrovasc Dis* 2001;11:59–64.
202. Santoro A, Giuliani S, Paolini S. Recurrent arteriovenous malformation in an adult. Case illustration. *J Neurosurg* 2000;93:1082.
203. Lindqvist M, Karlsson B, Guo WY, et al. Angiographic long-

term follow-up data for arteriovenous malformations previously proven to be obliterated after gamma knife radiosurgery. *Neurosurgery* 2000;46:803–810.
204. Sonstein WJ, Kader A, Michelsen WJ, et al. Expression of vascular endothelial growth factor in pediatric and adult cerebral arteriovenous malformations: an immunocytochemical study. *J Neurosurg* 1996;85:838–845.
205. Rodriguez-Arias C, Martinez R, Rey G, et al. Recurrence in a different location of a cerebral arteriovenous malformation in a child after radiosurgery. *Childs Nerv Syst* 2000;16:363–365.
206. Marks MP, Lane B, Steinberg GK, et al. Intranidal aneurysms in cerebral arteriovenous malformations: evalution and endovascular treatment. *Radiology* 1992;182:255–260.
207. Bhatnagar A, Flickinger JC, Kondziolka D, et al. An analysis of the effects of smoking and other cardiovascular risk factors on obliteration rates after arteriovenous malformation radiosurgery. *Int J Radiat Oncol Biol Phys* 2001;51(4):969–973.

10

ENDOVASCULAR THERAPY FOR ARTERIOVENOUS MALFORMATIONS

MICHAEL P. MARKS

Endovascular therapy of intracranial arteriovenous malformations (AVMs) is often used as part of a multimodal treatment plan that includes microsurgery and radiosurgery. In most cases, AVM embolization is done as an adjunctive therapy for these lesions and not used as the sole treatment. The endovascular therapist participating in the management of the patient with an AVM may have a number of potential goals to be achieved with endovascular treatment. These can include reduction in the flow through the AVM nidus, reduction in the size of the nidus, elimination of specific regions within the nidus and, less commonly, complete thrombosis of the AVM.

AVM embolization has undergone a steady improvement in the past decade, in large part owing to technologic advances in microcatheters and embolic agents used to treat these lesions. This chapter will focus on how endovascular therapy is used in the integrated management of the patient with AVM and the techniques for endovascular treatment. Much of the groundwork providing the basis for our management decisions, such as the natural history of the AVM and the use of surgery and radiosurgery in AVM treatment, were discussed in the previous chapter.

BACKGROUND

Hemorrhage

The goal of most AVM treatment plans is to achieve complete angiographic obliteration of the AVM. Treatment options for AVMs can include endovascular therapy, microsurgery, and stereotactic radiation. In many centers, currently, a multidisciplinary team approach is used to provide a combination of therapies. This is done to maximize the likelihood the AVM will be completely eradicated. Treatment plans are generally based on a concern that the AVM may bleed. Hemorrhage is the most common initial symptom of the patient with a brain AVM. Pooled data from 1,860 reported cases have suggested that 60% of patients with an AVM will come to medical attention with hemorrhage [1]. Retrospective studies have placed the annual risk of hemorrhage from AVMs at 2% to 4% per year, with hemorrhagic events resulting in a mortality rate of approximately 10% and a morbidity rate with the development of neurologic deficit of approximately 30% [2–4]. Additional retrospective data do suggest that the annual risk of bleeding is higher still in the patient who has had a previous hemorrhage [3,5,6]. A prospective study has suggested this is as high as 18% per year [7].

Angioarchitecture

There has been a considerable effort to evaluate the morphologic features of AVMs that may contribute to a poor natural history in the patient with AVM. The term *angioarchitecture* is often used to refer to these morphologic features that are readily demonstrable on a temporally resolved digital subtraction angiogram. These angioarchitectural elements include aneurysms in the region of the circle of Willis or more distally within the nidus of the AVM, the size of the AVM nidus, and observations regarding the feeding arteries and draining veins.

What characteristics of angioarchitecture can be observed angiographically that may result in a poor natural history, specifically bleeding from the AVM? Several studies have demonstrated deep venous drainage is a vascular characteristic that predisposes to a hemorrhage [8–11]. In addition, the finding of a single draining vein from the nidus conferred a higher risk of bleeding in some of these studies [8, 11]. The increased bleeding risk seen in the presence of a single draining vein has been explained on the basis of venous hypertension. It has also been suggested that acquired venous stenoses or kinking may also contribute to venous hypertension and increase the risk of bleeding [11]. Venous stenoses have not been found uniformly to influence the risk of bleeding, however, and these influences may be multifactorial. For example, in some patients collateral venous outflow patterns may be adequate to reduce the venous hypertension from a venous stenosis. In other patients, how-

M.P. Marks: Departments of Radiology and Neurosurgery, Stanford University Medical Center, Stanford, California.

ever, the collateral venous drainage may be inadequate, and the venous stenosis may result in venous hypertension and adversely influence the rate of hemorrhage.

The association between AVMs and intracranial aneurysms has been well documented. The incidence of coexisting aneurysms is found to vary in studies from 2.3% to 22.7% [12–23]. Several studies have reported a higher incidence of intracranial hemorrhage in patients with associated aneurysms [4,13,20,24]. Different types of aneurysms can be distinguished based on location. Aneurysms can be seen on the arteries of the circle of Willis or beyond the circle of Willis arising from arteries supplying the AVM. They may also be found immediately within the nidus itself as intranidal aneurysms. Many feel that the high flow and ensuing hemodynamic stress on feeding arteries leads to aneurysm formation. Therefore these aneurysms are often referred to as flow-related aneurysms. Support for this hemodynamic or flow-related theory comes from the observation that a high percentage of aneurysms are located on major feeding vessels to the AVM [22,25,26]. In the nidus itself, intranidal aneurysms have been shown to predispose to a high rate of hemorrhage (Fig. 10-1)[23,27,28]. These

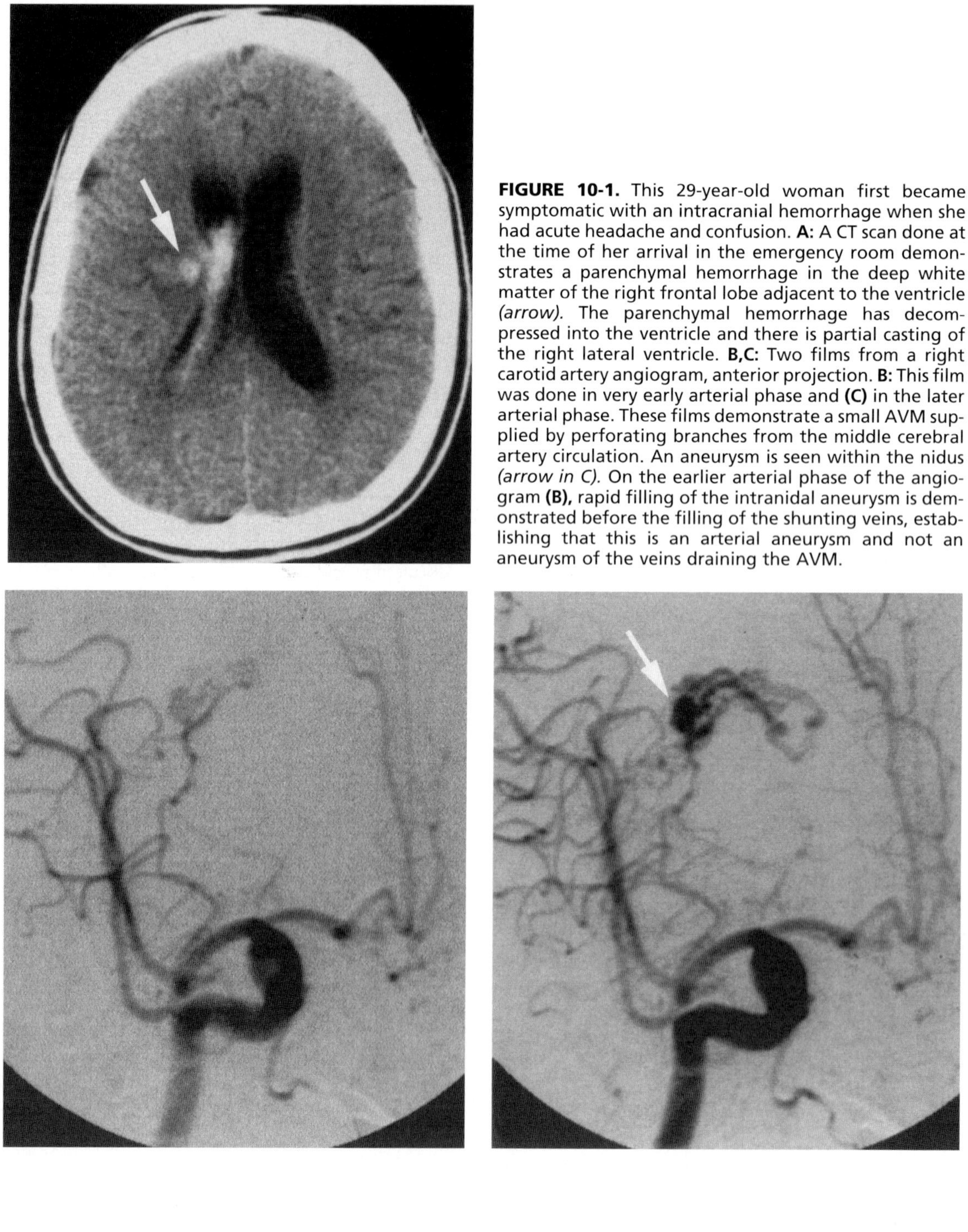

A B C

FIGURE 10-1. This 29-year-old woman first became symptomatic with an intracranial hemorrhage when she had acute headache and confusion. **A:** A CT scan done at the time of her arrival in the emergency room demonstrates a parenchymal hemorrhage in the deep white matter of the right frontal lobe adjacent to the ventricle *(arrow).* The parenchymal hemorrhage has decompressed into the ventricle and there is partial casting of the right lateral ventricle. **B,C:** Two films from a right carotid artery angiogram, anterior projection. **B:** This film was done in very early arterial phase and **(C)** in the later arterial phase. These films demonstrate a small AVM supplied by perforating branches from the middle cerebral artery circulation. An aneurysm is seen within the nidus *(arrow in C).* On the earlier arterial phase of the angiogram **(B),** rapid filling of the intranidal aneurysm is demonstrated before the filling of the shunting veins, establishing that this is an arterial aneurysm and not an aneurysm of the veins draining the AVM.

may not be readily distinguishable from true pseudoaneurysms that can be seen following an AVM hemorrhage. If one documents a rapid change in size of a contrast collection or the new appearance of a contrast collection following a hemorrhage, this may be more likely to represent a pseudoaneurysm. Pseudoaneurysms represent a communication with the lumen of the ruptured nidal vessel and a surrounding hematoma [29]. Changes in the size of these pseudoaneurysmal lesions have been demonstrated with serial angiography. Clearly these lesions are highly correlated with clinical bleeding and also represent a special therapeutic challenge because of the high risk of rebleeding [29].

AVM size—that is, the size of the nidus—can vary significantly. Evaluation of nidal size is certainly important in the overall planning for multimodal therapy, because it is a critical issue governing the likelihood of surgical resectability or radiosurgical success. Most surgical grading systems incorporate nidal size as a major variable in the evaluation of the patient with AVM [30–34]. Some investigators have observed that hemorrhages are more likely to occur with small AVMs [34,35]. Spetzler et al. evaluated feeding artery pressures and found that smaller AVMs had higher feeding artery pressures than larger AVMs, suggesting that these differences may explain the observation that small AVMs are more likely to bleed [35]. Other authors, however, have not found a relationship between bleeding frequency and small AVMs [7,8,21,36]. Indeed some series have even documented that larger AVMs are more likely to bleed [37, 38]. Feeding artery pressure (FAP) measurements have been evaluated as a separate physiologic marker for hemorrhage risk and have been shown to correlate with AVM bleeding [39–41]. The FAP has been shown by some investigators to correlate with AVM size [40]. Miyasaka et al. reported that small nidus size increases the risk of hemorrhage and that there is an inverse relationship between FAP and AVM size [40]. Duong et al., however, found that AVM size was not an independent predictor of hemorrhage, whereas the FAP was [41].

Are there vascular characteristics which can be identified angiographically that may reduce the risk of hemorrhage? Exclusively cortical venous drainage and venous recruitment have both been identified as characteristics of the venous drainage pattern which may protect against hemorrhage [9, 10]. Venous recruitment has been described as drainage seen through veins that would be considered unusual or not usually implicated in the drainage of the portion of the brain where the AVM nidus arises [10]. On the arterial side, the presence of anomalous arterial supply to the AVM has also been implicated as a vascular characteristic that is seen in patients with a decreased risk of hemorrhage. This anomalous supply is usually in the form of dilated transcortical or leptomeningeal arteries acting as collateral supply to the nidus and has been coined *angiomatous change* (Fig. 10-2) [42]. The term arises from the dilated leptomeningeal vessels often having an appearance that is similar to the AVM but does not make up a component of the nidus itself. Angiomatous change is likely to arise when feeding artery pressures are reduced to the nidus bed, and this characteristic is therefore thought to reflect a lower risk of hemorrhage from the AVM nidus.

Classification

A great deal of effort has been expended by various groups to develop classification schemes for cerebral AVMs. These systems are designed to create a scheme which will provide prognostic information for therapy. Many of the classification systems have concentrated on surgical therapy, although some have been designed to identify those patients who would be considered good candidates for endovascular therapy. Luessenhop and Gennarelli attempted to classify AVMs to determine the likelihood of operative success [43]. Valavanis and Yasargil developed a topographic classification of brain AVMs [44]. Surgical classifications have simplified the vascular characteristics that one needed to classify an AVM in an effort to streamline the evaluation system [32,33]. The surgical classification suggested by Spetzler and Martin [33] has become perhaps the most widely accepted grading system for AVM management. This simplified system which uses only three characteristics: lesion size, eloquence of the adjacent brain, and pattern of venous drainage, has proven easy to use and of clinical utility. This system assigns points for each of these three features (Table 10-1). The sum of these points adds up to the assigned grade so that AVMs are classified with grades of I through V. Lower-grade AVMs are generally considered resectable, so that a small AVM located in a noneloquent area with only superficial drainage would be a grade I AVM and more likely to be resectable without complications. High-grade AVMs, on the other hand, would have higher rates of complications. A grade V AVM, for example, would be a large lesion in an eloquent area that has deep venous drainage, and a complication would be more likely to occur at resec-

TABLE 10-1. SPETZLER-MARTIN GRADING SYSTEM

AVM Feature	Points
Size of nidus	
<3 cm (small)	1
3–6 cm (medium)	2
>6 cm (large)	3
Eloquence of surrounding brain	
Noneloquent	0
Eloquent	1
Venous drainage	
Superficial	0
Deep	1

From Spetzler RF, Martin NA. A proposed grading system for arteriovenous malformations. *J Neurosurg* 1987;65:476–483, with permission.

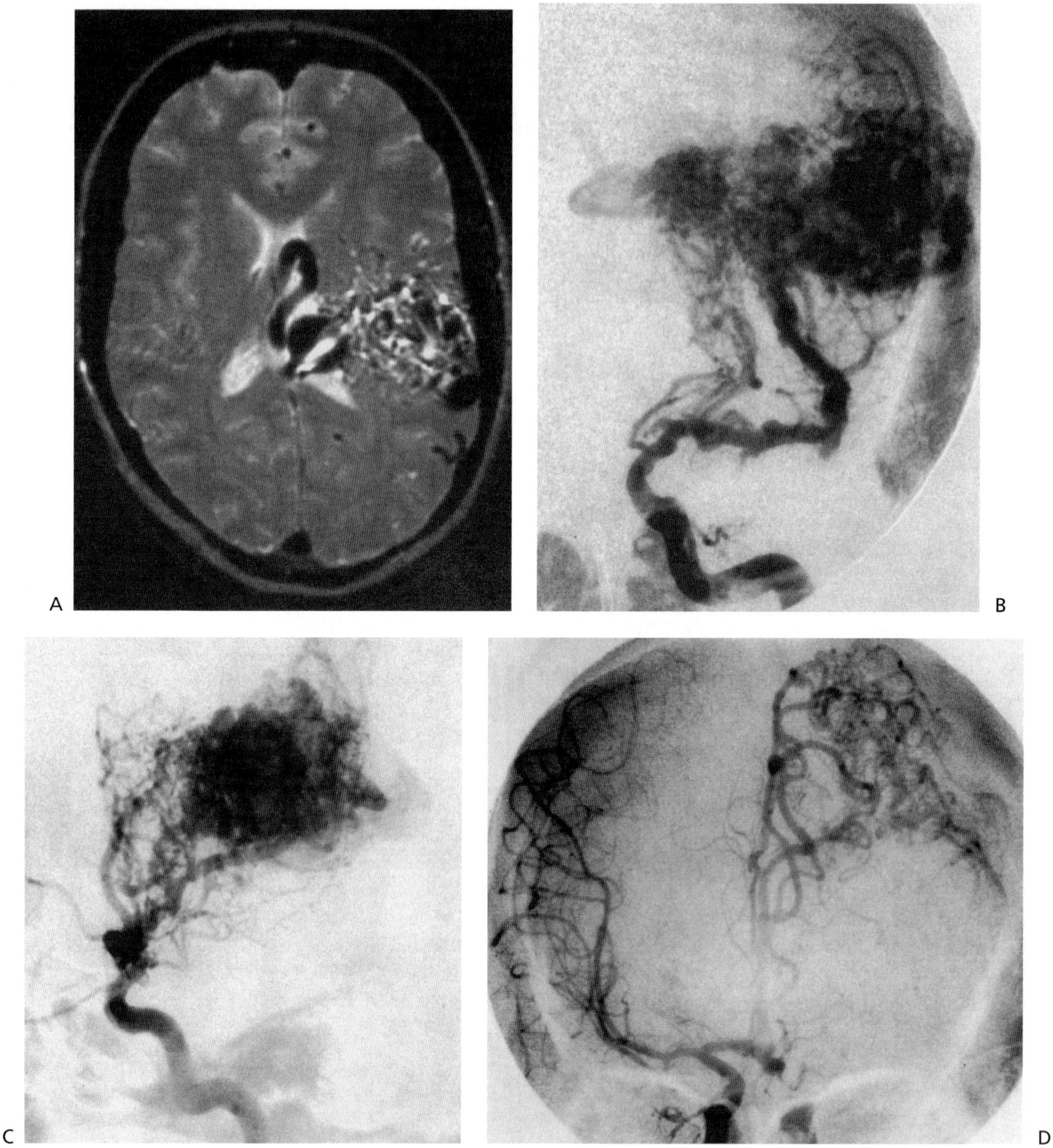

FIGURE 10-2. This 35-year-old woman had a long history of severe migraine headaches since childhood. At times these headaches were associated with episodes of numbness and weakness of the right side of the body which resolved. She had no history of a clinical hemorrhage. **A:** Axial T2-weighted image through the supratentorial brain demonstrates the large left frontoparietal AVM with central drainage. No evidence of prior hemorrhage was seen on this slice or the remainder of the MR study. **B,C:** Left internal carotid artery angiogram, anterior and lateral projections, respectively, demonstrate the large AVM. This wedge-shaped malformation extends from the cortex down to the ventricular surface and is fed by deep perforating arteries as well as opercular arteries from the middle cerebral artery circulation. *(Figure continues.)*

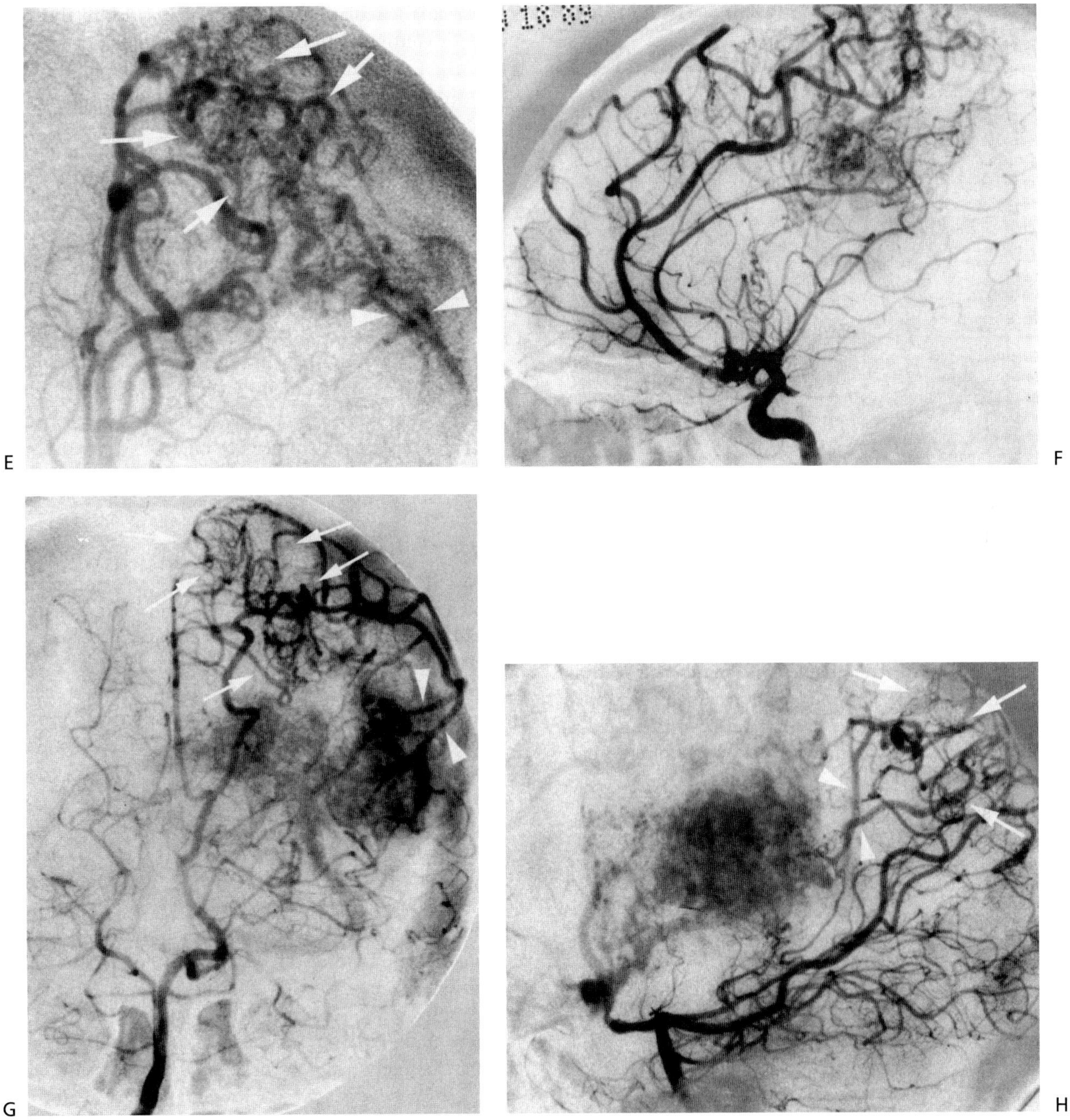

FIGURE 10-2. *Continued.* **D–F:** Selective views from a right internal artery carotid artery angiogram in the anterior projection **(D,E)** and the lateral projection **(F).** These studies demonstrate cross filling via the anterior communicating artery, with indirect supply via angiomatous change, to the AVM. The dilated vessels of the left anterior cerebral artery can be seen on both the lateral and anterior projections. The more magnified view from the anterior projection **(E)** demonstrates dilated arteries *(between arrows)* representing angiomatous change. These dilated leptomeningeal vessels supply the opercular arteries of the middle cerebral artery in a retrograde fashion *(arrowheads)* which then give additional indirect supply to the AVM nidus. **G,H:** Left vertebral angiogram, anterior and lateral projections, again demonstrates indirect supply via angiomatous change to the AVM. The left posterior cerebral artery is markedly dilated and gives rise to angiomatous change. This leptomeningeal collateral supply to the AVM is seen in the area between the arrows on both projections. The middle cerebral artery circulation then fills in a retrograde fashion *(arrowheads)* to supply the AVM.

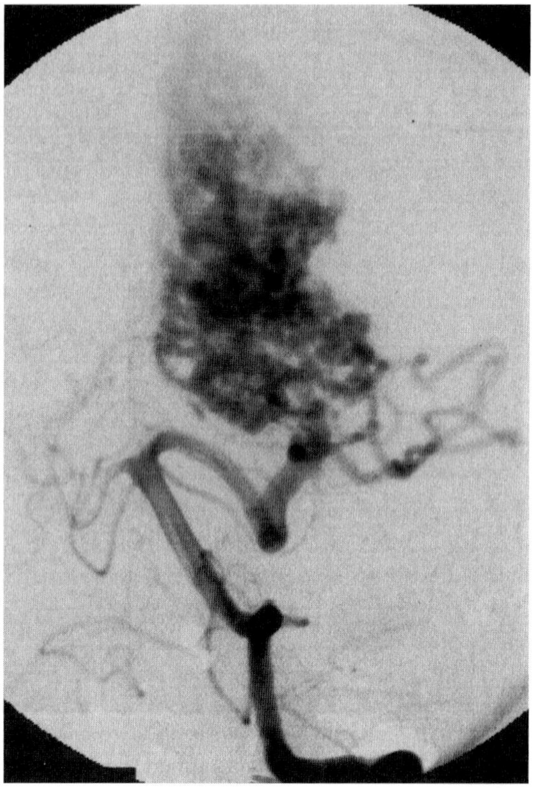
E

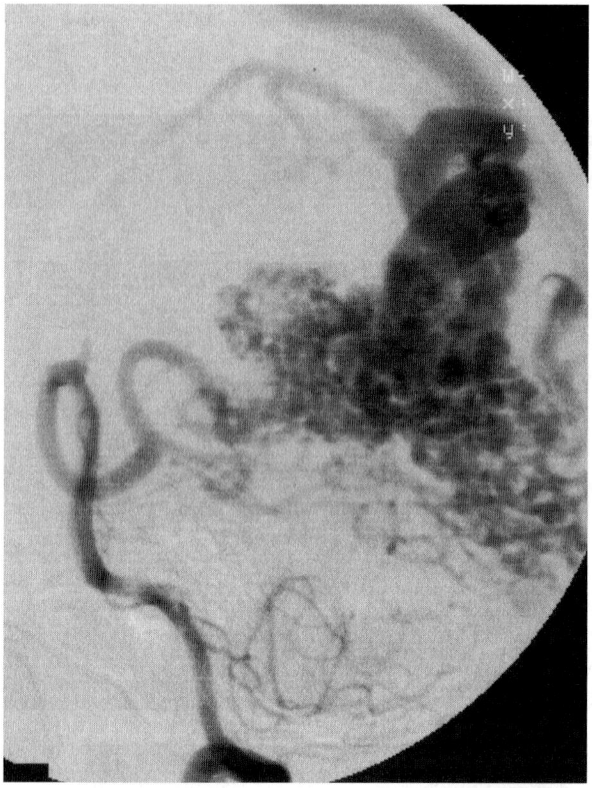
F

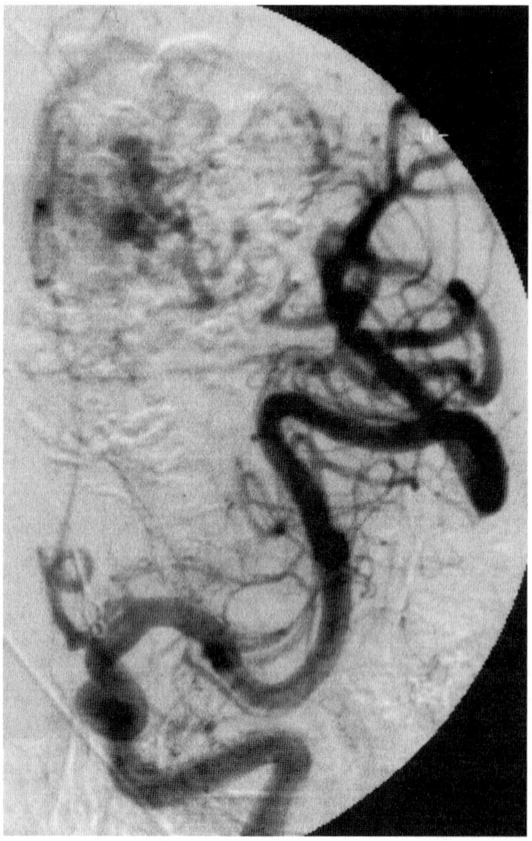
G

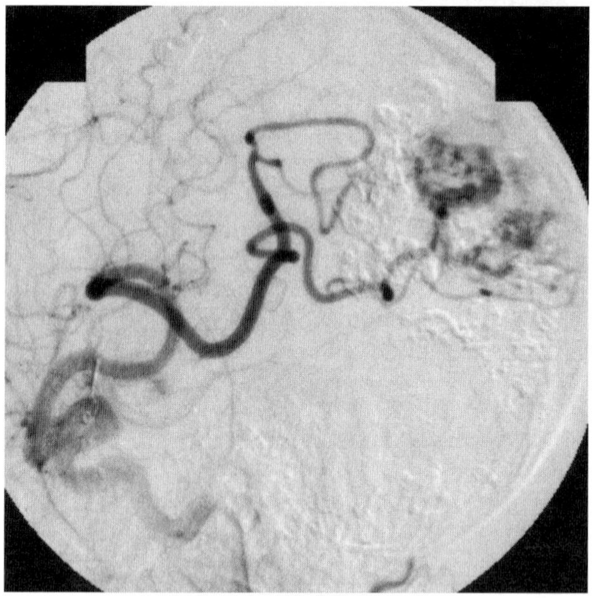
H

FIGURE 10-3. *Continued.* **E,F:** Left vertebral artery angiogram, anterior and lateral projections, respectively, demonstrates filling of the vascular malformation from branches of the posterior cerebral artery. There is some cortical venous drainage demonstrated. Because of the large size of the AVM and the combined supply from branches of the anterior, middle and posterior cerebral arteries, embolization was done to reduce the shunt flow prior to surgery. **G,H:** Left internal carotid artery, anterior and lateral projections, demonstrates markedly reduced size of the AVM nidus and decrease in the amount of shunt flow following staged embolization (compare with **C, D**). *(Figure continues.)*

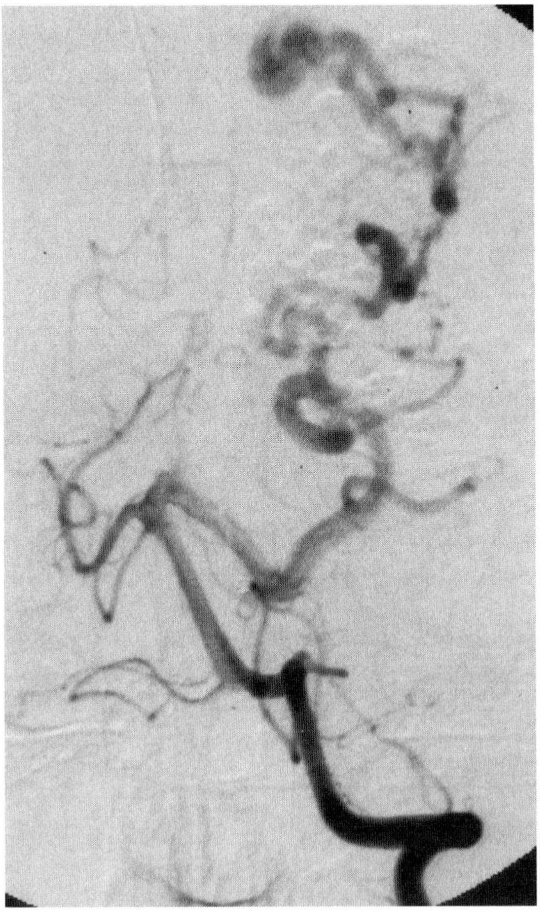

I

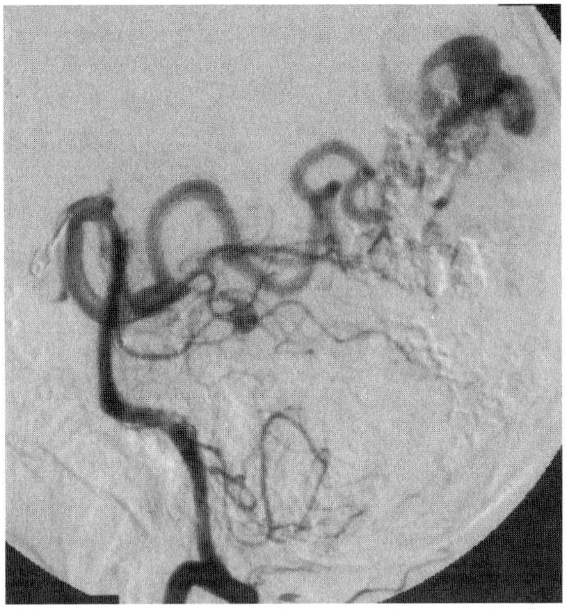

J

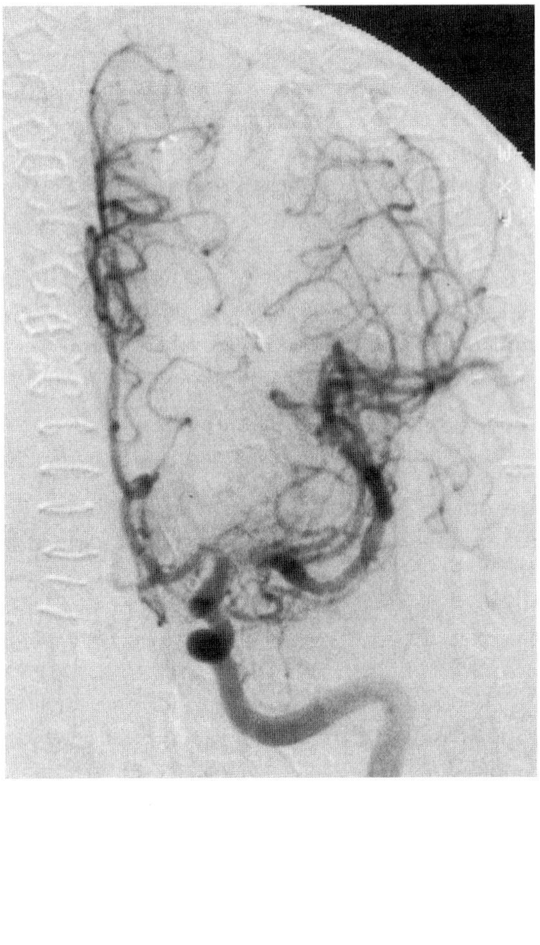

K

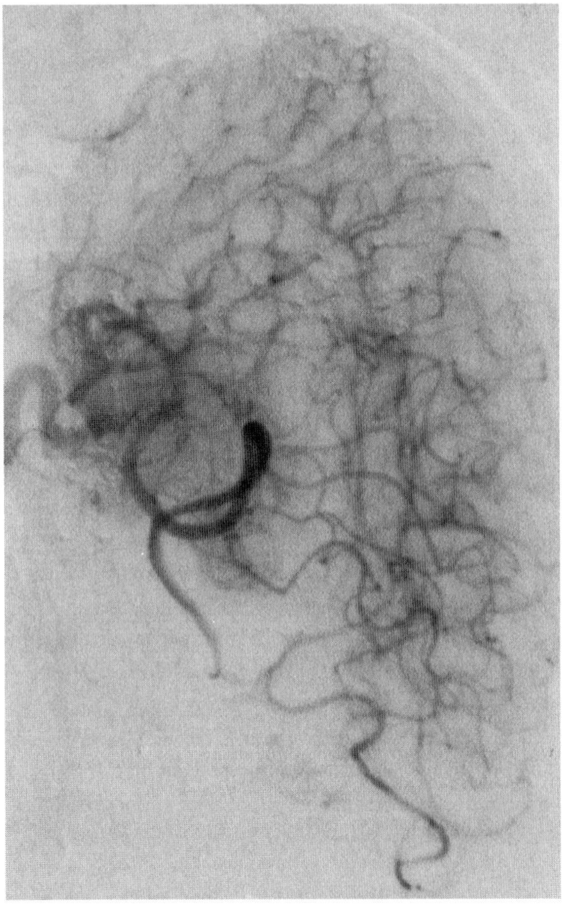

L

FIGURE 10-3. *Continued.* **I,J:** Left vertebral artery injection anterior and lateral projections demonstrate the nidus size and shunt flow has been markedly reduced after embolization (compare to **E, F**). **K,L:** Left internal carotid artery control angiogram in the anterior and lateral projections, respectively. This postoperative angiogram demonstrates complete excision of the remaining AVM shunt from this circulation. *(Figure continues.)*

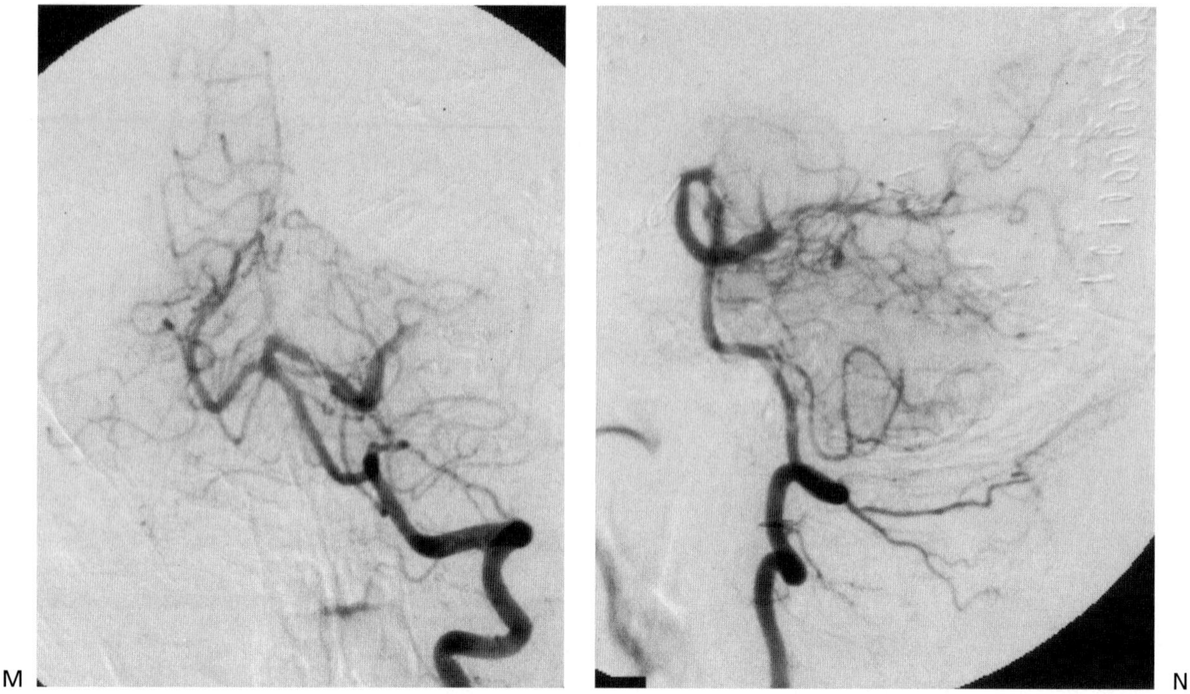

FIGURE 10-3. *Continued.* **M,N:** Left vertebral artery angiogram, anterior and lateral projections, respectively, done postoperatively also demonstrates that the component of the AVM nidus fed from the posterior cerebral artery has been effectively embolized and excised.

tion made AVMs of larger size and higher grade the surgical equivalent of lesions of smaller size and lower grade by reducing operative time, intraoperative blood loss, and making surgical complication rates and late neurologic outcome equivalent [60]. Viñuela et al. reported on the results of combined endovascular embolization and surgery in 101 cases [61]. These authors found that when the AVM was more than 75% obliterated by embolization, there was extensive thrombosis of draining veins and few subpial collateral vessels, which greatly facilitated surgical resection. However, embolic occlusion of less than 50% of the AVM nidus resulted in no change in the appearance or behavior of the nidus at the time of surgery, and in these cases the surgical resection was improved only if the embolization included feeders that were deep or relatively inaccessible. Pasqualin et al. performed a retrospective clinical comparison of AVMs with similar volumes (greater than 20 cm^3) treated with embolization plus surgery versus those treated by surgery alone. They showed that intraoperative bleeding was decreased in those patients treated by embolization, and the rate of new major deficits and death were less frequent in patients treated by embolization [62]. They concluded that the addition of embolization reduced the risk connected with surgical removal alone. A number of other authors have also reported that embolization helps to facilitate the surgery, decreases operative time, and reduces blood loss [59,63–68].

Preradiosurgical Embolization

The goals of preradiosurgical AVM embolization are somewhat different than those pursued in presurgical management. Most preradiosurgical embolization procedures are carried out to reduce the overall volume of the AVM nidus or to selectively treat an angioarchitectural element, such as an intranidal aneurysm, thought to be more prone to hemorrhage. Radiosurgery also may be used to treat a portion of the AVM that is not judged safe to treat after embolization or surgery when these procedures have left residual AVM (Fig. 10-4). Radiosurgical series have uniformly reported an inverse relationship between the AVM nidal size undergoing radiosurgery and the obliteration rates observed, regardless of the type of radiosurgery used [69–75]. Reports are quite variable in the method employed to measure AVM nidal size. They have variously used mean diameter, largest diameter, or one of a number of volume formulas. Regardless of the method used, a smaller nidal size at the time of initial radiotherapy results in improved obliteration rates. Radiosurgical treatment of an AVM nidus with a mean diameter that is less than 2.5 to 3 cm or that has a volume less than 10 cm^3 is generally more likely to produce such a complete obliteration.

Despite the theoretical advantages of performing embolization in advance of radiosurgery, precious few studies have reported the concerted efforts of the endovascular therapist and the radiosurgeon. Dawson et al. used particulate embo-

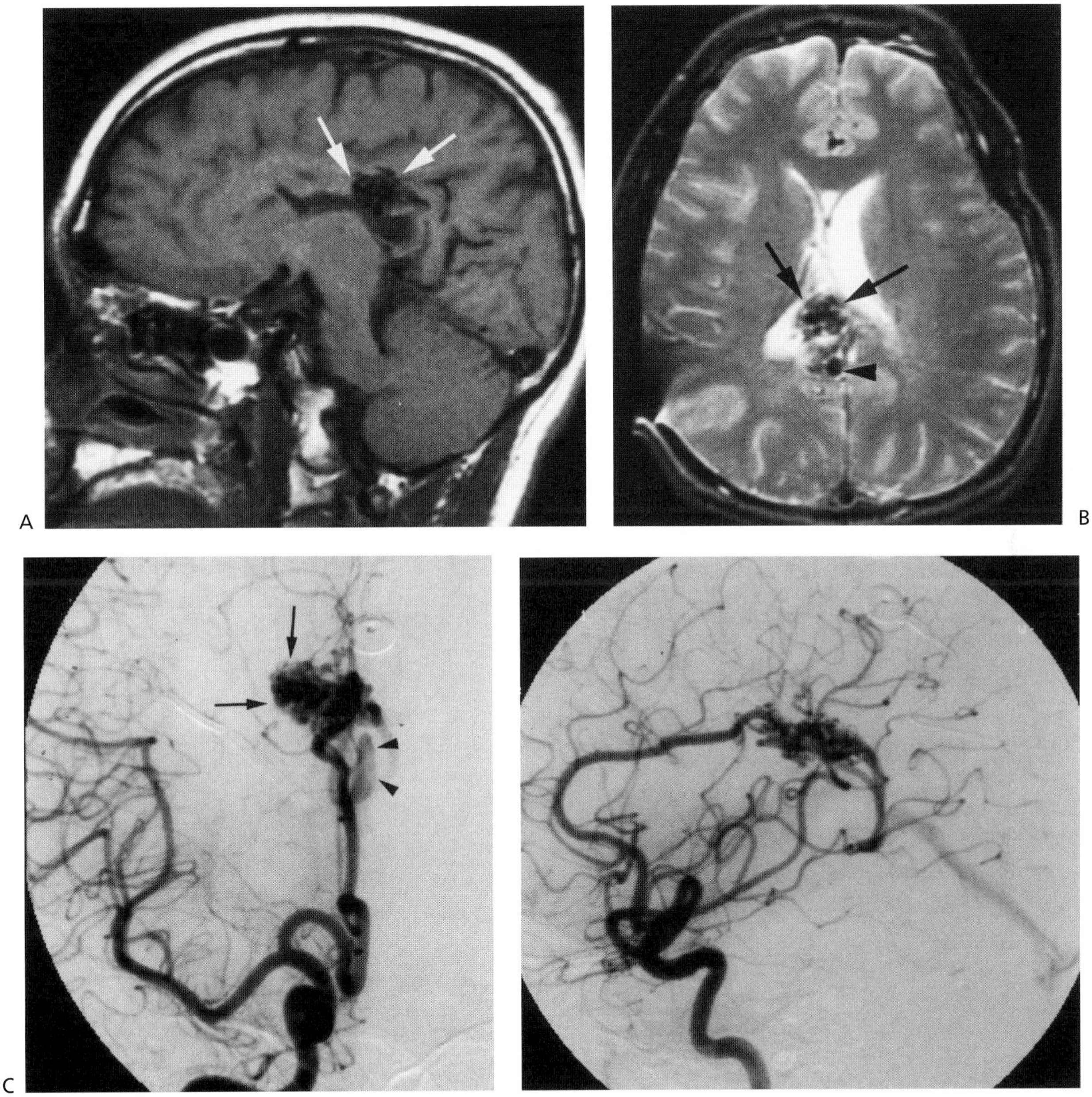

FIGURE 10-4. This 34-year-old man with an AVM in the splenium of the corpus callosum originally experienced an intracranial hemorrhage in his right parietal lobe and ventricles. He developed sensory changes in his left extremities and had some problems with his memory, but he was able to continue working full time after recovering from the hemorrhage. **A,B:** Sagittal **(A)** T1- and axial **(B)** T2-weighted MRIs demonstrate the nidus in the right splenium of the corpus callosum *(arrows)*. Drainage from the AVM was central, with a large draining vein going to the straight sinus *(arrowhead)*. **C,D:** Right internal carotid artery angiograms, anterior and lateral projections, respectively, demonstrate the AVM nidus *(arrows)* fed by the right anterior pericallosal artery. The nidus was noted to be exclusively on the right side of the midline. Central draining veins are also noted on this early arterial angiogram *(arrowheads)*. *(Figure continues.)*

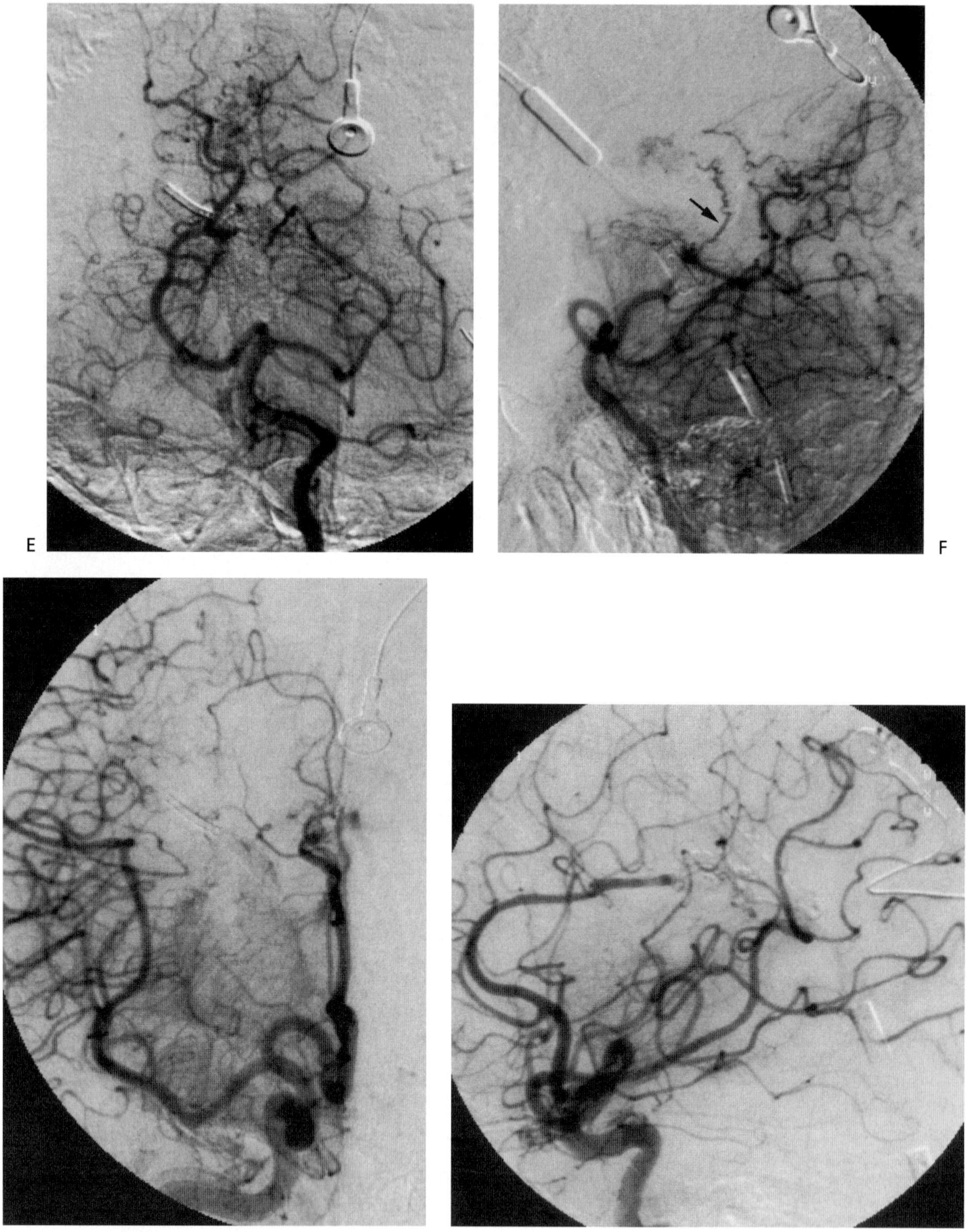

E F G H

FIGURE 10-4. *Continued.* **E,F:** Left vertebral artery angiogram, anterior and lateral projections, respectively, demonstrates slight filling of the AVM nidus from the posterior cerebral artery. The medial posterior choroidal artery *(arrow)* is the main artery from this circulation supplying the AVM nidus. **G,H:** Right internal carotid artery angiogram, anterior and lateral views, respectively, after embolization. The AVM was embolized with a microcatheter placed in the distal right pericallosal artery. Most of the AVM is obliterated with slight inflow into the AVM nidus remaining. *(Figure continues.)*

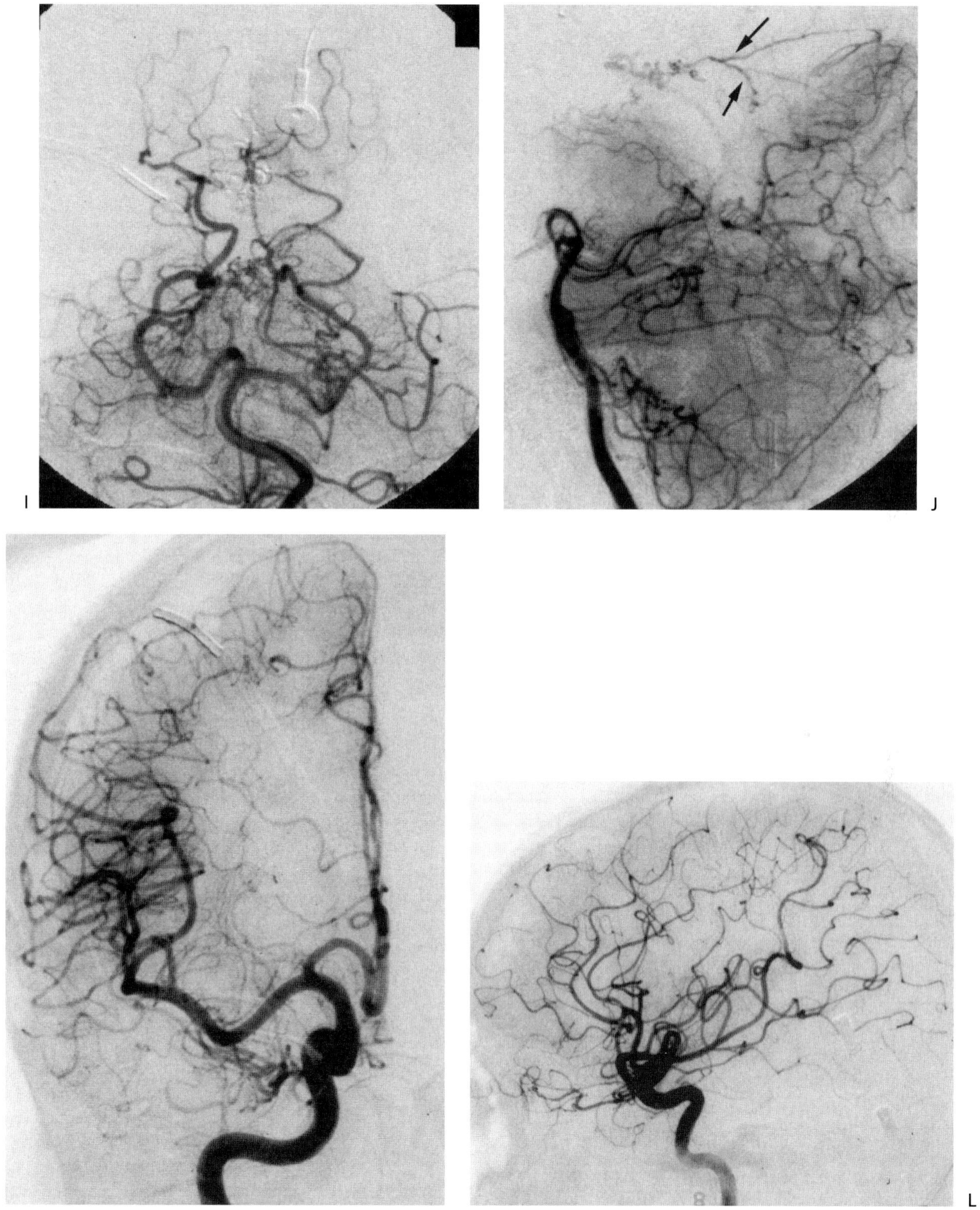

FIGURE 10-4. *Continued.* **I,J:** Left vertebral artery angiogram, anterior and lateral views, respectively, immediately after embolization demonstrates minimal collateral flow into the AVM nidus. The flow is coming from perisplenial branches from the posterior cerebral artery *(arrows).* Because the remaining live components of the AVM nidus were not felt to be safely treated by embolization, the patient was sent for radiosurgery. **K,L:** Right internal carotid angiogram, anterior and lateral views, respectively. This angiogram was performed 3 years after radiosurgery and shows complete obliteration of the AVM nidus. *(Figure continues.)*

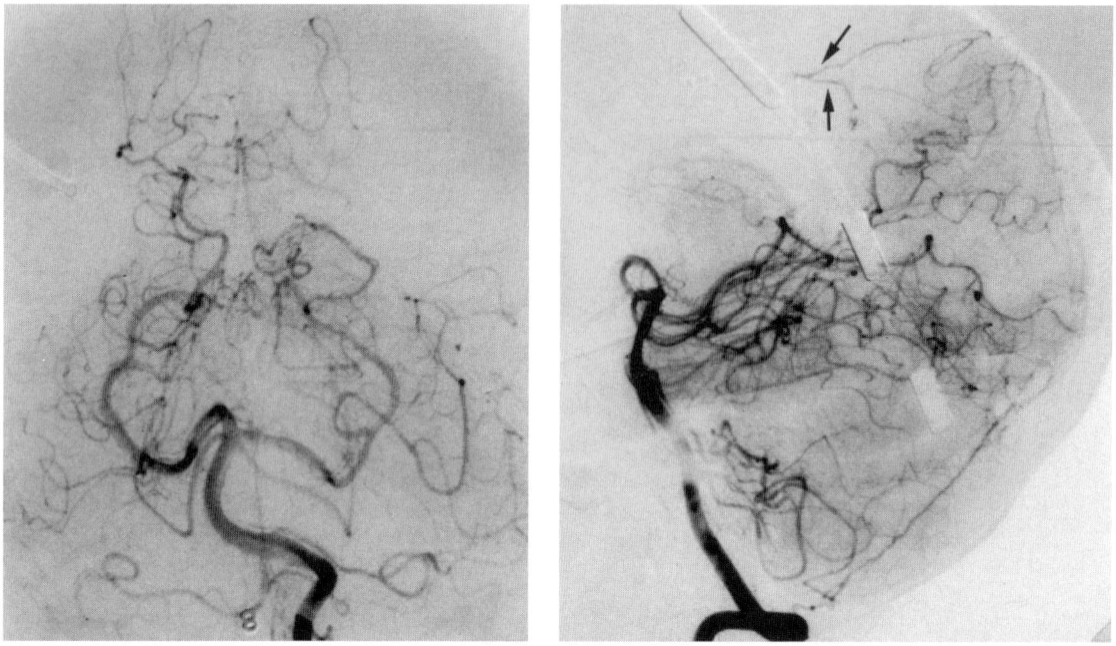

FIGURE 10-4. *Continued.* **M,N:** Left vertebral artery angiogram, anterior and lateral views, respectively. This angiogram was also obtained at the same time as the right internal carotid artery angiogram 3 years after radiosurgery and demonstrates no abnormal shunting in this circulation. The previously seen perisplenial branches *(arrows)* are still observed to fill but the nidal component is not observed.

lization in seven patients with larger AVMs [76]. Using a combination of polyvinyl alcohol (PVA) or silk, they achieved a 23.6% mean volume reduction following embolization. Their combined 1- and 2-year follow-up results after radiosurgery showed that, of seven AVMs, two were obliterated and two had greater than 98% volume reductions; three had minimal change in size. Guo et al. reported on the results of combined embolization and gamma knife radiosurgery in 46 patients [77]. Forty-three of the 46 patients had a decrease in the maximal diameter of the AVM nidus. This decrease varied from 5% to 71%. In addition, in 25 patients the original maximal nidus diameter of greater than 3 cm was reduced to less than 3 cm. Radiosurgical follow-up in this series was somewhat limited, with only 15 patients having follow-up angiograms after radiosurgery. In this group, five patients were observed to have undergone total obliteration and nine patients had partial obliteration.

Mathis et al. did a retrospective study of 24 patients with larger brain AVMs (greater than 3-cm diameter or greater than 10-cm^3 volume) who had undergone particulate embolization and stereotactic radiosurgery and were evaluated 2 or more years after the radiosurgery [78]. Twelve of the patients in the series (50%) had a complete obliteration. The authors found this to be essentially the same rate of obliteration achieved with AVMs that were initially under 4 to 10 cm^3, using the equivalent single-stage radiosurgery technique. Those patients with AVMs that were successfully obliterated using radiosurgery had a mean preembolization volume of 29 cm^3, which was reduced to 7.2 cm^3 after embolization; whereas those patients experiencing subtotal obliteration had a mean volume of 45 cm^3, which was reduced to 14 cm^3 after embolization. Three patients (12%) did demonstrate recanalization of embolized but not irradiated AVM segments on follow-up angiography.

Gobin et al. reported on the treatment of 125 patients with AVMs, with 96 of these patients ultimately undergoing combined embolization and radiosurgery [79]. AVMs of 14 of the patients in the study were completely occluded by embolization, and 15 patients were not considered candidates for radiosurgery for various reasons. Mean AVM volume for the entire study group was 18.6 cm^3 before embolization, and this was reduced to 6.2 cm^3 after embolization. Sixty-three of the 96 patients had follow-up after radiosurgery and in this group 41 (65%) had complete obliteration. Complications were seen in 14.4% of the patients and these were almost exclusively seen in those with Spetzler-Martin grade IV to V AVMs.

Embolization can also be performed after radiosurgery to assist in the multidisciplinary management of the patient with AVM who has failed to have a complete obliteration with radiosurgery. The goal here may be complete embolization of the AVM or further reduction in the size of the AVM to then facilitate additional radiosurgical or surgical management [80,81]. Pathologic evaluation of the AVMs that have undergone prior radiosurgery has demonstrated that they are somewhat less vascular and partially thrombosed, which appears to improve the success of both endovascular therapy and follow-up treatment with surgery [80, 81].

Curative and Palliative Embolization

Endovascular therapy can be used in certain selected circumstances as sole therapy. It may be the only treatment modality needed when one is able to obtain a complete angiographic occlusion of the AVM nidus, a curative embolization. It also can be used where an incomplete embolization is contemplated and no other therapies are being considered. This form of embolization is thought to slow the progression of symptoms in the patient with AVM and is considered a palliative embolization.

Curative embolization has had a more limited role when compared to embolization used as an adjunctive therapy to surgery or radiosurgery. Published series demonstrate that smaller AVMs with a smaller number of feeding pedicles are more likely to respond favorably to curative embolization alone. However, most series also report that AVMs with a smaller number of pedicles are not treated by embolization alone, and this likely reflects a referral bias. In a retrospective review by Viñuela et al. in 465 AVM embolizations performed at a single center, 45 patients (9.7%) had complete occlusion with embolization alone [82]. All of these were described as small AVMs fed by no more than four pedicles. These patients were treated with cyanoacrylate. Wikholm and colleagues reported a single-center series of patients treated between 1987 and 1993 [83]. These patients were also treated with cyanoacrylate. However, because of when the study was done, many of the patients were treated with older catheter technology, such as the calibrated-leak catheter. The avowed strategy of the authors was primarily to close the AVMs completely with embolization. Total occlusion of the AVM nidus was obtained in 20 patients (13.3%). Only 14 of the AVMs in this series had volumes of less than 4 cm^3, but 10 of these (71%) were totally occluded by embolization. In contrast, AVMs in the range of 4 to 8 cm^3 had a total occlusion rate of only 15%. Gobin et al. reported a total occlusion in 14 of 125 patients (11.2%) undergoing embolization in advance of radiosurgical treatment [79]. Total occlusion was seen in 9 of 56 (17%) AVMs smaller than 10 cm^3, while it was achieved in only 5 of 59 (8%) AVMs of 10 to 50 cm^3 and in none of 10 AVMs larger than 50 cm^3. None of the patients in this series had AVMs that were less than 4 cm^3. These authors also analyzed their outcomes on the basis of the number of arterial pedicles supplying the AVM nidus. Complete occlusion was seen in 33% of the nidi with one pedicle, 24% of those with two pedicles, 9% of those with three pedicles, and 3% of those with more than three pedicles. Valavanis and Yasargil report significantly higher rates of AVM obliteration than other authors [44]. These authors have identified a number of angioarchitectural features which they believe positively influence the likelihood of complete obliteration. These include the presence of direct and dominant feeders, the absence of perinidal angiogenesis, the presence of a monocompartmental nidus, and the presence of a pure fistulous nidus rather than a nidus with plexiform features. The authors also found that converging compartmental veins or a single nidal draining vein positively influenced complete obliteration. They used these angioarchitectural features to select a group of AVMs that were likely to undergo complete obliteration, and defined 182 of 387 cases in their series (47%) as being AVM appropriate for complete or curative embolization. Complete obliteration was achieved in 136 of these 182 cases (74.4%) which represented 35.1% of their entire series. In contradistinction to other authors, Valavanis and Yasargil believe the nidal size or volume and the number of feeding arteries does not significantly influence complete obliteration.

Palliative embolization has generally been applied to giant AVMs that are regarded to be unlikely to be curable using combined endovascular therapy with surgery or radiosurgery or both. The goal in this therapeutic approach may be to eliminate angioarchitectural elements that are the sites of repeated hemorrhage, such as intranidal aneurysms. In addition, some authors think that a reduction of AVM flow may slow the progression of some symptoms such as neurologic deficits or headaches. There have been a few scattered reports that neurologic deficits can be reversed with embolization, presumably by decreasing the degree of arterial steal or venous hypertension [84,85].

EMBOLIC MATERIALS

No discussion of AVM embolization would be complete without considering embolic materials used in the procedure. A variety of particulate and liquid agents have historically been available for AVM treatment. This aspect of AVM embolization (materials used for embolization) has undergone extensive change and is currently still in evolution. Liquid embolic agents have included cyanoacrylates, ethanol and, more recently, ethylene-vinyl alcohol copolymer (EVOH). Particulate agents have included PVA particles, silk, coils and, more recently, acrylic polymer microspheres.

Cyanoacrylates, usually in the form of NBCA, have become the most commonly used embolic agents for AVM treatment. NBCA polymerizes when it comes in contact with an ionic solution such as blood, so that it leaves the catheter in a liquid form and rapidly polymerizes within the circulation. Essentially, the cyanoacrylate monomer is a two-carbon ethylene group to which is attached a cyano group and an ester function (Fig. 10-5).

By varying the ester function on the cyanoacrylate monomer, one can control some of the physical properties of the material such as the polymerization rate, the heat produced

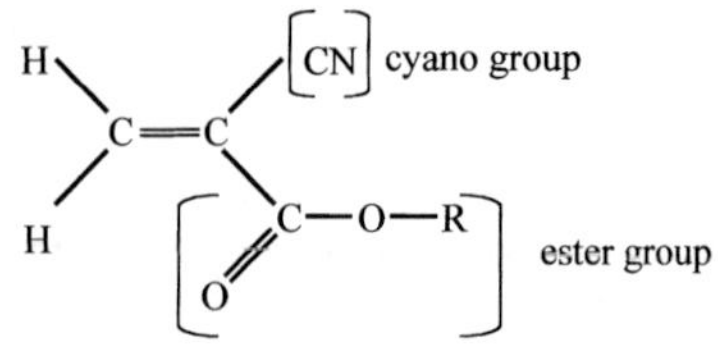

FIGURE 10-5. The cyanoacrylate monomer.

by polymerization, and the surface tension and viscosity of the material [86]. NBCA is currently the most widely used monomer (Fig. 10-6).

In an ionic environment an ion will join the β carbon of the ethyl group, freeing two electrons on the α carbon to then form with another monomer and initiate chain propagation. As the cyanoacrylate polymerizes, it forms a strongly bound chain which solidifies as an adhesive material, forming a cast of the vessel into which it has been introduced.

In earlier clinical use, isobutyl-2-cyanoacrylate (IBCA) was used extensively [63,65,87]. The manufacturer discontinued IBCA production after studies that showed that injection of large doses of IBCA into rat peritoneal cavities produced liver sarcoma [88–90]. More recently, NBCA has been approved in the United States by the Food and Drug Administration for the presurgical embolization of AVMs. To use the cyanoacrylate at the time of embolization, investigators have opacified the device, using either powdered metals such as tantalum or adding iodized oil such as ethiodized oil (Ethiodol) or lipiodol [91,92]. By adding varying amounts of iodized oil, investigators found that they could also alter the polymerization time and control the physical properties of the polymerized substance. In addition to physically occluding the vascular space, NBCA has been shown in experimental animals to cause a vasculitis which leads to chronic granulomatous change and fibrous tissue ingrowth [92]. Similar results have been seen when cyanoacrylates have been recovered from excised tissue specimens in humans [93–96]. Butyl-cyanoacrylates have now been in clinical use for approximately 25 years, and there is no data with this long history of human implantation to suggest that there is a significant risk of carcinogenesis.

Most practitioners currently use cyanoacrylate in a mixture with ethiodized oil, with cyanoacrylate having a final concentration of 20% to 50% of the embolic material. Practitioners may also add tantalum powder to this mixture to improve radiopacity. However, many practitioners find that the radiopacity of the 20% to 50% cyanoacrylate mixed with iodized oil alone is more than adequate to perform embolization. Cyanoacrylate polymerization time also can be prolonged with the use of glacial acetic acid [92], although it is not frequently used now. In general, the cyanoacrylates are considered to be stable and, along with the histologic reaction that ensues following their introduction intravascularly, they are thought to offer a permanent occlusion of the vessel [63,97]. In most cases in which an AVM recurs after cyanoacrylate embolization, it appears to be due to collateral supply revascularizing unembolized portions of the arteriovenous shunt rather than true recanalization of an embolized and occluded vessel [98]. True recanalization has, however, been reported with IBCA [99].

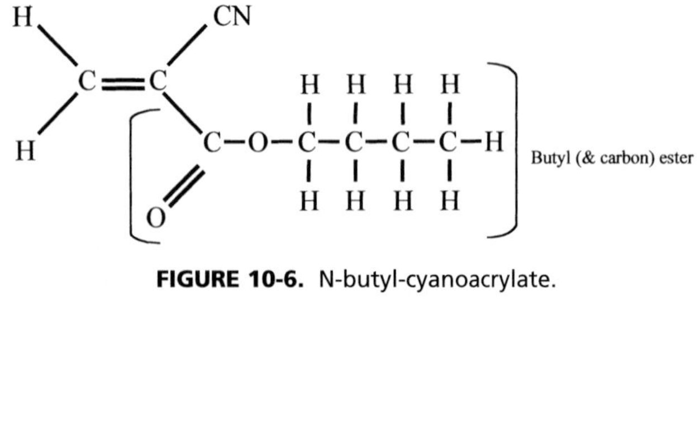

FIGURE 10-6. N-butyl-cyanoacrylate.

Ethanol has been used to treat peripheral vascular malformations with success [100–104]. Initially ethanol was used to treat brain AVMs in diluted mixtures that included contrast and particulates such as PVA [105]. More recently, ethanol has been reported as an embolic agent for brain AVMs in undiluted absolute form (98% ethanol) [106]. In this form, it is opacified by mixing it with metrizamide powder. When absolute ethanol contacts the vascular wall it causes denuding of the endothelial cells and fracturing of the blood vessel down to the level of the internal elastic lamina. With the occlusion of the capillary bed, infarction ensues in the target tissue. Yakes et al. have reported a series of 17 patients with brain AVMs treated using absolute ethyl alcohol [106]. Seven of the patients in this series had complete thrombosis of their AVMs with ethanol therapy, but complications occurred in eight patients. Many of these complications were transient and may well have resulted from the swelling that can be seen with ethanol embolization. Three patients in this series had subarachnoid hemorrhages after embolization, however, and two of these proved fatal. The use of pure ethanol opacified by metrizamide has also been reported to cause the intraventricular leakage of contrast from the choroid plexus [107]. This has been postulated to be due to injury to the choroidal epithelium by the ethanol or hyperosmolar contrast medium or both.

Embolic materials that use the solvent dimethyl sulfoxide (DMSO) have also been reported in small AVM embolization series [108–112]. These materials have included EVOH as well as cellulose acetate polymer (CAP). DSMO solutions can be made radiodense by the addition of a powder such as tantalum. Earlier reports suggested that AVMs embolized with DMSO as a solvent underwent severe inflammatory reactions and tissue damage including perivascular hemorrhage. Chaloupka et al. performed experiments using DSMO and EVOH in swine *rete mirabile* [113]. These initial studies demonstrated extensive infarction of the cerebral hemispheres and upper brainstem in the animals, thought to be due to vasospasm. In addition, some of the animals had subarachnoid hemorrhages and inspection of their cerebral arteries revealed microaneurysms caused by angionecrosis. Later work by Murayama et al. and Chaloupka et al. have suggested that low volumes of DSMO injected at a slower rate will not cause significant angionecrosis [114,115]. Recently, a small clinical AVM embolization series was reported [112], and EVOH and DSMO have begun to be evaluated in a clinical trial prior to approval by the Food and Drug Administration in the United States. Possible advantages over NBCA have been suggested for the EVOH in DMSO material because of its nonadhesive nature and slower time to solidify. It may be used for longer injection times, and it is thought that its use might reduce the risk of catheter gluing. With preliminary use in Europe, however, this material resulted in some catheters being retained in the cerebral vasculature after embolization. The inability to pull the catheter out after embolization may be due to a combination of vasospasm induced by the DSMO as well a mechanical hold that the material may have on the catheter as it refluxes from the catheter tip.

Particulate materials have also been used extensively in AVM embolization. These have included PVA, silk, embolization microspheres, and coils [116–120]. PVA has been used the most extensively of all the particulate materials. It has been shown to induce a foreign body reaction and promote angionecrosis [93]. It is generally mixed directly in a suspension of contrast material and has proven relatively easy to use. However, its use requires a guidewire-directed catheter rather than the potentially less traumatic flow-directed catheters used for liquid embolic treatment. In addition, and perhaps of the greatest concern, is that there is a high rate of true recanalization of shunt vessels observed after PVA occlusion [121,122]. Sorimachi et al. followed 36 patients embolized with PVA particles angiographically and found a 43% rate of AVM enlargement in the angiograms obtained more than 1 month after embolization [122]. In four of the five cases in their series with complete obliteration, nidi reappeared on follow-up angiograms. Some authors have suggested coil occlusion of the artery after PVA embolization to reduce recanalization [123]. Microspheres have also become available for particulate endovascular procedures [124]. They have been used to treat AVMs in the brain and spinal cord [119]. Because of their uniform size they reportedly clump less in the catheter and proximal vasculature.

TECHNIQUE FOR EMBOLIZATION

Patient Selection and Workup

Patients referred for endovascular AVM treatment are often candidates for some form of multimodal therapy. Patients who have small peripherally based AVMs may be considered for surgery alone. In general these are Spetzler-Martin grade I and II AVMs. Similarly, patients with small centrally located AVMs who are not considered good candidates for surgery may be treated with radiosurgery alone. The bulk of AVMs treated, however, qualify for multimodal therapy, such as embolization with surgery or radiosurgery. Occasionally all three modalities may be used to treat the larger AVM nidus.

All patients with AVMs at our institution are evaluated by a treatment planning team which includes a vascular neurosurgeon, an endovascular therapist, and a neurosurgeon guiding the radiosurgical treatment. Before therapy the patients have a comprehensive assessment which includes a history and neurologic examination. Prior imaging studies are evaluated. If these are not available, MRI is performed or, if there is a contraindication to MRI, CT scanning is done. These studies are evaluated for the size and precise location of the AVM nidus. They are also assessed for evidence of injury to the surrounding brain. This may include encephalomalacia or hemorrhage into the surrounding parenchyma. Many patients come with a complete angiogram for evaluation; however, if this is not available diagnostic angiographic studies are generally performed in advance of a final decision regarding the treatment plan.

The angiogram is evaluated for the location of the AVM as well as its size. Access to the AVM nidus via the arterial feeders is then assessed. The number of feeding arteries, the size of the feeders, and the access to the feeders are all evaluated. This assessment gives one an idea of how many pedicles may need to be individually catheterized for embolization and helps to determine in advance whether access to the AVM nidus will be difficult.

Evaluation of the arterial supply to the AVM nidus also includes a search throughout the intracranial vasculature for aneurysms. These may include saccular aneurysms on the vessels of the circle of Willis or at the more distal branch points of the intracranial vasculature. They may include intranidal aneurysms (aneurysms within the AVM nidus itself) or pseudoaneurysms. The importance of evaluating the angiogram for these various types of aneurysms was discussed in the angioarchitecture section of this chapter. Saccular aneurysms on the circle of Willis arteries or more distal arteries feeding the AVM are generally treated prior to the AVM embolization, due to the risk of aneurysmal rupture from catheter manipulation in the intracranial vasculature or alteration in the feeding artery pressure following embolization. These aneurysms may be treated using either a surgical or endovascular approach (Fig. 10-7). Pseudoaneurysms or intranidal aneurysms usually require endovascular attention in the early phases of embolization, again to reduce the risk of hemorrhage before further treatment (Fig. 10-8).

The venous system is assessed for the number of draining veins, the location of these draining veins, and the presence of venous occlusive disease. The number of draining veins may be important in deciding the hemorrhage risk of the patient and also is critical in understanding if there is an

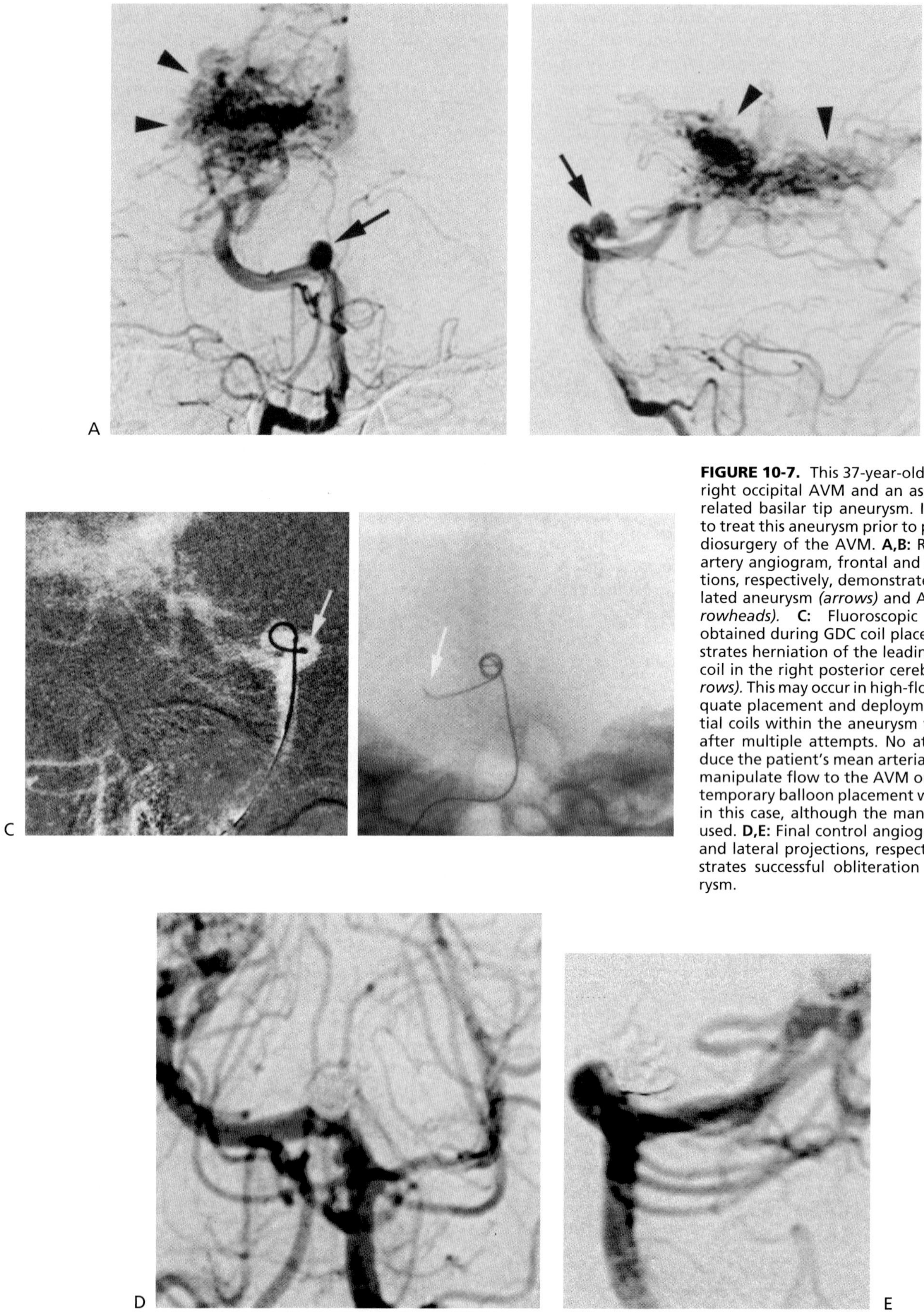

FIGURE 10-7. This 37-year-old woman had a right occipital AVM and an associated flow-related basilar tip aneurysm. It was decided to treat this aneurysm prior to performing radiosurgery of the AVM. **A,B:** Right vertebral artery angiogram, frontal and lateral projections, respectively, demonstrates the flow-related aneurysm *(arrows)* and AVM nidus *(arrowheads).* **C:** Fluoroscopic spot image obtained during GDC coil placement demonstrates herniation of the leading edge of the coil in the right posterior cerebral artery *(arrows).* This may occur in high-flow states. Adequate placement and deployment of the initial coils within the aneurysm was successful after multiple attempts. No attempts to reduce the patient's mean arterial pressure and manipulate flow to the AVM or occlude with temporary balloon placement was performed in this case, although the maneuvers can be used. **D,E:** Final control angiogram in frontal and lateral projections, respectively, demonstrates successful obliteration of the aneurysm.

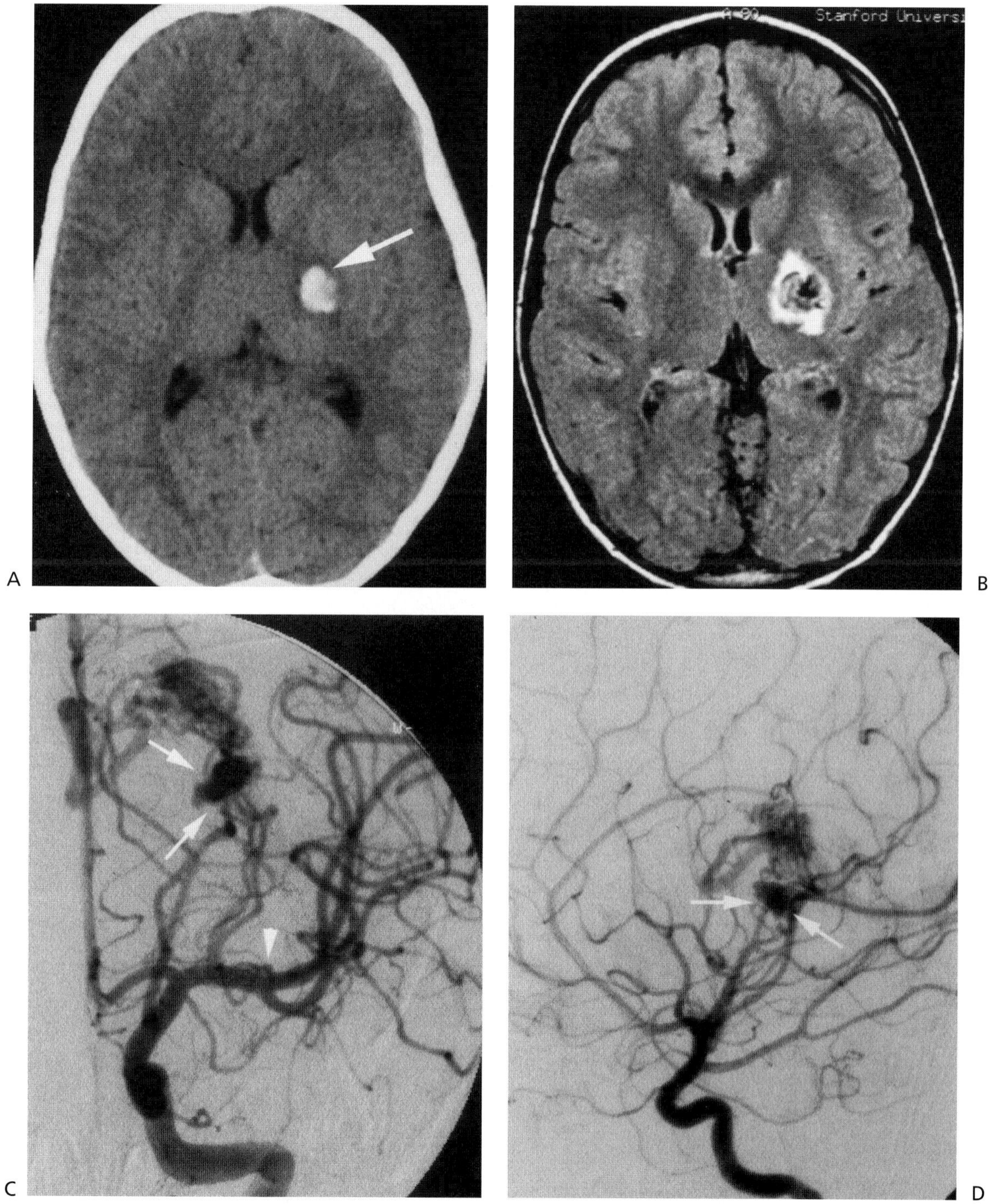

FIGURE 10-8. This 6-year-old girl developed an acute headache and became hemiparetic. **A:** CT scan done in the emergency room demonstrated a hemorrhage in the posterior limb of the left internal capsule *(arrow)*. **B:** Follow-up T1-weighted axial MRI demonstrates complex signal within the area of hematoma consistent with an AVM. A region of surrounding edema is noted. **C,D:** Left internal carotid artery angiogram, frontal and lateral projections, respectively, demonstrates a nidus in the left basal ganglia. An intranidal aneurysm was noted at the inferior margin of the nidus *(arrows)*. The nidus was supplied by a series of lenticulostriate arteries. The origin of the lenticulostriate artery supplying the intranidal aneurysm was seen to arise distally from the middle cerebral artery *(arrowhead)*. *(Figure continues.)*

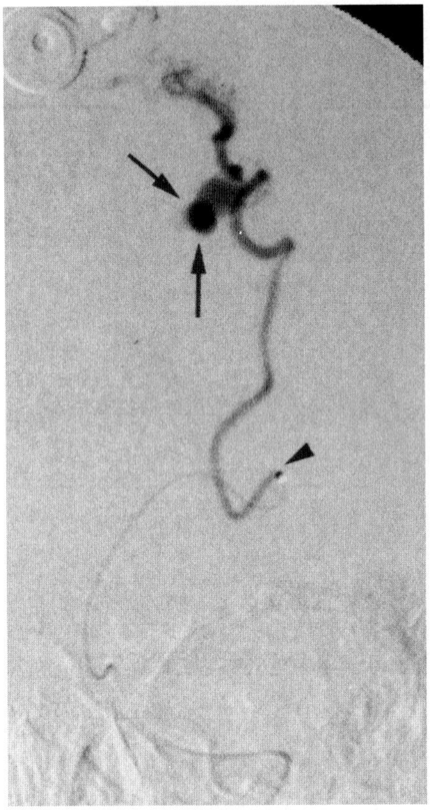

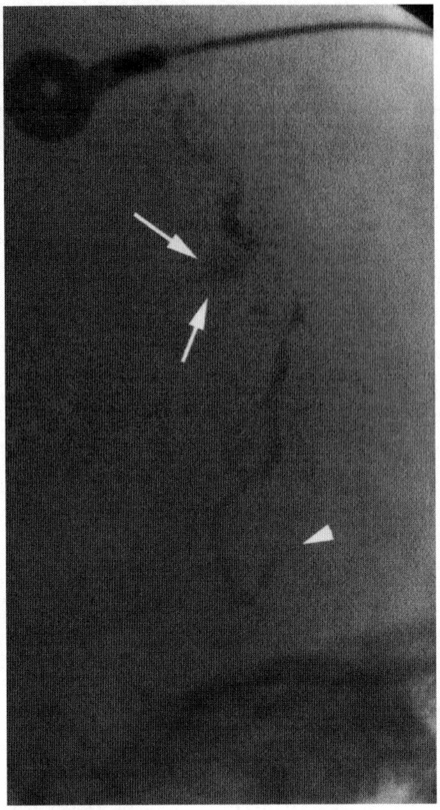

E,F

FIGURE 10-8. *Continued.* **E:** Superselective microcatheter angiogram in the lateral lenticulostriate artery supplying the AVM nidus and aneurysm *(arrows).* The catheter tip *(arrowhead)* sits beyond the origin of the lateral lenticulostriate artery. A dilute cyanoacrylate mixture was used to embolize this lenticulostriate branch (after electrophysiologic testing) in order to thrombose the aneurysm and embolize a portion of the AVM nidus. **F:** Glue cast demonstrating filling of the aneurysm *(arrows),* with the glue extending from where the microcatheter tip had been *(arrowhead).* **G,H:** Left internal carotid artery angiogram, anterior and lateral views, respectively, after embolization. This demonstrates continued filling of the nidus from other lenticulostriate branches with thrombosis of the intranidal aneurysm. The patient was sent for radiosurgery, having had this portion of the AVM nidus eliminated.

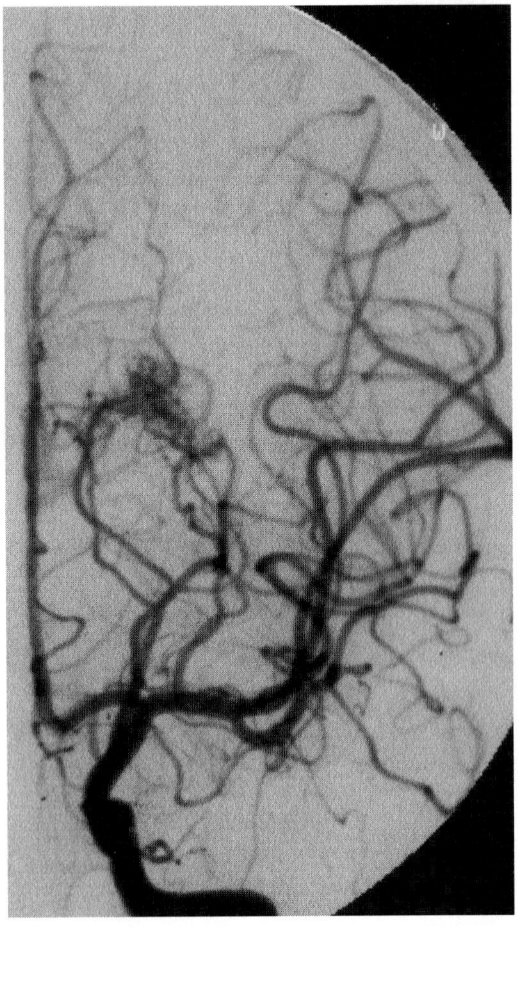

G

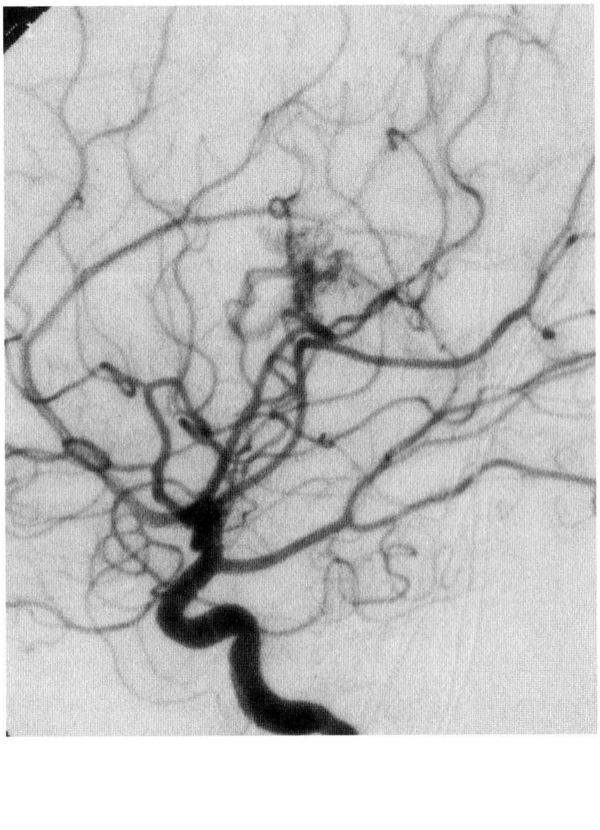

H

additional hemorrhage risk from a therapy such as endovascular treatment. A patient with a single draining vein presents a greater risk for venous occlusion during endovascular treatment that may lead to hemorrhage. In the treatment algorithm it is important to determine whether the location of the venous drainage is central, peripheral, or mixed. Those patients with central venous drainage have been shown to be at a higher risk for hemorrhage and at higher risk for complications from an intervention such as surgery. Finally, venous occlusive disease has also been linked to a greater risk of hemorrhage, and areas of critical stenosis in the venous system may represent an increased risk with the use of embolic material passing into them.

Embolization Procedure

All AVM endovascular procedures are currently performed in a biplane angiography suite. The patients are awake during the procedure in most cases, because this allows us to perform clinical physiologic testing prior to the AVM embolization. Exceptions to this rule include patients who are unable to lie still and children undergoing AVM embolization. Once any needed diagnostic angiograms are obtained, a coaxial system is used to introduce a microcatheter into the intracranial circulation. Embolization procedures are performed through a 5- or 6-French guide catheter because the newer, smaller diameter guide catheters have been made thin walled, allowing for ready introduction of the microcatheter and continued roadmapping through the guide catheter. The guide catheter receives a continuous flush with heparinized saline in a pressure bag. Guide catheters are kept extracranial in both the carotid and vertebral systems and generally placed at the C1-2 level. Once the guide catheter has been placed, a biplane roadmap is obtained and a specific arterial pedicle is selected for microcatheterization and subsequently embolization. The microcatheter is introduced into the guide catheter through a Y connector. Most of our embolization procedures are with liquid embolic material (NBCA) and a 1.5- or 1.8-French flow-directed catheter is therefore used in most cases to superselectively catheterize the intracranial circulation. At the time of introduction of the microcatheter, patients are systemically heparinized using 5,000 units heparin intravenously in a bolus, followed by 1,000-unit/hr boluses during the procedure. Protamine sulfate is kept in the room should there be any ensuing hemorrhagic complications so that the heparin can be reversed immediately.

If an intranidal or pseudoaneurysm is present, the pedicle supplying that portion of the AVM which contains the aneurysm generally is selected first. Larger pedicles are also treated earlier. With subsequent embolization procedures (using staging), when the flow in smaller pedicles has increased somewhat, these pedicles are then selected. Most commonly, the microcatheter is steamed into a hockey stick shape, with a distal tip of about 3 to 5 mm. This shape is used routinely for many of the pedicles arising from the middle cerebral artery circulation and vertebrobasilar circulation. In some cases, when a smaller arterial pedicle is designated for catheterization, the shape may be modified to include more or less bend in the distal tip. In addition, when the anterior cerebral artery circulation is slated for selective catheterization, an exaggerated C or U shape is often used to help the catheter flow into the A1 segment of the anterior cerebral artery. Without this shape the catheter often selects the middle cerebral artery from the superclinoid carotid artery.

The flow-directed catheter often can be guided into a specific intracranial branch by using a series of pulsed injections which help to retropulse the catheter and slip it into a desired branch. Recently, with the development of more easily torqued small-diameter wire, an 0.008- or 0.010-inch wire can be used to selectively catheterize some intracranial branches and help guide the microcatheter more precisely. We do not routinely use a guidewire, however, and prefer to use only flow direction if possible. The flow-directed catheter is initially introduced with a stiffening mandrel, which is gradually removed. The mandrel removal is started before the microcatheter leaves the end of the guide catheter. A guidewire is introduced only if we are unable to select a desired branch with repeated tries. We feel there is an added risk of perforation with introduction of the guidewire, particularly in the more distal portions of the intracranial circulation.

The microcatheter is placed at the margin of the nidus so that embolization of the vessels making up the actual fistulous communication can be achieved. Proximal positioning may lead to a higher risk of ischemic injury with the embolization, because supply to the capillary bed of the normal surrounding brain may be interrupted. When embolizing a high-flow fistula within the nidus, it is possible to pass the microcatheter directly on to the venous side of the arteriovenous fistula. In these cases one must be careful to maintain an adequate distance on the arterial side of the fistula to allow for complete embolization of the fistula without overly extensive embolization of the venous components of the nidus. When it is decided that adequate microcatheter position has been achieved, a selective digital subtraction angiogram is done through the microcatheter to evaluate the angioarchitecture of the nidus. At this time the flow characteristics through the shunt vessels are also evaluated. When performing this angiogram it is important to look for vessels which supply normal surrounding brain, because in most cases embolization of angiographically visible normal vessels is not desirable. Although wedging of the catheter is often considered advantageous, we have found that this often may not be achievable. Either the arterial vasculature is too dilated or the catheter position which allows for wedging results in embolization of only a minor portion of the nidus. Therefore, we often choose to embolize from a nonwedged position.

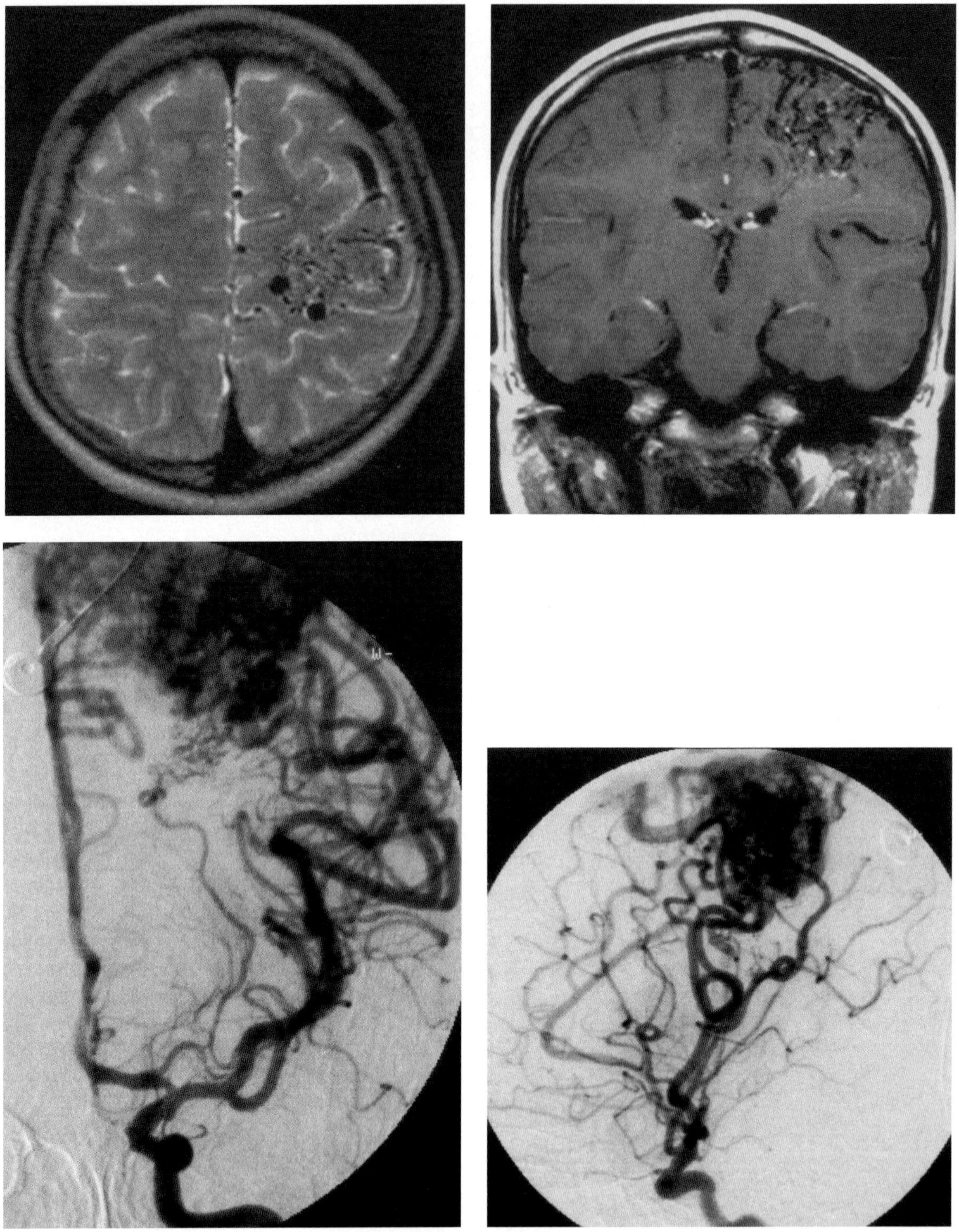

FIGURE 10-9. This 12-year-old girl experienced gradual-onset right hemiparesis and headache. She did not undergo embolization because of repeated positive somatosensory evoked potentials with amobarbital testing, despite numerous attempts to reposition the catheter in multiple feeding arteries. Despite this, the patient underwent Bragg-peak radiosurgery with significant nidal obliteration and no change in symptoms. **A,B:** Axial **(A)** T2- and coronal **(B)** T1-weighted MRIs demonstrate the patient's left frontal parietal AVM. **C,D:** Left internal carotid artery angiograms demonstrate the AVM with supply from both the anterior and middle cerebral artery circulations. *(Figure continues.)*

Once a superselective angiogram has been performed and we have confirmed that we are in a location to embolize the AVM nidus, the patient then undergoes superselective sodium amobarbital testing to determine if there are any electrophysiologic changes or changes in the clinical neurologic examination. We use 40 to 50 mg per pedicle. An independent neurologist does this testing. Neurophysiologic monitoring may include somatosensory evoked potentials, electroencephalogram and, in the posterior circulation, brainstem auditory evoked potentials [125]. This technique provides added information that may not be available from inspection of the superselective angiogram alone (Fig. 10-9) [126–128]. Some workers have abandoned clinical physiologic testing, citing as the most important reason that they wish to perform embolization exclusively in the anesthetized patient [129]. They feel general anesthesia eliminates problematic patient motion. We have not found that general anesthesia is necessary in our patients to reduce patient motion, and most of our patients are effectively treated with neuroleptics. There currently is no evidence that general anesthesia or intravenous sedation is safer, and this remains a matter of preference [130]. We also use physiologic monitoring with amobarbital testing (without corroborative physical examination) in a patient who requires general anesthesia, such as a child [131,132].

Once a decision has been made to perform an embolization based on the data obtained from the superselective angiogram and the physiologic testing, the embolic material is prepared. We usually use NBCA. This is mixed with lipiodol, and typical solutions range from 2:1 to 4:1 (lipiodol to NBCA). Generally enough solution is mixed to create a volume of 2 to 3 ml. The lipiodol is used to create radiopacity, and by varying the ratio one is able to slow polymerization time with increasing volumes of lipiodol. In general, a higher-flow AVM is treated with ratios of 2:1 to 3:1, while a slower-flow AVM is treated with ratios of 3:1 to 4:1. We have found that these more dilute solutions of glue allow for better nidal penetration. Concerns about overemboliza-

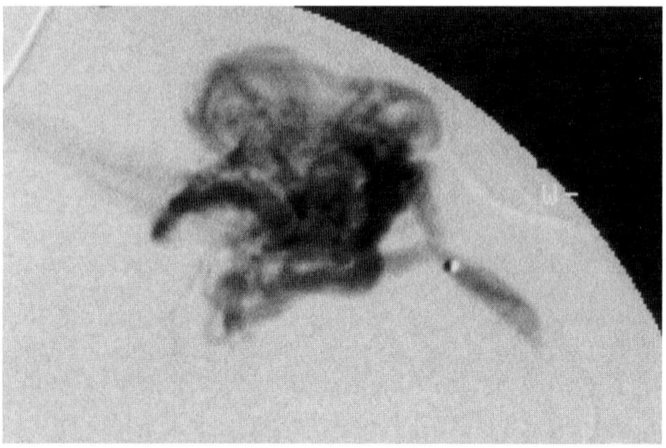

E

FIGURE 10-9. *Continued.* **E:** Superselective angiogram in one of the middle cerebral opercular feeders shows the microcatheter placed adjacent to the AVM nidus. Despite excellent placement in multiple feeding vessels, testing in this rolandic cortex AVM always showed positive results. **F:** Example of the positive results of the amobarbital test with somatosensory evoked potential monitoring (upper extremity). Note the initial amplitudes of the waveforms in the right extremities on the baseline study. These progressively flattened out 2 and 4.5 minutes after amobarbital administration. They returned to baseline amplitude height 10 minutes after amobarbital was given. *(Figure continues.)*

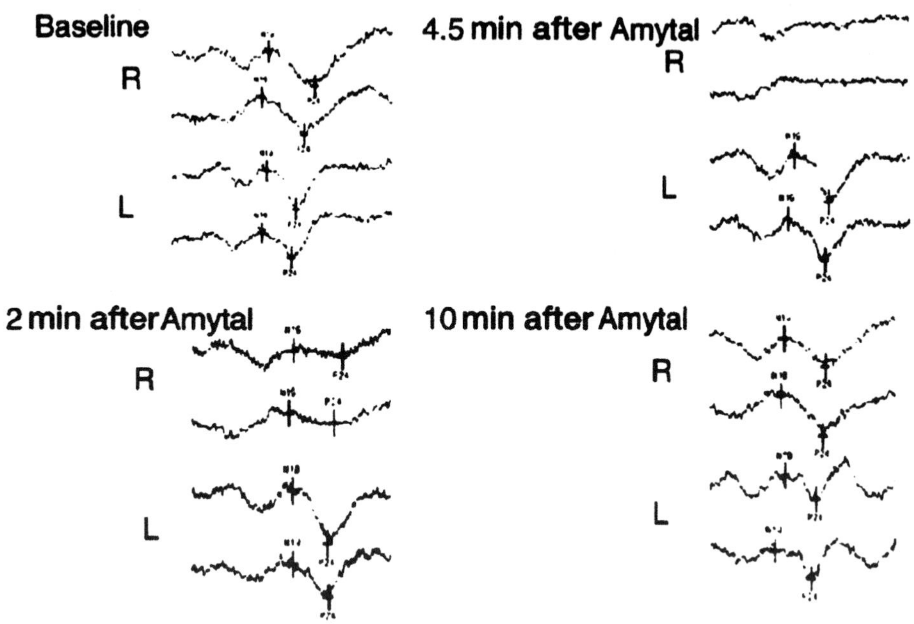

F

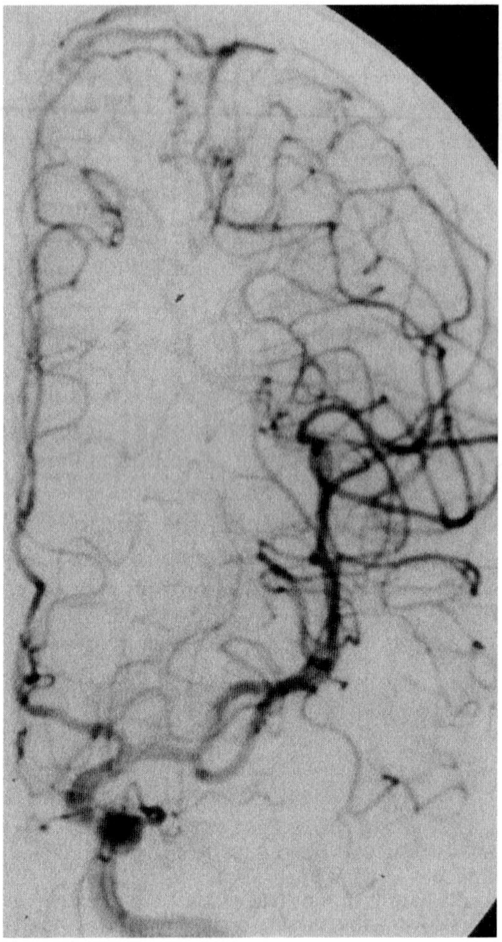

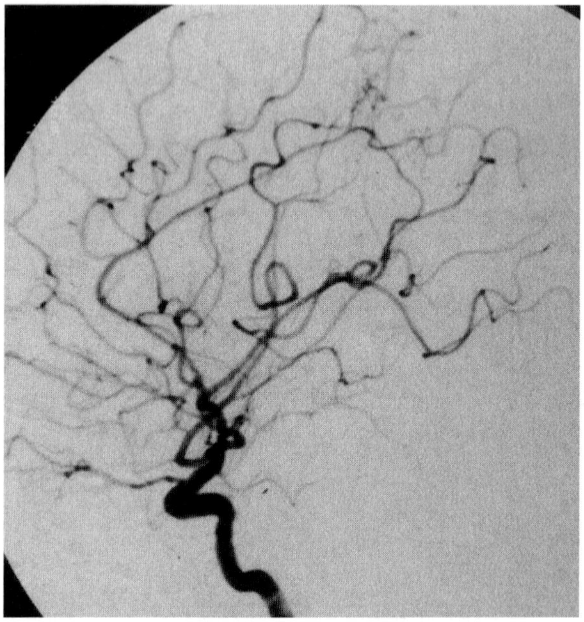

FIGURE 10-9. *Continued.* **G,H:** Left internal carotid artery angiogram, anterior and lateral views, respectively, from an outside institution 3 years after radiosurgery. This angiogram demonstrates extensive nidal obliteration. The small residual region of hypervascularity and early shunting will require repeat radiosurgical treatment. (**A, C,** and **F** from Paulsen RD, Steinberg GK, Norbash AM, et al. Embolization of rolandic cortex AVMs. *Neurosurgery* 1999;44:479–484, with permission.)

tion of material causing deposition on the venous side with more dilute solutions can be corrected by slowing the injection rate markedly to allow for polymerization to occur more proximally. If the fistulous communication is large and has very high flow, ratios as low as 0.5:1 to 1:1 may be used. On rare occasions, only a small amount of lipiodol is mixed so that almost-pure amounts of NBCA are injected directly. When this is desired, a slurry of lipiodol and tantalum powder is usually used to achieve radiopacity, because the small amounts of lipiodol added do not create adequate radiodensity. We have, however, stopped using tantalum in most cases, because we have found that the radiopacity of the lipiodol-NBCA mixture is adequate and the tantalum powder may clump and create occlusion in the microcatheter, inhibiting the embolization. Some authors have also suggested using hypotension when the shunt has very high flow, to improve glue deposition directly into the fistula [133].

All preparation of the NBCA for embolization is carried out at a separate table. The microcatheter is prepared by flushing it several times slowly with a 3-ml syringe filled with 5% dextrose solution. The proximal end of the catheter is washed with dextrose as well, and a towel is placed below the catheter to provide a clean working surface. With the catheter filled with dextrose, glue is then introduced with a 3-ml syringe. The glue is slowly injected in a full column, clearing first the dextrose within the catheter and then entering the circulation. Roadmapping is used so that the glue can be clearly visualized. A projection is chosen that allows one to readily see the length of the distal catheter to ensure that there is not significant reflux of glue during the injection. The goal of the embolization is to fill the vessels of the nidus up to the area of the draining vein. When glue passes through the nidus and is observed to begin to fill the drain vein the embolization is stopped. The embolization is done by two physicians. The physician injecting embolic material indicates that the catheter should be pulled. The catheter is immediately pulled from the circulation through the guide catheter by a second physician. Many practitioners withdraw on the syringe to create negative pressure, because they feel that this may prevent embolization of glue that could be adherent to the distal tip of the microcatheter. Usually two to four pedicles are embolized per session. We do not seek to achieve complete nidus embolization in one session and often stage embolization sessions approximately

1 week or more apart. This is thought to reduce the risk of venous stasis and normal pressure breakthrough bleeding. Larger AVMs may require as many as three to five staged embolization sessions.

At the conclusion of the embolization procedure, heparin is reversed with protamine sulfate. Usually vasodilators such as sodium nitroprusside or esmolol hydrochloride are administered to maintain the mean arterial pressure in the range of 65 to 75 mm Hg. This is done for the first 24 hours after a procedure when the risk of hemorrhagic complication is felt to be the highest. Patients are also treated postprocedure with steroids, and at discharge they are placed on a 1-week tapering dose. This is done to minimize edema that may ensue following the inflammatory response seen

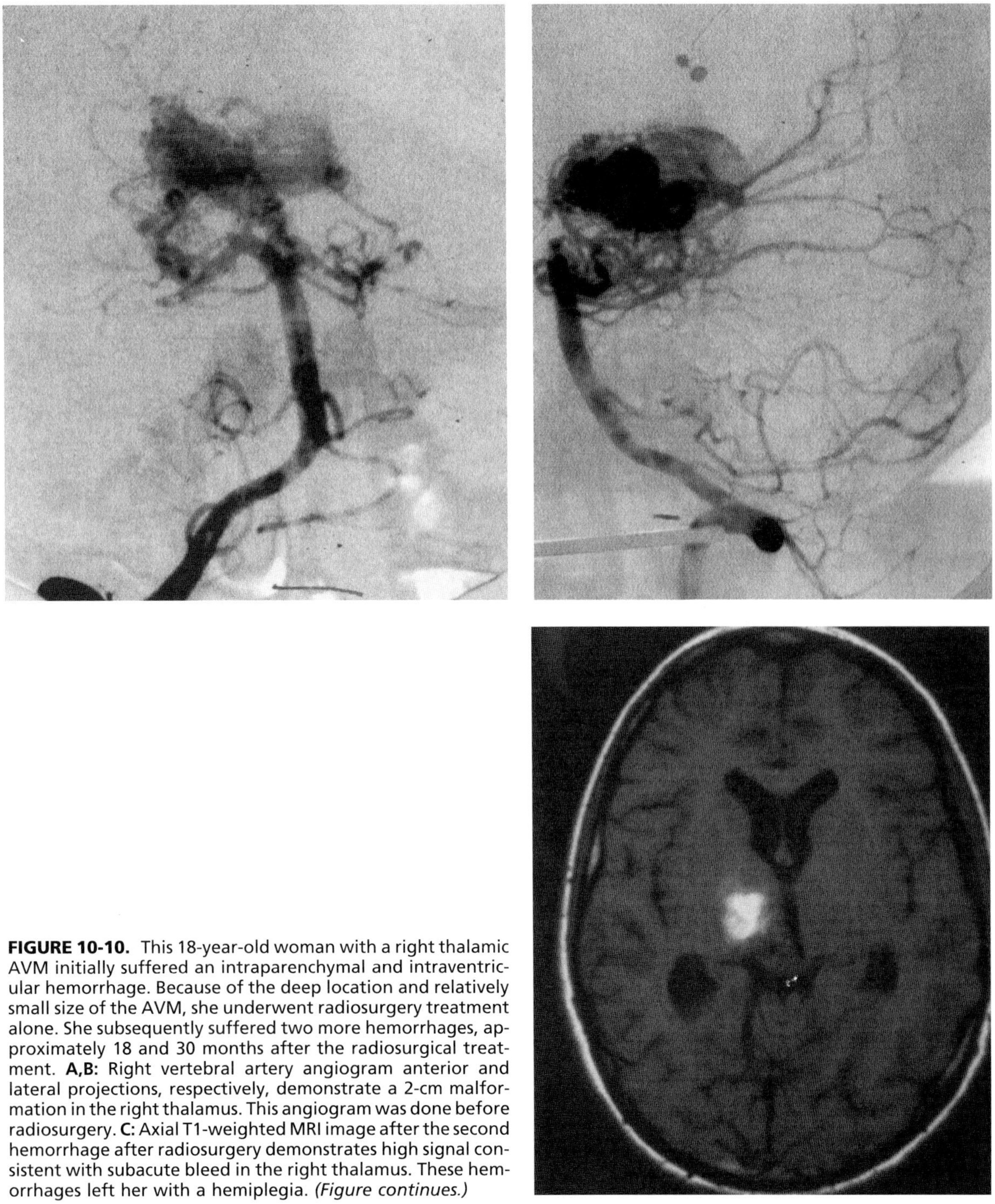

A B C

FIGURE 10-10. This 18-year-old woman with a right thalamic AVM initially suffered an intraparenchymal and intraventricular hemorrhage. Because of the deep location and relatively small size of the AVM, she underwent radiosurgery treatment alone. She subsequently suffered two more hemorrhages, approximately 18 and 30 months after the radiosurgical treatment. **A,B:** Right vertebral artery angiogram anterior and lateral projections, respectively, demonstrate a 2-cm malformation in the right thalamus. This angiogram was done before radiosurgery. **C:** Axial T1-weighted MRI image after the second hemorrhage after radiosurgery demonstrates high signal consistent with subacute bleed in the right thalamus. These hemorrhages left her with a hemiplegia. *(Figure continues.)*

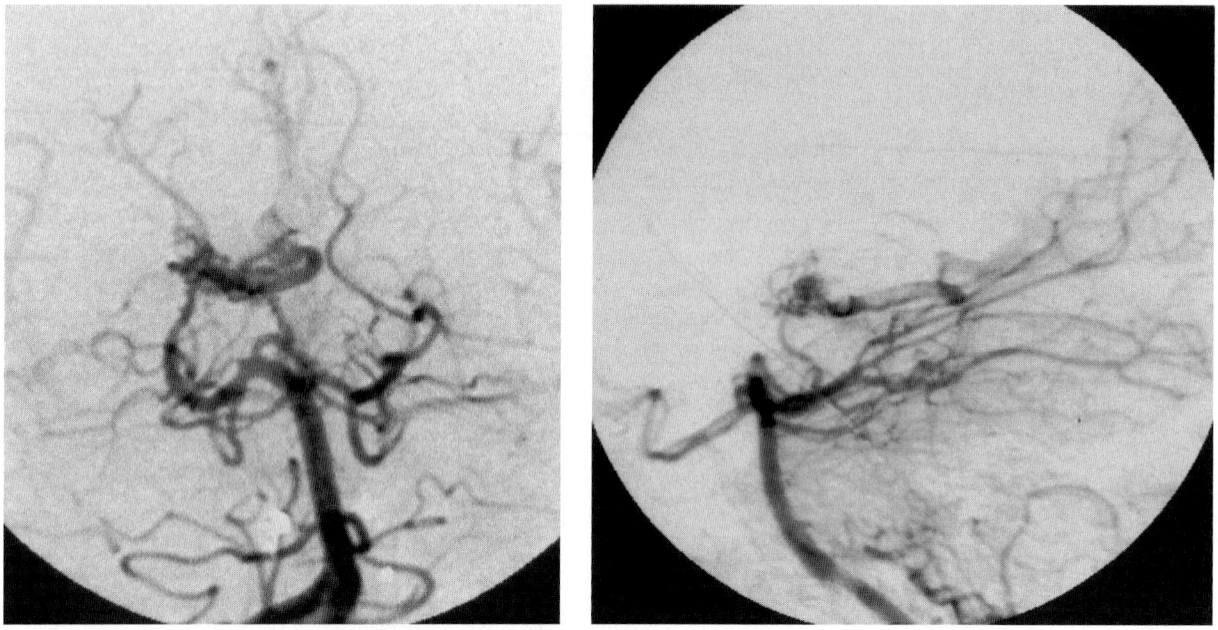

D E

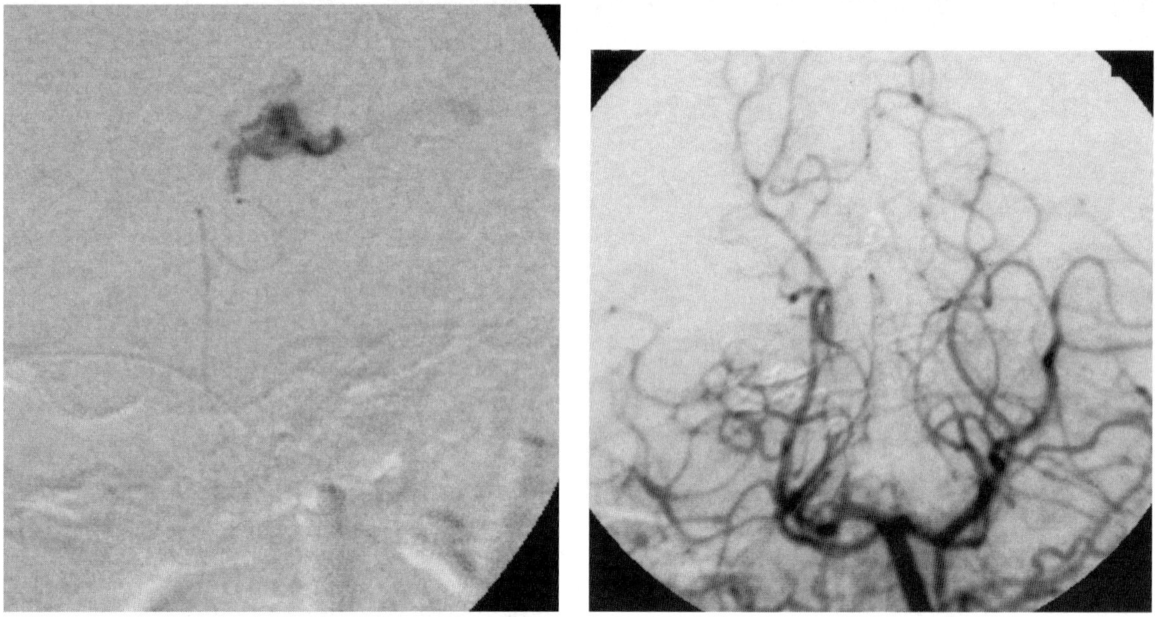

F G

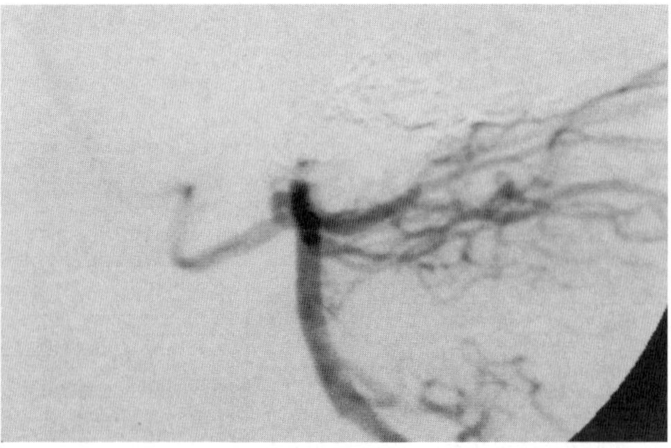

H

FIGURE 10-10. *Continued.* **D,E:** Right vertebral angiogram anterior and lateral projections, respectively. This angiogram was performed approximately 3 years after the first radiosurgical treatment. It demonstrates significant residual AVM supplied by thalamoperforating arteries. The patient underwent two staged embolization procedures cannulating four separate perforating branches that supplied the AVM. **F:** Superselective angiogram lateral projection with the microcatheter placed in a thalamoperforater. This demonstrates filling of the distal portion of the thalamoperforater with adequate purchase to prevent reflux into the posterior cerebral artery. Compare this with the lateral angiogram **(E)**. **G,H:** Right vertebral angiogram, anterior and lateral projections, respectively, demonstrates complete obliteration of the AVM nidus with no evidence of venous shunting. The patient was followed with angiography about 24 months after this, which showed continued obliteration.

with intravascular NBCA and occlusion of blood flow to portions of the AVM nidus.

Complications

Any of the complications seen with cerebral angiography can occur during the angiographic evaluation of the patient undergoing endovascular therapy. The most serious (and frequent) complications of endovascular therapy, however, occur as a direct result of the embolization procedure. These complications can be grouped into two general categories, those that are ischemic and those that are hemorrhagic.

In general, ischemic complications are the direct result of thromboembolic occlusion from embolic material in vessels supplying the normal capillary bed of the brain. This may result from embolization of normal capillary beds distal to the catheter or may occur from reflux of embolic material proximally down the catheter shaft and into normal vasculature. The complication of unappreciated embolization distal to the catheter can be minimized by proper attention to the preembolization superselective angiogram and physiologic testing. Reflux down the catheter should generally be minimized by the endovascular therapist. In addition, it is incumbent upon the person injecting embolic material to be aware of any branches proximal to the catheter tip and the distance that embolic material would have to reflux to enter those branches. Clearly, one should avoid allowing embolic material to reflux into those branches which have not been as carefully evaluated by superselective angiography or physiologic testing, because the risk of occlusion of these branches is unknown. Some branch points may clearly lead to normal vasculature. This is true, for instance, when embolizing in a dilated perforating artery from major branches of the circle of Willis, where reflux leads directly into a large artery of the circle. Here it is incumbent upon the operator to ensure that there is adequate purchase in the perforating artery being embolized, so that reflux is not likely to result in passage of embolic material into the larger parent artery (Fig. 10-10).

Hemorrhagic complications may occur as a result of rupture within a portion of the AVM nidus after embolization or perforation in the feeding arteries supplying the AVM. The risk of hemorrhage due to vessel perforation has been reduced significantly with the introduction of flow-directed catheters. Previously, guidewire-directed catheter perforation was more commonly reported [134,135]. The use of small 0.008- and 0.010-inch guidewires in the usually flow-directed catheters may still result in arterial perforation. For this reason we tend to minimize their use. In general, perforations of this sort result in subarachnoid hemorrhage, and in the awake patient this can be more acutely recognized. The perforation is confirmed by evidence of contrast extravasation. Some authors have recommended introducing coils across the perforation site to assist with halting bleeding [134]. In general, we have found that reversing the heparin immediately and allowing the spasm induced by the trauma and normal clotting function to act results in a rapid cessation of bleeding.

Hemorrhage from the AVM nidus itself may result from compromise to venous outflow; however, the etiology of the hemorrhage is not always discernible. Other possible sites for hemorrhage, such as intranidal aneurysms and pseudoaneurysms, should be addressed early in the embolization process. Care should be exercised during the embolization to avoid causing venous occlusion. This is particularly true when a single draining vein is observed to exit the nidus (Fig. 10-11).

How frequent are serious complications from AVM embolizations? Frizzel and Fisher performed an analysis in 1995 reviewing morbidity and mortality rates for AVM em-

A
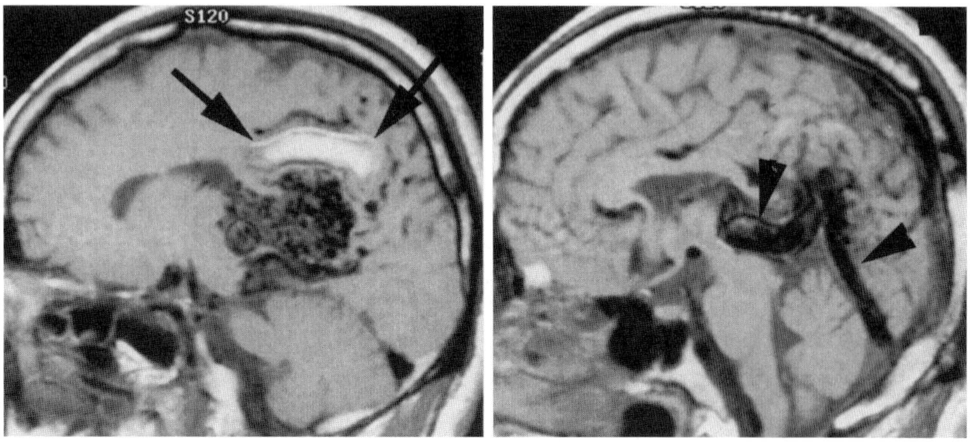

FIGURE 10-11. This 40-year-old man developed an intraparenchymal hemorrhage. Workup demonstrated a left hemispheric paramedian AVM. **A:** Left of midline *(left)* and midline *(right)* sagittal T1-weighted MRIs depict the AVM nidus with an overlying intraparenchymal hemorrhage. The bleed is hyperintense consistent with methemoglobin *(arrows).* Enlarged flow void consistent with dilated draining galenic venous system is demonstrated *(arrowheads). (Figure continues.)*

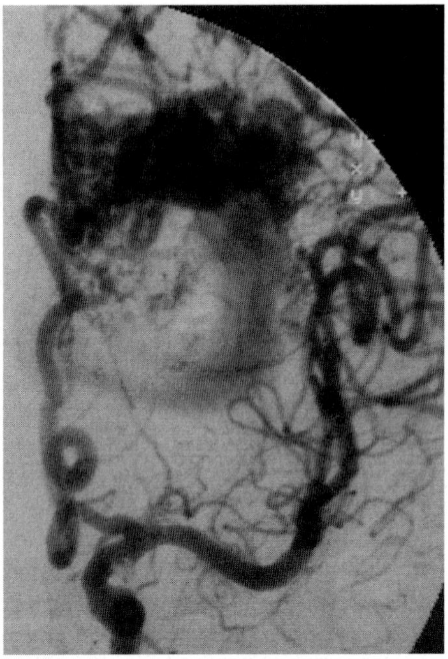

B

FIGURE 10-11. **B–D:** Left internal carotid artery angiogram in anterior **(B)** and lateral **(C,D)** projections confirms the findings noted at cross-sectional imaging. **D:** A magnified view in the early venous phase. The dominant venous egress is via the enlarged vein of Galen and straight sinus *(arrowheads).* **E:** Unsubtracted image from a left ICA injection after the patient's second staged transarterial embolization with NBCA demonstrates radiopaque cyanoacrylate within the AVM nidus *(arrows)* as well as within the straight sinus *(arrowheads).*

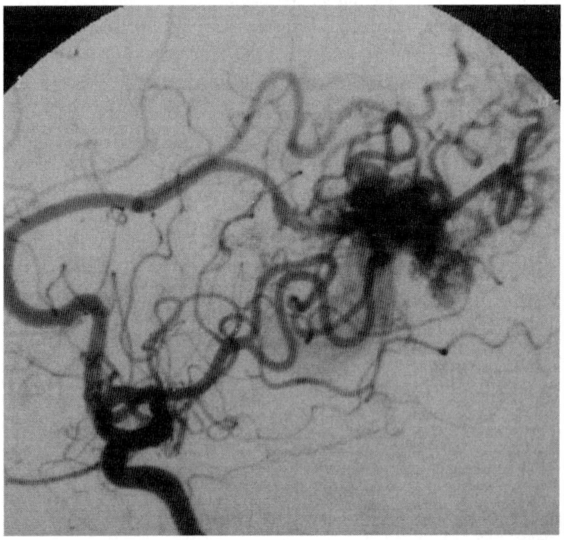

C

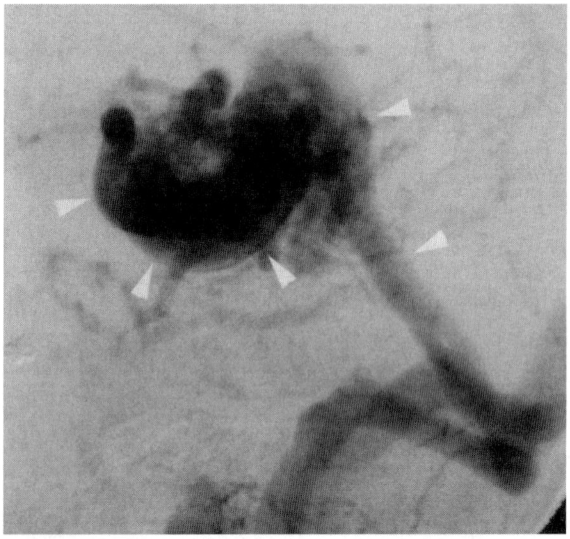

D

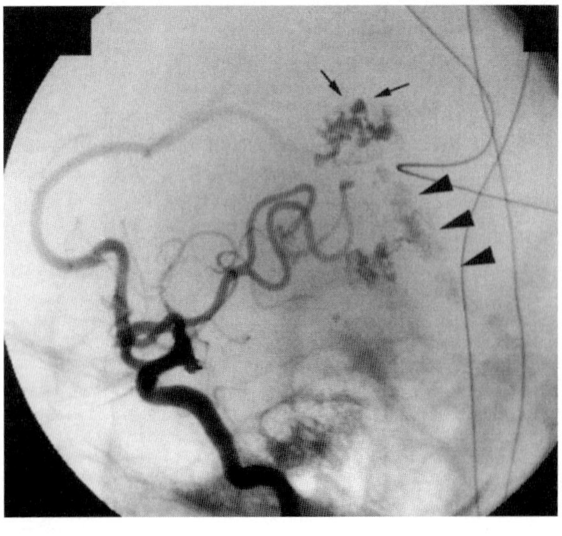

E

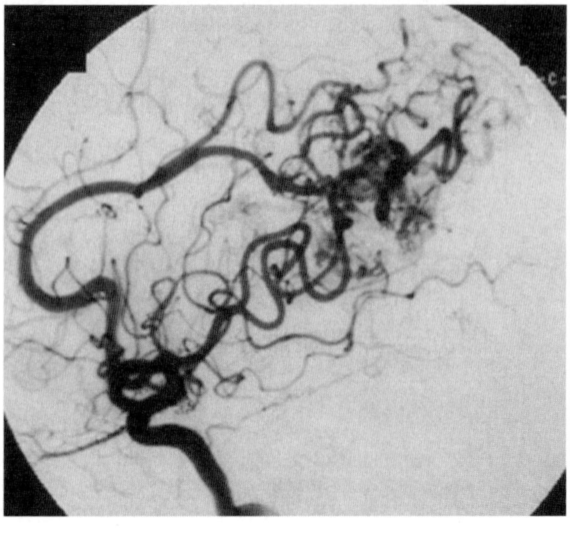

F

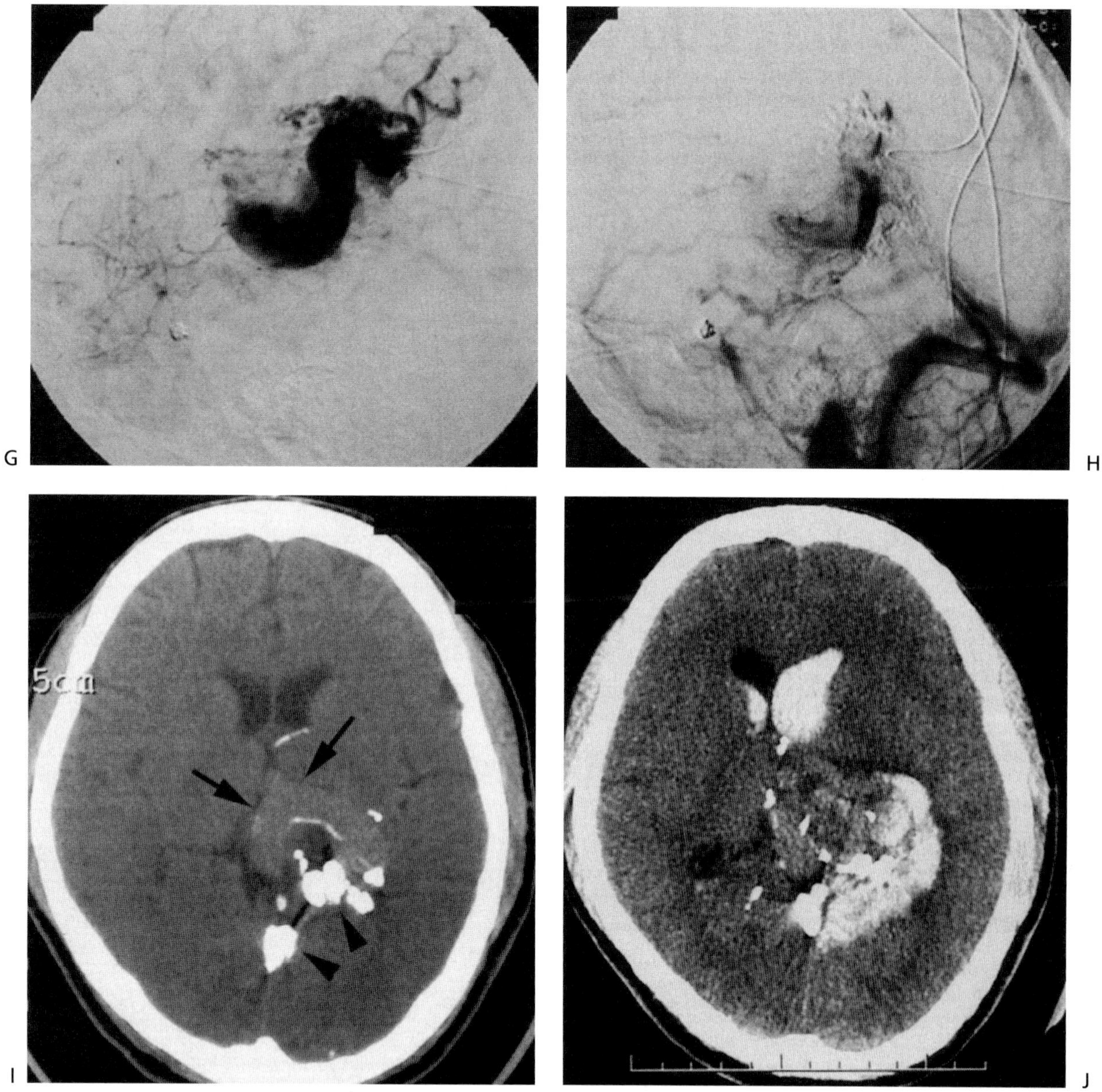

FIGURE 10-11. *Continued.* **F–H:** Left internal carotid angiogram, lateral projection, in the arterial **(F)** and venous phases **(G,H)** demonstrates obliteration of a significant portion of the AVM nidus. However, there is significantly delayed venous flow due to presence of NBCA within the vein of Galen and straight sinus. **I:** After the procedure, the patient was admitted to the intensive care unit, where his mean arterial pressure was controlled pharmacologically for 48 hours. The patient remained asymptomatic throughout this time. Noncontrast axial CT images through the level of the straight sinus demonstrate the enlarged draining vein *(arrows)* as well as embolization material within the distal portion of the vein and the straight sinus *(arrowheads).* This CT scan was performed after the procedure as per routine post–AVM embolization protocol Apparent hypodensity within the occipital lobes, particularly the left, is due to beam hardening artifact. **J:** Axial CT noncontrast image 72 hours after embolization, when the patient suddenly lost consciousness, demonstrates intraparenchymal and intraventricular hemorrhage with significant left-to-right midline shift. The patient eventually expired secondary to complications from this intracranial hemorrhage.

bolization reported in the literature during the preceding 35 years [136]. This analysis reported the results of embolization in 1,264 patients. Overall there was a permanent morbidity rate of 8% and temporary morbidity rate of 10% in this series. A mortality rate was 1% for the entire series and 2.1% for those AVMs that underwent embolization before 1990. Similar results have been seen with a larger series of patients reported since 1995 [63,79,132,137,138].

REFERENCES

1. Mast H, Mohr JP, et al. "Steal" is an unestablished mechanism for the clinical presentation of cerebral arteriovenous malformation. *Stroke* 1995;26:1215–1220.
2. Ondra SL, Troupp H, George ED, et al. The natural history of symptomatic arteriovenous malformations of the brain: a 24-year follow-up assessment. *J Neurosurg* 1990;73:387–392.
3. Crawford PM, West CR, Chadwick DW, et al. Arteriovenous malformations of the brain: natural history in unoperated patients. *J Neurol Neurosurg Psychiatry* 1986;49:1–10.
4. Wilkins RH. Natural history of intracranial vascular malformations: a review. *Neurosurgery* 1985;16:421–430.
5. Marks MP, Bracci P, Steinberg GK. Natural history of cerebral AVMs correlated with angiographic risk factors of hemorrhage. Paper presented at: American Society of Neuroradiology 31st Annual Meeting; May 16–20, 1993; Vancouver, BC, Canada.
6. Pollock BE, Flickinger JC, Lunsford LD, et al. Factors that predict the bleeding risk of cerebral arteriovenous malformations. *Stroke* 1996;27:1–6.
7. Mast H, Young WL, Koennecke HC, et al. Risk of spontaneous haemorrhage after diagnosis of cerebral arteriovenous malformation. *Lancet* 1997;350:1065–1068.
8. Albert P, Salgado H, Polaina M, et al. A study on the venous drainage of 150 cerebral arteriovenous malformations as related to hemorrhagic risks and size of the lesion. *Acta Neurochir (Wien)* 1990;103:30.
9. Marks MP, Lane B, Steinberg G, et al. Hemorrhage in intracerebral AVMs: angiographic determinants. *Radiology* 1990;176: 807–813.
10. Nataf F, Meder JF, Roux FX, et al. Angioarchitecture associated with haemorrhage in cerebral arteriovenous malformations: a prognostic statistical model. *Neuroradiology* 1997;39:52–58.
11. Miyasaka Y, Yada K, Ohwada T, et al. An analysis of the venous drainage system as a factor in hemorrhage from arteriovenous malformations. *J Neurosurg* 1992;76:239–243.
12. Anderson RM, Blackwood W. The association of arteriovenous angioma and saccular aneurysm of the arteries of the brain. *J Pathol Bacteriol* 1959;77:101–110.
13. Batjer H, Suss RA, Samson D. Intracranial arteriovenous malformations associated with aneurysms. *Neurosurgery* 1986;18: 29–35.
14. Boyd-Wilson JS. The association of cerebral angiomas with intracranial aneurysms. *J Neurol Neurosurg Psychiatry* 1966;22: 218–223.
15. Brown RD, Wiebers DO, Forbes GS. Unruptured intracranial aneurysms and arteriovenous malformations: frequency of intracranial hemorrhage and relationship of lesions. *J Neurosurg* 1990;73:859–863.
16. Deruty R, Mottolese C, Soustiel J, et al. Association of cerebral arteriovenous malformation and cerebral aneurysm: diagnosis and management. *Acta Neurochir (Wien)* 1990;107:133–139.
17. Kondziolka D, Nixon BL, Lasjaunias P, et al. Cerebral arteriovenous malformations with associated arterial aneurysms: hemodynamic and therapeutic considerations. *Can J Neurol Sci* 1988; 15:130–134.
18. Lasjaunias P, Piske R, TerBrugge K, et al. Cerebral arteriovenous malformations (CAVM) and associated arterial aneurysms (AA): analysis of 101 CAVM cases with 37 AA in 23 patients. *Acta Neurochir (Wien)* 1988;91:29–36.
19. Locksley HB. Report on the cooperative study of intracranial aneurysms and subarachnoid hemorrhage. Section V, part 1. Natural history of subarachnoid hemorrhages, intracranial aneurysms and arteriovenous malformations—based on 6,368 cases in the cooperative study. *J Neurosurg* 1966;25:219–222.
20. Miyasaka K, Wolpert SM, Prager RJ. The association of cerebral aneurysms, infundibula and intracranial arteriovenous malformations. *Stroke* 1982;13:196–203.
21. Patterson JH, McKissock WA. A clinical survey of intracranial angiomas with special reference to their mode of progression and surgical treatment: a report of 110 cases. *Brain* 1956;79: 233–266.
22. Suzuki J, Onuma T. Intracranial aneurysms associated with arteriovenous malformations. *J Neurosurg* 1979;50:742–746.
23. Turjman F, Massoud T, Viñuela F, et al. Aneurysms related to cerebral arteriovenous malformations: superselective angiographic assessment in 58 patients. *AJNR Am J Neuroradiol* 1994; 15:1601–1605.
24. Thompson RC, Steinberg GK, Levy RP, et al. The management of patients with arteriovenous malformations and associated intracranial aneurysms. *Neurosurgery* 1998;43:202–211.
25. Okamoto S, Handa H, Hashimoto H. Location of intracranial aneurysms associated with cerebral arteriovenous malformation: statistical analysis. *Surg Neurol* 1984;22:335–340.
26. Perret G, Nishioka H. Report of the cooperative study of intracranial aneurysms and subarachnoid hemorrhage. Section VI. Arteriovenous malformations: an analysis of 545 cases of cranioocerebral arteriovenous malformations and fistulae reported to the cooperative study. *J Neurosurg* 1966;25:467–490.
27. Marks MP, Lane B, Steinberg GK, et al. Intranidal aneurysms in cerebral arteriovenous malformations evaluation and endovascular treatment. *Radiology* 1992;183:355–360.
28. Willinsky R, Lasjaunias P, TerBrugge K, et al. Brain arteriovenous malformations. Analysis of the angio-architecture in relationship to hemorrhage. *J Neuroradiol* 1988;15:225–237.
29. Garcia-Monaco R, Rodesch G, Alvarez H, et al. Pseudoaneurysms within ruptured intracranial arteriovenous malformations: diagnosis and early endovascular management. *AJNR Am J Neuroradiol* 1993;14:315–321.
30. Luessenhop AJ, Rosa L. Cerebral arteriovenous malformations. Indications for the results of surgery, and the role of intravascular techniques. *J Neurosurg* 1984;60:14–22.
31. Pelletieri L, Carlsson CA, Grevsten SS, et al. Surgical versus conservative treatment of intracranial arteriovenous malformations: a study in surgical decision making. *Acta Neurochir (Wien)* 1979[Suppl]29:1–86.
32. Shi Y, Chen X. A proposed scheme for grading intracranial AVMs. *J Neurosurg* 1986;65:484–489.
33. Spetzler RF, Martin NA. A proposed grading system for arteriovenous malformations. *J Neurosurg* 1987;65:476–483.
34. Graf CJ, Perret GE, Torner JC. Bleeding from cerebral arteriovenous malformations as part of their natural history. *J Neurosurg* 1983;37:331–337.
35. Spetzler RF, Hargraves RW, McCormick PW, et al. Relationship of perfusion pressure and size to risk of hemorrhage from arteriovenous malformations. *J Neurosurg* 1992;76:918–923.
36. Karlsson B, Lindquist C, Johansson A, et al. Annual risk for the first hemorrhage from untreated cerebral arteriovenous malformations. *Minim Invas Neurosurg* 1997;40:40–46.
37. Hirai S, Mine S, Yamakami I, et al. Angioarchitecture related

to hemorrhage in cerebral arteriovenous malformations. *Neurol Med Chir (Toyko)* 1998[Suppl]38:165–170.
38. Jomin M, Lesoin F, Lozes G. Prognosis for arteriovenous malformations of the brain in adults based on 150 cases. *Surg Neurol* 1985;23:362–366.
39. Norbash AM, Marks MP, Lane B. Correlation of pressure measurements with angiographic characteristics predisposing to hemorrhage and steal in cerebral arteriovenous malformations. *AJNR Am J Neuroradiol* 1994;15:809–813.
40. Miyasaka Y, Kurata A, Irikura K, et al. The influence of vascular pressure and angiographic characteristics on haemorrhage for arteriovenous malformations. *Acta Neurochir (Wien)* 2000;142: 39–43.
41. Duong HD, Young WL, Vang MC, et al. Feeding artery pressure and venous drainage pattern are primary determinants of hemorrhage from cerebral arteriovenous malformations. *Stroke* 1998;29:1167–1176.
42. Marks MP, Lane B, Steinberg G, et al. Vascular characteristics of intracerebral arteriovenous malformations in patients with clinical steal. *AJNR Am J Neuroradiol* 1991;12:489–496.
43. Luessenhop AJ, Gennarelli TA. Anatomic grading of supratentorial arteriovenous malformations for determining operability. *Neurosurgery* 1977;1:30–35.
44. Valavanis A, Yasargil MG. The endovascular treatment of brain arteriovenous malformations. *Adv Tech Stand Neurosurg* 1998; 24:131–214.
45. Hamilton MG, Spetzler RF. The prospective application of a grading system for arteriovenous malformations. *Neurosurgery* 1994;34:2–7.
46. Richling B, Killer M. Endovascular management of patients with cerebral arteriovenous malformations. *Neurosurg Clin N Am* 2000;11:123–145.
47. Luessenhop AJ, Spence WT. Artificial embolization of cerebral arteries: report of use in a case of arteriovenous malformation. *JAMA* 1960;172:1153–1155.
48. Luessenhop AJ, Kachmann R, Shevlin W, et al. Clinical evaluation of artificial embolization in the management of larger cerebral arteriovenous malformations. *J Neurosurg* 1965;23: 400–417.
49. Luessenhop AJ, Presper JH. Surgical embolization of cerebral arteriovenous malformations through internal carotid and vertebral arteries: long-term results. *J Neurosurg* 1975;42:443–451.
50. Wolpert SM, Stein BM. Catheter embolization of intracranial arteriovenous malformations as an aid to surgical excision. *Neuroradiology* 1975;10:73–85.
51. Wolpert SM, Stein BM. Factors governing the course of emboli in the therapeutic embolization of cerebral arteriovenous malformations. *Radiology* 1979;131:125–131.
52. Russell EJ, Levy JM. Direct catheter redirection of a symptomatic errant intracranial Silastic sphere embolus. *Radiology* 1987; 165:631–633.
53. Hilal SK. Endovascular treatment of arteriovenous malformations of the central nervous system. In: Wilson CB, ed. *Intracranial arteriovenous malformations.* Baltimore: Williams & Wilkins, 1988:259–273.
54. Kerber C. Intracranial cyanoacrylate: a new catheter therapy for arteriovenous malformation [Letter]. *Invest Radiol* 1975;10: 536–538.
55. Serbinenko FA. Balloon catheterization of occlusion of major cerebral vessels. *J Neurosurg* 1974;41:125–145.
56. Kerber C. Balloon catheter with a calibrated leak. *Radiology* 1976;120:547–550.
57. Kikuchi T, Strother CM, Boyer M. New catheter for endovascular interventional procedures. *Radiology* 1987;165:870–871.
58. Dion JE, Duckwiler GR, Lylyk P, et al. Progressive suppleness Pursil catheter: a new tool for superselective angiography and embolization. *AJNR Am J Neuroradiol* 1989;10:1068–1070.
59. DeMerritt JS, Pile-Spellman J, Mast H, et al. Outcome analysis of preoperative embolizations with N-butyl cyanoacrylate in cerebral arteriovenous malformations. *AJNR Am J Neuroradiol* 1995;16:1801–1807.
60. Jafar JJ, David AJ, Berenstein A, et al. The effect of embolization with N-butyl-cyanoacrylate prior to surgical resection of cerebral arteriovenous malformations. *J Neurosurg* 1993;78:60–69.
61. Viñuela F, Dion JE, Duckwiler G, et al. Combined endovascular embolization and surgery in the management of cerebral arteriovenous malformations: experience with 101 cases. *J Neurosurg* 1991;75:856–864.
62. Pasqualin A, Scienza R, Cioffi F, et al. Treatment of cerebral arteriovenous malformations with a combination of preoperative embolization and surgery. *Neurosurgery* 1991;3:358–368.
63. Debrun GM, Aletich V, Ausman JI, et al. Embolization of the nidus of brain arteriovenous malformations with n-butyl-cyanoacrylate. *Neurosurgery* 1997;40:112–121.
64. Spetzler RF, Martin NA, Carter LP, et al. Surgical management of large AVMs by stages embolization and operative excision. *J Neurosurg* 1987;67:17–28.
65. Pelz DM, Fox AJ, Viñuela F, et al. Preoperative embolization of the brain AVMs with isobutyl-2-cyanoacrylate. *AJNR Am J Neuroradiol* 1988;9:757–764.
66. Deruty R, Pelissou-Guyotat C, Mottolese C, et al. The combined management of cerebral arteriovenous malformations: experience with 100 cases and review of the literature. *Acta Neurochir (Wien)* 1993;123:101–112.
67. Grzyska U, Westphal M, Zanella F. A joint protocol for the neurosurgical and neuroradiologic treatment of cerebral arteriovenous malformations: indications, technique and results in 76 cases. *Surg Neurol* 1993;40:476–484.
68. Fournier D, TerBrugge KG, Willinsky R, et al. Endovascular treatment of intracerebral arteriovenous malformations: experience in 49 cases. *J Neurosurg* 1995;75:228–233.
69. Steinberg GK, Fabrikant JI, Marks MP, et al. Stereotactic heavy-charged particle Bragg-peak radiation for intracranial arteriovenous malformations. *N Engl J Med* 1990;323:96–101.
70. Lunsford LD, Kondziolda D, Flickinger JC, et al. Stereotactic radiosurgery for arteriovenous malformations of the brain. *J Neurosurg* 1991;75:512–524.
71. Colombo F, Pozza F, Chiergo G, et al. Linear accelerator radiosurgery of cerebral arteriovenous malformations: an update. *Neurosurgery* 1994;34:14–21.
72. Friedman WA, Bova FJ, Mendenhall WM. Linear accelerator radiosurgery for arteriovenous malformations: the relationship of size to outcome. *J Neurosurg* 1995;82:180–189.
73. Karlsson B, Lindquist C, Steiner L. Prediction of obliteration after gamma knife surgery for cerebral arteriovenous malformations. *Neurosurgery* 1997;40:425–431.
74. Pollock BE, Flickinger JC, Lunsford LD, et al. Factors associated with successful arteriovenous malformation radiosurgery. *Neurosurgery* 1998;42:1239–1244.
75. Schlienger M, Atlan D, Lefkopoulos D, et al. LINAC radiosurgery for cerebral arteriovenous malformations: results in 169 patients. *Int J Radiat Oncol Biol Phys* 2000;46:1135–1142.
76. Dawson RC, Tarr RW, Hecht ST, et al. Treatment of arteriovenous malformations of the brain with combined embolization and stereotactic radiosurgery: results after 1 and 2 years. *AJNR Am J Neuroradiol* 1990;11:857–864.
77. Guo WY, Wikholm B, Karlsson C, et al. Combined embolization and gamma knife radiosurgery for cerebral arteriovenous malformations. *Acta Radiol* 1993;34:600–606.
78. Mathis JA, Barr JD, Horton JA, et al. The efficacy of particulate embolization combined with stereotactic radiosurgery for treat-

ment of large arteriovenous malformations of the brain. *AJNR Am J Neuroradiol* 1995;16:299–306.
79. Gobin YP, Laurent A, Merienne L, et al. Treatment of brain arteriovenous malformations by embolization and radiosurgery. *J Neurosurg* 1996;85:19–28.
80. Marks MP, Lane B, Steinberg GK, et al. Endovascular treatment of cerebral arteriovenous malformations following radiosurgery. *AJNR Am J Neuroradiol* 1993;14:297–303.
81. Steinberg GK, Change SD, Levy RP, et al. Surgical resection of large incompletely treated intracranial arteriovenous malformations following stereotactic radiosurgery. *J Neurosurg* 1996; 84:920–928.
82. Viñuela F, Duckwiler G, Guglielmi G. Contribution of interventional neuroradiology in the therapeutic management of brain arteriovenous malformations. *J Stroke Cerebrovasc Dis* 1997;6:268–271.
83. Wikholm G, Lundqvist C, Svendsen P. Embolization of cerebral arteriovenous malformations. Part I. Technique, morphology, and complications. *Neurosurgery* 1996;39:448–459.
84. Fox AJ, Girvin JP, Viñuela F, et al. Rolandic arteriovenous malformations: improvement in limb function by IBC embolization. *AJNR Am J Neuroradiol* 1985;6:575–582.
85. Kusske JA, Kelly WA. Embolization and reduction of the "steal" syndrome in cerebral arteriovenous malformations. *J Neurosurg* 1974;40:313–321.
86. Vinters HV, Galil KA, Lundie MJ, et al. The histotoxicity of cyanoacrylates. *Neuroradiology* 1985;27:279–291.
87. Viñuela F, Fox AJ, Pelz D, et al. Angiographic follow-up of large cerebral AVMs incompletely embolized with isobutyl-2-cyanoacrylate. *AJNR Am J Neuroradiol* 1986;7:919–925.
88. Berenstein A, Hieshima G. Clinical versus experimental use of isogutyl-2-cyanoacrylate [Letter]. *J Neurosurg* 1987;67: 318–319.
89. Samson D, Marshall D. Carcinogenic potential of isobutyl-2-cyanoacrylate [Letter]. *J Neurosurg* 1986;65:571–572.
90. Samson D, Marshall D. The use of isobutyl-2-cyanoacrylate in embolization [Letter]. *Surg Neurol* 1987;28:319.
91. Cromwell LD, Kerber CW. Modification of cyanoacrylate properties for therapeutic embolization. *AJR Am J Roentgenol* 1979;132:799–801.
92. Brothers MF, Kaufmann JCE, Fox AJ, et al. n-Butyl 2-cyanoacrylate: substitute for IBCA in interventional neuroradiology—histopathologic and polymerization time studies. *AJNR Am J Neuroradiol* 1989;10:777–786.
93. Germano IM, Davis RL, Wilson CB, et al. Histopathological follow-up study of 66 cerebral arteriovenous malformations after therapeutic embolization with polyvinyl alcohol. *J Neurosurg* 1992;76:607–614.
94. Vinters HV, Debrun G, Kaufmann JCE, et al. Pathology of arteriovenous malformations embolized with isobutyl-2-cyanoacrylate (bucrylate). *J Neurosurg* 1981;55:819–825.
95. Vinters HV, Lundie MJ, Kaufmann JCE. Long-term pathological follow-up of cerebral arteriovenous malformations treated by embolization with bucrylate. *N Engl J Med* 1986;314:477–483.
96. Schmeitzer JS, Chang BS, Madsen P, et al. The pathology of arteriovenous malformations of the brain treated by embolotherapy. II. Results of embolization with multiple agents. *Neuroradiology* 1993;35:468–474.
97. Wikholm G. Occlusion of cerebral arteriovenous malformations with N-butyl-cyanoacrylate is permanent. *AJNR Am J Neuroradiol* 1995;16:479–482.
98. Fournier D, TerBrugge K, Rodesch G, et al. Revascularization of brain arteriovenous malformations after embolization with bucrylate. *Neuroradiology* 1990;32:497–501.
99. Rao VRK, Mandalam KR, Gupta AK, et al. Dissolution of isobutyl-2-cyanoacrylate on long-term follow-up. *AJNR Am J Neuroradiol* 1989;10:135–141.
100. Takebayashi S, Hosaka M, Ishizula E, et al. AVMs of the kidneys: ablation with alcohol. *AJR Am J Roentgenol* 1988;150: 587–590.
101. Yakes WF, Luethke JM, Merland JJ, et al. Ethanol embolization of arteriovenous fistulas: a primary code of therapy. *J Vasc Interv Radiol* 1990;1:89–96.
102. Mourao GS, Hodes JE, Gobin YP, et al. Curative treatment of scalp AV fistulas by direct puncture and embolization with absolute alcohol. *J Neurosurg* 1991;75:634–637.
103. Yakes WF. Extremity venous malformations: diagnosis and management. *Semin Interven Radiol* 1994;11:332–339.
104. Berthelsen B, Fogdestam I, Svendsen P. Venous malformations of the face and neck. *Acta Radiol Diagn (Stockh)* 1986;27: 149–155.
105. Lylyk P, Viñuela F, Vinters HV, et al. Use of a new mixture for embolization of intracranial vascular malformations. Preliminary experimental experience. *Neuroradiology* 1990;32: 304–310.
106. Yakes WF, Krauth L, Eckund J, et al. Ethanol endovascular management of brain arteriovenous malformations: initial results. *Neurosurgery* 1997;40:1145–1154.
107. Phatouros CC, Halbach VA, Malek A, et al. Intraventricular contrast medium leakage during ethanol embolization of an arteriovenous malformation. *AJNR Am J Neuroradiol* 1999;20: 1329–1332.
108. Taki W, Yonekawa Y, Iwata H, et al. A new liquid material for embolization of arteriovenous malformations. *AJNR Am J Neuroradiol* 1990;11:163–168.
109. Terada T, Nakamura Y, Nakai K, et al. Embolization of arteriovenous malformations with peripheral aneurysms using ethylene, vinyl alcohol copolymer: report of three cases. *J Neurosurg* 1991;75:655–660.
110. Tokunaga K, Kinugasa K, Kawada S, et al. Embolization of cerebral arteriovenous malformations with cellulose acetate polymer: a clinical, radiological, and histological study. *Neurosurgery* 1999;44:981–990.
111. Kimura H, Fukushima T, Utsunomiya H, et al. Clinicopathological comparative evaluation of HEMA-MMA and EVAL embolization in arteriovenous malformations. *Surg Cereb Stroke* 1997;25:452–457.
112. Jahan R, Murayama Y, Gobin YP, et al. Embolization of arteriovenous malformations with Onyx: clinicopathological experience in 23 patients. *Neurosurgery* 2001;48:984–997.
113. Chaloupka JC, Viñuela F, Vinters HV, et al. Technical feasibility and histopathologic studies of ethylene vinyl copolymer (EVAL) using a swine endovascular embolization model. *AJNR Am J Neuroradiol* 1994;15:1107–1115.
114. Murayama Y, Viñuela F, Uloa A, et al. Nonadhesive liquid embolic agent for cerebral arteriovenous malformations: preliminary histopathological studies in swine *rete mirabile*. *Neurosurgery* 1998;43:1164–1175.
115. Chaloupka JC, Huddle DC, Alderman J, et al. A reexamination of the angiotoxicity of superselective injection of DMSO in the swine *rete* embolization model. *AJNR Am J Neuroradiol* 1999; 20:401–410.
116. Schumacher M, Horton JA. Treatment of cerebral arteriovenous malformations with PVA. *Neuroradiology* 1990;33:101–105.
117. Purdy PD, Batjer HH, Risser RC, et al. Arteriovenous malformations of the brain: choosing embolic materials to enhance safety and ease of excision. *J Neurosurg* 1992;77:217–222.
118. Nakstad PH, Nornes H. Superselective angiography, embolisation and surgery in treatment of arteriovenous malformations of the brain. *Neuroradiology* 1994;36:410–413.
119. Beaujeux R, Laurent A, Wassef M, et al. Trisacryl gelatin micro-

spheres for therapeutic embolization. II. Preliminary clinical evaluation in tumors and arteriovenous malformations. *AJNR Am J Neuroradiol* 1996;17:541–548.

120. Soong HK, Eskridge JM, Chung EC, et al. Preoperative embolization of cerebral arteriovenous malformations with silk sutures: analysis and clinical correlation of complications revealed on computerized tomography scanning. *J Neurosurg* 2000;92:955–960.
121. Nichols DA, Fufenacht DA, Jack CR, et al. Embolization of spinal dural arteriovenous fistula with polyvinyl alcohol particles: experience in 14 patients. *AJNR Am J Neuroradiol* 1992;13:933–940.
122. Sorimachi T, Koike T, Takeuchi S, et al. Embolization of cerebral arteriovenous malformations achieved with polyvinyl alcohol particles: angiographic reappearance and complications. *AJNR Am J Neuroradiol* 1999;20:1323–1328.
123. Nakstad PH, Bakke SJ, Halld JK. Embolization of intracranial arteriovenous malformations and fistulas with polyvinyl alcohol particles and platinum fibre coils. *Neuroradiology* 1992;34:348–351.
124. Bendszus M, Klein R, Burger R, et al. Efficacy of trisacryl gelatin microspheres versus polyvinyl alcohol particles in the preoperative embolization of meningiomas. *AJNR Am J Neuroradiol* 2000;21:255–261.
125. Lopez JR. Intraoperative neurophysiological monitoring. *Int Anesthesiol Clin* 1996;34:33–54.
126. Peters KR, Quisling RG, Gilmore R, et al. Intraarterial use of sodium methohexital for provocative testing during brain embolotherapy. *AJNR Am J Neuroradiol* 1993;14:171–174.
127. Rauch RA, Viñuela F, Dion J, et al. Preembolization functional evaluation in brain arteriovenous malformations: the superselective Amytal test. *AJNR Am J Neuroradiol* 1992;13:303–308.
128. Rauch RA, Viñuela F, Dion J, et al. Preembolization functional evaluation in brain arteriovenous malformations: the ability of superselective Amytal test to predict neurologic dysfunction before embolization. *AJNR Am J Neuroradiol* 1992;13:309–314.
129. Aletich VA, Debrun GM. Intracranial arteriovenous malformations: the approach and technique of cyanoacrylate embolization. In: Connors JJ, Wojack C, eds. *Interventional neuroradiology.* Philadelphia: WB Saunders, 1999:240–258.
130. Manninen PH, Gignac EM, Gelb AW, et al. Anesthesia for interventional neuroradiology. *J Clin Anesth* 1995;7:448–452.
131. Paulsen RD, Steinberg GK, Norbash AM, et al. Embolization of rolandic cortex arteriovenous malformations. *Neurosurgery* 1999;44:479–484.
132. Paulsen RD, Steinberg GK, Norbash AM, et al. Embolization of basal ganglia and thalamic arteriovenous malformations. *Neurosurgery* 1999;44:991–996.
133. Pile-Spellman J, Young W, Joshi S, et al. Adenosine-induced cardiac pause for endovascular embolization of cerebral arteriovenous malformations: technical case report. *Neurosurgery* 1999;44:881–886.
134. Halbach V, Higashida R, Dowd C, et al. Management of vascular perforations that occur during neurointerventional procedures. *AJNR Am J Neuroradiol* 1991;12:319–327.
135. Purdy PD, Batjer HH, Samson D. Management of hemorrhagic complications from preoperative embolization of arteriovenous malformations. *J Neurosurg* 1991;74:205–211.
136. Frizzel RT, Fisher WS. Cure, morbidity and mortality associated with embolization of brain arteriovenous malformations: a review of 1246 patients in 32 series over a 35 year period. *J Neurosurg* 1995;85.
137. Wallace RC, Flom RA, Khayata MH, et al. The safety and effectiveness of brain arteriovenous malformation embolization using acrylic and particles: the experience of a single institution. *Neurosurgery* 1995;37:606–615.
138. Lundqvist C, Wikholm G, Svendsen P. Embolization of cerebral AVMs. Part II. Aspects of complications and late outcome. *Neurosurgery* 1996;39:460–469.

Endovascular and Percutaneous Therapy of the Brain and Spine, edited by Michael P. Marks and Huy M. Do.
Lippincott Williams & Wilkins, Philadelphia © 2002.

11

ENDOVASCULAR THERAPY FOR DURAL ARTERIOVENOUS FISTULAS

JOHN C. CHALOUPKA

Vascular malformations that produce arteriovenous (AV) shunting within the dura mater and its associated venous connections (both cortical and epidural) constitute a special category of cerebrovascular disease. They frequently can produce either ischemic or hemorrhagic complications of the central nervous system. These AV shunting lesions of the dura are quite distinct from the archetypal arteriovenous malformations (AVMs) and pial arteriovenous fistulas (AVFs) of the brain on multiple histopathologic, pathogenetic, and clinicobiologic criteria, and therefore should be considered a separate clinical entity [1–8]. It is generally acknowledged that dural arteriovenous fistulas (or malformations) are acquired lesions, which characteristically develop in middle to late adulthood [4,6,9–11].

These AV shunting malformations of the dura have been variably called dural arteriovenous anomalies [12,13], dural arteriovenous malformations [3,14–16], and dural arteriovenous fistulas (DAVFs) [1,2,7,12,17,18]. These various names are at least partly a reflection of the uncertainty regarding their pathogenesis [7]. Some authors have therefore suggested that dural arteriovenous fistulous malformation (AVFM) would be a more accurate descriptor of these lesions [19]. Regardless of the pathologic etiology of these lesions, it has been generally agreed that the fundamental pathoanatomical unit of the malformation is an arteriovenous fistula. For this reason it is preferable to refer to these malformations as DAVFs for the sake of clarity and uniformity [7].

The clinical manifestations of DAVFs depend upon a combination of factors that relate to the precise anatomical location, angioarchitecture, and pathophysiologic consequences of a given lesion. Symptoms may range from a seemingly innocuous, yet irritating, subjective pulsatile bruit, to a catastrophic cerebral hemorrhage or venous infarction. Many DAVFs are asymptomatic and are only incidentally discovered when patients are being evaluated for unrelated problems. Even asymptomatic lesions may possess significant pathoanatomical or clinicobiologic features that portend a more aggressive natural history (and therefore demand aggressive therapeutic intervention despite the lack of symptoms).

The diagnosis and management of DAVFs has evolved substantially over the last decade. With the advent of safer and more effective percutaneous microcatheterization used for intracranial navigation and embolization, there has been an increasing reliance upon endovascular therapy as the first (and often only) line of treatment. This has come about because of numerous concurrent developments in technology and technique such as improvements in microcatheter and embolic technology, microcatheterization technique, and radiographic angiography equipment.

BACKGROUND

Epidemiology

DAVFs may occur in all ages from neonates to the very aged. Literature reviews have shown that the peak age at discovery for DAVFs is in the fifth and sixth decades [20, 21]. There is an overall higher incidence in women (female-to-male ratios in the range of 2:1), particularly with DAVFs of the cavernous and transverse sigmoid sinuses [21–24]. Although still comparatively uncommon, an increasing number of DAVFs are being discovered in infants and children [15,22,25]. These pediatric DAVFs tend to be more complex, usually consisting of multifocal fistulas with higher-flow AV shunting, and therefore higher probability of exhibiting more aggressive clinical manifestations (e.g., congestive heart failure, hypertensive venopathy, hydrocephalus) than many adult DAVFs. Even prospective antenatal diagnosis of fetal DAVFs in utero is occasionally possible, as recently reported by Levine et al. [26].

The true incidence of DAVFs is difficult to determine. Earlier case series reported from large single tertiary academic centers estimated that DAVFs represented only 10% to 15% of all cerebral malformations diagnosed with cathe-

J.C. Chaloupka: Departments of Radiology and Neurosurgery, University of Iowa Hospitals and Clinics, Iowa City, Iowa.

ter angiography [27,28]. With the advent of better diagnostic tools and more effective (and safer) endovascular surgical techniques, many centers have had a significant increase in cases well above these original estimates. One of the fundamental problems with estimating incidence of these malformations is related to referral bias. The incidence of DAVFs may have been significantly underestimated in the past owing to a combination of factors. First, many DAVFs are either minimally symptomatic or completely asymptomatic [12], which results in underreporting. Furthermore, patients with stable DAVFs frequently have been managed conservatively in a community practice setting and therefore are not referred to specialized neurovascular centers for diagnosis and treatment. Because of the protean manifestations of these malformations, it is also not uncommon for the correct diagnosis to be missed.

A variety of conditions have been described that may occur in association with DAVFs. Numerous reports have described the association between thrombosis or thrombophlebitis of a dural sinus and the development of a DAVF [16,23,29–34] with the implication that there is a direct causal relationship (i.e., thrombosis leads to development of a DAVF). However, this phenomenon has been clearly documented in only a minority of patients [5,16,23,30,31, 35]. Furthermore, many authors have also reported occasional instances of spontaneous thrombosis occurring in a dural sinus previously involved with a DAVF [9,30,31,35, 36], which confuses the issue of pathogenesis. Other associated conditions that have been described include prior craniotomy [37], intracranial infection [31], trauma [16,38], sinusitis [31], pregnancy and postparturition [18,24,39], remote surgery [18,31], previous anatomical abnormalities in a dural sinus [16,23], and Rendu-Osler-Weber syndrome [31]. Few studies have reported the actual proportion of sequential cases of DAVFs that occur with a putative etiologic association. The largest published series of 205 cases reported by Cognard et al. [5] noted a clearly defined etiologic factor in only 26% of cases. Such etiologic factors included cranial trauma, recent craniotomy (within 1 year), otitis media, mastoiditis, lower extremity thrombophlebitis, general surgery, or angiographically proven dural sinus thrombosis.

Pathogenesis

Several theories of pathogenesis have been suggested over the last three decades. At one time it was widely believed that DAVFs are congenital or developmental anomalies of the dural vasculature, similar to cerebral AVMs [13–15, 25]. There was little factual support for this theory other than the observed similarities in dysplastic changes of the dural vasculature to those of cerebral AVMs and the occasional DAVF detected in infants. Some authors still contend that the complex and deep DAVFs encountered in both infants and adults may be congenital in origin [9], although strong embryologic and pathoanatomical support for this theory is lacking.

During the last two decades, the preponderance of evidence indicates that most DAVFs are acquired lesions. As stated earlier, it has been suggested often that spontaneous thrombosis of a major dural sinus may be the fundamental precipitating event leading to a DAVF. Many authors have theorized that occlusion of a portion of the dural sinus can lead to opening of preexisting physiologic AV shunts within the dura. These low-pressure shunts within the microvascular bed subsequently may recruit additional meningeal arterial supply through the rich collateral microarterial network within the dura [13,18,23,29,31]. Another variation of this theme has been proposed by Picard et al. [30], who suggested that DAVFs may arise from disruption of thin-walled microvenous pouches within the dura, creating microscopic AV fistulas. This disruption may occur from an event which modifies the AV gradient within the dura, such as an episode of localized dural thrombosis.

Although prior dural sinus thrombosis is indeed a plausible mechanism for the development of DAVFs and is supported by limited documentation, such a theory fails to account for the many patients who have had no evidence of prior dural sinus thrombosis or thrombophlebitis and for those patients who have had numerous other associated conditions (e.g., inflammation, infection, craniotomy). The role of preexisting dural AV shunts [40,41] in the pathogenesis of DAVFs is unconfirmed. A few investigators have proposed that dural venous hypertension or ischemia may have a critical putative role in the pathogenesis of DAVFs [8,34,42], although the precise relationship between venous hypertension and the formation of these fistulous connections has not been elucidated.

It has been postulated that DAVFs may result as a direct consequence of pathologic neoangiogenesis within the dura [4]. This notion of abnormal new blood vessel formation or growth producing a DAVF was actually first implied in the classic paper of Houser et al. [23], who suggested that indigenous dysplastic dural vessels present within the sinus develop further and establish a direct artery-to-sinus communication. Although not stating it outright, Sundt and Piepgras [32] also implied possible neoangiogenic mechanisms in the pathogenesis of DAVFs when hypothesizing that the organization of thrombus within a dural sinus establishes dural blood supply with the potential for communicating with the patent portion of the sinus.

A wide range of cellular processes are known to trigger growth of new microvasculature into normal and pathologic tissues. Many of these stimuli are actually the same conditions that have been described in association with DAVFs. For example, it has been well documented that both acute and chronic inflammatory cells (which are invariably present in organizing thrombus, infections, traumatized tissues, and so forth) secrete various cytokinin and mitogenic factors (e.g., transforming growth factor beta [TGF-beta], platelet-derived growth factor [PDGF], basic fibroblast growth factor [bFGF], vascular endothelial growth factor [VEGF]), which can be potent stimulators of neoangiogenesis. Within the last decade, several basic and translational research studies have shown that one of the most potent stimulators of angiogenesis is ischemia [43–47]. This observation fits well with previous theories proposing a link between cerebral venous hypertension or ischemia, or both, and the pathogenesis of DAVFs. One of the earliest studies to link these types of growth factors to pathologic neoangiogenesis was in patients with moyamoya disease, in which immunohistochemical staining showed increased local production of bFGF [46,48].

A variety of local or remote events may promote angiogenesis in the dura. This includes associated conditions such as dural sinus thrombosis, thrombophlebitis, infection, aseptic inflammation, and trauma. These initiating events can stimulate production of angiogenic factors directly or indirectly from various sources (e.g., inflammatory cells, platelets, endothelium, etc.). Although several putative growth factors may be involved, the most potent known angiogenic factor, VEGF, is a likely candidate, because it already has been shown to have critical roles in normal and pathologic angiogenesis [11]. However, it is also likely that some additional set of conditions or factors occurring locally within the affected dura is required for the genesis and propagation of the DAVF. These can be additional angiogenic cofactors, local environmental influences (e.g., venous hypertension, local hyperemia, ischemia), and very likely genetic influences or susceptibilities.

The actual mechanics of fistula formation via angiogenesis can be envisioned easily. Usually, angiogenesis in mature tissues is initiated through so-called *budding* or *sprouting* of neovasculature from existing capillary beds. Such budding and proliferation of the rich microvascular network within the inner strata of the dura could eventually extend into the more superficial layers containing the plexus of microscopic dural venous channels. These venous channels are not true three-layered veins, but rather thin-walled endothelial lined grooves that are likely susceptible to ingrowth of the budding neovasculature, resulting in the creation of numerous AV fistulas. Stimulation of neoangiogenesis within the inner dura can also explain the recruitment of pial arterial supply and apparent growth of some DAVFs [4,11].

Recently a few animal and human studies have provided strong supporting evidence of this theory by demonstrating elevated expression of various angiogenic growth factors, including VEGF and bFGF, within DAVFs [33,49–51]. However, demonstration of high levels of such growth factors within a lesion does not, in itself, prove causation. Indeed, increased production of various angiogenic factors may be a result (rather than a cause) of the DAVF. However, recently a more direct linkage between angiogenic growth factors and the *de novo* pathogenesis of a DAVF was reported by our group in a large animal model designed to study the effects of direct local stimulation of angiogenesis [52]. Using a surgically implantable hydrogel polymeric release technique, adsorbed VEGF delivered into a segment of the superior sagittal sinus (SSS) consistently produced DAVFs in swine that were confirmed on conventional angiographic and histopathologic studies [52]. This finding still must be viewed as preliminary, however, requiring more carefully designed and controlled studies to confirm a causal relationship [11]. Clinical studies that more carefully evaluate expression of growth factors (e.g., VEGF, bFGF, PDGF, and angiopoietin-1) and their corresponding receptor targets will be needed to confirm the associations and help better define cellular mechanisms of pathogenesis.

Pathophysiology

The shunting of arterial blood flow and pressure into the intracranial and pericranial venous system is the fundamental pathophysiologic process of most DAVFs. Unlike cerebral AVMs, ischemic complications of DAVFs in the brain and cranial nerves are usually not related to arterial steal phenomenon from the AV shunting [32]. Arterialization of the major dural sinus or cortical veins, or both, result in elevated pressure and blood flow disturbances (turbulence). In an acute or subacute setting, this can cause unfavorable alterations in the net pressure gradients across the capillary beds of the brain, resulting in interstitial exudation, edema, congestion, and eventual venous obstructive ischemia. If this continues to progress, cerebral infarction with or without hemorrhage ensues. Conversely, if the dominant venous drainage pathways of the dural sinus system are gradually recruited for venous drainage of the DAVF, global chronic intracranial hypertension and hydrocephalus may occur instead. The mechanism of this process is presumed to be long-standing diminished resorption of interstitial fluid and cerebrospinal fluid produced by chronically elevated intracranial venous pressure. It also has been observed that in some cases the combination of intracranial hypertensive venopathy and disturbed blood flow patterns can lead to progressive venoocclusive disease in the cortical veins and dural sinuses by a yet-to-be well-defined mechanism. Experimental and pathologic studies have shown reactive neointimal proliferation in vessels subjected to superphysiologic blood flow or increased shear [53,54], while other studies have shown that endothelia possess a complex array of intracellular mechanisms for transducing mechanical forces that likely influence not only their alignment in a flow field, but also growth and repair of the intimal lining [55]. The progressive venoocclusive disease seen in association with some DAVFs (particularly pediatric and complex or multifocal types) eventually cannot be adequately compensated for by venous rerouting, thereby resulting in widespread cerebral edema, ischemia, and infarction.

The natural history of DAVFs is as varied as their clinical manifestations. A few reports have suggested that a variable percentage of these lesions (18% to 50%) may undergo spontaneous resolution [38,56–58], although large prospective population-based studies are again lacking to substantiate these estimates. Many DAVFs may also remain clinically stable over a long period of time [16,21,22,59]. This benign clinical behavior in a relatively large proportion of malformations has led many clinicians to recommend conservative or expectant management in so-called nonaggressive DAVFs [4,10,60,61].

A subset of DAVFs will cause serious, acute, or progressive clinical syndromes that warrant definitive treatment. A wide spectrum of clinical manifestations of aggressive DAVFs is possible. Extensive or high-flow DAVFs (e.g., multifocal, SSS, deep venous or galenic types) can produce intraparenchymal hematoma, venous infarction, dementia, ataxia, seizures, and ischemic demyelination. Vision loss can occur as a consequence of orbital congestive (or hypertensive) venopathy from aggressive cavernous or inferior petrosal sinus DAVFs, producing retinal ischemia, optic nerve ischemia, subretinal effusions, retinal detachment, or intractable open angle glaucoma. Ophthalmoplegia owing to cranial nerve dysfunction (most commonly affecting the sixth and third cranial nerves) may be the result either of mass effect from intracavernous or orbital apex varices or, more commonly, from venous ischemia of the cranial nerve vasa nervosum.

In infants with DAVFs, global intracranial hypertensive venopathy can be compounded by progressive multifocal dural sinus and cortical venous thrombosis. If inadequate rerouting of venous drainage occurs in these cases, progressive neurologic and cognitive deterioration will usually develop, following a very similar natural history to vein of Galen malformations manifesting in infancy. This syndrome is characterized by progressive ischemia and edema of the subcortical and deep periventricular white matter, selective neuronal infarction of cortex, and deposition of dystrophic calcifications in the affected area [62].

Classification

Dural arteriovenous fistulas have been classified by the specific locations of the fistulas. Although this approach is simple and useful for descriptive localization and general anatomical therapeutic planning, it may be inadequate for defining the clinical behavior, prognosis, and response to therapy of a particular lesion. Probably the single most important determinant of DAVF behavior is based on the venous outflow pattern of the lesion. Thus, most modern classification schemes incorporate this information to provide overall greater guidance for clinical diagnosis and therapeutic planning.

Perhaps the most well recognized classification system specific to DAVFs is that developed by Djindjian et al. [17, 18]. This system categorizes a lesion into one of the following four types: type I DAVFs are characterized by normal antegrade drainage into a venous sinus or meningeal vein, type II lesions drain into a sinus with reflux into adjacent sinuses or cortical vein, type III DAVFs drain directly into cortical veins with resultant retrograde flow into the cerebral venous compartment, and type IV DAVFs have drainage directly into a venous pouch (venous lake, venous ectasia). They concluded from their study that type I DAVFs were benign, with each sequential type having more aggressive characteristics. In particular the type III and IV DAVFs were considered the most dangerous, with the former being associated with venous infarction and hemorrhage of the brain, and the latter being associated with subarachnoid or subdural hemorrhage from rupture of the associated venous lakes. Since introduction of the Djindjian classification of DAVFs in 1978, several other studies have been published in the literature attempting to correlate certain features of DAVFs with the likelihood of associated hemorrhage or other specific neurologic complications [29,69,70].

With the advent of more effective endovascular therapeutic techniques, a means of predicting lesion risk and management strategies emerged. Cognard et al. [5] developed a classification system derived from a modified version of that published by Djindjian et al. [17,18]. In their scheme, they defined five types of DAVFs that are based exclusively upon the pattern of venous outflow. As such, type I DAVFs were characterized by normal antegrade flow into the affected dural sinus. Type II lesions were associated with an abnormal direction of venous drainage within the affected dural sinus. These lesions could be further categorized into three subtypes: type IIa lesions with retrograde flow solely into the sinus or sinuses, type IIb lesions with retrograde venous drainage into the cortical veins only, and type IIa + b lesions with retrograde drainage into sinuses and cortical veins. Type III DAVFs drained directly into cortical vein(s) without venous ectasia, whereas type IV DAVFs had drainage into cortical veins with venous ectasia greater than 5 mm in diameter and 3 times larger than the diameter of the draining vein. A DAVF was considered to be type V when drainage was into spinal perimedullary veins. Correlation with their clinical data yielded the following conclusions: type I DAVFs can be considered benign, and treatment is usually not necessary, except possibly for symptom palliation; type IIa lesions are best treated with arterial embolization; type IIb and IIa + b lesions usually require both transarterial and transvenous embolization for effective treatment. For lesions of type III through V, aggressive transarterial and occasionally transvenous embolization aimed at complete occlusion of the fistula is necessary, and frequently may need to be supplemented with surgical techniques in eliminating the dangerous cortical venous drainage.

Other classification systems for DAVFs have been devised that focus on putative mechanisms of development. For example, Mironov [65] developed a classification scheme based on his theories of pathogenesis, which assumed that the propensity for the development of dural sinus thrombosis is central and is dependent on the location and flow volume of the fistula. This classification model described the following five types of DAVF: type I were DAVFs of the dural sinuses, type II included DAVFs of the cavernous sinus, type III were DAVFs of the galenic venous system, type IV involved the venous plexus of the skull base, and type V were DAVFs of the parasinusal cortical veins. From their data they concluded that the morphologic development of DAVFs appears to be dependent on the volume of flow in the venous recipient and that pronounced development of pathologic AV shunts takes place at the level of the large basal dural sinuses [65].

Other classification schemes have been proposed [19, 66] which are simplifications or other modifications of the Djindjian and Cognard classification systems.

DIAGNOSIS

A careful clinical history and physical examination will often suggest a DAVF is present. This is particularly true for certain common anatomical sites for DAVFs, such as the cavernous sinus and the sigmoid sinus. The former frequently shows the classic signs and symptoms of orbital hypertensive venopathy, which include pulsatile exophthalmos, chemosis, conjunctival injection, and episcleral venous dilatation. DAVFs of the cavernous sinus may also manifest with open-angle glaucoma, optic neuropathy, and ocular paresis secondary to cranial nerve palsies (most commonly affecting the sixth and third cranial nerves). Dural arteriovenous fistulas of the sigmoid sinus or combination of sigmoid and transverse sinuses most frequently cause pulsatile tinnitus. Other common symptoms and signs related to this anatomical site of AV shunting include headaches, retroauricular pain, and an objective bruit on auscultation (also occasionally on palpation). Less commonly associated clinical manifestations include vertigo, lower cranial nerve palsies (e.g., hypoglossal, Horner syndrome), and hearing loss.

It must be emphasized that a high index of suspicion should be maintained for the possibility of a DAVF when confronted with an unexplainable constellation of neurologic complaints and deficits. This is particularly true in patients with nonspecific symptoms such as headaches, dizziness, memory loss, dementia, and seizures. These patients will often undergo an extensive workup without obtaining a diagnosis. Certain other clinical scenarios should also raise one's suspicion of a DAVF. For example, an intracranial hemorrhage in any patient that cannot be explained on the basis of trauma, hypertension, or the usual common hemorrhagic cerebrovascular lesions (i.e., aneurysms, AVMs, cavernous malformations), should be suspected of being the result of a DAVF with cortical venous drainage. Another example is in patients who develop either apoplectic or progressive myelopathy, who may be harboring a DAVF of the posterior fossa with descending spinal perimedullary venous drainage [59]. Unexplained communicating hydrocephalus in children and intracranial venous thrombosis in children and adults are other situations in which a DAVF should be considered in the differential diagnosis. Nonaneurysmal subarachnoid hemorrhage (more commonly confined to the posterior fossa) may also develop in patients with posterior fossa and cranial base, deep, or galenic DAVFs with cortical venous drainage [31,67].

Modern diagnostic imaging also plays a pivotal role in diagnosis and therapeutic planning, although many pitfalls and limitations still exist that must be recognized. The diagnosis may be suspected from nonspecific or indirect findings obtained by imaging. Magnetic resonance imaging (MRI) studies may show dilated flow voids, occluded dural sinuses, or abnormal curvilinear, serpiginous, or dural enhancement [68,69]. Some authors have advocated the use of spin-echo MRI as the procedure of choice for detection of the complications of DAVF, such as infarct or hemorrhage [69]. Magnetic resonance angiography (MRA) has also been used for the detection of certain types of DAVF. Ikawa et al. have employed three-dimensional time-of-flight (3-D TOF) detection and diagnosis of carotid-cavernous fistulas by demonstrating abnormal flow in the superior ophthalmic vein [70]. They conclude that DAVFs of the cavernous sinus often can be diagnosed by MRA through demonstration of abnormally dilated draining veins. Phase-contrast MRA can be used to demonstrate the direction of flow in the draining sinuses and veins [71]. The prospective accuracy of MRI and MRA in detecting DAVFs has not been rigorously evaluated. Recent experience has demonstrated that these imaging modalities have a disappointingly low sensitivity and specificity [72].

The gold standard for diagnosis of DAVFs remains catheter cerebral angiography. This study should include selective injections of the internal carotid, external carotid (including the ascending pharyngeal artery), and vertebral arteries. Lesions suspected to be localized to the craniocervical junction may also require selective injections of the thyrocervical and costocervical trunks to visualize the ascending and deep cervical arteries, respectively. Catheter angiography permits accurate demonstration of the anatomical site of involvement of AV shunting, arterial supply, and venous drainage, and prevailing hemodynamics. This information is useful for both prognostication of natural history and proper therapeutic planning [4,6,73].

TREATMENT

The decision to treat a particular DAVF should weigh the potential risks and benefits of a single or multiple modality approach, as opposed to either the severity of active symptoms or the long-term prognosis based upon angioarchitecture (e.g., Cognard type III to V DAVFs) and anatomical location (e.g., deep venous or galenic DAVF). Clearly some DAVFs are likely to exhibit relatively benign clinical behavior related to inherent low shunt flow and progressive spontaneous occlusion of the involved dural sinus, the latter often leading to spontaneous resolution [16,38,56–58]. Some DAVFs may remain hemodynamically and clinically stable for extended periods [16,20,21], although prospective prediction of this benign clinical course is questionable. In the past, it had been argued that owing to this apparent benign behavior, patients exhibiting either mild or stable symptoms, and so-called nonaggressive angiographic features should be managed expectantly or conservatively [9, 10,31]. For the most part, a variable percentage of DAVFs occurring in the cavernous sinus and sigmoid sinus are more likely to fall into this category and thus have been the main types of lesions (by anatomical site) managed conservatively. However, over the last decade busy clinical practices have experienced so-called *paradoxical clinicoradiologic features* or *paradoxical aggressive clinical behavior* (i.e., sudden, unpredictable onset of aggressive clinical course) in patients with such DAVFs being managed expectantly [35,74]. With the advent of safer and more effective endovascular surgical techniques over the last several years, the threshold for undertaking both palliative and curative therapeutic embolization for DAVFs of the cavernous and transverse sinuses has been substantially lowered.

In general, aggressive treatment of DAVFs should be considered in any clinical scenario that threatens to produce a permanent injury to the central nervous system (including cranial nerves), vision, or is life-threatening. As outlined earlier, threats to neurologic function largely depend on the severity of pathophysiologic derangements that are related to AV shunting.

Patients who develop either intracranial hemorrhage or ischemic stroke from aggressive DAVFs are at greatest risk for serious permanent neurologic morbidity and mortality. Patients who develop large intraparenchymal hematomas that produce cerebral herniation will require emergent surgical evacuation first. DAVFs otherwise discovered in hemorrhagic or ischemic stroke should be approached by urgent endovascular surgical intervention. Early recurrent hemorrhage or progressive neurologic deterioration after the first hemorrhage is a major problem in such patients, carrying an estimated incidence of 35% in the first 2 weeks and an overall poorer prognosis (death and severe neurologic morbidity) [75–77]. Other neurologic sequelae demanding prompt intervention include seizures, global central nervous system depression, hydrocephalus, intractable severe headaches, and myelopathy [78,79].

The deterioration of visual acuity by a DAVF may be the consequence of a variety of pathophysiologic processes, including venous hypertensive ischemic optic neuropathy, retinal edema and detachments, uncontrollable glaucoma, or severe corneal edema. Other orbital or ocular complications of cavernous DAVFs that should prompt stronger consideration of therapeutic intervention include disfiguring exophthalmos, progressive ophthalmoplegia, and intractable retroorbital pain.

Several equally important angiographic features portending an aggressive clinical course mandate aggressive and definitive treatment. These features include deep venous or galenic drainage, tentorial or superior petrosal sinus involvement, generalized progressive dural sinus thrombosis with extensive cortical venous rerouting, multiplicity, and recruitment of cortical venous drainage [1,29,38,57,58,75, 80–84]. The last two findings on angiography are particularly ominous, because previous studies [2,29,31] have shown that there is a high incidence (40% to 95%) of intracranial hemorrhage and venous infarction in untreated patients.

Endovascular surgical management of DAVFs has become more widely considered a primary therapeutic modality for most DAVFs, and in those complex or difficult access lesions that may require multimodal intervention (e.g., embolization followed by surgical disconnection, embolization followed by stereotactic radiosurgery) is still usually the first line of attack. Traditionally, it has been convenient to broadly divide endovascular surgical techniques for the treatment of DAVFs into transarterial and transvenous approaches.

Transarterial embolization techniques developed for DAVFs were viewed in terms of the degree of penetration (i.e., proximal versus distal) into the site of AV shunting (which has been referred to often as the nidus in an analogous fashion to cerebral AVMs) and the permanence of the embolic agent. Proximal occlusion has generally been discouraged with the exception of being advocated only for preoperative devascularization, while distal transarterial occlusion was necessary for primary palliative or occasionally curative therapy. The permanence of the embolic agent has been, and continues to be, a critical issue in terms of durability of an endovascular operation intended for definitive treatment. Particulate embolization suspensions (mostly consisting of varying size polyvinyl alcohol [PVA] particles) have been and, at many centers continue to be, a popular agent for transarterial embolization of DAVFs. The major advantages of PVA embolization are its relatively undemanding technical requirements (in terms of both purchase of the microcatheter and the preparation and delivery of the suspension), favorable short-term histotoxicity, and safety profile. There are major disadvantages and shortcomings of PVA embolization of DAVFs, including the often transitory nature of vascular occlusion, inability to occlude larger-caliber fistulous channels, need for using predominantly larger-caliber guidewire-directed microcatheters, higher risk of serious inadvertent pulmonary embolization [85], and higher failure rate to achieve optimal devascularization [86].

With the advent of improved endovascular technologies (e.g., microcatheters, microguidewires, embolics), and the maturation of embolization techniques using liquid embolic agents, these paradigms have changed [86]. As a consequence of superior microcatheter technology and techniques, the goal is to achieve maximal distal access with the intention of performing nidal embolization of the DAVF whenever possible. Increasing numbers of lesions may be cured definitively with transarterial embolization alone. Transarterial embolization of the meningeal supply to certain types of DAVFs (e.g., transverse sigmoid sinus, most type III and IV lesions, and deep or galenic) is preferred as the first line of attack, owing to one or more factors including technical ease, lower risks of technical and clinical complications, enhanced efficacy, or lack of facile access for a transvenous approach.

Transarterial embolization alone for many types of DAVFs is frequently either unnecessary (e.g., cavernous sinus lesions) or inadequate for definitive treatment owing to one or more of the following reasons: (a) primary transvenous embolization may be technically easier, safer, and either equivalent or superior to comparable transarterial approaches for certain anatomical sites, (b) some lesions derive meningeal supply from branches of the intracranial circulation that cannot be accessed or embolized safely, (c) a plethora of external carotid artery (ECA) meningeal supply may be present, consisting of innumerable plexiform branches that cannot be accessed satisfactorily, and (d) overt or occult dangerous external carotid artery–internal carotid artery (ECA-ICA) or external carotid artery–vertebral artery (ECA-VA) anastomoses often exist, which may preclude safe and effective transarterial embolization.

Consequently, for a number of DAVFs endovascular intervention requires the use of transvenous embolization techniques. Such techniques are typically directed at achieving a segmental therapeutic occlusion of the involved dural sinus or occlusion of the directly recruited cortical vein. When contemplating such transvenous therapeutic embolizations of a dural sinus or cortical vein, two fundamental principles must be applied for optimal technical and clinical outcomes. First and foremost, a critical assessment is needed of an individual patient's tolerance to occlusion of a major dural sinus or cortical vein that is involved with a DAVF. As a rule of thumb, if it is possible to identify normal venous pathways of the brain that are using the involved dural sinus or cortical vein as a conduit, then there may be significant risk of intolerance to permanent occlusion. The notable exception to this rule, however, is with cavernous DAVFs, in which the cavernous sinus can be occluded therapeutically with impunity.

If there is evidence of venoocclusive disease associated with the DAVF (i.e., types IIb through V venous drainage), then transvenous embolization is usually, but not always, safer. However, for certain types of DAVFs, such as those affecting the transverse sigmoid sinus, deep venous, galenic, complex, and SSS, it may be difficult to judge confidently if therapeutic occlusion of a major intracranial venous pathway will be tolerated. As a general rule, normal cortical veins draining directly into or in close proximity to an affected segment of sinus may cause venous ischemia and infarction if transvenous embolization is performed. Therefore, a rigorous effort must be made prospectively to identify these cortical veins. In many situations this may be accomplished by performing either simultaneous or sequential selective injections of the pial and meningeal circulation obtained in the same angiographic projection. Careful evaluation of the early and late phases of these angiograms usually reveals at least the major normal cortical veins and their attachments to the dural sinus system. The most important major veins to identify in such an analysis include Labbé, Trolard, internal cerebral, Galen, superficial middle cerebral, lateral cerebellar, precentral cerebellar, and vermian.

It is also possible to perform provocative testing with temporary balloon occlusion of the diseased portion of the dural sinus [4,35], although no validated protocols articulating technical approaches and important functional assessments (e.g., duration of occlusion, adjunctive imaging studies) have yet been developed. Cognard et al. recently reported only a single case out of their extensive institutional experience of successful provocative testing in a patient who developed hemiparesis shortly after temporary balloon occlusion of a portion of the SSS affected by a DAVF [35].

The second guiding principle of transvenous embolotherapy of DAVFs is to ensure complete exclusion of the involved dural sinus (or other intracranial venous pathway) from the remaining normal intracranial venous pathways. The specific sites of fistulous communication must be identified and targeted precisely for complete therapeutic occlusion (Fig. 11-1). In such cases, it is preferable to leave intentionally an adequate amount of arterial supply to the DAVF to permit road mapping and serial reevaluation as the diseased venous segment is obliterated. It is important to avoid simple trapping and partial embolization of the involved segment of dural sinus, because this can lead to diversion of shunt flow into normal cerebral venous pathways and ultimately result in conversion of the DAVF into a more dangerous and aggressive disease. This principle also applies

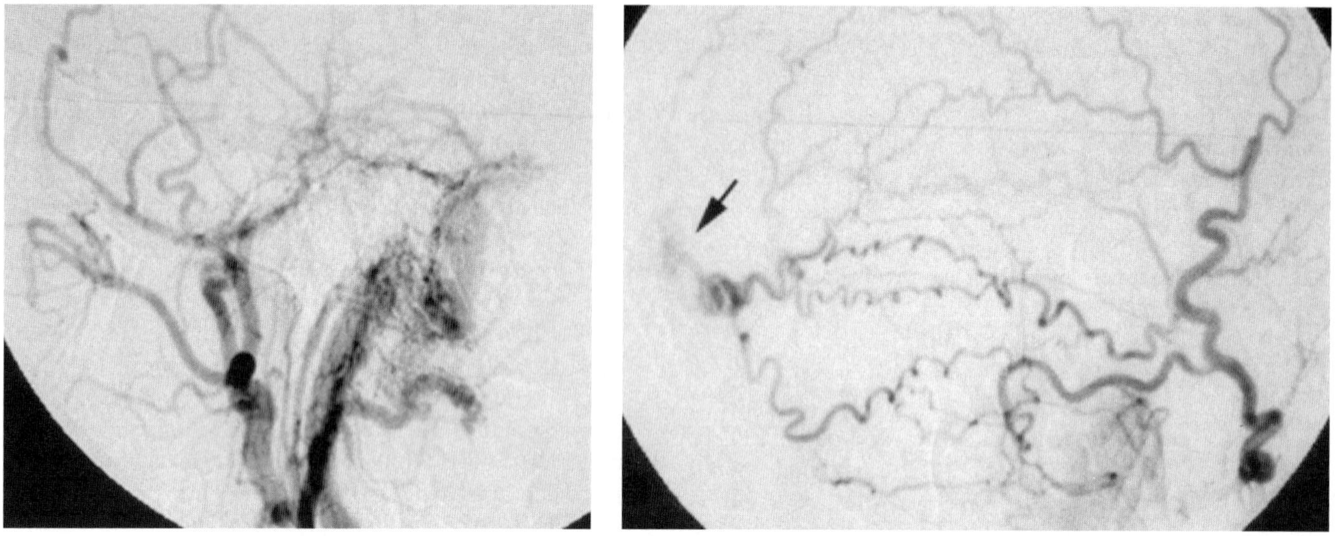

A B

FIGURE 11-1. This 45-year-old woman had intractable headaches and severe pulsatile tinnitus. She had originally developed mild-to-moderate pulsatile tinnitus, when she sought treatment at her local hospital. She was found to have a type1 DAVF of the transverse sigmoid sinus that was treated incompletely with particulate transarterial embolization (complicated by an ischemic facial nerve palsy). **A,B:** Right external carotid artery angiogram lateral projection **(A)** and superselective left occipital artery angiogram **(B)** show extensive recurrence of the DAVF via numerous feeders directly from RECA branches. The *arrow* in **(B)** shows the site of left occipital communication. There was also indirect supply from the LECA and ascending cervical artery (not shown). *(Figure continues.)*

when attempting curative transarterial, intranidal embolization of type III through V lesions, in which it is critical to intentionally fill the recipient venous channel with cyanoacrylate to ensure a permanent cure of the fistula [35].

Although endovascular techniques are generally preferred for first-line treatment, an operative approach in some instances is either the preferred or only method of treatment for certain DAVFs. In the past this was true for DAVFs of the anterior cranial fossa, which often are supplied by ethmoidal branches of the ophthalmic artery. Although these branches are now more readily approachable with modern microcatheterization techniques [6,31], there may be relatively higher risk and technical difficulty to consider. A subfrontal exposure provides relatively easy access to the ethmoidal feeders and involved draining vein(s). Thus, the operation enjoys a high success and low complication rate [87]. In the past, conventional teaching suggested that successful surgical treatment of DAVFs involving a major dural sinus would require either resection or fulguration of the entire segment of involved dural sinus and surrounding dura. Such approaches have enjoyed variable success and failure, often carrying significant risk of morbidity and mortality due to difficulties in achieving hemostasis from the extensive vascularity of the surrounding dura, bone, and subcutaneous tissues [32]. More recently, open surgical management has focused on performing functional disconnection of DAVFs from their dangerous cortical venous drainage, which has been met with better technical and clinical outcomes [7].

Some DAVFs refractory to combined endovascular and open surgical management may be treated with stereotactic radiosurgery, although the published experience with such a treatment modality remains very limited. The few reported series have been in mostly cavernous lesions with heterogeneous clinical and demographic characteristics. In these reports success rates varying as high as 75% to 80% for so-called low-flow DAVFs of the cavernous sinus, and as low as 20% for higher-flow and noncavernous DAVFs, were recorded [88–90]. Because of this limited experience it is widely held currently that stereotactic radiosurgery should be reserved as a secondary modality after endovascular and open surgical approaches have been exhausted or entertained.

TECHNIQUE FOR ENDOVASCULAR TREATMENT

General Considerations

It has become customary to be prepared to perform therapeutic embolization at the time of planned diagnostic catheter angiography whenever possible. Such an approach has certain strengths and weaknesses that have to be balanced. The major disadvantages are the postponing of the gold

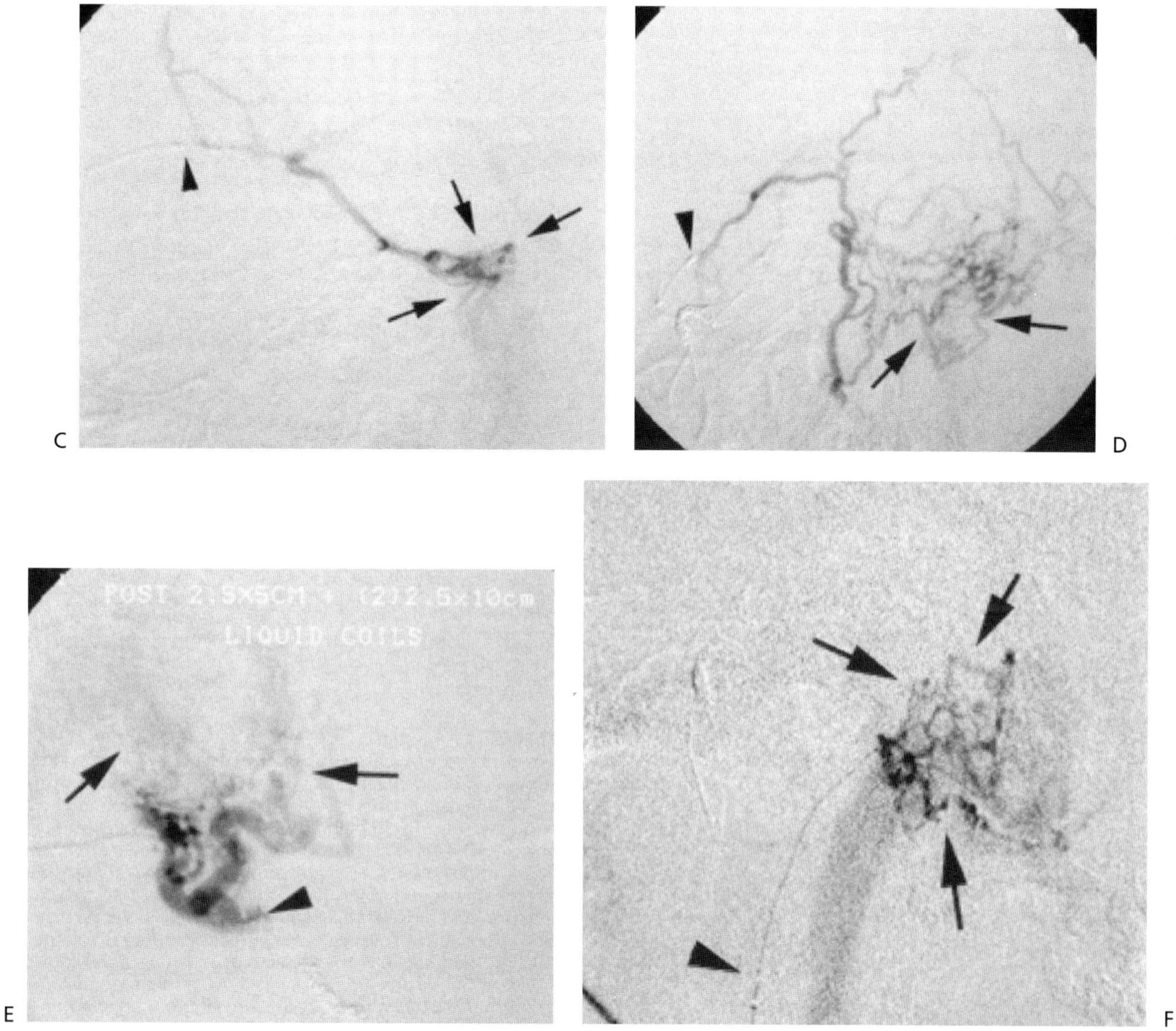

FIGURE 11-1. *Continued.* **C–F:** Superselective angiograms of the posterior auricular **(C)**, middle meningeal **(D)**, occipital **(E)**, and ascending pharyngeal **(F)** arterial feeders, respectively, show the extensive multicompartmental supply to the DAVF (*arrowheads* show catheter tips, *arrows* show portions of arteriovenous arcade). These feeders, as well as others, were serially embolized with aliquots of 4:1 ethiodized oil-to-NBCA mixture. Unfortunately, owing to the extensive collateral revascularization of the DAVF after previous particulate embolization, complete angiographic obliteration of the fistula was not possible with superselective transarterial acrylic embolization alone. *(Figure continues.)*

standard confirmatory exam until the actual time of planned intervention. This denies the operators a chance to more leisurely absorb and interpret the anatomical and hemodynamic data obtained from the catheter angiograms, which is essential for therapeutic planning. The major advantages, though, include reducing the potential risk of morbidity associated with repeated conventional angiography, increasing patient satisfaction, and reducing overall costs. Furthermore, basic information needed for general therapeutic planning can be obtained from the good-quality noninvasive imaging (particularly MRI and MRA). Therefore, prior to seeing a patient with a DAVF in our clinic, we insist on having these noninvasive imaging studies performed to facilitate and streamline the remaining diagnostic workup and the actual therapeutic recommendations and planning among our neurovascular team.

In the past the majority of patients referred for endovascular therapeutic embolization of their DAVFs have had the procedure performed under awake sedation, typically using intermittent small doses of intravenous fentanyl (25 to 50 μg) and midazolam (0.5 to 1.0 mg). However, with the increased use of superselective wedged intranidal injec-

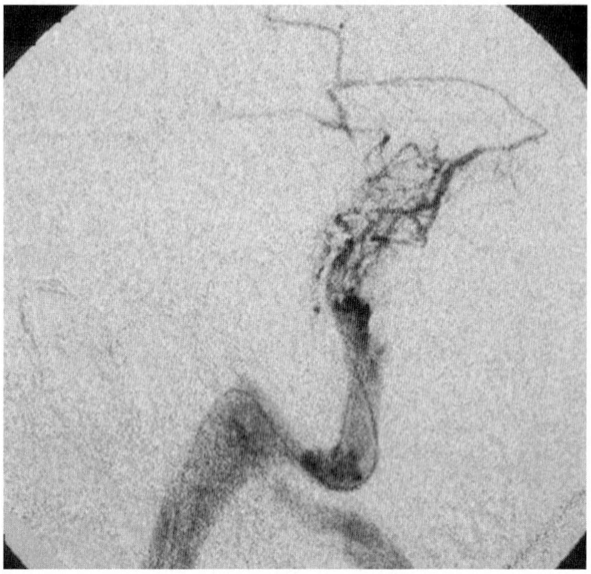

G

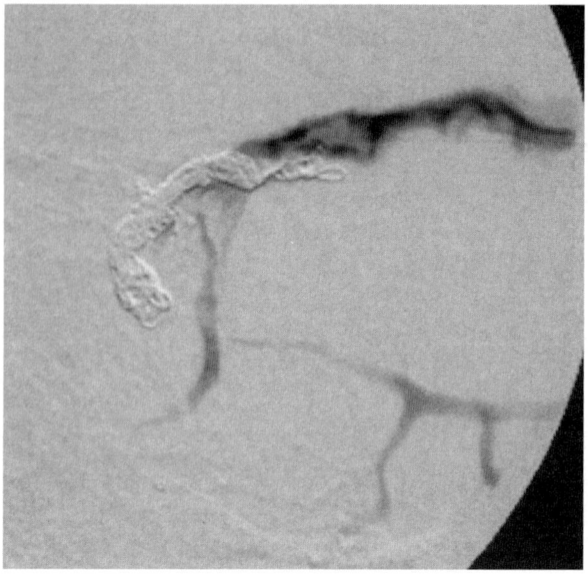

H

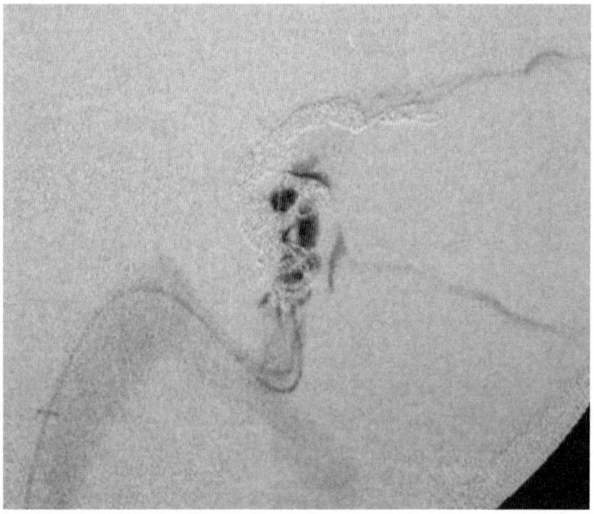

I

FIGURE 11-1. *Continued.* **G–I:** Dural sinus venograms, via retrograde transvenous catheterization lateral projections, show first the recipient parallel venous compartment of the DAVF adjacent to the transverse sigmoid sinus junction **(G)**. Note the retrograde filling of distal middle meningeal feeding branches and cortical venous reflux (type 2b DAVF). **H:** This compartment was filled completely with varying sized detachable coils. Subsequently the transverse sigmoid sinus junction and most of the sigmoid sinus were occluded using both detachable coils (GDC system) and fibered nonretrievable (Tornado system) microcoils **(I,J)**. **K:** Lateral final control left external carotid angiogram shows complete obliteration of the DAVF. A 6-month follow-up angiogram confirmed durable occlusion of the fistula.

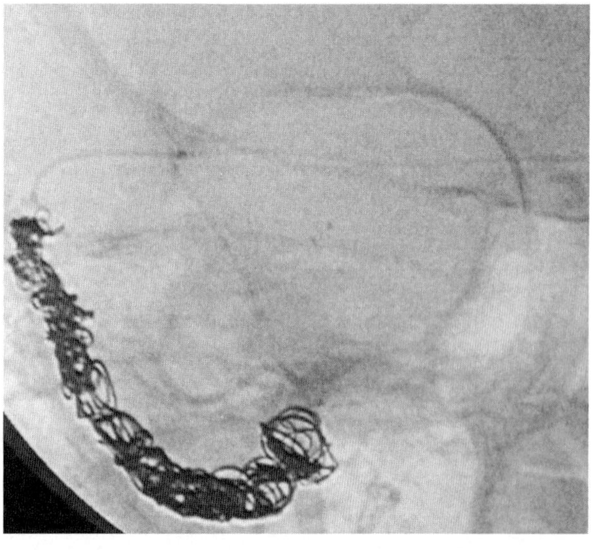

J

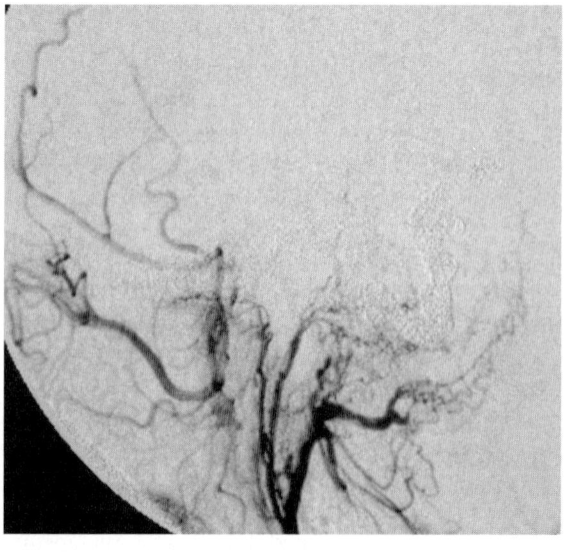

K

tions of acrylic, and aggressive transvenous catheterization of the dural sinuses and cortical veins, more rigorous manipulation of microcatheters is now often required. These types of manipulations invariably elicit severe (although usually transient) headaches, making it increasingly more difficult to ensure patient comfort during these frequently lengthy sessions. Therefore, general anesthesia has become necessary in some cases. There are also other important advantages of performing DAVF embolotherapy under general anesthesia, including better hemodynamic monitoring and manipulation of the patient (e.g., artificial hypotension to slow shunt flow during embolization), lack of voluntary and involuntary motion, enhanced patient compliance, and better intensive care capability to manage preembolization complications (e.g., intracranial hemorrhage). These advantages must be balanced against a few important disadvantages, including potential risk of morbidity associated with repeated intubation, risk of repeated general anesthesia, and inability to assess functional significance of the surrounding brain.

To minimize potential thromboembolic complications of endovascular surgery, we perform most of the embolizations under systemic heparinization, typically starting with an intravenous bolus of 5,000 units of heparin sulfate, followed by additional hourly boluses of 1,000 units for the next 3 to 4 hours. All flush solutions (usually normal saline) used for perfusing arterial sheaths and guiding catheters are also heparinized (1,000 to 3,000 units/liter). On the few occasions when a recent intracranial hemorrhage has occurred from a DAVF, no systemic anticoagulation is used, although all flush solutions remain heparinized.

With the development of better second- and third-generation reinforced thin-walled guiding catheters designed specifically for neuroendovascular applications, it is now standard practice to place either a 5- or 6-French (Fr.) guiding catheter into the appropriate cervical artery for subsequent coaxial microcatheterization. These new guiding catheters have a braided wall that resists kinking but possesses a relatively large inner lumen to facilitate coaxial device delivery and continuous flushing with heparinized saline. Most of these guiding catheters come with preformed curves, which allows for relatively easy access into the great vessels through direct guidewire-assisted catheterization in relatively nontortuous aortic arches. In cases of increased vessel tortuosity, these guiding catheters usually can be positioned properly by exchange guidewire technique (typically with a 300-cm hydrophilic coated 0.035-inch nitinol guidewire [Glidewire, Terumo, Japan]). To maximize optimal "pushability" of the various microcatheters used for superselective catheterization, the guiding catheter is positioned as close as technically feasible to the skull base for intracranial catheterization, and variably up the external carotid trunk or proximal internal maxillary artery as needed. Recently, with the increasing use of carotid stent-assisted angioplasty, 90-cm-long 7- or 6-Fr. vascular sheaths inserted through a common femoral can be used as an alternative to the above-mentioned guiding catheters. More commonly, these long sheaths have been used effectively as an adjunct for more secure access into very tortuous and dolicoectatic cervical arteries, using the so-called *triaxial catheterization method.*

A considerable variety of technologically sophisticated microcatheters are now available for both transarterial and transvenous DAVF embolization. These microcatheters can be broadly divided into three categories as follows: guidewire-directed, flow-directed, and hybrid (i.e., possessing mixed properties of the first two groups). Much of the current success of endovascular surgery in effectively treating DAVFs can be linked to the dramatic enhancements made in these microcatheters (e.g., variable stiffness monoextrusion polymers, metallic or polymeric braiding, polytetrafluoroethylene [PTFE] inner lumen coatings, hydrophilic outer coatings) that now permit fairly routine ultrasuperselective catheterization of many more arterial feeding pedicles than was possible just 10 years ago. The selection of a particular microcatheter depends upon several objective and subjective performance factors that likely vary considerably from operator to operator.

With recent developments in the design and availability of hydrophilic flow-directed microcatheter (FDMC) technology, there has been a shift toward increased use of these devices for transarterial management of DAVFs. Currently, it is now feasible to approach all intracranial meningeal arterial supply (e.g., posterior meningeal artery, meningeal branches of the SCA, artery of Davidoff and Schechter, and meningohypophyseal trunk) and many very distal and small ECA feeders to a DAVF (e.g., terminal branches of the occipital and superficial temporal arteries, transmastoidal branches of the occipital artery) with one or more of the new generation 1.8- or 1.5-Fr. FDMCs (e.g., Spinnaker, Target Therapeutics of Boston Scientific; FlowRider, Micro Therapeutics; Magic Olive, Balt).

The overriding rationale for using these FDMCs is to achieve purchase into the most distal portion of feeding pedicles, permitting wedged positioning of the microcatheter tip. This is highly desirable, because wedged positioning essentially translates to operator-dependent flow regulation within the nidal compartment supplied by the catheterized feeder, permitting a more controlled, distal permeation of the targeted vasculature with liquid embolic agents. This very distal positioning of the microcatheter often prove crucial to the success of embolization techniques that rely on flow-control delivery of the liquid embolic agent (Figs. 11-2 and 11-3). Wedged positioning usually can be confirmed on angiography in which the observed flow rate of injected contrast appears to be entirely dependent on the rate of applied pressure from the syringe injection. Repeated test injections are often needed to ensure that significant proximal reflux does not occur.

Navigating the FDMCs into these very distal positions may be difficult owing to one or more of the following

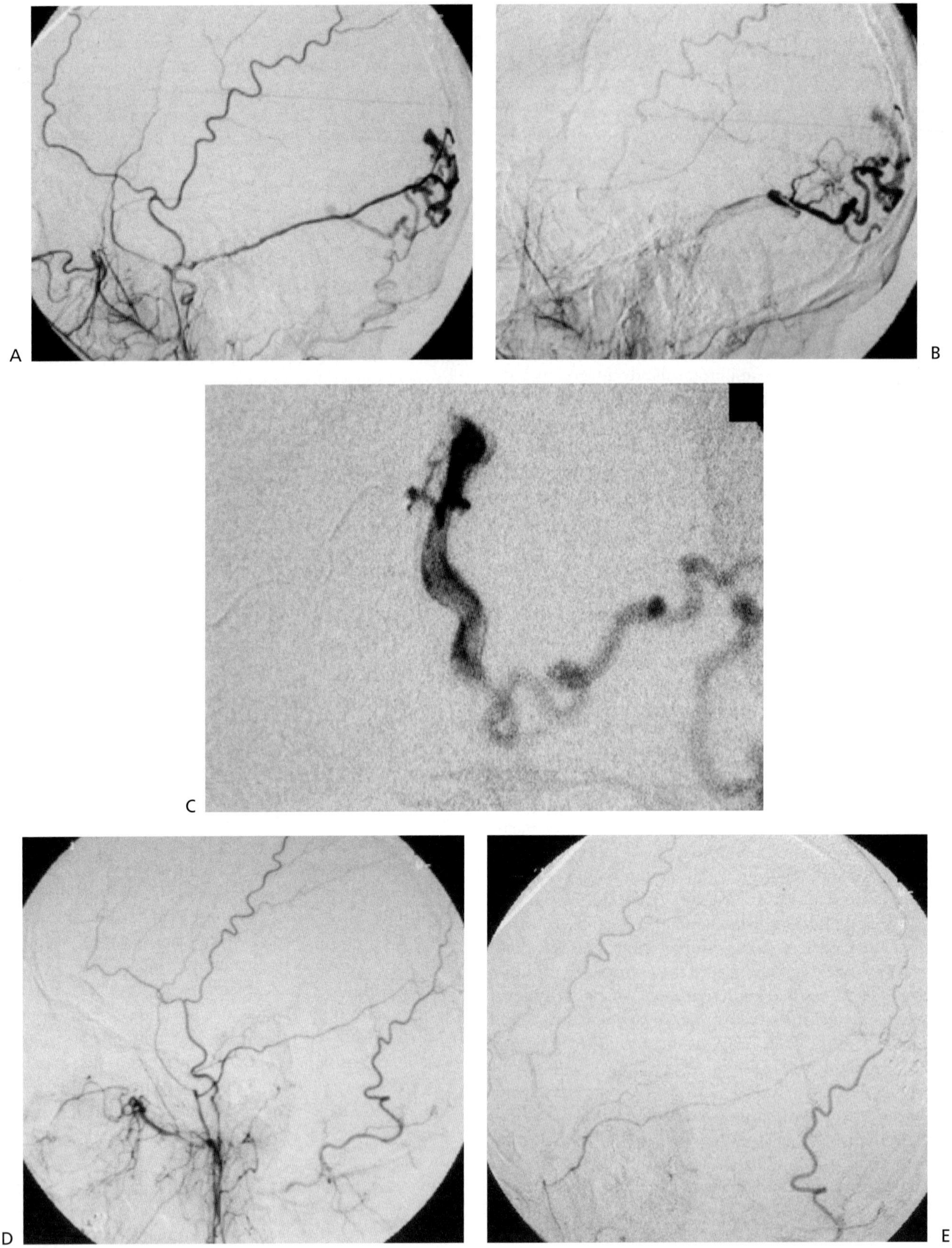

situations: (a) increased tortuosity of the intracranial vasculature, (b) unfavorable angle of origin of a targeted branch, (c) increasingly diminishing caliber of a feeding artery that approximates the outer diameter of the microcatheter, and (d) lack of sufficient AV shunt flow to facilitate flow navigation. Although the enhanced elasticity of the FDMCs makes them highly desirable for superselective catheterization of small and tortuous arteries, their pushability into these vessels is often suboptimal owing to their inherent lack of longitudinal rigidity. This problem can be overcome with one or more of the following adjunctive techniques. With the advent of the newer hydrophilic coated 0.009- to 0.012-inch microguidewires (e.g., Mirage 0.009, Quicksilver 10, Micro Therapeutics; Mizzen HiSupport, Target-Boston Scientific; Gold Tip, Meditech-Terumo) it is now technically possible to increase the pushability performance of FDMCs to that typically seen with conventional over-the-wire braided microcatheters. Owing to a combination of tapered grind profiles and hydrophilic coating, these newer 0.009- to 0.011-inch microguidewires reduce friction encountered during coaxial manipulation through the inner lumen of many FDMCs, permitting more distal placement of the guidewire. Consequently, it is now feasible to place these microguidewires to not only the very distal tip of a FDMC, but sufficiently beyond it in very distal or tortuous intracranial arteries [86,91]. The most popular maneuver now used is to initially advance the guidewire through at least the proximal two-thirds to three-fourths of the FDMC, followed by slow simultaneous advancement of both devices through sharp turns and distal tortuosity of the targeted arterial territory [91,92]. Usually the guidewire is permitted to advance slightly faster than the FDMC, in which the distal tip of the former reaches within approximately 1 cm of the end of the microcatheter. At this point the guidewire is then withdrawn slowly without any additional pushing of the FDMC, and additional advancement of the microcatheter frequently occurs.

A few modifications of the above-described technique for superselective catheterizations of difficult to access vasculature may prove useful. These maneuvers can be classified as either guidewire assisted (which includes the previously described maneuver) or guidewire directed. For the guidewire-assisted techniques, we routinely place the tip of the microguidewire approximately 1 cm beyond the tip of the FDMC. Initially, both the microguidewire and microcatheter are advanced as a unit for as long as possible. Subsequently, some additional resistance from unfavorable vascular tree geometry is encountered. At this point the microguidewire is initially withdrawn 5 to 8 mm while fixing the FDMC in position, followed immediately by re-advancing both devices as a unit to as close as possible to the targeted distal feeding pedicle or nidal vessel. Finally, slow withdrawal of the microguidewire is performed, in which additional advancement of the distal tip of the FDMC may occur. These maneuvers can be repeated as needed to achieve the desired purchase for embolization.

In some situations the guidewire-assisted maneuvers are insufficient to reach the targeted vessel, most commonly as a result of very unfavorable branch origin angulation or other geometric constraints (e.g., 360-degree loops). For such situations the above-mentioned maneuvers can be modified into a guidewire-directed technique, basically consisting of torque manipulation of the microguidewire into the desired branch followed by advancement of the FDMC. However, unlike conventional guidewire-directed microcatheter technique, the FDMC typically will not advance over a fixed microguidewire (i.e., "stripping"). To advance the FDMC, the previously described technique of initial gradual withdrawal of the microguidewire followed by immediate simultaneous advancement of both devices is used.

Use of conventional over-the-wire microcatheters is preferable for many ECA branch superselective catheterizations (e.g., proximal occipital branches, ascending pharyngeal, posterior auricular, and middle meningeal arteries). Currently, our preference is to use the sub–2-Fr. braided micro-

FIGURE 11-2. A 52-year-old right-handed man experienced abrupt onset of a severe left-sided occipital headache and subsequent loss of right visual fields in both eyes. Workup at his local hospital revealed a large intraparenchymal hemorrhage of the left occipital lobe, which was managed conservatively. A catheter angiogram later revealed a DAVF of the dorsal falx tentorial complex near the torcula, supplied by bilateral middle meningeal and occipital arteries. **A,B:** Lateral selective right external carotid angiogram lateral projection in early **(A)** and late **(B)** arterial phases shows a type III DAVF, with congested cortical venous drainage centered around the lateral occipital pole. Supply is from both the posterior division of the middle meningeal artery and transosseous dural branches of the occipital artery. Selective left external carotid injection (not shown) showed a mirror image pattern of arterial supply to the DAVF. **C:** Superselective wedged injection of the terminal portion of the posterior division of the right middle meningeal artery shows the arteriovenous arcade around the recipient cortical vein. From this position a very slow injection of 4:1 ethiodized oil-to-NBCA mixture was used to not only permeate the arteriovenous arcade but also to fill the recipient cortical vein. **D,E:** Right **(D)** and left **(E)** external carotid artery angiograms, lateral projections, confirm complete obliteration of the DAVF. This case illustrates the ability to obliterate definitively the reciprocal arterial supply to a DAVF through a single superselective wedged injection of cyanoacrylate.

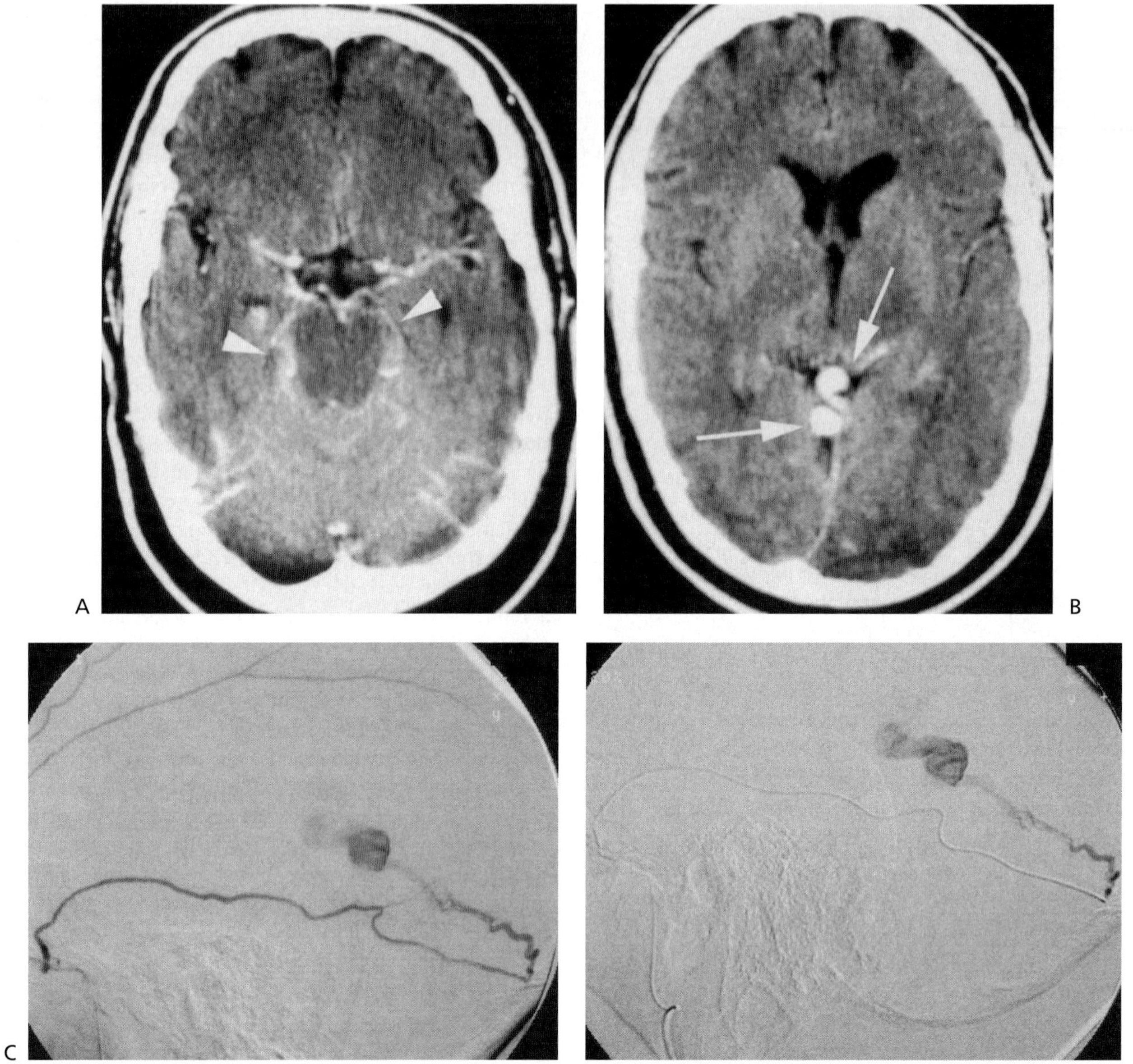

FIGURE 11-3. This 53-year-old man had gradual onset of diplopia, memory problems, and somnolence. **A,B:** Contrast-enhanced CT of the brain at the level of the mesencephalon **(A)** and diencephalon **(B)** shows diffuse swelling and edema associated with perimesencephalic enhancement and mild ectasia of the vein of Galen. **C,D:** Left middle meningeal artery angiograms show a type III DAVF of the galenic system. With the microcatheter in a wedged ultrasuperselective position, a 4:1 ethiodized oil-to-NBCA embolic mixture was injected into the fistula. Unfortunately, the recipient vein could not be completely casted with cyanoacrylate. *(Figure continues.)*

catheters that accept either a 0.014- or 0.010-inch microguidewire (e.g., 1.9- or 1.7-Fr. Prowler, Cordis Neurovascular). These catheters possess excellent pushability and trackability profiles, owing to their reinforced walls, inability to kink, and inner lumen lining with PTFE. The major disadvantages of these microcatheters are their added distal tip stiffness (which increases the risk of dissection or perforation) and poor response to steam shaping and poor memory. In situations in which these disadvantages are a sufficient concern for increased risk of complications or technical failure, it is preferable to use a softer, unbraided hydrophilic microcatheter (FasTracker 18 or 10, Target-Boston Scientific) that has excellent response to steam shaping and excellent memory. As is usually the case, there is a

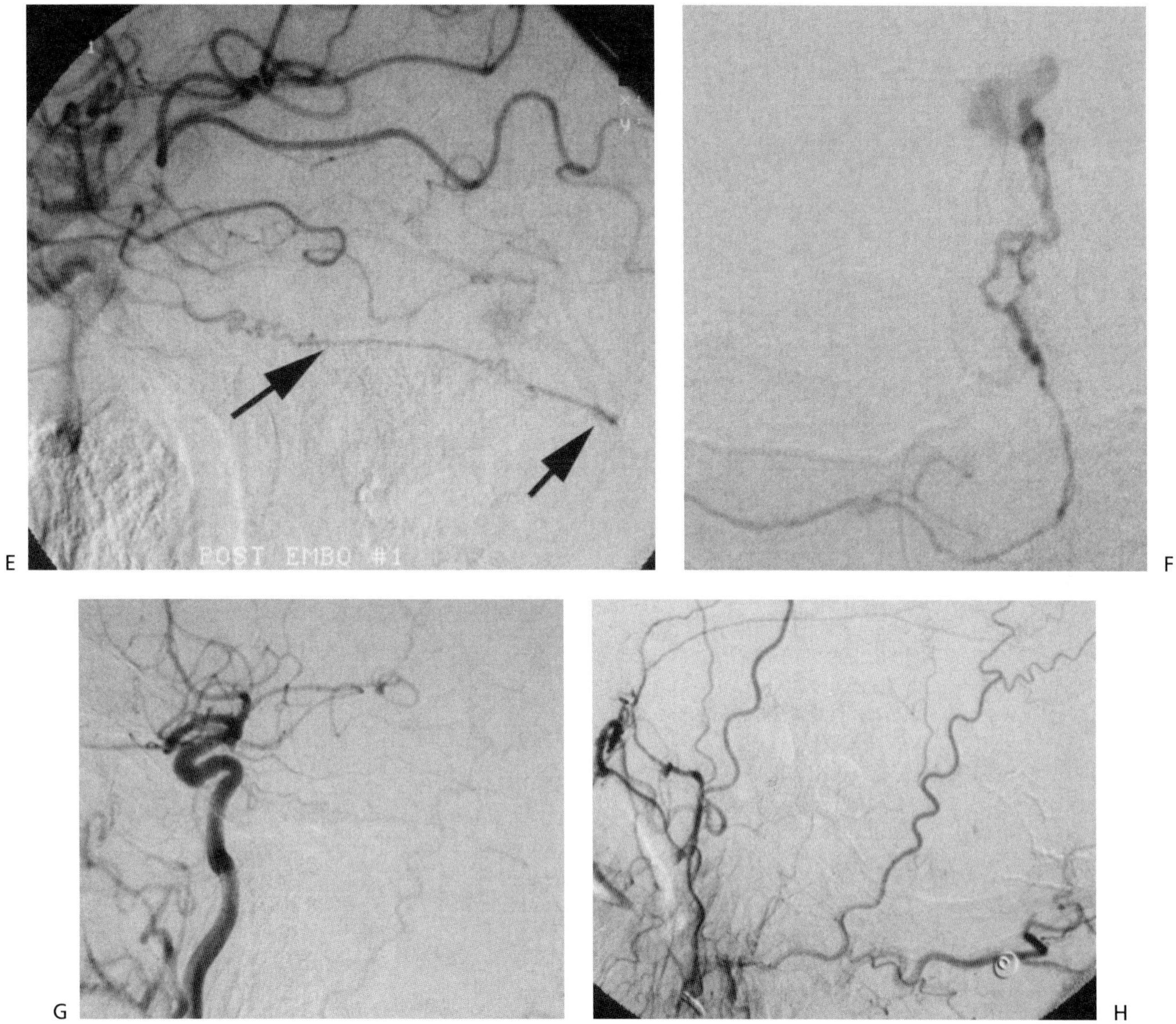

FIGURE 11-3. *Continued.* **E:** Left internal carotid artery angiogram shows persistent flow to the DAVF via the marginal tentorial artery. **F:** Superselective angiogram of the distal left posterior meningeal artery also shows reciprocal supply to the DAVF. Again, a very slow injection of a 4:1 ethiodized oil-to-NBCA mixture was used to permeate the remaining DAVF nidus. **G,H:** Control angiograms from selective left internal and left external carotid arteries show complete angiographic obliteration of the DAVF. A 6-month follow-up angiogram confirmed complete obliteration. This case also illustrates the ability to definitively obliterate DAVFs through reciprocal feeders using ultrasuperselective wedge injection of cyanoacrylate.

substantial trade-off of poorer pushability, increased risk of kinking, and more rapid delamination of these types of microcatheters.

Embolic Materials

Since the first published description of therapeutic embolization of a DAVF in the early 1970s [17], a considerable variety of materials and devices deliverable through microcatheters have been used with varying safety and efficacy. Therapeutic transarterial embolization with particulates (e.g., PVA, microfibrillar collagen, and gel foam), liquid silicone, ethyl alcohol, various nonretrievable and retrievable platinum microcoils, and cyanoacrylates [3,6,9,35,56, 58,60,93–96] all have been described. As noted earlier, transarterial embolization of DAVFs with PVA, either alone or in conjunction with subsequent endovascular operations (e.g., transvenous embolization) or surgical resection, has been used extensively for over two decades. However, the use of this temporary embolic suspension will likely be supplanted by liquid embolic embolization with the currently available liquid adhesives. In addition, newer liquid nonadhesive copolymers, such as ethylene-vinyl alcohol and cellulose acetate, are being developed and evaluated for transarterial embolization [97–101], and may supplant liquid adhesives, owing to their easier technical requirements and more predictable performance characteristics.

Therapeutic embolization of DAVFs with cyanoacrylic liquid adhesives has been performed for two decades, although the efficacy of the technique has evolved within the last several years as a result of the development of better glue formulations [96,102–105]), advances in microcatheter and microguidewire technologies [4,106–109], and better delivery techniques [6,35,86,91,92]. Liquid adhesive intranidal embolization with N-butyl cyanoacrylate (NBCA) currently provides a level of enhanced efficacy and safety that cannot be matched by other materials and techniques. The effective use of liquid adhesives requires tremendous personal commitment, training, and experience, owing to a combination of the more rigorous technical demands in preparation and delivery of the embolic agent, and its relatively unforgiving nature for technical error. Even in skilled and experienced hands, NBCA suspensions with ethiodized oil and tantalum powder exhibit a certain degree of unpredictability with regard to important physical and chemical properties (e.g., polymerization rate, binding, and viscosity), making it a less than ideal embolic agent [98,104,110–112].

Transvenous embolization of DAVFs also has become an essential tool in the therapeutic armamentarium of endovascular surgeons. A variety of embolic materials, including detachable balloons, liquid adhesives, silk suture, copper wire, and platinum and stainless steel coils, have been tried and used successfully for transvenous embolization of DAVFs [9,31,113–115]. In particular, nonretrievable platinum microcoils (e.g., Tornado, Cook; Target) and larger stainless steel coils (e.g., Gianturco and Hilal coils, Cook), which can be delivered through either microcatheters or standard diagnostic angiographic catheters, have been and to some degree continue to be the preferred embolic devices. However, since the advent of detachable platinum coil technology over the last decade (e.g., Guglielmi detachable coil [GDC], Target-Boston Scientific; spherical and helical detachable coils, Micrus), these devices have become increasingly important for transvenous embolization. These retrievable and detachable coils are particularly useful in situations in which a high degree of precision is needed for depositing the embolic device within a targeted segment of the affected dural sinus or cortical vein. This is also true of difficult access targets (e.g., absent or hypoplastic inferior petrosal sinus, marginal sinus, adjacent cortical veins), whereby only a small-caliber microcatheter (e.g., 1.7- or 1.8-Fr.) can be navigated into the proper position. Furthermore, the ability to reposition and retrieve these coils makes them especially useful when there is unstable or marginal access to the targeted venous compartment. Finally, retrievable and detachable coil technology is extremely useful (if not essential) for performing transvenous embolizations of DAVFs with exceptionally high shunt flow, permitting the operator to test the behavior of the coils exposed to the torrent of blood flow without the risk of inadvertent and uncontrolled migration.

The preparation and formulation of the liquid adhesive embolic mixture we use is an iterative adaptation of previously described mixtures of cyanoacrylate, iodized oil, and inert metallic powders [99,96,105,111,116]. In the past we used a medical grade formulation of NBCA (Histoacryl Blue, Braun), which was permitted only on a compassionate use basis. Recently Cordis Neurovascular Systems was able to obtain Food and Drug Administration approval of their formulation of NBCA after successful completion of a multicenter randomized clinical trial to demonstrate equivalent safety compared to PVA embolization of brain AVMs. Consequently, we are now routinely using this formulation of cyanoacrylate for most transarterial embolizations of high-flow vascular malformations. We have noted some significant differences in physical behavior between Histoacryl and Trufill NBCA. Most important of these is the characteristically longer polymerization times seen with the latter, in which relative differences in the rate of polymerization varied from two- to fourfold [117,118]. Depending on the technique used for delivery of the acrylic embolic suspension, this difference could be advantageous (e.g., for flow-arrest intranidal embolization) or problematic (e.g., free-flow injections).

Consistency and reliability require a fairly rigid and ritualized routine for preparing the liquid adhesive embolic mixture. This ensures the highest degree of uniformity of the suspension and minimizes potential adverse technical outcomes, such as premature polymerization, component separation, and metallic powder precipitation, that are not infrequently encountered. When mixing the components of the suspension, we use a well-cleaned, sterile "shot" glass to permit better continuous visual monitoring of the material prior to its aspiration into a syringe. Typically 0.1 to 0.2 cc of powdered tantalum is placed within one side of the bottom of the mixing container (which is kept slightly tilted), followed by injection of iodized oil (Ethiodol, Savage Labs, Melville, NY) or iodized oil (Lipidiol). These components are mixed steadily with a needle cap, while the NBCA is being drawn into another 1-ml syringe. While keeping the mixing container partially tilted, the NBCA is injected slowly into the tantalum-oil suspension through a 21-gauge needle that is submerged within the suspension. The resulting three-component embolic suspension is then mixed thoroughly, until immediately before the embolization is to be performed. At that time, the mixture is slowly aspirated through a 23-gauge needle (which minimizes aggregation of tantalum particles) into a solvent-resistant 1-ml Luer-Lok syringe.

A few different types of conventional and so-called hybrid techniques of liquid adhesive injection are used, which has been driven by the changing technical requirements and performance of transarterial embolization of high-flow vascular malformations [86]. Traditionally, liquid adhesive embolization has been classified into either "full-column" [92, 119] or "sandwich" [6,120,121] injection techniques. The former has been classically used for wedged injection embolizations, through the use of a relatively large volume of embolic mixture (typically between 1 and 3 ml), injected slowly and continuously through the microcatheter. In contrast, the sandwich delivery technique originally was developed for "free-flow" injections of relatively small aliquots of the cyanoacrylate mixture that would ideally be pushed through the microcatheter in a closely confined bolus. Either type of injection techniques can be modified to effectively deliver liquid adhesive mixtures in a wide spectrum of flow conditions that are encountered during cerebral AVM embolization.

The sandwich technique, which consists of flushing and filling the microcatheter dead space with a 10% dextrose solution, may prove very useful for free-flow liquid embolization. This solution acts as an ion buffer by formation of hydration shells around the dextrose molecules, thus diminishing free movement of hydroxyl ions that may initiate anionic polymerization of the NBCA monomer. The liquid adhesive mixture is then placed or "loaded" typically within two plastic appliances (a three-way and a one-way stopcock) and the hub of the microcatheter, being introduced by a separate 1-ml Luer-Lok syringe through the three-way stopcock. When embolization is to be performed, another 1-ml Luer-Lok syringe filled with 10% dextrose is attached to the other port of the three-way stopcock, permitting pushing of the interposed bolus of liquid adhesive through and eventually out of the microcatheter.

By estimating various parameters such as the rate of flow, distance to the targeted pathology, and volume of vasculature within the lesion, the operator can estimate the appropriate polymerization time and volume of the bolus needed to optimally occlude the targeted nidus and feeding pedicle without excessive filling of the venous drainage of the cerebral AVM. Polymerization times can be modified significantly by changing the ratio of iodized oil to NBCA, with increasing ratios resulting in significantly longer polymerization times. The precise timing of polymerization derived from a particular formulation of liquid adhesive that results in occlusion of the targeted vasculature generally is not possible, owing to the multitude of parameters that likely affect this process (e.g., flow rate, injection rate, inadvertent mixing with dextrose solution; mixing with blood; size, length, and tortuosity of feeding arteries; number and configuration of nidal vessels) [86,104,117]. Only a few studies have attempted to quantify the actual rate of polymerization of medical grade cyanoacrylates (i.e., isobutyl cyanoacrylate and N-butyl cyanoacrylate) using either indirect optical density measurements within small aliquots of plasma or *in vivo* animal models [96]. Although some degree of quantification was possible with the simple bench top *in vitro* tests, showing nonlinear variability of polymerization time related to varying ratios of acrylic, iodized oil, and acetic acid, the data derived from these studies was not directly transferable to clinical practice. Therefore, the utility of such measurements is of questionable value, because the various above-mentioned anatomical and hemodynamic parameters that influence polymerization time and binding of a given liquid adhesive mixture in a real clinical setting have not been taken into account [104,117].

In some situations a modified free-flow delivery of liquid adhesive can be performed using a full-column injection. As with the sandwich technique, preembolization flushing and subsequent loading of the microcatheter with 10% dextrose is essential to prevent premature polymerization of the cyanoacrylate as it traverses the microcatheter. In this technical modification the liquid adhesive mixture needs to be injected relatively rapidly to overcome the intrinsic pulse-pressure gradient within the catheterized vessel. A good preconceived estimate of the volume of embolic agent needed to fill the intravascular space of the targeted vessels completely is essential for successful execution, as well as an operator's ability to modify rapidly the pressure and rate of injection of the embolic agent as rapid changes in flow are visualized under continuous fluoroscopy. This particular technique requires considerable practice and experience.

For wedged flow-controlled embolizations, both the sandwich and full-column delivery techniques may be used. When it is estimated that the targeted compartment will require a relatively small volume of embolic agent, it may be preferable to use the sandwich technique. In contrast, when larger targeted vascular volumes are anticipated it is preferable to use the full-column delivery technique to ensure that enough volume of embolic agent is delivered. In either type of delivery technique, longer polymerization times are desirable. For such wedge injection embolizations, the ratio of ethiodized oil to NBCA is in the range of 3:1 to 5:1. Interestingly, the flow-controlled injection techniques are best performed with extremely slow rates of injection, in which injection times of 30 to 40 seconds are typical, and may be up to 1 to 2 minutes. Some degree of reflux past the tip of the microcatheter is inevitable and is generally used as an end-point indicator of the embolization. With the advent of the new hydrophilic coatings on most contemporary microcatheters, inadvertent bonding of the microcatheter tip to the vessel is much less likely to occur [122].

These injection times are orders of magnitude greater than the polymerization times that had been measured by prior *in vitro* bench top experiments. Therefore, it is likely that alternative physical mechanics must be in effect to explain this phenomenon. Based on *in vitro* experiments of polymerization and bonding mechanics [117,118,123], we have hypothesized that during wedged injection conditions, the minute targeted vasculature is flooded with the liquid adhesive mixture. In such a situation, there is little availability or mixing of electron donor species to initiate polymerization, except at the perimeter of the advancing embolic bolus (where it contacts the inner wall of the vessel). Consequently, a thin outer skin of polymer is formed that contains an inner liquid embolic mixture (unpolymerized cyanoacrylate). This thin skin is easily ruptured by the rise in intraluminal pressure generated by slow injection through a syringe, resulting in continuing propagations of the embolic bolus into multiple nidal vessels.

It is generally accepted that embolization with liquid adhesives is less likely to develop recanalization and is more likely to reach the site of fistulous communication [6,91, 92,120,121], although recanalization of vessels embolized with acrylic mixtures has been reported occasionally [71]. The likelihood of a durable embolization with liquid adhesives probably increases when superselective microcatheterization is performed to achieve wedged flow-control conditions, or when relatively large volumes are delivered in modified free-flow conditions. In such cases complete casting of not only the targeted nidal vasculature, but also the most proximal associated draining veins, is desirable to minimize the chance of thrombus resorption and recanalization.

Adjunctive Management and Techniques

The major potential neurologic complications of endovascular surgical management of DAVFs include hemorrhage, cerebral ischemic injury (both arterial and venous), cerebral edema from venous congestion, cranial nerve injuries (ischemic and compressive), and direct neurotoxicity (induced by contrast media or degradation products of cyanoacrylate). In considering these most commonly encountered complications, a simple prophylactic cerebroprotective regimen for patients undergoing cerebral AVM embolization is suggested. This regimen is aimed at minimizing neuronal ischemia or injury related to some of the more important common pathways of pathogenesis, including the calcium ischemic cascade, membrane destabilization, inflammatory injury, alternating depolarization and repolarization instabilities, and microvascular homeostasis. An exhaustive review of the pathoetiologic mechanisms and putative therapies is beyond the scope of this chapter. The interested reader should refer to some recent excellent reviews on the topic [8,124–127]. There remains controversy regarding the actual efficacy of these measures due to lack of properly designed clinical studies. Consequently, these management paradigms have been implemented variably from center to center, resulting in a lack of consensus on what is considered the standard of practice for endovascular therapeutic procedures.

Because many of the newer pharmacologic therapies directed at various mechanisms of neuronal ischemia and injury remain investigational or unproven (e.g., NMDA and non-NMDA antagonists, antioxidants, free radical scavengers, nitric oxide inhibitors, etc.), there is in reality only a limited repertoire of agents that can be used presently. It is likely, however, that within the next 5 years additional effective therapies will become available that can be added to or will supplant currently used agents.

The regimen we use is similar to the one used for preemptive cerebral protection for brain AVM embolization [86]. Just prior to the start of each embolization session, the patient is premedicated with 10 mg dexamethasone (Decadron) intravenously, 60 mg nimodipine orally, and an anticonvulsant (typically a loading dose of 18mg/kg phenytoin intravenously). If postembolization reactive edema is anticipated, or if there is preexisting venous congestion or hemorrhage, or both, osmotic diuresis is initiated with mannitol or hypertonic saline. For uncomplicated cases the dexamethasone is tapered rapidly (typically at 6-, 4-, and 2-mg intervals) over a period of 24 to 48 hours, while the nimodipine is administered for 48 hours at 60 mg every 4 hours. When osmotic diuretics are used, they are typically administered for no longer than 48 hours. The anticonvulsant therapy is maintained for an extended period that typically lasts for a minimum of 3 months in patients without clinical seizures, and at least 1 year in patients who have suffered seizures before or during their treatment.

In addition to the above cerebroprotective regimen, a variety of other medications are administered during and after an embolization session. Although there has been a trend toward performing more of the cerebral AVM embolizations under general anesthesia, many patients still undergo the procedure under awake sedation. In these cases a modified neuroleptanalgesic regimen is used, consisting of intermittent dosages of midazolam (1 to 2 mg loading, 0.5 mg every 1 to 2 hours maintenance) and fentanyl (25 to 50 μg loading). Additional doses of analgesics (usually fentanyl 25 to 50 μg, or morphine sulphate 2 to 3 mg intravenously every hour) are frequently administered as needed to ameliorate episodic headaches that typically are associated with either rigorous superselective navigation or rapid withdrawal of the microcatheter following cyanoacrylate injection. With the frequent occurrence of intense headaches combined with the need of repeat administration of short-acting opiates, episodic nausea and vomiting may be encountered. Therefore prophylactic or reactive administration of rapidly acting antiemetics, such as promethazine (12.5 to 25 mg intramuscularly), prochlorperazine (5 to 10 mg orally or rectally), trimethobenzamide (200 mg intramuscularly, orally, or rectally), or dimenhydrinate (50 mg orally), is often needed. Finally, with the administration of corticosteroids, it is also necessary to administer an ulcer prophylaxis regimen, typically using a histamine-2 blocker, ranitidine (150 mg orally twice a day) or cimetidine (300 mg intravenously every 8 hours).

Blood pressure management may also be beneficial in reducing hemorrhagic complications during and immediately after therapeutic embolization of DAVFs associated with cortical venous reflux or direct drainage. Dysfunctional autoregulation in regions of the brain affected by venous ischemia or prior hemorrhage are predisposed to perfusion breakthrough edema and hemorrhage. In most cases, patients treated with nimodipine as part of the standard cerebroprotective cocktail will have a slight-to-mild decrease in their baseline systemic blood pressure, which is usually sustained during the length of the embolization session. However, some patients (particularly those undergoing treatment under awake sedation or those with underlying hypertension) may develop significant rises in blood pressure, which need to be corrected promptly. In many cases readministration of sedation and analgesia will correct the problem. Short-acting antihypertensives that can be administered by rapid intravenous infusion, such as labetalol (10 to 20 mg intravenously, initial dose), esmolol (500 μg/kg over 1 minute loading, 50 μg/kg over the next 4 minutes), and hydralazine (10 to 60 mg intravenously) should be tried first. If the hypertension remains intractable, it may be necessary to start a continuous infusion of nitroprusside (0.5 to 8 μg/kg per minute).

Special Clinical and Technical Considerations of Selected Dural Arteriovenous Fistulas

Sigmoid Transverse Sinuses

The sigmoid transverse sinus (STS) has been reported to be the most frequently encountered location for DAVF [3, 4,9,10,30,35]. Lesions occurring in the approximate anatomical region of these contiguous major dural sinuses have been lumped together, mostly for the sake of simplifying their classification and their relatively uniform clinical features (i.e., nearly all patients develop subjective pulsatile tinnitus). In reality, these DAVFs are very heterogeneous with regard to precise anatomical localization (e.g., exclusive involvement of the sigmoid sinus or the transverse sinus versus involvement of both sinuses), angioarchitecture, and pattern of normal intracranial venous drainage. These variables profoundly influence not only the clinical behavior and natural history but also the technical difficulties and risks associated with endovascular surgical management. For example, many of the DAVFs that involve the sigmoid sinus exclusively have less extensive ECA supply (that in turn may be more effectively treated by transarterial embolization alone), and a lower risk of complication associated with transvenous embolization. Conversely, DAVFs with exclusive involvement of the dominant (usually right) transverse sinus are likely to have more extensive arterial supply and be associated with a relatively higher risk of transvenous embolization complications.

Fortunately, most DAVFs of the STS complex are not associated with actual or potential risk of serious neurologic sequelae. Therefore, in these cases, indications for endovascular management are dictated by the severity and duration of symptoms. The most common complaints that ultimately lead to intervention are severe pulsatile tinnitus or intractable headaches, or both, that interfere substantially with quality of life. A careful risk-benefit analysis is advisable in these latter situations, because patients with such subjective complaints may be unwilling to accept even transient neurologic complications related to therapy. In stark contrast, STS DAVFs that exhibit either overt or potential aggressive clinical behavior generally have been considered less frequently encountered. As described earlier, the basic pathophysiologic mechanism responsible for many of these complications can be related to the consequences of diversion of arterialized shunt flow into cortical veins. Transient ischemic attacks, cerebrovascular accident, intracerebral hemorrhage, subarachnoid and subdural hemorrhage, progressive motor deficits, ataxia, memory dysfunction, visual disturbances, and seizures have all been reported to occur in association with aggressive STS DAVFs [13,14,16,20, 23,29,31] (Fig. 11-4). Rarely, neurologic deficits may be due to either generalized intracranial venous hypertension (particularly in association with intracranial venoocclusive disease) or mass effect from a large varix. The actual proportion of these more aggressive lesions encountered in a given clinical practice is likely highly dependent on referral bias.

As previously discussed, endovascular surgical treatment of STS DAVFs can be accomplished by both transarterial and transvenous approaches. Owing to a combination of superior microcatheterization technology and improvements in liquid embolization techniques, we increasingly favor aggressive transarterial approaches as the first (and not infrequently only) mode of therapy (Fig. 11-5). This is in direct contrast to conventional teaching less than a decade ago, when it was uniformly recognized that transarterial embolization of such malformations rarely, if ever, resulted in definitive treatment. This belief to a large extent was linked to the acknowledged lack of permanent occlusion achieved when particulate embolization of a STS DAVF is performed (which has been the popular mode of therapy here in the United States). Consequently, in the past, indications for transarterial embolization have been limited to cases of palliative reduction of shunt flow or in preparation for a planned transvenous occlusion of the involved segment of dura. In many cases, however, the latter may not be necessary owing to the effectiveness of transvenous embolization used alone.

The blood supply to STS DAVFs can be quite variable, although most commonly transmastoidal branches of the

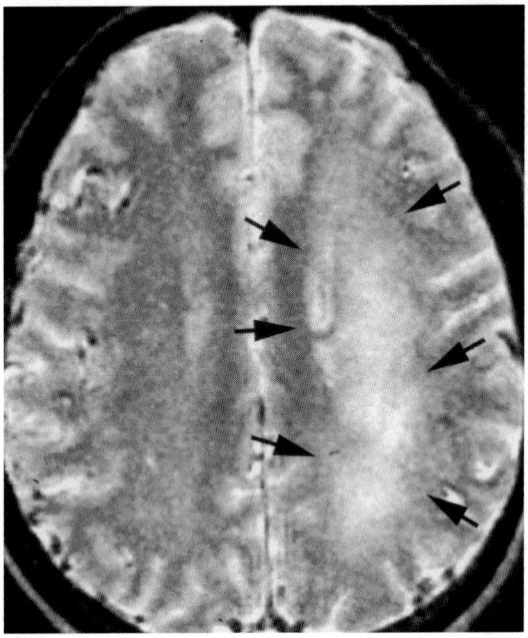

A

FIGURE 11-4. This 69-year-old man was referred for an MRI study of the brain. His family reported that, over the past few months, he was becoming very slow to understand things, progressively lethargic and confused, and his speech was clipped and slow. Workup demonstrated bilateral STS DAVFs. **A:** Pretreatment axial T2-weighted MRI at the level of the centrum semiovale demonstrates extensive white matter edema in the left hemisphere *(arrows).* **B,C:** Anterior projections from a left external carotid artery angiogram in early arterial and mid-venous phases, respectively. This demonstrates a left sigmoid sinus fistula with multiple sites of fistulous communication. The sigmoid jugular outflow is thrombosed and there is retrograde filling of the left transverse sinus to the level of the Torcular. **B:** From here drainage is into the straight sinus *(arrow).* **C:** Multiple cortical veins were noted to fill from the transverse sinuses bilaterally and the straight sinus *(arrows).* (type IIb). Note that the right transverse sinus is also disconnected from normal outflow. The site of the more proximal fistulous communication in the sigmoid sinus is marked by an *arrowhead* in Fig. 11-8C. **D:** Superselective injection of the left occipital artery lateral projection demonstrating the fistula in the left sigmoid sinus *(arrowhead).* Reflux drainage into the vein of Labbé and straight sinus *(arrows)* are noted on this early phase of the angiogram. **E:** Left external carotid artery angiogram late venous phase lateral projection. This late venous phase of the external carotid artery angiogram demonstrates extensive flow into the superior sagittal sinus *(arrows)* from a plethora of cortical veins. *(Figure continues.)*

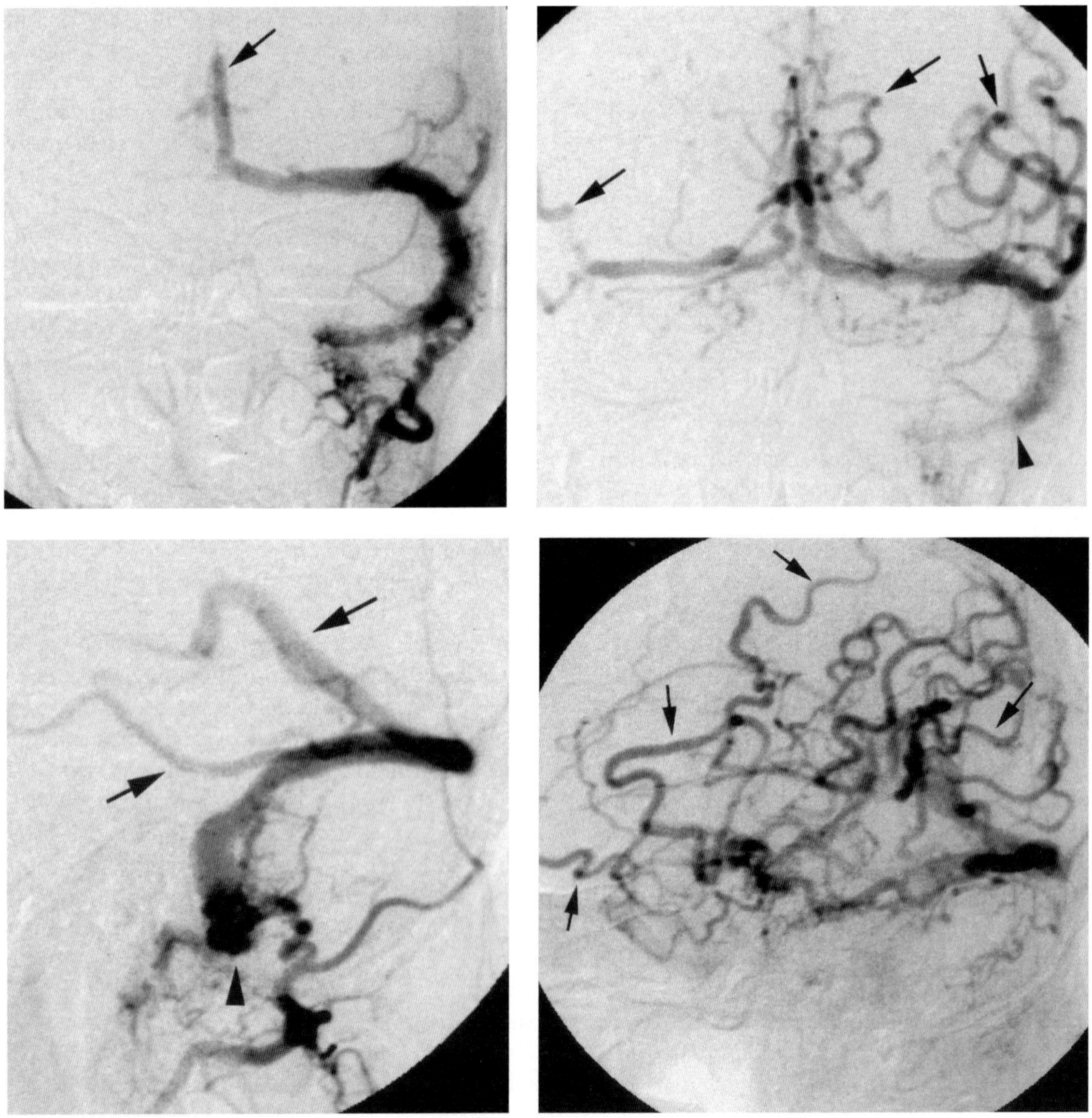

B C

D E

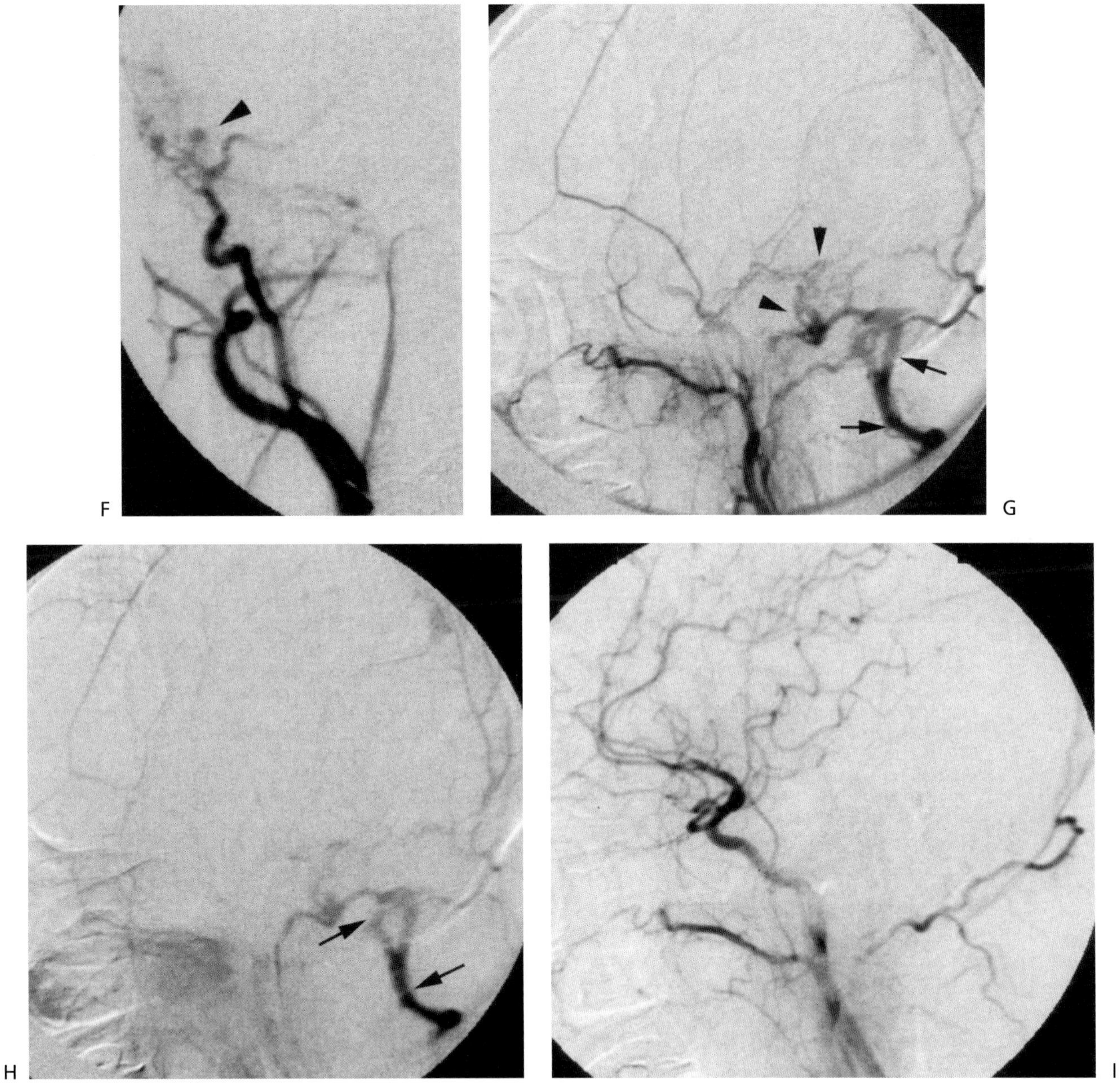

FIGURE 11-4. *Continued.* **F:** Right external carotid artery angiogram early arterial phase. This demonstrates a contralateral right sigmoid sinus fistula *(arrowhead)* **G,H:** Right external carotid artery angiogram lateral projection from midarterial and late venous phases, respectively, demonstrates the sigmoid sinus fistula *(arrowheads)* **(G).** The drainage is noted to go via transosseus veins into extraossesus muscular veins *(arrows).* This right hemispheric drainage is very different from the cortical venous drainage of the left hemisphere and accounts for the asymmetry in the venous hypertensive edema seen more exclusively in the left hemisphere on the MRI. The patient underwent superselective catheterization of the arterial supply to both the right and left fistulas. Dilute ethiodized oil-to-NBCA liquid embolization was performed selectively in all of the feeding branches. **I:** Right common carotid artery control angiogram lateral projection postembolization demonstrates that there is no filling of the right STS DAVF. *(Figure continues.)*

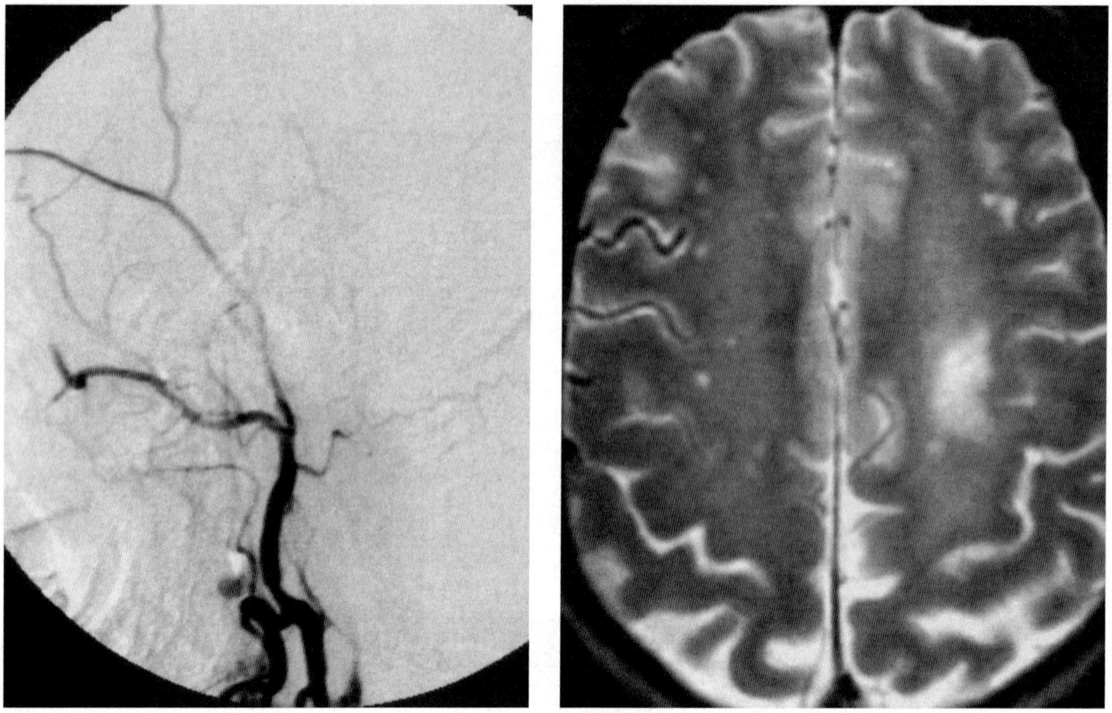

J K

FIGURE 11-4. *Continued.* **J:** Left external carotid artery control angiogram lateral projection post embolization demonstrates there is no filling of the left STS fistula. **K:** Axial T2-weighted MRI obtained approximately 3 months after therapy at the same level as the MRI shown in **(A).** A residual area of high signal is noted in the left hemisphere white matter. This was thought to represent an area of deep white matter infarct. The marked asymmetry in the white matter signal between the left and right hemispheres has significantly improved. The patient was reported by his family to be markedly improved. At follow-up in clinic he was observed to be alert and appropriate and had normal language function. (From Michael P. Marks and Huy M. Do, unpublished material, with permission.)

occipital and posterior auricular arteries, as well as posterior division branches of the middle meningeal artery, are dominant suppliers. Other commonly encountered feeders may arise from the neuromeningeal trunk of the ascending pharyngeal artery, posterior meningeal branch of the vertebral artery, and the marginal tentorial artery of Bernasconi and Casanari. Effective and durable transarterial embolization is highly dependent on successful delivery of a permanent liquid embolic agent into the actual "nidus" of the DAVF (i.e., site of microfistulous connections within the dura). Therefore, the ultimate success of transarterial embolization of STS DAVFs is linked to important anatomical and angioarchitectural characteristics of the lesion. Factors that favor definitive treatment of STS DAVFs with exclusively transarterial embolization include isolated involvement of the sigmoid sinus, fewer major feeding pedicles (<5), shorter

FIGURE 11-5. A 38-year-old man abruptly experienced focal motor and complex seizures after suffering from moderate headaches weeks before. An MRI of the brain showed right temporal lobe edema and abnormal cortical vascularity (not shown). **A,B:** Selective right external carotid artery angiograms, lateral projection, in early and late phases, respectively, show a type IIb DAVF affecting a partially thrombosed transverse sigmoid sinus complex. The DAVF is supplied by numerous feeders from the occipital, posterior auricular, ascending pharyngeal, and middle meningeal arteries. Note the extensive congested cortical venous drainage over the temporal lobe on the late phase of the angiogram *(arrows),* **(B). C,D:** Stage 1 transarterial embolization. Superselective angiograms of two major feeding branches of the occipital artery show multicompartmental supply to the DAVF. **E:** These occipital feeders, as well as those from the posterior auricular, were embolized serially with aliquots of 4:1 iodized oil-to-NBCA mixture. Note the small quantity of glue that was placed inadvertently within two of the draining cortical veins *(arrowheads).* **F:** Lateral control angiogram from selective right external carotid angiogram shows residual DAVF supplied by branches of the middle meningeal artery *(arrows). (Figure continues.)*

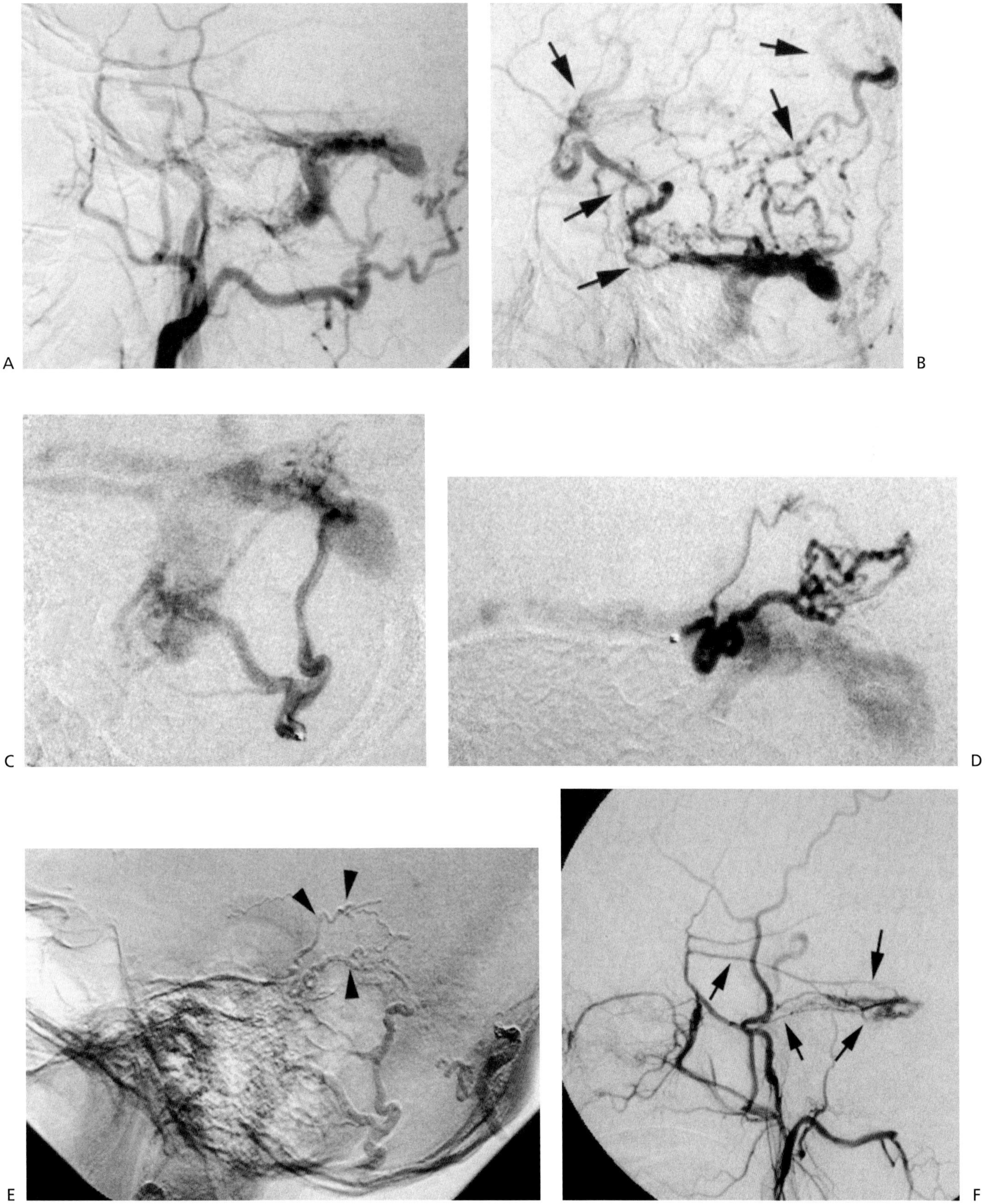
A
B
C
D
E
F

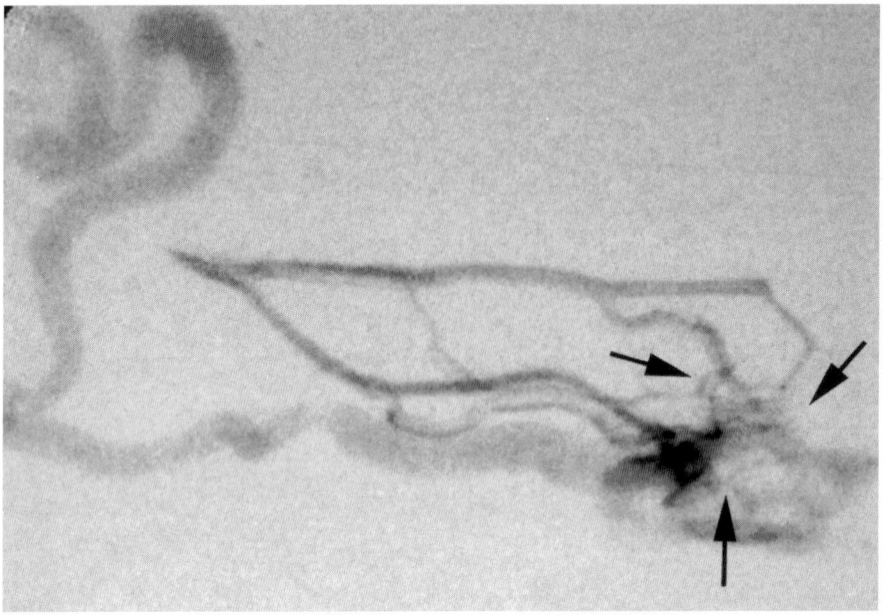

G

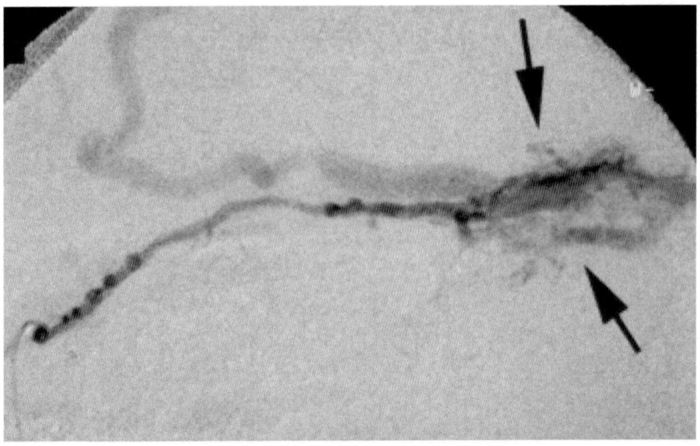

H

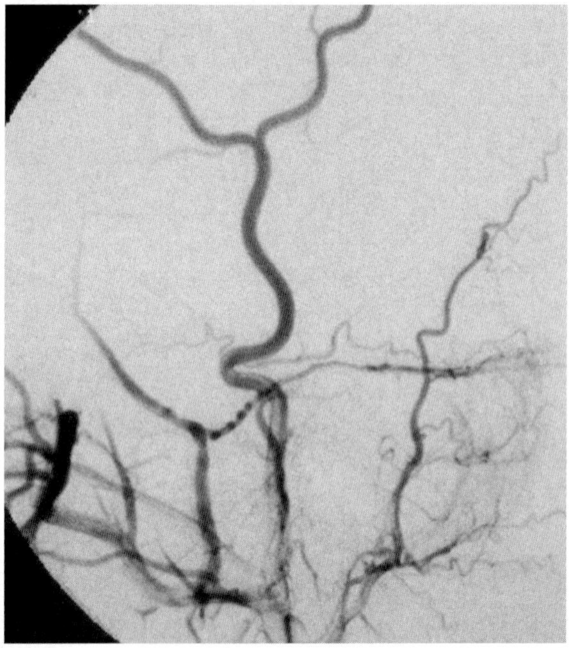

I

FIGURE 11-5. *Continued.* **G,H:** Stage 2 transarterial embolization. Superselective angiograms of the posterior division **(G)** and petrosal branch **(H)** of the middle meningeal artery, lateral projections, show arterial supply to the DAVF. Through these feeders, very slow injections of 4:1 iodized oil-to-NBCA mixture were used to permeate the DAVF nidus. **I:** Final control right external carotid angiogram, lateral projection, shows complete obliteration of the DAVF. A 7-month follow-up angiogram confirmed durable occlusion of the DAVF.

lengths of sinus involvement (<2 cm), and coexistent dural sinus occlusive disease (Fig. 11-6).

When definitive cure of a STS DAVF is mandatory, it is still often necessary to occlude the affected portion(s) of the dural sinus. Unfortunately, there are inherent risks associated with such intentional occlusions, which relate to loss of normal venous outflow of portions of the brain. If it is uncertain whether the diseased segment of dural sinus is acting as a conduit for normal venous drainage, then a balloon test occlusion of the dural sinus can be performed to evaluate potential tolerance to permanent occlusion. However, the reliability of this provocative test is questionable at best (see Superior Sagittal Sinus section). In situations where the STS complex is deemed essential for normal cerebral venous drainage, endovascular stenting may be considered to maintain the patency of the sinus as a downstream conduit and possibly simultaneously ablate the microfistulas within the wall of the affected dural sinus [128]. Otherwise, open surgical disconnection of cortical venous drainage and local fulguration may be the only option for a definitive cure.

The relatively large diameter of the STS complex, combined with the torrent of shunted blood flow often associated with these DAVFs, has posed some significant technical challenges and limitations when attempting transvenous embolization. In the past, many advocated use of larger-caliber platinum and stainless steel coils compatible with 0.018- to 0.035-inch catheters. However, these pushable coils can deploy unpredictably through the delivery catheter and migrate into unintended sites (e.g., normal adjacent dural sinus, lungs). This is particularly true when the coils are not sized properly. In an attempt to minimize this problem, correct sizing of coils can be assisted by placing either an external radiopaque marker of known dimensions (e.g., dime) near the STS complex [31], placing a guiding catheter with known outer diameter in the field of digital subtraction angiography acquisition, or the use of quantitative digital subtraction angiography available with most new biplane neuroangiography equipment. It is often highly preferable to, at the very least, start and finish transvenous embolizations of any dural sinus with the currently available detachable platinum coil systems (GDC, Target-Boston Scientific; ACT-PMS, Micrus). Use of these systems permits repositioning, better sizing, and generally tighter packing than the nondetachable fibered coils, adding safety and precision to the procedure.

Once transvenous embolization has been initiated, it is imperative to occlude completely the involved segment of sinus in order to avoid diversion of shunt flow into normal cortical veins. To accomplish this goal it is critical to perform very tight packing of the dural sinus with sequentially smaller coils in a given segment targeted for therapeutic occlusion. This strategy is similar to the current endovascular surgical technique applied to occluding intracranial aneurysms. Mixing the detachable coils with the more thrombogenic nondetachable coils may be a good compromise for occluding large segments of the STS complex, whereby the enhanced safety and precision of the transvenous occlusion

A

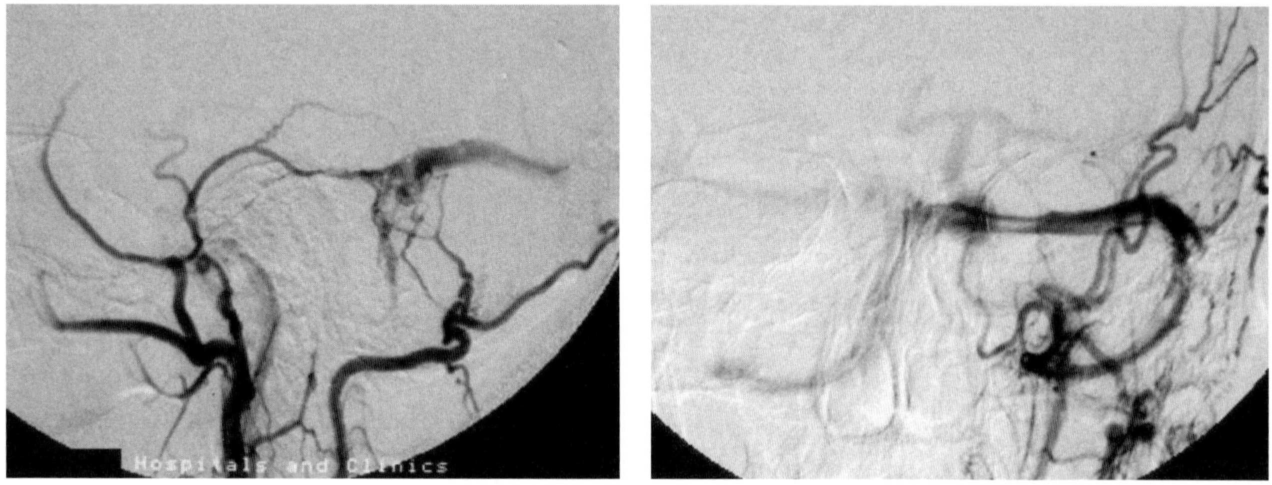

B

C

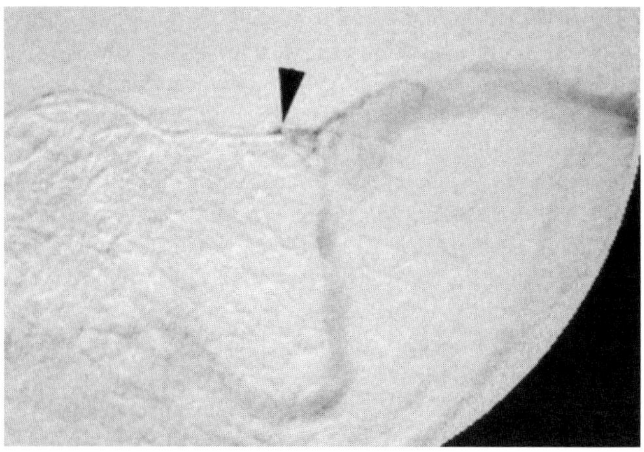

FIGURE 11-6. A 50-year-old woman with a 3-year history of initially mild pulsatile tinnitus. At the time she sought medical care she underwent a diagnostic angiogram at another institution, which showed a type I DAVF of the transverse sigmoid sinus junction. Expectant management was recommended. She subsequently presented for treatment with progressive severe headaches and worsening of her pulsatile tinnitus. **A,B:** Selective left external carotid angiograms, anterior and lateral projections, respectively, show a DAVF of the transverse sigmoid sinus complex with associated partial sinus thrombosis and retrograde sinus venous drainage (type IIa). Arterial supply is the petrosal branch of the middle meningeal artery and transmastoidal branches of the occipital artery. **C:** Superselective angiogram, lateral projection, of the terminal portion of the middle meningeal artery petrosal branch, shows the plexiform fistulous connections to the dural sinus. *Arrowhead* marks catheter tip. This was embolized with a 4:1 iodized oil-to-NBCA mixture. *(Figure continues.)*

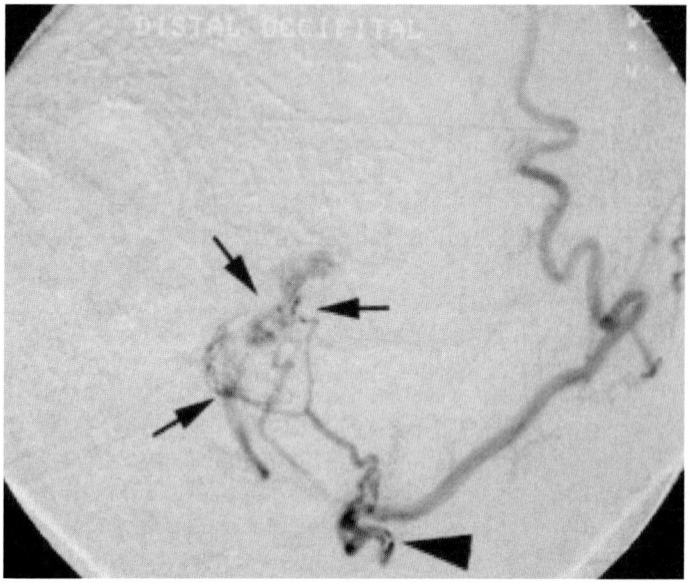

D

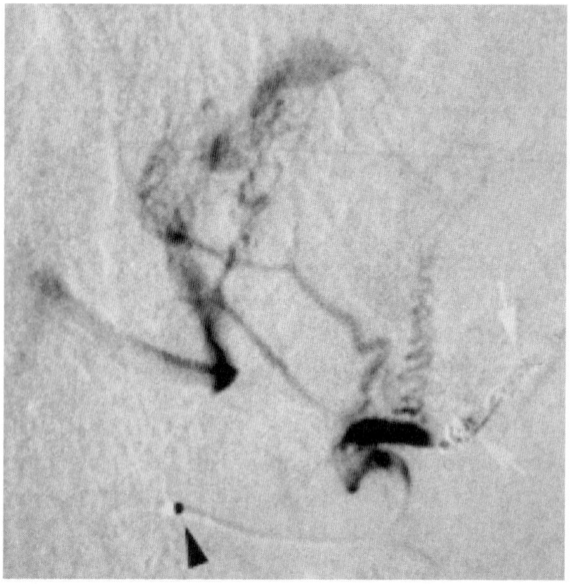

E

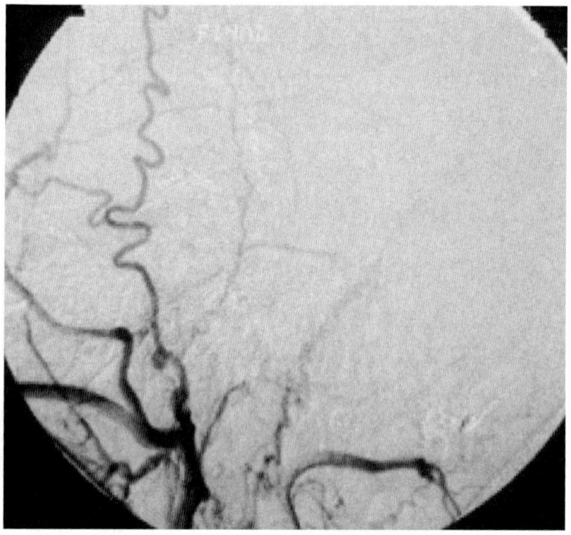

F

FIGURE 11-6. *Continued.* **D,E:** Superselective serial angiograms of the occipital artery show the transmastoidal supply to the DAVF (*arrowheads* mark catheter tip). *Arrows* demonstrate sites of fistulous communication in the arteriovenous arcade. Distal protection of the occipital artery territory downstream was achieved by placement of injectable soft platinum microcoils (Liquid Coils) seen in **(E)**. This subsequently permitted slow injection of another aliquot of 4:1 iodized oil-to-NBCA mixture to achieve distal nidal permeation. **F:** Control right external carotid angiogram, lateral projection, shows complete obliteration of the DAVF. A 6-month follow-up angiogram showed durable obliteration of the fistula.

can be preserved at the beginning and end of the endovascular operation, while the segment between can be more economically occluded with coils that are more likely to promote rapid thrombosis. Partial transarterial embolization in conjunction with transvenous embolization may also be helpful in slowing the degree of AV shunting, which in turn promotes complete thrombosis of the dural sinus [9,30,31]. Alternative transvenous approaches are also possible, including cervical internal jugular venipuncture, cannulation of the contralateral STS complex, and direct puncture of the diseased segment of dural sinus after craniotomy.

We have found that limited occlusion of shorter segments of not only the sigmoid sinus, but also the transverse sinus, is uniformly better tolerated than extensive obliteration of most or all of the STS complex, owing to the smaller risk of inadvertent occlusion of normal cortical venous drainage pathways into the STS complex (see Fig. 11-1). Such a strategy often permits empiric preservation of normal major venous pathways, such as the vein of Labbé and transverse cerebellar veins connected to the transverse sinus. This is useful when angiographic analysis of the relationship between normal cortical venous drainage of the brain and venous drainage of the DAVF is equivocal. Again, this tolerance to therapeutic occlusion is substantially dependent on adequate alternative venous drainage pathways (e.g., codominant contralateral STS, preexisting chronic dural sinus occlusive disease with collateral rerouting). On occasion a venous pouch can be identified, which acts as the initial venous drainage site for the fistula. Occlusion of this venous pouch alone may allow for preservation of much of the normal brain venous drainage (Fig. 11-7).

Despite adherence to these technical guidelines, poor technical and clinical outcomes may occur occasionally. For example, despite apparent complete obliteration of the af-

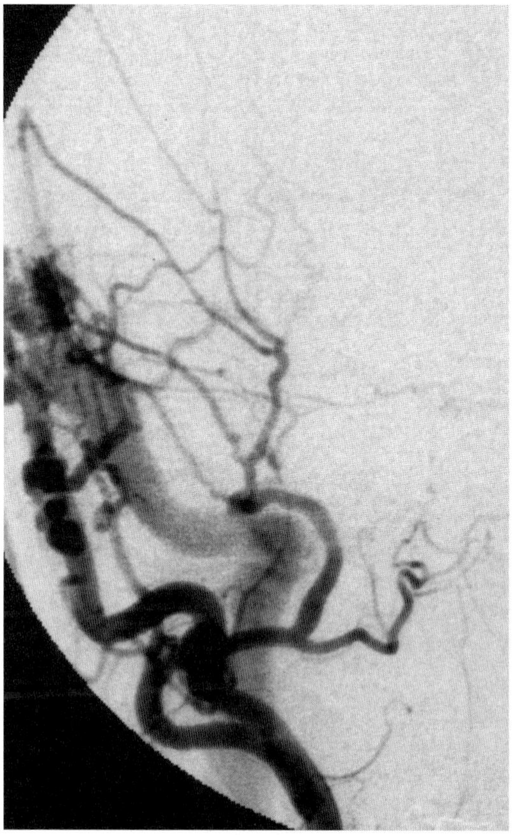

A

FIGURE 11-7. This 43-year-old man had an episode of transient left arm numbness and a near syncopal episode. He was found to have a high-flow retromastoid dural fistula and a dissection of the right internal carotid artery with severe stenosis. Endovascular treatment of the high-flow fistula was followed by anticoagulation for his carotid dissection. **A–C:** Right external carotid artery angiograms, anterior, lateral, and magnified lateral projections, respectively. They demonstrate a high-flow fistula with supply from middle meningeal artery branches and branches of the occipital artery. These arteries come to a central fistulous site **(B).** The fistulous communication was noted to attach to an irregular pouch adjacent to the dural sinus in the region of the transverse sigmoid sinus junction *(arrows).* Branches of the right internal carotid and right vertebral arteries were also noted to supply this high-flow fistula (not shown). *(Figure continues.)*

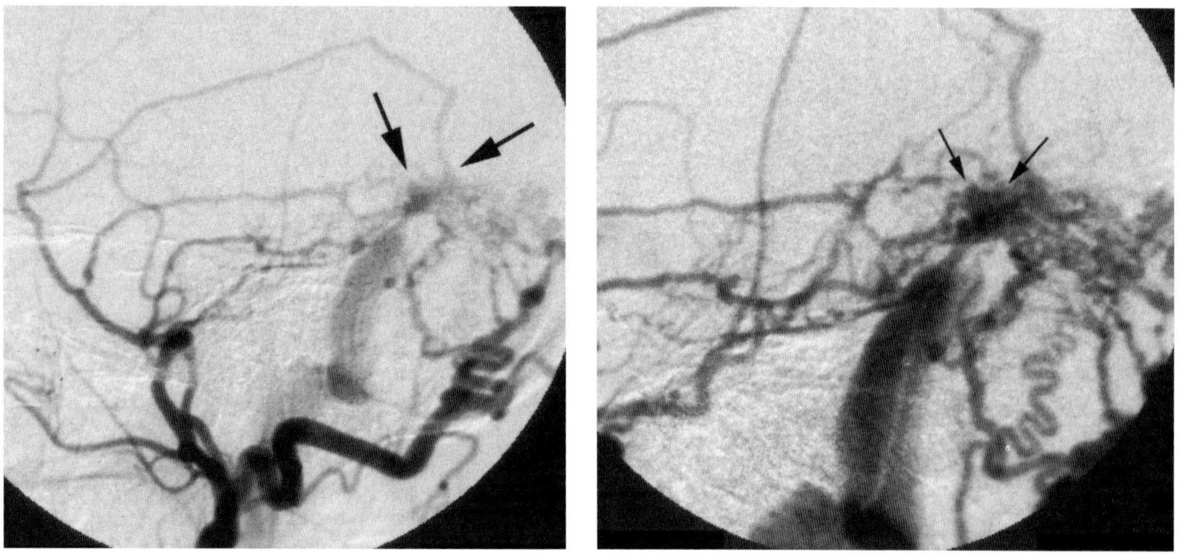

B C

fected STS complex via transvenous embolization, persistence of the DAVF may occur as a result of venous drainage rerouting from within the wall of the sinus (see Fig. 11-1). Such a development usually is associated with cortical venous rerouting, resulting in venous infarction and hemorrhage. Prospective identification of this unusual pattern of venous rerouting within the dura should prompt immediate consideration of either aggressive transarterial liquid adhesive embolization, if feasible, or craniotomy with fulguration and surgical disconnection.

Superior Sagittal Sinus

Isolated involvement of the SSS and or the torcular herophili, with or without recruitment of adjacent cortical veins, is unusual [4,30,31]. These lesions may have a higher than

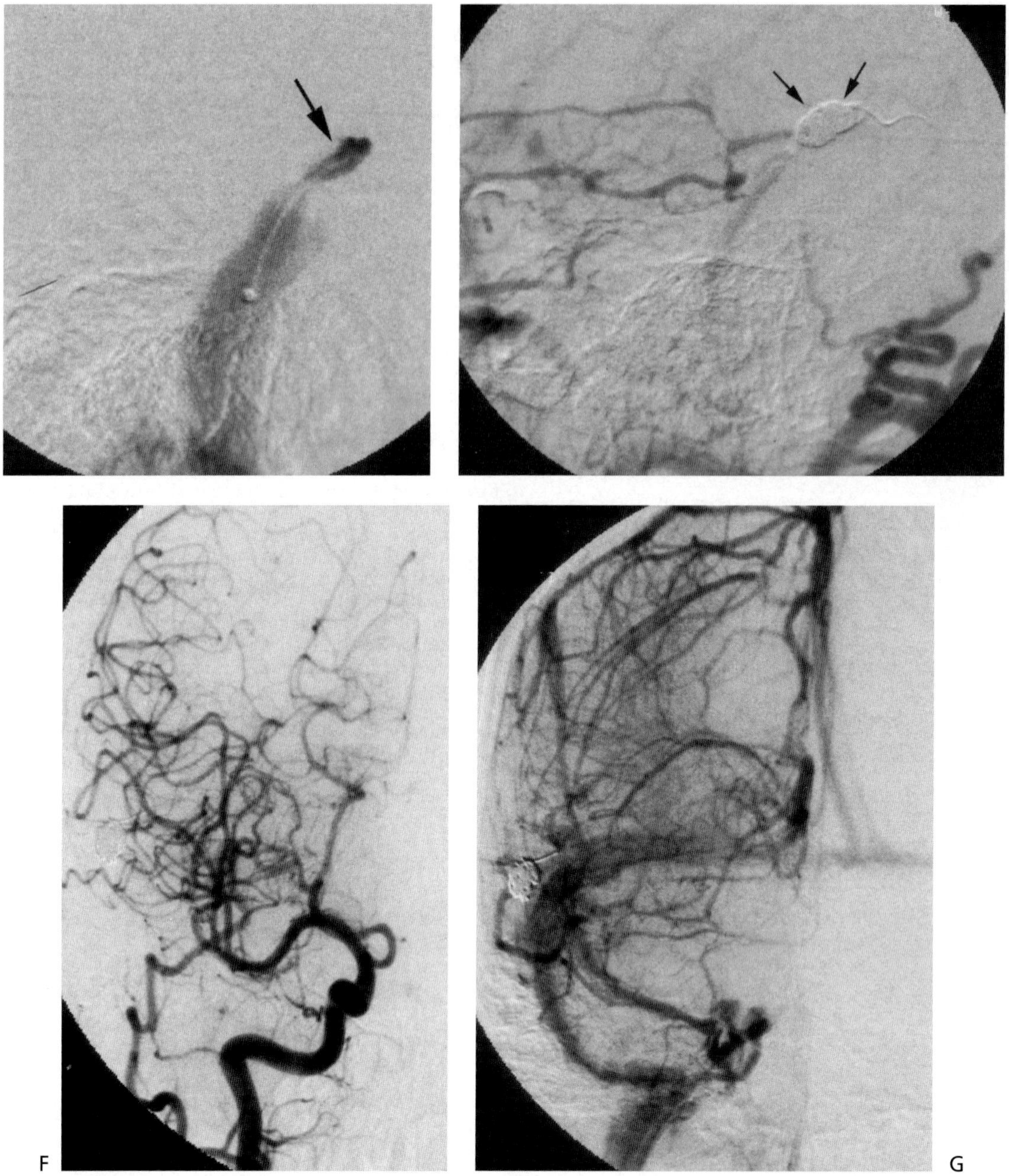

D E F G

FIGURE 11-7. *Continued.* **D:** Venogram lateral projection. The venous pouch *(arrow)* was entered selectively using a microcatheter. A stenosis at the outflow site of the venous pouch enabled coil packing to be selectively performed locally in the pouch preserving flow in the sigmoid sinus. **E:** Right external carotid artery angiogram, lateral projection, late arterial phase, following packing with GDC. The coils were tightly packed into the venous pouch, occluding venous outflow from the fistula. *(Figure continues.)*

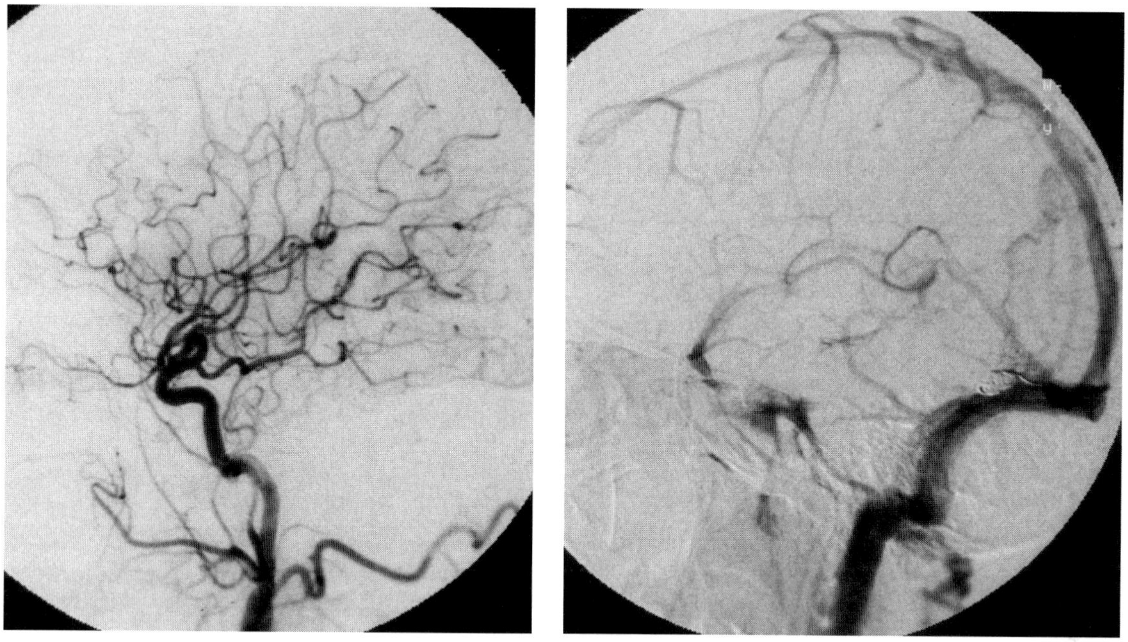

H I

FIGURE 11-7. *Continued.* **F–I:** Right common carotid artery control angiograms, anterior and lateral projections, in the midarterial **(F,H)** and late venous **(G,I)** phases. This control angiogram demonstrates the tightly packed coil mass with no filling of the fistula. On the venous phase of the angiogram **(G,I)**, the coil mass is distinct from the transverse sigmoid sinus and there is free flow within the normal dural sinuses. (From Michael P. Marks and Huy M. Do, unpublished material, with permission.)

usual association of prior trauma [31] and are more likely to produce an aggressive clinical course [29,31]. Patients frequently have severe headaches and intracranial hemorrhage (up to 50%). The latter can manifest as subdural, subarachnoid, and intraparenchymal hemorrhage. Occasionally patients will suffer either nonhemorrhagic stroke (i.e., venous infarction) or dementia [14,31]. The propensity of SSS DAVFs to exhibit aggressive behavior has been attributed to their greater likelihood of having associated (or exclusive) cortical venous drainage and partial dural sinus thrombosis (resulting in localized or diffuse intracranial venous hypertension). Most DAVFs of the SSS occur in the middle third of the sinus (Fig. 11-8).

Endovascular treatment of SSS DAVFs is often challenging, typically requiring multistaged percutaneous and occasionally direct-exposure approaches. The key to success for managing this group of DAVFs is through superior ultrasuperselective catheterization of the dominant arterial feeding pedicles. Usually, standard percutaneous transfemoral catheterization techniques will permit distal purchase into the middle meningeal, superficial temporal, and occipital arteries that invariably provide the major meningeal arterial supply to these lesions. With distal positioning, the probability of successfully depositing liquid embolics into the fistulas increases greatly. In order for such microcatheterizations to succeed, it is critical to first obtain distal purchase of the major ECA branch connecting to the feeders (i.e., internal maxillary and occipital arteries) with a 5-Fr. braided guiding catheter. This provides a more stable platform for advancing the microcatheter into the often tortuous and relatively small feeding pedicles that are a considerable distance from the major ECA branches. Ultrasuperselective catheterization of these branches has been enhanced particularly by the use of the smaller 1.5-Fr. hydrophilic coated FDMCs in combination with 0.009- or 0.010-inch hydrophilic coated microguidewires (as described in detail earlier). An important technical note to emphasize is that frequently the transosseous branches of the superficial temporal and occipital arteries form anastomotic arcades with the middle meningeal artery, resulting in reciprocal blood supply to the dura. Intentional proximal occlusion of one or more of the arterial inputs to these arcades can accentuate blood flow from a dominant feeding artery, which subsequently can be targeted by superselective catheterization for nidal embolization. We use very dilute suspensions of liquid adhesives (4:1, ethiodol:NBCA) with a very slow injection (60 to 90 seconds), similar to those performed for nidal embolization of brain AVMs [86]. Such a technique usually permits excellent permeation into fistulous communications, resulting in a higher likelihood of definitive cure. Despite better technique and technology, ultrasuperselective catheterization into the most distal portions of the superficial temporal, occipital, and middle meningeal arteries at times still is not possible. In such cases free-flow injections of small boluses of dilute NBCA suspensions using the sandwich technique may achieve the desired effect. However, owing to the in-

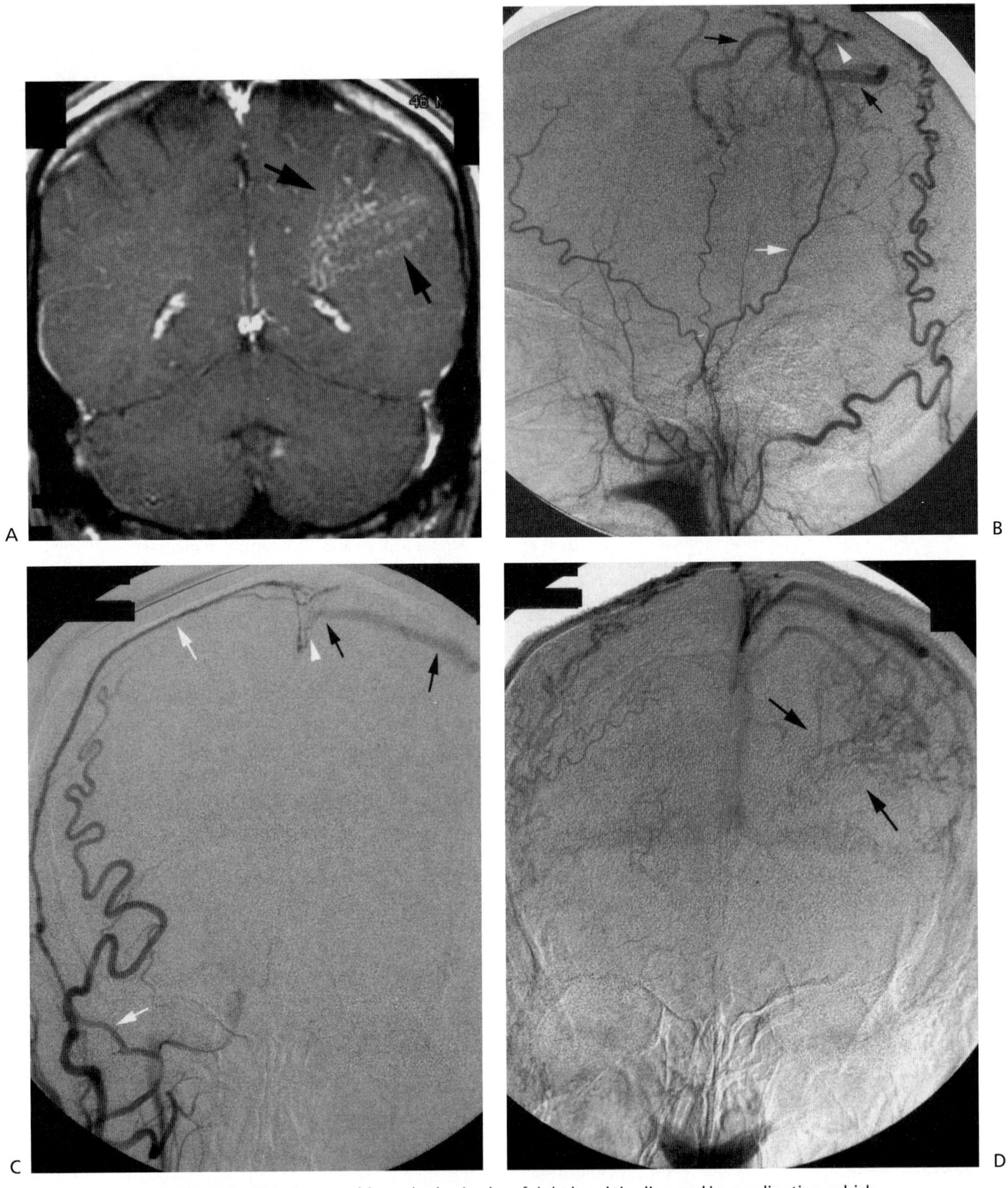

FIGURE 11-8. This 46-year-old man had episodes of right hand tingling and incoordination, which led to a workup with pre- and postcontrast MRIs. **A:** Pretreatment T1-weighted coronal MRI (following gadolinium administration). This demonstrates a series of contrast-enhanced vessels *(arrows)* that are dilated medullary veins draining into the subependymal venous system. **B–D:** Right external carotid artery angiogram, lateral projection midarterial phase **(B)**, anterior projection midarterial phase **(C)**, and anterior projection late venous phase **(D)**. This demonstrates a superior sagittal sinus fistula with drainage exclusively into a cortical vein *(black arrows)*, **(B,C)**. This type III fistula is fed by branches of the superficial temporal artery *(white arrows)* and a hypertrophied occipital artery. The site of the fistulous communication is marked with a *white arrowhead* **(C)**. Retrograde filling of the cortical vein gives rise to drainage into the medullary and subependymal venous complex *(arrows)* **(D)**, which compares with the contrast-enhanced structures seen on the MRI study **(A)**. *(Figure continues.)*

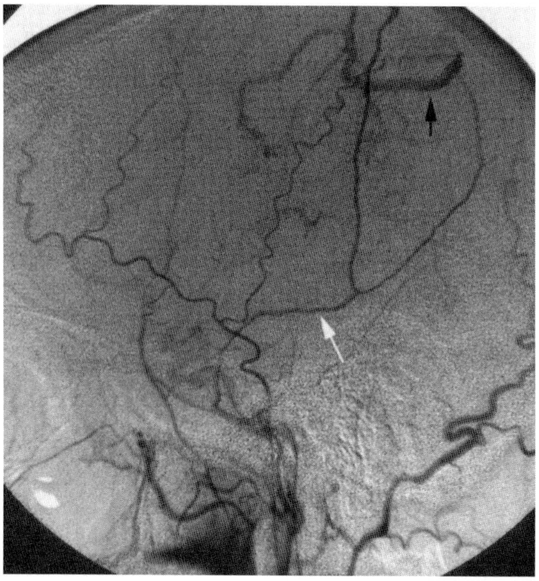

E

FIGURE 11-8. *Continued.* **E–G:** Left external carotid artery angiograms, midarterial phase lateral projection **(E)**, midarterial phase anterior projection **(F)**, and late venous phase anterior projection **(G)**. There is a similar pattern to the one seen from the right external carotid artery angiogram with prompt filling of the cortical vein *(black arrows)* **(F)**. Also noted is the filling of the medullary veins of the left hemisphere *(black arrows)* **(G)**. A prominent portion of the supply is from the middle meningeal artery *(white arrows)* **(E,F)**. The site of the fistula is the same as that demonstrated by the right external carotid artery injection *(white arrowhead)* **(F)**. *(Figure continues.)*

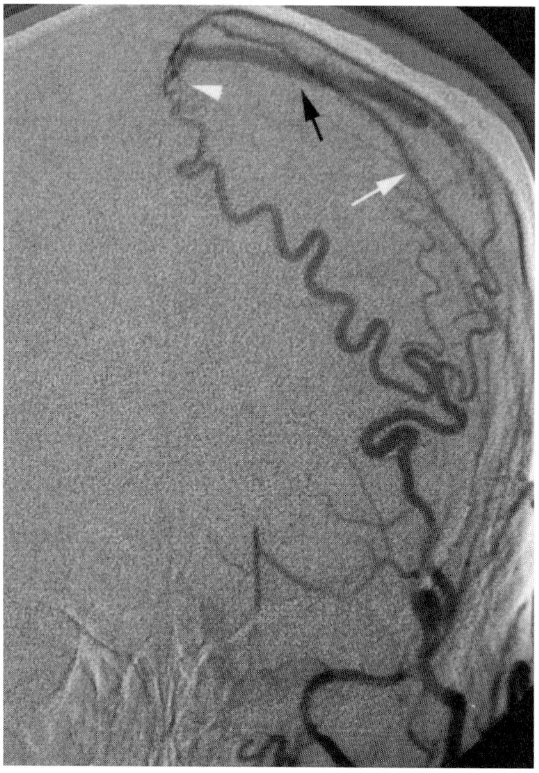

F

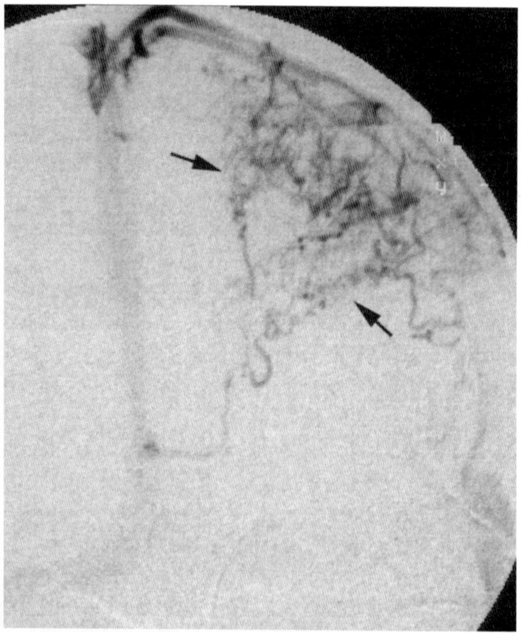

G

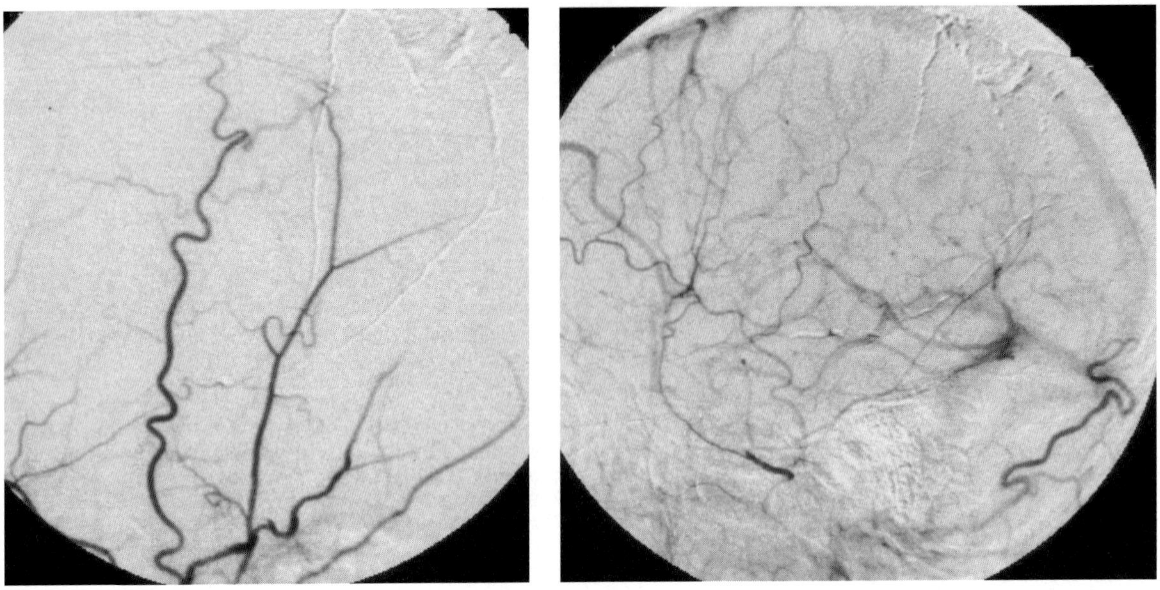

H I

FIGURE 11-8. *Continued.* Embolization of the external carotid artery feeders with dilute mixtures of ethiodized oil-to-NBCA were performed bilaterally. **H:** Right external carotid artery control angiogram, midarterial phase lateral projection, demonstrates no filling of the fistula following embolization. **I:** Left external carotid artery control angiogram, midvenous phase lateral projection, demonstrates no filling of the fistula following embolization. (From Michael P. Marks and Huy M. Do, unpublished material, with permission.)

creased tortuosity and plexiform distal arborization of the feeding pedicles, precise deposition of liquid adhesive into the actual fistulas may be difficult and may result in undesirable occlusion of other branches or distal venous penetration.

Depending on the precise anatomical location and functional status of the surrounding normal dural sinuses, transvenous embolization may be performed successfully without catastrophic sequelae. However, in general, such an approach carries a higher-than-average risk of cerebral infarction or hemorrhage owing to the brain's intolerance to acute occlusion of the SSS. Conventional neurosurgical doctrine has indicated that, as a rule, the anterior one-third of the SSS usually can be safely occluded, whereas the posterior two-thirds of the SSS cannot. Certainly in the case of a normal, unobstructed SSS with low venous pressures, such a rule will apply for most patients. However, DAVFs of the SSS typically are associated with chronic venous hypertension, cortical venous rerouting, and variable occlusive disease of the affected segment of the sinus. Therefore, therapeutic occlusion of these more posterior segments of the SSS can be well tolerated much more frequently than conventional wisdom would predict. This was first confirmed by Halbach et al. in 1988 [94] and later by others. Short segments (1 to 2 cm) of the middle portion of the SSS could be occluded safely in preexisting sinus occlusive disease and venous rerouting (Fig. 11-9).

Deep Venous and Galenic System

Deep venous DAVFs are a somewhat heterogeneous group defined by their venous drainage into the vein of Galen or its major tributaries or both (e.g., basal vein of Rosenthal, precentral cerebellar vein, superior vermian veins). The specific fistulous sites can be highly variable however, including the vein of Galen, strait sinus, tentorium cerebelli, falx cerebelli, and posterior falx cerebri. Combined involvement of these sites may be encountered as well. Some authors have advocated distinguishing between lesions involving primarily the tentorium cerebelli from those occurring in the other anatomical sites, owing to the characteristic involvement of the superior petrosal sinus for the former [31]. This seems justified not only on an anatomical basis, but also in terms of strategies for endovascular surgical management (particularly transvenous approaches).

Deep venous and galenic DAVFs are among the most frequently encountered subtypes associated with aggressive clinical behavior [29]. Patients commonly suffer catastrophic intracranial hemorrhage, brainstem ischemia, infarction, and edema, or dementia. Severe headaches, ataxia, and vertigo are also often reported [9,67]. It is generally believed that these DAVFs are more likely to have an aggressive clinical course because of their frequent association with deep venoocclusive disease and recruitment of cortical venous drainage.

Owing to the poor prognosis of untreated DAVFs occurring within this region, timely and aggressive therapeutic intervention is warranted, despite the potentially greater risks of iatrogenic complications. Unfortunately, notwithstanding the many advances in endovascular surgical technique and technology, deep venous and galenic DAVFs remain among the most difficult and challenging subtypes to

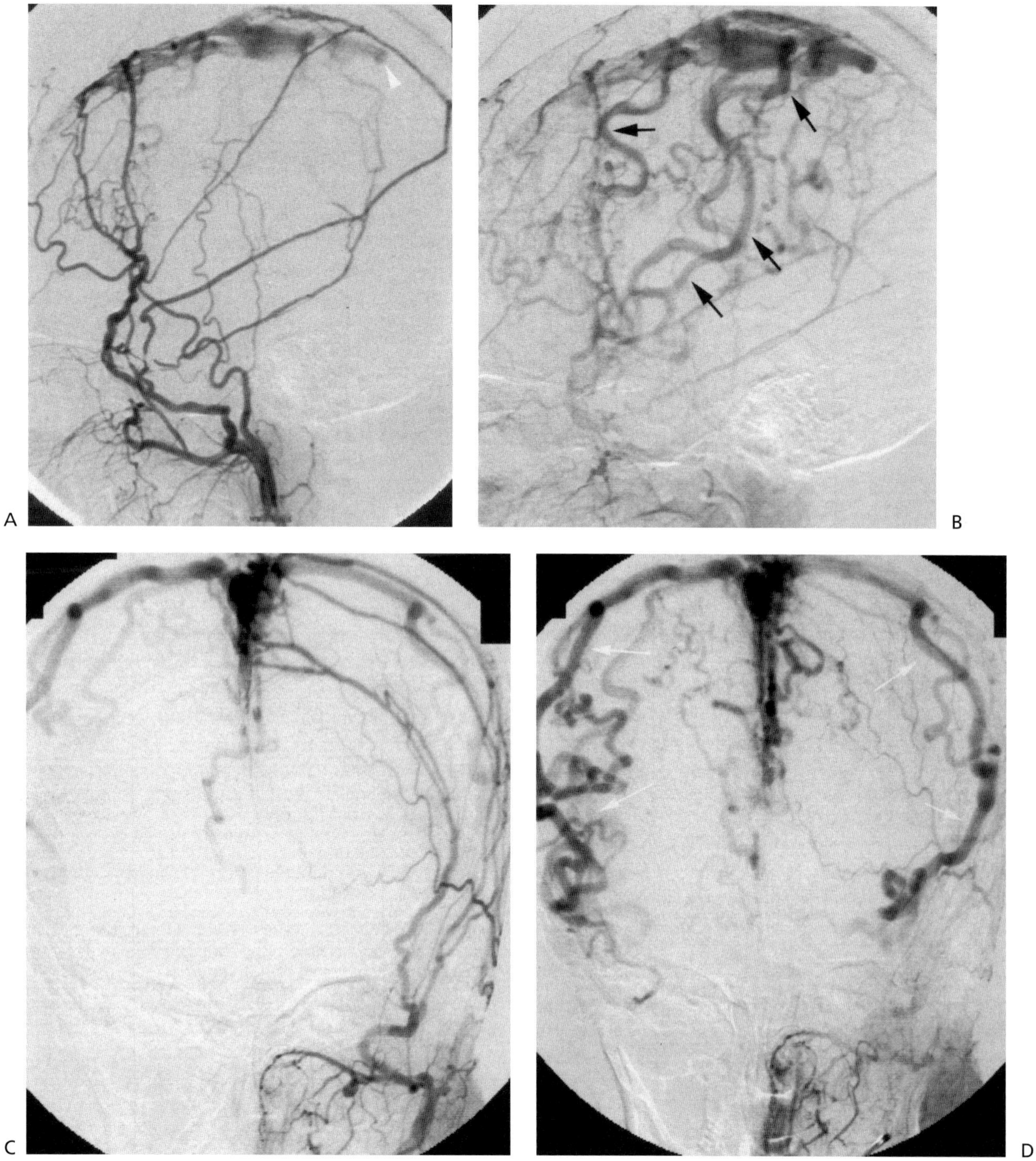

FIGURE 11-9. This 28-year-old woman experienced a bruit in her right ear for about a year. She sought medical attention after she began experiencing right-sided facial numbness and right temporal headaches along with episodes of right-handed weakness. **A,B:** Right external carotid artery angiograms, lateral projection, arterial phase and midvenous phase, respectively. There is an extensive fistula of the middle third of the superior sagittal sinus supplied by multiple branches of the middle meningeal and superficial temporal artery. Note that the outflow from the distal portion of the sinus is occluded *(arrowhead)* **(A).** The egress from this occluded segment of the superior sagittal sinus is via a multitude of retrograde draining cortical veins *(arrows)* **(B). C,D:** Left external carotid artery angiograms, anterior projection, midarterial phase and midvenous phase, respectively. This demonstrates supply similar to the superior sagittal sinus fistula from the left side shown here in the anterior projection. The superficial cortical veins draining this fistula are seen draped over both hemispheres *(arrows)* **(D).** *(Figure continues.)*

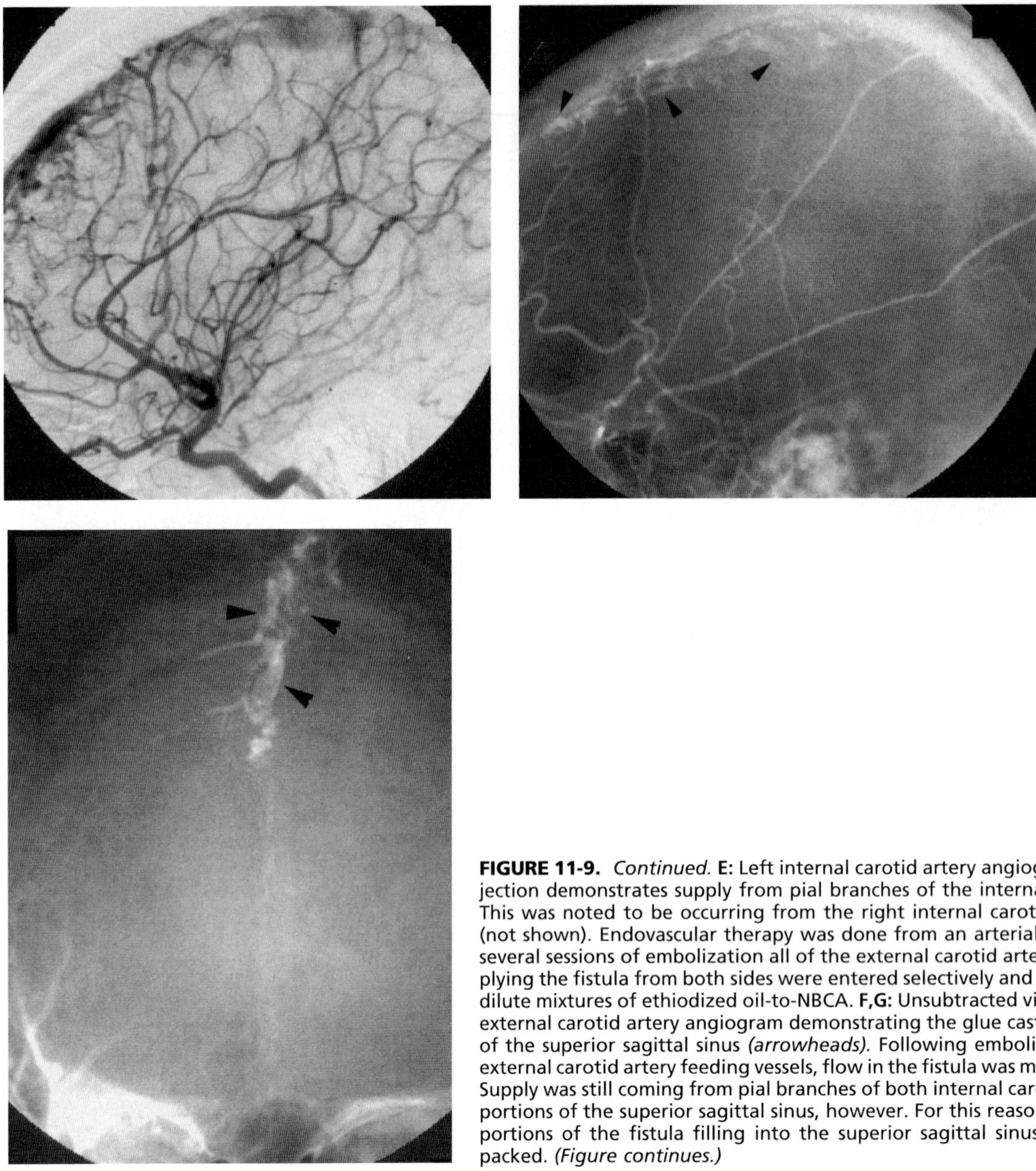

E F G

FIGURE 11-9. *Continued.* **E:** Left internal carotid artery angiogram lateral projection demonstrates supply from pial branches of the internal carotid artery. This was noted to be occurring from the right internal carotid artery as well (not shown). Endovascular therapy was done from an arterial approach. Over several sessions of embolization all of the external carotid artery branches supplying the fistula from both sides were entered selectively and embolized using dilute mixtures of ethiodized oil-to-NBCA. **F,G:** Unsubtracted views from a right external carotid artery angiogram demonstrating the glue cast within portions of the superior sagittal sinus *(arrowheads).* Following embolization of all the external carotid artery feeding vessels, flow in the fistula was markedly reduced. Supply was still coming from pial branches of both internal carotid arteries into portions of the superior sagittal sinus, however. For this reason, the remaining portions of the fistula filling into the superior sagittal sinus were surgically packed. *(Figure continues.)*

manage optimally. As a rule, these malformations tend to recruit a plethora of bilateral meningeal arterial supply from numerous extracranial and intracranial territories. This includes extensive reciprocal supply through the posterior falx via multiple branches of the middle meningeal, occipital, and superficial temporal arteries (see Fig. 11-2), posterior meningeal branch of the vertebral artery, and tentorial or falcine branches of the anterior and posterior cerebral arteries. Lesions that primarily affect the tentorium cerebelli also may derive significant supply from the marginal tentorial and lateral clival branches of the meningohypophyseal artery and the petrosal branch of the middle meningeal artery.

As with other anatomical sites, superselective microcatheterization as distally as possible is highly desirable. This increases the operator's ability to deliver dilute liquid adhesive into the actual fistulous connections. As noted earlier, intentional less distal embolization of either minor or more difficult to reach reciprocal feeding arteries may enhance the operator's ability to achieve optimal permeation of the nidus from another accessed feeding pedicle. In such scenarios we prefer to use very slow, wedged injections of 4:1 dilutions of NBCA. Owing to the extensive reciprocal blood supply, multiple staged transarterial embolizations invariably are needed to significantly reduce the high-flow AV

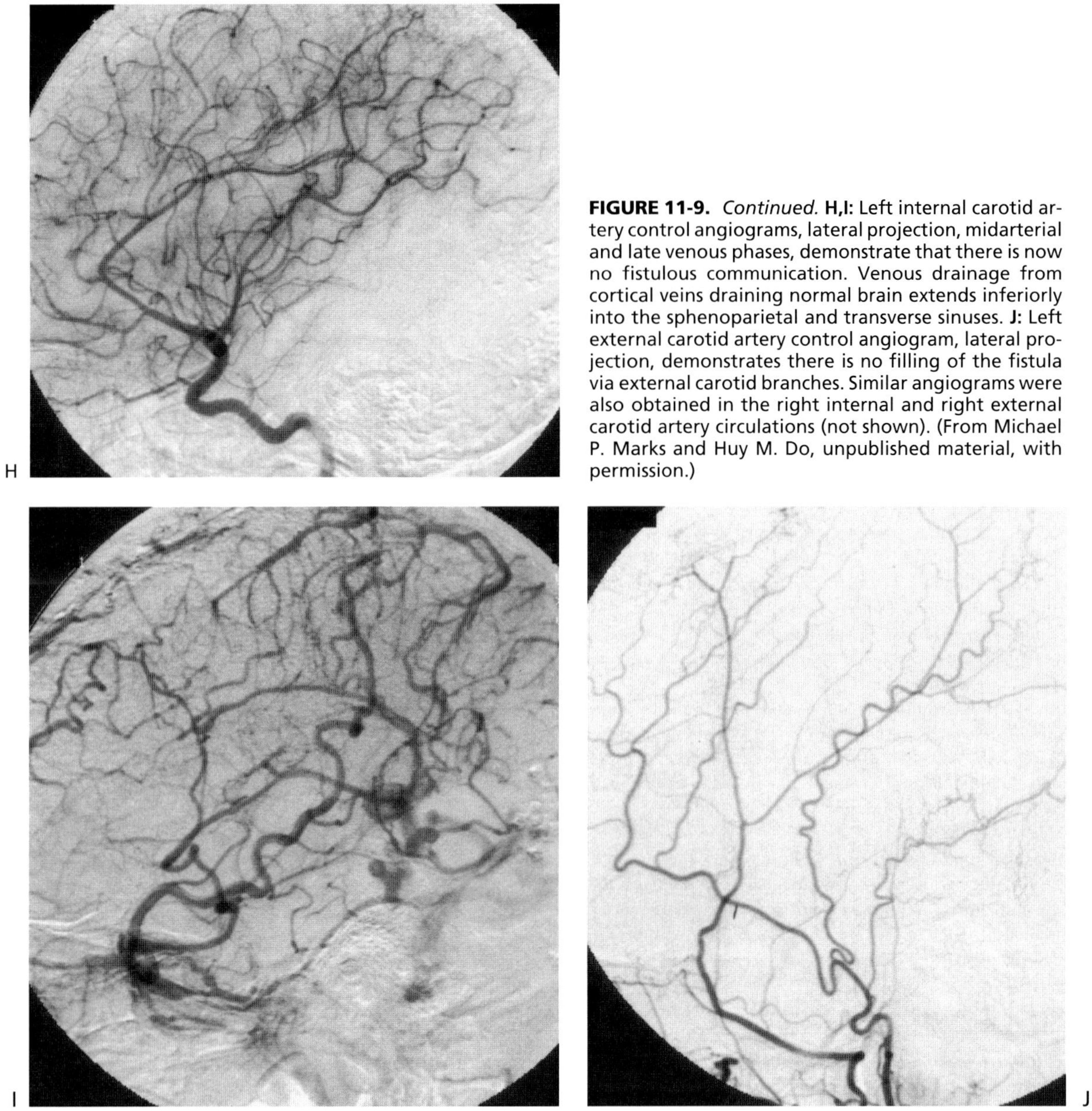

FIGURE 11-9. *Continued.* **H,I:** Left internal carotid artery control angiograms, lateral projection, midarterial and late venous phases, demonstrate that there is now no fistulous communication. Venous drainage from cortical veins draining normal brain extends inferiorly into the sphenoparietal and transverse sinuses. **J:** Left external carotid artery control angiogram, lateral projection, demonstrates there is no filling of the fistula via external carotid branches. Similar angiograms were also obtained in the right internal and right external carotid artery circulations (not shown). (From Michael P. Marks and Huy M. Do, unpublished material, with permission.)

shunting that characteristically occurs with these lesions. With the implementation of these more aggressive transarterial approaches, occasionally deep venous and galenic DAVFs may be effectively treated by this mode of embolization alone. Such success is likely linked to the presence of a more limited arterial supply, favorable anatomy of major feeders for ultrasuperselective microcatheterization, and significant coexistent durovenous occlusive disease.

Definitive endovascular surgical treatment of most deep venous and galenic DAVFs requires additional transvenous embolization despite the use of aggressive transarterial approaches. Ideally in such cases, prospective identification of normal cerebral venous drainage sharing the deep system draining the DAVF is highly desirable. However, in practice, unequivocal demonstration of this phenomenon on cerebral angiography can be particularly difficult. Furthermore, owing to the potential increased fragility of the deep venous tributaries to arterialized pressure and manipulation of microcatheter systems, temporary balloon test occlusion of the vein of Galen is not advisable.

REFERENCES

1. Castaigne P, Bories J, Brunet P, et al. Fistules arterio-veineuses de la dure-mere. *Ann Med Interne (Paris)* 1975;126:813–817.
2. Castaigne P, Bories J, Brunet P, et al. Les fistules arterioveineuses meningees pures a drainage veineux cortical. *Rev Neurol* 1976; 132:169–181.
3. Lasjaunias P, Berenstein. Dural arteriovenous malformations (DAVMs). In: *Surgical neuroangiography 2.*New York: Springer Verlag, 1987:273–315.
4. Chaloupka JC. Endovascular therapy of dural arteriovenous fistulae. *Semin Interv Radiol* 1994;11:1–13.
5. Cognard C, Gogin YP, Pierot L, et al. Cerebral dural arteriovenous fistulas: clinical and angiographic correlation with a revised classification of venous drainage. *Radiology* 1995;194: 671–680.
6. Chaloupka JC, Putman CM. Endovascular therapy for surgical diseases of the cranial base. *Clin Plast Surg* 1995;22:417–450.
7. Chaloupka JC, Huddle DC. Classification of cerebral vascular malformations. *Neuroimaging Clin N Am* 1998;8:295–321.
8. Welch KMA, Caplan LR, Reis DJ, et al., eds. *Primer on cerebrovascular diseases.* New York: Academic Press, 1997.
9. Duckwiler G. Dural arteriovenous fistula. *Neuroimaging Clin N Am* 1992;291–307.
10. Lownie SP. Intracranial dural arteriovenous fistulas: endovascular therapy. *Neurosurg Clin N Am* 1994;5:449–458.
11. Chaloupka JC, Marx WF, Kallemes DF. Dural arteriovenous fistulae: pathophysiology and proposed therapies. *J Neurosurg* 2001;94:858–860.
12. Aminoff MJ, Kendall BE. Asymptomatic dural vascular anomalies. *Br J Radiol* 1973;46:662–667.
13. Aminoff MJ. Vascular malformations of the central nervous system. In: Mulliken JB, Young AE, eds. *Vascular birthmarks, hemangiomas and malformations.* Philadelphia: WB Saunders, 1988:286–290.
14. Hunt WE. Dural arteriovenous malformations. In: Wilson CB, Stein BM, eds. *Intracranial arteriovenous malformations.* Baltimore: Williams & Wilkins, 1984:222.
15. Albright AL, Latchaw RE, Price RA. Posterior dural arteriovenous malformations in infancy. *Neurosurgery* 1983;13: 129–135.
16. Chaudhary M, Sachdev VP, Cho Sh, et al. Dural arteriovenous malformation of the major venous sinuses: an acquired lesion. *AJNR Am J Neuroradiol* 1982;3:13–19.
17. Djindjian R, Cophignon J, Theron J. Embolization by superselective arteriography from the femoral route; review of 60 cases: technique, indications, complications. *Neuroradiology* 1973;6: 20–26.
18. Djindjian R, Merland JJ. *Superselective arteriography of the external carotid artery.* New York, Springer, 1978:405–412.
19. Borden JA, Wu JK, Shucart WA. A proposed classification for spinal and cranial dural arteriovenous fistulous malformations and implications for treatment. *J Neurosurg* 1995;82:166–179.
20. Obrador S., Soto M, Silvela J. Clinical syndromes of arteriovenous malformations of the transverse-sigmoid sinus. *J Neurol Neurosurg Psychiatry* 1975;38:436–451.
21. Fermand M, Reizine D, Melki JP, et al. Long term follow-up of 43 pure dural arteriovenous fistulae (AVF) of the lateral sinus. *Neuroradiology* 1987;29:348–353.
22. Newton TH, Hoyt WF. Dural arteriovenous shunts in the region of the cavernous sinus. *Neuroradiology* 1970;1:71–81.
23. Houser OW, Campbell JK, Campbell RJ, et al. Arteriovenous malformation affecting the transverse sinus—an acquired lesion. *Mayo Clin Proc* 1979;54:651–661.
24. Toya S, Shiobara R, Izumi J, et al. Spontaneous carotid-cavernous fistula during pregnancy or in the postpartum stage. *J Neurosurg* 1981;54:352–356.
25. Pang D, Kerber C, Biglan AW, et al. External carotid-cavernous fistula in infancy: case report and review of the literature. *Neurosurgery* 1981;8:212–217.
26. Levine D, Barnes PD, Madsen JR, et al. Central nervous system abnormalities assessed with prenatal magnetic resonance imaging. *Obstet Gynecol* 1999;94:1011–1019.
27. Newton TH, Cronqvist S. Involvement of dural arteries in intracranial arteriovenous malformations. *Radiology* 1968;93: 1071–1078.
28. Nagasawa S, Yamamoto T, Ogata M. Intracerebral arteriovenous malformation angiographically resembling a dural malformation. *Surg Neurol* 1979;12:411–416.
29. Awad IA, Little JR, Akrawi WP, et al. Intracranial dural arteriovenous malformations: factors predisposing to an aggressive neurological course. *J Neurosurg* 1990;72:839–850.
30. Picard L, Bracard S, Moret J, et al. Spontaneous dural arteriovenous fistulas. *Semin Interv Radiol* 1987;4:219–240.
31. Halbach VV, Higashida RT, Hieshima GB, et al. Endovascular therapy of dural fistulas. In: Viñuela F, Dion JE, Halbach VV, eds. *Interventional neuroradiology: endovascular therapy of the central nervous system.* New York: Raven Press, 1992:29–50.
32. Sundt TM, Piepgras DG. The surgical approach to arteriovenous malformations of the lateral and sigmoid dural sinuses. *J Neurosurg* 1983;59:32–39.
33. Terada T, Higashida RT, Halbach VV, et al. The role of angiogenic factor bFGF in the development of dural AVFs. *Acta Radiol* 1996;138:877–883.
34. Amautovic KI, Al-Mefty O, Angtuaco E, et al. Dural arteriovenous malformations of the transverse/sigmoid sinus acquired from dominant sinus occlusion by a tumor: report of two cases. *Neurosurgery* 1998:42:383–388.
35. Cognard C, Houdart E, Casaasco AE, et al. Endovascular therapy and long term results for intracranial dural arteriovenous fistulae. In: Conners JJ, Wojack JC, eds. *Interventional neuroradiology: strategies and practical approaches.* Philadelphia: WB Saunders, 1999:199–214.
36. Bitoh S, Sakaki S. Spontaneous cure of dural arteriovenous malformation of the posterior fossa. *Surg Neurol* 1970;12:111–114.
37. Watanabe A, Takahara Y, Ibuchi Y, et al. Two cases of dural arteriovenous malformation occurring after intracranial surgery. *Neuroradiology* 1984;26:375–380.
38. Halbach VV, Hieshima BG, Higashida RT, et al. Carotid cavernous fistulae: indications for urgent treatment. *AJNR Am J Neuroradiol* 1987;8:627–633.
39. Chaloupka JC, Goller D, Goldberg RA, et al. True anatomic compartmentalization of the cavernous sinus in a patient with bilateral cavernous dural arteriovenous fistulae: an unusual diagnostic and therapeutic challenge. *J Neurosurg* 1993;79: 592–595.
40. Kerber CW, Newton TH. Macro and micro vasculature of the dura mater. *Neuroradiology* 1973;6:175–179.
41. Rowbotham GF, Little E. Circulations of the cerebral hemispheres. *Br J Surg* 1965;52:8–24.
42. Terada T, Higashida RT, Halbach VV, et al. Development of acquired fistulas in rats due to venous hypertension. *J Neurosurg* 1994;80:884–889.
43. Cao Y, Linden P, Shima D, et al: *In vivo* angiogenic activity and hypoxia induction of heterodimers of placenta growth factor/ vascular endothelial growth factor. *J Clin Invest* 1996;98: 2507–2511.
44. Folkman J. Seminars in medicine of the Beth Israel Hospital,

Boston: clinical applications of research on angiogenesis. *N Engl J Med* 1995;333:1757–1763.
45. Folkman J, DAmore PA. Blood vessel formation: what is the molecular basis? *Cell* 1996;87:1153–1155.
46. Takahashi Y, Yamamoto T, Abe T, et al. The cerebrospinal fluid in patients with moyamoya disease spontaneous occlusion of circle of Willis contains high level of basic fibroblast growth factor. *Neurosci Lett* 1993;160:214–216.
47. Yoshimoto T, Houkin K, Takahashi A, et al. Angiogenic factors in moyamoya disease. *Stroke* 1996;27:2160–2165.
48. Hoshimaru M, Takahashi JA, Kikuchi H, et al. Possible roles of basic fibroblast growth factor in the pathogenesis of moyamoya disease: an immunohistochemical study. *J Neurosurg* 1991;75: 267–270.
49. Hamada Y, Goto K, Inoue T, et al. Histopathological aspects of dural arteriovenous fistulas in the transverse-sigmoid sinus region in nine patients. *Neurosurgery* 1997;40:452–456.
50. Lawton MT, Jacobowitz R, Spetzler RF. Redefined role of angiogenesis in the pathogenesis of dural arteriovenous malformations. *J Neurosurg* 1997;87:267–274.
51. Uranishi R, Nakase H, Sakaki T. Expression of angiogenic growth factors in dural arteriovenous fistula. *J Neurosurg* 1999; 91:781–786.
52. Chaloupka JC, Huddle DC, Alderman JS. Local induction of angiogenesis within the walls of a dural sinus results in the creation of dural arteriovenous fistulae: demonstration by a polymeric release implantation model in swine. *J Neurosurg* 1999; 90:194a(abst).
53. Pile-Spellman JM, Baker KF, Liszczak TM, et al. High flow angiopathy: cerebral blood vessel changes in experimental chronic arteriovenous fistula. *AJNR Am J Neuroradiol* 1986;7: 811–815.
54. McCormick WF. The pathology of vascular (arteriovenous) malformations. *J Neurosurg* 1966;24:807–816.
55. Malek AM, Izumo S. Control of endothelial gene expression by flow. *J Biomech* 1995;28:1515–1528.
56. Courtheoux P, Labbé D, Hamel C, et al. Treatment of bilateral spontaneous dural carotid-cavernous fistulas by coils and sclerotherapy. *J Neurosurg* 1987;66:468–470.
57. Grossman RI, Sergott RC, Goldberg HI, et al. Dural malformations with ophthalmic manifestations: results of particulate embolization in seven patients. *AJNR Am J Neuroradiol* 1985;6: 809–813.
58. Viñuela F, Fox AJ, Debrun GM, et al. Spontaneous carotid-cavernous fistulas: clinical, radiological, and therapeutic considerations. *J Neurosurg* 1984;60:976–984.
59. Gobin YP, Rogopoulos A, Aymard A, et al. Endovascular treatment of intracranial dural arteriovenous fistulas with spinal perimedullary venous drainage. *Neurosurgery* 1992;77:718–723.
60. Halbach VV, Higashida RT, Hieshima GB, et al. Endovascular therapy of dural fistulas. In: Viñuela F, Dion JE, Halbach VV, eds. *Interventional neuroradiology: endovascular therapy of the central nervous system.* New York: Raven Press, 1992:29–50.
61. Davies MA, TerBrugge K, Willinsky R, et al. The validity of classification for the clinical presentation of intracranial dural arteriovenous fistulas. *J Neurosurg* 1996;85:830–837.
62. Garcia-Monaco R, Lasjaunias P, Berenstein A. Therapeutic management of vein of Galen aneurysmal malformations. In: Viñuela F, Dion JE, Halbach VV, eds. *Interventional neuroradiology: endovascular therapy of the central nervous system.* New York: Raven Press, 1992:113–127.
63. Lasjaunias P, Chiu M, Brugge KT, et al. Neurological manifestations of intracranial dural arteriovenous malformations. *J Neurosurg* 1986;64:724–730.
64. Malik G, Pearce J, Ausman J, et al. Dural arteriovenous malformations and intracranial hemorrhage. *Neurosurgery* 1984;15: 332–338.
65. Mironov A. Classification of spontaneous dural arteriovenous fistulas with regard to their pathogenesis. *Acta Radiol* 1995;36: 582–592.
66. Lalwani AK, Dowd CF, Halbach VV. Grading venous restrictive disease in patients with dural arteriovenous fistulas of the transverse/sigmoid sinus. *J Neurosurg* 1993;7:11–15.
67. Halbach VV, Higashida RT, Hieshima GB, et al. Treatment of dural fistulas involving the deep cerebral venous system. *AJNR Am J Neuroradiol* 1989;10:393–399.
68. Elster AD, Chen MY, Richardson DN, et al. Dilated intercavernous sinuses: an MR sign of carotid-cavernous and carotid-dural fistulas. *AJNR Am J Neuroradiol* 1991;12:641–645.
69. Osborn AG. Intracranial vascular malformations. In: *Diagnostic neuroradiology.* St Louis: Mosby, 1994:284–329.
70. Ikawa F, Uozumi T, Kiya K, et al. Diagnosis of carotid-cavernous fistulas with magnetic resonance angiography demonstrating the draining veins utilizing 3-D time-of-flight and 3-D phase contrast techniques. *Neurosurg Rev* 1996;19:7–12.
71. Fournier D, TerBrugge K, Rosesh G, et al. Revascularization of brain arteriovenous malformations after embolization with bucrylate. *Neuroradiology* 1990;32:497–501.
72. Putman CM, Chaloupka JC, Kalyanpur A, et al. Pitfalls and limitations in the MRI/MRA diagnosis of DAVF: an examination of discordant findings with conventional angiography. 34th Annual Meeting of the American Society of Neuroradiology, June 1996.
73. Hu WY, TerBrugge KG. The role of angiography in the evaluation of vascular and neoplastic disease in the external carotid artery circulation. *Neuroimaging Clin N Am* 1996;6:625–644.
74. Dare AO, Chaloupka JC, Mayer PL, et al. Paradoxical clinicoradiologic features of a cavernous dural arteriovenous malformation: a limitation of expectant management. *Int J Clin Neurosci* 1997;4:8–10.
75. Findlay JM, Miekle BW. Fatal rebleeding from a dural arteriovenous malformation of the posterior fossa: case report with pathological examination. *Can J Neurol Sci* 1994;21:67–71.
76. Nabors NW, Azzam CJ, Albanna FJ, et al. Delayed postoperative dural arteriovenous malformations: report of two cases. *J Neurosurg* 1987;66:768–822.
77. Duffau H, Lopes M, Janosevic V, et al. Early rebleeding from intracranial dural arteriovenous fistulas: report of 20 cases and review of the literature. *J Neurosurg* 1999;90:78–84.
78. Iwama T, Hashimoto N, Takagi Y, et al. Hemodynamic and metabolic disturbances in patients with intracranial dural arteriovenous fistulas: positron emission tomography evaluation before and after treatment. *J Neurosurg* 1997;86:806–811.
79. Ito M, Sonokawa T, Mishina H, et al: Reversible dural arteriovenous malformation-induced venous ischemia as a cause of dementia: treatment by surgical occlusion of draining dural sinus: case report. *Neurosurgery* 1995;37:1187–1192.
80. Viñuela F, Dion JE, Halbach VV, eds. *Interventional neuroradiology: endovascular therapy of the central nervous system.* New York: Raven Press, 1992.
81. Barnwell SL, Halbach VV, Dowd CF, et al. Multiple dural arteriovenous fistulas of the cranium and spine. *AJNR Am J Neuroradiol* 1991:12:441–445.
82. Barnwell SL, Halbach VV, Higashida RT, et al. Complex dural arteriovenous fistulas: results of combined endovascular and neurosurgical treatment in 16 patients. *J Neurosurg* 1989;71: 352–358.
83. Ishii K, Goto K, Ihara K, et al. High risk dural arteriovenous

fistulae of transverse and sigmoid sinuses. *AJNR Am J Neuroradiol* 1988;8:1113–1121.
84. Vdyasager C. Persistent embryonic veins in the arteriovenous malformations of the dura. *Acta Neurochir (Wien)* 1979;48: 199–215.
85. Kline JN, Ryals TJ, Galvin JR, et al. Pulmonary embolization and infarction. An iatrogenic complication of transcatheter embolization of a cerebral arteriovenous malformation with polyvinyl alcohol sponge. *Chest* 1993;103:1293–1295.
86. Chaloupka JC. Preoperative endovascular therapeutic embolization of cerebral arteriovenous malformations. In: Awad IA, Jafar JJ, Rosenwasser RH. *Vascular malformations of the central nervous system.* Philadelphia: Lippincott–Raven, 1999.
87. Martin NA, King WA, Wilson CB, et al. Management of dural arteriovenous malformations of the anterior cranial fossa. *J Neurosurg* 1990;72:692–697.
88. Hirai T, Korogi Y, Baba Y, et al. Dural carotid cavernous fistulas: role of conventional radiation therapy. Long-term results with irradiation, embolization, or both. *Radiology* 1998:207: 423–430.
89. Lewis AI, Tomsick TA, Tew JM Jr. Management of tentorial dural arteriovenous malformations: transarterial embolization combined with stereotactic radiation or surgery. *J Neurosurg* 1994;81:851–859.
90. Guo WY, Pan DH, Wu HM, et al. Radiosurgery as an alternative for dural arteriovenous fistulas of the cavernous sinus. *AJNR Am J Neuroradiol* 1998;19:1081–1087.
91. Aletich VA, Debrun GM, Koenigsberg R, et al. Arteriovenous malformation nidus catheterization with hydrophilic wire and flow-directed catheter. *AJNR Am J Neuroradiol* 1997;18: 929–935.
92. Debrun GM, Aletich V, Ausman JI, et al. Embolization of the nidus of brain arteriovenous malformations with n-butyl cyanoacrylate. *Neurosurgery* 1997;40:112–119.
93. Halbach VV, Higashida RT, Hieshima BG, et al. Transvenous embolization of direct carotid cavernous fistulas. *AJNR Am J Neuroradiol* 1988;9:741–747.
94. Halbach VV, Higashida RT, Hieshima GB, et al. Treatment of dural arteriovenous malformations involving the superior sagittal sinus. *AJNR Am J Neuroradiol* 1988;9:337–343.
95. Berenstein A. Flow-controlled silicone fluid embolization. *AJR Am J Roentgenol* 1980;134:1213–1218.
96. Brothers MF, Kaufmann JCS, Fox AJ, et al. N-Butyl 2-cyanoacrylate: substitute for IBCA in interventional neuroradiology—histopathologic and polymerization time study. *AJNR Am J Neuroradiol* 1989;10:777–786.
97. Taki W, Yonekawa Y, Iwata H, et al. A new liquid material for embolization of arteriovenous malformations. *AJNR Am J Neuroradiol* 1990;11:163–168.
98. Chaloupka JC, Viñuela F, Vinters HV, et al. Technical feasibility and histopathologic studies of ethylene vinyl copolymer (EVAL) using the swine endovascular embolization model. *AJNR Am J Neuroradiol* 1994;15:1107–1115.
99. Sadato A, Taki W, Ikada Y, et al. Experimental study and clinical use of poly(vinyl acetate) emulsion as liquid embolisation material. *Neuroradiology* 1994;36:634–641.
100. Chaloupka JC, Huddle DC, Alderman J, et al. A re-examination of the angiotoxicity of superselective injection of DMSO in the swine *rete* embolization model. *AJNR Am J Neuroradiol* 1999; 45:650–656.
101. Jahan R, Murayama Y, Gobin YP, et al. Embolization of arteriovenous malformations with Onyx: clinicopathological experience in 23 patients. *Neurosurgery* 2001;48:984–995.
102. Gyurko G, Szucs J, Ezsely F, et al. Use in vascular surgery of the tissue adhesive Histoacryl. *Acta Chir Hung* 1974;15:353–360.
103. Debrun G, Lacour P, Caron JP, et al. Detachable balloon and calibrated-leak balloon techniques in the treatment of cerebral vascular lesions. *J Neurosurg* 1978;49:635–649.
104. Kailasnath P, Chaloupka JC. Quantitative assessment of the binding mechanics of NBCA: preliminary *in-vitro* results. *Interv Neuroradiol* 1997;3[Suppl 1]:102.
105. Spiegel S, Viñuela F, Fox AJ. Adjusting the polymerization time of IBCA. *AJNR Am J Neuroradiol* 1985;6:461–463.
106. Debrun G, Lacour P, Caron JP, et al. Treatment of arteriovenous fistulas and of aneurysms using an inflatable and releasable balloon. Experimental principles. Application to man. *Nouv Presse Med* 1975;4:2315–2318.
107. Higashida RT, Hieshima BG, Halbach VV. Advances in the treatment of complex cerebrovascular disorders by interventional neurovascular techniques. *Circulation* 1991;83: 1196–1206.
108. Katada K, Sano H, Katoh Y, et al. Ethyl 2-cyanoacrylate as an embolic agent for cranial arteriovenous malformations. An experimental study. *Acta Radiol Suppl* 1986;369:623–626.
109. Kerber CW, Bank WO, Manelfe C. Control and placement of intracranial microcatheters. *AJNR Am J Neuroradiol* 1980;1: 157–159.
110. Berenstein AB, Choi IS, Kupersmith MJ, et al. Complications of endovascular embolization in 202 patients with cerebral AVMs. *AJNR Am J Neuroradiol* 1989;10:876(abst).
111. Dion JE, Mathis JM. Cranial arteriovenous malformations. The role of embolization and stereotactic surgery. *Neurosurg Clin N Am* 1994;5:459–474.
112. Pelz DM, Lownie SP, Fox AJ, et al. Symptomatic pulmonary complications from liquid acrylate embolization of brain arteriovenous malformations. *AJNR Am J Neuroradiol* 1995;16:19–26.
113. Monsein LH, Debrun GM, Miller NR, et al. Treatment of dural carotid-cavernous fistulas via the superior ophthalmic vein. *AJNR Am J Neuroradiol* 1991;12:435–439.
114. Debrun G, Lacour P, Viñuela F, et al. Treatment of 54 traumatic carotid-cavernous fistulas. *J Neurosurg* 1981;55:678–692.
115. Mullan S. Treatment of carotid-cavernous fistulas by cavernous sinus occlusion. *J Neurosurg* 1979;50:131–144.
116. Viñuela F, Fox AJ, Debrun G, et al. Pre-embolization superselective angiography in the treatment of brain arteriovenous malformations with isobutyl-2-cyanoacrylate. *AJNR Am J Neuroradiol* 1984;5:765–769.
117. Kailasnath P, Chaloupka JC. Quantitative assessment of polymerization-binding mechanics of cyanoacrylates: model development and validation. *AJNR Am J Neuroradiol* 2001 *(in press).*
118. Chaloupka JC, Peters SS, Weigele JB. Quantitative analysis of liquid polymers. 2001 Joint Meeting of the AANS/CNS Cerebrovascular Section and ASITN. February 2001.
119. Lasjaunias P, Manelfe C, TerBrugge K, et al. Endovascular treatment of cerebral arteriovenous malformations. *Neurosurg Rev* 1986;9:265–275.
120. Viñuela F. Update on intravascular functional evaluation and therapy of intracranial arteriovenous malformations. *Neuroimaging Clin N Am* 1992;2:279–289.
121. Viñuela F, Mombela L, Roach M, et al. Stenotic and occlusive disease of the venous drainage system of deep brain AVMs. *J Neurosurg* 1985;63:180–184.
122. Mathis JM, Evans AJ, DeNardo AJ, et al. Hydrophilic coatings diminish adhesion of glue to catheter: an *in vitro* simulation of NBCA embolization. *AJNR Am J Neuroradiol* 1997;18: 1087–1091.
123. Kailasnath P, Chaloupka JC. Quantitative assessment of the binding mechanics of NBCA: preliminary *in-vitro* results. *Interv Neuroradiol* 1997;3[Suppl 1]:102.
124. Hoff JT. Cerebral protection. *J Neurosurg* 1986;65:579–584.
125. Krause GS, White BC, Aust SD, et al. Brain cell death following

ischemia and reperfusion: a proposed biochemical sequence. *Crit Care Med* 1988;16:714–726.

126. Levy ML, Rabb C, Couldwell WT. Protection of the neuronal pool. In: Apuzzo MLJ, ed. *Brain surgery: complication avoidance and management.* New York: Churchill Livingstone. 1993; 857–873.
127. Martin NA, ed. Neurosurgical intensive care. *Neurosurg Clin N Am* 1994;4:573–849.
128. Murphy K, Gailloud P, Venbrux A, et al. Endovascular treatment of grade IV transverse sinus dural arteriovenous fistula by sinus recanalization, angioplasty, stent placement; technical case report. *Neurosurgery* 2000;46:497–500.

12

CAROTID-CAVERNOUS FISTULAS

THOMAS A. TOMSICK

Carotid-cavernous fistulas (CCFs) are arteriovenous communications between the carotid artery or its branches and the cavernous sinus (CS), classically resulting in Dandy's clinical triad of pulsatile exophthalmos, chemosis, and bruit.

CCFs have been historically classified by (a) etiology (spontaneous or posttraumatic), (b) flow rate (high or low flow), and (c) angioarchitecture (direct fistulas with a connection between the ICA itself and the CS, and indirect or dural arteriovenous fistulas between meningeal arteries and the CS). The term *carotid-cavernous fistula* generically is applied to both direct and dural types, a throwback to preangiography days when the importance of distinguishing between the two was not appreciated and the distinction not easily made.

Selective arteriography has allowed distinction of the different angioarchitectural types. Barrow distinguished four types of CCFs depending on arterial supply as follows:

Type A: direct communications between the internal carotid artery (ICA) and the CS, usually with high flow rates. Types B, C, and D: dural arteriovenous fistulas (DAVFs) fed by the meningeal arteries of the ICA or the external carotid artery (ECA) or both. Type B fistulas are relatively uncommon and are supplied only by dural branches of the ICA. Type C fistulas are supplied solely by dural branches of the ECA. The most common dural fistula, type D, is supplied by meningeal branches of both the ICA and ECA [1]. We have subclassified the latter into D1 or D2, depending on unilateral or bilateral supply, respectively [2].

BACKGROUND

Direct Fistula

Etiology and Pathology

Direct fistulas, type A, are most commonly traumatic and are more commonly seen in a younger male population, usually due to motor vehicle accidents or penetrating injuries [9]. Approximately 20% of type A CCFs may be spontaneous, due to rupture of either cavernous ICA aneurysms or weakened ICA vessel walls coursing through the CS [10].

Parkinson described the typical pathology of a traumatic type A CCF, a short endotheliolized opening between the ICA and any one of the adjacent variable lateral sellar venous channels that he envisioned enclosed by the dura of the CS. He suggested two types of traumatic CCFs, tears of the ICA and tears of the meningeal vessels that originate from the cavernous segment [11], theorizing that the branches may be more likely to be torn with fractures because they are in intimate contact with bone throughout much of their course. It is postulated that the movement of the artery during trauma, with fixation at the proximal petrosphenoid ligament just beyond the lacerum segment, may create sufficient wall tension to stretch and tear the ICA.

Van Dellen draws on the concept that CCFs are part of a continuum of the arterial injury. He suggests that certain arterial wall tears allow false aneurysms to form [12], so that a true CCF may not always occur when the arterial tear does not breach the venous walls but rather compresses them, but a pseudoaneurysm results instead. Small pseudoaneurysms are as easily explained, however, by incomplete transmural tears, in contradistinction to a complete wall tear into a venous sinusoid with fistula formation.

Debrun described the site of CCF origin by dividing the cavernous ICA into five arbitrary segments, finding the most common site of occurrence at the proximal horizontal portion of the ICA near the artery of the inferior CS (40%) [13]. Following this, they occur with decreasing frequency at the junction of the horizontal and posterior vertical ascending cavernous segment (28%), at the origins from the posterior vertical ascending segment itself (20%), and in a few cases CCFs occur distally near the anterior genu and clinoidal segment (12%). Our own series and that of Helmke demonstrated a slight variance in ostium locations compared to Debrun's series [14,15].

Direct type A flow rates are variable and depend on the size of the ostium and the nature of the venous drainage compartments available. Complete steal of ICA flow to the

T.A. Tomsick: Department of Neuroradiology, University Hospital, Cincinnati, Ohio.

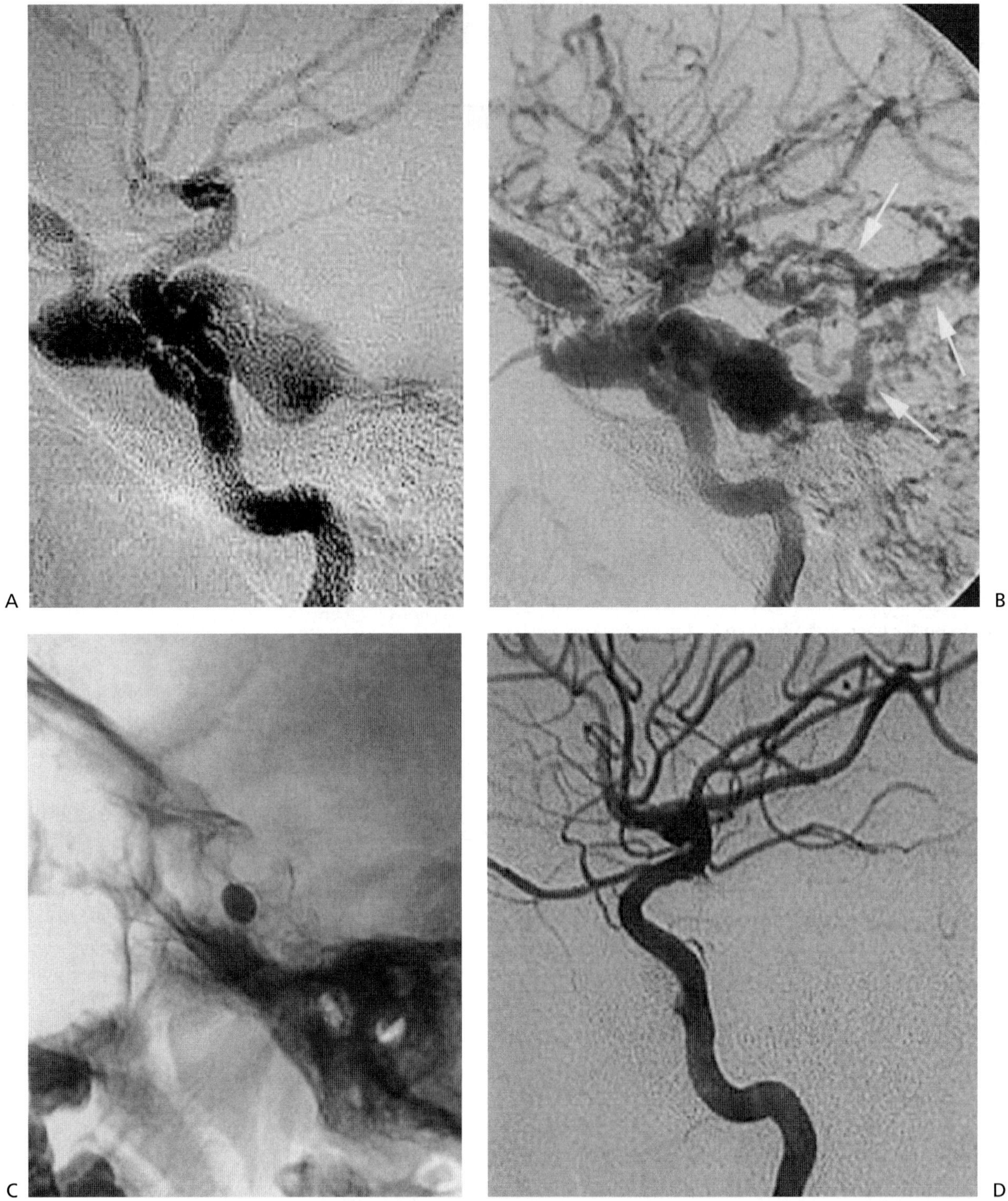

FIGURE 12-1. This 11-year-old child was brought for evaluation 2 months following head injury with bilateral CN VI paresis, bruit, and arterialization of the conjunctiva. **A:** The early arterial image demonstrates a traumatic type A CCF with 3-mm ostium, minimal dilation of the proximal venous channel, and greater distention of the draining CS, with aneurysmal dilation of the posterior cavernous–superior petrosal sinus connection. **B:** Later image demonstrates dilation of the CS, superior petrosal sinus, and pial cortical venous drainage *(arrows)*. **C:** A single 0.5-cc detachable silicone balloon inflated to 0.15 cc with metrizamide 200 mg/dl was detached in the proximal venous channel just beyond the fistula ostium. **D:** CCF closure following balloon placement. Fourteen-month follow-up magnetic resonance angiography demonstrated a small asymptomatic "venous bulge."

CCF occurs in approximately 5% of cases at diagnosis. Most fistula ostia are holes of 2.6 mm [13]. These are typically small enough to be treated with detachable balloons of 0.28-cc mean volume, equivalent to balloon inflation to 7 mm × 9 mm dimensions (Figs. 12-1 and 12-2). Bilateral traumatic CCFs occur in approximately 1% to 2% of patients with traumatic CCFs [16,17].

Spontaneous type A CCFs are more common in an older, female population, although reports in children have appeared [18,19]. Spontaneous type A fistulas generally have been ascribed to rupture of a cavernous aneurysm or spontaneous rupture of a congenitally weakened, arteriosclerotic, or arteriopathic artery. Fibromuscular dysplasia with or without ICA dissection [20,21], and arteriopathy of Ehlers-Danlos syndrome or pseudoxanthoma elasticum, are also known to predispose to spontaneous type A CCFs [22–24]. Patients with these problems are difficult to evaluate and treat by the usual intraarterial methods due to arterial tortuosity and vascular fragility created by the qualitative and quantitative collagen deficiency [25].

Clinical Features

With traumatic CCFs, an intracranial bruit may be audible immediately or may first be identified only when patients awaken and complain of a noise. Other soft tissue swelling from head trauma initially may delay recognition of the typical ophthalmologic signs. Bruit and eye signs may develop in a delayed fashion as well. On the other hand, with

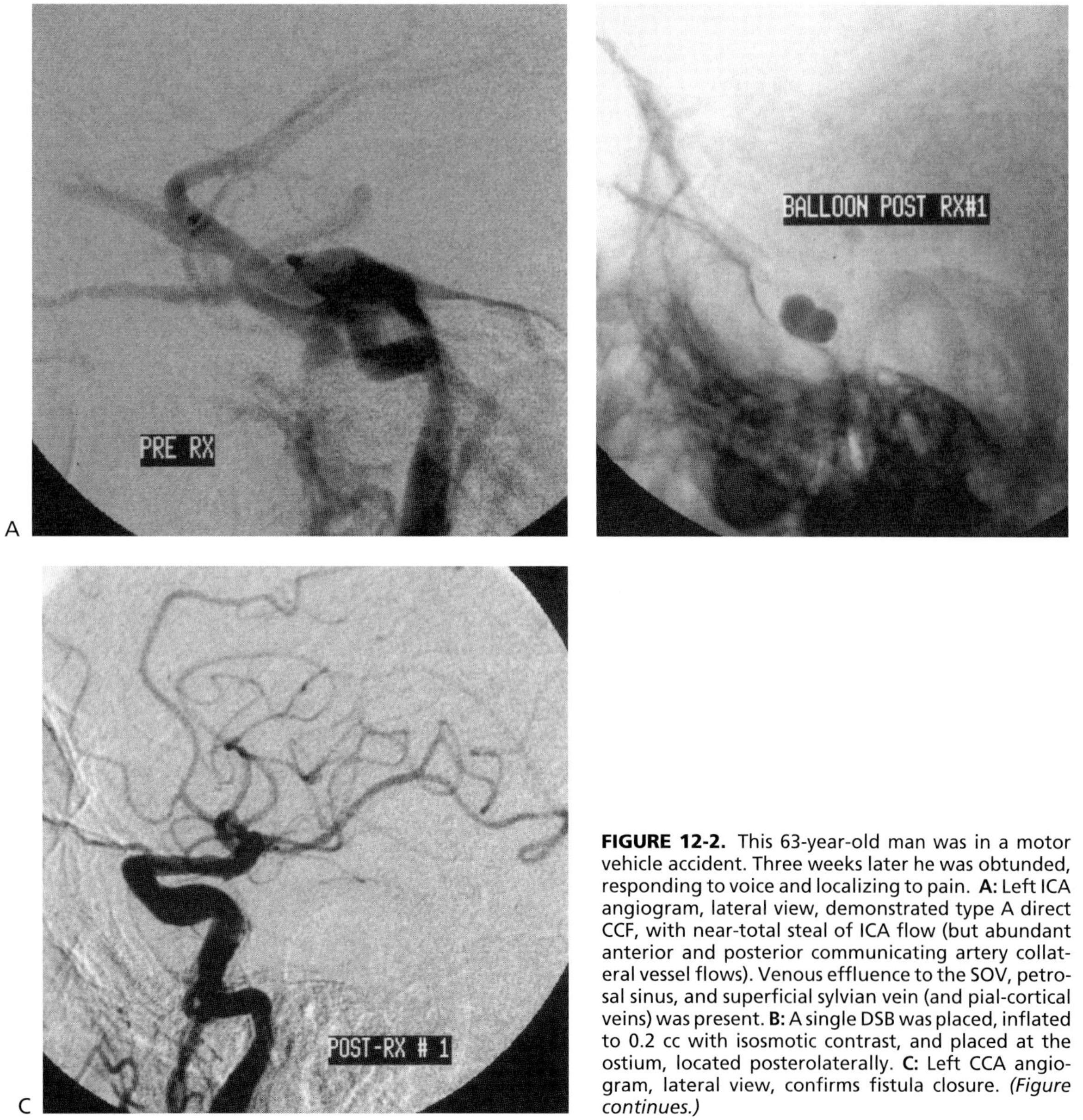

FIGURE 12-2. This 63-year-old man was in a motor vehicle accident. Three weeks later he was obtunded, responding to voice and localizing to pain. **A:** Left ICA angiogram, lateral view, demonstrated type A direct CCF, with near-total steal of ICA flow (but abundant anterior and posterior communicating artery collateral vessel flows). Venous effluence to the SOV, petrosal sinus, and superficial sylvian vein (and pial-cortical veins) was present. **B:** A single DSB was placed, inflated to 0.2 cc with isosmotic contrast, and placed at the ostium, located posterolaterally. **C:** Left CCA angiogram, lateral view, confirms fistula closure. *(Figure continues.)*

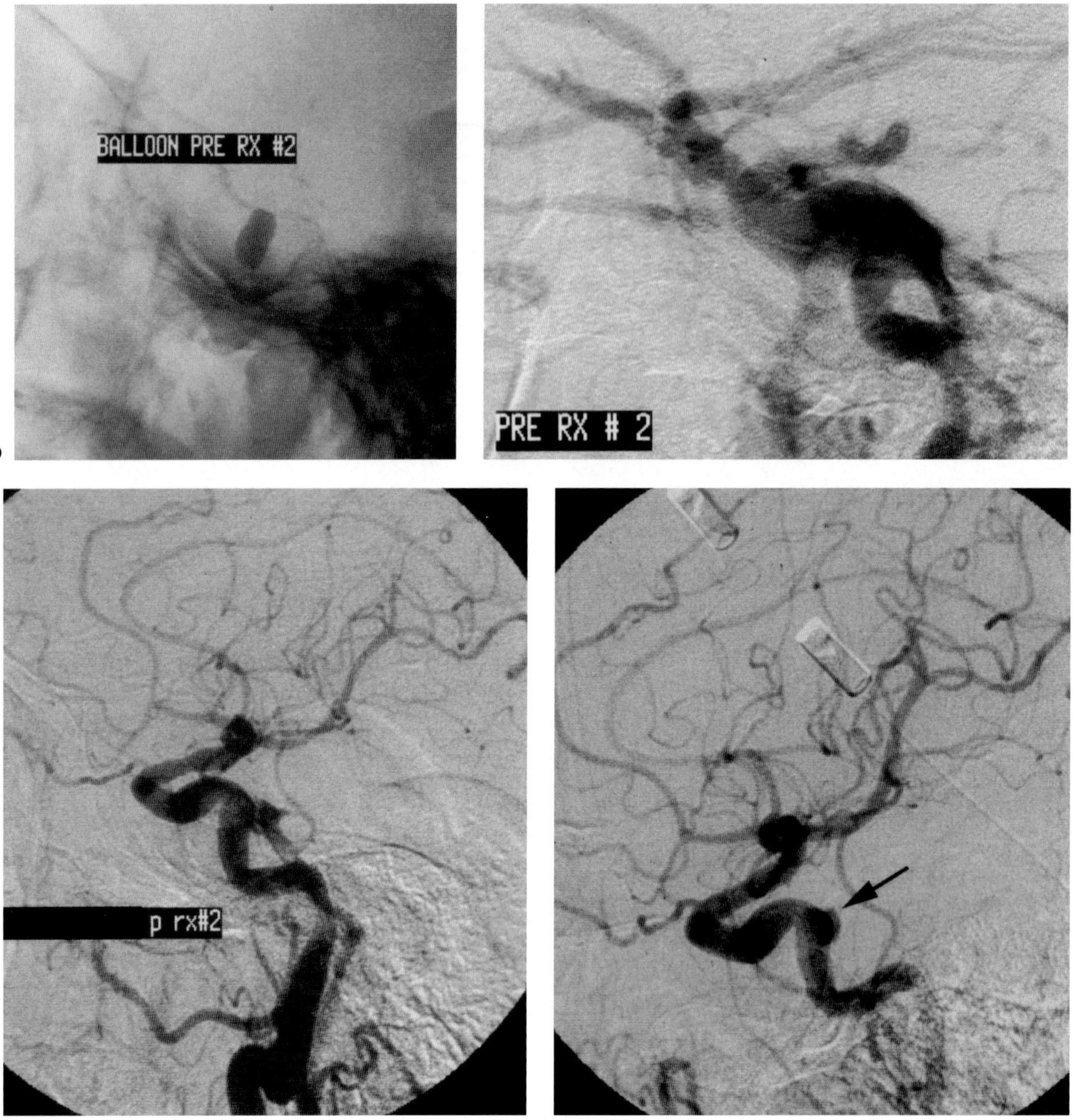

FIGURE 12-2. *Continued.* **D:** The bruit reappeared the next morning, and a digital skull image demonstrated balloon movement. **E:** Repeat left CCA angiogram, lateral view, confirmed fistula reoccurrence. **F:** Left CCA angiogram, lateral view, after placement of second DSB (0.2 cc) demonstrates minimal flow to the inferior petrosal sinus. **G:** Left CCA angiogram 3 months later confirmed interval CCF closure, with a small venous bulge at the fistula site *(arrow).*

aneurysmal rupture of spontaneous CCFs, more rapid development of pain, chemosis, and proptosis is the rule.

Noninvasive imaging may be performed as the first step in clinical evaluation, and the imaging changes have been well described by Cornelius. They include dilated CS and superior ophthalmic vein (SOV); dilated secondary-draining pial veins; proptosis, soft tissue edema, and swelling of retrolobare fat and periorbita; edema and hemorrhage of the brain; abnormal flow signal in the CS on magnetic resonance angiography [26].

Neurophthalmologic sequelae occur in the vast majority of patients as proptosis (up to 90%), conjunctival arterialization and chemosis (up to 90%), corneal damage, diplopia (at least 50%), pain (25%), trigeminal nerve (cranial nerve V [CN V]) dysfunction, elevated intraocular pressure, and visual loss (up to 50%) (Fig. 12-3). Ophthalmologic findings of proptosis, chemosis, and arterialization of the conjunctiva may be unilateral, bilateral (due to intercommunicating CS drainage), or may exist only on the side opposite the fistula. Intracerebral and subarachnoid hemorrhage related to venous hypertension in CCFs may be life-threatening.

Five percent of patients will develop intracranial hemorrhage, and 1% to 2% will manifest life-threatening epistaxis. Epistaxis can be either acute or remote from the initial trauma due to rupture of a pseudoaneurysmal CS varix. Generalized increased intracranial pressure and venous hypertension of the brain(stem) can occur spontaneously or can be related to treatment that shuts off pathways of venous effluence [27,28]. In our treatment series of 150 type A CCFs, we witnessed total visual loss in 1.5%, coma due to venous hypertension of the brainstemin 1.5%, intracerebral hemorrhage in 2%, venous hypertension with neurologic deficit and CT-demonstrated brain edema in 2%, and life-threatening epistaxis in 2% prior to treatment. We have documented neurologic symptoms due to steal phenomenon only once in our experience, that due to a 40-year-old fistula treated initially by ICA ligation [29–31].

Angiography

Selective angiography determines the size and location of the direct fistula ostium; presence or absence of aneurysm, pseudoaneurysm, or venous sinus varix; pattern of venous drainage including pial venous drainage; collateral arterial supply to the involved ICA; and excludes the presence of an associated dissection or other traumatic injury. Angiography should include injection of both common carotid arteries (CCAs), the ipsilateral ICA and ECA, contralateral ICA with ipsilateral carotid compression, and vertebral artery

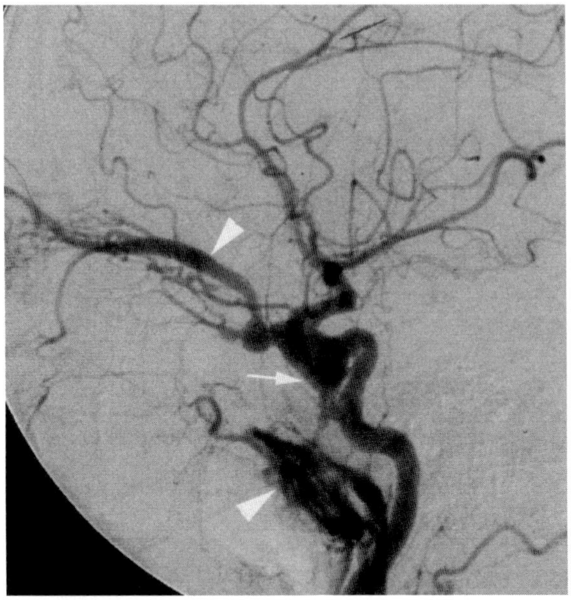
A

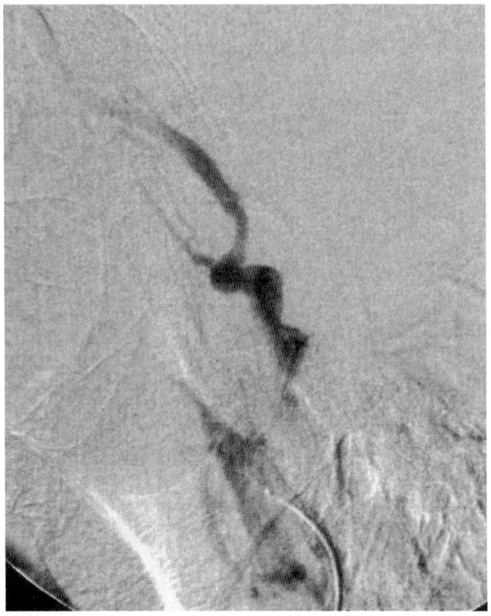
B

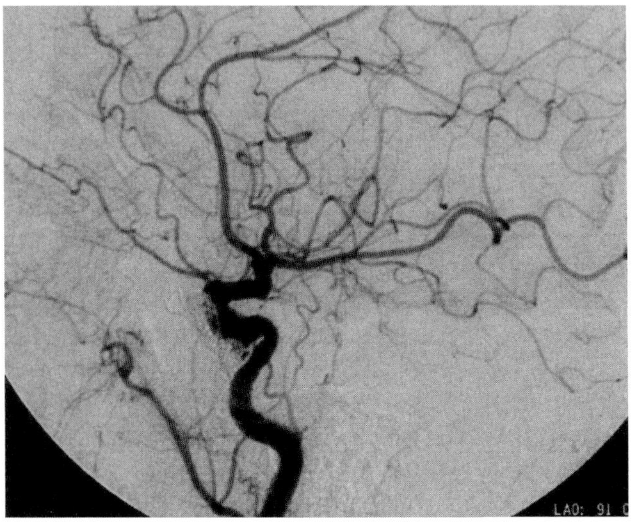
C

FIGURE 12-3. This 71-year-old woman was in an auto accident 4 weeks previously with chest trauma, but no head injuries. She experienced rapid progression of pain, bruit, and remarkable chemosis, proptosis, visual loss (light perception only), and intraocular pressure of 40 mm Hg over the past 5 days. **A:** Left CCA arteriogram, lateral view, demonstrates a direct CCF arising from the inferior C4 segment of the ICA just beyond the tight curve of the posterior cavernous genu *(arrow),* with venous effluence via an attenuated SOV and pterygoid plexus *(arrowhead).* **B:** A 0.5-cc DSB mounted on a heat-shaped Tracker-18 catheter, with 0.010-inch guidewire placed through a rotating hemostatic valve, was placed coaxially into the ICA but would not enter the fistula. A double-catheter technique was not attempted. **A:** Rapid Transit catheter was introduced through a 7-Fr. Berenstein catheter via the left jugular, facial veins, and pterygoid plexus into the CS. Contrast injection confirmed restricted venous effluence through distal narrowing of the SOV. **C:** The SOV was disconnected first, and the anterior CS subsequently packed, with a 7 cm × 30 cm standard GDC-18, and fibered GDCs (2 mm × 6 mm, 2 mm × 5 mm, 2 mm × 4 mm, and 2 mm × 3 mm), with CCF occlusion.

with ipsilateral carotid compression [3]. The contralateral CCA arteriogram is performed to exclude a carotid stenosis or dissection, preexisting aneurysm or traumatic pseudoaneurysm, or contralateral CCF. A contralateral carotid injection with ipsilateral compression (or temporary balloon occlusion) determines patency of the anterior communicating artery as a source for collateral supply. Spontaneous cross filling due to a fistulous steal eliminates the necessity of the latter maneuver.

The appearance of the opacifying CS (or the venous plexus of the lateral compartment of the CS [4]) varies between patients, appearing channel-like (see Fig. 12-1A), pseudoaneurysmal (see Fig. 12-2A), or as a network of interconnecting sinusoids. If the fistula ostium is not adequately visualized, a carotid occlusion arteriogram should be considered. The ICA can be catheterized and ipsilateral common carotid compression applied below the catheter tip; contrast is injected at 1 ml per second at one or two frames per second to slowly opacify the ICA and fistula. A double-lumen balloon catheter can be used wherein the balloon is inflated and contrast is injected via the distal lumen with similar injection rates and imaging, allowing slow opacification of the ICA below the fistula, with entry into the fistula contrasted by hemodilution of flow from retrograde filling of the ICA above the fistula [5–7].

The Huber maneuver (vertebral artery injection with

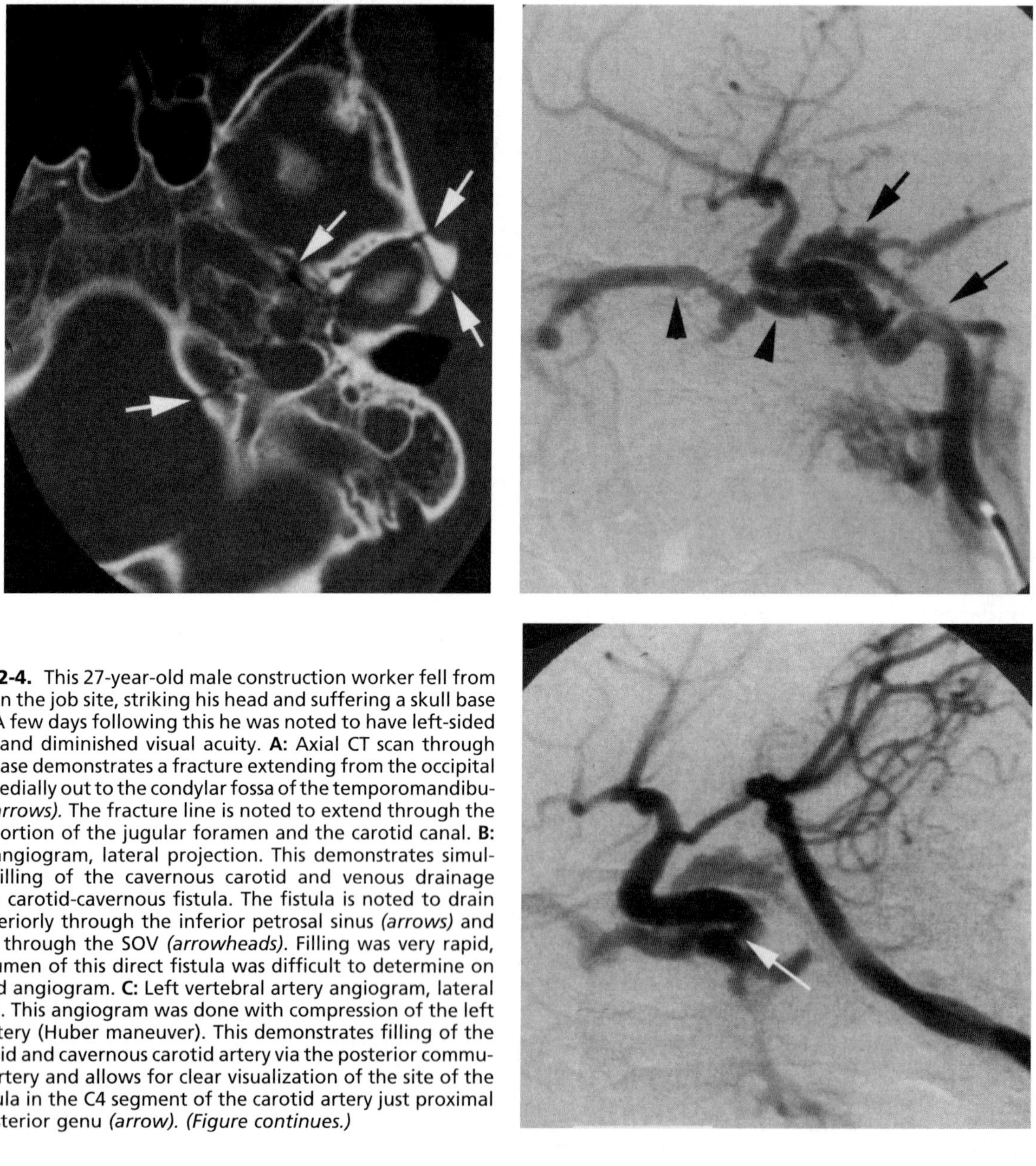

A B C

FIGURE 12-4. This 27-year-old male construction worker fell from a height on the job site, striking his head and suffering a skull base fracture. A few days following this he was noted to have left-sided proptosis and diminished visual acuity. **A:** Axial CT scan through the skull base demonstrates a fracture extending from the occipital condyle medially out to the condylar fossa of the temporomandibular joint *(arrows).* The fracture line is noted to extend through the anterior portion of the jugular foramen and the carotid canal. **B:** Left ICA angiogram, lateral projection. This demonstrates simultaneous filling of the cavernous carotid and venous drainage through a carotid-cavernous fistula. The fistula is noted to drain both posteriorly through the inferior petrosal sinus *(arrows)* and anteriorly through the SOV *(arrowheads).* Filling was very rapid, and the lumen of this direct fistula was difficult to determine on the carotid angiogram. **C:** Left vertebral artery angiogram, lateral projection. This angiogram was done with compression of the left carotid artery (Huber maneuver). This demonstrates filling of the supraclinoid and cavernous carotid artery via the posterior communicating artery and allows for clear visualization of the site of the direct fistula in the C4 segment of the carotid artery just proximal to the posterior genu *(arrow). (Figure continues.)*

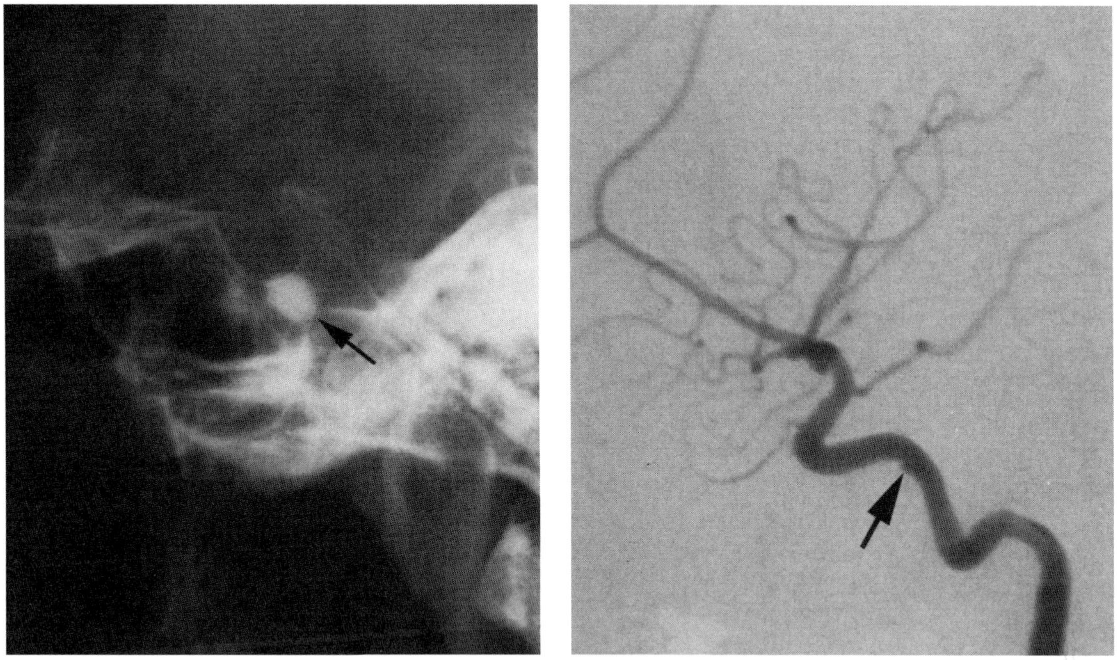

D E

FIGURE 12-4. *Continued.* **D:** Lateral radiograph of the skull immediately following treatment. A single detachable silicone balloon was placed in the CS just beyond the ostium of the fistula and inflated with isosmotic contrast *(arrows).* **E:** Left ICA angiogram, lateral projection, following treatment demonstrates a small venous bulge *(arrow)* at the fistula site with complete closure of the fistula. (From Michael P. Marks and Huy M. Do, unpublished material, with permission.)

ipsilateral carotid compression) results in retrograde filling of the ipsilateral posterior communicating artery to the cavernous-carotid artery segment with direct filling of the fistula (Fig. 12-4) [8]. This maneuver may also demonstrate the rare double fistula. Venous drainage patterns are variable and best correlate with patients' symptoms. Patients with SOV drainage typically have ocular signs and symptoms. Patients with petrosal venous drainage tend to have cranial nerve paresis. Exaggerated pial-cortical venous drainage predisposes to intracranial hemorrhage, increased intracranial pressure, or neurologic deterioration.

Indirect Fistulas

Etiology and Pathology

Indirect (type B,C, or D) CCFs, also sometimes called dural CCFs, have a predilection for spontaneous occurrence in postmenopausal females. Hypertension and diabetes have been suggested as predisposing factors. Dural CCFs may represent a collateral response to a thrombosis of the CS and may be a manifestation of a thrombotic tendency that may lead to multiple AVFs (Fig. 12-5) [86–88]. Trauma is less commonly associated with a symptomatic type B, C, or D CCF [89].

We have discovered a few asymptomatic traumatic dural CCFs (usually type B) during angiography for other indications. Congenital dural AVFs have been reported in infants as young as 5 weeks of age.

The prevalence of types B–D dural AVFs of the CS is uncertain. Frequency in a referral population does not define its occurrence in the general population.

It is probable that minimally affected patients are not referred to endovascular centers and do not enter databases, although most embolization treatment series do include a number of such patients managed conservatively.

Clinical Features

Kurata emphasized that Dandy's classic triad of CCF (exophthalmos, bruit, and conjunctival chemosis) were present in less than 50% of his 12 patients, and cranial nerve paresis was the only finding in five [93]. A wide variation in specific symptoms and signs has been reported [94]. At the time of diagnosis, the incidence of signs and symptoms, when noted, in 260 reviewed cases was pain (40%), red eye (90%), proptosis (89%), bruit (39%), decreased visual acuity (32%), increased intraocular pressure (83%), and double vision or cranial nerve paresis (68%). The diplopia is usually horizontal due to abducent nerve (CN VI) paresis (50%), with oculomotor (CN III) and trochlear nerve (CN IV) dysfunction less common. A mechanical ptosis is often

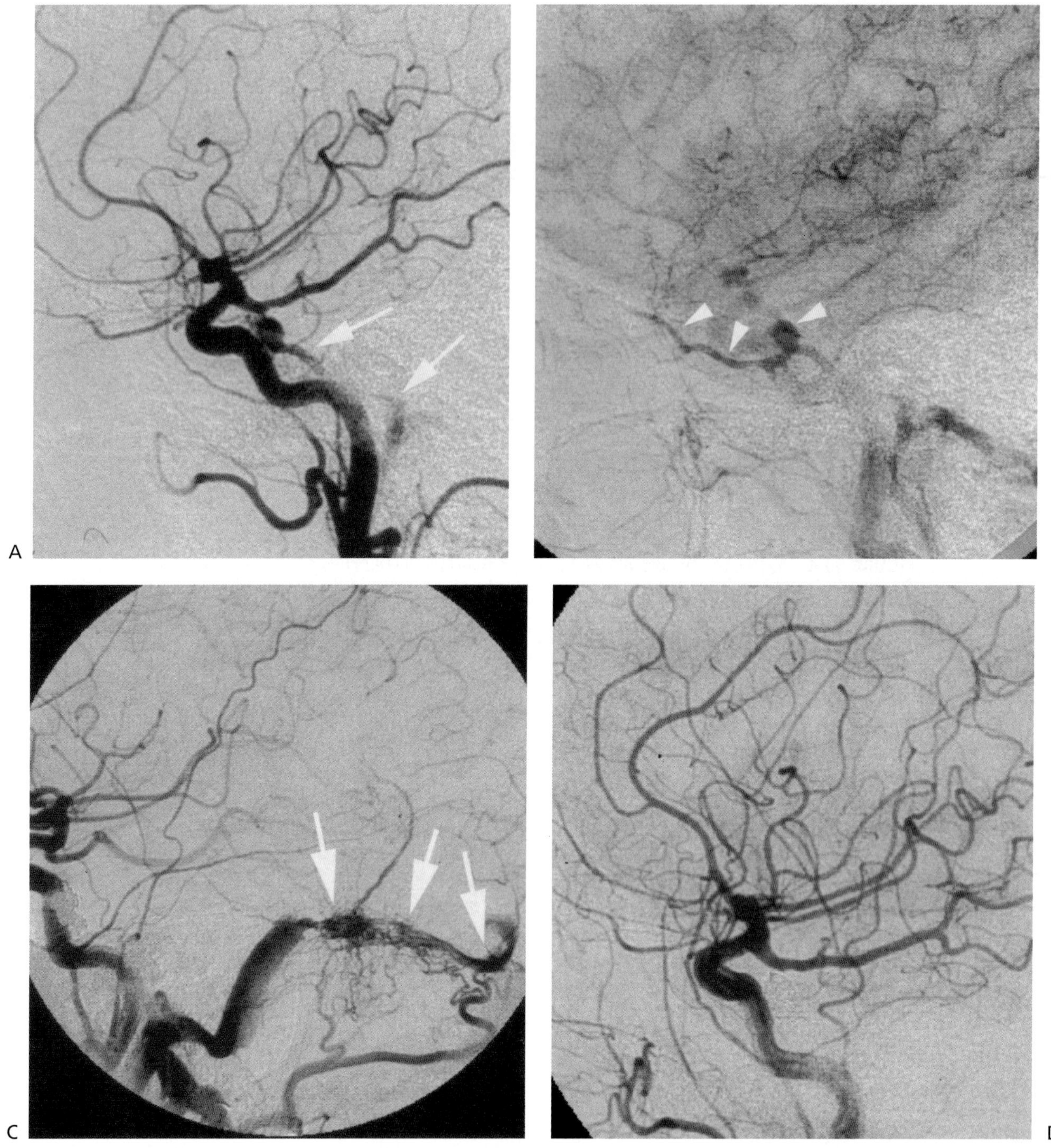

FIGURE 12-5. This 72-year-old woman developed eye pain, chemosis, minor proptosis, and noise in her left ear. **A,B:** Right CCA angiogram, lateral view, demonstrates a type D dural arteriovenous fistula of the CS, with early petrosal (*arrows* in A) and late attenuated superior ophthalmic (*arrowheads* in B) venous drainage. **C:** Left CCA angiogram, lateral view, demonstrates a dural arteriovenous fistula to the left transverse sinus *(arrows)*. **D:** Right CCA angiogram, lateral view, posttreatment. The right internal jugular vein was catheterized with a 6-Fr. Envoy catheter, and a Rapid Transit microcatheter was passed into the posterior cavernous–petrosal junction, and the sinus, and the fistulous flow was occluded with 36 cm of GDC coils. The transverse sinus fistula was treated with particle embolization and stereotactic radiosurgery, with complete closure of both AVF at follow-up angiography.

found in inflamed eyes, and pupillary signs due to iris ischemia may make interpretation of oculomotor nerve dysfunction less reliable [95]. Facial numbness due to trigeminal nerve (CN V) dysfunction is much less common than with type A CCFs. Facial nerve paresis may develop rarely, probably secondary to increased venous pressure [96].

Third, fourth, and sixth cranial nerve pareses are most commonly on the side of the fistula, although they may be bilateral or even on the side opposite the fistula due to flow to the opposite CS from connecting channels (Fig. 12-6). Cranial nerve pareses may occur in the absence of chemosis, proptosis, and red eye if the venous drainage is directed posteriorly toward the SOV. The specific cause of cranial nerve paresis remains conjectural and may be multifactorial, related to venous congestion, venous compression, or less likely ischemia due to arterial steal from the meningohypophyseal and inferior CS arterial supply to the nerves.

Bilateral arterial supply or bilateral drainage or both do not equate with bilateral fistulas, which are uncommon. It may be difficult to distinguish between single or multiple fistulas in lesions with higher flow and bilateral ECA and ICA contribution (type D2).

Unlike high-flow type A fistulas, most spontaneous typeB–D CCFs will improve, and many heal, during medical management. Patients with headache, visual deterioration, high intraocular pressure, and optic disc changes refractory to medication, progressive diplopia, or unusual cosmetic deformity will usually be evaluated further and offered endovascular treatment in hopes of accelerating the healing process. Nukui reported complete regression of signs and symptoms in 18 of 19 patients with dural CCFs over 6-month to 6- to 8-year observation periods, with marked improvement noted in one additional patient [97]. Sasaki and Nukui reviewed the clinical course of 26 patients (which may have included the previous 19) and further documented the temporal changes of signs and symptoms over the period of observation. Nineteen of the 26 patients underwent spontaneous regression. Complete disappearance of symptoms occurred within 6 months in five, within 6 to 12 months in four, within 1 to 2 years in four, and in more than 2 years in six. Moderate to marked improvement occurred in five additional patients, and two patients were still symptomatic after 1.0 and 9.6 years. Conversely, signs and symptoms increased within 1 month in five patients, within 6 months in nine, and in more than 6 months in six.

Exacerbations and remissions of signs and symptoms is a hallmark of the disease process because the CS thromboses,

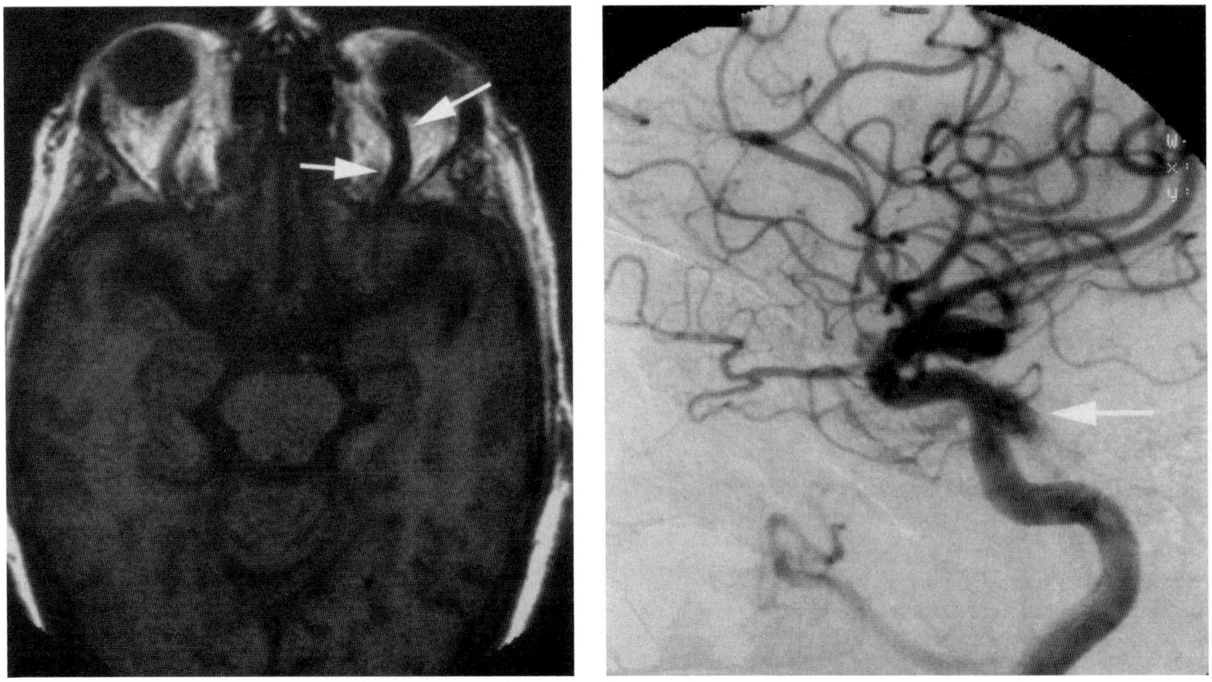

A B

FIGURE 12-6. This 70-year-old woman developed bilateral chemosis and proptosis starting several months previously. Her ophthalmologic exam demonstrated decreased visual acuity in the right eye, and her right fundus was described as grossly abnormal with edema of the optic nerve, hemorrhages, and exudates throughout the retina consistent with a central retinal vein occlusion. She also had bilateral sixth cranial nerve palsies. **A:** Axial T1-weighted MRI image through the level of the orbits. MRI demonstrated bilateral proptosis and an enlarged SOV on the left *(arrow)*. **B:** Right ICA angiogram demonstrates an indirect carotid-cavernous fistula, which was supplied by small branches of the posterior trunk and inferiolateral trunk from the C4 segment of the cavernous-carotid artery. The posterior portion of the CS was noted to fill on the arterial phase on this angiogram *(arrow)*. *(Figure continues.)*

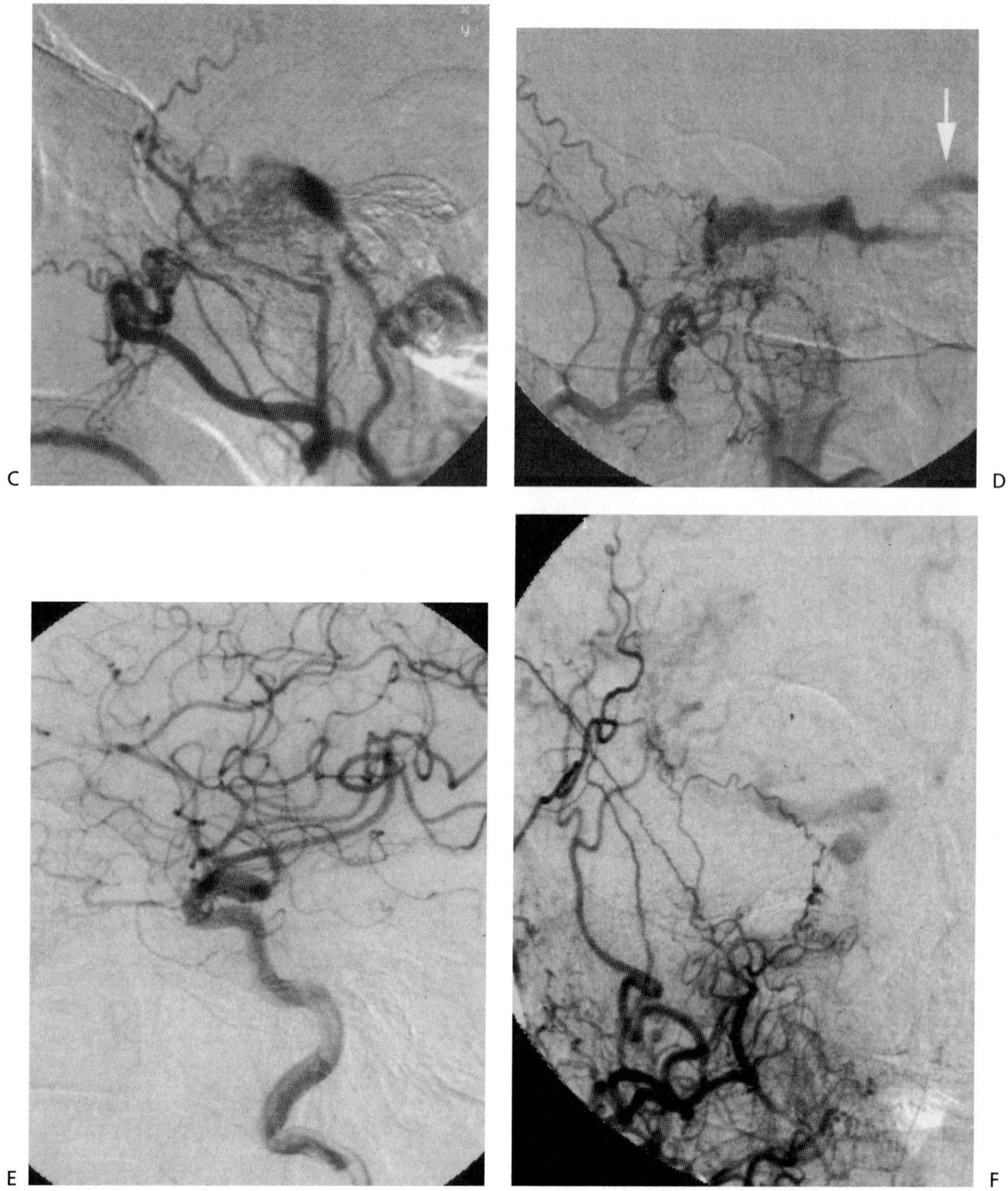

FIGURE 12-6. *Continued.* **C,D:** Right ECA angiogram, lateral and anterior projections, respectively. This demonstrated filling of the right CS via the branches of the middle meningeal artery and distal internal maximal artery, including the arteries in the foramen rotundum and the pterygoid canal. The venous drainage is seen to cross the clival plexus in the midline and drain out via the left SOV *(arrow).* There was no drainage on the right via the inferior petrosal sinus or SOV. These findings were consistent with the patient's physical examination, which demonstrated evidence of a right central vein occlusion and proptosis in the left eye from this indirect fistula on the right. The patient underwent embolization with PVA particles treating the middle meningeal and distal internal maxillary supply. This reduced the flow significantly to the fistula. She was then placed on a regimen of manual compression of the right carotid artery for 6 weeks. **E:** Right ICA angiogram, lateral view, late arterial phase. This angiogram done 6 weeks after the embolization therapy and following manual compression demonstrates there is not filling of the fistula from the vessels of the ICA. **F:** Right ECA angiogram, anterior projection. This angiogram, also done 6 weeks following embolization and manual compression therapy, demonstrates no filling of the fistula from ECA branches. The patient's proptosis and chemosis, as well as the patient's visual acuity in the right eye, had significantly improved by that time. (From Michael P. Marks and Huy M. Do, unpublished material, with permission.)

and venous flow is shunted in different directions. CCF thrombosis may lead paradoxically to increased ophthalmologic signs and symptoms as blood flow is redirected during the occlusive process. Secondary routes of venous effluence may close, rendering residual drainage routes less compliant and shunting flow toward potentially more dangerous venous drainage.

Thrombosis of the CCF may be accompanied by thrombosis of the superior ophthalmic and retinal veins, and vision may be lost while the fistula "heals" [62,98–102]. Redirected flow following partial thrombosis may also be toward the brain through pial veins, with the dangers of venous hypertension or hemorrhage. Venous drainage may also be directed toward spinal pial venous drainage, causing myelopathy [103].

Subarachnoid or intracerebral hemorrhage complicating dural CCFs has been reported uncommonly but, as expected, always associated with cerebral venous drainage, usually demonstrated with lesser ophthalmic and petrosal drainage [104,105]. Of our patients with types B–D CCFs, we have encountered no patients with hemorrhage prior to, during, or following management, with approximately 20% known to have had pial venous cortical drainage. Therefore, pial-cortical drainage in and of itself does not constitute the urgent requirement for treatment that may be warranted in direct, high-flow type A CCFs.

Angiography and Diagnosis

The goal in evaluation of type B, C, or D CCFs is to determine location of the fistula, arterial supply and entry point, and pattern of venous drainage including pial venous drainage. Lasjaunias described the angiographic evaluation of the CS, which includes selective ICA, ipsilateral vertebral, proximal, and distal internal maxillary artery, and the ascending pharyngeal artery. Contralateral ICA and ECA injection is also required for CCF evaluation. ECA arterial supply to types C and D fistulas includes the middle meningeal artery, accessory meningeal artery, distal internal maxillary artery (including the artery of foramen rotundum and the vidian artery), and ascending pharyngeal artery [90].

ICA arterial supply to types B and D fistulas includes the meningohypophyseal artery, the artery to the inferior CS (lateral mainstem), and McConnell's capsular arteries [91]. Contralateral dural branches of the ICA and ECA often supply these complex fistulas, and we call this a type D2 supply pattern.

Arterial supply is often complex and needs to be studied in detail prior to transarterial embolization or even venous sinus packing. Angiographic demonstration of dangerous congenital variants, including ophthalmic, meningeal, vidian artery and artery of the foramen rotundum to ICA branch; ascending pharyngeal artery to cavernous and petrous carotid artery; and occipital artery communication to the ICA or the vertebral artery, historically important in the era of arterial embolization, has become less critical in the current era of venous-side therapeutic occlusion [92].

The exact site of the fistula needs to be identified if transvenous embolization is attempted, so that the fistulous connection is totally overlaid with coils and therefore does not redirect flow toward other venous outflow pathways. Identification of the SOV, inferior petrosal sinus (IPS), and pterygoid plexus drainage is important because these are the primary routes for transvenous embolization.

TECHNIQUE FOR ENDOVASCULAR TREATMENT

Direct Fistulas

Spontaneous closure of a symptomatic traumatic direct CCF is uncommon [32]. In our experience, only 3 of 150 symptomatic traumatic type A CCFs have resolved spontaneously without any attempt at treatment, one low-flow and two high-flow lesions. It must be remembered that spontaneous disappearance of ocular signs and bruit do not necessarily indicate closure of a high-flow type A direct fistula. Pial venous or petrosal sinus drainage may persist following SOV occlusion, with altered turbulence effects even diminishing previously audible bruits.

In treatment decisions the likelihood of spontaneous closure, then, must be weighed against the presence or absence of function-threatening neurologic and ophthalmologic signs, taking into consideration arteriographic demonstration of high-risk features of CS varix, pseudoaneurysm, and cortical venous drainage [33,34].

Arterialized cortical venous flow, however, is a relatively common phenomenon with type A CCF (see Figs. 12-1A and 12-2A). Of 90 type A CCF arteriograms available for recent review, 29 (32%) exhibited middle cerebral or sylvian venous drainage, and 24 (26%) anterior pontomesencephalic, lateral mesencephalic, petrosal, or cerebellar venous drainage, up to 3 years posttrauma. Although hemorrhage or sequelae of venous hypertension occur only in the presence of pial venous drainage, these complications occur with a relatively low incidence. Two of 29 (7%) patients with middle cerebral vein or sylvian venous drainage developed hemorrhage. Neither patient had SOV drainage and one had petrosal drainage. Lack of the latter two venous outflow pathways is a greater predictor of hemorrhage risk. Two of 23 patients (8%) with posterior fossa pial venous drainage developed coma. Pial venous drainage, in and of itself, is not a predictor of a hemorrhage and need not call for emergent treatment.

Balloon occlusion of CCFs has become the treatment of choice, because the possibility and likelihood of placing a single balloon with immediate closure of the fistula is relatively high (see Figs. 12-1, 12-2, and 12-4) [35,36]. Balloon availability and balloon characteristics have been well-described by Monsein [37]. The Target Therapeutics detachable silicone balloon (DSB) is the only detachable balloon approved for use in the United States. It is the descendant of the Hieshima and Interventional Therapeutics Corporation's DSB. The DSB is supplied in multiple dimensions and volumes from 0.5 to 1.0 cc. The Debrun latex detachable balloon (LDB), which set the standard for CCF treatment, is still in use, although not approved by the Food and Drug Administration.

Balloon occlusion can be performed relatively rapidly, and the end result reasonably predicted, in approximately 50% of individuals (see Fig. 12-2). Other treatment choices have evolved, however, including "pushable" fibered, or electronically or mechanically detachable coil occlusion (see Fig. 12-3). Direct surgical approaches need be used rarely [38,39]. Reported success rates of detachable balloon CCF occlusion from the literature have been relatively high, with 89% success rates reported in large series [13,40–52] and 98% success with the Hieshima DSB [53,54]. The largest single-case series has just been published by Wu et al. It included 482 patients with traumatic CCF, with 462 improved, and no deaths related to treatment, from 1986 to 1998, using a variety of balloons, coils, and cyanoacrylate adhesive, preserving the ICA in 84% [55]. Many other small case report series exist. Technical or clinical success indicators will vary according to our ability to (a) close the fistula, (b) preserve ICA flow, and (c) improve patients' signs and symptoms. These procedural, technical, and clinical success rates may vary inversely if one is willing to accept less ICA preservation by the transarterial route.

Initially, technically unsuccessful procedures, repeated with a different selection of detachable balloon (DB) sizes or different technical maneuvers (such as a double-balloon technique) [56,57] or devices, may subsequently be successful. DB procedures might be "unsuccessful" and stopped in favor of alternative transvenous or operative methods when balloon placement may appear unsafe, or ICA preservation appears unlikely, decreasing the transarterial DB fistula occlusion technical success rate (see Fig. 12-3). Success, then, need not focus so much on procedural and technical success but more on management success. This means treating the CCF by the best method for the individual patient, with ICA preservation a primary, although not necessarily absolute, focus. New coil methods may increase ICA preservation, but large series confirming such are not yet available.

In our early series of 100 patients, preserving ICA flow in 67 patients, single DBs initially were used for CCF occlusion and ICA patency in 52 patients, with inflation volumes of 0.1 to 0.8 cc [51]. Average single-balloon volume was 0.28 cc, equivalent to 7 mm × 9 mm inflation dimensions.

Multiple balloons may be required for fistula-only occlusion in approximately 25% of such patients, and we used up to four balloons of 2.1-cc total volume in one patient.

With patient improvement the indicator of success, Kupersmith compared 16 measurable ophthalmologic physical exam parameters prior to and following therapy [46], and found improvement in 88% of individual abnormal findings and reversion to normal in 75%.

This mirrors our experience that patients usually improve markedly, but each and every sequela of the disease may not normalize. For instance, sixth cranial nerve paresis may be due to direct traumatic nerve injury at the time of initial trauma and not be subject to improvement by CCF treatment. Blindness caused by direct optic nerve injury will not reverse. Blindness due to ocular ischemia or deceased retinal perfusion rarely, if ever, can be reversed [58].

Our long-term clinical follow-up of 88 CCFs treated with DBs from 1979 to 1993 included 47 of 58 (81%) treated with LDB (mean 10.0, range 5.9 to 15.5 years) and 28 of 30 (93%) treated with DB (mean 4.0, range 1.0 to 6.6 years). No other late recurrent symptoms of ophthalmologic or cerebral sequelae of CCFs treated with LDB or DSB were discovered, and none has subsequently become evident [76]. It is our practice to inform patients that the artery tear site can never be normal again, but the scar left behind may have a small bulge or scar aneurysm that will likely cause no trouble in later years.

Overall success rates and complications in the spontaneous and traumatic groups are generally similar, although several caveats in the former should be emphasized. Rupture of an aneurysm with a relatively wide neck is probably a relative contraindication for fistula-only closure with contrast-filled DB, insofar as the risk of delayed balloon prolapse back into the ICA must be considered high. Balloons may pull back into the ICA at detachment or prolapse back into and occlude the ICA with larger traumatic ostia as well, and may even dilate the ostium in doing so [59]. We experienced one delayed DSB balloon deflation which led to major cerebral infarction 6 weeks following treatment in an elderly patient. ICA CCF occlusion is an acceptable technique with CCFs due to wide-neck aneurysm rupture, if adequate collateral reserve is documented. Availability of a permanent solidifying material, such as hydroxyethyl methacrylate (HEMA), might recommend its use as a balloon-filling agent in attempts to preserve ICA flow with wide-necked ostia. Guglielmi detachable coil (GDC) electrothrombosis may be a better alternative in some of these cases, although wide-neck aneurysms are also less assuredly occluded with this technique [60]. Again, placement of a stent plus intraaneurysmal and fistula coils has proven a useful adjunct, and may someday be the treatment of choice prospectively when this circumstance is encountered. It remains unclear if venous compartment coil packing, with patent neck and ostium, is an adequate treatment for most patients.

CCF closures may occur following unsuccessful attempts at balloon occlusion. Balloon manipulation at the ostium, or within the CS, may somehow stimulate thrombosis. Carotid compression for type A CCFs may be useful as an initial adjunctive method, but it triggers thrombotic occlusion much less frequently than with dural CCFs [61]. Thrombotic process may be so exuberant as to create CS or SOV thrombosis or both, with all flow initially directed toward thrombosing ophthalmic veins, creating a pressurized, less compliant system that leads to more florid orbital and ocular changes than the wide open fistula, itself, caused [62].

Preservation of ICA flow is the goal in every procedure but cannot always be accomplished safely. Overall ICA patency rates in the literature with LDB, in series larger than five patients, was 69%. Higashida reported ICA patency rates of 88% with the Interventional Therapeutics Corporation's silicone balloon. ICA occlusion may be mandatory for severe ICA injury or a very large ostium (Figs. 12-7 and 12-8).

If the fistula ostium is initially too large, it is unlikely that any combination of balloons will recreate a presenting surface at the fistula ostium that is sufficiently without threat for pseudoaneurysm formation or thromboembolism, so we feel ICA occlusion is acceptable under that circumstance. If the fistula cannot be closed completely, a small amount of residual flow is acceptable, as long as it is not redirected toward a dangerous drainage pattern in expectation that thrombosis will supervene following the procedure (see Fig. 12-2). Carotid compression following partial closure may stimulate further thrombosis. Patients with incomplete closure must be monitored with noninvasive imaging or repeat arteriography for subsequent increase in bruit or potential redirection of flow into more dangerous effluence patterns.

It is clear that type A high-flow CCFs can be treated effectively and safely, although not with impunity, with detachable balloons. Other devices, such as GDC or pushable fibered coils, are proving useful as well (see Figs. 12-3, 12-7, and 12-8) [78,79]. In fact, if a draining venous channel is clearly detailed and wider than the ostium, controlled coil placement using a 5- or 6-Fr. guide catheter may be preferable to DSB placement through an 8-Fr. system. However, with a wide ostium the risk of coils prolapsing back into the ICA must be considered great, so coil use may be limited [79,80]. Temporary placement of a balloon within the ICA at the fistula ostium has been shown to be useful in coil occlusion of direct CCFs, similar to the balloon-assist technique for wide-neck aneurysms [81]. Coil availability makes innovative approaches more feasible (see Fig. 12-7 and 12-8). Coil use has safety limitations as well, and deaths have already occurred in patients with coil-treated CCFs [82,83]. The combined use of balloons and coils may have a place in management, but balloon integrity in contact with a coil mass must be examined before this can be recommended [84,85]. Stents may be developed that

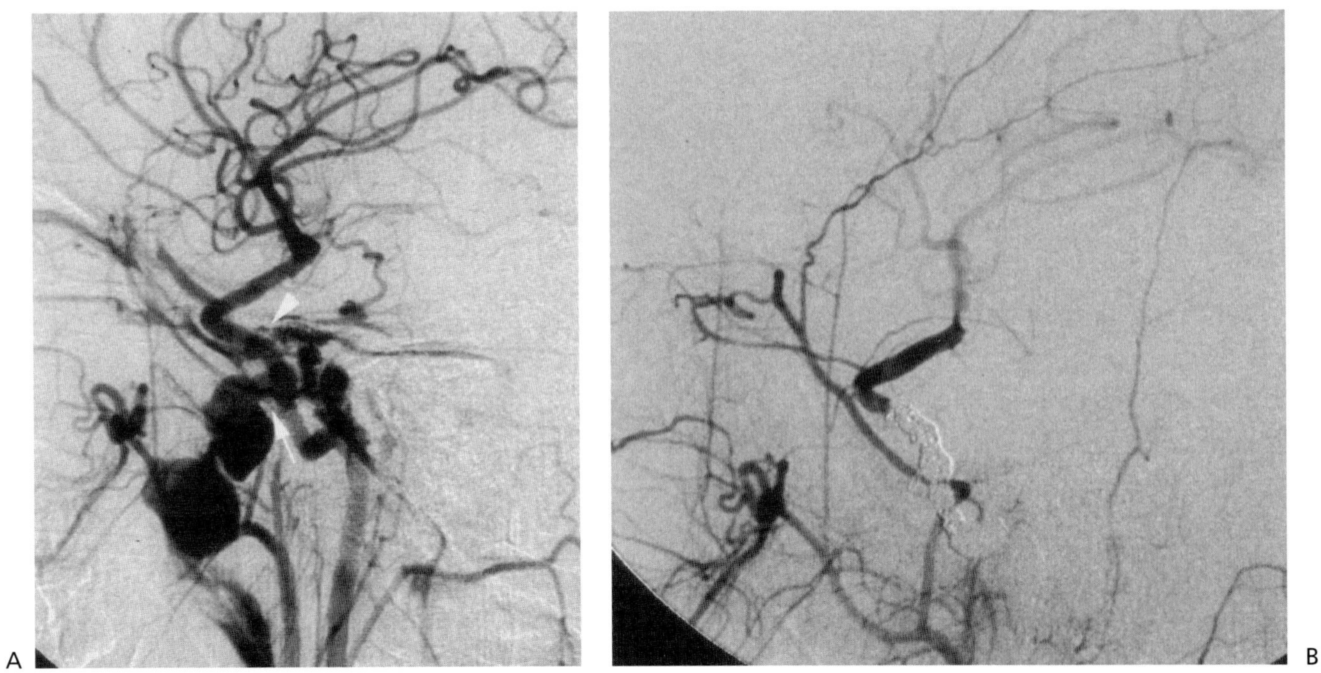

FIGURE 12-7. This 16-year-old boy was in an motor vehicle accident and was comatose. He developed life-threatening epistaxis. **A:** Left CCA angiogram, lateral view, demonstrates a proximal tear of the ICA at the lacerum segment, with rupture into the nasopharynx *(arrow),* and a more distal direct type A CCF from the horizontal segment of the ICA *(arrowhead).* **B:** Proximal flow arrest was obtained by placing a 0.5-cc nondetachable silicone balloon with 0.010-inch guidewire through a 5-Fr. sheath, floating it from the aortic arch into the left ICA for proximal flow arrest, then placing GDCs and fibered GDCs and fibered pushable coils through a Rapid Transit microcatheter from the horizontal C4 ICA to the horizontal C2 segment. Left CCA injection demonstrates trapping of the fistula ostium and the arterial tear, and bleeding ceased.

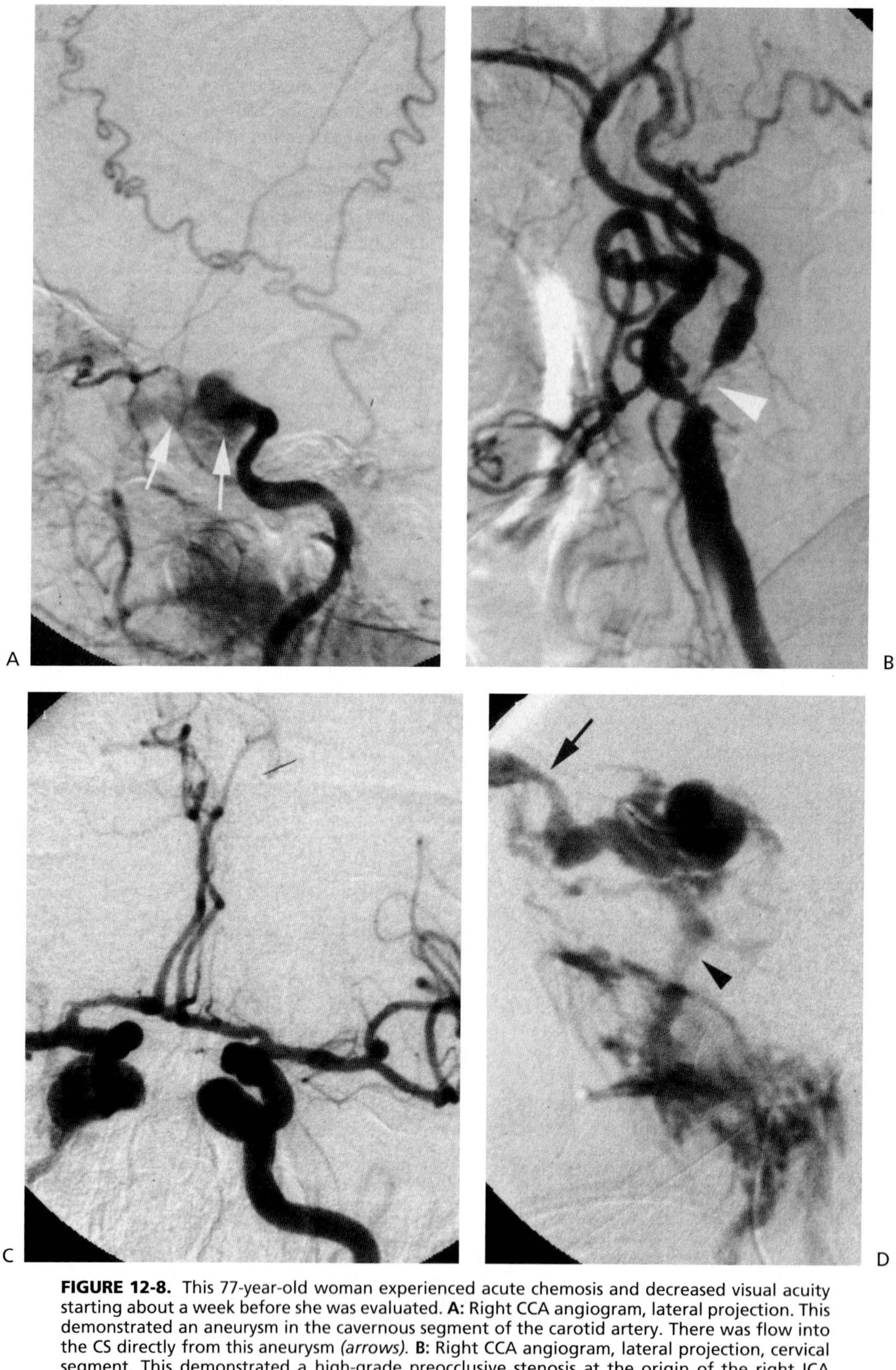

FIGURE 12-8. This 77-year-old woman experienced acute chemosis and decreased visual acuity starting about a week before she was evaluated. **A:** Right CCA angiogram, lateral projection. This demonstrated an aneurysm in the cavernous segment of the carotid artery. There was flow into the CS directly from this aneurysm *(arrows).* **B:** Right CCA angiogram, lateral projection, cervical segment. This demonstrated a high-grade preocclusive stenosis at the origin of the right ICA *(arrowhead).* **C:** Left ICA angiogram, anterior projection. This demonstrated rapid cross filling across the anterior communicating artery into the right carotid circulation, with flow down the supraclinoid carotid into the cavernous-segment aneurysm. **D:** Right ICA angiogram, venous phase, lateral projection. The venous drainage was via the SOV *(arrow)* and the pterygoid plexus *(arrowhead).* No filling of the inferior petrosal sinus was seen. Attempts were made to cannulate the nonfilling inferior petrosal sinus, which proved unsuccessful. *(Figure continues.)*

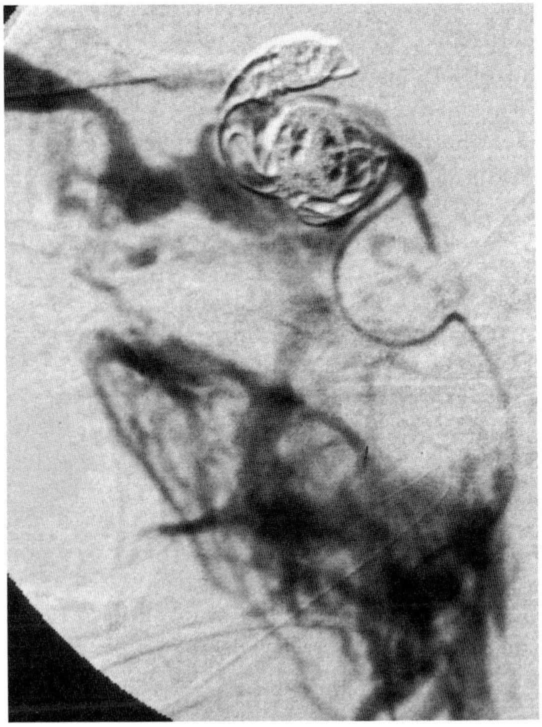

E

FIGURE 12-8. *Continued.* **E:** Right ICA angiogram, venous phase, lateral projection. Because the CS fistula filled from the supraclinoid carotid artery in a retrograde fashion as well as from the cervical carotid, it was felt that the best therapeutic approach to treatment was trapping of the fistula by coiling a portion of the supraclinoid carotid artery and the aneurysm and closing the severely stenosed carotid artery. Balloon occlusion was not attempted because of the severe stenosis of the proximal ICA. A 0.014-inch microcatheter was passed through the stenosis into the supraclinoid carotid artery, and GDC coils were used to occlude both the supraclinoid and cavernous portions of the carotid artery. This angiogram was done midway through the coiling procedure. **F:** Right CCA angiogram with reflux into the subclavian and vertebral artery, lateral projection. This angiogram was obtained after the coiling procedure was completed, showing that there is no filling of the fistula. **G:** Left ICA angiogram, anterior projection. This angiogram was obtained immediately following the coiling procedure, demonstrating continued filling of the intracranial carotid circulation with no filling of the aneurysm or carotid-cavernous fistula site. (From Michael P. Marks and Huy M. Do, unpublished material, with permission.)

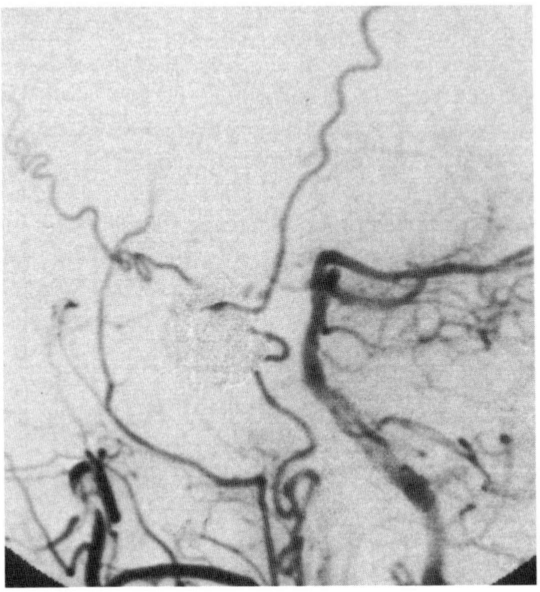

F

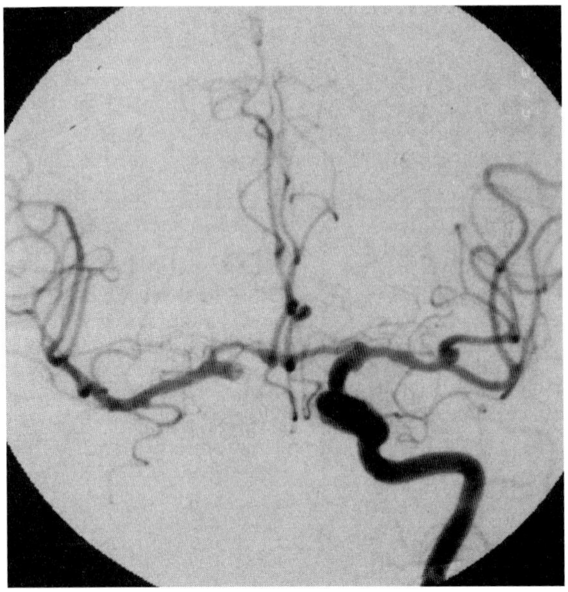

G

allow parent artery preservation in wide-neck CCFs, and early stent placement with CS coil packing may well prove to be the treatment of choice for such lesions.

It is important to point out that ICA occlusion should be accompanied by total occlusion of the fistula ostium, so that collateral flow to C4 branches and to the ICA and fistula does not occur. Three or more balloons are required for CCF ICA occlusion, to guarantee against an unexpected deflation or balloon advancement and guarantee adequate occlusive effect [66].

Fistula occlusion has been accomplished by navigating through the vertebrobasilar circulation, through a collateral posterior communicating artery to the ICA and CS to attempt CCF closure with embolization with coils, or even acrylic placement performed by that route [67,68]. Direct puncture of the CS through the superior orbital fissure for embolization can also be performed [69].

Premature detachment of the hand-tied latex balloon is most uncommon [45,46,70]. Premature detachment of the silicone balloon was reported by Interventional Therapeutics Corporation in July of 1987 in 1.8% of uses in treating CCFs. Balloons should be advanced gently with partial inflations and deflations to the level of the ostium. When the balloon diameter approximates the lumen diameter of the ICA, it is more likely to be stripped off the catheter.

Mounting a valved balloon on an appropriate shapeable microcatheter (e.g., Tracker-18, 12-cm tip) which accepts a torqueable guidewire is a useful technique to advance balloons more safely in tortuous vessels, so as to not have to maximally inflate the balloon to depend on its flow-guided characteristics to advance it to the fistula [71]. Traction must not be exerted on an inflated valved balloon which could then detach, although well-tied LDBs withstand considerably greater manipulation.

Care must be exerted when a balloon is removed and retracted into the guide catheter. A valved balloon may be detached inadvertently if it must be retracted into the introducing catheter for removal, when the blunt balloon base impacts the catheter tip. Moving a coaxial catheter up to the balloon base may prevent this problem. Some consideration should be given to removing the entire system from the carotid artery prior to balloon retraction.

We have experienced LDB premature deflation within 24 hours in only one patient, requiring repeat treatment. Partial thrombosis of the CS and SOV, as well as high volumes of contrast material used, may have contributed to the thrombosis in this patient. Although portions of the communicating venous compartment of the CS likely thrombose following CCF occlusion, the sinus may still be opacified by normal venous flow after balloon placement, and symptomatic venous thrombosis with vision loss has been reported in only one other case [72]. Premature deflation of isosmotic contrast–filled DSBs was reported in 16 of 370 (4.3%) balloons used in treating CCFs as reported by International Therapeutics Corporation in 1993. The DSB is responsive to osmotic gradients and must be filled with near-isosmotic contrast, such as iohexol 180 mg %. We experienced one delayed, yet premature, deflation of a DSB in one elderly patient, likely with an aneurysm causing CCF, with balloon deflation (or rupture) and prolapse into the ICA and MCA at 3 months posttreatment. The risks of balloon placement with aneurysmal ostia, in which the margins of safety for position maintenance are reduced, is emphasized.

Prolapse of a detached balloon into the ICA may be related to a relatively wide ostium but shallow sinus, an underlying aneurysm with wide neck, unrecognized partial deflation, or actual balloon dilation of the CCF ostium. We have tested for potential prolapse in several patients by first introducing a nondetachable balloon, trying to occlude the fistula, and then putting gentle traction on the balloon to see if it moves back into the ICA too easily, as might be experienced at the time of balloon traction detachment.

Movement or advancement of balloons within the CS may also occur, again perhaps related to partial balloon deflation, or merely an attempt by the balloon to assume a position of least tension in the sinus space (see Fig. 12-2). Balloon deflation may allow movement or advancement, and DSBs are less likely to deflate minimally than LDBs. This may allow fistulas to reopen, or change the direction of venous shunting. When detachable balloons deflate minimally or shift only slightly, it is unlikely that additional balloons can be placed through the ostium until some further balloon deflation or movement occurs. Repeat treatment is therefore likely futile, unless sufficient space is created for additional placement; observation is in order, waiting to determine whether the fistula will close on its own or whether balloon deflation will lead to CCF enlargement, allowing a second treatment attempt. It must be kept in mind that partial closures may allow the CCF to return with a different pattern of venous drainage with the adverse implications previously discussed. Treatment by transvenous methods to occlude a residual or recurrent CCF may be indicated when early thrombosis does not occur [65]. When sphenoid bone fractures render the CS walls more compliant, balloon movement within the CS may also occur.

Complication rates from the LDB literature suggest neurologic complication rates of 6.7%. Intraprocedural ischemic complications may occur due to thromboembolism from catheter systems or be due to balloon deflation and movement problems just discussed. Anticoagulation for procedures should be mandatory, even if a nonemergent procedure must be delayed to allow its administration. Although most procedures can be performed quickly with single balloon use, others unpredictably may require longer catheterization times, increasing the risk of thromboembolism in a patient who has not been heparinized. We use intravenous heparin, maintaining activated clotting time at 2- to 3-times baseline with hourly heparin boluses.

Understandably, cerebral ischemia is a risk following purposeful ICA occlusion, but it has not occurred acutely in any of our 40 purposeful ICA balloon occlusions for CCFs (age range 12 to 80 years) or during long-term clinical follow-up. Very few of the ischemic complications reported in the literature were due to purposeful ICA occlusion. It is very likely that CCFs lend themselves better to ICA occlusion than do unclippable aneurysms [73]. CCFs begin to recruit collateral flow to the involved ICA distribution, so that by the time ICA balloon occlusion is performed, collateral flow may be better established. In addition, CCFs tend to occur in a younger population that is more likely to tolerate ICA occlusion. We recently performed our first bypass graft prior to ICA occlusion for CCF in a patient who had a mild asymmetry on single photon emission computed tomography (SPECT) during balloon occlusion test (BOT), with no anterior communicating, and only a small posterior communicating artery, collateral flow.

Paresis of cranial nerves III, IV, V, and VI may occur following CCF closure, usually when a large number of balloons or large volumes of single balloons are used. Preexisting third cranial nerve pareses usually improved, but sixth cranial nerve pareses present from the time of trauma usually do not resolve, based on our long-term follow-up of patients treated since 1979. These are likely due to traumatic injuries to the nerve itself and not due to progressive compression by dilated vascular structures.

Debrun reported 30% transient ophthalmoparesis following LDB treatment, usually due to sixth cranial nerve dysfunction. He suggested that filling large detachable balloons with permanent solidifying agents, rather than contrast material with a mass effect that will diminish as a balloon deflates, is more likely to lead to permanent cranial nerve dysfunction. Development of cranial nerve paresis in a delayed manner following treatment does suggest that a pseudoaneurysm may be developing as a balloon deflates or moves (see below) [72].

Pseudoaneurysms may develop from the ostium and CS as latex balloons deflate. Debrun et al. reported a 60% occurrence of "venous pouches" or false aneurysms in preserved ICAs in their original report of 54 patients [13]. Pseudoaneurysm development with deflating LDBs and even DSBs filled with isosmotic contrast is well documented (see Fig. 12-1D). LDB-related pseudoaneurysms are usually asymptomatic and will decrease in size with time. Early symptomatic pseudoaneurysm with pain and increasing ophthalmoparesis will require a second treatment and may well require parent artery occlusion, however. Small pseudoaneurysms occur even in patients with spontaneous closure [74,75].

We have encountered no infections with detachable balloon placement, in spite of simultaneous orbital infections. We give antibiotics (cefazolin [Ancef] 1 g every 8 hours for three doses) for prolonged or complicated treatments.

Halbach et al. reported two occurrences of normal perfusion pressure breakthrough phenomenon, one following surgical occlusion in a CCF present for 23 years, the second during balloon occlusion in a CCF present for 7 years, and minimized the effects of the latter episode with subtotal, graded occlusion [77]. Balloon placement may close off posterior drainage but redirect flow toward the SOV, with acute pressure changes and even intraorbital hemorrhagic consequences [63]. Intracerebral hemorrhage may be caused by redirection of flow toward the sphenoparietal sinus and cortical veins [64,65].

Chronic fistulas may lead to local steal of blood, even creating ischemic symptoms. This local ischemia creates local hypotension and chronic arteriolar dilation with loss of normal autoregulation. When a fistula is closed, by whatever means, the chronically dilated vessels cannot respond to regulate flow, and cerebral edema or hemorrhage may supervene.

Indirect or Dural Fistulas

Any treatment plan must take into account the usual course of events in the natural history of the disease process. The natural healing potential of a dural CCF may be accelerated with digital (manual) compression of the carotid artery. Higashida suggested that simultaneous carotid and jugular compression be used to diminish arterial pressure and flow while increasing venous pressure, thus equalizing arteriovenous pressure gradients, causing stasis and stimulating thrombosis (see Fig. 12-6).

Transvenous embolization with coil packing has become the treatment of choice for dural CCFs (see Fig. 12-5) [106]. This can be accomplished via retrograde or transjugular catheterization of the inferior petrosal sinuses, the SOV, or the pterygoid plexus [107]. Transfemoral transvenous approaches may be facilitated by placement of a 70-cm, 7- or 8-Fr. sheath or catheter into the internal jugular vein; a 90- to 100-cm, 4- or 5-Fr. coaxial guide catheter in the inferior petrosal sinus or facial vein; and a microcatheter into the CS. Coil placement should disconnect the fistula from the draining veins, working from distal to proximal, trying to guarantee that the fistulous entry point is effectively trapped. Selected type A CCFs may be treated in similar fashion. Complex flow patterns may occur within the CS, making treatment planning complex.

Puncture of the angular vein or facial vein with a micropuncture needle and ultrasonographic guidance, with retrograde catheterization of the SOV and CS, has been performed successfully by Denardo and Scott (A. Denardo, J. Scott, personal communication, 1997). Direct surgical cannulation of the SOV in the anterior orbit is also a useful approach [108,109].

Meyers recently reviewed the experience at the University of California at San Francisco of 135 indirect CCF patients managed between 1986 and 2000. Of these, 90% of patients were clinically cured, and 97% exhibited good recovery when treated by endovascular methods; 2.3% suffered a procedure related complication; and 3% persisted with a moderate or severe disability (P. Meyers, personal communication, 2001).

Transarterial embolization techniques historically have led to fewer immediate cures of dural CCFs, but they may be useful when venous access is not available, or following incomplete resolution of fistulas following transvenous occlusion (see Fig. 12-6) [110]. Pial venous drainage may represent an obstacle to adequate management by arterial occlusive techniques, because particulate emboli may pass through some shunts to stimulate thrombosis of cortical veins.

Stereotactic radiosurgery remains an extremely useful technique in therapy for dural CCFs that are not threatening vision loss immediately, although fistula resolution may take 12 months or longer, not unlike spontaneous resolution. Typically we may choose to treat an older patient with stereotactic radiosurgery unless vision is threatened or signs and symptoms are disabling [111,112].

REFERENCES

1. Barrow D, Spector R, Landman J, et al. Classification and treatment of spontaneous carotid cavernous sinus fistulas. *J Neurosurg* 1985;62:248–256.
2. Ernst RJ, Tomsick TA. Classification and angiography of carotid cavernous fistulas. In: Tomsick T, ed. *Carotid cavernous fistula.* Cincinnati, OH: Digital Educational Publishing, 1997: 13–22.
3. Debrun G. Management of traumatic carotid-cavernous fistulas. In: Viñuela F, ed. *Interventional neuroradiology: endovascular therapy of the central nervous system.* New York: Raven Press, 1992:107–112.
4. Parkinson D. Anatomy of the lateral sellar compartments (cavernous sinus). In: Schmilek HH, Sweet WB, eds. *Operative neurosurgical techniques.* Philadelphia: WB Saunders, 1995: 479–492.
5. Berenstein A, Kricheff I. Balloon catheters for investigation of carotid cavernous fistulas. *Radiology* 1979;132:762–764.
6. Cares H, Roberson G, Grand W, et al. A safe technique for the precise localization of carotid cavernous fistulas during balloon obliteration. *J Neurosurg* 1978;49:146–149.
7. Mehringer C, Heishima G, Grinnell V, et al. Improved localization of carotid cavernous fistula during angiography. *AJNR Am J Neuroradiol* 1982;3:82–84.
8. Huber P. A technical contribution to the exact angiographic localization of carotid cavernous fistulas. *Neuroradiology* 1976; 10:239–241.
9. Locke CE. Intracranial arteriovenous aneurysm or pulsating exophthalmos. *Ann Surg* 1924;80:1–24.
10. Tomsick TA. Type A (direct) CCF: etiology, prevalence, and natural history. In: Tomsick T, ed. *Carotid cavernous fistula.* Cincinnati, OH: Digital Educational Publishing, 1997:35–38.
11. Parkinson D. Transcavernous repair of a carotid-cavernous fistula: a case report. *J Neurosurg* 1967;26:420–424.
12. Van Dellen JR. Intracavernous traumatic aneurysms. *Surg Neurol* 1980;13:203–207.
13. Debrun G, Lacour P, Viñuela F, et al. Treatment of 54 carotid-cavernous fistulas. *J Neurosurg* 1981;55:678–692.
14. Tomsick TA. Type A (direct) CCF: etiology, prevalence, and natural history. In: Tomsick T, ed. *Carotid cavernous fistula.* Cincinnati, OH: Digital Educational Publishing, 1997:43.
15. Helmke K, Kruger O, Laas R. The direct carotid-cavernous fistula: a clinical, pathoanatomical and physical study. *Acta Neurochir (Wien)* 1994;127:1–5.
16. Higashida RT, Halbach VV, Tsai FY, et al. Interventional neurovascular treatment of traumatic carotid and vertebral lesions: results in 234 cases. *AJR Am J Roentgenol* 1989;153:577–582.
17. Lewis AI, Tomsick TA, Tew JM. Management of 100 consecutive direct carotid-cavernous fistulas: results of treatment with detachable balloons. *Neurosurgery* 1995;36:239–244.
18. Gossman MD, Berlin AJ, Weinstein MA, et al. Spontaneous direct carotid-cavernous fistula in childhood. *Ophthal Plast Reconstr Surg* 1993;9:62–65.
19. Debrun G, Viñuela F, Fox AJ, et al. Indications for treatment and classification of 132 carotid-cavernous fistulas. *Neurosurgery* 1988;22:285–289.
20. Numaguchi Y, Higashida RT, Abernathy JM, et al. Balloon embolization in carotid-cavernous fistula in fibromuscular dysplasia. *AJNR Am J Neuroradiol* 1987;8:380–382.
21. Hieshima GB, Cahan LD, Mehringer CM, et al. Spontaneous arteriovenous fistulas of cerebral vessels in association with fibromuscular dysplasia. *Neurosurgery* 1986;18:454–458.
22. Taki W, Nakahara I, Nishi S, et al. Pathogenetic and therapeutic considerations of carotid-cavernous sinus fistulas. *Acta Neurochir (Wien)* 1994;127:6–14.
23. Bradac GB, Bender A, Curio G, et al. Report of two spontaneous direct carotid-cavernous fistulas. *Neuroradiology* 1985;27: 436–439.
24. Kashiwaga S, Tsuchida E, Goto K, et al. Balloon occlusion of a spontaneous carotid-cavernous fistula in Ehlers-Danlos syndrome type IV. *Surg Neurol* 1993;39:187–190.
25. Horowitz MB, Purdy PD, Valentine RJ, et al. Remote vascular catastrophes after neurovascular interventional therapy for type-4 Ehlers-Danlos syndrome. *AJNR Am J Neuroradiol* 2000;21: 974–976.
26. Cornelius RS. CCF: imaging evaluation. In: Tomsick T, ed. *Carotid cavernous fistula.* Cincinnati, OH: Digital Educational Publishing, 1997:23–31.
27. Teng MH, Chang T, Pan DH, et al. Brainstem edema: an unusual complication of carotid-cavernous fistula. *AJNR Am J Neuroradiol* 1991;12:139–142.
28. Wilms G, Peene P, Herpels V, et al. Balloon embolization of carotid-cavernous fistula. Fatal cavernous sinus and brain stem venous thrombosis by balloon migration. *Rofo Fortschr Geb Rontgenstr Neuen Bildgeb Verfahr* 1992;156:393–395.
29. Iida K, Uozumi T, Arita K, et al. Steal phenomenon in a traumatic carotid-cavernous fistula. *J Trauma* 1995;39:1015–1017.
30. Nahlovsky I, Petr F, Malec R, et al. The steal syndrome in carotid-cavernous fistula. *Cesk Neurol Neurochir* 1985;48: 403–405.
31. Cheng TS, Lee JD, Suh JH, et al. Increased cerebral perfusion after detachable balloon embolization of carotid cavernous fistula on technetium-99m-HMPAO brain SPECT. *J Nucl Med* 1993;34:1987–1989.
32. Francis PM, Flom RA, Zabramski JM, et al. Treatment of carotid-cavernous fistula: Part I. *Interv Neuroradiol BNI Quarterly* 1991;7:2–8.
33. Halbach VV, Hieshima GB, Higashida RT, et al. Carotid-cavernous fistulae: indications for urgent treatment. *AJR Am J Roentgenol* 1987;149:587–593.
34. d'Angelo VA, Monte V, Scialfa G, et al. Intracerebral venous hemorrhage in "high risk" carotid-cavernous fistula. *Surg Neurol* 1988;30:387–390.
35. Debrun GM. Type A CCF: latex balloon treatment. In: Tomsick T, ed. *Carotid cavernous fistula.* Cincinnati, OH: Digital Educational Publishing, 1997:107–114.
36. Tomsick TA. Type A CCF: transarterial balloon occlusion. In: Tomsick T, ed. *Carotid cavernous fistula.* Cincinnati, OH: Digital Educational Publishing, 1997:115–143.
37. Monsein LH. Detachable balloons. In: Tomsick T, ed. *Carotid cavernous fistula.* Cincinnati, OH: Digital Educational Publishing, 1997:95–106.
38. VanLoveren HR, Tauber M, Lewis AI, et al. Direct surgical treatment of carotid cavernous fistula. In: Tomsick T, ed. *Carotid cavernous fistula.* Cincinnati, OH: Digital Educational Publishing, 1997:83–93.
39. Tu YK, Liu HM, Hu SC. Direct surgery of carotid cavernous fistulae and dural arteriovenous malformations of the cavernous sinus. *Neurosurgery* 1997;41:798–806.
40. Barrow D, Fleischer AS, Hoffman JC. Complications of detachable balloon catheter technique in the treatment of traumatic intracranial arteriovenous fistulas. *J Neurosurg* 1982;56: 396–403.
41. Mickle JP, Quisling RG. Balloon embolization of high-flow traumatic arteriovenous fistulae to the brain. *J Fla Med Assoc* 1982;69:767–774.

42. Peters JLM. Treatment of 20 direct carotid cavernous fistula. *Diagn Imaging* 1983;52:137–140.
43. Benati A, Maschio A, Perini S, et al. Treatment of post-traumatic carotid-cavernous fistula using a detachable balloon catheter. *J Neurosurg* 1980;53:784–786.
44. Negoro M, Kageyama N, Isiguchi T. Cerebovascular occlusion by catheterization and embolization: clinical experience. *AJNR Am J Neuroradiol* 1983;4:362–365.
45. Kendall B. Results of treatment of AVF with the Debrun technique. *AJNR Am J Neuroradiol* 1983;4:405–408.
46. Kupersmith MJ, Berenstein A, Flamm E, et al. Neuroophthalmologic abnormalities and intravascular therapy of traumatic carotid cavernous fistulas. *Ophthalmology* 1986;93:906–912.
47. Berthelsen B, Svendsen P. Treatment of direct carotid-cavernous fistulas with detachable balloons. *Acta Radiol* 1987;28: 683–691.
48. Scialfa G, Valsecchi F, Scotti G. Treatment of vascular lesions with balloon catheters. *AJNR Am J Neuroradiol* 1983;4: 395–398.
49. Corradino G, Gellad FE, Salcman M. Traumatic carotid-cavernous fistula. *South Med J* 1988;81:660–663.
50. Santhosh J, Rao VR, Ravimandalam K, et al. Endovascular management of carotid cavernous fistulae: observation on angiographic and clinical results. *Acta Neurol Scand* 1993;88: 320–326.
51. Lewis AI, Tomsick TA, Tew JM Jr. Management of 100 direct carotid-cavernous fistulas: results of treatment with detachable balloons. *Neurosurgery* 1995;36:239–245.
52. Brosnahan D, McFadzean RM, Teasdale E. Neuro-ophthalmic features of carotid cavernous fistulas and their treatment by endoarterial balloon embolization. *J Neurol Neurosurg Psychiatry* 1992;55:553–556.
53. Bell J. Personal communication: Interventional Therapeutics Corp, 1993.
54. Higashida R, Halbach V, Tsai FY, et al. Interventional neurovascular treatment of traumatic carotid cavernous fistula with detachable balloon. *AJR Am J Roentgenol* 1989;153:577–582.
55. Wu Z, Zhang Y, Yang X, et al. Treatment of carotid cavernous fistulas. *Interv Neuroradiol* 2000;6:277–289.
56. Masaryk TJ, Perl J, Wallace RC, et al. Detachable balloon embolization: concomitant use of a second safety balloon. *AJNR Am J Neuroradiol* 1999;20:1103–1106.
57. Teng MMH, Chang CYC, Chiang J, et al. Double-balloon technique for embolization of carotid cavernous fistulas. *AJNR Am J Neuroradiol* 2000;21:1753–1756.
58. Brodsky MC, Hoyt WF, Halbach VV, et al. Recovery from total monocular blindness after balloon embolization of carotid-cavernous fistula. *Am J Ophthalmol* 1987;104:86–87.
59. Graeb DA, Robertson WD, Lapointe JS, et al. Avoiding intraarterial balloon detachment in the treatment of posttraumatic carotid-cavernous fistulae with detachable balloons. *AJNR Am J Neuroradiol* 1985;6:602–605.
60. Guglielmi G, Viñuela F, Briganti F, et al. Carotid-cavernous fistula caused by a ruptured intracavernous aneurysm: endovascular treatment by electrothrombosis with detachable coils. *Neurosurgery* 1992;31:591–597.
61. Higashida RT, Hieshima GB, Halbach VV, et al. Closure of carotid cavernous fistulae by external compression of the carotid artery and jugular vein. *Acta Radiol Suppl* 1986;369:580–583.
62. Knudtzon K. A remarkable case of pulsating exophthalmos in an old patient who recovered spontaneously after bilateral aseptic thrombosis of the cavernous sinus. *Acta Ophthalmol* 1950;28: 363–369.
63. Lasjaunias P, Berenstein A. *Arteriovenous fistulas (AVFs). Surgical neuroangiography.* Vol 2. New York: Springer-Verlag, 1990:202.
64. Dohrmann PJ, Batjer HH, Samson D, et al. Recurrent subarachnoid hemorrhage complicating a traumatic carotid-cavernous fistula. *Neurosurgery* 1985;17:480–483.
65. Halbach VV, Higashida RT, Dowd CF, et al. Treatment of carotid-cavernous fistulas associated with Ehlers-Danlos syndrome. *Neurosurgery* 1990;26:1021–1027.
66. Phatouros CC, Cartmill M, Ashpole RD, et al. Transmural migration of an intracavernous carotid detachable balloon used to control surgically induced hemorrhage. *Neuroradiology* 1998; 40:338–340.
67. Garcia-Cervignon E, Bien S, Laurent A, et al. Treatment of a recurrent traumatic carotid cavernous fistula: vertebro-basilar approach after surgical occlusion of the internal carotid artery. *Neuroradiology* 1988;30:355–357.
68. Debrun GM, Ausman JI, Charbel FT, et al. Access to the cavernous sinus through the vertebral artery: technical case report. *Neurosurgery* 1995;37:144–147.
69. Teng MM, Lirng JF, Chang T, et al. Embolization of carotid cavernous fistula by means of direct puncture through the superior orbital fissure. *Radiology* 1995;194:705–711.
70. Wilms G, Peene P, Nowe G, et al. Angiographic diagnosis and treatment of post-traumatic carotid cavernous fistula. *Bull Soc Belge Ophtalmol* 1989;231:83–89.
71. Wessbecher F, Hartling RP, Nieves M, et al. Treatment of carotid-cavernous fistulas: a new balloon delivery system. *AJNR Am J Neuroradiol* 1992;13:331–332.
72. Debrun G. Treatment of carotid cavernous and vertebral fistulas. In: Smith R, ed. *Vascular malformations and fistulas of the brain.* New York: Raven Press, 1982:197–230.
73. Larson JF, Tew JM, Tomsick TA, et al. Treatment of aneurysms of the internal carotid artery by intravascular balloon occlusion: long-term follow-up of 58 patients. *Neurosurgery* 1995;36: 23–30.
74. Osborne A. *Intracranial aneurysms. Diagnostic neuroradiology.* St Louis: Mosby Year Book, 1994:27.
75. Graves VB, Strother CK, Weinstein JM, et al. Giant intracavernous aneurysm after spontaneous thrombosis of a carotid-cavernous fistula. *AJNR Am J Neuroradiol* 1988;9:595–597.
76. Lewis AI, Tomsick TA, Tew JM, et al. Long-term results in direct carotid-cavernous fistulas after treatment with detachable balloons. *J Neurosurg* 1996;84:400–404.
77. Halbach VV, Higashida RT, Hieshima GB, et al. Normal perfusion breakthrough occurring during treatment of carotid and vertebral fistulas. *AJNR Am J Neuroradiol* 1987;8:751–756.
78. Barnwell SL, O'Neill OR. Endovascular therapy of carotid-cavernous fistulas. *Neurosurg Clin N Am* 1994;5:485–495.
79. Kuether TA, O'Neill OR, Nesbit GM, et al. Direct carotid-cavernous fistulas after trigeminal balloon microdecompression gangliolysis: case report. *Neurosurgery* 1996;39:853–856.
80. Bavinzski G, Killer M, Gruber A, et al. Treatment of post-traumatic carotico-cavernous fistulae using electrolytically detachable coils: technical aspects and preliminary experience. *Neuroradiology* 1997;39:81–85.
81. Morris PP. Balloon reconstructive technique for the treatment of a carotid cavernous fistula. *AJNR Am J Neuroradiol* 1999; 20:1107–1109.
82. Jensen ME, Mathis JM, Evans AJ, et al. Non-aneurysmal uses for the Guglielmi detachable coil. Paper presented at: RSNA Annual Meeting; 1995; Chicago, IL.
83. Siniluoto T, Seppanen S, Kuurne T, et al. Transarterial embolization of direct CCF with Guglielmi detachable coils. *AJNR Am J Neuroradiol* 1997;18:519–523.
84. Evans AJ, Jensen ME, Mathis JM, et al. The Guglielmi detachable coil in the treatment of arteriovenous fistulae. *Interv Neuroradiol* 1996;2:201–207.
85. White RI, Pollak JS, Wirth JA. Pulmonary arteriovenous mal-

formations: diagnosis and transcatheter embolotherapy. *J Vasc Interv Radiol* 1996;7:787–804.
86. Houser OW, Campbell JK, Campbell RJ, et al. Arteriovenous malformation affecting the transverse dural venous sinus—an acquired lesion. *Mayo Clin Proc* 1979;54:651–661.
87. Graeb DA, Dolman CL. Radiological and pathological aspects of dural arteriovenous fistulas: a case report. *J Neurosurg* 1986; 64:962–967.
88. Mironov A. Pathogenetical consideration of spontaneous dural arteriovenous fistulas (DAVFs). *Acta Neurochir (Wien)* 1994; 131:45–48.
89. Komiyama M, Nakajima H, Nishikawa M, et al. Traumatic carotid cavernous sinus fistula: serial angiography studies from the day of trauma. *AJNR Am J Neuroradiol* 1998;19: 1641–1644.
90. Lasjaunias P. Arteriography of the head and neck: normal functional anatomy of the external carotid artery. In: Bergeron RT, ed. *Head and neck imaging excluding the brain.* St Louis: Mosby, 1984:344–354.
91. Halbach V, Higashida R, Heishma G, et al. Endovascular therapy of dural fistulas. In: Viñuela F, ed. *Interventional neuroradiology. Endovascular therapy of the central nervous system.* New York: Raven Press, 1992:29–49.
92. Lasjaunias P, Berenstein A. *Dangerous vessels. Functional anatomy of craniofacial arteries in surgical neuroangiography.* Vol I. Berlin, Heidelberg: Springer-Verlag, 1987:239–244.
93. Kurata A, Takano M, Tokiwa K, et al. Spontaneous carotid cavernous fistula presenting only with cranial nerve palsies. *AJNR Am J Neuroradiol* 1993;14:1097–1101.
94. Tomsick T, Dural CCF. Etiology, prevalence, and natural history. In: Tomsick T, ed. *Carotid cavernous fistula.* Cincinnati, OH: Digital Educational Publishing, 1997:57–73.
95. Leonard TJ, Moseley IF, Sanders MD. Ophthalmoplegia in carotid cavernous sinus fistula. *Br J Ophthalmol* 1984;68: 128–134.
96. Moster ML, Sergott RC, Grossman RI. Dural carotid-cavernous sinus vascular malformation with facial nerve paresis. *Can J Ophthalmol* 1988;23:27–29.
97. Sasaki H, Nukui H, Kaneko M, et al. Long-term observations in cases with spontaneous carotid-cavernous fistulas. *Acta Neurochir (Wien)* 1988;90:117–120.
98. Grossman RI, Sergott RC, Goldberg HI, et al. Dural malformations with ophthalmic manifestations: results of particulate embolization in seven patients. *AJNR Am J Neuroradiol* 1985;6: 809–813.
99. Sergott RC, Grossman RI, Savino PJ, et al. The syndrome of paradoxical worsening of dural-cavernous sinus arteriovenous malformations. *Ophthalmologica* 1987;94:205–212.
100. Miki T, Kyoske N, Saitoh Y, et al. Matas procedure in the treatment of spontaneous carotid cavernous sinus fistula: a complication of retinal hemorrhage. *No Shinkei Geka* 1988;16: 971–976.
101. Suzuki Y, Kase M, Yokoi M, et al. Development of central retinal vein occlusion in dural carotid-cavernous fistula. *Ophthalmologica* 1989;199:28–33.
102. Bianchi-Marsoli S, Righi C, Ciasca P, et al. Low dose heparin therapy for dural cavernous sinus fistulas. *Neuroradiology* 1996; 38:15(abst).
103. Lasjaunias P, Chiu M, TerBrugge K, et al. Neurological manifestations intracranial dural arteriovenous malformations. *J Neurosurg* 1986;64:724–730.
104. Kawakami K, Someda K, Inagaki T, et al. Subarachnoid hemorrhage and spontaneous closure in idiopathic carotid-cavernous fistula. Case report. *Neurol Med Chir (Toyko)* 1987;27: 990–994.
105. Watanabe A, Ishii R, Suzuki Y, et al. The cerebral circulation in cases of carotid cavernous fistula. *Neuroradiology* 1990;32: 108–113.
106. Halbach VV, Dowd CF, Higashida RT, et al. Transvenous coil treatment of CCF. In: Tomsick T, ed. *Carotid cavernous fistula.* Cincinnati, OH: Digital Educational Publishing, 1997: 163–175.
107. Jahan R, Gobin YP, Glenn B, et al. Transvenous embolization of a dural arteriovenous fistula of the cavernous sinus through the contralateral pterygoid plexus. *Neuroradiology* 1998;40: 189–193.
108. Monsein LH, Miller NR, Debrun GM. Treatment of CCF via the superior ophthalmic vein: detachable balloon occlusion. In: Tomsick T, ed. *Carotid cavernous fistula.* Cincinnati, OH: Digital Educational Publishing, 1997:177–182.
109. Tomsick TA, Kulwin DR. Treatment of CCF via the superior ophthalmic vein; coil occlusion. In: Tomsick T, ed. *Carotid cavernous fistula.* Cincinnati, OH: Digital Educational Publishing, 1997:183–188.
110. Viñuela F, Duckwiler G, Guglielmi G. CCF: types B, C, D arterial embolization. In: Tomsick T, ed. *Carotid cavernous fistula.* Cincinnati, OH: Digital Educational Publishing, 1997: 155–161.
111. Gaskill-Shipley MF. Radiation therapy for CCF. In: Tomsick T, ed. *Carotid cavernous fistula.* Cincinnati, OH: Digital Educational Publishing, 1997:189–194.
112. Link MJ, Coffey RL, Nichols DA, et al. The role of radiosurgery and particulate embolization in the treatment of dural arteriovenous fistula. *J Neurosurg* 1996;84:804–809.

Endovascular and Percutaneous Therapy of the Brain and Spine, edited by Michael P. Marks and Huy M. Do.
Lippincott Williams & Wilkins, Philadelphia © 2002.

13

ENDOVASCULAR THERAPY FOR INTRACRANIAL TUMORS

RAM CHAVALI
MARY E. JENSEN
IN SUP CHOI

Endovascular techniques have steadily gained acceptance and play an increasing role in the treatment and palliation of head and neck and intracranial tumors. Endovascular embolization of vascular tumors is now considered a standard preoperative procedure. The concept and description of functional vascular anatomy of the head and neck by pioneering interventional neuroradiologists widened the scope and safety of endovascular procedures immensely. This has been coupled with advancements in the tools we use, including embolic materials and imaging equipment, which have reduced the risk related to endovascular procedures significantly. All of the changes have occurred in concert with ever-increasing abilities of neurosurgeons and skull base surgeons to remove advanced deep-seated vascular tumors.

Today's technology and the dissemination of the concept of functional vascular anatomy of the head and neck allow most of these procedures to be done with minimal risk when the operator has appropriate training. Cross-pollination of the many medical, basic science, and industrial subspecialties now invigorates the field even more, and with advances on the horizon such as biodegradable occlusion materials which can be impregnated with various biologically active materials, including gene therapy agents, the future is ever brighter for the practitioner and, more importantly, the patient.

Although nothing can replace solid clinical training, this chapter will give the interventionist a well-grounded review in the background, strategies, and approaches to preoperative and palliative embolization for intracranial tumors.

R. Chavali: Department of Interventional Neuroradiology, Lahey Clinic Medical Center, Burlington, Massachusetts.

M.E. Jensen: Departments of Radiology and Neurosurgery, University of Virginia Health Sciences Center, Charlottesville, Virginia.

In Sup Choi: Department of Radiology, Tufts University School of Medicine, Boston, Massachusetts, and Department of Interventional Neuroradiology, Lahey Clinic Medical Center, Burlington, Massachusetts.

Intracranial tumors which can benefit from preoperative embolization include (extraaxial) meningioma, hemangiopericytoma, paraganglioma, neurogenic tumors, esthesioneuroblastomas, malignant bone tumors, and primary or metastatic malignancies of the central nervous system (CNS). Of intraaxial tumors, hemangioblastoma and choroid plexus tumors are amenable to preoperative embolization, while aggressive glial cell tumors, specifically glioblastoma multiforme, have been treated with intraarterial chemotherapeutic agents without significant improvement in survival rates. This chapter will discuss salient features of intracranial lesions typically treated with endovascular therapy, strategies in treatment, and potential complications. The reader is also referred to Chapter 14 for a discussion of endovascular treatment of extracranial tumors, because many of these lesions overlap with primarily intracranial tumors and extend into the intracranial space.

BACKGROUND

Meningiomas

Meningiomas are the most frequently encountered extraaxial masses. Meningiomas are slow-growing, well-encapsulated, generally benign tumors arising from arachnoid cap cells and account for 13% to 18% of all intracranial neoplasms [1]. Highly vascular tumors that derive their rich blood supply from the dura, these lesions are seen most frequently in middle-aged women but can occur at any age in either sex. Other factors may be related to their etiology, because the incidence is increased in patients previously irradiated for head and neck pathology and in persons afflicted with type 2 neurofibromatosis [2].

The anatomical location of meningiomas parallels that of the arachnoid villi and, in decreasing frequency, appears over the convexities (Fig. 13-1), along the sphenoid wing (Fig. 13-2), in the olfactory groove (Fig. 13-3), adjacent to the sella, and within the posterior fossa [3]. Any meningo-

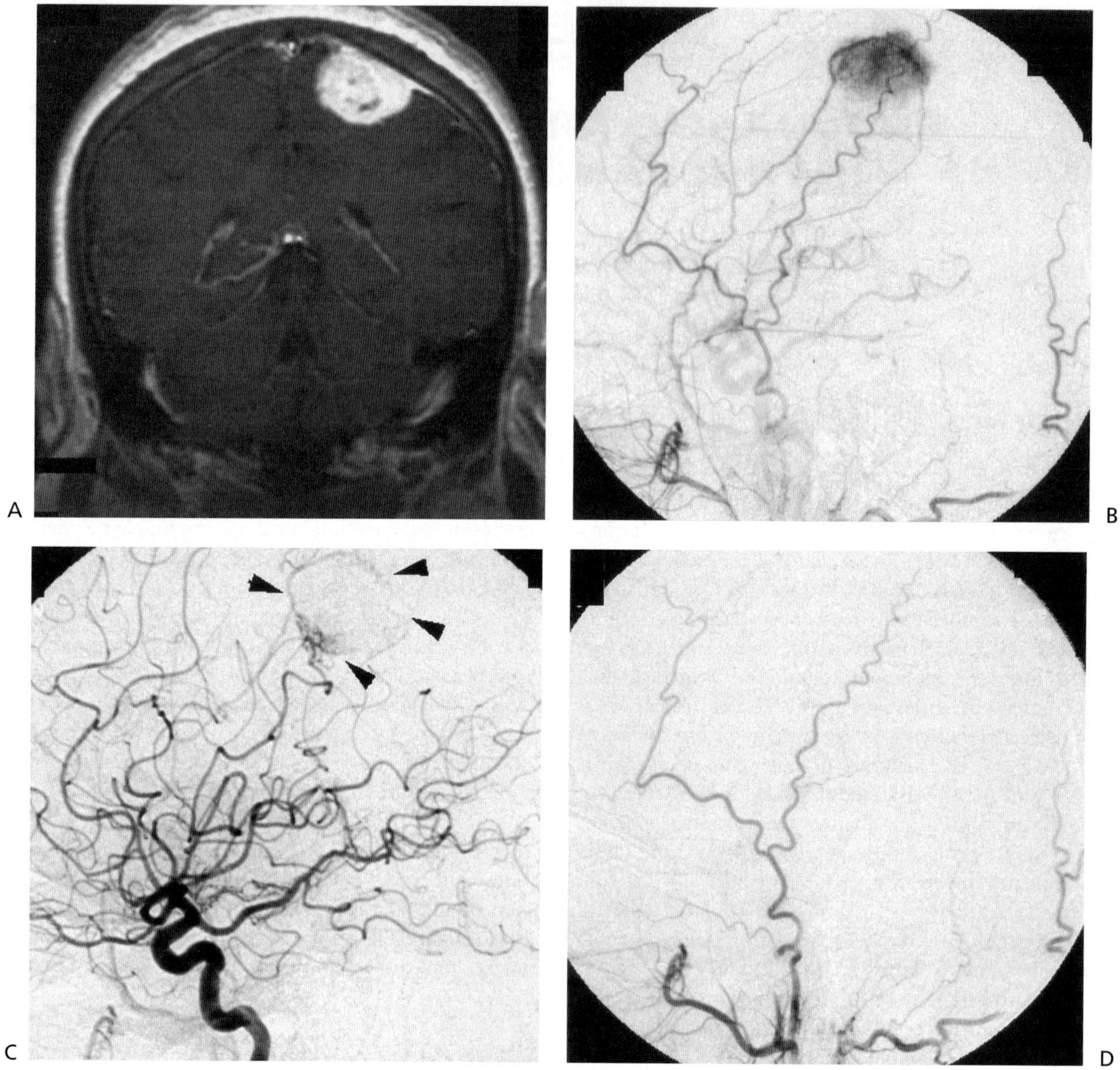

FIGURE 13-1. **A:** Coronal postcontrast MR shows an enhancing dural-based extraaxial mass impinging on the left parietal cortex, consistent with a convexity meningioma. **B:** Injection of the ECA demonstrates the enlarged MMA filling the densely staining tumor. **C:** A lateral ICA study shows small pial branches feeding the periphery of the tumor. **D:** Following PVA embolization, no tumor blush is identified.

epithelial cell, however, can give rise to this tumor, explaining the intracranial, choroidal, intradiploic, spinal, or ectopic location. Arachnoid membranous tissue along the cranial nerves as well as the dural fibroblasts serve as sources of these typically slow-growing tumors [4–6]. As intraventricular masses related to the choroid plexus, they are most common within the lateral ventricles.

Symptoms vary and may include headache, seizures, progressive motor impairment, or dementia. Intratumoral hemorrhage, with a sudden increase in volume, may mimic a stroke. Tumors involving the skull base often appear as isolated cranial nerve dysfunction or palsy, or as transient ischemic attacks if the carotid artery is compromised [7].

On pathologic examination these tumors are well circumscribed with a focal dural attachment, project inward from the subdural surface, and cause compression but not invasion (except in malignant form) of the adjacent brain. Invasion of the dura and dural sinuses is common and the tumor may incite underlying bony hyperostosis. Intratumoral hemorrhage is rare and associated with angiomatous or intraventricular forms, and necrosis is reserved for the very large, malignant, or embolized tumors. Occasionally

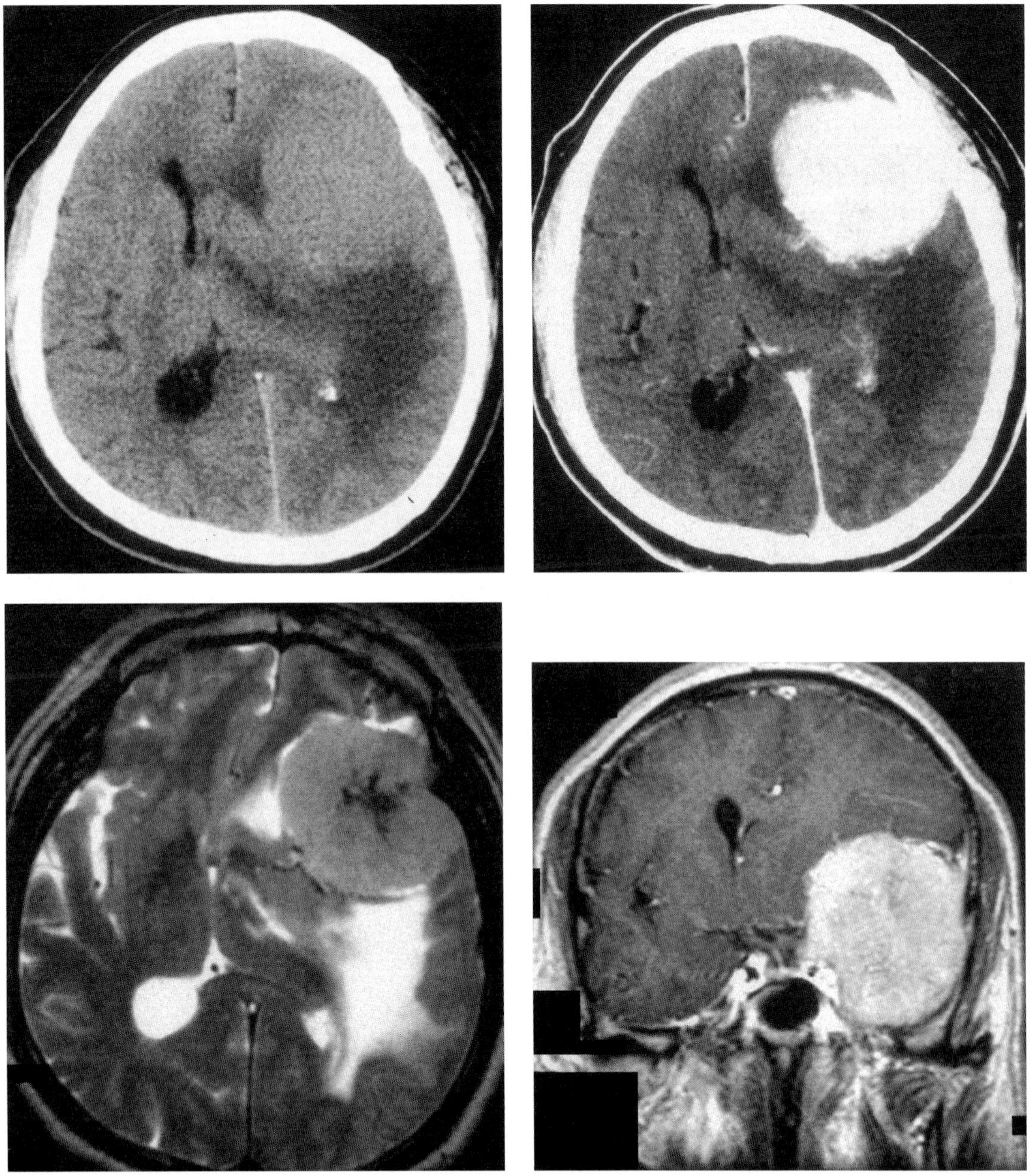

A B C D

FIGURE 13-2. A,B: Pre and post-contrast CT respectively demonstrating a large middle cranial fossa mass extending upward into the frontal lobe region. **C,D:** T_2-weighted axial and T_1-weighted coronal post-contrast MR respectively. Tumor is isodense to gray matter and is easily identified following contrast enhancement. Note T2 hypointensity characteristic of meningioma. Extraaxial nature can best be appreciated on coronal enhanced T1 images. *(Figure continues.)*

the appearance is one of a diffuse, carpet-like growth over the dura, referred to as *meningioma en plaque* [3].

Most meningiomas have a classic appearance on computed tomography (CT)—that of an isodense or slightly hyperdense, sharply marginated mass that abuts the dura and enhances homogeneously. Tiny punctate calcifications are common; nodular or dense calcification is less likely. Adjacent bone may demonstrate thickening or blistering of the cortex, or bony erosion from pressure or infiltration.

Contrast-enhanced magnetic resonance imaging (MRI) provides better detection and morphologic characterization of these tumors than CT. Multiplanar imaging and the absence of beam-hardening artifact from bone allow detection of the dural attachment regardless of location and demonstrate adjacent neurologic structures. Cortical displacement is more apparent because of its superior gray-white contrast. MRI is also preferable to CT in evaluating involvement of regional blood vessels because of the differences between tumor signal intensity and signal flow void.

Diagnostic angiography provides a wealth of information

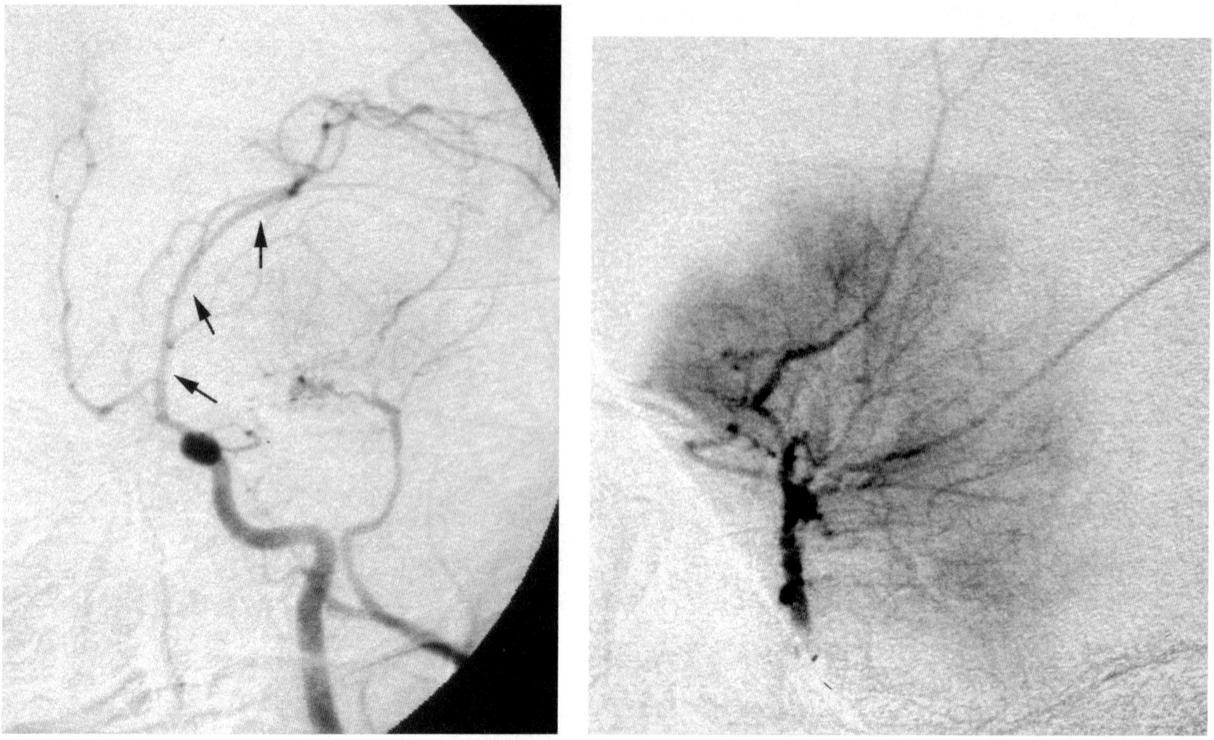

E F

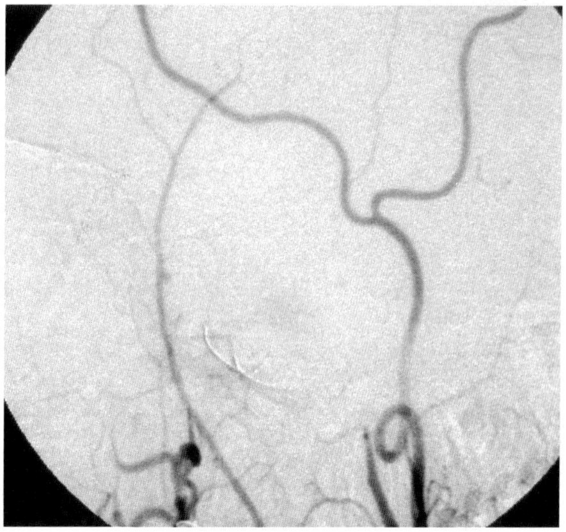

G

FIGURE 13-2. *Continued.* **E:** Left CCA injection anteroposterior view demonstrates mass effect with uplifting and draping of MCA branches *(arrows).* **F:** Selective left middle meningeal injection lateral view demonstrates vascularity of tumor. **G:** Successful devascularization following PVA and coil embolization of middle meningeal supply seen on final left distal ECA control study.

prior to surgical resection. The examination is tailored to the location of the tumor and the pertinent vascular anatomy. Selective injection of appropriate vessels reveals the arterial supply, tumor vascularity, and dural attachment site, arterial displacement or encasement and collateral supply, regional venous anatomy and patency of dural sinuses, and dangerous anastomoses. An area of particular interest is at the orbital apex, where the anterior division of the middle meningeal artery (MMA) makes a sharp turn to run posteriorly. It is at this location where the meningolacrimal or recurrent meningeal branch may communicate with the ophthalmic artery, and a magnified study of the orbit during MMA injection is recommended. Common angiographic findings in meningiomas include hypertrophied meningeal vessels that branch into a sunburst pattern after penetrating the tumor (see Fig. 13-3), a dense, homogeneous blush which persists into the late venous phase, recruitment of pial supply to the periphery of larger lesions (see Figs. 13-1 and 13-3), and prolonged venous drainage [8]. *En plaque* tumors are, as a rule, smaller and less vascular.

Complete surgical removal is the optimal treatment for these histologically benign tumors. Radiation therapy is considered during the postoperative period if the lesion proves to be malignant upon pathologic examination. Fol-

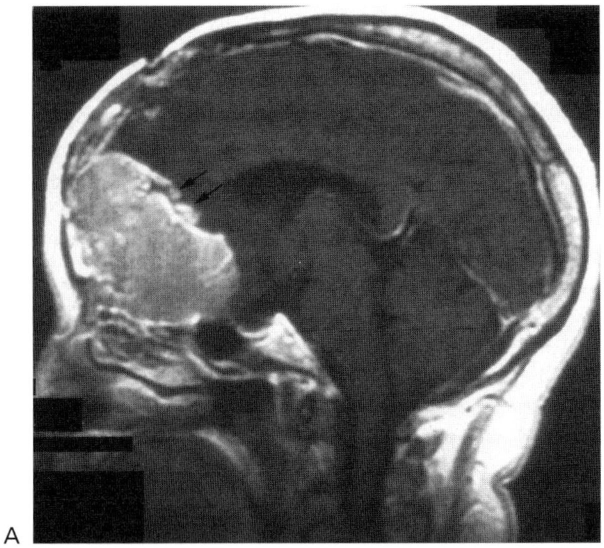

FIGURE 13-3. **A:** Sagittal contrast-enhanced MRI shows a large extraaxial mass arising from the olfactory groove with posterior displacement of the frontal lobes and congestion of adjacent veins *(arrows)*. **B,C:** Anteroposterior **(B)** and lateral **(C)** injections of the common carotid artery show the typical sunburst pattern of the neovascularity, arising from ethmoidal branches of the right IMA and ophthalmic artery, and from regional pial branches. The ACA is displaced superiorly and posteriorly by the mass. PVA embolization of the IMA and ophthalmic artery was performed. **D,E:** Final anteroposterior **(D)** and lateral **(E)** angiograms show marked decrease in the tumor blush, with the residual staining from fine pial feeders.

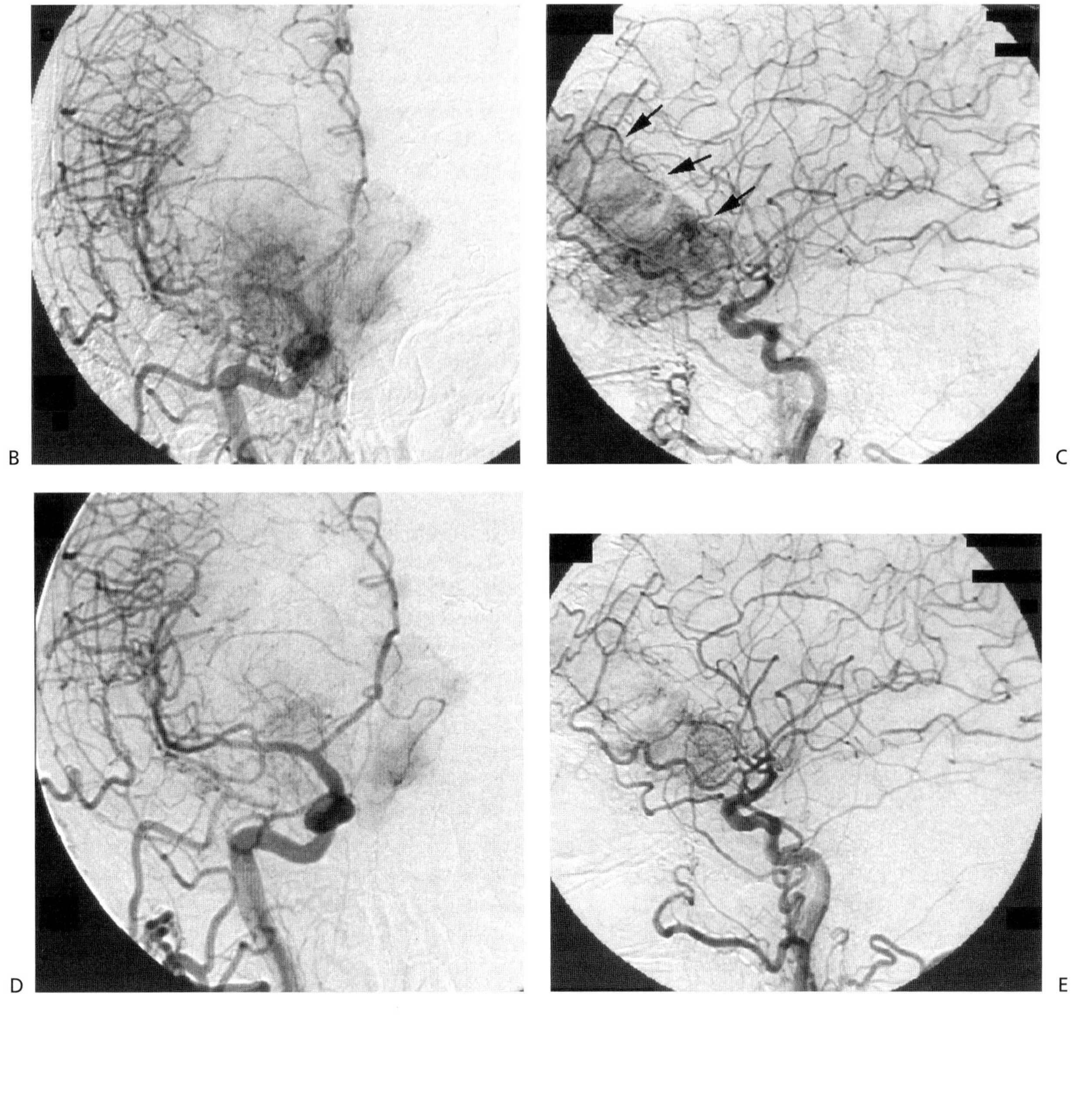

lowing partial resection of a benign tumor, radiotherapy is indicated when the risk of resection of an eventual recurrence is judged excessive. Other candidates include the patient with multiply recurrent tumors for whom repeat surgery is not indicated and the progressively symptomatic patient with an inoperable tumor [9].

Although much of the literature supports reduction of blood loss and ease of tumor removal following treatment [8,10–12], controversy remains. In a recent prospective study of 60 patients, Bendszus et al. [13] found that only complete tumor embolization had a statistically significant effect on blood loss. In another study, Oka et al. [14] concluded that blood loss was significantly less in skull base tumors 6 cm or smaller. In short, presurgical embolization is often based entirely upon the surgeon's preference. Tumors which present a more formidable surgical challenge (e.g., skull base lesions, tumors with dural sinus or skull involvement, or large tumors with significant edema) may well benefit from embolization [15]. Embolization may also decrease the likelihood of tumor recurrence by producing necrosis at the site of dural attachment [8].

The vascular supply to meningiomas can be relatively predictable based on the location. Parasagittal, high convexity, and falx cerebri meningiomas receive supply from ipsilateral middle meningeal and artery of the falx cerebri, with collateral supply from corresponding contralateral arteries. Frontal convexity and anterior falcine meningiomas may receive contributions from branches of the anterior ethmoidal or anterior falcine branches of the ophthalmic artery. Meningiomas originating along the tentorium recruit supply from marginal tentorial artery and inferolateral trunk. The artery of the falx cerebelli is the main supply to lesions near the straight sinus and torcular herophili. Dural supply to skull base tumors include the ethmoidal, falcine, cavernous, clival, and tentorial branches, which arise from a combination of larger vessels.

A large meningioma may recruit additional pial supply. Pial feeders may supply the periphery, or capsule, of the tumor, but these vessels are often not amenable to embolization. There is no direct correlation with the size of the tumor and pial supply, although in our experience there appears to be a trend. Bitzer et al. suggested pial supply may be associated with the development of peritumoral vasogenic edema seen in some patients [16].

Complete angiographic evaluation requires visualization of some or all of the following arteries: the internal carotid artery (ICA), ophthalmic artery, internal maxillary artery (IMA), accessory meningeal artery, MMA, ascending pharyngeal artery, and occipital artery. Lesions involving the posterior fossa necessitate injection of the vertebral artery with its anterior and posterior meningeal branches.

Many skull base meningiomas, particularly those adjacent to or in the midline, exhibit a dominant internal carotid, ophthalmic, or vertebral artery supply, making adequate embolization difficult but not impossible. Advances in microcatheter and microguidewire technology allow more efficient and safer selective catheterization and embolization of small or tortuous branches arising from intracranial arteries. Reports of successful ophthalmic artery embolization [17,18] show that treatment of this vessel can be performed safely. The catheter tip is placed distal to the central retinal artery. Larger particles (500 to 1000 μm) or microcoils are usually chosen. Provocative testing with both amobarbital (Amytal) and lidocaine may demonstrate visual changes, indicating a positive test and negating treatment [17]. Visual loss has been described when Gelfoam powder was used [18]; therefore, very small particles should be avoided.

The meningohypophyseal trunk and inferolateral trunk are also amenable to selective catheterization, although the origins of both are small and arise at an acute angle. Entry into the orifice with a guidewire is often possible, but advancement of the microcatheter can be difficult, posing considerable risk of vascular perforation. Tenuous tip position may result in reflux of embolic material into the cerebral circulation. These risks are minimized if soft-tipped microcatheters and microguidewires are used in conjunction with road mapping techniques [19].

Catheter tip position will often determine the embolic agent used. The closer to the entrance of the tumor, the less likely is reflux; hence, very small particles or liquid agents may be selected [19]. When these agents are employed in branches supplying cranial nerves, provocative testing with lidocaine is recommended, although false-negative results have been reported. For most preoperative patients, polyvinyl alcohol (PVA) in the 250- to 350-μm range is adequate. Embolization is discontinued when delayed "washout" and loss of tumor blush is noted. Complete stasis in the arterial feeder may be attained with microcoil placement to prevent recanalization. In summary, the same principles of external carotid artery (ECA) branch embolization apply, with the understanding that the tiniest of refluxes can result in devastating consequences for the patient.

In those tumors in which the feeding branch cannot be catheterized adequately, proximal embolization with a safety balloon inflated distal to the feeders can be performed as previously described (Fig. 13-4) [20]. Another treatment option is direct puncture of the tumor, either percutaneously or at the time of surgical exposure (using intraoperative angiography), followed by instillation of liquid embolic material [21].

Prior to embolization, patients are often placed on corticosteroids to minimize the effects of anticipated tumor swelling. Resection is usually performed within 2 to 5 days, allowing optimal tumor shrinkage and softening while discouraging recruitment of collateral blood supply or recanalization of embolized vessels. Waiting longer than 10 days may negate the benefits of the embolization.

Embolization of recurrent tumors may be difficult or complex because of altered vascular anatomy. The arterial supply may become predominantly pial in origin, or less accessible dural, cutaneous, or transosseous vessels may be recruited. Small dural collateral vessels around the site of surgical ligation of larger vessels can foil reembolization, because larger embolic agents are unable to pass through to the tumor bed.

Complications of meningioma embolization are uncommon, similar to those of other head and neck tumors, and include cranial nerve palsies, blindness, and stroke. Embolization of scalp vessels or normal meningeal branches with small particles can result in necrosis or poor healing. Intratumoral, subdural, and subarachnoid hemorrhage during embolization have also been reported (see Fig. 13-4) [22,23]. Possible causes include sudden changes in blood flow that resulted in rupture of pathologic vessels, or from rupture as a result of high injection pressure. However, one must keep in mind that in experienced hands the expected complication rate is approximately 1% and the advantages described above usually outweigh the risks.

Hemangiopericytomas

Accounting for less than 2% of all soft tissue sarcomas [24, 25], hemangiopericytomas are highly vascular tumors which arise from the immature smooth muscle cells surrounding capillaries, called pericytes [24,26–28]. When intracranial

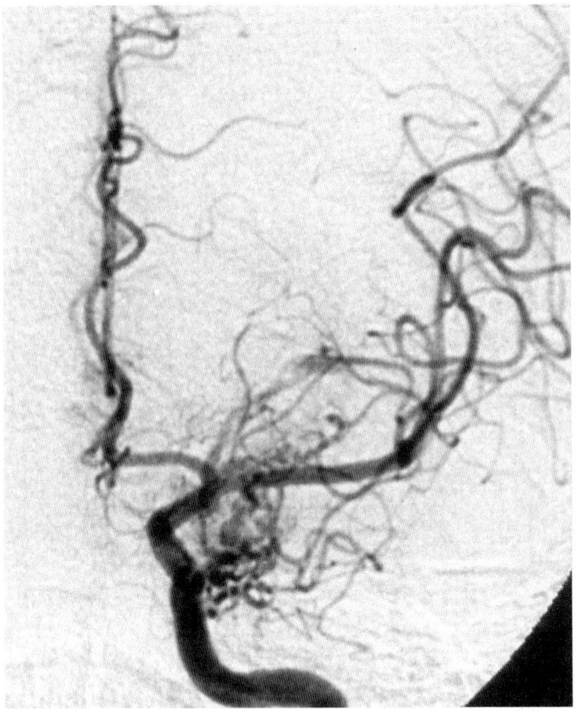

A

FIGURE 13-4. This elderly woman with a recurrent sphenoid wing meningioma was referred for preoperative embolization. **A–C:** The meningohypophyseal trunk feeders **(A,B)** were too small to access directly, so a temporary balloon was floated past their origins and inflated **(C).** *(Figure continues.)*

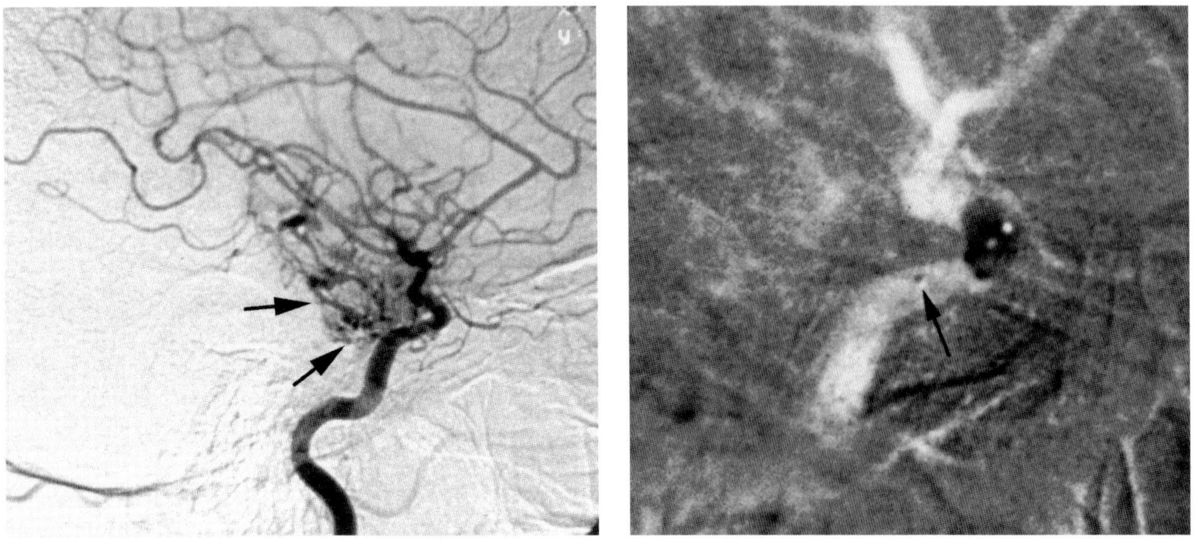

B C

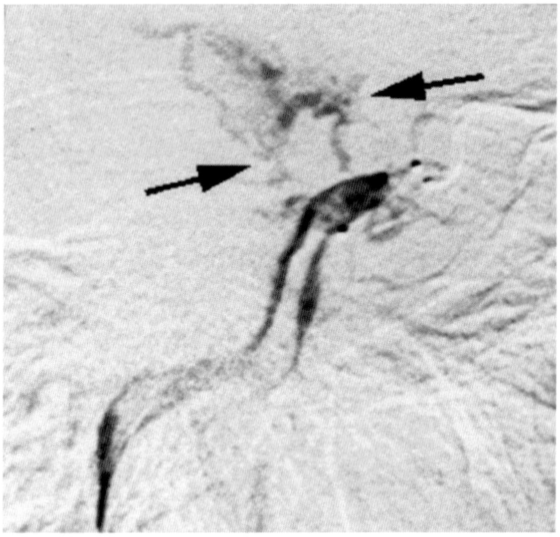

D

FIGURE 13-4. *Continued.* **D:** Embolization with small PVA (50 to 150 μm) via a second microcatheter placed in the proximal genu of the cavernous segment was performed with marked decrease in the tumor blush noted. After balloon deflation, no distal emboli were identified and the patient remained unchanged neurologically. A repeat angiogram was done later when she experienced right-sided weakness. **E:** It showed no evidence of a distal embolus, but there was acute elevation of the MI segment indicating mass effect. **F:** An emergent head CT showed hemorrhage into the tumor bed, and she was taken to the operating room.

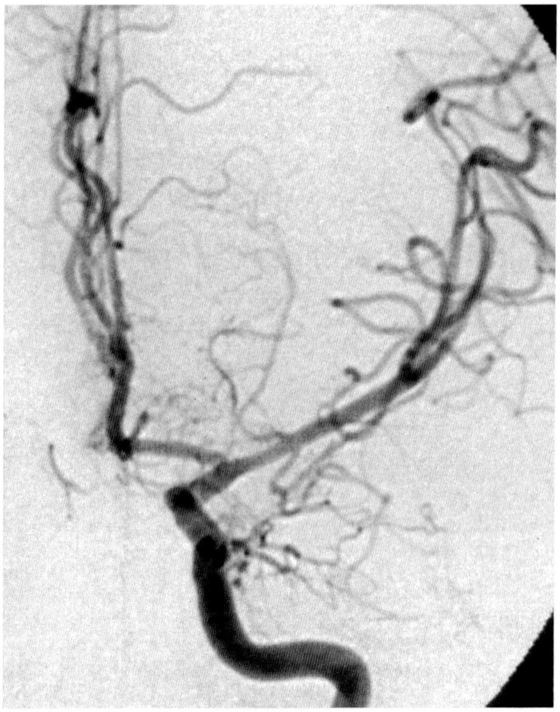

E

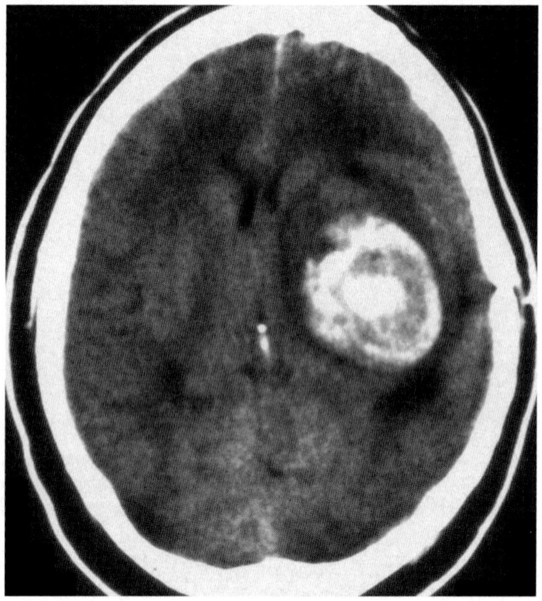

F

in origin, these lesions account for less than 1% of all CNS tumors [28]. Overall, 25% arise in a head and neck location, particularly in the nose, mouth, nasopharynx, and paranasal sinuses [24,29].

Meningeal-based hemangiopericytomas show a slight male predominance in a slightly younger population than patients with meningiomas, and their location parallels that of meningiomas [27,28]. Extracranial lesions do not demonstrate a sex predilection and are seen in all ages, with a peak incidence in the fifth decade [26]. The average duration of symptoms is 11 months with intracranial tumors [28]. Supratentorial masses cause headache, papilledema, and hemiparesis, whereas infratentorial tumors predispose the patient to gait disturbances and ataxia [28]. The most common course of extracranial lesions is a painless mass of varying size that demonstrates progressive enlargement [26]. Nasal tumors frequently cause epistaxis and nasal obstruction; local pain, swelling, and headache are reported also [29]. Physical examination shows the tumor to be firm and circumscribed, occasionally nodular, with no overlying skin changes [26].

Meningeal hemangiopericytomas are considered by some authors to represent a subtype of angioblastic meningiomas [28] and by others as a distinctly different histologic tumor

[30]. Soft tissue or bone tumors have an identical histologic appearance to their meningeal counterparts. Tumor behavior and pathologic appearance may not coincide, with histologically benign lesions demonstrating a malignant clinical course. More than one-half of patients experience local and distant recurrences [26], with most metastases located in the bone or lungs. Nasal hemangiopericytomas are more benign in nature when compared with their intracranial counterparts, but recurrences have been observed in up to 23% of cases, with metastases seen in 3.5% [29].

On plain radiographic films, localized pressure erosion or bony destruction adjacent to the soft tissue mass can be seen, and metastatic lesions have an osteolytic appearance [26]. CT examination shows intracranial tumors to be isodense, or slightly hyperdense, ill-defined heterogeneous masses that demonstrate enhancement. Extensive peritumoral edema, absence of calcifications, and nonenhancing cystic areas are also noted. MRI shows an isointense mass on T1 which becomes hyperintense on T2, in addition to edema, central necrosis, and cyst formation, giving rise to heterogeneous signal [31].

Angiography of intracranial lesions demonstrates a vascu-

A

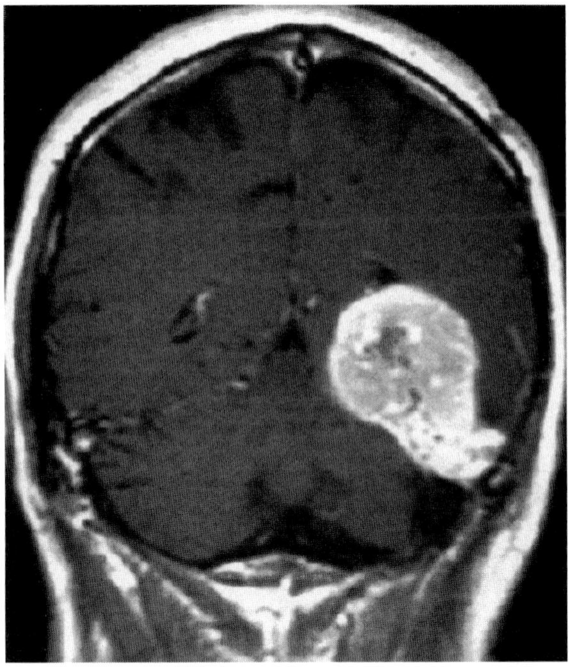

FIGURE 13-5. A: Coronal T_1-weighted contrast-enhanced MRI shows a large dural-based, inhomogeneously enhancing mass arising from the left tentorium. Areas of signal void within the tumor correspond to enlarged feeding vessels. **B,C:** Anteroposterior **(B)** and lateral **(C)** vertebral angiograms show enlarged, tortuous intratumoral vessels fed by the posterior temporal branch of the posterior cerebral artery (PCA) *(arrowheads)*. Venous shunting is identified along the anterior and superior rim. Because of the increased flow, a flow-directed catheter was positioned in the posterior temporal artery. As the catheter was advanced distally, contrast injection showed extravasation of contrast, indicating vessel perforation. *(Figure continues.)*

B

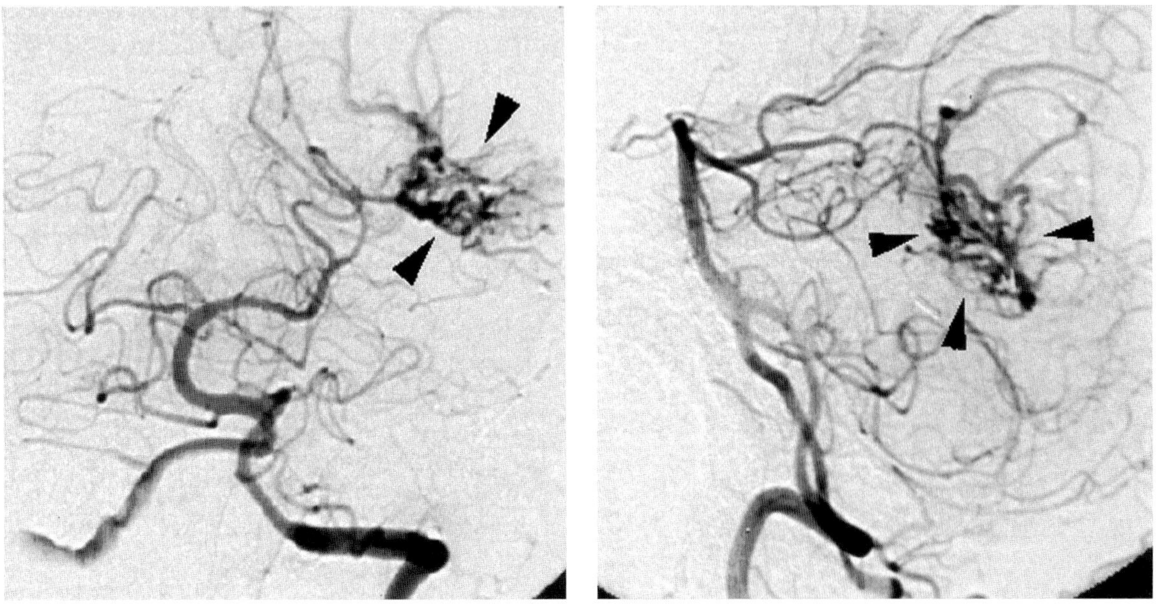

C

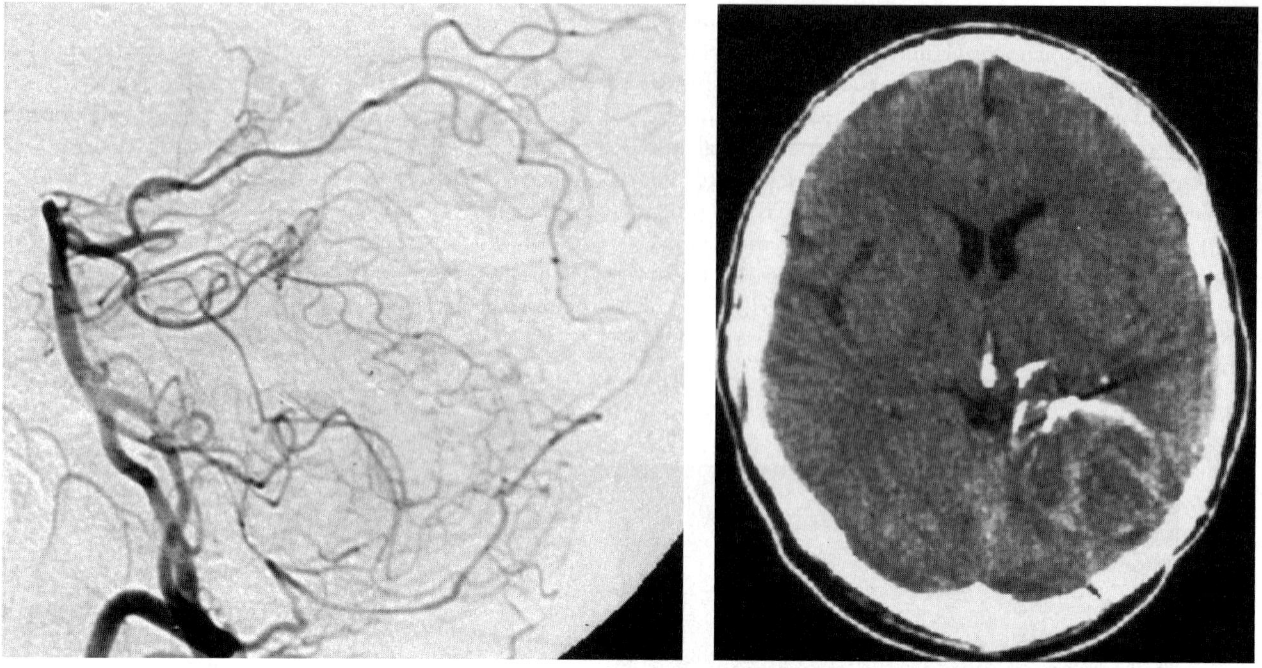

FIGURE 13-5. *Continued.* **D:** The branch was embolized with NBCA, resulting in occlusion of the feeding artery. **E:** A posttreatment CT scan demonstrates the high-density NBCA and a rim of contrast extravasation medially and anteriorly.

lar mass that fills rapidly and drains slowly, and may have intradural (Fig. 13-5) or mixed intradural-extradural blood supply (Fig. 13-6). In many cases, the ICA contributes significantly and is the only arterial supply for one-half of the cases [28]. Small corkscrew vessels are often noted, leading to an intense, uniform, well-demarcated tumor blush [26].

Surgical removal is the primary therapy for these tumors and is complicated by tumor vascularity [27] and a high rate of local recurrence and metastasis. Postresection irradiation of the tumor site increases survival rates by 50% [26]. Preliminary results with radiosurgery have demonstrated dramatic early shrinkage of small- and medium-sized intracranial hemangiopericytomas that have recurred or developed after previous surgery or radiation therapy or both [32].

As with other vascular tumors, presurgical embolization has been shown to be effective in hemostatic control during removal [27,33]. Intracranial lesions with exuberant pial supply pose the most difficult challenge because the technical difficulty and complication rate are increased. Superselective studies followed by provocative testing using a short-acting barbiturate will confirm correct catheter placement prior to embolization. In high-flow lesions, flow-directed catheters may be of use but limit the embolic choices to liquid agents, such as alcohol or N-butyl-2-cyanoacrylate (NBCA), or very small particles (50 to 150 μm). Extracranial lesions are embolized in a manner similar to that described for the other head and neck tumors. Direct puncture with installation of a liquid agent also has been described.

Hemangioblastomas

These uncommon tumors actually are benign CNS tumors of unknown histogenetic etiology. They account for 2% of all primary CNS tumors. Patients can suffer from headache, disequilibrium, nausea, vomiting, and vertigo. These are tumors of adults, most commonly occurring between the third and fifth decades, with mean age of 39. They are very rare in children [35]. Most occur sporadically, but between 10% and 20% are associated with von Hippel-Lindau (VHL) syndrome, a hereditary phakomatosis with autosomal dominance but incomplete penetrance. Multiple hemangioblastomas are pathognomonic for VHL, and CNS hemangioblastomas eventually develop in 44% of patients with VHL. Approximately 90% of hemangioblastomas occur within the posterior fossa, usually within the cerebellum. Other less common locations include the spinal cord (3% to 13%), medulla (2% to 3%), and rarely in a supratentorial location (1.5%) [36]. Hemangioblastomas are highly vascular lesions that are the cause of death in 82% of those with VHL. They are, however, eminently curable, making these patients strong surgical candidates and thus also candidates for preoperative embolization.

Hemangioblastomas are well-circumscribed masses.

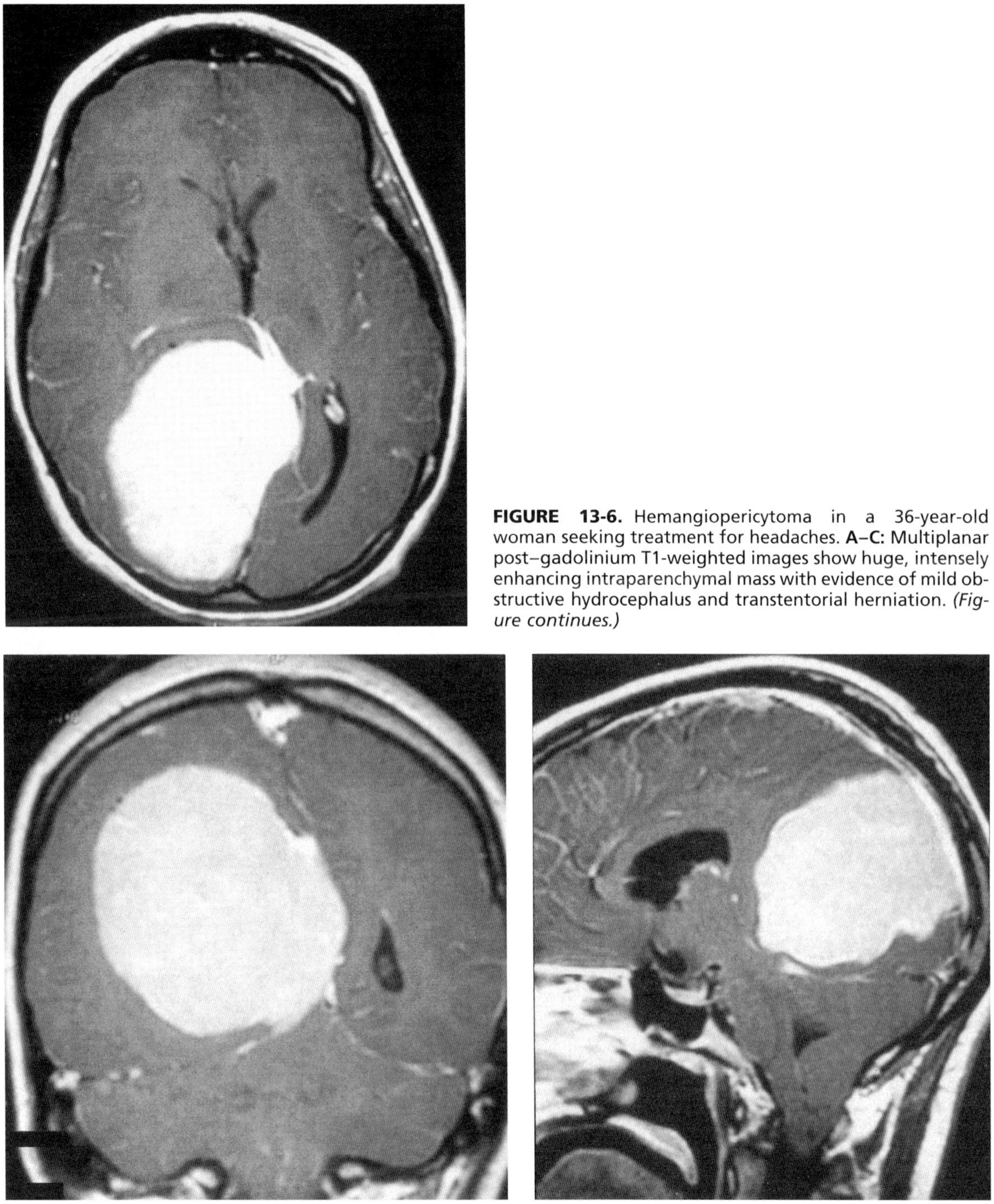

A B C

FIGURE 13-6. Hemangiopericytoma in a 36-year-old woman seeking treatment for headaches. **A–C:** Multiplanar post–gadolinium T1-weighted images show huge, intensely enhancing intraparenchymal mass with evidence of mild obstructive hydrocephalus and transtentorial herniation. *(Figure continues.)*

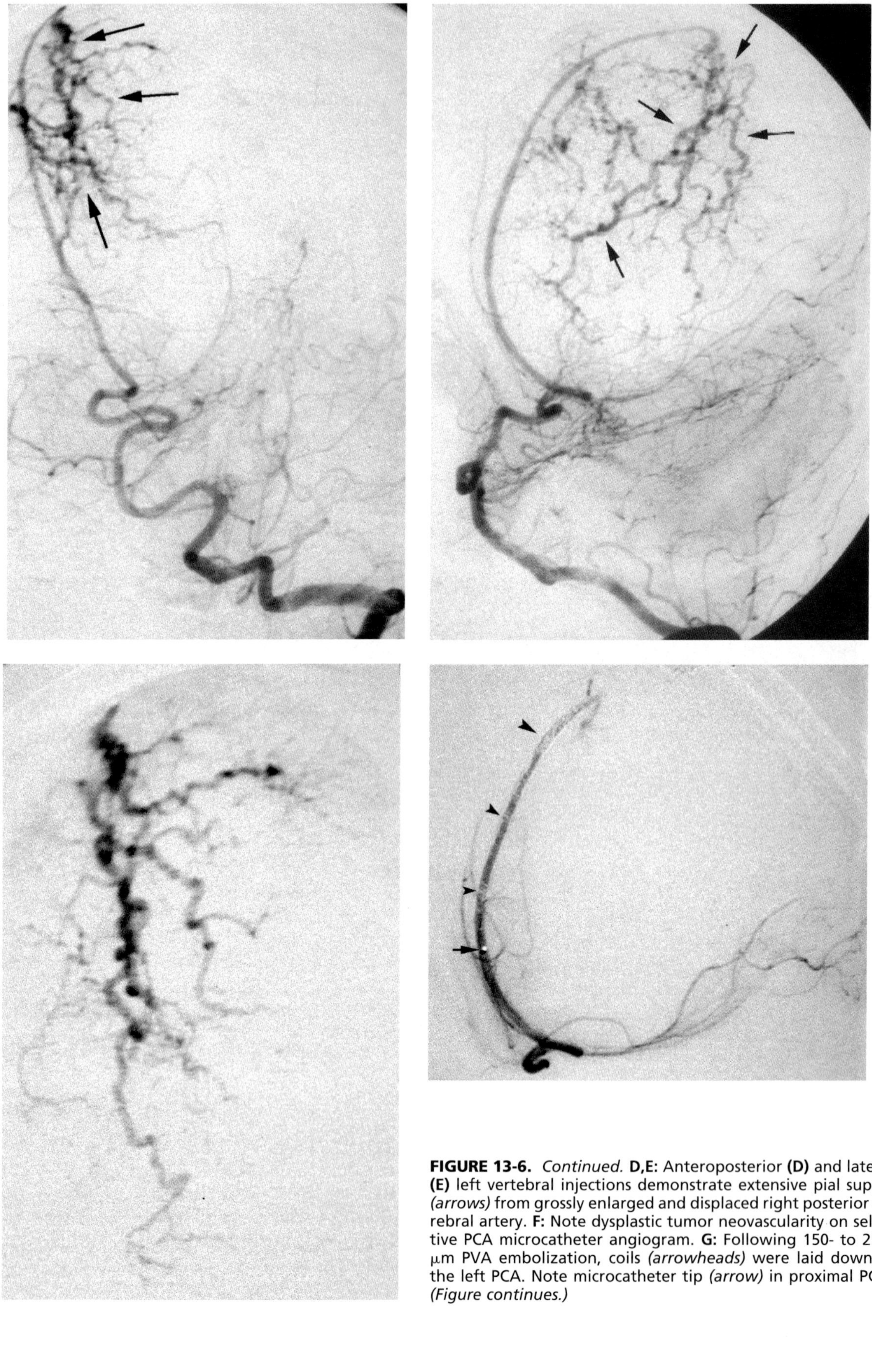

D E F G

FIGURE 13-6. *Continued.* **D,E:** Anteroposterior **(D)** and lateral **(E)** left vertebral injections demonstrate extensive pial supply *(arrows)* from grossly enlarged and displaced right posterior cerebral artery. **F:** Note dysplastic tumor neovascularity on selective PCA microcatheter angiogram. **G:** Following 150- to 250-μm PVA embolization, coils *(arrowheads)* were laid down in the left PCA. Note microcatheter tip *(arrow)* in proximal PCA. *(Figure continues.)*

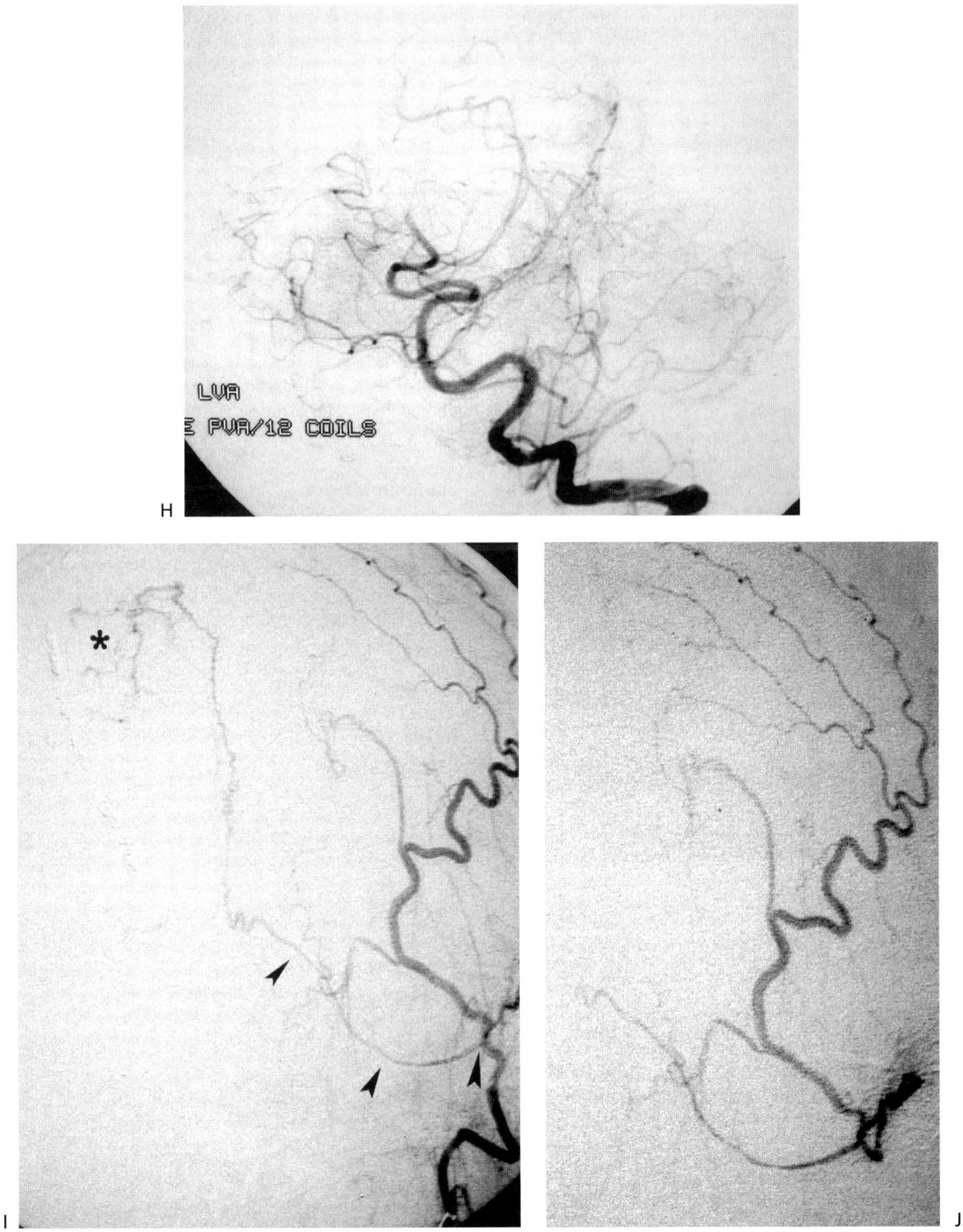

FIGURE 13-6. *Continued.* **H:** Left vertebral injection after PVA and coil embolization demonstrates no significant residual pial supply. **I:** Left occipital artery injection reveals posterior meningeal artery *(arrowheads)* supply to tumor *(asterisk).* **J:** This too was embolized with PVA particles and a single coil.

About 60% are cystic masses with a mural nodule that usually abuts a pial surface, and the remaining 40% are solid. Microscopically, the tumors are somewhat heterogeneous, composed of both endothelial cells and pericytes or of interstitial stromal cells. The former usually predominate. Densely packed thin-walled vessels varying in type from capillary to cavernous are seen within the nodule, and the cyst wall usually represents compressed brain or reactive gliosis [37].

Imaging characteristics include a low-density cyst with a strongly enhancing mural nodule on contrast CT. Calcification is rarely noted. On MRI, the cyst is slightly hyperintense to CSF on T1-weighted images and hyperintense on T2-weighted images (Fig. 13-7). The tumor nodule is more variable on MRI but demonstrates intense enhancement following gadolinium administration. Serpentine flow voids can also be seen frequently on T2-weighted sequences. On angiography, the common pattern for a tumor with a cyst is a large avascular mass with a solid component that has intense and prolonged vascular staining. Arteriovenous shunting is usually not seen. The solid components are relatively homogeneous and well-defined masses. If small cystic components are present within the tumor nodule, then a "Swiss cheese" appearance can be seen (see Fig. 13-7).

Typically, hemangioblastomas within the posterior fossa are supplied primarily by the AICA and PICA, with additional supply from the superior cerebellar arteries [38]. Those within the inferior cerebellum can receive supply from lateral spinal arteries. Additionally, because of their location, they are able often to recruit dural supply from posterior meningeal or dural branches of the vertebral artery [39]. The feeders usually are significantly dilated and end in the tumor. Those with more than one feeder also demonstrate multicompartmental angioarchitecture and, if a tumor boundary is ill-defined or not seen where expected, one should look for an as yet unopacified additional supply. Draining veins are seen late in the venous phase of the angiogram and usually are dilated. Small tumors usually have only one draining vein, whereas larger tumors may have multiple draining veins.

Because the pial vessels supplying hemangioblastomas are dilated and end in tumor, these lesions often are ideal candidates for preoperative embolization. Indeed, the fragility of the tumor margins makes operating on these neoplasms quite difficult for the surgeon. Again, as for the other vascular tumors, we can impact positively and significantly on intraoperative blood loss and operative time, improving the patient's overall risk profile.

The catheter tip should be as close to the tumor as possible and beyond any normal pial branches. To ensure intratumoral penetration of particles, maintenance of antegrade flow is preferable, so catheter wedging should be avoided. PVA or NBCA glue are both reasonable choices depending on anatomy, catheter position, and surgeon preference. Small particles starting at 150 to 250 μm are ideal for penetration and devascularization. The advantage of NBCA is that both tumor and feeding vessels can be occluded simultaneously without the same concern for vessel rupture or reflux that may occur with particle embolization if there are sudden flow and pressure changes.

Navigation and embolization of the more delicate pial vessels requires greater operator experience than that required for the external system. Vasospasm can occur. Serious unnecessary thromboembolic complications can also result from lack of meticulous technique in flushing of the guide catheter and the microcatheter. High-resolution angiographic equipment is even more critical for frequent monitoring of the embolization and ensuring patency of all distal branches. Particular attention must be paid to any changes in flow and pressure which might lead to subsequent embolic material reflux and stroke or vessel rupture.

Intraarterial Chemotherapy for Brain Tumors

Because many chemotherapeutic agents cannot pass the blood-brain barrier, the intraarterial administration of chemotherapy has revolutionized the treatment of solid brain tumors. The intact tight junctions of the blood-brain barrier will not allow most chemotherapeutic agents to pass. This hurdle can be overcome by the use of osmotic disruption. When the cells of the capillary endothelium are exposed to a hyperosmolar solution of mannitol the cells shrink, causing the tight junctions to be pulled apart for a short time. This allows an increase in the amount of chemotherapy subsequently delivered to the tumor and surrounding areas, perhaps by as much as 100 times [40]. This technique was pioneered in the 1980s by Neuwelt et al. at the Oregon Health Sciences University, which is now the coordinating center for the national Blood-brain Barrier Pro-

FIGURE 13-7. Hemangioblastoma in a 22-year-old man with VHL syndrome. **A,B:** Sagittal T1-weighted post–gadolinium-enhanced images reveal typical intensely enhancing, well-defined tumor nodules in the left cerebellum and tonsil *(arrowhead).* Note flow void *(arrows)* at superior aspect of the tumor in **(A). C:** Left vertebral angiogram reveals enlarged feeders from AICA *(small arrow)* and PICA *(large arrow)* and classic "Swiss cheese" architecture with lack of opacification anteriorly of the large nodule. Note smaller vermian and other cerebellar lesions *(arrowhead).* **D:** There is prolonged parenchymal opacification long into the venous phase. **E:** Following PVA and coil embolization of feeding arteries, no significant residual supply to large lesion was left, making subsequent surgical resection quite easy with minimal blood loss.

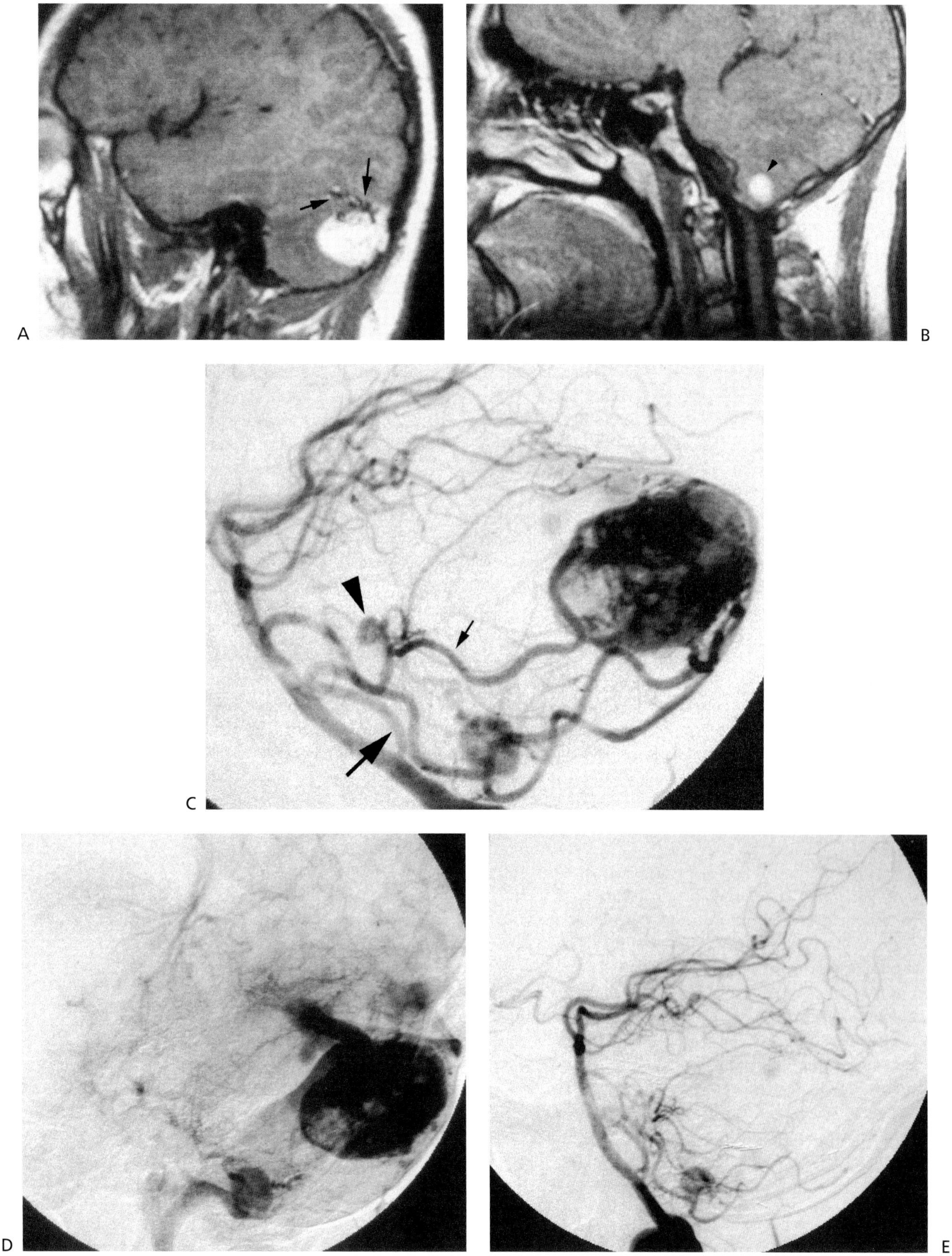
A
B
C
D
E

gram (BBBP). The program has designed protocols for the treatment of both primary and metastatic tumors of the brain.

The use of a multidisciplinary team, including the endovascular specialist, a neurooncologist, an anesthesiologist, and skilled nurses in a step-down unit, experienced in this technique can decrease the periprocedural morbidity and mortality in this fragile population.

General anesthesia is administered, because osmotic disruption of the blood-brain barrier is painful. A urinary catheter is inserted and output measured to monitor fluid balance. This is followed by the intravenous infusion of some chemotherapeutic agents, because these agents must be metabolized into an active form *in vivo.* Intravenous chemotherapy is administered prior to the osmotic disruption, so that the bulk of the active agent can be delivered for the entire duration of the opening of the tight junction.

Catheter placement is confirmed by angiography, and the appropriate volume of a 25% mannitol solution is infused via a mechanical pump at a rate of 3 to 12 ml/sec for a 30-second period. Suggested recommendations are to use 125 ml of this solution for an anterior circulation lesion, and 80 ml for a posterior circulation tumor [40]. Immediately following mannitol infusion, any intraarterial chemotherapeutic agents administered by this route are infused over 10 minutes. Superselective catheter placement was performed initially because of a concern over ocular complications. This led to the finding that superselective (supraophthalmic) catheter placement was fraught with a significantly increased risk of neurologic complications. Superselective placement does, however, have benefit in treating resistant tumors and in severe hematologic toxicity [41]. Gobin et al. have shown improvement with changes in rate and volume *(vide infra).* Catheter placement must be as selective as possible, allowing for infusion to a 3-cm margin beyond the visualized CT abnormalities, where pathologic studies have long shown that tumor cells exist. Nitrosoureas and platinum-containing chemotherapeutic agents have shown the greatest effect of all antimitotic agents used in the past two decades. Carmustine (BiCNU), nimustine (ACNU), and carboplatin trials are ongoing.

To document the extent of blood-brain barrier disruption, nonionic contrast is administered intravenously immediately following the osmotic infusion and prior to the intraarterial chemotherapy infusion. Immediately following the conclusion of both the intravenous and intraarterial infusions, a CT scan is obtained; this must not be delayed beyond 1 hour after the disruption. Generally, the procedure is performed 1 or 2 days per month [42].

There are risks associated with this procedure. The infusion is painful and thus must be carried out with general anesthesia and all the attendant risks thereof. In addition, focal motor seizures may occur in 3% to 7% of patients, as may stroke [43]. Transient asystole has also been reported in 1.5% of patients [40]. Visual complications can arise from periorbital vasoconstriction from the mannitol infusion or endarteritis from the chemotherapeutic agents or their solvents. Nimustine and carboplatin are better tolerated by the optic system. Heparin and steroids given prior to the procedure and continuing until 48 hours postprocedure can reduce these complications. In patients with preexisting deficits, more than one-half experience a transient worsening of these deficits, which may last for up to 72 hours [40,42]. Other complications, such as dissections, may be related directly to the catheterization itself. This has been seen in 5% of patients reported by the BBBP consortium. In addition there are the hematologic and renal toxicities of the various chemotherapeutic agents.

To evaluate these adverse events systematically, Gobin et al. retrospectively reviewed results of 462 procedures performed in 113 patients enrolled in six intraarterial chemotherapy protocols [44]. Specifically, they were concerned that much of the neurotoxicity was based upon excessive dosage administered, because it was calculated using intravenous dosage guidelines. They correctly postulated that in intraarterial infusions the brain is exposed to the chemotherapeutic agents during the first pass. Based upon their results, they developed the concept of hemispheric dosage, which allows for calculation of the dose of the chemotherapeutic agents based on cerebral vascular territory. In addition, they used a pulsatile injection technique and a superselective injection to further minimize the uninvolved areas exposed to the chemotherapy. These techniques are now considered standard for this procedure.

Intraarterial chemotherapy has been shown to be practical and can be performed with a reasonably low complication rate. The concept of selective delivery of drugs has major merit both in terms of the concentrations achieved at the tumor site and in terms of minimizing systemic effects. Although overall outcomes may not have changed significantly since the introduction of intraarterial chemotherapy, they do show promise. With the continued development of targeted, specific chemotherapeutic agents and our improving control of blood-brain barrier manipulation, outcomes may well improve.

TECHNIQUE FOR TREATMENT

The indications and method of endovascular treatment are determined by the goal of therapy. Embolization procedures should be decided upon in a multidisciplinary fashion with the neurosurgeon or otolaryngologist or both. The patient and family must be aware of all alternatives, including no treatment. This discussion is facilitated by an explanation of the natural history of the lesion. The preoperative goal is to devascularize the operative bed so as to reduce blood loss, operative time, and difficulty. Our task is to make the patient's risk in the subsequent operation safer by selectively obliterating the pathologic vasculature while preserving vessels supplying surrounding normal tissues. If the embolization is being performed for palliation or to improve mass effect temporarily in an otherwise "nonsurgical" patient, then the materials used for the embolization will be modified some to accommodate the depth of penetration desired. As a general rule, however, tumor embolization should be regarded as a preoperative measure rather than an alternative to surgery.

Vascular intracranial and skull base tumors, which derive nourishment from surgically inaccessible arteries, and those tumors which have encased or invaded supplying vessels such as the ICA are ideally suited to endovascular intervention. CT and MRI without and with contrast are complementary with respect to evaluating bone and soft tissue characteristics, respectively. MRI is excellent for determining not only size and location but also whether there is involvement of vascular structures, both arterial and venous, because of multiplanar imaging capability and flow-imaging techniques. Although there is a strong relationship between enhancement on CT or MRI and tumor vascularity, this is not 100% correlated. High-quality selective angiographic assessment remains the gold standard to determine arterial supply, angioarchitecture, venous drainage and vascular displacement, and encasement by tumor mass. This information is of great importance to the operating surgeon.

Although the histologic spectrum of tumors that can be treated is wide, one can generalize that those extraaxial tumors, such as meningiomas, supplied by the external carotid system are best suited to embolization. The technical difficulties and associated risks involved in pial vessel embolization generally do not favor intracranial embolization of tumors supplied in this fashion. However, tumors such as hemangioblastomas and choroid plexus tumors characterized by dilated feeding arteries ending in the tumor may also be ideal lesions for embolization.

We usually perform diagnostic angiography and embolization procedures concomitantly. Exceptions to this rule may occur if there is a question of the vascularity of the tumor or involvement of the major vessels, wherein a balloon test occlusion is requested prior to temporary or permanent occlusion. Therefore in most cases, unless there is contraindication, the patient is scheduled for general anesthesia delivered by endotracheal tube or laryngeal mask. General anesthesia allows for less patient movement and leads to significantly less vasospasm in the external carotid system, which in turn makes for an overall safer and more efficient procedure. Because risk is directly correlated with length of any procedure, this strategy may be of great benefit. The advantage of the laryngeal mask technique is that induction and reversal are impressively rapid and smooth. The disadvantage is functional testing for the external carotid system is not done and we rely upon anatomy and angioarchitecture for embolization.

Catheterization

We routinely place a 6- or 7-French (Fr.) introducer sheath, suturing it securely, for the subsequent numerous catheterizations needed for proper mapping and embolization. For pediatric patients, the size of the catheter is downsized to a 4- or 5-Fr. system. The common femoral artery access site is the preferred approach. If this is unavailable, axillary or even radial punctures can be performed as an alternative. Brachial artery cannulation and direct puncture of the carotid arteries should be avoided, because the risk for complicating dissection, thrombosis, and hemorrhage are well documented.

The standard diagnostic catheter we choose for neuroangiography is a 5-Fr. Berenstein (Merit Medical) catheter and the preferred basic guide catheter is an MPC Envoy (Cordis). These gently angled nontapered catheters are excellent for most patients, allowing continuous flushing around 0.038-inch guidewires and microcatheters. For those vessels particularly difficult to catheterize due to excessive aortic and general vascular tortuosity, a reverse-curve catheter such as a Simmons-type catheter is very useful. Envoy catheters also are supplied with a Simmons shape. We find these braided catheters have excellent "body," providing a stable platform from which to work coaxially, and are relatively atraumatic to the vessel wall. The large lumen of these guide catheters comes at the cost of having a very thin wall, however, and they should be handled accordingly. Because of the thin wall, the lumen may be compressed into an oval shape if stressed, and as such must be placed in a secure position prior to subsequent microcatheter introduction. Our standard guidewire is the 0.038-inch Glidewire (Terumo), a hydrophilic angled wire. In tortuous anatomy this may be somewhat too stiff, so a long, tapered "floppy" guidewire is used. These hydrophilic guidewires are more trackable than conventional ones. A torque device is used to steer the wire.

A wide selection of microcatheters are now available for superselective catheterization. They range in size from 1.0- to 2.6-Fr. diameters, with varying stiffness for pushability and hydrophilicity for reaching distal targets. In general, the largest-bore catheter that will allow distal navigation without occluding the target vessel should be chosen. This allows the widest choice of material for the subsequent embolization. Some microcatheters are braided for reinforcement and support. They all can be steam shaped, using a shaping mandril, as necessary. Microguidewires have also become specialized and varied with respect to flexibility, support, size, and shape. They range in size from 0.010- to 0.018-inch diameters. Although a wide selection may be useful for specific needs, most neurointerventionists become accustomed to using a more limited combination of microcatheter and microguidewires for the vast bulk of the work. In our experience, the best catheterization control and flexibility for external carotid embolizations is achieved with a 0.010- or 0.014-inch Prowler microcatheter (Cordis) in combination with an Agility 10 Soft (Cordis) microguidewire. Occasionally, when vessels are hypertrophied, we use the larger Rapid Transit microcatheter. The advantage of this catheter is that the inner lumen is of the greatest bore and allows embolization with large particles without as great a threat of catheter occlusion. Following a difficult catheterization, there are few more frustrating experiences than having the microcatheter become plugged with PVA particles. Thus, constant diligence in regular flushing of the catheter and more frequent rinsing of the hub with saline following particle deposition is necessary. Constant-flush systems for the guide catheter using heparinized saline are also mandatory to prevent unnecessary thromboembolic complications in these lengthy procedures.

When balloon test occlusion is needed, our standard balloon occlusion catheter is the Medi-tech (Boston Scientific, Natick, MA) OB 5/2/100, a 5-Fr. double-lumen 100-cm end-hole catheter with a mounted, nondetachable silicone balloon. The balloon measures 2 cm in length and inflates to 8 mm in diameter. No guide catheter system is required and the tip beyond the balloon is quite short, minimizing chances for intimal injury. Diligence must be exercised in removing any air from the system prior to introduction into the vasculature. The balloon is inflated with a nonionic contrast agent diluted 1:1 with saline.

When only a more proximal microcatheter position can be achieved, placement of a temporary occlusion balloon in the parent vessel distal to the origin of the artery directly supplying the tumor may help to enhance flow within the supplying vessel. In addition, a balloon catheter can be used to occlude flow within a vertebral artery or ICA to protect against distal embolization.

Embolization

Coils, particles, and liquid agents are available for occlusion of the target vascular territory. Liquid agents are more permanent and occlusive, but they can be more difficult to control and have a greater inherent risk. Particles are the preferred embolization material for preoperative embolization and, if properly sized, can reach the intratumoral vasculature. We will touch upon the salient features of each of the commonly used embolic agents.

PVA particles are the most commonly used particulate embolic agents. These particles are somewhat irregular in shape. They are packaged in varying sizes, sorted from approximately 50 to 1,200 μm in roughly 1,000-μm increments. PVA is inert, nonresorbable, and insoluble. PVA acts by initially plugging vessels and then causes a mild inflammatory response, leading to a giant cell foreign body reaction and thrombosis. Recanalization will take place within a few weeks to months; however, PVA is an effective preoperative embolic agent. These particles constitute a permanent agent in that they are not biodegraded; however, their occlusion cannot be considered permanent.

Particles are mixed with contrast to provide opacity and are injected under roadmap fluoroscopy. During fluoroscopy one must be sure to visualize the sites of potentially dangerous anastomoses. Particles penetrate according to size and travel to their intended sites of occlusion in the flow of blood. The concentration and rate of injection are inversely proportional to the depth of penetration. Slower injection with a dilute suspension of small particles will result in the deepest penetration. In addition to PVA particles, Gelfoam powder or gelatin sponge particles (Embospheres) can be used.

A danger that must be kept in mind is that of vessel rupture when particles are forcibly injected after outflow is occluded. One must pay close attention to the hemodynamics of the vessel being embolized because they can change very rapidly. With this in mind, we use 1-ml syringes to suspend and inject the particles.

With the microcatheter in good position, manual test injections with contrast only are performed to (a) gauge the amount, rate, and force required to deliver particles accurately to the target and (b) determine the force which will produce reflux. As embolization progresses and the sump effect diminishes, the rate of injection should diminish and caution increase. When flow becomes sluggish, the embolization is usually stopped. To keep particles in suspension, we continuously rotate the syringe while injecting under fluoroscopic roadmap conditions. The chances of reflux are greater when embolizing branches within the initial segment of the ECA (such as carotid body tumors), and within extradural carotid (C4, C5 segment) and vertebral musculospinal branches. For these branches, if the risk is deemed acceptable, temporary balloon inflation should be considered, and embolization proceeded with warily and stopped while antegrade flow still persists but is sluggish [45,46].

Transarterial embolization using Gelfoam sponge has been widely used since the mid-1970s. Gelfoam is supplied either in powder form or sheets of varying thickness which can be cut to size. This gelatin material is resorbable, with a biologic effectiveness of somewhere between 7 and 21 days. The powder comes in a size of 40 to 60 μm and reaches the precapillary level of the tumor microvasculature. This can produce significantly greater tumor necrosis than the larger PVA particles. Tumors such as meningiomas, with small-caliber neovascularity without significant arteriovenous shunting, are ideally suited to this material. One must be extremely cautious when using Gelfoam powder, because the precapillary and capillary beds of normal tissues, including cranial nerves, can be occluded leading to permanent neurologic deficits. These small particles can also pass through ECA-ICA anastomoses, causing ischemic stroke, or into the ophthalmic artery, causing blindness. The complication of scalp necrosis has also been seen. Diminished wound healing, especially when subsequent reconstructive surgery is contemplated, should be considered a relative contraindication to the use of Gelfoam powder. More commonly used are the Gelfoam sheets, which can be cut with a scalpel into small pledgets, rolled, and injected through the microcatheter to occlude the proximal pedicle at the end of an embolization. Alternatively, these Gelfoam "torpedoes" can be used initially to temporarily occlude dangerous anastomoses prior to particle embolization.

Trisacryl gelatin microspheres (Embospheres, Biosphere Medical), consisting of a new hydrophilic, collagen-coated nonabsorbable material, have been approved recently as an embolic agent by the Food and Drug Administration. These microspheres are much more uniform in size and are smooth in shape when compared to PVA particles. As with Gelfoam powder, these particles can achieve very distal penetration and are best suited to those tumors without arteriovenous shunting (e.g., meningiomas). Bendszus et al. recently described their prospective experience in the preoperative embolization of meningiomas with Embospheres and compared the results with those achieved with standard PVA particles [47]. They found the newer Embospheres to have significantly greater distal penetration on histopathologic study and were associated with significantly less blood loss intraoperatively. The degree of necrosis within the tumor was insignificant. Embospheres may enjoy an advantage over PVA particles in that catheter blockage is less likely to occur.

Metallic coils are made of stainless steel or platinum for optimal radiographic opacity and may be made more thrombogenic by the attachment of Dacron fibers to them. One significant limitation with stainless steel coils, when compared with platinum coils, is that they are strongly ferromagnetic, leading to difficulties in interpreting subsequent MRI studies. Platinum coils, on the other hand, are less thrombogenic (even when fibered) and more radiopaque. Coils are available in a variety of configurations including straight, curved, helical, tornado, vortex, and complex. They are extruded from the tip of the microcatheter with the aid of a coil pusher and remain permanently in position. They are used largely for occlusion of a feeding branch following particulate embolization. They also may be used at the beginning of embolization to occlude a dangerous anastomosis, giving protection against inadvertent cerebral embolization. Soft low-friction, injectable platinum coils (Berenstein liquid coils, Boston Scientific) can be used to occlude a vessel more distally, because they can be propagated further downstream by the injection. These types of coils may be useful in reducing rapid flow prior to liquid embolic embolization with NBCA. Pushable coils cannot be repositioned easily beyond the microcatheter tip.

NBCA was recently granted Food and Drug Administration approval as an occlusion device. This is a stable nonabsorbable liquid polymerizing agent that is mixed with an oil-based contrast material (ethiodized oil [Ethiodol]) and tantalum powder for greater opacity. Because it polymerizes upon contact with any ionic solution or blood, it requires great care and skill in handling. The polymerization rate is retarded by dilution with ethiodized oil. Occlusion of peripheral and proximal vessels may occur almost simultaneously. It is therefore recommended that if NBCA is used for tumoral embolization, the polymerization time be delayed significantly to allow penetration into the intratumoral vasculature. Ischemic necrosis of normal tissue and premature polymerization with consequent gluing of the catheter tip in the artery are known complications.

Absolute, or dehydrated, ethyl alcohol (Abbott Laboratories) is a potent cytotoxic agent, inducing anoxic cell damage, protein precipitation, and fibrinoid necrosis of the intima. Subsequent thrombosis is permanent. Because of its low viscosity and potential for complete necrosis, this embolic agent should be used with great care. A higher incidence of complicating cranial nerve deficits and normal tissue infarction is the cost of using this agent. Alcohol use in our practice is limited to the extremely rare cases of malignant tumors wherein only tumor vessels are selected distal to any normal branch. A slow infusion technique with a 1-ml syringe is used with frequent examination of the remaining vascularity to avoid any possibility of reflux. It is possible to mix absolute ethanol with a 30% solution of PVA suspension. The cytotoxic effect is diminished; however, the mechanical occlusion provided by the particles allows prolonged contact time of the ethanol with the endothelium, giving a synergistic effect toward tumor necrosis.

Other liquid embolic agents are currently under investigation and may expand our armamentarium. Neuracryl (Prohold Technologies), a new cyanoacrylate (2-hexyl cyanoacrylate), is under clinical investigation in the United States and Europe. It is characterized by less adhesiveness and cohesiveness, but greater viscosity, than NBCA. As such it is more predictable and allows catheter withdrawal even after partial polymerization. Onyx (Micro Therapeutics) is a DMSO-associated hydrogel that is easily injectable, forming an amorphous substance when exposed to water or blood. The material is not adhesive, so longer injection durations are possible.

Functional Anatomy and Critical Anastomoses

A thorough understanding of the functional vascular anatomy is a prerequisite to performing endovascular therapy. The traditional description of the ECA as a single vascular tree with a branching pattern supplying a fixed territory is not completely accurate. Rather, fixed territories can be "collected" by any of a fixed set of arteries which, in turn, are collected into major arterial trunks. There is extreme variability in the vascular supply of critical structures. Vascular pedicles can have multiple embryologic origins. Any anatomical region is essentially in a state of hemodynamic equilibrium between two or more vascular pedicles.

The ECA-ICA anastomoses are the remains of embryologic arterial feeders to neural crest tissues. In the adult these anastomoses are important because they continue to supply the cranial and upper cervical nerves. ECA-VA (vertebral artery) anastomoses represent the remains of the network of arteries supplying the embryonic metameres. Thus, the location of the transosseous vessels at the skull base and the persistent ECA-ICA and ECA-VA anastomoses remain a major path for unintended, off-target embolization. The areas that contain these potential anastomoses must be specifically and deliberately included in the radiographic field whenever embolization is performed. As a corollary, when embolizing a lesion within a certain territory, or field, one should cone down to exclude all but the target and the area of all potential dangerous anastomoses.

Lack of opacification of a certain anastomosis does not mean that it is not present, only that the present hemodynamic balance does not favor its visualization. This emphasizes the need for selective rather than global angiograms to delineate all important anatomy. Moreover, because distal runoff is diminished during embolization, a sudden increase in pressure can lead to flow reversal within these anastomoses, a potential disaster for the unsuspecting interventionist. Continuous monitoring of the flow dynamics is therefore very important.

The concept of functional vascular anatomy, then, allows a defined angiographic protocol to be used when the location of a lesion is known. Thus modern CT and MRI aid greatly in topographic analysis to streamline the subsequent angiographic examination. Specific dangerous vessels of the ECA, their cranial nerve contributions, and the most commonly encountered ECA-ICA anastomoses are summarized below.

In the region of the cavernous segment of the ICA, the IMA has anastomoses to the cavernous carotid artery via the MMA, accessory meningeal artery, and artery of foramen rotundum. The MMA via its cavernous branch can supply V2 and the gasserian ganglion. The accessory meningeal artery passing through the foramen ovale can supply V2, V3, and the masseteric division of V. The artery of foramen rotundum can also supply V2.

The superior division of the ascending pharyngeal artery (APA) through its lateral (carotid) branch can supply the gasserian ganglion as well as the pericarotid sympathetic plexus. The jugular branch of the APA gives rise to lateral clival branches, and the hypoglossal branch gives rise to the medial clival branches. These supply the lower cranial (IX, X, XI) and twelfth cranial nerves, respectively.

Slightly inferiorly, the petrous segment of the ICA anastomoses with the IMA through the anterior tympanic artery and vidian artery supplying the chorda tympani and vidian nerve, respectively. Moreover, the APA can form an anastomosis to the petrous ICA via the mandibular branch of the superior pharyngeal artery and through the inferior tympanic artery supplying the Jacobson nerve (CN IX) within the Jacobson canal. Finally, the stylomastoid branch of the posterior auricular or occipital artery anastomoses with the petrous ICA whilst giving supply to the vasa nervorum of the intratemporal cranial nerve (CN VII) within the temporal bone.

Overlying the orbit, and best monitored in the lateral plane, are anastomoses between the IMA and the ophthalmic artery. An orbital branch of the infraorbital artery passes through the inferior orbital fissure. A meningo-ophthalmic branch of the MMA passes through the foramen of Hyrtl. In addition, a recurrent meningeal branch of the MMA courses through the superior orbital fissure. There also may be a transmalar branch of the anterior deep temporal artery which can supply orbital contents.

Posteriorly, dangerous anastomoses also exist between the extracranial circulation and the vertebral artery. The occipital and vertebral arteries have anastomosing branches at the C1 and C2 cervical space levels supplying the respective cervical roots. The neuromeningeal trunk of the APA, from its hypoglossal division (supplying CN XII), gives rise to the odontoid arch system which, in turn, sends a branch to the C3 space anastomosing with the vertebral artery. Yet another independent musculospinal artery directly connects the APA and the ascending cervical artery at the C4 level. One cervical level above, at C3, the ascending cervical, in turn, connects to the vertebral artery at the foramen transversarium. There is another anterior anastomotic artery at C4 between the ascending cervical and vertebral arteries. The posterior deep cervical artery has anastomotic arteries to the vertebral artery at C2 and C3 spaces and, as mentioned earlier, anastomoses with the occipital artery. Finally, a direct C4 collateral vessel exists between the ECA trunk and the ascending cervical artery.

The presence of any anastomosis does not, in and of itself, preclude embolization. One must, however, be aware of their existence in order to adjust embolization techniques. The safest procedure involves positioning the catheter tip well beyond the level of anastomosis. Strategies may also include using particles of larger caliber than the anastomotic artery (typically 300 μm of particles will suffice), temporary occlusion of the carotid or vertebral artery at the level of the anastomotic artery, and coil or Gelfoam pledget occlusion of the anastomosis. Anastomoses can also aid in the embolization procedure. For instance, an occlusion balloon inflated proximally can impose flow reversal within an anastomosis to assist in particle flow toward the target.

Complications

Reflux from the ECA to the ICA and vertebral arteries, or antegrade embolization through anastomoses, can result in cerebral infarction, blindness, or cranial nerve palsies. Forceful injection into a restricted system (e.g., with catheter wedged in a terminal vessel or after flow is significantly reduced toward the end of an embolization) can result in vessel rupture. As already mentioned, one must be careful not to occlude cutaneous branches (superficial temporal artery, posterior auricular artery, or occipital artery), especially within the planned craniotomy or reconstructive site, for fear of poor postoperative wound healing. Dissection can occur while manipulating the microcatheter or microguidewire, although with technical improvements and experience this risk continues to decline.

Biplane digital subtraction angiography with good road mapping should be considered a minimal angiographic standard to make these often-intense procedures as efficient and rapid as possible. Careful coning, filtering, and pulse fluoroscopy, as well as appropriate shielding, should be used at all times to minimize radiation hazards both to patient and staff.

It must be kept foremost in one's mind that as a preoperative maneuver, every effort should be undertaken to keep the morbidity of the embolization process to near zero, so as to decrease the overall risk to the patient who still has another procedure to endure. With proper technique and experience, the procedure-related stroke rate should be less than 1%.

Preoperative Venous Occlusion

Carrier et al. described preoperative detachable coil occlusion of venous anastomoses leading to significant reduction in blood loss for surgery of the jugular bulb [48]. Retrograde hemorrhage during and following surgery for tumor involving the jugular foramen or jugular bulb is a known difficulty with lesions of the skull base. Transvenous occlusion of venous tributaries including the inferior petrosal sinus, anterior and posterior condylar veins, and the posterior cervical anastomosis can be performed to minimize venous blood loss during subsequent surgery. Careful study of the associated normal cerebral venous egress is mandatory so as to not occlude functioning venous pathways with a consequent potentially disastrous venous infarct.

Percutaneous Direct Embolization

Casasco et al. initially described direct percutaneous devascularization of a craniofacial tumor in 1994 and since have developed the technique of direct intratumoral embolization using NBCA or dehydrated alcohol [49]. This represents a significant contribution to the preoperative devascularization of the skull base tumor that has significant supply from internal carotid or vertebral sources, wherein an endovascular route is more fraught with difficulties and may not be possible for technical reasons. For those who have no endovascular approach because of prior surgical clipping, this may represent the only tool left in the armamentarium of the interventionist. The technique begins with critical review of cross-sectional imaging in both coronal and axial planes to plan an approach, either transnasal, transoral (transbuccal), precondylar, or via direct puncture of the overlying skin, when the abnormality is subcutaneous.

The procedure is performed under direct biplane fluoroscopic control to reach areas supplied even by difficult pial branches. For superficial lesions, 19- or 21-gauge butterfly needles are used. For anterior skull base tumors, a transnasal route can be used with a 20-gauge spinal needle or a 21-gauge Chiba needle, which is introduced through the nostril under the inferior nasal turbinate and directed to the tumor parallel to the hard palate. For tumors in the pterygomaxillary region, the precondylar route is used with a coaxial technique. A 16-gauge needle is initially inserted anterior to the mandibular condyle, from lateral to medial to the tumor's surface, at which point an 18- or 20-gauge needle is used for embolization. Glomus tumors, and neuromas, and occasionally meningiomas, in which the jugular foramen is enlarged, can be approached via a retropetrosal approach. The needle is inserted between the tip of the mastoid (ipsilateral) and mandibular ramus and angled superiorly, medially, and posteriorly, so that on lateral view the needle is parallel to the posterior wall of the second cervical vertebra.

Extent, location, and shape of tumor are first evaluated on cross-sectional imaging. Corticosteroids are used for premedication, administered 1 day preoperatively and continued for 1 day after the procedure. Under general anesthesia, a diagnostic angiogram is performed and the arterial catheter is left within the appropriate vessel to monitor the progress of devascularization. Also, if there is direct carotid supply, a temporary balloon catheter is used to occlude the respective origins so as to prevent inadvertent reflux of glue into the carotid (or vertebral as appropriate) circulation. This is not done for ophthalmic or supraophthalmic carotid supply wherein the procedure is considered contraindicated.

Once the needle is placed, as described above, reflux of blood should be observed if in the tumor, and contrast is injected gently to confirm intratumoral location. If there is opacification of an arterial pedicle, this will help with averting potential problems with subsequent embolization, usually performed with 50% NBCA (1 : 1, NBCA : Ethiodol) mixed with tantalum under slow, masked digital subtraction angiographic control. The injection is stopped for any arterial or venous pedicle opacification. Five to ten depositions are usual, and the needles are left in place as a guide for the next puncture. Absolute alcohol is used palliatively for inoperable tumors. Regular angiographic monitoring is done through the indwelling catheter following each injection. In their series of 56 patients treated, Casasco et al. reported either complete or greater than 80% devascularization in all, with significant improvement of the surgical time and blood loss [49]. For those in whom palliative therapy was performed, there was significant reduction or total disappearance of mass effect in all cases. Metastases treated with alcohol had recurrences at 6 months. Benign tumors had longer follow-up without recurrence.

Complications include local pain which is responsive to analgesics, transient cranial nerve palsies, and into the ICA. In the Casasco et al. series, two patients had ICA reflux. One patient experienced blindness as a result of occlusion of the ophthalmic artery and the other had a fatal middle cerebral artery stroke [49].

REFERENCES

1. Russell DS, Rubinstein LJ. *Pathology of tumors of the nervous system.* Baltimore: Williams & Wilkins, 1977:65–100.
2. Rachlin JR, Rosenblum ML. Etiology and biology of meningiomas. In: Al-Mefty O, ed. *Meningiomas.* New York: Raven Press, 1991:27–35.
3. Chou SM, Miles JM. The pathology of meningiomas. In: Al-Mefty O, ed. *Meningiomas.* New York: Raven Press, 1991:37–57.
4. Buetow MP, Burton PC, Smirniotopolos JG. Typical, atypical, and misleading features in meningioma. *Radiolgraphics* 1991;11: 1087–1100.
5. Russell DS, Rubinstein LJ. *Pathology of tumors of the nervous system,* 5th ed. Baltimore: Williams & Wilkins, 1989.
6. Osborne AG. *Diagnostic neuroradiology.* St Louis: Mosby Year Book, 1994.
7. Rengachary SS, Suskind DL. Meningiomas in the elderly and asymptomatic meningiomas. In: Al-Mefty O, ed. *Meningiomas.* New York: Raven Press, 1991:153–159.
8. Manelfe C, Lasjaunias P, Ruscalleda J. Preoperative embolization of intracranial meningiomas. *AJNR Am J Neuroradiol* 1986;7: 963–972.
9. Guthrie BL, Carabell SC, Laws ER Jr. Radiation therapy for intracranial meningiomas. In: Al-Mefty O, ed. *Meningiomas.* New York: Raven Press, 1991:255–261.
10. Dean BL, Flom RA, Wallace RC, et al. Efficacy of endovascular treatment of meningiomas: evaluation with matched samples. *AJNR Am J Neuroradiol* 1994;15:1675–1680.
11. Wakhloo AK, Juengling FD, Velthoven VV, et al. Extended preoperative polyvinyl alcohol microembolization of intracranial meningiomas: assessment of two embolization techniques. *AJNR Am J Neuroradiol* 1993;14:571–582.
12. Macpherson P. The value of pre-operative embolisation of meningioma estimated subjectively and objectively. *Neuroradiology* 1991;33:334–337.
13. Bendszus M, Rao G, Burger R, et al. Is there a benefit of preoperative meningioma embolization? *Neurosurgery* 2000;47: 1306–1311.
14. Oka H, Kurata A, Kawano N, et al. Preoperative superselective embolization of skull-base meningiomas: indications and limitations. *J Neurooncol* 1998;40:67–71.
15. Latchaw RE. Preoperative intracranial meningioma embolization: technical considerations affecting the risk-to-benefit ratio. *AJNR Am J Neuroradiol* 1993;14:583–586.
16. Bitzer M, Wokel L, Luft AR, et al. The importance of pial blood supply to the development of peritumoral edema in meningiomas. *J Neurosurg* 1997;87:368–373.
17. Lefkowitz M, Giannotta SL, Hieshima G, et al. Embolization of neurosurgical lesions involving the ophthalmic artery. *Neurosurgery* 1998;43:1298–1303.
18. Terada T, Kinoshita Y, Yohote H, et al. Preoperative embolization of meningiomas fed by ophthalmic branch arteries. *Surg Neurol* 1996;45:161–166.
19. Robinson DH, Song JK, Eskridge JM. Embolization of meningohypophyseal and inferolateral branches of the cavernous internal carotid artery. *AJNR Am J Neuroradiol* 1999;20:1061–1067.
20. Theron J, Cosgrove R, Melanson D, et al. Embolization with temporary balloon occlusion of the internal carotid or vertebral arteries. *Neuroradiology* 1986;28:246–253.
21. Chaloupka JC, Mangla S, Huddle DC, et al. Evolving experience with direct puncture therapeutic embolization for adjunctive and palliative management of head and neck hypervascular neoplasms. *Laryngoscope* 1999;109:1864–1872.
22. Kallmes DF, Evans AJ, Kaptain GJ, et al. Hemorrhagic complications in embolization of a meningioma. case report and review of the literature. *Neuroradiology* 1997;39:877–880.
23. Hayashi T, Shojima K, Utsunomiya H, et al. Subarachnoid hemorrhage after postoperative embolization of a cystic meningioma. *Surg Neurol* 1987;27:295–300.
24. Cosentino CM, Poulton TB, Esguerra JV, et al. Giant cranial hemangiopericytoma: MR and angiographic findings. *AJNR Am J Neuroradiol* 1993;14:253–256.
25. Lorigan JG, David CL, Evans HL, et al. The clinical and radiologic manifestations of hemangiopericytoma. *AJR Am J Radiol* 1989;153:345–349.
26. Yaghmai I. Angiographic manifestations of soft-tissue and osseous hemangiopericytomas. *Radiology* 1978;126:653–659.
27. Chin LS, Rabb CH, Hinton DR, et al. Hemangiopericytoma of the temporal bone presenting as a retroauricular mass. *Neurosurgery* 1993;33:728–731.
28. Guthrie BL, Ebersold MJ, Scheithauer BW, et al. Meningeal hemangiopericytoma: histopathological features, treatment, and long-term follow-up of 44 cases. *Neurosurgery* 1989;25:514–521.
29. Weber W, Henkes H, Metz KA, et al. Haemangiopericytoma of the nasal cavity. *Neuroradiology* 2001;43:183–186.
30. Kabus D, Sidhu GS, Wieczorek RL, et al. Metastatic meningioma. Hemangiopericytoma or angioblastic meningioma? *Am J Surg Pathol* 1993;17:1144–1150.
31. Parker DR, Rabinov JD. Neuroradiology case of the day. Case 2: recurrent meningeal hemangiopericytoma. *AJR Am J Radiol* 1991;156:1307–1313.
32. Coffey RJ, Cascino TL, Shaw EG. Radiosurgical treatment of recurrent hemangiopericytomas of the meninges: preliminary results. *J Neurosurg* 1993;78:903–908.
33. Abdel-Fattach HM, Adams GL, Wick MR. Hemangiopericytoma of the maxillary sinus and skull base. *Head Neck* 1990;12: 77–83.
34. George B, Casasco A, Deffrennes D, et al. Intratumoral embolization of intracranial and extracranial tumors: technical note. *Neurosurgery* 1994;35:771–774.
35. Neumann HPH, Eggert HR, Scheremet R, et al. Central nervous system lesions in von Hippel Lindau syndrome. *J Neurol Neurosurg Psychiatry* 1992;55:898–901.
36. Ho VB, Smirniotopoulos JG, Murphy FM, et al. Radiologic-pathologic correlation: hemangioblastoma. *AJNR Am J Neuroradiol* 1992;13:1343–1352.
37. Burger PC, Scheithauer BW, Vogel FS. *Surgical pathology of the nervous system and its coverings,* 3rd ed. New York: Churchill Livingstone, 1991:193–437.
38. Vazquez-Anon V, Botella C, Beltran A, et al. Preoperative embolization of solid cervicomedullary junction hemangioblastoma. *Neuroradiology* 1997:39:86–89.
39. Tampieri, D, Leblanc R, TerBrugge K. Preoperative embolization of brain and spinal hemangioblastomas. *Neurosurgery* 1993;33: 502–505.
40. Neuwelt EA. *Implications of the blood-brain barrier and its manipulation.* Vols 1 and 2. New York: Plenum Press, 1989.
41. Chirac J. Intra-arterial chemotherapy for central nervous system tumors. In: Connors JJ, Wojak JA, eds. *Interventional neuroradiology.* Philadelphia: WB Saunders, 1999:368–374.

42. Doolittle ND, Miner ME, Hall WA, et al. Safety and efficacy of a multicenter study using intraarterial chemotherapy in conjunction with osmotic opening of the blood-brain barrier for the treatment of patients with malignant brain tumors. *Cancer* 2000; 88:637–647.
43. Wolpert SM. Superselective therapy for cerebral gliomas. In: Valavanis A, ed. *Interventional neuroradiology.* Berlin: Springer, 1993:151–157.
44. Gobin YP, Cloughesy TF, Chow KL, et al. Intraarterial chemotherapy for brain tumors by using a spatial dose fractionation algorithm and pulsatile delivery. *Radiology* 2001;218:724–732.
45. Valavanis A. Interventional neuroradiology for head and neck surgery. In: Cummings CW, Fredrickson JM, Harker LA, et al., eds. *Otolaryngology—head and neck surgery. Update II.* St Louis: Mosby–Year Book, 1990:206–223.
46. Choi IS, Tantivatana J. Endovascular diagnosis and management. In: Arriaga MA, Day JD, eds. *Neurosurgical issues in otolaryngology: principles and practice.* Philadelphia: Lippincott Williams & Wilkins, 1999:75–93.
47. Bendszus M, Klien R, Burger R, et al. Efficacy of trisacryl gelatin microspheres versus polyvinyl alcohol particles in the preoperative embolization of meningiomas. *AJNR Am J Neuroradiol* 2000;21: 255–261.
48. Carrier DA, Arriaga MA, Gorum MJ, et al. Preoperative embolization of anastomoses of the jugular bulb: an adjuvant in jugular foramen surgery. *AJNR Am J Neuroradiol* 1997;18:1252–1256.
49. Casasco AE, Houdart E, Jhaveri HS, et al. Percutaneous direct embolization of head and neck vascular tumors. In Connors JJ, Wojak JA, eds. *Interventional neuroradiology.* Philadelphia: WB Saunders, 1999:338–345.

Endovascular and Percutaneous Therapy of the Brain and Spine, edited by Michael P. Marks and Huy M. Do.
Lippincott Williams & Wilkins, Philadelphia © 2002.

14

ENDOVASCULAR AND PERCUTANEOUS THERAPY FOR EXTRACRANIAL TUMORS

MARY E. JENSEN

Evaluation and treatment of pathologic processes involving the extracranial head, neck, and skull base are the bread and butter of many interventional neuroradiology services. Endovascular procedures have been safely and effectively used for the provocative testing of regional blood supply, presurgical embolization of vascular tumors, palliation of pain or neurologic dysfunction, and emergency treatment of uncontrollable hemorrhage. This chapter focuses on the therapeutic strategies and techniques used by the interventional neuroradiologist in the treatment of the more common neoplasms affecting the head and neck. The reader is also referred to the previous chapter for a discussion of the treatment of intracranial tumors, because some of these lesions may extend into and beyond the skull base.

BACKGROUND

Juvenile Nasal Angiofibromas

Juvenile nasal angiofibromas are highly vascular, locally aggressive, benign hamartomas of the nasopharyngeal region, occurring primarily in adolescent males. Constituting 0.5% of all head and neck tumors [1,2], they are the most common benign tumors of the nasopharynx [3,4]. Despite their histology, however, juvenile nasal angiofibromas may demonstrate a malignant clinical course because of their anatomically complex location, their ability to extend intracranially, and their high degree of vascularity, which can result in fatal hemorrhage [5,6]. The most frequent symptom complex is progressive nasal obstruction, followed by recurrent, often severe, epistaxis [3]. The tumor appears as a grayish red, smooth-surfaced mass arising from the posterior lateral wall of the nasopharynx, which may ulcerate with increasing size [5]. Tumor growth is submucosal and lobulated, spreading along the path of least resistance through various fissures, foramina, and ostia [1,6]. Involvement of adjacent structures may result in sinus obstruction, facial deformity, proptosis, blindness, cranial nerve palsies, or hearing loss. The diagnosis usually is made on the basis of the patient's history, clinical examination, and cross-sectional imaging. Biopsy is neither necessary nor indicated, because massive uncontrollable hemorrhage may ensue [7].

Radiographic evaluation often includes computed tomography (CT), magnetic resonance imaging (MRI), and angiography, and is key for tumor staging and surgical planning [8–10]. In operative candidates, the anatomical location of the tumor often determines the surgical approach. Tumor location and extent, bony involvement, and sinus obstruction or invasion are easily depicted on axial and coronal CT [6]. A nasopharyngeal mass with extension into the pterygopalatine fossa is noted in 90% of patients, and anterior bowing of the posterior wall of the maxillary sinus commonly is identified. Obstruction of ostia results in sinus opacification. Tumor expansion causes pressure erosion or remodeling of adjacent bone (Fig. 14-1).

Whereas CT is superior in visualizing bony detail, magnetic resonance (MR) is better at delineating the intracranial and extracranial boundaries of tumor extension. The typical MR appearance is one of a low-to-intermediate signal intensity mass on all sequences with homogeneous enhancement. MR can also differentiate tumor extension into the paranasal sinuses from inflammatory or obstructive changes. Often linear flow voids are seen on MR and reveal the vascular nature of this tumor [11,12].

Angiography shows the typical appearance of homogenous blush in a reticulated pattern that persists into the venous phase (Fig. 14-2; see Fig. 14-1) [2,3]. The portion of the tumor located within the nasopharynx is most often supplied by the pterygopalatine portion and the distal branches of the internal maxillary artery (IMA). When the tumor extends posteriorly into the sphenoid sinus or skull base, the ascending pharyngeal artery (see Figs. 14-1 and

M.E. Jensen: Departments of Radiology and Neurosurgery, University of Virginia Health Sciences Center, Charlottesville, Virginia.

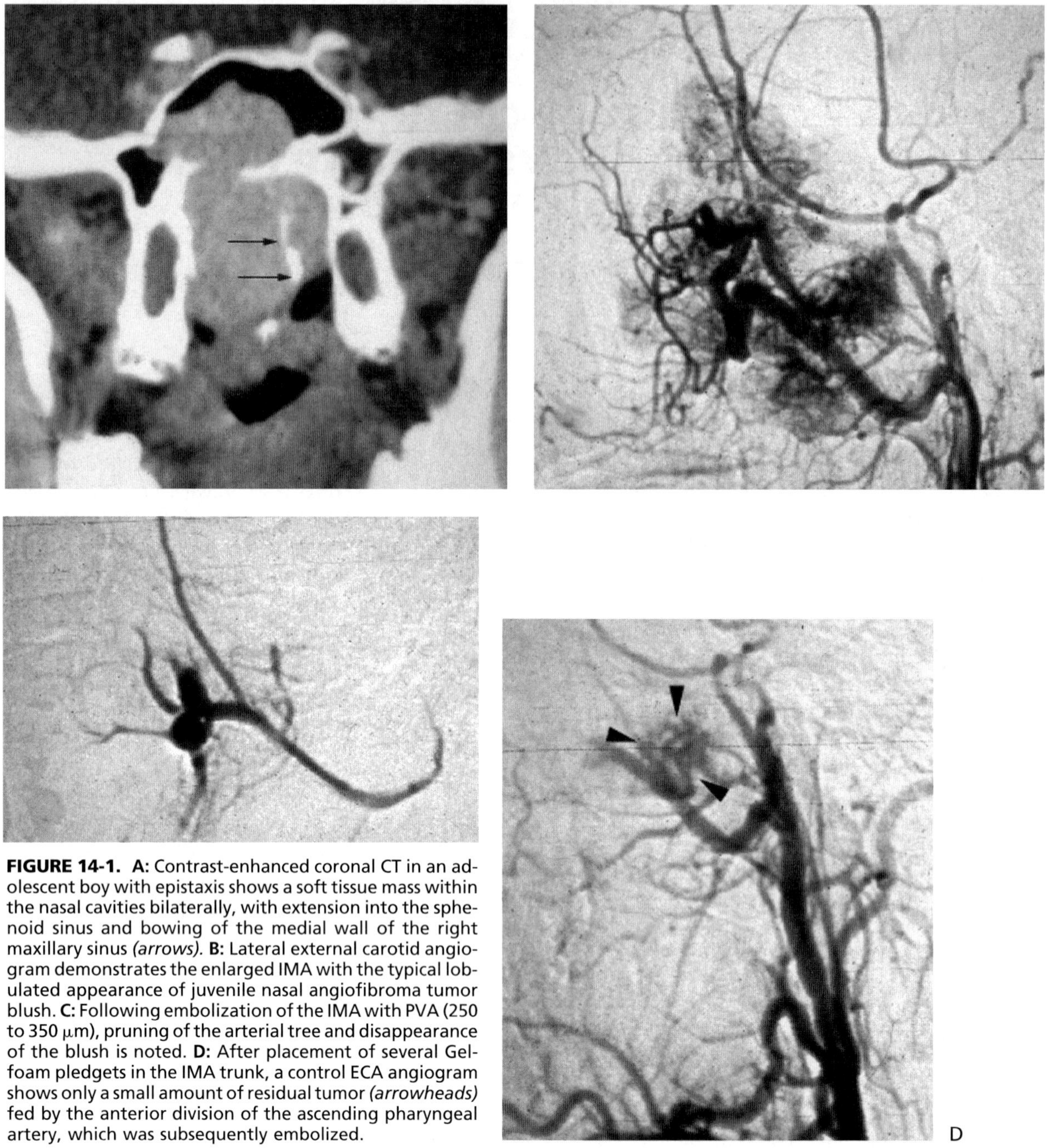

A B C D

FIGURE 14-1. A: Contrast-enhanced coronal CT in an adolescent boy with epistaxis shows a soft tissue mass within the nasal cavities bilaterally, with extension into the sphenoid sinus and bowing of the medial wall of the right maxillary sinus *(arrows)*. **B:** Lateral external carotid angiogram demonstrates the enlarged IMA with the typical lobulated appearance of juvenile nasal angiofibroma tumor blush. **C:** Following embolization of the IMA with PVA (250 to 350 μm), pruning of the arterial tree and disappearance of the blush is noted. **D:** After placement of several Gelfoam pledgets in the IMA trunk, a control ECA angiogram shows only a small amount of residual tumor *(arrowheads)* fed by the anterior division of the ascending pharyngeal artery, which was subsequently embolized.

14-2) and petrosal and cavernous branches of the internal carotid artery (ICA) (Fig. 14-3) may be recruited. Tumors involving the anterior septal area may be fed by the facial artery or the distal IMA. Extension into the orbit or skull base may stimulate recruitment of branches from the ICA, the middle meningeal or accessory meningeal artery, or the ophthalmic artery. In cases in which the tumor reaches or crosses the midline, examination of the contralateral vascular supply is necessary.

Surgical removal is the treatment modality of choice for extracranial disease, with radiation therapy reserved for intracranial extension or unresectable residual or recurrent disease [6,10,12–14]. Other therapeutic regimens have been reported [2,15] and include chemotherapy, cryotherapy, electrocoagulation, injection of sclerosing agents, and treatment with a testosterone receptor blocker (flutamide) [16]. Although rare, spontaneous regression of these tumors has been noted [17,18] and may be linked to the hormonal dependency of this tumor [18].

The surgical approach is based upon tumor location [19],

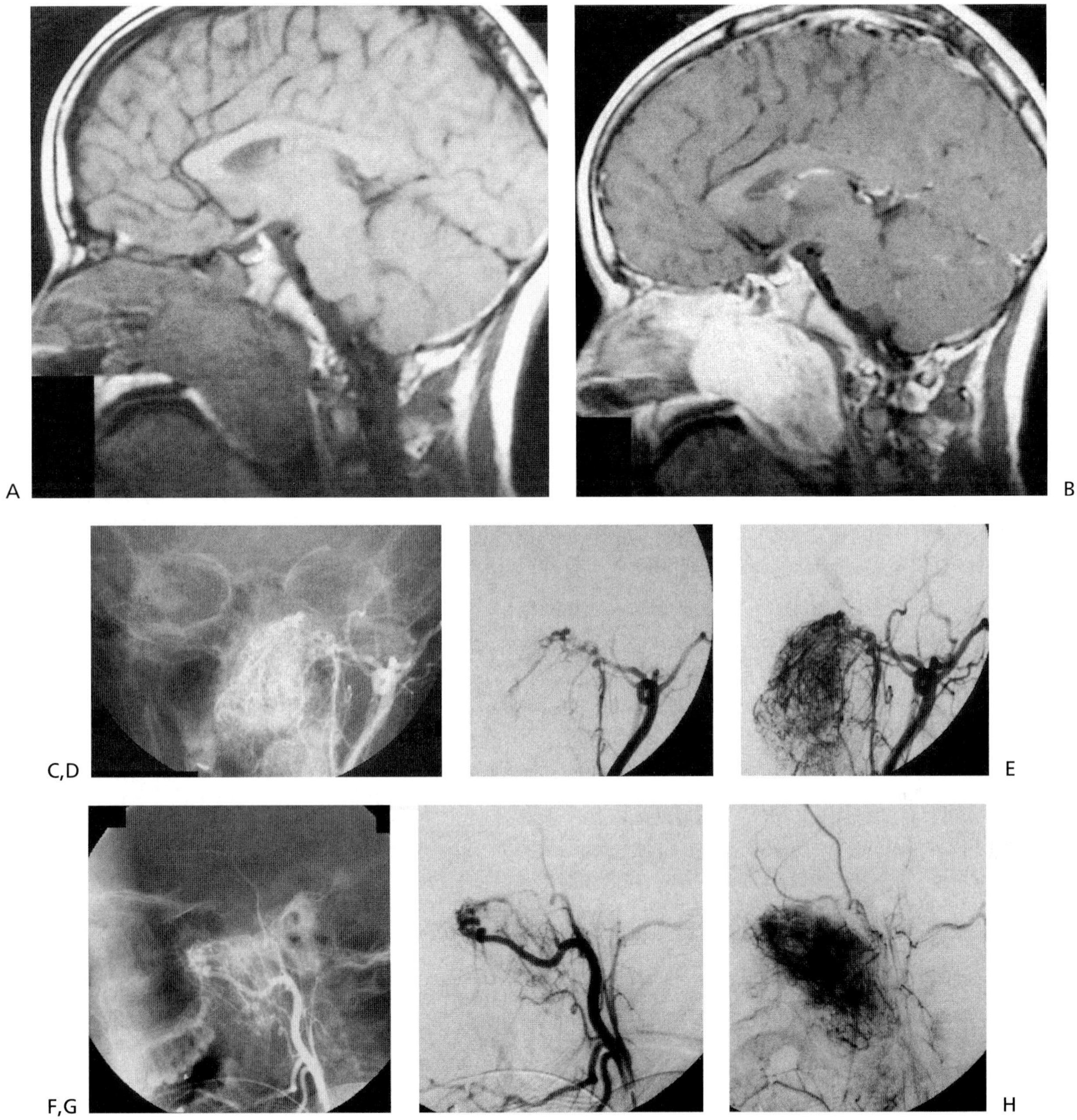

FIGURE 14-2. A: This image shows a teenage male with epistaxis. **A,B:** Sagittal MRI pre- and postcontrast shows the typical appearance of a juvenile nasal angiofibroma. The study demonstrates a large nasopharyngeal mass with extension into the sphenoid sinus on the postcontrast study. There is homogeneous enhancement of the tumor. Focal areas of lower signal suggest the vascular nature of the tumor. **C–E:** Pretreatment left ECA angiogram, anterior projection, shows the vascular anatomy in unsubtracted mode **(C)** and the early and late arterial phases **(D,E),** respectively. **F–H:** Pretreatment left ECA angiogram, lateral projection, again demonstrates the vascular anatomy in the unsubtracted mode in the early and later arterial phases, respectively. This tumor was supplied by proximal and distal branches of the IMA as well as the ascending pharyngeal artery. Typical blush of juvenile nasal angiofibroma is noted. *(Figure continues.)*

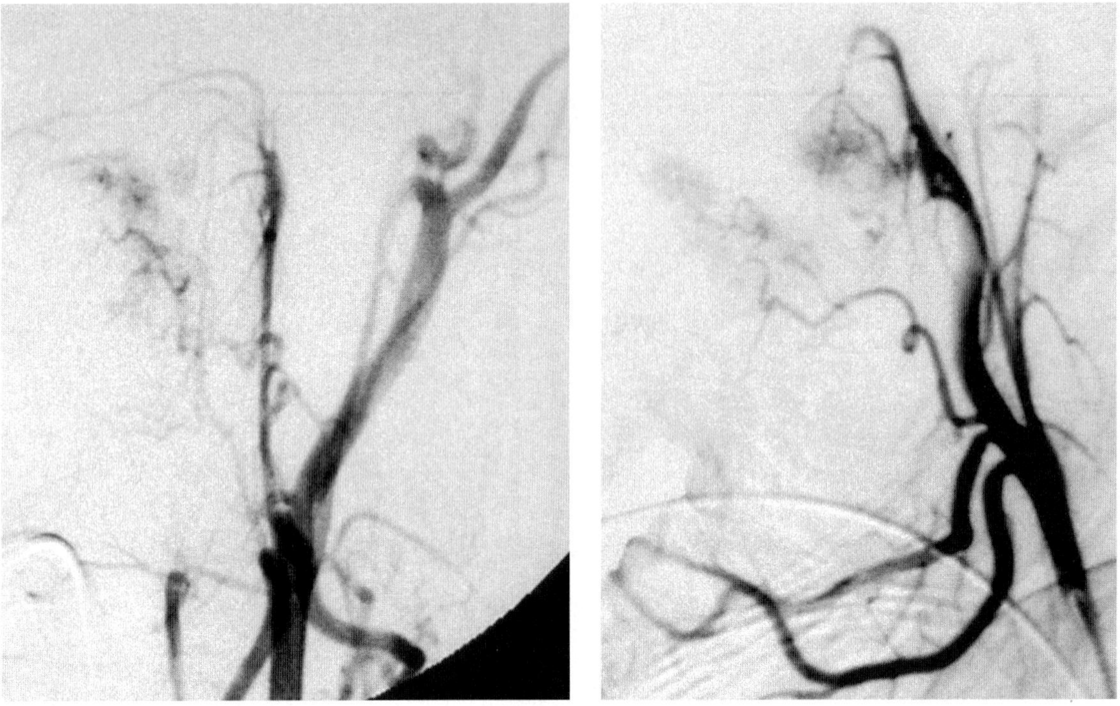

I J

FIGURE 14-2. *Continued.* **I,J:** Postembolization anterior and lateral left ECA angiograms. The IMA branches were embolized with PVA with marked diminution in the blood supply to the tumor and disappearance of the tumor blush. Continued supply from the ascending pharyngeal and ascending palatine artery is still noted. (From Michael P. Marks and Huy M. Do, unpublished material, with permission.)

tumor stage [7,20], effectiveness of the embolization [19], and the surgeon's preference; adequate exposure is essential for complete removal of the lesion. Endoscopic management of small and medium-sized tumors is technically possible after preoperative embolization [20]. Blood loss, the most common surgical complication, may contribute to incomplete removal and additional morbidity and mortality. Although preoperative estrogen administration has been used in the past to induce involution, a risk of testicular damage remains [14]. Surgical ligation of the external carotid artery (ECA) or IMA may reduce hemorrhage, but the regional collateral supply often makes this approach ineffectual and can hinder subsequent procedures by stimulating recruitment of ICA or vertebral feeders [21].

Transcatheter embolization is now the accepted and desirable means of preoperative tumor devascularization, effectively reducing blood loss and improving surgical exposure [2,6,8–10,13,15,22]. Moulin et al. [23] demonstrated a statistically significant difference in blood loss between embolized and nonembolized surgical groups with high-grade tumors. The benefit of embolization in patients with low-grade tumors was less clear cut. Embolization is performed at the same time as the diagnostic angiogram, usually 2 to 5 days prior to surgery (see Figs. 14-1 and 14-2) [2,14,22]. Most of the tumor mass is supplied by ECA branches unless extensive skull base or intracranial extension has occurred. Usually there is little to be gained by embolization of ICA feeders; however, in larger tumors embolization of these vessels may change an inoperable lesion into an operable one [15]. Standard transcatheter embolization of ECA branches using polyvinyl alcohol (PVA) particles and Gelfoam pledgets is usually performed, although some authors have advocated the use of tissue adhesive [24]. Techniques for treatment of tumors fed by ICA branches include distal vascular protection with a temporary balloon followed by proximal embolization, superselective catheterization of larger feeding vessels, or percutaneous direct puncture [25] (see Fig. 14-3). The risks of ICA embolization significantly exceed that of external carotid procedures, and the risk-to-benefit ratio must be carefully weighed for each individual. Direct puncture offers an alternative to the transarterial approach with the potential for decreased risk of intracranial embolization, provided that the embolic material is not pushed retrograde into the feeding branches [25].

Radiotherapy is reserved for poor surgical candidates, recurrent or residual disease which is deemed inoperable, or large, massively invasive tumors in which surgical removal may threaten vision or require carotid artery resection [1, 7,10,13,14]. Potential complications include brainstem dysfunction, long-term cranial neuropathies, and secondary malignancies of the head and neck [7]. Embolization has been used as an adjunctive therapy in patients treated with

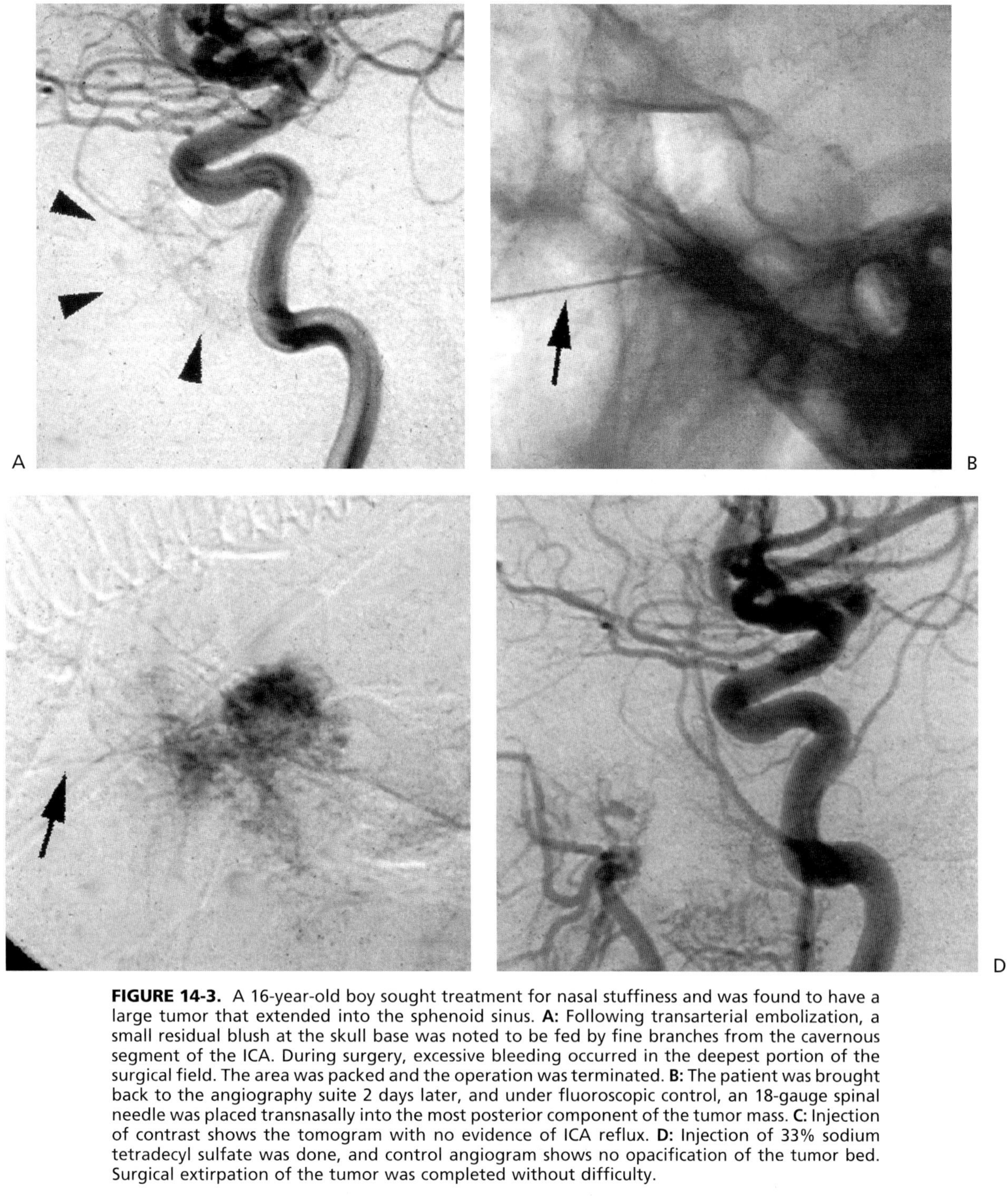

FIGURE 14-3. A 16-year-old boy sought treatment for nasal stuffiness and was found to have a large tumor that extended into the sphenoid sinus. **A:** Following transarterial embolization, a small residual blush at the skull base was noted to be fed by fine branches from the cavernous segment of the ICA. During surgery, excessive bleeding occurred in the deepest portion of the surgical field. The area was packed and the operation was terminated. **B:** The patient was brought back to the angiography suite 2 days later, and under fluoroscopic control, an 18-gauge spinal needle was placed transnasally into the most posterior component of the tumor mass. **C:** Injection of contrast shows the tomogram with no evidence of ICA reflux. **D:** Injection of 33% sodium tetradecyl sulfate was done, and control angiogram shows no opacification of the tumor bed. Surgical extirpation of the tumor was completed without difficulty.

irradiation who demonstrated residual mass, with good results [13].

Paragangliomas

Paragangliomas, also known as chemodectomas or glomus tumors, are derived from neural crest cells which are located along the aortic arch and brachiocephalic vessels [26]. They are benign, highly vascular tumors which are capable of local invasion and may exhibit histologically aggressive behavior toward adjacent nerves [27]. In decreasing order of frequency, they are located in the temporal bone (glomus tympanicum and jugulare tumors [Fig. 14-4]), the carotid bifurcation (carotid body tumors [Fig. 14-5]), and the naso- or oropharyngeal carotid space (glomus vagale tumors [Fig. 14-6]). Rarely, these tumors are found elsewhere in the head and neck region and the pulmonary tree [26]. These less common locations can include the paranasal sinuses, larynx, orbit and sphenopalatine fossa. Multiplicity of tumors is estimated to occur with an incidence of approximately 10% in nonfamilial cases, while synchronous lesions may be seen in 25% to 50% of familial cases [26,28,29]. Women are affected 4 to 6 times more commonly than men, and occurrence peaks between the fifth and sixth decades of life.

Patients with jugulotympanic paragangliomas often ex-

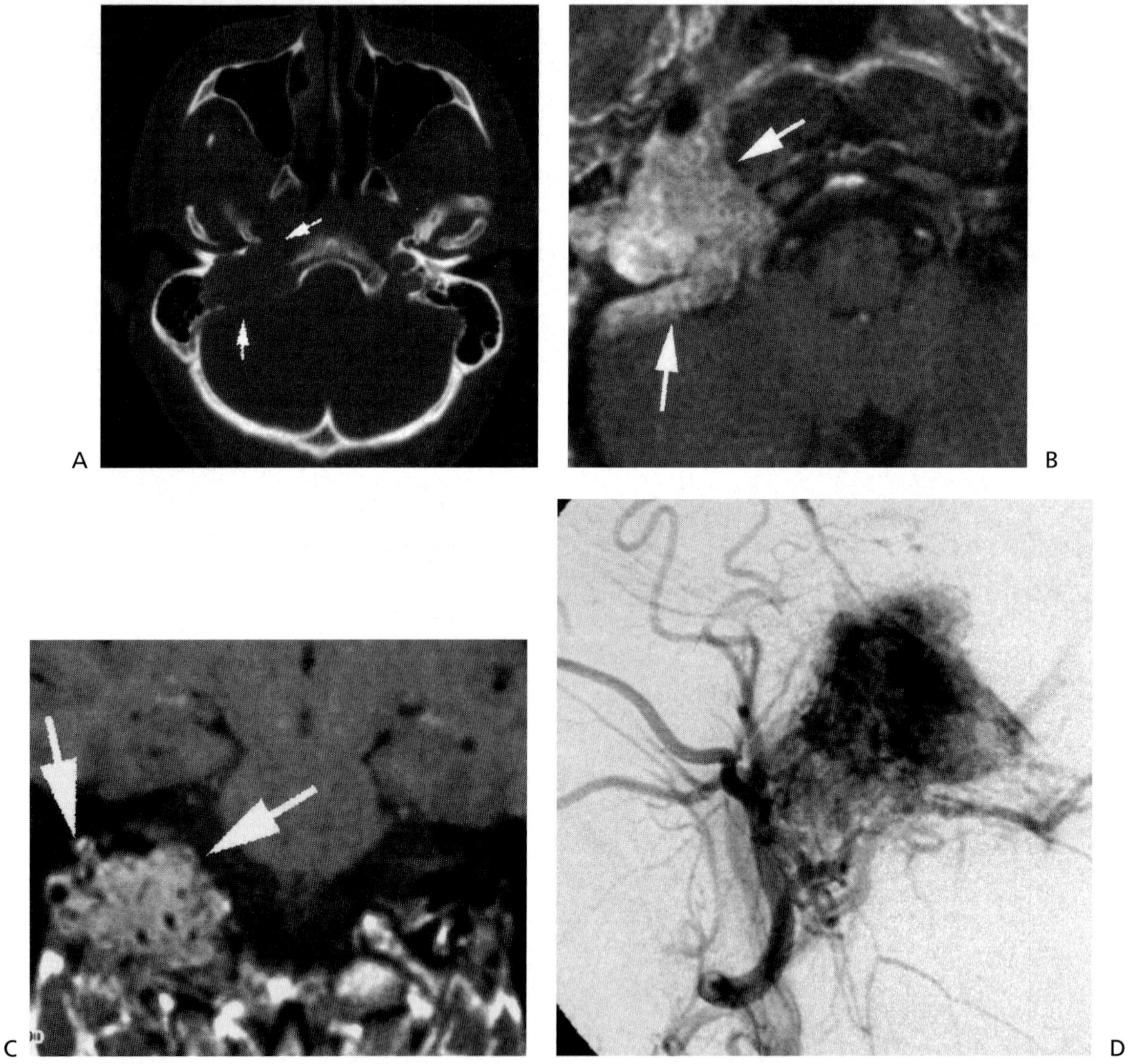

FIGURE 14-4. This middle-aged man developed right-sided tinnitus and multiple cranial nerve palsies. **A:** Axial CT scan shows erosion of the right jugular foramen and jugular spine and involvement of the carotid canal and clivus. **B:** A corresponding T2-weighted MR image shows a lobulated, speckled-appearing mixed signal mass that abuts the carotid artery anteriorly and the cerebellum posteriorly, and extends medially into the hypoglossal canal. **C:** Coronal T1-weighted images demonstrate the signal voids from intratumoral vascularity. **D:** Lateral ECA angiography shows dense tumor blush with shunting into the inferior petrosal sinus and retrograde into the right transverse sinus. *(Figure continues.)*

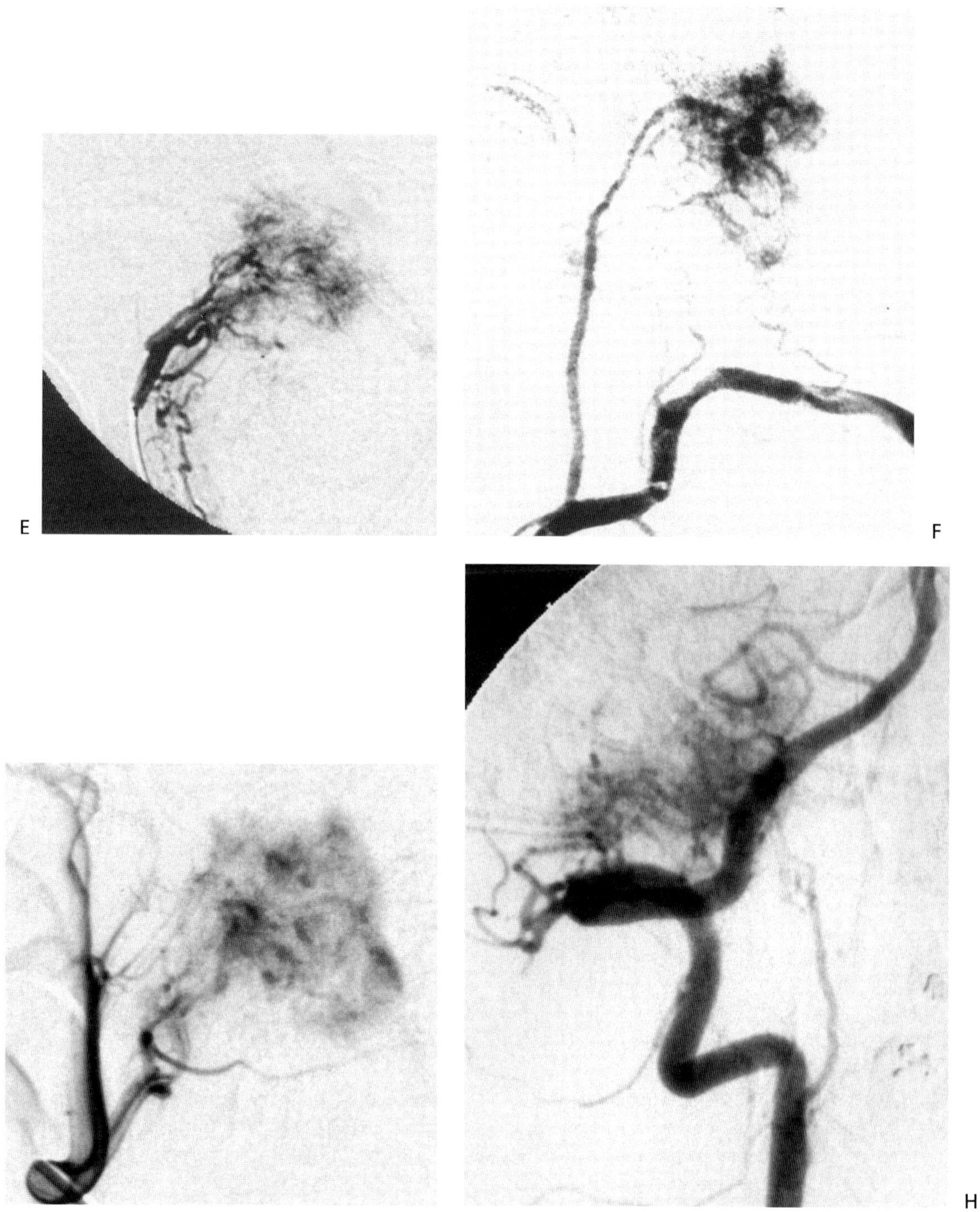

FIGURE 14-4. *Continued.* **E–G:** Superselective angiography shows multiple compartments including the inferior tympanic branch of the ascending pharyngeal artery **(E),** the stylomastoid branch of the occipital artery **(F),** and the posterior auricular artery **(G).** All branches were embolized with PVA (250 to 350 μm). **H:** Injection of the right vertebral artery shows multiple muscular branches supplying the lesion. *(Figure continues.)*

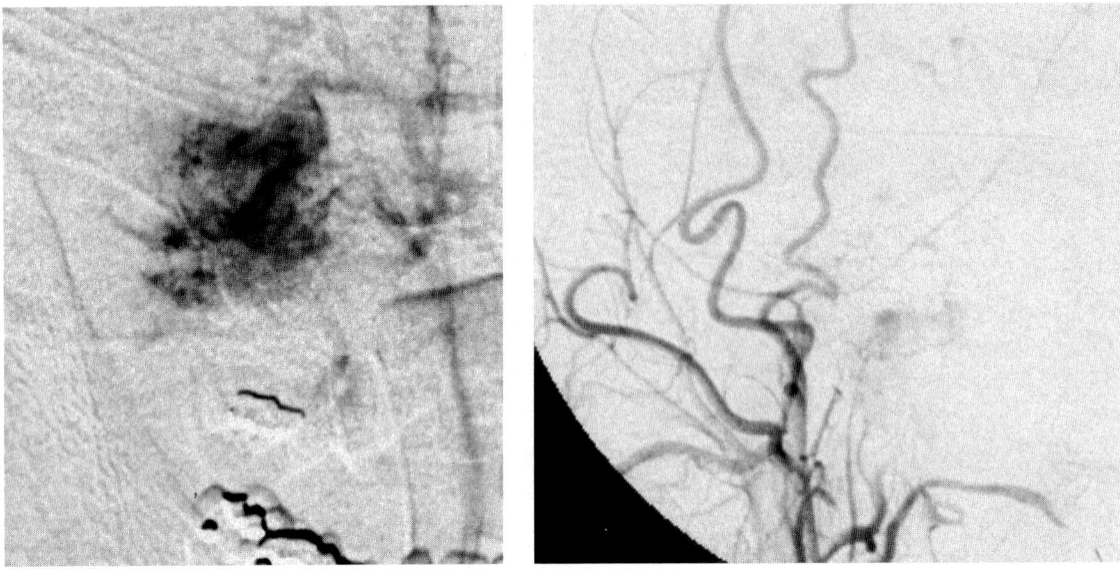

I J

FIGURE 14-4. *Continued.* **I:** A C3 branch was large enough to catheterize selectively and embolize with PVA. **J:** Final postembolization ECA study shows near-complete obliteration of this portion of the tumor.

perience conductive hearing loss, pulsatile tinnitus, or progressive cranial nerve palsies. Otoscopic examination may reveal a bluish aural polyp. Biopsy is contraindicated because aberrant vascular structures (e.g., carotid artery, jugular bulb) may manifest in a similar manner, and extensive hemorrhage can occur [30]. Most carotid body and glomus vagale tumors are asymptomatic, often identified incidentally on physical exam as a palpable neck mass. Dysphagia, hoarseness secondary to vagal paralysis, or Horner syndrome from sympathetic chain involvement may be initial symptoms. Compression of anatomical structures or skull base extension can occur with larger tumors, and neural invasion is often discovered at surgery. One to three percent of all lesions may exhibit catecholamine secretion, manifesting as palpitations, headache, facial flushing, and labile blood pressure [26,28].

Macroscopically these tumors are encapsulated, lobulated masses, ranging in color from tan to purple-red, spongy in texture, and hemorrhagic in appearance [26]. At the skull base, these slow-growing tumors have a propensity to expand along pathways of least resistance, spreading through the air cells and neurovascular foramen to extend beyond the temporal bone. Vagale tumors can engulf or invade the nerve, making preservation of function during surgery difficult. Carotid body lesions often adhere to the carotid adventitia, complicating surgical resection and obscuring visualization of regional cranial nerves. There is a small incidence of malignant degeneration with these tumors. Even though local invasion is common, metastatic disease is infrequent, with a 4% incidence in jugulotympanic tumors and 19% in intravagale paragangliomas [26, 29,31].

Therapeutic planning is based upon the information obtained by the radiographic evaluation, which usually includes cross-sectional imaging and angiography, and occasionally ultrasonography. Evaluation of tumor size, location, and extent, identification of synchronous lesions, assessment of intracranial extension, and determination of tumor angioarchitecture and major vascular involvement are issues which need to be addressed prior to selection of the appropriate therapy [28,32].

Axial and coronal CT of the temporal bone with bone and soft tissue windows allows comprehensive radiographic evaluation, with particular attention to the tympanic cavity and the bony walls separating it from the carotid canal and the jugular fossa [32–35]. Erosion of the jugular plate indicates the presence of a glomus jugulare tumor (see Fig. 14-4), and its boundaries, relationship to the carotid artery and facial nerve, and intracranial extension can be ascertained with CT [32]. Distinct homogeneously enhancing masses within the carotid space causing vascular displacement are indicative of glomus vagale or carotid body tumors. MR defines the tumor–vessel relationships and intracranial involvement better than CT. Large feeding vessels may be identified on MR as serpiginous signal voids (see Figs. 14-4 and 14-6) interspersed among areas of high signal intensity from tumoral hemorrhage, giving a salt-and-pepper appearance [35]. Carotid body tumors may demonstrate blood flow within a solid, slightly heterogeneous mass on pulsed Doppler analysis [36].

Diagnostic angiography demonstrates the angioarchitecture and blood supply of the tumor, in addition to revealing synchronous lesions and providing a vascular map for preoperative embolization or provocative testing [32]. Typi-

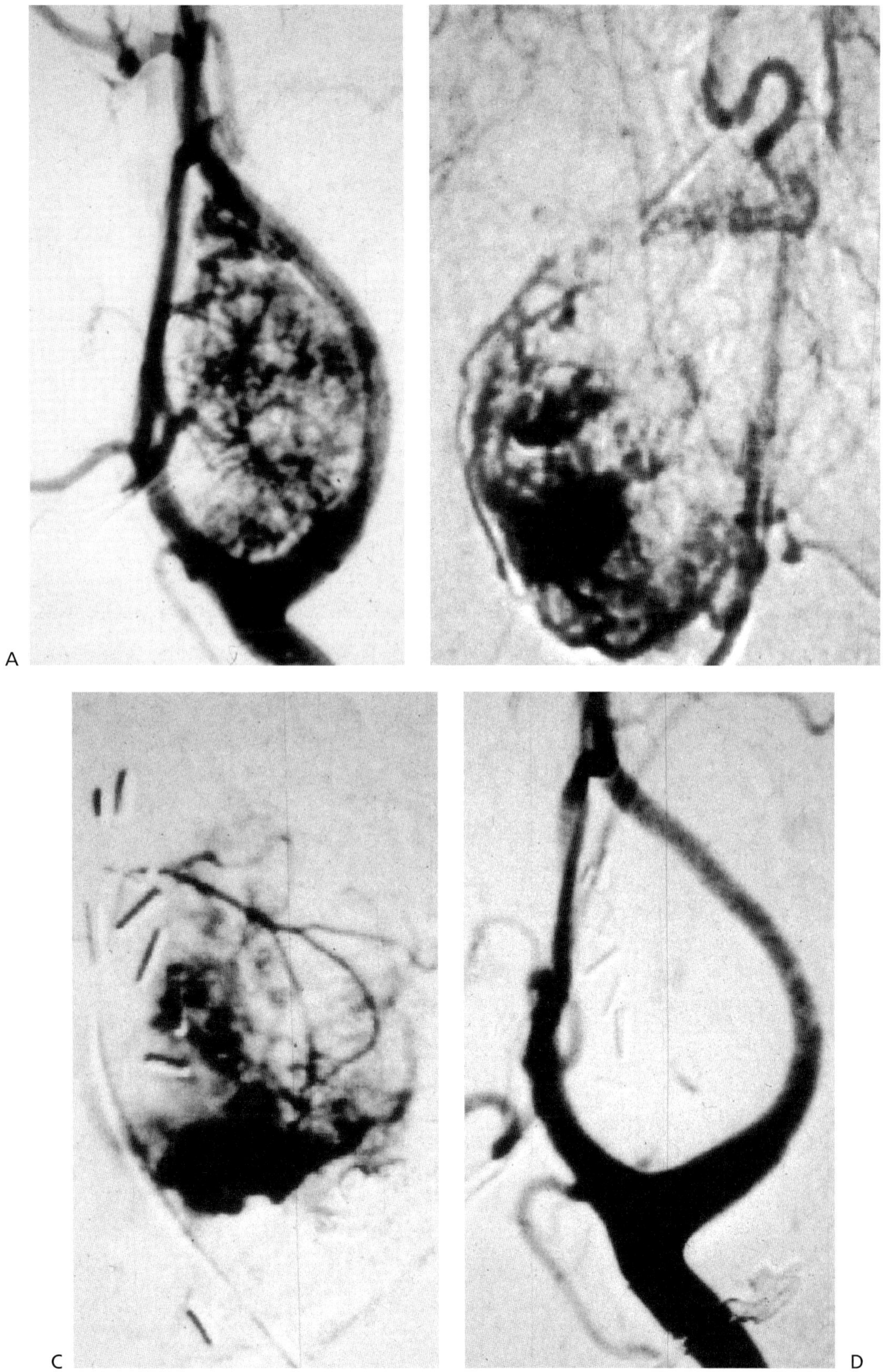

FIGURE 14-5. **A:** Lateral common carotid study shows splaying of the bifurcation vessels caused by a large, inhomogeneously staining mass consistent with a carotid body tumor. **B,C:** Superselective studies reveal a feeder arising from the posterior division of the ascending pharyngeal **(B)** and a muscular branch of the occipital artery **(C)**. **D:** Following embolization with particles, the tumor has been completely devascularized. The surgical clips are from removal of the synchronous, contralateral lesion.

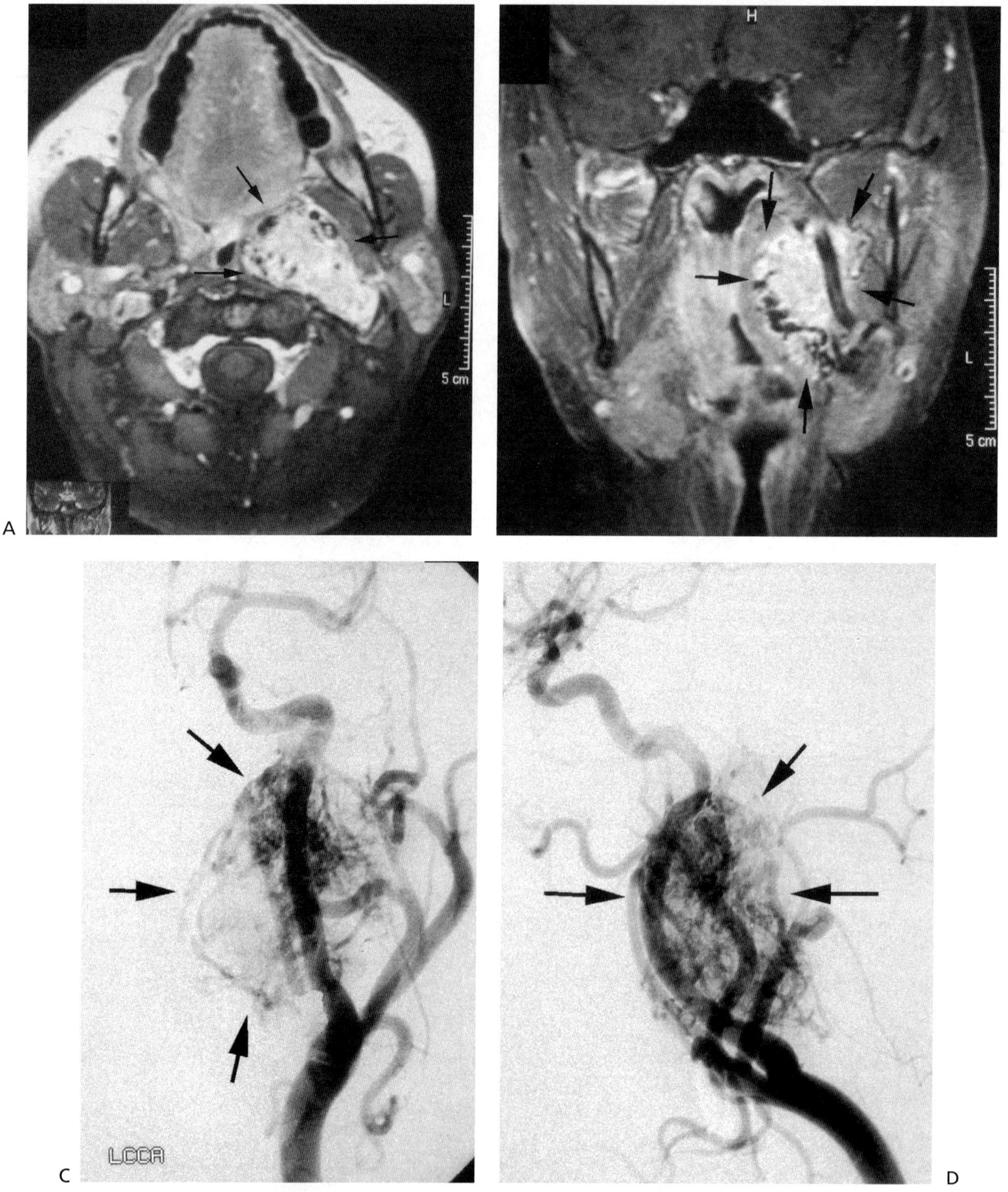

FIGURE 14-6. Glomus vagale tumor in a 52-year-old woman with onset of hoarseness and dysphasia. **A,B:** Axial and coronal postcontrast MRI images demonstrate a large mass *(arrows)* displacing both the left external and ICA anteriorly with mass effect in the oral pharynx. **C,D:** Left common carotid artery angiograms, anteroposterior and lateral projections, respectively, confirm the intense tumor blush *(arrows)* and the mass effect on both the external and ICA with anterior displacement of both structures. *(Figure continues.)*

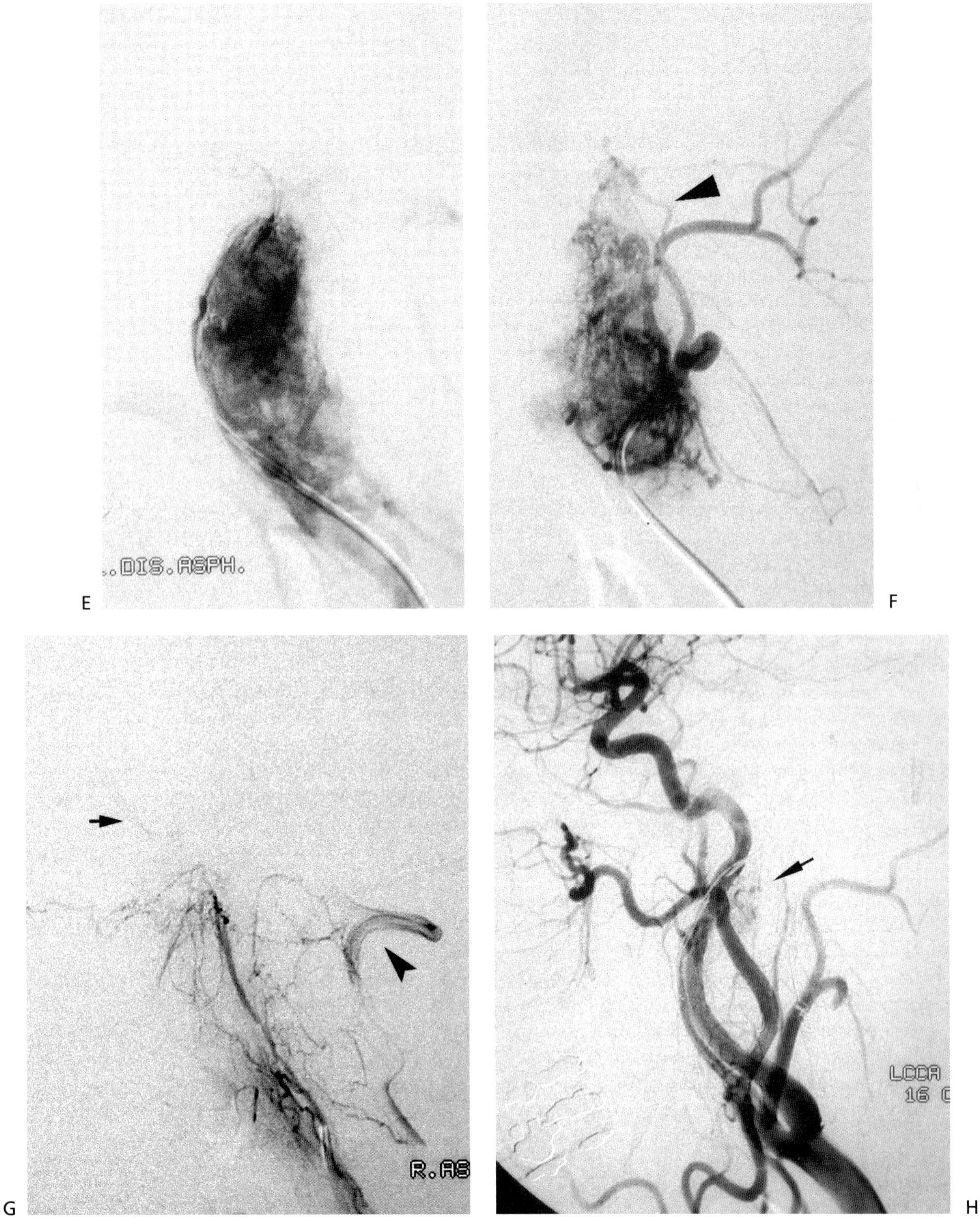

FIGURE 14-6. *Continued.* **E,F:** Selective injections of the ascending pharyngeal **(E)** and occipital artery **(F)** demonstrate extensive tumor supply from the stylomastoid artery, which was also noted on the occipital artery injection *(arrowhead).* **G:** Contralateral ascending pharyngeal artery angiogram, lateral projection, demonstrates that there is no supply to the tumor from this artery. This injection, however, nicely demonstrates dangerous anastomoses to both the carotid artery *(arrow)* and the vertebral artery *(arrowhead).* **H:** Control left common carotid artery angiogram following selective PVA and coil embolization of the arterial supply from the external carotid circulation. There is minimal residual tumor vascularity seen *(arrow).* (From R. Chavali and I.S. Choi, unpublished material, with permission.)

cally these tumors are highly vascular and exhibit dense staining. In addition, arteriovenous shunting is commonly observed (see Fig. 14-4). Cardiovascular collapse may follow injection of contrast into hormonally active lesions.

Typical arterial feeders to glomus jugulare and tympanicum tumors include the inferior tympanic branch of the ascending pharyngeal artery, the stylomastoid branch of the occipital artery, the posterior auricular artery, the petrosal branch of the middle meningeal artery, and the anterior tympanic branch of the IMA [37]. In larger tumors invading the skull base, petrous and cavernous branches of the ICA or muscular or intracranial branches of the vertebral artery may be recruited [38] (see Fig. 14-4).

Carotid body tumors arise from the posteromedial aspect of the carotid bifurcation and tend to displace the ICA posteriorly (see Fig. 14-5). The ascending pharyngeal artery is the most common feeding vessel identified, although larger lesions may recruit supply from adjacent ECA branches (e.g., muscular branches of the occipital artery, the ascending cervical artery, and unnamed branches of the carotid bifurcation). Glomus vagale tumors are located superior to the bifurcation and posterior to the ICA, thus pushing it anteriorly (see Fig. 14-6). Vascular supply similar to that of carotid body tumors is noted, although bifurcation branches are usually not involved.

Superselective studies reveal the tumoral angioarchitecture, dividing lesions into single or multiple compartment types. With single-compartment lesions, injection of any feeder results in opacification of the entire tumor. In multicompartmental lesions, injection of any feeder reveals only that component of the tumor; therefore the entire tumor is visualized only after every feeding vessel is studied. The embolization strategy will depend upon the type of angioarchitecture encountered.

Controversy concerning optimal management of paragangliomas continues with vocal proponents of radiation therapy [20] and surgical removal [28,31] stating their cases in the literature. The development of high-resolution radiographic imaging, microsurgical techniques, and transarterial embolization have made surgery the preferred management technique [28,30,31,39]. However, emphasis is placed on an individualized treatment plan based on patient age, general health, symptom complex, and information provided by the diagnostic investigation. Surgical cure is desirable in younger patients with appropriate-sized tumors when an excellent long-term functional outcome is expected, while radiation therapy is reserved for tumor control in the older patient or palliation of symptoms caused by an unresectable lesion [27,28,40]. Observation of the asymptomatic elderly patient or one who is not suited to surgery is another option [28,41].

Many surgeons promote a multidisciplinary approach which includes preoperative embolization, because improved visualization and reduced morbidity and blood loss during resection has been noted [31,39,42–44]. Smaller carotid body and glomus vagale tumors may not require embolization, although a statistically significant difference in operative blood loss has been shown in treated carotid body tumors with diameters exceeding 3 cm [31,39,42,45].

Small to medium-sized particulate embolization is performed in a manner similar to that described for other head and neck tumors. In the case of single-compartment tumors, the entire lesion may be embolized through one feeding vessel, preferably one with a paucity of collaterals and distant from the carotid bifurcation, thereby minimizing the risk of embolic introduction into the intracranial circulation. Multicompartmental tumors require selective catheterization and embolization of each individual feeder (see Figs. 14-4 and 14-5). If ICA or vertebral artery territory supply requires treatment, selective catheterization of the feeding artery or distal placement of a protective balloon is required. If the operative plan includes sacrifice of the vessel, presurgical occlusion of the artery in conjunction with embolization may be performed using detachable balloons. It is important to note that complete obliteration of all tumor blush is not required to provide effective devascularization [42], and an overzealous approach to therapy may increase the risk of complications.

Even when embolization is deemed unnecessary, provocative testing of the carotid circulation may be indicated when carotid shunting or resection is anticipated. Temporary balloon occlusion of the parent artery during diagnostic angiography may identify a subset of patients who will not tolerate transient interruption of the carotid supply, forewarning the surgeon prior to tumor removal [28].

As in the treatment of other head and neck tumors, stroke is a potential major complication. The posterior circulation is at greatest risk because of the rich angioanastomotic network found at the C2-3 level between muscular branches of the vertebral artery and the ascending pharyngeal and occipital arteries, which often supply the tumor (Fig. 14-6). Cranial nerve palsy is a risk [46]. The facial nerve is especially vulnerable, because its vascular supply mimics that used by jugulotympanic tumors.

Schwannomas

Schwannomas are usually solitary lesions that arise from the neural sheath of cranial, spinal, or peripheral nerves. In most cases they are benign but malignant neoplasms have been reported, occurring *de novo* or arising from irradiated benign lesions. There has been confusion in the literature regarding the terminology used when referring to these tumors. The current literature does distinguish between neurilemmoma (schwannoma) and neurofibroma on a histologic basis, with neuroma referring to the exaggerated cellular response to injury formed at the site of a severed nerve [47].

These relatively uncommon lesions occur mainly in the central nervous system, but 13% arise from various locations in the head and neck, especially within the lateral cervical

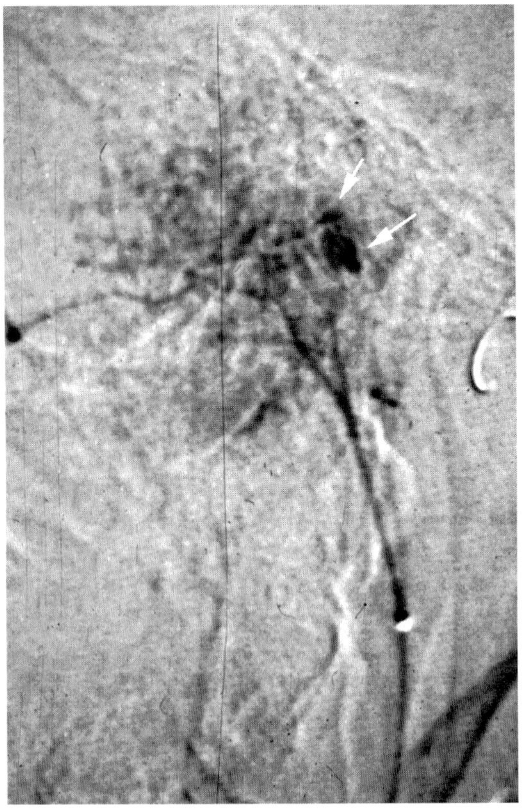

FIGURE 14-7. This superselective injection of the ascending pharyngeal artery in a patient with an acoustic schwannoma shows a mildly hypervascular mass with puddling of contrast material.

region. Females in the third and fourth decades of life are most often affected. The clinical picture varies, depending upon the size, location, specific nerve involved, and presence or absence of malignancy [48].

CT scanning shows a uniformly hypodense mass which enhances peripherally, leaving a central mottled lucency [49]. Contrast-enhanced MRI shows a smoothly contoured, enhancing lesion with variable internal cystic formation.

A degree of variability is noticed in the angiographic pattern, which can range from a vascular to nonshunting hypervascular mass exhibiting tortuous vessels and puddling of contrast material (Fig. 14-7). The arterial supply is recruited from regional vessels of which external carotid branches are the most common [50].

Neuroforaminal schwannomas are often fed by dural muscular branches of the vertebral artery, and skull base lesions can parasitize branches of the cavernous carotid, ophthalmic, and vertebral arteries. Hypervascular tumors may be suitable for preoperative embolization using protocols and techniques similar to those already described [51].

Hemangiomas

Hemangiomas are slowly growing, benign hamartomas, usually discovered incidentally on radiographs or at autopsy. Most are noted to arise from the thoracic and lumbar vertebrae, but occasionally the cervical spine is involved. Although the majority remain clinically silent, these tumors can produce pain and, rarely, spinal cord compression [52–54]. Impingement of the cord may be secondary to epidural extension of the tumor, narrowing of the spinal canal from bony hypertrophy, compression fracture of the vertebral body or, rarely, epidural hemorrhage [55].

Characteristically, plain radiographs demonstrate a prominent vertical trabeculation pattern (resembling corduroy cloth) or coarse honeycomb appearance, within a vertebral body of decreased density. The cortex may be thinned with bulging of the margins, but it remains intact unless extension into the paraspinal or epidural spaces occurs. Axial CT images show the striations in cross-section, with an intervening stroma of soft tissue or fat, giving the bone a polka dot or honeycomb pattern (Fig. 14-8) [56,57].

Tumors that compress the spinal cord are most likely to arise from the midthoracic region, involve the entire vertebral body, extend into the neural arch, and demonstrate an expanded, indistinct cortical margin with irregular trabeculae and an extraosseous soft tissue mass [52]. The addition of intrathecal contrast outlines tumor extension into the epidural space and its effect upon the neural axis. In profoundly involved vertebral bodies, collapse may occur.

Unlike most bony lesions, the intraosseous portions of vertebral hemangiomas demonstrate a mottled, increased signal intensity on both T1 and T2 MRI sequences, with intervening, scattered low-to-isointense areas corresponding to the trabeculations. Correlation with histopathologic sections indicates that the shortened T1 signal reflects the adipose-laden stroma interspersed between thin-walled vessels and bony trabeculae. The increased signal on T2 images is less easily explained and may arise from the more cellular components of the tumor. Extraosseous tumor is composed mainly of angiomatous and fibrous elements, accounting for an intermediate soft tissue signal on T1 and an increased signal on T2 [56].

Selective angiography of asymptomatic hemangiomas shows minimal hypervascularity with no extension of the vascular image outside the vertebra. In contrast, compressive lesions may demonstrate dilated feeding arteries, extreme hypervascularity with dense, homogeneous staining (see Fig. 14-8), and opacification extending beyond the normal hemivertebral territory to involve the entire body, the paraspinal soft tissues, or the extradural space [52].

The treatment of symptomatic vertebral hemangiomas is varied and controversial. Therapeutic modalities include transarterial embolization, direct puncture embolization, surgical resection, radiotherapy, or a combined approach. Most authors agree that surgical biopsy or resection should not be performed without preoperative embolization (see Fig. 14-8) [53,54,58–61]. Particulate embolization of regional feeders is most commonly used, although preoperative percutaneous injection of methylmethacrylate into the

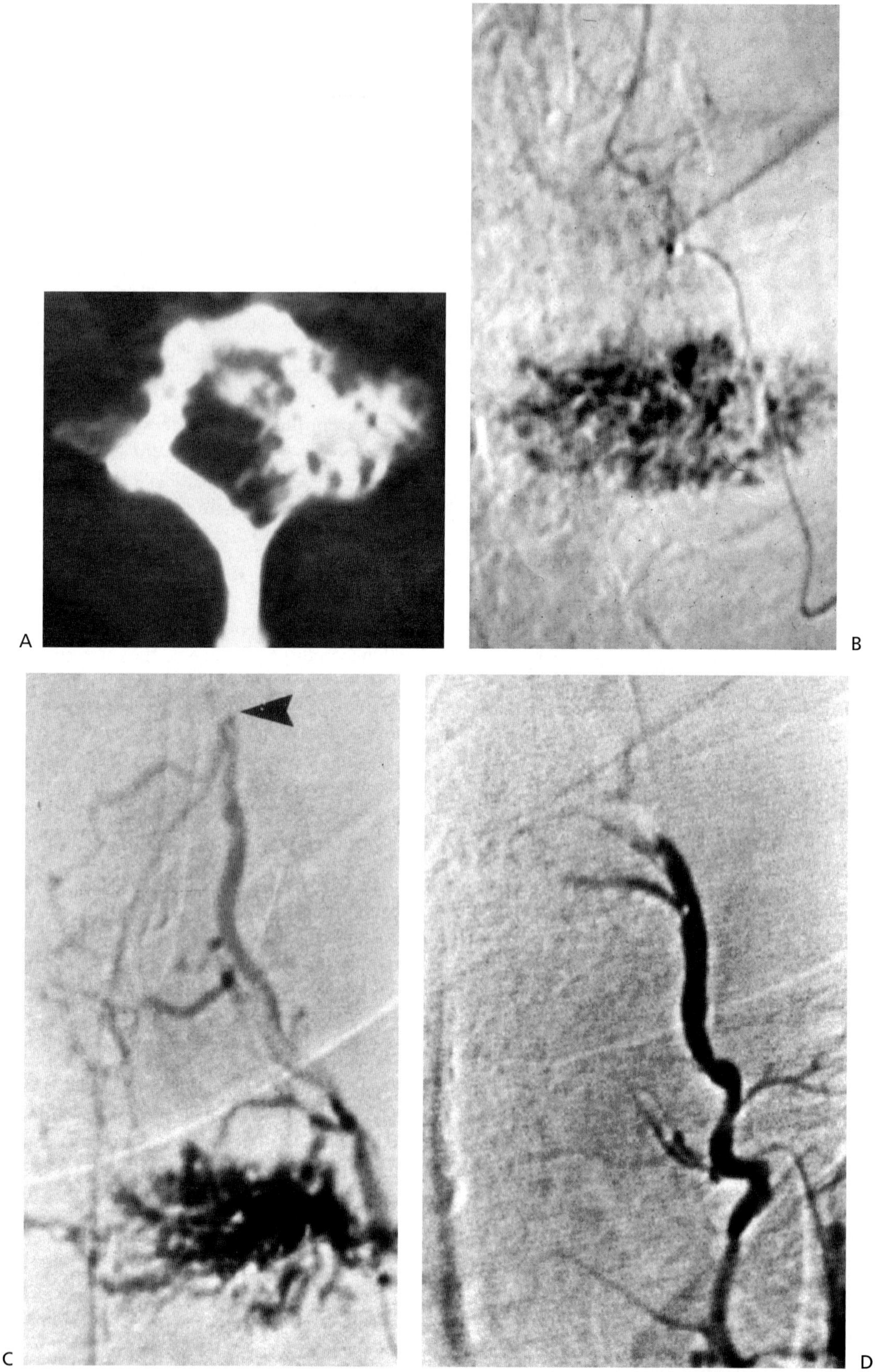

vertebral body and N-butyl-2-cyanoacrylate (NBCA) into the neural arch has been described [62]. Transcatheter embolization alone may alleviate acute neurologic decompensation from spinal cord compression [52,63,64], but relief may be only transient [58]. Excellent pain palliation has also been achieved with embolization alone in a small number of cases [53,54,65], although few long-term studies are available [66]. The risk of vertebral body embolization is very low provided that the regional vascular supply to the cord is identified and avoided. Arterial feeders to the cervical vertebrae or cervicothoracic junction or both may arise from the vertebral arteries, the thyrocervical and costocervical trunks, and the supreme intercostal arteries, and all should be included in the angiographic evaluation when indicated.

Tumors with inaccessible blood supply may benefit from direct puncture embolization. Slow instillation of small amounts (12 ml or less) of absolute ethanol has been shown to devascularize symptomatic hemangiomas with preservation of the trabecular support and vertebral stability [67]. However, injection of larger amounts (40 to 50 ml) of absolute alcohol may cause osteonecrosis with resultant vertebral collapse [68].

Treatment of painful vertebral hemangiomas without epidural extension by intraoperative [59] or percutaneous vertebroplasty is an alternative to transarterial embolization or radiotherapy [69]. With this procedure, the vertebral body is injected, under fluoroscopic control, with a fast-curing acrylic cement that has been opacified with metallic powder or barium sulfate. The aim is to achieve a near-immediate analgesic effect by providing strengthening and consolidation of the vertebral body.

Opinions vary regarding radiotherapy. Some investigators feel the risk of radionecrosis outweighs the questionable benefits. Others consider radionecrosis unlikely at fractionated doses of less than 40 Gy and have found good results in patients whose symptoms are moderate, slowly progressive, or limited to pain [53,58,59]. With total vertebral involvement, laminectomy in conjunction with radiotherapy has demonstrated a 93% recovery rate without recurrence in one series [70]. If surgery is contraindicated, the patient may benefit from embolization prior to radiotherapy [58].

Aneurysmal Bone Cysts

Aneurysmal bone cysts are benign, expansile, vascular bony tumors found in children, adolescents, and young adults [71]. Constituting 1.4% of all bone tumors, they occur in the spine in up to 20% of cases [72,73]. Early symptoms include pain and swelling, and vertebral lesions are often accompanied by paresis and sensory abnormalities of the extremities [73,74]. The classic plain film radiographic appearance consists of an expansile osteolytic lesion with a well-defined transition zone and a peripheral shell of thin cortical bone [71]. Multiple internal septations are often present [74]. In vertebral tumors, the epicenter is located in the neural arch with extension to the vertebral body via the pedicles in 60% of patients [73]. Encroachment on the spinal canal is common [71], and some lesions extend to contiguous vertebrae.

CT may show a thin rim of calcium not evident on plain radiographs, and is useful in identifying calcified tumor matrix characteristic of other primary bone or soft tissue tumors. MRI demonstrates the extent of the tumor and its relationship to the adjacent thecal sac and neural structures (Fig. 14-9), while both CT and MR imaging may show fluid–fluid levels within the lesion caused by layering of solid blood components [71]. Other findings noted with aneurysmal bone cysts include septations within the lesion which may be enhanced, and signal characteristics of low intensity on T1 images and high intensity on T2 images [73,75].

Arteriovenous shunting, diffuse tumor staining in the late arterial phase, and indistinct pools of contrast in cystic areas are common angiographic findings (see Fig. 14-9) [76], yet none is necessarily characteristic for an aneurysmal bone cyst [72]. These lesions often lack a true major feeding vessel, and distinct arterial feeders or draining veins may or may not be identified [72,77].

Complete surgical excision of the tumor is the most effective, and preferred, method of treatment although problematic in challenging locations such as the sacrum, spine or pelvis, or in large lesions. If excision would cause severe disability, curettage (intralesional excision) with bone grafting may be performed. Although an overall recurrence rate of 19% following curettage has been reported [74], lesions in the vertebrae had a lower rate than those in the long bones. Radiotherapy has been used to treat inoperable lesions or to alleviate pain, but tumor recurrence and complications such as radiation-induced myelopathy and sarcomatous change have been reported [72,76,78].

Transarterial embolization has been described as preparatory for surgical resection [71,72,75,79] (see Fig. 14-9), for

FIGURE 14-8. This 45-year-old woman had neck pain and an expansile lesion of the C7 vertebral body. **A:** CT scan shows a honeycomb appearance of the left vertebral body, pedicle, transverse process, and lamina, with encroachment on the spinal canal. **B:** Selective injection of the ascending cervical artery shows dense reticulated tumor blush arising from small muscular branches. **C:** Normal tissue distal to the tumor was protected with a Gelfoam pledget *(arrowhead)* followed by particulate embolization. **D:** No residual blush is detected.

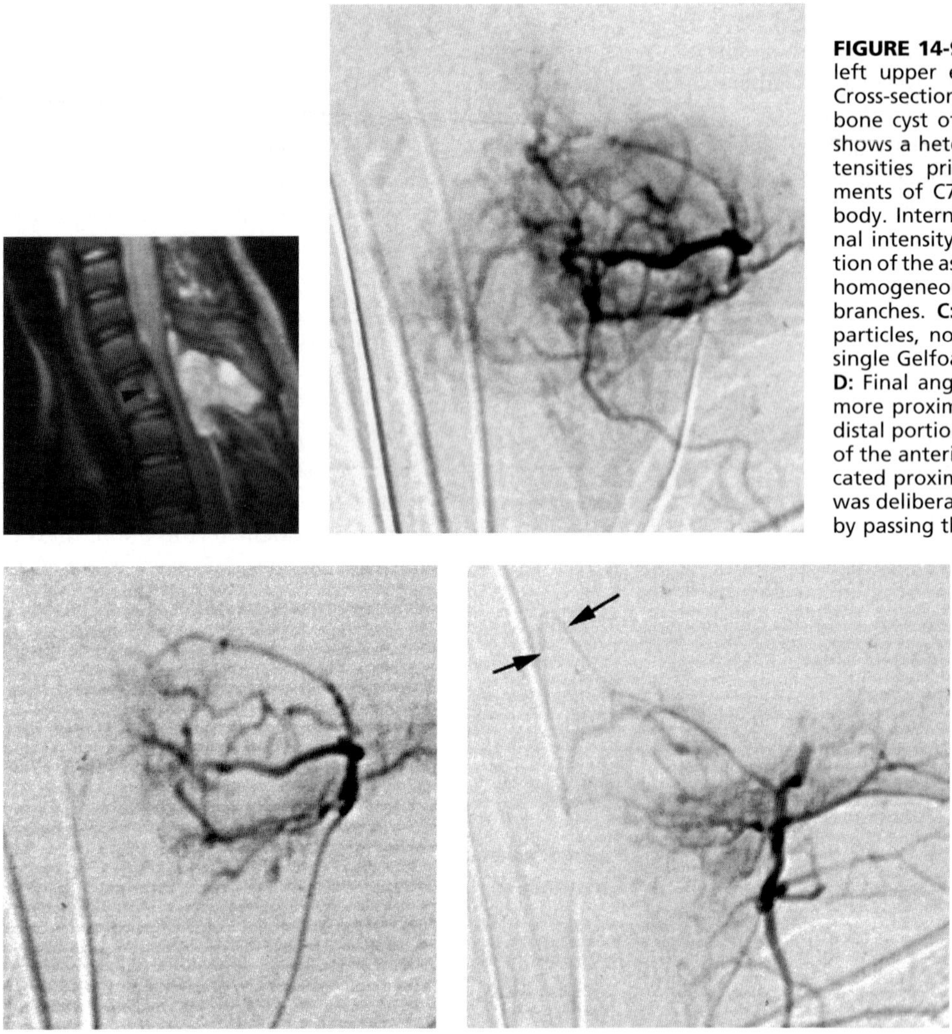

FIGURE 14-9. This 9-year-old girl demonstrated left upper extremity numbness and weakness. Cross-sectional imaging revealed an aneurysmal bone cyst of C7. **A:** Proton density sagittal MRI shows a heterogeneous mass of mixed signal intensities primarily involving the posterior elements of C7, with extension into the vertebral body. Internal septations separate the high–signal intensity cystic areas. **B:** Superselective injection of the ascending cervical branch shows a fine, homogeneous tumor blush from multiple small branches. **C:** Following embolization with PVA particles, no significant tumor blush remains. A single Gelfoam pledget was placed in the vessel. **D:** Final angiogram with the microcatheter in a more proximal position shows truncation of the distal portion of the artery. Also seen is a branch of the anterior spinal artery *(arrows)* that was located proximal to the tumor neovascularity, and was deliberately excluded from the embolization by passing the microcatheter distal to its origin.

treatment of clinical symptoms [77,80], and as definitive therapy [71,80–82]. Embolization may be considered as the treatment of choice when the tumor extent is such that total excision or radical curettage would be too risky, reconstruction would be difficult, or operative morbidity might involve neural elements or compromise the stability of the spine [81].

Transarterial embolization is feasible provided that an adequate vascular supply is present and there are no spinal cord branches identified. In several reports [71,76,79,81], presurgical embolization with PVA or Gelfoam was noted to aid tumor excision by decreasing blood loss and improving visualization. In several small series, vertebral tumors were treated palliatively with PVA particles [71,77,81], Gelfoam sponge [80], ethanol [77], or a combination of agents [83]. Pain control and partial or complete regression of the tumor was noted in the majority of patients [71,77,83,84]. Regression was determined by cessation of growth or tumor shrinkage and radiographic evidence of progressive ossification. In addition to particulate and liquid embolic agents, the use of coils has also been described. Prior to tumor embolization, coils have been placed distal to vessels supplying the tumor in order to protect the normal, distal vascular bed [77,79,83]. Coils have also been used for proximal vessel occlusion following tumor embolization to enhance the extent and duration of the peripheral arterial occlusion [77, 40,83]. The presence of coils may interfere with attempts at repeat embolization [77,81] by limiting access to the main feeding vessel. This situation can be circumvented by the use of Gelfoam pledgets instead of coils.

Percutaneous injection of aneurysmal bone cysts involving the cervical spine and mandible have been reported [85]. The cystic spaces were filled with Ethibloc (Ethicon, Hamburg, Germany), a radiopaque fibrosing agent composed of alcohol and vegetable protein. Follow-up studies demonstrated tumor shrinkage and progressive ossification. Injection of calcitonin has also been described as being effective in some cases, resulting in tumor regression [86].

Embolization of aneurysmal bone cysts using particulate agents is associated with a morbidity in the range of 0 to 2%. The complication rate increases when liquid agents are used, particularly ethanol [83]. Complications associated with the use of ethanol consist mainly of inducing ischemia in adjacent neural structures or causing tissue necrosis from leakage of material outside of the tumor confines. Local pain, fever, and nausea have also been observed during the first few days after any embolization procedure [77]. Some authors [81,87] advocate the use of provocative testing with sodium amobarbital (Amytal) and the monitoring of somatosensory evoked potentials during embolization, especially when liquid agents are used.

Remission of clinical symptoms generally occurs within days to weeks after embolization, with evidence of ossification apparent within 2 to 4 months [77,79]. The reappearance of pain is a major indicator of recurrent tumor growth [77] and additional embolizations may be performed as necessary.

Other rare tumors, such as osteoblastomas [88,89], osteoid osteomas [90], and giant cell tumors [91] may exhibit vascularity and can be embolized in a manner to that used for hemangiomas or aneurysmal bone cysts.

Metastatic Bone Tumors

Certain metastatic tumors are highly vascular in nature, particularly primary renal or thyroid malignancies. Other metastases may exhibit varying degrees of neovascularity including lesions that originate from breast, hepatocellular, and squamous cell primaries. Many reports on the surgical resection of vascular metastases recommend preoperative embolization to decrease blood loss and improve visibility at the surgical site [91–95]. In one series, the major perioperative complications were related to excessive blood loss in patients who did not undergo preoperative embolization [93].

Reports attempting to quantify the actual amount of blood loss are scarce. Gellad et al. [94] described 24 patients who underwent surgical decompression of vascular vertebral metastases. Twenty patients were treated with preoperative embolization and had an average blood loss of 1,850 ml during surgery. The four patients without preoperative embolization had an average blood loss of greater than 3,500 ml. Olerud et al. [95] found that the average blood loss in surgery performed after embolization was decreased by 67%. In a series by Broaddus et al. [91] the estimated blood loss in seven of nine surgical procedures in patients who were embolized preoperatively ranged from 300 to 800 ml. No transfusions were required in these patients. More extensive resections in two other patients necessitated postoperative transfusion despite preoperative embolization. In this series, microfibrillar collagen (20 to 180 μm) was used as the embolic agent. Adequate embolization can be performed with particles 150 to 250 μm in size with similar beneficial effects, while lowering the risk of inadvertent spinal cord embolization. Spinal metastases often derive their blood supply from branches of the vertebral artery. When *en bloc* excision of the tumor is anticipated, the surgeon may request permanent occlusion of the vertebral artery prior to surgery (Fig. 14-10). In such situations, detachable balloons may be used to trap the segment of vessel that is to be removed. After passage of the test occlusion, the more distal balloon is detached. Any feeders located proximal to the balloon can be embolized from the vertebral artery stump, provided no spinal cord supply is present. A second balloon is then placed proximal to the lesion and detached. Excessive manipulation of the vessel during surgery, particularly if the vertebral segment is low and the occlusion is fresh, may result in displacement of the proximal balloon into the subclavian artery [96].

In patients for whom surgery is not an option, embolization has been shown to be an effective palliative measure to aid in pain control, relieve nerve root or cord compression [97], and slow tumor growth. In some instances, increased calcification following embolization suggesting partial bone healing has been noted [98].

The embolization techniques for treatment of metastatic lesions are similar to those described for primary bone tumors. The anterior spinal artery must be identified and avoided. In presurgical cases, embolization is usually performed with particulate agents. Surgical removal of the tumor should be done as soon as possible following the embolization procedure to minimize the recanalization of embolized vessels or the opening of collaterals. For palliative measures, a tumoricidal or chemotherapeutic agent may be mixed with other embolic materials or used alone to aid in tumor shrinkage.

Direct puncture embolization may be effective in cases in which the tumor and spinal cord share the same arterial supply [99]. For preoperative lesions, liquid or particulate agents or soft embolic materials such as NBCA should be used so as to not interfere with the surgical resection. Direct puncture and installation of methylmethacrylate (vertebroplasty) to stabilize compression fractures and reduce pain has been very successful [69,100–102]. To avoid neural or vascular structures, needle placement can be done under fluoroscopic control or CT guidance.

A rare but potentially devastating complication associated with vertebral body embolization is acute tumoral edema which causes neurologic dysfunction, necessitating immediate surgical decompression. Postprocedural observation for 24 hours in an intensive care unit is recommended. In those patients embolized for pain palliation, vertebral body collapse can occur over several weeks. Certain precautions, such as the use of external bracing or avoiding activities that increase axial loading of the spine, should be employed.

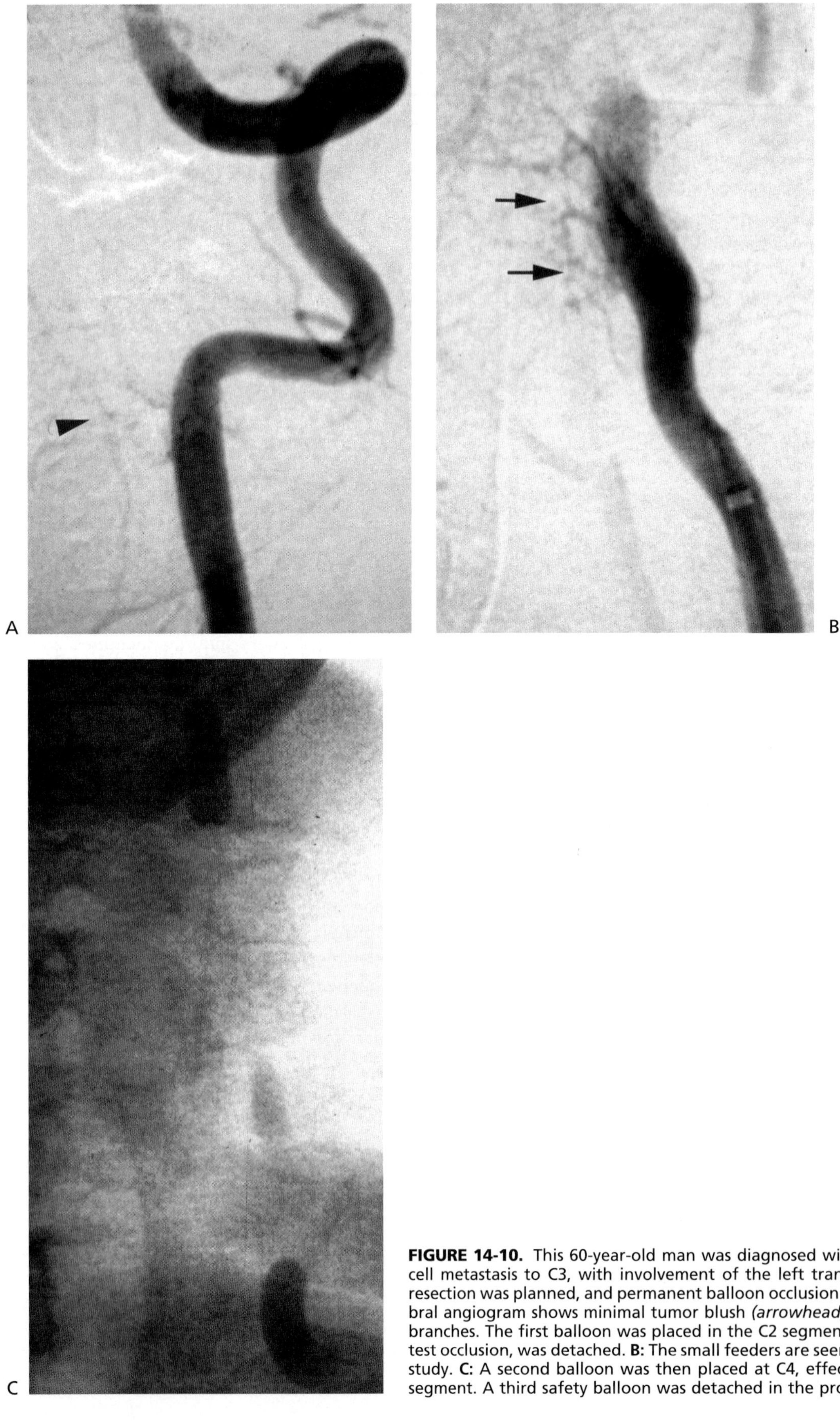

FIGURE 14-10. This 60-year-old man was diagnosed with a hypovascular squamous cell metastasis to C3, with involvement of the left transverse foramen. An *en bloc* resection was planned, and permanent balloon occlusion was requested. **A:** Left vertebral angiogram shows minimal tumor blush *(arrowhead)* arising from small regional branches. The first balloon was placed in the C2 segment and, following a successful test occlusion, was detached. **B:** The small feeders are seen better on the postocclusion study. **C:** A second balloon was then placed at C4, effectively trapping the affected segment. A third safety balloon was detached in the proximal vertebral artery.

TECHNIQUE FOR EMBOLIZATION

Every therapeutic strategy is patient specific, dictated by the nature of the lesion, the symptoms and clinical examination, and the desired outcome. Rarely is embolization a curative treatment for head and neck tumors; instead, endovascular procedures usually fulfill an adjunctive role, either presurgical or palliative [103–111]. It is the interventionist's responsibility to discuss the appropriate options and relative risks of the embolization procedure with the referring clinician to optimize the treatment plan.

In most cases, the primary goal of embolization is tumor devascularization through the promotion of thrombosis within its vascular bed without compromising circulation to normal tissue. In potentially resectable lesions, embolization facilitates the surgical approach by reducing blood loss, thereby decreasing the need for transfusion and shortening the operative time. A drier surgical field provides improved visualization, manipulation, and dissection of the lesion and adjacent tissues. In some cases, embolization allows extirpation of otherwise inoperable lesions by occluding inaccessible or unresectable portions of the tumor.

With palliative procedures, embolization may result in shrinkage of the lesion, decompression of adjacent structures, improved neurologic function, and decreased pain. Endovascular therapy also can be combined with chemotherapy or radiation to treat unresectable tumors.

Provocative testing may be a required element of the embolization or a complementary procedure to the diagnostic angiogram. Identification of patients with inadequate collateral circulation aids the surgeon in operative planning, particularly when parent artery clamping or sacrifice is anticipated.

Vascular Supply to the Head and Neck

Prior to undertaking endovascular intervention, a thorough understanding of the neurovascular anatomy is necessary because of the abundance of anatomical variations, collateral supply, and territorial anastomoses found in the cervical region. The blood supply to tumors involving the head and neck is derived from regional vascularity and is provided primarily by branches of the ECA with recruitment of vertebral, internal carotid, thyrocervical, or costocervical branches as these territories become involved. Tumors adjacent to the brain may parasitize regional pial blood supply as they enlarge. Lesions of the cervical spine draw their blood supply from the vertebral artery and the ascending cervical and deep cervical arteries of the thyrocervical trunk. Parent vessels may also supply nervous tissue, either directly (e.g., an anterior spinal artery branch arising from the ascending cervical artery) or by collateral channels.

Prevention of serious complications requires knowledge and recognition of territorial anastomoses. With head and neck neoplasms, the most common dangerous anastomoses involve communication of the ICA or vertebral arteries with the ascending pharyngeal, occipital, middle meningeal, accessory meningeal, and distal internal maxillary arteries. Likewise, the middle meningeal, internal maxillary, superficial temporal, and facial arteries can all anastomose with the ophthalmic artery, which may result in blindness or stroke. These important collaterals may not be recognized on the initial angiogram or they may open as the blood flow changes during embolization. It is essential that the interventionist has a complete knowledge of these pathways, performs careful, flow-directed embolization, and does frequent check angiograms to prevent inadvertent embolization of the brain or orbit.

In addition to providing collateral circulation, the external carotid system is the primary blood supply to many of the cranial nerves. Palsies of cranial nerves V, VII, IX, X, XI, or XII may result from inappropriate embolization of the feeding branches to the vasa nervorum. Selection of suitable embolic materials and provocative testing when necessary will assist in avoidance of this complication.

Patient Selection and Preparation

Appropriate candidates for endovascular or percutaneous therapy are patients with symptomatic vascular neoplasms that may benefit from embolization, either prior to surgical resection or for palliation. When obtaining informed consent, a description of the proposed therapy and its attendant risks, benefits, and alternatives are discussed thoroughly with the patient and family. In children or uncooperative adults, or during procedures in which extreme pain is anticipated (such as with alcohol injection), general anesthesia is often required. General anesthesia precludes the ability to examine the patient neurologically and may therefore preclude the immediate identification of complications.

All patients should undergo a baseline neurologic evaluation by a qualified nurse and physician prior to the procedure. Most patients are sedated with a combination of antianxiety medication such as midazolam (Versed), and an analgesic such as fentanyl. Continuous physiologic monitoring (electrocardiogram, blood pressure, and oxygen saturation) must occur throughout the procedure. Systemic heparinization of the patient after placement of the sheath reduces the risk of thrombus formation on guiding catheters and within the coaxial system. Intermittent neurologic evaluation, particularly during the embolization, allows monitoring of the patient's mental status and neurologic function.

Following embolization, acute tumor swelling or, rarely, hemorrhage within the tumor bed may occur. This may lead to acute neurologic decompensation with large or critically located lesions. Therefore postprocedural management should include a 24-hour stay in a suitable intensive care unit with frequent neurologic evaluations. Intravenous steroids may be administered in patients with large tumors or extensive edema. Many patients are receiving steroids prior to embolization. If symptoms worsen after the procedure, a transient increase in the dosage is recommended. For patients who have not been taking steroids but have large tumors located adjacent to the brain or spinal cord, 6 to 10 mg of dexamethasone (Decadron) may be given immediately prior to embolization, followed by a rapid taper over the ensuing 24 to 48 hours. Mannitol is a drug frequently used in the treatment of increased intracranial pressure or spinal cord compression. Discussion with the neurosurgical team should be done prior to mannitol administration because emergency surgical decompression may be the more appropriate therapy. A 1.0-g/kg bolus of mannitol followed by a second bolus of 0.25 to 0.50 g/kg is the usual dosage [112]. Mild symptoms such as localized pain or headache also may occur and usually respond to nonsteroidal antiinflammatory agents, but small doses of narcotics may occasionally be necessary.

Diagnostic Angiography

High-quality diagnostic angiography is mandatory prior to embolization. All procedures are recorded using high-resolution digital subtraction angiography (DSA). DSA is preferred over cut-film technology due to its superior contrast resolution, the availability of road mapping functions, pixel shifting capabilities to minimize motion artifact, and near-instant review of angiographic runs.

The angiographic evaluation of a tumor's arterial supply is guided by its location and size, as seen on cross-sectional imaging, and expected direct and collateral supply. Extracranial tumors that are located laterally and peripherally may require only ipsilateral injection of the ECA. Conversely, large, invasive tumors that cross the midline and have deep components will require examination of the ipsilateral and contralateral ICA and ECA. The vertebral artery and the thyrocervical and costocervical trunks will be evaluated in posteriorly located lesions.

There is no specific order in which the vessels are studied; however, the operator should plan the evaluation so that the maximal amount of information is obtained in the shortest amount of time. Completion of the diagnostic study in an efficient, stepwise manner leaves the bulk of the procedure time for embolization, and patient cooperation is best early in the treatment before fatigue and discomfort set in.

Vascular access is obtained generally via the common femoral artery. A 5- or 6-French (Fr.) vascular sheath is placed and connected to pressurized heparinized saline flush (4,000 units of heparin per 1,000 ml normal saline). If temporary balloon occlusion testing is anticipated, a larger sheath (7 to 8 Fr.) will be needed, because balloon-tipped catheters require large-lumen guiding catheters. The diagnostic angiography catheter may be used as a guiding catheter for the embolization, provided that the lumen is of sufficient size (0.035-inch or larger internal diameter) to accept standard microcatheters. However, adequate injection around the microcatheter for road mapping purposes is usually not possible with tapered diagnostic catheters. Conversely, a guiding catheter may be used for the diagnostic angiogram, but it may be more likely to induce vasospasm as the tip is thin walled and nontapered, making it relatively sharp.

The use of isoosmolar nonionic media (iodixanol [Visipaque]), particularly for ECA injections, will decrease discomfort substantially in sensitive patients. Performing contrast injections by hand, instead of by a mechanical injector, is another way to decrease procedure time.

Provocative Testing

Many of the cranial nerves receive their blood supply from ECA branches. For example, the facial nerve obtains supply from the petrosal branch of the middle meningeal artery, the stylomastoid branch of the occipital artery, the stylomastoid branch of the posterior auricular artery, or some combination thereof. Embolization of these vessels using very small particles or liquid agents may place the patient at risk for facial nerve palsy if the capillary blood flow and collateral blood supply are blocked. Provocative testing with lidocaine offers a functional test of the capillary bed prior to the embolization of an agent that could result in permanent damage [113]. Ten to 30 mg of lidocaine is injected intraarterially into the vessel to be treated, followed by neurologic evaluation for regional cranial nerve dysfunction. If testing induces a deficit, the catheter tip is repositioned distal to the feeding vessel, or an embolic agent larger than the vasa nervorum (150 to 200 μm) is used to avoid a permanent deficit.

A similar test for retinal function using lidocaine can be performed when treating the ophthalmic artery or its collateral supply [114]. Pharmacological testing of the spinal cord with lidocaine and a short-acting barbiturate has also been described [115] but if positive at the cervical level may result in respiratory failure, and therefore is not recommended.

Patients undergoing prolonged temporary occlusion of the parent artery during surgery or embolization should have provocative testing of the ICA or vertebral artery collateral supply performed using a test occlusion catheter positioned in a straight, nondiseased, extracranial portion of the vessel [116,117]. If the surgeon is anticipating resection of the vessel during surgery, then balloon occlusion testing is performed at the site of the surgical ligation. If this point is above the skull base, a permanently attached silicone or latex balloon mounted on a microcatheter is used for the test (Fig. 14-11) instead of the more rigid double-lumen catheter [118].

Regardless of the system used, immediately prior to balloon inflation the patient is fully heparinized to prevent clot formation on the balloon or within the dead space distal to the balloon. If a double-lumen system is used, contrast is

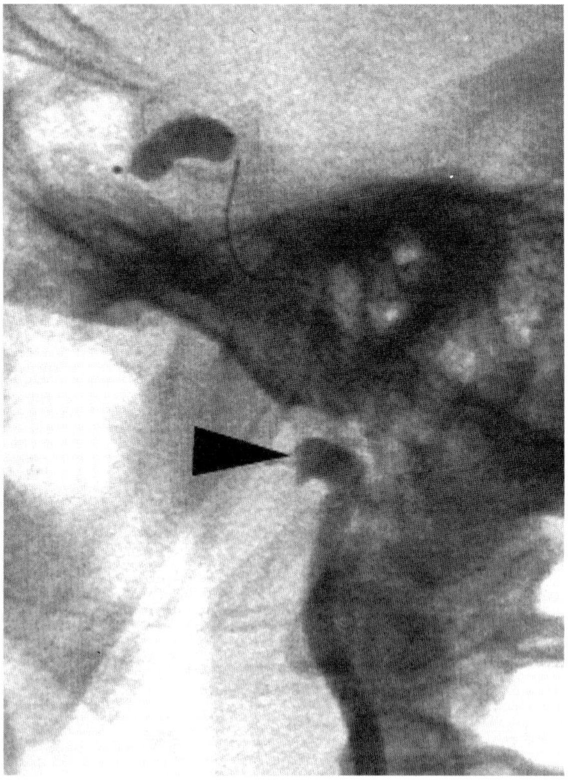

FIGURE 14-11. A hand-tied latex balloon attached to a microcatheter is used to temporarily occlude the ICA during provocative testing. The balloon is positioned in the horizontal segment of the cavernous carotid artery, proximal to the ophthalmic artery origin. Stasis of the contrast column *(arrowhead)* indicates complete occlusion of the vessel.

injected through the distal lumen while the balloon is inflated, until flow arrest is observed. Another method is to inflate the balloon while the distal lumen is attached to a pressure monitoring device, and inflation is terminated when damping of the arterial wave form is seen. In either case, complete occlusion should be confirmed by the presence of a stagnant contrast column when contrast is injected through the distal lumen. The injection port is infused with a slow infusion of heparinized saline flush during the testing phase. If saline is infused too rapidly, partial or total replacement of oxygenated blood within the ophthalmic artery may produce signs and symptoms of ocular ischemia, including orbital pain and uniocular visual loss [119]. These findings may be interpreted as a false-positive occlusion test or may falsely indicate a thromboembolic complication.

Because microcatheter balloon systems do not have a lumen distal to the balloon, contrast is injected through the guiding catheter, and complete occlusion of the vessel is achieved when the contrast column is static below. Perceived disadvantages of this system are the inability to infuse saline during the test occlusion or to record stump pressures. In theory, the lack of a continuous saline infusion may increase the risk of thrombus formation distal to the balloon; however, the literature does not support this assertion [118].

Once the balloon is inflated and vascular occlusion is confirmed, neurologic testing is performed immediately and every 5 minutes thereafter, for a total of 30 minutes, to rule out immediate or delayed cerebral ischemia. Occasionally, electroencephalographic monitoring during balloon occlusion testing of the ICA is performed on patients who cannot be tested clinically. Follow-up stable xenon-enhanced CT blood flow imaging or single photon emission computed tomography (SPECT) imaging can provide additional information about regional cerebral blood flow [120–122]. Following balloon deflation, a control angiogram is done of the balloon inflation site and the intracranial circulation to exclude vascular damage and distal emboli.

Embolization Materials

A variety of catheters, guidewires, and embolic agents are available for use in the treatment of head and neck neoplasms [123–127], and a brief outline is included in this discussion. When using coaxial systems involving microcatheters, the guiding catheter acts as an introducer, and its tip is positioned in the origin of the major artery that supplies the lesion. A side-arm adaptor is placed on the guiding catheter hub, and the microcatheter is advanced through the rotating hemostatic valve into the guiding catheter lumen. A three-way stopcock is attached to the side arm on the adaptor and a continuous heparinized saline infusion is attached to one of the stopcock ports. When the stopcock valve is flushing, the dead space between the guiding catheter and the microcatheter is infused with heparinized saline. The second port is used for the intermittent injection of contrast material through the guiding catheter for serial angiograms or road mapping, without disturbing the placement of the microcatheter.

The microcatheter is advanced over a steerable guidewire; negotiation of the tortuous ECA vessels for superselective placement of the catheter requires the torque and support that a guidewire provides. Even though some tumors are highly vascular, the regional blood flow is not increased enough in neoplasms to make use of flow-directed catheters practical. In addition, the internal diameter of wire-directed catheters is typically larger than that of their flow-directed counterparts, making them compatible with a wider variety of embolic agents. Steerable microcatheters are also used for mounting hand-tied or detachable microballoons on the distal tip for temporary balloon testing or permanent vascular occlusion; some flow-directed microcatheters have tip modifications that allow the same options.

In some cases, direct percutaneous puncture of the tumor can be done, using an 18- to 22-gauge spinal needle for injection of a liquid embolic agent.

Commonly used particulate agents include PVA (Contour; Target Therapeutics, Fremont, CA), microfibrillar collagen (Avitene; Alcon, Woburn, MA), and gelatin powder or shaved gelatin sponge (Gelfoam; Upjohn, Kalamazoo, MI). Liquid embolic materials include tissue adhesives (NBCA [Trufill]; Cordis, Miami Lakes, FL), dehydrated alcohol (Tera Pharmaceuticals, Buena Park, CA), and hypertonic glucose and sodium tetradecyl sulfate (Sotradecol; Elkins-Sinn, Cherry Hill, NJ). Occasionally, larger mechanical embolic agents such as Gelfoam pledgets, platinum microcoils (Target Therapeutics), and silicone (Target Therapeutics) or latex balloons (Laboratories Nycomed, Paris, France) may be used for protection of distal vascular territories or as terminal occlusive devices after use of more penetrating agents.

In many cases, the desired outcome can be achieved with several different embolic agents. Factors affecting the choice of an embolic agent include the therapeutic goal, location of the tumor, size of the feeding vessel, position of the catheter tip, blood flow characteristics, the presence and location of dangerous anastomoses, and operator experience. The risk-to-benefit ratio should factor heavily into the selection of the agent used. For example, the greatest penetration of a tumor bed is achieved by liquid agents or very small particles, such as gelatin powder. However, these agents carry an increased risk of tissue necrosis or injury to neurologic tissue. Particles of 150 to 350 μm provide adequate distal penetration while sparing the vasa nervorum of cranial nerves and the capillary bed of adjacent scalp and soft tissues. Thus, in situations in which temporary hemostasis is desired (e.g., preoperative embolization), the use of medium-sized particles makes more sense than a liquid agent.

Embolization Procedure

The desired end point of embolization is selective deposition of embolic agent inside the tumor bed with sparing of the adjacent normal tissues. The radiographic appearance will be one of tumor blush obliteration with preservation of the main arterial trunk. To achieve this goal, meticulous technique is of paramount importance, especially during catheter manipulation and the injection of embolic material [128]. After identification of the arterial supply, the microcatheter is advanced into each feeding vessel and a magnified study is performed to define the angioarchitecture, evaluate the tumor neovascularity, and identify dangerous anastomoses. Excessive guidewire or catheter manipulation, or wedging of the catheter tip, may induce vasospasm, altering blood flow to the lesion and preventing safe and effective embolization [128]. Vasospasm often reverses following removal of the catheter or guidewire. Severe situations may require the application of topical nitroglycerin or intraarterial vasodilators such as papaverine.

To allow the operator to monitor the progress of the embolization, particles are suspended and delivered in contrast material [129]. Liquid agents also can be opacified with contrast material, although dilution of the agent will occur. The addition of tantalum powder to tissue adhesives renders them fluoroscopically visible.

In most instances, the embolic agent is injected by hand into the arterial stream in small, pulsed aliquots. Tissue adhesive is the exception; it is either injected as a continuous column, or as a bolus sandwiched between dextrose aliquots. The operator monitors the flow of the embolic agent away from the catheter tip and into the tumor bed, evaluating for reflux of the embolic material around the catheter tip or stagnation of flow in the feeding vessel. Frequent control angiograms during the embolization are necessary, because collateral branches may be seen only after the resistance in the tumor neovascularity has been increased by partial embolization. The embolization is complete when the tumor blush is no longer visualized. During this process, care is taken not to wedge the catheter tip, because forcible injection into a closed system can result in vessel rupture or in the opening of previously unseen anastomoses [130], with inadvertent embolization of normal adjacent tissue or the intracranial circulation.

Larger anastomoses or side branches feeding normal tissue are excluded in one of three ways, (a) the catheter tip is placed distal to the orifice of the branch and no reflux occurs (see Fig. 14-9), (b) proximal embolization is done using particles larger than the branch lumen (Fig. 14-12), or (c) the proximal lumen of the branch is blocked with a gelatin sponge pledget or platinum microcoil, followed by particulate embolization in the main trunk of the feeding vessel.

In some instances, an artery that feeds a tumor from its proximal portion also supplies normal tissue from its distal aspect. In this situation, the microcatheter is advanced to a point distal to the tumor branch takeoff, and the normal vascular territory is protected with a gelatin sponge pledget or microcoil. The catheter tip is then withdrawn to a point proximal to the tumor branches and embolization is performed (see Fig. 14-8).

After tumor bed embolization, the proximal portion of the main feeding vessel may be occluded using a gelatin sponge pledget to further promote thrombosis and prevent early recanalization (see Fig. 14-9). The microcatheter tip is placed at the site of embolization and flushed with heparinized saline. To construct a pledget, a Gelfoam sponge pad is flattened with the cylindrical portion of a 10-ml syringe, and 1-mm by 3-mm strips are cut with a razor blade. The pledgets are rolled tightly and placed within the Luer-Lok stem of a 1-ml syringe filled with contrast. The syringe is attached to the hub and the pledget is quickly injected into the microcatheter. Continued pressure on the syringe results in expulsion of the pledget into the vessel, evidenced by the appearance of contrast and the sudden ease of injection. If the injection is not performed quickly, the pledget can swell in the microcatheter, resulting in catheter blockage or rupture. Multiple pledgets can be injected until vessel occlusion is seen. Dissolution of the pledget occurs within several days to 6 weeks, reestablishing flow to the excluded territory. The pledget may appear as a filling defect within

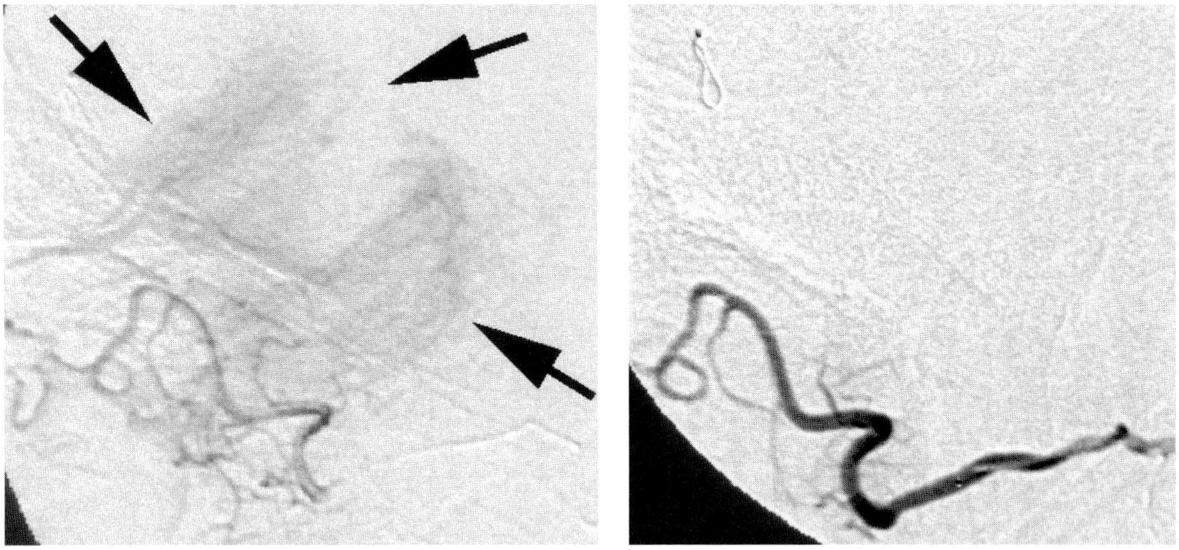

A B

FIGURE 14-12. Lateral view of the ophthalmic artery shows dense tumor blush supplying an olfactory groove meningioma. **A:** Attempts to place the microcatheter tip distal to the central retinal artery were unsuccessful, so embolization was performed using large particles (PVA, 500 to 700 μm). **B:** Following embolization, the tumor blush is no longer seen; the patient's vision remained unchanged.

the static contrast column. Microcoils have been used for this purpose also, but permanent vascular occlusion may occur, impeding reembolization in cases of tumor recurrence. Microcoils are more suitable than Gelfoam pledgets when placement of the agent must be very precise and reflux must be avoided at all costs (Fig. 14-13). Because microcoils are placed with a pushing device, their deposition is accurately controlled, unlike that of the injected pledget. Presurgical embolization should not consist of proximal vascular ligation alone, because this will result only in an opening of collateral channels with continued blood supply to the tumor and no tumor bed embolization.

Primary tumor location within the skull base or extension of tumor into this region may recruit supply from small branches of the ICA or vertebral arteries. The orifices of these feeders are usually too small to select with a microcatheter. If superselective embolization is precluded, embolization can be performed from the parent artery provided that an occlusion balloon is inflated distal to the distal-most feeding artery. A permanently attached silicone or latex balloon mounted on the end of a microcatheter is floated to a point distal to the tumor feeders and inflated, using the same protocol as for a provocative test occlusion. Once the patient has passed the test, a second microcatheter is advanced into the parent artery and positioned proximal to the tumor feeders. Embolization is performed through the second catheter until the tumor blush is eliminated. To prevent escape of residual embolic agent into the intracranial circulation, copious flushing of the dead space proximal to the balloon prior to balloon deflation is mandatory. This flushing is done through the microcatheter and the guiding catheter. The balloon is then deflated, and a neurologic exam and a check angiogram of the intracranial circulation are performed to rule out distal embolization.

When the parent artery is to be sacrificed during surgery, the previously described procedure can be done with detachable balloons. Instead of deflating the balloon following embolization, the balloon is detached and additional safety balloon(s) placed in the proximal portion of the parent artery (see Chapter 7).

When neither selective catheterization nor parent artery occlusion is desired or indicated, some tumors may be treated by direct puncture, either percutaneously (Fig. 14-14) or intraoperatively. Chaloupka et al. [131] reported excellent results using this technique in 24 patients with head and neck tumors. Early in their experience, patients initially underwent standard microcatheter transarterial embolization followed by direct puncture angiography and embolization. As the investigators gained experience, later patients were treated predominantly or exclusively via direct puncture. Tissue adhesive was injected in most patients, although absolute ethanol was also used. Advantages of the direct puncture approach include delivery of the agent to the capillary bed with a more complete embolization, establishment of a good cleavage plane, staining of the tumor allowing ready identification of pathology from normal tissue, and a low complication rate. Disadvantages include the possibility of retrograde reflux through feeders into the parent artery, the need for general anesthesia for intraprocedural pain management, and passage of a large embolization needle (16 to 20 gauge) through regions containing vital neurovascular structures. If needed, the tumor may be punctured under

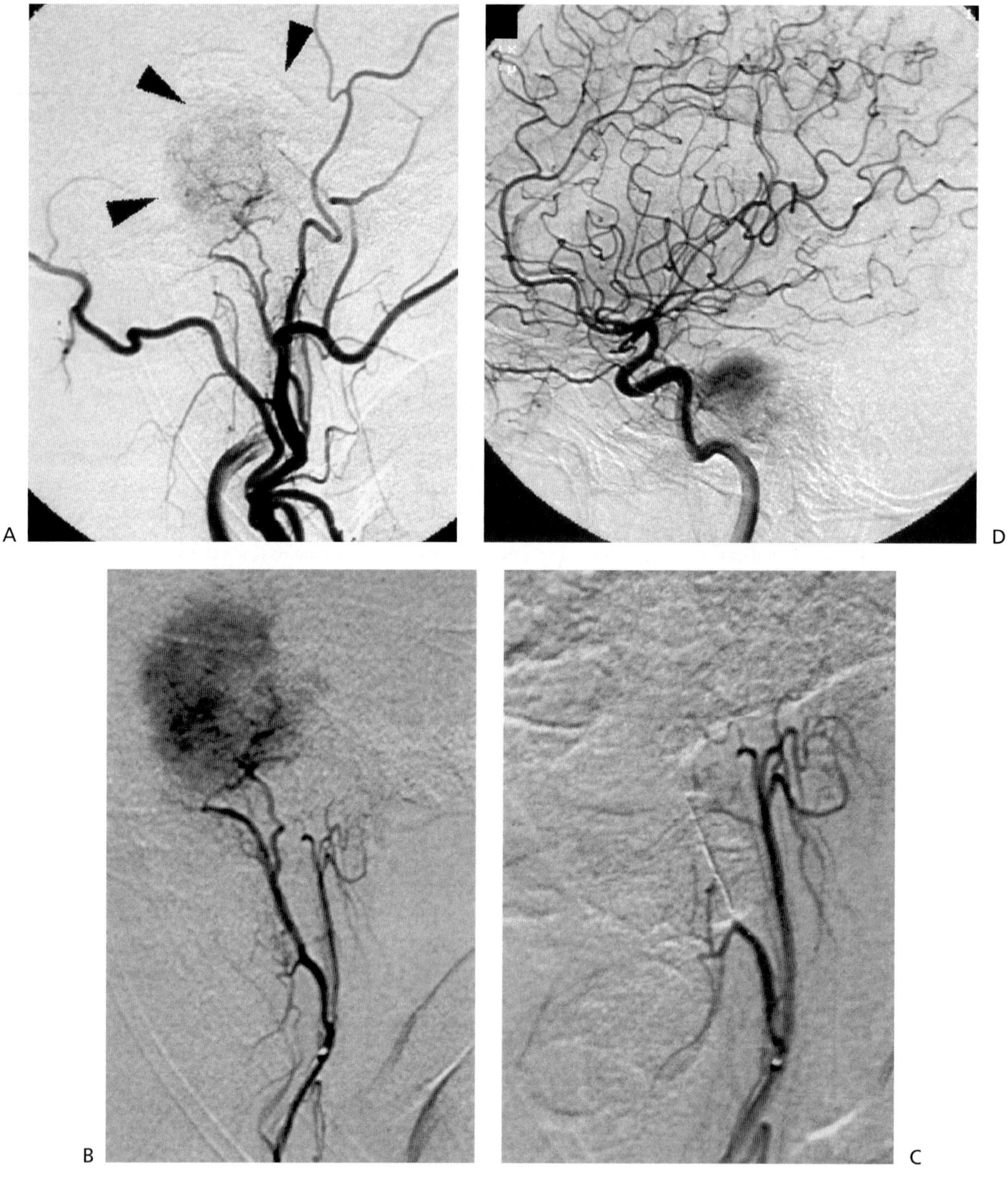

FIGURE 14-13. A,B: Lateral injection of the ECA **(A)** in a patient with a petrous apex meningioma demonstrates tumor blush arising from the posterior division of the ascending pharyngeal artery **(B). C:** Following particulate embolization, the main trunk of the posterior division was occluded using straight coils. **D:** Lateral injection of the ICA shows enlarged meningohypophyseal trunk branches filling a significant portion of the tumor. These branches were too small to catheterize selectively.

FIGURE 14-14. This 55-year-old man had a renal cell metastasis to C2 which caused extreme cervical pain and left arm weakness. The metastasis was fed by multiple small muscular branches of both vertebral arteries. **A:** Direct puncture of the tumor with an 18-gauge spinal needle was performed, and contrast injection shows significant tumor blush with no reflux into the vertebral artery. **B:** Following injection of a 33% solution of sodium tetradecyl sulfate, the control angiogram from the left vertebral artery shows the central avascular area corresponding to the preembolization "tumorogram."

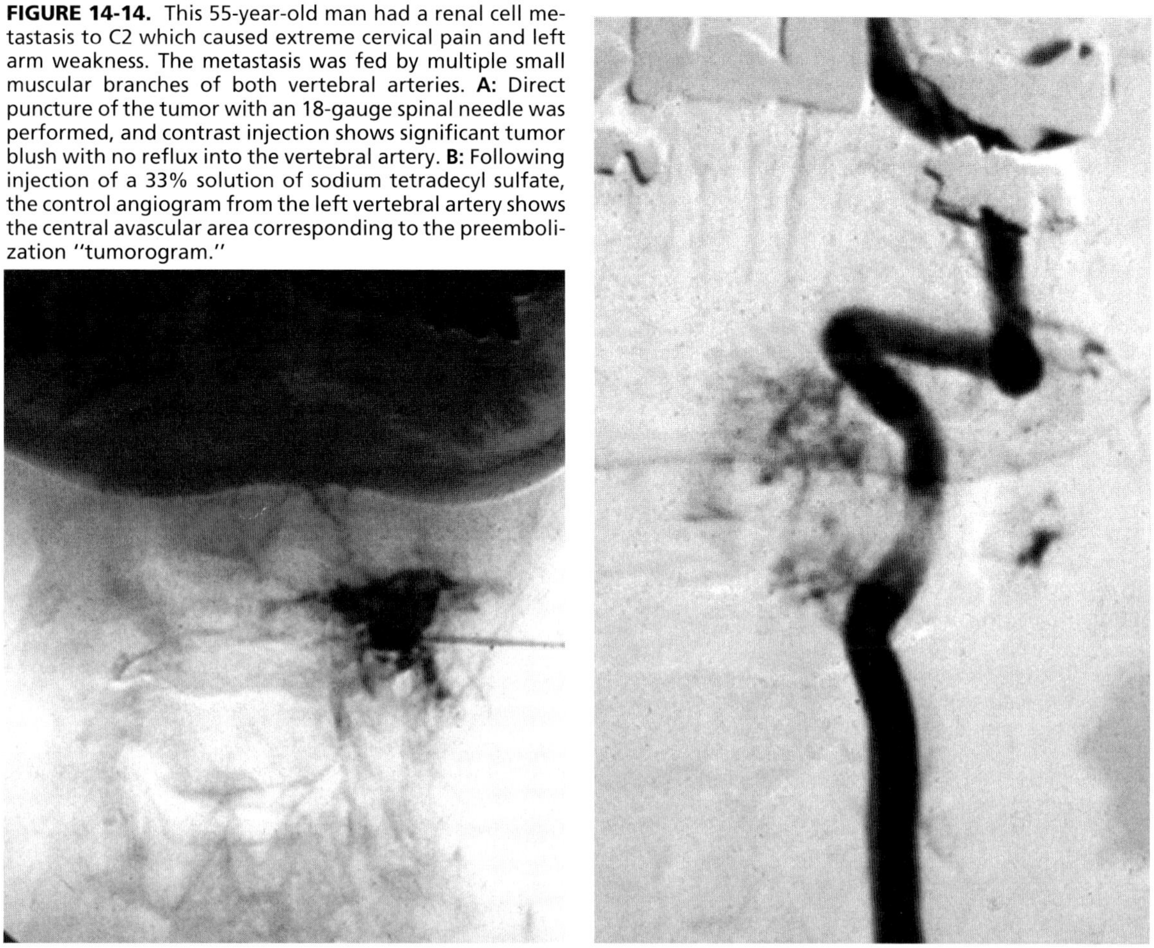

A B

CT guidance and the patient transferred to the fluoroscopy suite for treatment. Although this approach shows promise, particularly as a palliative treatment, further study is necessary before safety and long-term efficacy can be measured.

Complications

Embolization of most head and neck tumors carries a very low morbidity and mortality rate (less than 1%) when performed by an experienced interventionist [103–111]. Minor adverse effects are much more common; some patients experience transient mild fever, facial pain, headache, and trismus, all of which are self-limiting. Care must be taken to avoid the distal branches of the scalp, because poor skin healing may occur. If embolization is performed in these vessels, the main trunks distal to the tumor feeder should be protected first with reabsorbable embolic material such as gelatin sponge pledgets. More severe complications, including cranial nerve palsies [132], blindness [133], and stroke may occur, but most of these mishaps are due to inappropriate embolic agent selection, reflux of the emboli into the internal carotid circulation, or failure to recognize dangerous anastomoses [22]. Rare events include aspiration pneumonia due to aggravation of preexisting cranial nerve dysfunction [132], pulmonary embolism from migration of embolic material to the lungs [132], hemorrhage into the tumor bed [134], and carotid sinus syndrome during manipulation of the carotid sinus [135].

REFERENCES

1. Mehra YN, Mann SBS, Dubey SP, et al. Computed tomography for determining pathways of extension and a staging and treatment system for juvenile angiofibromas. *Ear Nose Throat J* 1989; 68:576–589.
2. Davis KR. Embolization of epistaxis and juvenile nasopharyngeal angiofibromas. *AJNR Am J Neuroradiol* 1986;7:953–962.
3. Buetow PC, Smirniotopoulos JG, Wenig BM. Pediatric sinonasal tumors. *Appl Radiol* 1993;22:21–28.
4. Edner G, Anniko M, Hindmarsch T, et al. Balloon embolization of the sphenopalatine artery in a case of a juvenile angiofibroma. *Arch Otorhinolaryngol* 1982;234:225–233.
5. Weprin LS, Siemers PT. Spontaneous regression of juvenile nasopharyngeal angiofibroma. *Arch Otolaryngol Head Neck Surg* 1991;117:796–799.
6. Bryan NR, Sessions RB, Horowitz BL. Radiographic management of juvenile angiofibromas. *AJNR Am J Neuroradiol* 1981; 2:157–166.

7. Gantz B, Seid AB, Weber RS. Nasopharyngeal angiofibroma. *Head Neck* 1992;14:67–71.
8. Paris J, Guelfucci B, Moulin G, et al. Diagnosis and treatment of juvenile nasopharyngeal angiofibromas. *Eur Arch Otorhinolaryngol* 2001;258:120–124.
9. Radkowski D, McGill T, Healy GB, et al. Angiofibroma. Changes in staging and treatment. *Arch Otolaryngol Head Neck Surg* 1996;122:122–129.
10. Ungkanont K, Byers RM, Weber RS, et al. Juvenile nasopharyngeal angiofibroma: an update of therapeutic management. *Head Neck* 1996;18:60–66.
11. Som PM. Clinical radiology quiz. *Am J Otolaryngol* 1990;11: 355–356.
12. Deschler DG, Kaplan MJ, Boles R. Treatment of large juvenile nasopharyngeal angiofibroma. *Otolaryngol Head Neck Surg* 1992;106:278–284.
13. Fields JN, Halverson KJ, Devineni VR, et al. Juvenile nasopharyngeal angiofibroma: efficacy of radiation therapy. *Radiology* 1990;176:263–265.
14. Gullane PJ, Davidson J, O'Dwyer T, et al. Juvenile angiofibroma: a review of the literature and a case series report. *Laryngoscope* 1992;102:928–933.
15. Garcia-Cervigon E, Bien S, Rufenacht D, et al. Pre-operative embolization of naso-pharyngeal angiofibromas. *Neuroradiology* 1988;30:556–560.
16. Gates GA, Rice DH, Koopmann CF, et al. Flutamide-induced regression of angiofibroma. *Laryngoscope* 1992;102:641–644.
17. Jacobsson M, Petruson B, Ruth M, et al. Involution of juvenile nasopharyngeal angiofibroma with intracranial extension: a case report with computed tomographic assessment. *Arch Otolaryngol* 1989;115:238–239.
18. Dohar JE, Duvall AJ. Spontaneous regression of juvenile nasopharyngeal angiofibroma. *Ann Otol Rhinol Laryngol* 1992;101: 469–471.
19. Fagan JJ, Snyderman CH, Carrau RL, et al. Nasopharyngeal angiofibromas: selecting a surgical approach. *Head Neck* 1997; 19:391–399.
20. Jorissen M, Eloy P, Rombaux P, et al. Endoscopic sinus surgery for juvenile nasopharyngeal angiofibromas. *Acta Otorhinolaryngol Belg* 2000;54:201–219.
21. Siniluoto TMJ, Luotonen JP, Tikkakoski TA, et al. Value of pre-operative embolization in surgery for nasopharyngeal angiofibroma. *J Laryngol Otolaryngol* 1993;107:514–521.
22. Lasjaunias P. Nasopharyngeal angiofibromas: hazards of embolization. *Neuroradiology* 1980;136:119–123.
23. Moulin G, Chagnaud C, Gras R, et al. Juvenile nasopharyngeal angiofibroma: comparison of blood loss during removal in embolized group versus nonembolized group. *Cardiovasc Intervent Radiol* 1995;18:158–161.
24. Gruber A, Bavinzski G, Killer M, et al. Preoperative embolization of hypervascular skull base tumors. *Minim Invasive Neurosurg* 2000;43:62–71.
25. Tranbahuy P, Borsik M, Herman P, et al. Direct intratumoral embolization of juvenile angiofibroma. *Am J Otolaryngol* 1994; 15:429–435.
26. Gulya AJ. The glomus tumor and its biology. *Laryngoscope* 1993;103:7–15.
27. Carrasco V, Rosenman J. Radiation therapy of glomus jugulare tumors. *Laryngoscope* 1993;103:23–27.
28. Jackson CG. Diagnosis for treatment planning and treatment options. *Laryngoscope* 1993;103:17–22.
29. McPherson GAD, Halliday AW, Mansfield AO. Cervical paragangliomas: diagnosis and management in 25 patients. *Br J Surg* 1989;76:33–36.
30. O'Leary MJ, Shelton C, Giddings NA, et al. Glomus tympanicum tumors: a clinical perspective. *Laryngoscope* 1991;101: 1038–1043.
31. LaMurgalia GM, Fabian RL, Brewster CD, et al. The current surgical management of carotid body paragangliomas. *J Vasc Surg* 1992;15:1038–1045.
32. Curtin HD. Radiologic approach to paragangliomas of the temporal bone. *Radiology* 1984;150:837–838.
33. Lo WWM, Solti-Bohman G, Lambert PR. High-resolution CT in the evaluation of glomus tumors of the temporal bone. *Radiology* 1984;150:737–742.
34. Chakeres DW, LaMasters L. Paragangliomas of the temporal bone: high-resolution CT studies. *Radiology* 1984;150: 749–753.
35. Olsen WL, Dillon WP, Kelly WM, et al. MR imaging of paragangliomas. *AJR Am J Radiol* 1987;148:201–204.
36. Derchi LE, Serafini G, Rabbia C, et al. Carotid body tumors: US evaluation. *Radiology* 1992;182:457–459.
37. Moret J, Delvert G, Lasjaunias P. Vascular architecture of tympanojugular glomus tumor. Its application regarding therapeutic angiography. *J Neuroradiol* 1982;9:237–260.
38. Jordan CE, Newton TH. Internal carotid artery supply to temporal bone chemodectomas. *Neuroradiology* 1975;8:253–257.
39. Ward PH, Liu C, Viñuela F, et al. Embolization: an adjunctive measure for removal of carotid body tumors. *Laryngoscope* 1988; 98:1287–1291.
40. Somasundar P, Krouse R, Hostetter R, et al. Paragangliomas: a decade of clinical experience. *J Surg Oncol* 2000:74:286–290.
41. Wax MK, Briant DR. Carotid body tumors: a review. *J Otolaryngol* 1992;21:277–285.
42. Robison JG, Shagets FW, Beckett WC Jr, et al. A multidisciplinary approach to reducing morbidity and operative blood loss during resection of carotid body tumor. *Surg Gynecol Obstet* 1989;168:166–170.
43. Liapis CD, Evangelidakis EL, Papavassiliou VG, et al. Role of malignancy and preoperative embolization in the management of carotid body tumors. *World J Surg* 2000;24:1526–1530.
44. Wang SJ, Wang MB, Barauskas TM, et al. Surgical management of carotid body tumors. *Otolaryngol Head Neck Surg* 2000;123: 202–206.
45. Tikkakoski T, Luotonen J, Leinonen S, et al. Preoperative embolization in the management of neck paragangliomas. *Laryngoscope* 1997;107:821–826.
46. Marangos N, Schumacher M. Facial palsy after glomus jugulare tumor embolization. *J Laryngol Otol* 1999;113:268–270.
47. Batsakis JG. *Tumors of the head and neck,* 2nd ed. Baltimore: Williams & Wilkins, 1979:313–326.
48. Gore DO, Rankow R, Hanford JM. Peripharyngeal neurilemmoma. *Surg Gynecol Obstet* 1956;103:193.
49. Silver AJ, Mawad ME, Hilal SK, et al. Computed tomography of the carotid space and related cervical spaces. Part II: neurogenic tumors. *Radiology* 1984;150:729–735.
50. Moscow NP, Newton TH. Angiographic features of hypervascular neurinomas of the head and neck. *Radiology* 1975;114: 635–640.
51. Abramowitz J, Dion JE, Jensen ME, et al. Angiographic diagnosis and management of head and neck schwannomas. *AJNR Am J Neuroradiol* 1991;12:977–984.
52. Laredo J, Reizine D, Bard M, et al. Vertebral hemangiomas: radiologic evaluation. *Radiology* 1986;161:183–189.
53. Raco A, Ciappetta P, Artico M, et al. Vertebral hemangiomas with cord compression: the role of embolization in five cases. *Surg Neurol* 1990, 34:164–168.
54. Picard L, Bracard S, Roland J, et al. Embolization of vertebral hemangiomas. Technique, indications, results. *Neurochirurgie* 1989;35:289–293.
55. Schnyder P, Fankhauser H, Mansouri B. Computed tomogra-

phy in spinal hemangioma with cord compression. Report of two cases. *Skeletal Radiol* 1986;15:372–375.
56. Ross JS, Masaryk TJ, Modic MT, et al. Vertebral hemangiomas: MR imaging. *Radiology* 1987;165:165–169.
57. Price HI, Batnitzky S. The computed tomographic findings in benign diseases of the vertebral column. *Crit Rev Diagn Imaging* 1985;24:39–89.
58. Nguyen JP, Djindjian M, Gaston A, et al. Vertebral hemangiomas presenting with neurologic symptoms. *Surg Neurol* 1987; 27:391–397.
59. Nicola N, Lins E. Vertebral hemangioma: retrograde embolization-stabilization with methyl methacrylate. *Surg Neurol* 1987; 27:481–486.
60. Jayakumar PN, Vasudev MK, Srikanth SG. Symptomatic vertebral haemangioma: endovascular treatment of twelve patients. *Spinal Cord* 1997;35:624–628.
61. Ng VW, Clifton A, Moore AJ. Preoperative endovascular embolization of a vertebral hemangioma. *J Bone Joint Surg Br* 1999; 79:808–811.
62. Cotten A, Deramond H, Cortet B, et al. Preoperative percutaneous injection of methyl methacrylate and N-butyl cyanoacrylate in vertebral hemangiomas. *AJNR Am J Neuroradiol* 1996;17: 137–142.
63. Gross CE, Hodge CJ, Binet EF, et al. Relief of spinal block during embolization of a vertebral body hemangioma. *J Neurosurg* 1976;45:404–406.
64. Hekster REM, Luyendijk W, Tan TI. Spinal cord compression caused by vertebral hemangioma relieved by percutaneous catheter embolization. *Neuroradiology* 1972;3:160–164.
65. Silva ML, Brunelle F. Embolisation of vascular lesions of the spinal column in childhood: a report of three cases. *Neuroradiology* 1996:38;809–811.
66. Hekster RE, Endtz LJ. Spinal-cord compression caused by vertebral haemangioma relieved by percutaneous catheter embolisation: 15 years later. *Neuroradiology* 1987;29:101.
67. Heiss JD, Doppman JL, Oldfield EH. Brief report: relief of spinal cord compression from vertebral hemangioma by intralesional injection of absolute ethanol. *N Engl J Med* 1994;331: 508–511.
68. Heiss JD, Doppman JL, Oldfield EH. Treatment of vertebral hemangioma by intralesional injection of absolute ethanol. *N Engl J Med* 1996;334:1340.
69. Deramond H, Depriester C, Toussaint P, et al. Percutaneous vertebroplasty. *Semin Musculoskelet Radiol* 1997;1:285–296.
70. Nguyen JP, Djindjian M, Pavlovitch JM, et al. Vertebral hemangioma with neurologic signs. Therapeutic results. Survey of the French Society of Neurosurgery. *Neurochirurgie* 1989;35: 299–303, 305–308.
71. Cory DA, Fritsch SA, Cohen MD, et al. Aneurysmal bone cysts: imaging findings and embolotherapy. *AJR Am J Radiol* 1989; 153:369–373.
72. Dysart SH, Swengel RM, van Dam BE. Aneurysmal bone cyst of a thoracic vertebra. *Spine* 1992;17:846–848.
73. Caro PA, Mandell GA, Stanton RP. Aneurysmal bone cyst of the spine in children. MRI imaging at 0.5 tesla. *Pediatr Radiol* 1991;21:114–116.
74. DeDios AM, Bond JR, Shives TC, et al. Aneurysmal bone cyst: a clinicopathologic study of 238 cases. *Cancer* 1992;69: 2921–2931.
75. Sullivan RJ, Meyer JS, Dormans JP, et al. Diagnosing aneurysmal and unicameral bone cysts with magnetic resonance imaging. *Clin Orthop* 1999;366:186–190.
76. Disch SP, Grubb RL, Gado MH, et al. Aneurysmal bone cyst of the cervicothoracic spine: computed tomography evaluation of the value of preoperative embolization. *Neurosurgery* 1986; 19:290–293.
77. DiChristofaro R, Biagini R, Boriani S, et al. Selective arterial embolization in the treatment of aneurysmal bone cyst and angioma of bone. *Skeletal Radiol* 1992;21:523–527.
78. Adamsbaum C, Kalifa G, Seringe R, et al. Direct Ethibloc injection in benign bone cysts: preliminary report on four patients. *Skeletal Radiol* 1993;22:317–320.
79. Konya A, Szendroi M. Aneurysmal bone cysts treated by superselective embolization. *Skeletal Radiol* 1992;21:167–172.
80. Chuang VP, Soo CS, Wallace S, et al. Arterial occlusion: management of giant cell tumor and aneurysmal bone cyst. *AJR Am J Radiol* 1981;136:1127–1130.
81. DeRosa GP, Graziano GP, Scott J. Arterial embolization of aneurysmal bone cyst of the spine. *J Bone Joint Surg Am* 1990; 72:777–780.
82. Boriani S, Delure F, Campanacci L, et al. Aneurysmal bone cyst of the mobile spine. *Spine* 2001;26:27–35.
83. Rossi C, Ricci S, Boriani S, et al. Percutaneous transcatheter arterial embolization of bone and soft tissue tumors. *Skeletal Radiol* 1990;19:555–560.
84. Szendroi M, Cser I, Konya A, et al. Aneurysmal bone cyst. A review of 52 primary and 16 secondary cases. *Arch Orthop Trauma Surg* 1992;11:318–322.
85. Guibaud L, Herbreteau D, Dubois H, et al. Aneurysmal bone cysts: percutaneous embolization with an alcoholic solution of zein: series of 18 cases. *Radiology* 1998;208:369–373.
86. Szendroi M, Antal I, Liska GY, et al. Calcitonin therapy of aneurysmal bone cysts. *J Cancer Res Clin Oncol* 1992;119: 61–65.
87. Papagelopoulos P, Currier B, Shaughnessy S, et al. Aneurysmal bone cyst of the spine. Management and outcome. *Spine* 1998; 23:621–628.
88. Kroon HM, Schurmans J. Osteoblastoma: clinical and radiologic findings in 98 new cases. *Radiology* 1990;175:783–790.
89. Ohkawa M, Fujiwara N, Tanabe M, et al. Benign osteoblastoma of the temporal bone. *AJNR Am J Neuroradiol* 1997;18: 324–326.
90. Crouzet G, Mnif J, Vasdev A, et al. Osteoid osteoma of the spine: radiological aspects and value of arteriography: four cases. *J Neuroradiol* 1989;16:145–159.
91. Broaddus WC, Grady MS, Delashaw JB Jr, et al. Preoperative superselective arteriolar embolization: a new approach to enhance resectability of spinal tumors. *Neurosurgery* 1990;27: 755–759.
92. King GJ, Kostuik JP, McBroom RJ, et al. Surgical management of metastatic renal carcinoma of the spine. *Spine* 1991;16: 263–271.
93. Sundaresan N, Choi IS, Hughes JE, et al. Treatment of spinal metastases from kidney cancer by presurgical embolization and resection. *J Neurosurg* 1990;73:548–554.
94. Gellad FE, Sadato N, Numaguchi Y, et al. Vascular metastatic lesions of the spine: preoperative embolization. *Radiology* 1990; 76:683–686.
95. Olerud C, Johsson H Jr, Lofberg AM, et al. Embolization of spinal metastases reduces preoperative blood loss. 21 patients operated on for renal cell carcinoma. *Acta Orthop Scand* 1993; 64:9–12.
96. Kallmes D, Cloft H, Chadduck J, et al. Percutaneous deflation of a vertebral artery occlusion balloon that migrated to the axillary artery. *J Vasc Interv Radiol* 1997;8:809–812.
97. O'Reilly GV, Kleefield J, Klein LA, et al. Embolization of solitary spinal metastases from renal cell carcinoma: alternative therapy for spinal cord or nerve root compression. *Surg Neurol* 1989; 31:268–271.
98. Soo CS, Wallace S, Chuang VP, et al. Lumbar artery embolization in cancer patients. *Radiology* 1982;145:655–659.
99. Chiras J, Cognard C, Rose M, et al. Percutaneous injection of

an alcoholic embolizing emulsion as an alternative preoperative embolization for spine tumor. *AJNR Am J Neuroradiol* 1993; 14:1113–1117.

100. Kaemmerlen P, Thiesse P, Bouvard H, et al. Percutaneous vertebroplasty in the treatment of metastases. Technic and results. *J Radiol* 1989;70:557–562.
101. Weill A, Chiras J, Simon JM, et al. Spinal metastases: indications for and results of percutaneous injection of acrylic surgical cement. *Radiology* 1996;199:241–247.
102. Cotten A, Dewatre F, Cortet B, et al. Percutaneous vertebroplasty for osteolytic metastases and myeloma: effects of the percentage of lesion filling and the leakage of methyl methacrylate at clinical follow-up. *Radiology* 1996;200:525–530.
103. Latchaw RE, Gold LH. Polyvinyl foam embolization of vascular and neoplastic lesions of the head, neck, and spine. *Radiology* 1979;131:669–679.
104. TerBrugge KG, Lasjaunias P, Chiu MC. Super-selective angiography and embolization of skull base tumors. *Can J Neurol Sci* 1985;12:341–344.
105. Valvanis A. Preoperative embolization of the head and neck: indications, patient selection, goals, and precautions. *AJNR Am J Neuroradiol* 1986;7:943–952.
106. Russell EJ. Functional angiography of the head and neck. *AJNR Am J Neuroradiol* 1986;7:927–936.
107. Theron J, Cosgrove R, Melanson D, et al. Embolization with temporary balloon occlusion of the internal carotid or vertebral arteries. *Neuroradiology* 1986;28:246–253.
108. Mehta BA, Jack CR Jr, Boulos RS, et al. Interventional neuroradiology: Henry Ford Hospital experience with transcatheter embolization of vascular lesions in the head, neck, and spine. *Henry Ford Hosp Med J* 1986;34:19–30.
109. Forbes G, Earnest F, Jackson IT, et al. Therapeutic embolization angiography for extra-axial lesions in the head. *Mayo Clin Proc* 1986;61:427–441.
110. Platzbecker H, Kohler K. Embolization in the head and neck region. *Acta Radiol Suppl* 1991;377:25–26.
111. Jensen ME. Endovascular treatment of vascular pathology of the head and neck. *Semin Interv Radiol* 1994;11:21–36.
112. Greenberg J. *Handbook of head and spine trauma.* New York: Marcel Dekker, 1993:227.
113. Horton JA, Kerber CW. Lidocaine injection into external carotid branches: provocative test to preserve cranial nerve function in therapeutic embolization. *AJNR Am J Neuroradiol* 1986; 7:105–108.
114. Horton JA, Dawson RC. Retinal wada test. *AJNR Am J Neuroradiol* 1988;9:1167–1168.
115. Doppman JL, Girton M, Oldfield EH. Spinal wada test. *Radiology* 1986;161:319–321.
116. Gonzalez CF, Moret J. Balloon occlusion of the carotid artery prior to surgery for neck tumors. *AJNR Am J Neuroradiol* 1990; 11:649–652.
117. Mathis JM, Barr JD, Horton JA. Therapeutic occlusion of major vessels, test occlusion and techniques. *Neurosurg Clin N Am* 1994;5:393–401.
118. Meyers PM, Thakur GA, Tomsick TA. Temporary endovascular balloon occlusion of the internal carotid artery with a nondetachable silicone balloon catheter: analysis of technique and cost. *AJNR Am J Neuroradiol* 1999;20:559–564.
119. Russell EJ, Goldberg K, Oskin J, et al. Ocular ischemic syndrome during carotid balloon occlusion testing. *AJNR Am J Neuroradiol* 1994;15:258–262.
120. Erba SM, Horton JA, Latchaw RE, et al. Balloon test occlusion of the internal carotid artery with stable xenon/CT cerebral blood flow imaging. *AJNR Am J Neuroradiol* 1988;9:533–537.
121. Monsein LH, Jeffrey PJ, van Heerden BB, et al. Assessing adequacy of collateral circulation during balloon test occlusion of the internal carotid artery with ^{99m}Tc-HMPAO SPECT. *AJNR Am J Neuroradiol* 1991;12:1045–1051.
122. Peterman SB, Taylor A Jr, Hoffman JC Jr. Improved detection of cerebral hypoperfusion with internal carotid balloon test occlusion and ^{99m}Tc-HMPAO cerebral perfusion SPECT imaging. *AJNR Am J Neuroradiol* 1991;12:1035–1041.
123. Berenstein A, Kricheff II. Catheter and material selection for transarterial embolization: technical considerations. I. Catheters. *Radiology* 1979;132:619–630.
124. Berenstein A, Kricheff II. Catheter and material selection for transarterial embolization: technical considerations. II. Materials. *Radiology* 1979;132:631–639.
125. Kunstlinger F, Brunelle F, Chaumont P, et al. Vascular occlusive agents. *AJR Am J Radiol* 1981;136:151–156.
126. Lasjaunias P, Berenstein A. Technical aspects of surgical neuroangiography. In: *Surgical neuroangiography.* Vol 1. Berlin: Springer-Verlag, 1987:1–56.
127. Dion JE. Principles and methodology. In: Viñuela F, Halbach VV, Dion JE, eds. *Interventional neuroradiology.* New York: Raven Press, 1992:1–15.
128. Kerber CW. Flow-controlled therapeutic embolization: a physiologic and safe technique. *AJR Am J Radiol* 1980;134:557–561.
129. Kerber CW. Catheter therapy: fluoroscopic monitoring of deliberate embolic occlusion. *Radiology* 1977;125:538–540.
130. Seeger JF, Gabrielsen TO, Latchaw RE. Some technique-dependent patterns of collateral flow during cerebral angiography. *Neuroradiology* 1974;8:149–155.
131. Chaloupka JC, Mangla S, Huddle DC, et al. Evolving experience with direct puncture therapeutic embolization for adjunctive and palliative management of head and neck hypervascular neoplasms. *Laryngoscope* 1999;109:1864–1872.
132. Bentson J, Rand R, Calcaterra T, et al. Unexpected complications following therapeutic embolization. *Neuroradiology* 1978; 16:420–423.
133. Mames RN, Snady-McCoy L, Guy J. Central retinal and posterior ciliary artery occlusion after particle embolization of the external carotid artery system. *Ophthalmology* 1991;98: 527–531.
134. Kallmes DF, Evans AJ, Kaptain GJ, et al. Hemorrhagic complications in embolization of a meningioma: case report and review of the literature. *Neuroradiology* 1997;39:877–880.
135. Eskridge JM, Harris AB, Finch L, et al. Carotid sinus syndrome and embolization procedures. *AJNR Am J Neuroradiol* 1993; 14:818–820.

Endovascular and Percutaneous Therapy of the Brain and Spine, edited by Michael P. Marks and Huy M. Do.
Lippincott Williams & Wilkins, Philadelphia © 2002.

15

CERVICOFACIAL VASCULAR ANOMALIES

PATRICIA E. BURROWS

Treatment of cervicofacial vascular anomalies is challenging, due both to technical limitations and incomplete understanding of their biology. Best results are achieved within multidisciplinary vascular anomalies centers, where practitioners are familiar with the complexities of diagnosis and treatment, and are able to offer up-to-date therapy. Recent developments in the field of vascular anomalies include discoveries regarding underlying genetic defects, identification of uncommon clinical variants, and recognition of new associations between vascular birthmarks and other developmental anomalies and effects. Appropriate treatment requires that the correct diagnosis is made. The biologic classification of vascular anomalies proposed by Mulliken and Glowacki consists of two major categories: tumors (hemangioma, hemangioendothelioma, and angiosarcoma) and vascular malformations (Table 15-1) [1]. This classification is supported by clinical, histologic, histochemical, and biochemical differences [1-4], as well as by angiography and modern cross-sectional imaging [5–11] and, in some instances, genetics [12]. Hemangiomas are proliferative endothelial cell tumors that typically are discovered in infancy, grow rapidly during the first year of life, and involute spontaneously. Vascular malformations are considered developmental anomalies and are further classified according to the channel abnormalities (arterial [AM], arteriovenous [AVM], capillary [CM], venous [VM], lymphatic [LM], combined malformation) or flow characteristics (high flow, low flow). The lesions can be distinguished readily by characteristic imaging findings on computed tomography (CT), magnetic resonance imaging (MRI), and angiography [5–8,11,13]. Interventional radiologic techniques, such as embolization and direct intralesional sclerosant injection, play an important role in the management of vascular anomalies [9, 14–21].

P.E. Burrows: Department of Radiology, Children's Hospital, Boston, Massachusetts.

BACKGROUND

Patient Evaluation and Imaging

On arrival, patients are evaluated in a multidisciplinary clinic whenever possible. Most anomalies can be diagnosed clinically. In questionable cases, application of a continuous-wave Doppler probe is a quick, inexpensive way to distinguish between low-flow and high-flow lesions. Likewise, ultrasonography can be used to characterize many of the superficial lesions.

Those patients with uncertain diagnosis or clinical indications for treatment are usually evaluated further by MRI. MRI protocol for vascular anomalies includes spin-echo sequences (T1-weighted sequences without and with intravenous gadolinium, and T2-weighted sequences), and gradient recall–echo sequences or magnetic resonance (MR) angiography to document the presence or absence of high-flow vessels [6,13,22,23]. MR venography is useful in slow-flow lesions, to identify anomalies of the facial and intracranial veins.

Ultrasonography, when combined with color Doppler imaging and Doppler spectral analysis of vascular channels, can be used to predict the tissue content and flow characteristics of vascular anomalies [10].

CT with intravenous contrast enhancement can be substituted for MRI, but it is generally less reliable in predicting tissue content and flow characteristics. Where MRI is available, CT is used to define osseous involvement and to demonstrate calcification (phleboliths).

Catheter angiography is generally reserved for patients in whom the specific diagnosis is not clear after noninvasive imaging (MRI), or patients who are undergoing transcatheter embolization. Angiographic findings are generally highly specific for the composition of hemovascular anomalies, but the extent of some lesions, especially low-flow malformations, may be much better seen with MRI.

Direct percutaneous cannulation and contrast injection into VMs, with angiographic filming (closed system venography), is usually performed at the same time as sclerother-

TABLE 15-1. BIOLOGIC CLASSIFICATION OF VASCULAR ANOMALIES

Vascular Tumors
Hemangiomas
Infantile
Proliferating
Involuting
Involuted
Congenital
Rapidly involuting
Noninvoluting
Kaposiform hemangioendothelioma
Angiosarcoma
Vascular Malformations
High flow
Arteriovenous malformations
Arteriovenous fistulas
Low flow
Capillary malformations
Venous malformations
Lymphatic malformations
Combined

apy (direct intralesional sclerosant injection). This technique most precisely delineates the angioarchitecture of low-flow vascular malformations.

Hemangiomas

Hemangiomas are the most common tumors of infancy, occurring in 12%. They are present at birth in only 40% of patients, often as a faint macular stain [2]. They are more common in females, whites, and premature infants. They usually appear within the first 1 to 3 months of life and demonstrate a phase of rapid growth due to endothelial cell proliferation. The proliferative phase usually levels off at about 9 or 10 months of age and is followed by a much slower phase of involution, which may take up to 10 years to be completed. Involution may occur much faster in congenital hemangiomas [24]. The clinical appearance of a hemangioma depends upon its depth and whether the lesion is in its proliferating or involuting phase. Superficial hemangiomas involving the skin surface have a characteristic strawberry-like appearance. Deep lesions may have normal overlying skin, or a bluish hue reflecting the draining veins. Hemangiomas are usually warm and may occasionally be pulsatile. During involution, the lesions become softer and less pulsatile, related to fibrofatty replacement.

In the proliferating phase, imaging findings include well-circumscribed, lobulated, uniformly enhancing lesions with dilated feeding and draining vessels. On MRI spin-echo sequences, the lesions are typically isointense or hypointense to muscle on T1-weighted imaging, and moderately hyperintense on T2-weighted imaging, with a lobulated configuration. Flow voids are seen within and around the mass on spin-echo images. Gradient imaging or MR angiography, demonstrates high-flow vessels. The hallmark of the hemangioma is the presence of an enhancing, homogeneous parenchymal mass, with evidence of high-flow vessels (Fig. 15-1). The presence of associated cerebrovascular and cerebral abnormalities should be established prior to treatment. Intravenous contrast injection is important to rule out malignant tumors and other masses that resemble hemangiomas.

Sonography, with Doppler interrogation, also demonstrates a parenchymal mass with high-flow vessels (low arterial resistance and increased venous velocity). Angiography is necessary only if embolization is considered and characteristically demonstrates a hypervascular mass with a dense, prolonged capillary blush and dilated feeding and draining vessels. During and after involution, the lesions become progressively replaced by fatty tissue, which is most readily demonstrated on CT.

Infrequent associated anomalies in patients with cervicofacial hemangiomas include cystic posterior fossa malformations, bifid sternum, right aortic arch, coarctation of the aorta, ocular and auricular anomalies, and intracranial arterial anomalies (e.g., persistent trigeminal artery, hypoplastic internal carotid artery) (Table 15-2) [25,26]. The term *PHACE syndrome* has been proposed to incorporate the association between *p*osterior fossa anomalies, facial *h*emangiomas, *a*rterial and *a*uricular anomalies, *c*ardiovascular defects, and *e*ye abnormalities [26]. A strong female predilection has also been noted in this neuroectodermal syndrome. Acute cerebrovascular occlusive disease, similar to idiopathic moyamoya phenomenon, has been seen in a small number of patients [27].

The differential diagnosis of hemangioma in an infant with a soft tissue mass and skin discoloration includes infantile fibrosarcoma, rhabdomyosarcoma, neurofibroma, nasal glioma, and vascular malformation. MRI features are usually distinguishable from hemangioma, but if there is any concern about the possibility of malignancy, biopsy is recommended.

Specific treatment of hemangiomas includes systemic or intralesional corticosteroids, angiogenesis inhibitors such as interferon, chemotherapy (vincristine or cyclophosphamide), radiotherapy, and laser and arterial embolization [9, 28,29]. Because most hemangiomas involute spontaneously with a satisfactory result, specific treatment is generally indicated only in endangering forms or locations, including ocular, airway, hepatic, and disseminated hemangiomas, and those associated with ulceration or congestive cardiac failure. Arterial embolization is rarely needed but is useful in patients with high-output cardiac failure or bleeding that is not responsive to medical management (Figs. 15-1 and 15-2). Early primary excision is advisable in some situations (e.g., hemangioma of the eyelid or scalp). Usually, plastic surgery is delayed until involution has occurred, to minimize the resulting scar. Central nervous system involvement

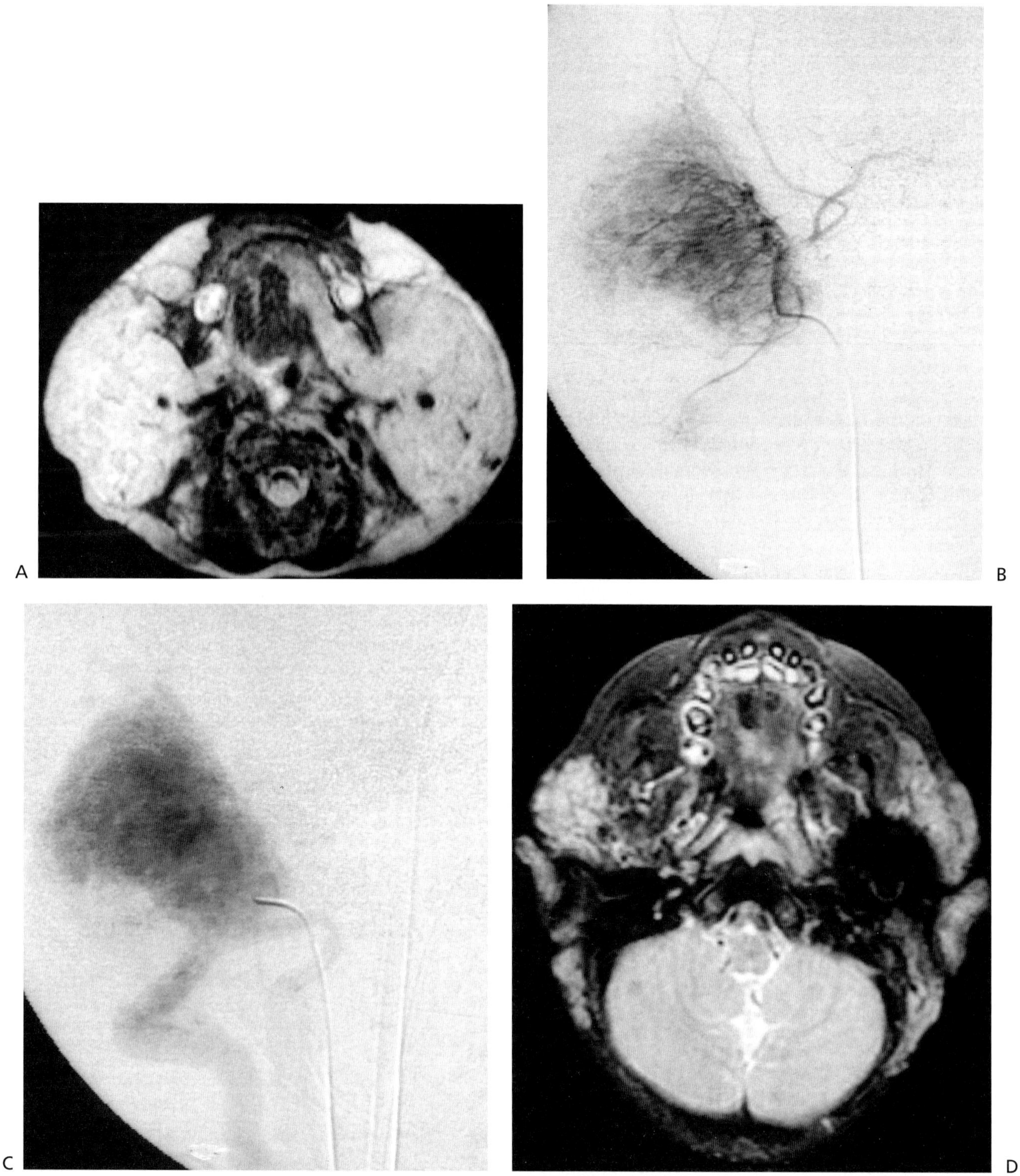

FIGURE 15-1. Embolization of bilateral parotid hemangiomas because of the development of mild congestive heart failure. **A:** Axial T2-weighted MR prior to embolization shows the large bilateral hyperintense masses with large vascular flow voids indicating draining veins. **B,C:** Right external carotid angiogram, arterial and parenchymal phases, frontal digital subtraction angiography shows a characteristic capillary blush of an infantile hemangioma, with a dense parenchymal stain and markedly dilated draining veins. The lesions were superselectively embolized with particles. The patient was also treated with interferon-α. **D:** Axial T2-weighted MRI 4 months after embolization shows significant regression of the hemangiomas.

TABLE 15-2. ASSOCIATIONS WITH HEMANGIOMAS

Female gender
White race
Prematurity
Sternal cleft
Right aortic arch
Coarctation of the aorta
Cervicocranial arterial anomalies (e.g., persistent trigeminal artery)
Intracranial arterial occlusions and aneurysms
Cystic malformations of the posterior fossa
Ocular and auricular anomalies
Spinal dysraphism
Genitourinary anomalies

is uncommon and is generally seen in contiguity with facial lesions, or in patients with disseminated hemangiomatosis.

Patients with Kasabach-Merritt syndrome demonstrate marked decrease in platelet counts (usually less than 10,000), with or without low levels of fibrinogen and other coagulation factors, due to consumption within the lesion. The soft tissue mass is usually kaposiform hemangioendothelioma, not infantile hemangioma [30]. Clinically, the lesions are most common on the trunk and extremities and usually present a characteristic rapid enlargement with edematous, purple skin discoloration. Imaging studies typically demonstrate high-flow, diffuse soft tissue masses with surrounding edema. These lesions are notoriously difficult to treat, but the coagulopathy resolves with successful treatment or spontaneous involution of the lesion. Pharmacologic treatment, similar to that used for hemangiomas, usually is tried first. If this fails, embolization may be performed, to try to improve the platelet count or prior to surgical resection. Clinical improvement does not always occur after embolization and, if it does, is usually transient. Intralesional sclerosant injection has been found to be useful in selected cases.

Vascular Malformations

Vascular malformations are errors of vascular morphogenesis. Although generally considered to be present at birth, they may be initially inapparent, becoming evident or symptomatic later in life. In general, they grow in proportion to the growth of the affected child but may increase in size secondary to hemodynamic changes such as increased blood flow (resulting in vessel elongation and dilatation), obstruction, or thrombosis. The evolution of individual lesions, especially high-flow lesions, may be stimulated by various factors including hormonal change (accelerated growth, puberty, pregnancy), trauma (including surgery and possibly embolization), and infection.

Vascular malformations are classified according to the channel abnormalities present and flow characteristics (see Table 15-1). High-flow vascular malformations include arteriovenous fistulas (AVFs), which have direct arteriovenous connection without intervening nidus, and AVMs, which consist of a plexiform collection of vessels (nidus) between feeding arteries and draining veins. Clinically, fast-flow lesions are characterized by increased temperature, soft tissue enlargement, and bruit or continuous sound on auscultation. Low-flow vascular malformations include CMs, VMs, LMs, and combined malformations.

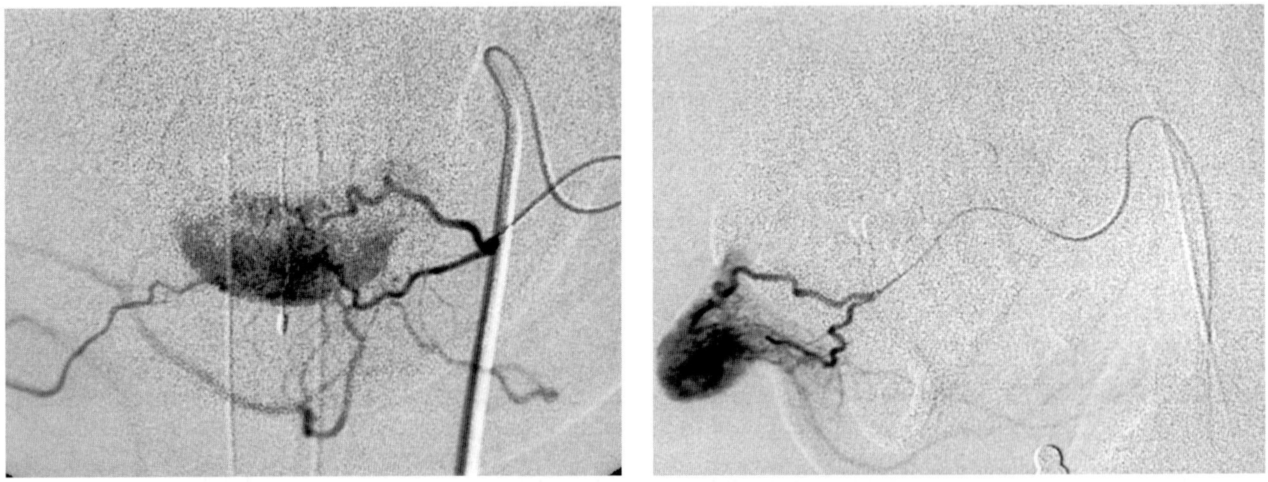

A B

FIGURE 15-2. Residual labial hemangioma in a 3-year-old girl. There was clinical confusion about the diagnosis, because the lesion had not regressed well on steroid treatment and was thought possibly to represent an AVM. Left inferior labial arteriogram, using a microcatheter, frontal **(A)** and lateral **(B)** projections, digital subtraction technique, shows the characteristic homogeneous parenchymal blush of a hemangioma, along with the dilated draining veins. The lesion was embolized with small particles and a contour resection was carried out on the following day. The histologic diagnosis of resected tissue confirmed the diagnosis of hemangioma.

Arteriovenous Malformations

Soft tissue (extracranial) AVM is rarely discrete but rather behaves more as a "field defect" in the head and neck, often crossing contiguous tissue planes. Except for extremely high-flow lesions, which may cause cardiac overload in infancy, most AVMs are asymptomatic in the first one to two decades of life. Clinical findings include local hyperthermia, pulsations, thrill, and bruit. The use of continuous-wave Doppler in the examining room is often helpful in detecting the vascular shunt before it is audible with a stethoscope. Evolution of these lesions often seems to be precipitated by hormonal factors (puberty, pregnancy, hormone therapy), trauma, infection, or surgery. A combination of arterial steal and venous hypertension results in tissue ischemia, ultimately leading to pain and skin ulceration, often associated with severe bleeding. Dental AVMs (e.g., those involving the maxilla, mandible, and oral cavity) are particularly dangerous, often associated with life-threatening hemorrhage related to tooth eruption, dental infection, and dental extraction. The Schobinger classification is useful to characterize the clinical stage of an AVM [31]. In stage I, cutaneous AVM initially demonstrates a superficial blush and warmth, with arteriovenous shunting detectable by continuous-wave Doppler. As it evolves, the color intensifies and tortuous, tense veins appear (stage II, expansion). Dystrophic changes, ulceration, bleeding, and persistent pain follow and characterize stage III. Cardiac overload (stage IV) may develop. In stages III and IV tissue damage is usually irreversible.

These lesions are characterized on CT, MRI, and ultrasonography by the presence of dilated feeding and draining vessels. The intervening nidus may or may not be visible, depending on the size of the channels. Unlike hemangioma, the lesion should not have an associated parenchymal mass, but some signal abnormalities, possibly related to a fibrofatty matrix or edema, may be evident on MRI. CT and MRI frequently show increased thickness of fat, increased size, and sometimes signal abnormality of affected muscle, and bony changes that include sclerosis, lytic defects, and signal change.

Angiography demonstrates variable degrees of arterial dilation and tortuosity, arteriovenous shunting, and dilated draining veins. In older patients, feeding arteries may have aneurysms. Discrete AVFs may be present within diffuse AVMs. Especially in young children, a discrete nidus often is not demonstrable.

Treatment of AVMs remains problematic. Most AVMs are not curable by existing techniques. Pharmacologic therapy is not useful. Surgical resection, after embolization, often combined with the use of tissue expanders and free flaps for resurfacing, is the standard of care but is associated with a high clinical recurrence rate [31]. Treatment must be planned carefully to avoid stimulating progression and interfering with future management. Close follow-up is essential, because AVMs may extend, especially after surgical intervention, into tissue that initially does not appear to be involved. Proximal ligation or embolization of feeding vessels must be avoided (Figs. 15-3 and 15-4). Superselective arterial embolization, using permanent embolic materials, may be indicated to decrease symptoms such as swelling, pain, bleeding, and ischemic ulceration [16,18,32,33]. Embolization with 100% ethanol has been proposed as an ablative procedure (Figs. 15-4 and 15-5) [34,35].

Treatment options correlate with clinical staging. Endovascular therapy is not feasible in stage I, because there is not enough shunting to distinguish AVM from normal tissue. In stages II and III, embolization can be used as the primary mode of treatment, or it can be performed prior to surgical resection [14,19,34–38].

A retrospective review of 81 patients with extracranial AVMs of the head and neck reported a 69% clinical "cure" rate for surgical excision (Schobinger clinical stages I and II) and a 62% cure rate for more extensive lesions incorporating embolotherapy prior to surgery [31]. Although it is generally acknowledged that preoperative embolization is helpful in minimizing blood loss, there is minimal published data regarding the effectiveness of primary embolization.

Arteriovenous Fistulas

Congenital cervicofacial AVFs are infrequently associated with high-output cardiac failure in neonates or young infants; most are diagnosed due to the presence of an audible bruit or pulsatile mass when physical examination is performed. They are most common in the neck but may occur in the deep face, scalp, or orbit. Congenital AVF is curable by appropriate endovascular procedures [9] and should generally be treated at the time of diagnosis.

Capillary Malformations

CMs involving the skin surface include port wine stain and telangiectasia. Facial port wine stains are often associated with progressive thickening of the skin and subcutaneous layers as well as overgrowth of the underlying facial skeleton, often resulting in facial asymmetry and dental malocclusion. Although most port wine stains are isolated vascular anomalies, they may signal an underlying deep vascular malformation or a more complex dysmorphogenesis. Approximately 1% to 2% of patients with port wine stains have Sturge-Weber syndrome. CM is often the predominant cutaneous element in combined vascular malformations. Currently, pulsed dye laser techniques are the standard treatment for isolated CMs. They are usually not effective in patients with combined vascular anomalies.

Venous Malformations

VMs have a variable clinical picture, depending upon depth and extent. Genetic defects related to Tie-2 receptor func-

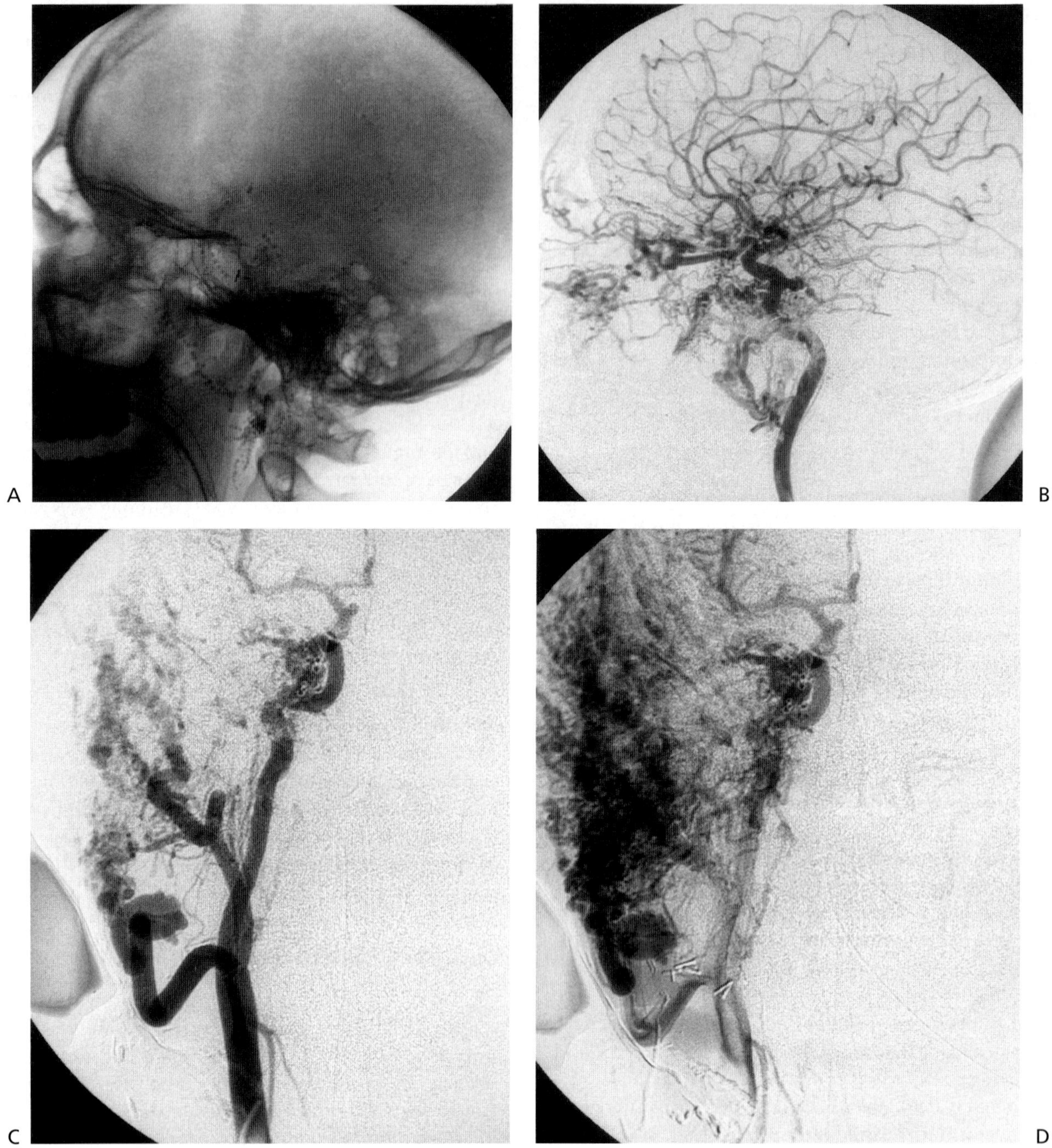

FIGURE 15-3. Schobinger stage III AVM of the right side of the face in a 20-year-old man who had undergone numerous embolization procedures as a child, as well as partial resection and resurfacing with a free flap. **A:** Lateral radiograph of the skull shows the microbeads throughout branches of the right external carotid artery. **B:** Lateral right internal carotid angiogram, digital subtraction technique, shows extensive collateral vessels from the ophthalmic and internal carotid arteries supplying the face and the facial AVM. **C,D:** Right common carotid angiogram, frontal projection, digital subtraction, showing the extensive residual intramuscular AVM. The patient underwent further surgery with a reasonably good result.

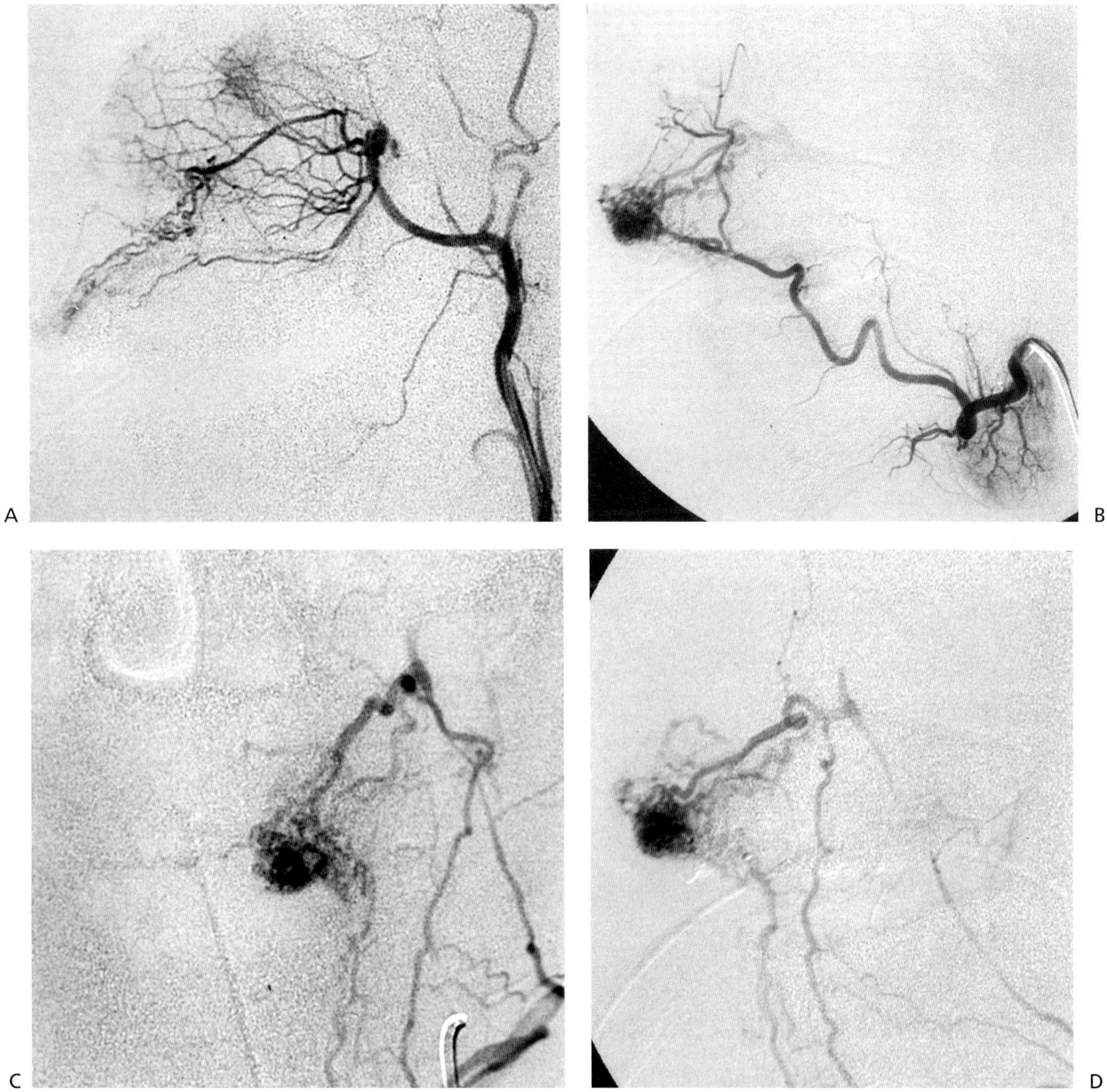

FIGURE 15-4. Focal AVM of the left upper lip, recurrence after prior surgical resection, in a 25-year-old woman. This has been treated by arterial and superselective embolization with absolute ethanol, in two stages, with a good result. **A:** Initial left distal external carotid angiogram shows some arterial supply from the infraorbital branch of the internal maxillary artery. **B:** Initial left lateral facial arteriogram shows a focal AVM in the left upper lip supplied by the superior labial artery and some alar branches. **C,D:** Selective angiography in the left superior labial artery, using a microcatheter, frontal and lateral projections, respectively, shows opacification of most of the AVM, as well as a normal-size continuation of the superior labial artery across the midline. Note the prominent draining veins. This vessel was embolized slowly, using absolute ethanol, with manual compression of the right side of the lip and the draining veins. *(Figure continues.)*

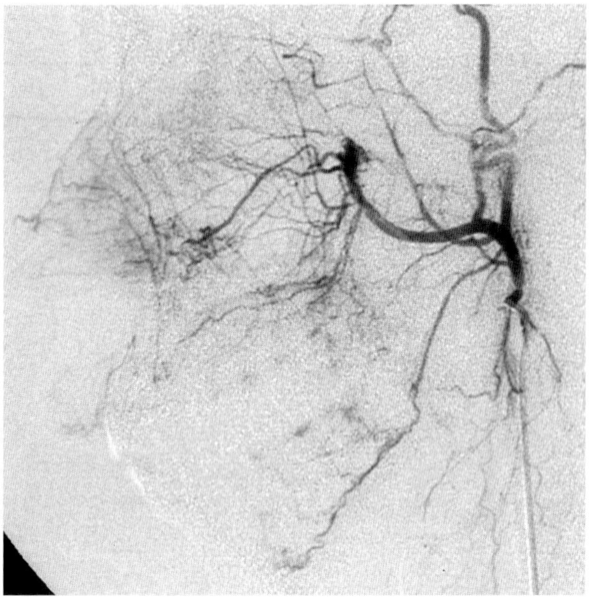
E

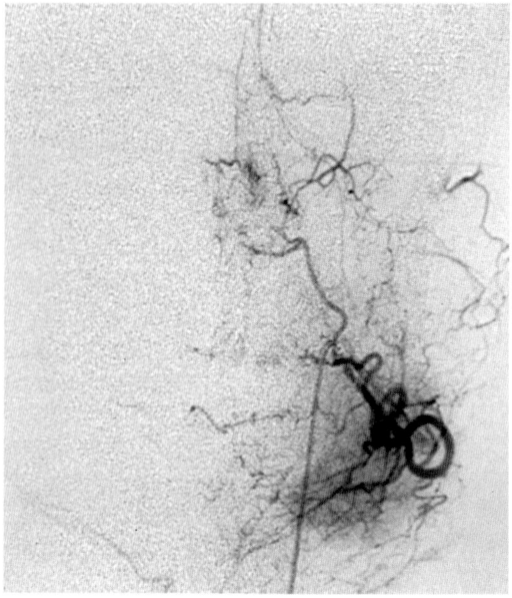
F

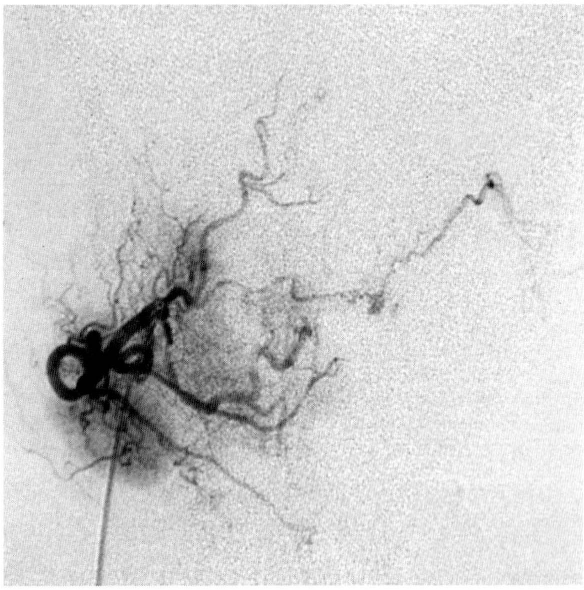
G

FIGURE 15-4. *Continued.* **E:** Repeat distal left external carotid angiogram, lateral projection, 9 months following embolization shows obliteration of the infraorbital arterial supply to the AVM. **F:** Left facial arteriogram, anterior projection, also shows no residual supply from the previously embolized left superior labial or ala arteries. **G:** Right facial arteriogram, anterior projection, shows a small arteriovenous fistula supplied by the right superior labial artery. **H:** Superselective contrast injection into the distal right superior labial artery with a microcatheter shows an AVM in the left side of the upper lip, draining into the originally seen veins. This site was embolized carefully with a small amount of absolute ethanol. **I:** Right facial arteriogram, following the second ethanol embolization, shows apparent control of the AVM. The soft tissue swelling regressed well, and the patient has required no further treatment.

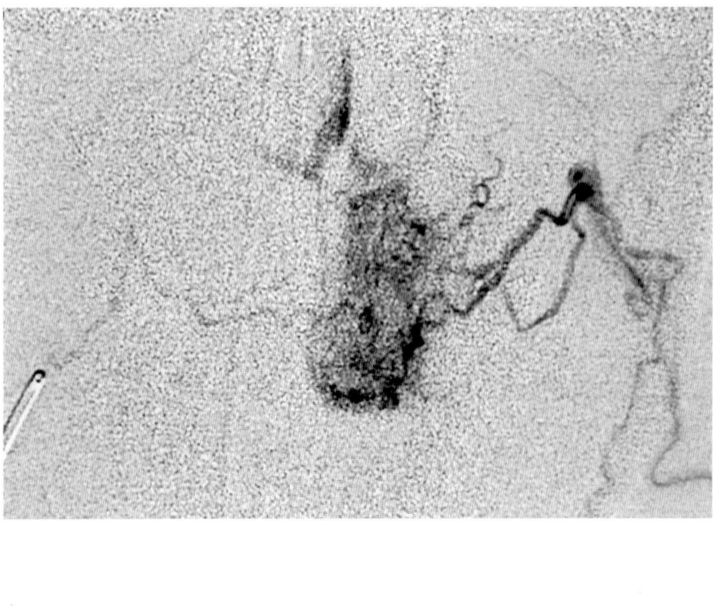
H

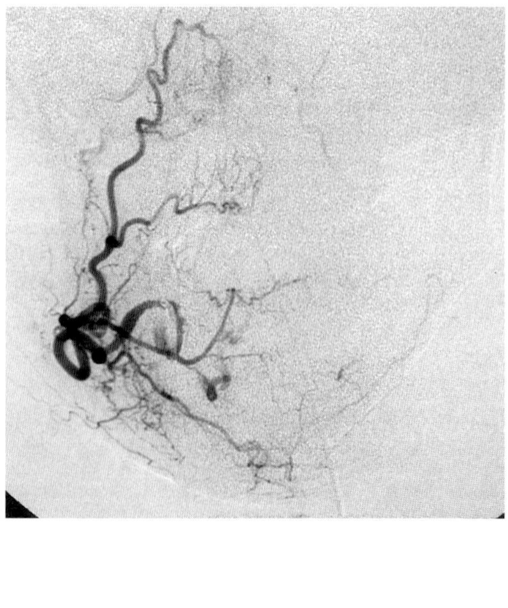
I

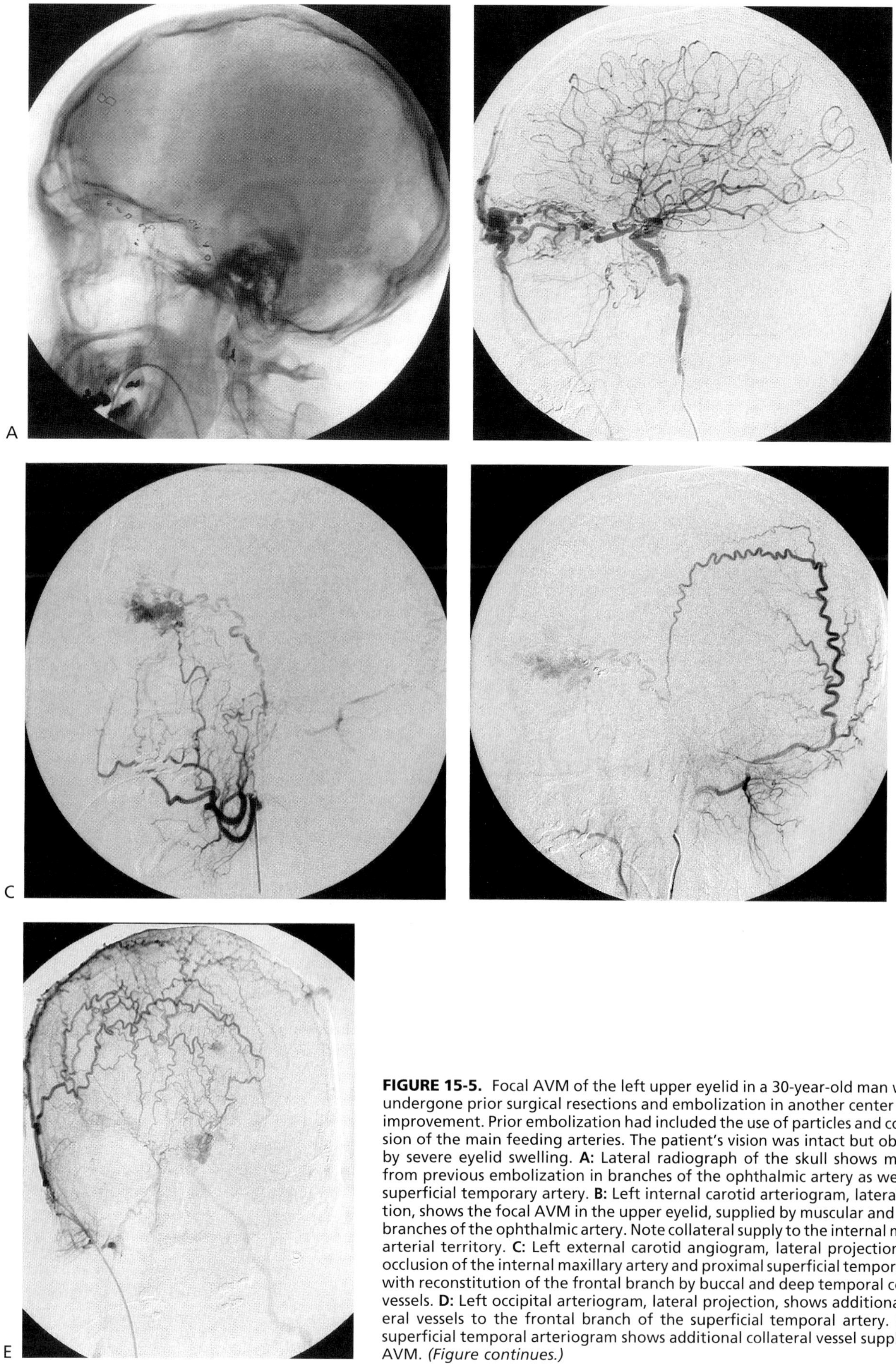

FIGURE 15-5. Focal AVM of the left upper eyelid in a 30-year-old man who had undergone prior surgical resections and embolization in another center without improvement. Prior embolization had included the use of particles and coil occlusion of the main feeding arteries. The patient's vision was intact but obstructed by severe eyelid swelling. **A:** Lateral radiograph of the skull shows microcoils from previous embolization in branches of the ophthalmic artery as well as the superficial temporary artery. **B:** Left internal carotid arteriogram, lateral projection, shows the focal AVM in the upper eyelid, supplied by muscular and lacrimal branches of the ophthalmic artery. Note collateral supply to the internal maxillary arterial territory. **C:** Left external carotid angiogram, lateral projection, shows occlusion of the internal maxillary artery and proximal superficial temporal artery with reconstitution of the frontal branch by buccal and deep temporal collateral vessels. **D:** Left occipital arteriogram, lateral projection, shows additional collateral vessels to the frontal branch of the superficial temporal artery. **E:** Right superficial temporal arteriogram shows additional collateral vessel supply to the AVM. *(Figure continues.)*

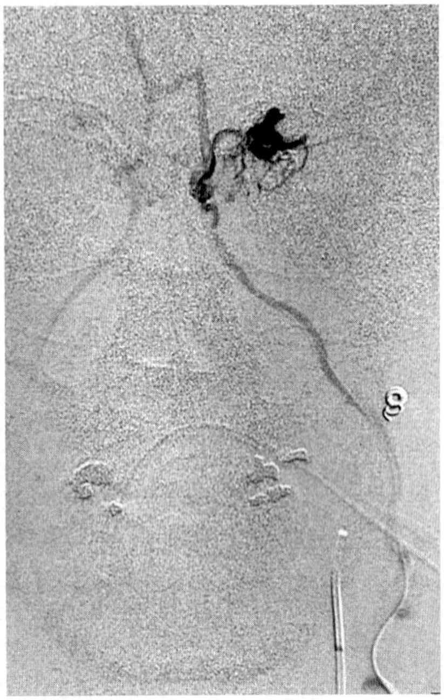

F

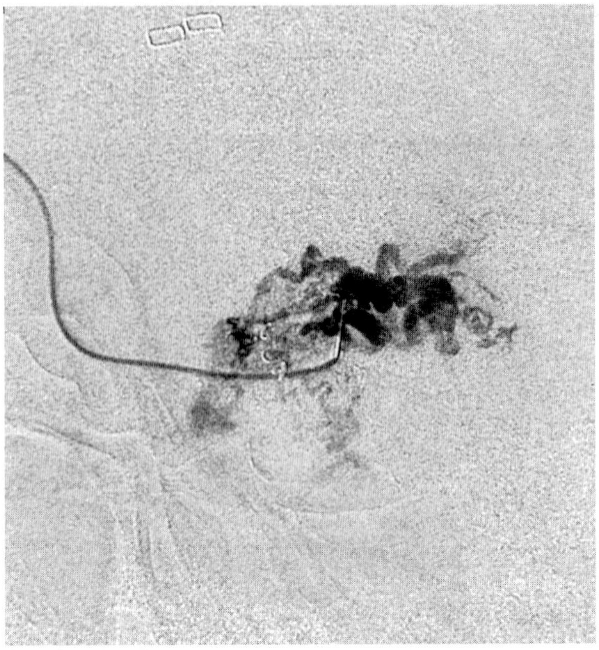

G

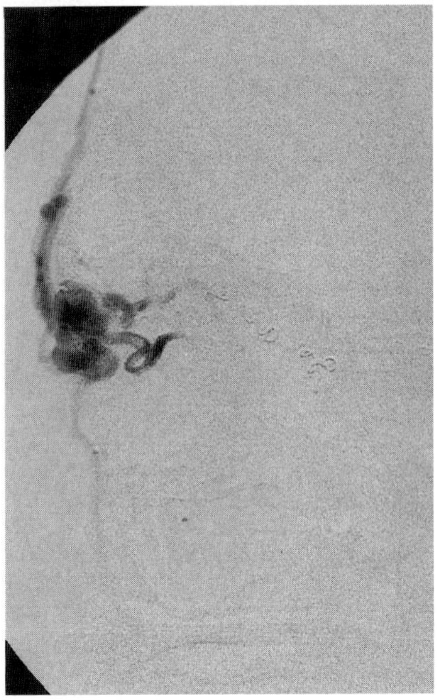

H

FIGURE 15-5. *Continued.* **F:** Attempted retrograde transfemoral catheterization of the nidus via the left facial vein, frontal projection. There is inadequate filling of the nidus for effective embolization. **G:** Direct contrast injection into the draining veins of the AVM, frontal projection. This site was injected with ethanol while arterial inflow from the superficial temporal artery was compressed manually. **H:** Selective catheterization of a supraorbital branch of the ophthalmic artery, lateral projection, shows direct AVF. This vessel was embolized with 5-mm fibered platinum microcoils followed by ethanol. *(Figure continues.)*

tion, associated with defective formation of the smooth muscle of the media, have been identified [12,39]. The lesions are typically soft and compressible and distend with Valsalva maneuver or venous compression. Many of these lesions appear as spongy collections of venous channels having variable communications with adjacent veins. Alternatively, some VMs represent varicosities or dysplasias of small and large venous channels. They may contain phleboliths. The overlying skin, when involved, is blue or purple in color. Most VMs are symptomatic with pain and swelling. Lesions involving the oral cavity may bleed, but this usually is not life-threatening. VMs can involve the airway, either intrinsically or by local compression. Extensive facial VMs are associated with intracranial developmental venous anomalies [40]. Midline facial VMs may be associated with intracranial venous anomalies and sinus pericranii.

MRI is the imaging modality of choice; characteristic findings include focal or diffuse collections of high T2 signal, often containing identifiable spaces of variable size separated by septations [5,6]. Small fluid–fluid levels may be

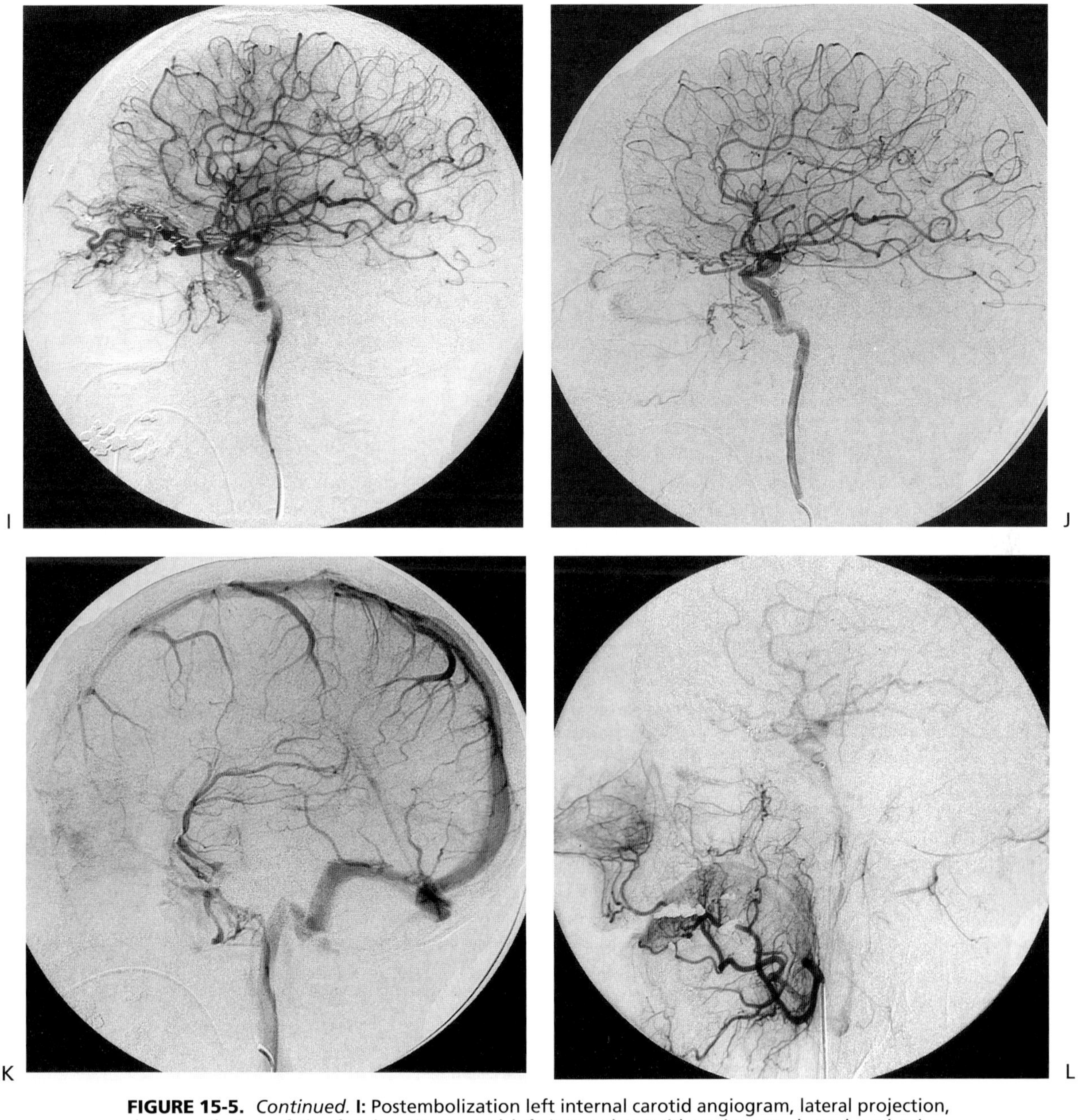

FIGURE 15-5. *Continued.* **I:** Postembolization left internal carotid angiogram, lateral projection, shows occlusion of the fistula. **J,K:** Control left internal carotid angiogram, lateral projection, arterial and venous phases, respectively, 2 months after the second ethanol embolization shows no residual AVM. *(Figure continues.)*

visible. Phleboliths may be evident as areas of signal void which are most prominent on gradient images. Flow-sensitive images demonstrate no high-flow vessels within or around the lesions. Contrast administration results in variable enhancement and is important for distinguishing VMs from LMs. Angiography is not necessary for diagnosis but typically shows either no filling of the malformation or delayed opacification of sinusoidal spaces with or without dysplastic draining veins. A small percentage of VMs have associated AVFs. Direct percutaneous cannulation of the malformation with contrast injection typically shows the interconnecting spaces and draining veins.

Treatment includes the use of aspirin (to decrease thrombosis), sclerotherapy, and surgical excision. Angiogenesis inhibitors are not effective. The erroneous diagnosis of cavernous hemangioma often leads to inappropriate treatment with drugs or even radiotherapy. Direct injection of sclerosant drugs, most commonly sodium tetradecyl sulfate (STS) or absolute ethanol, results in thrombosis and gradual shrinkage of the malformation and, in most vascular anoma-

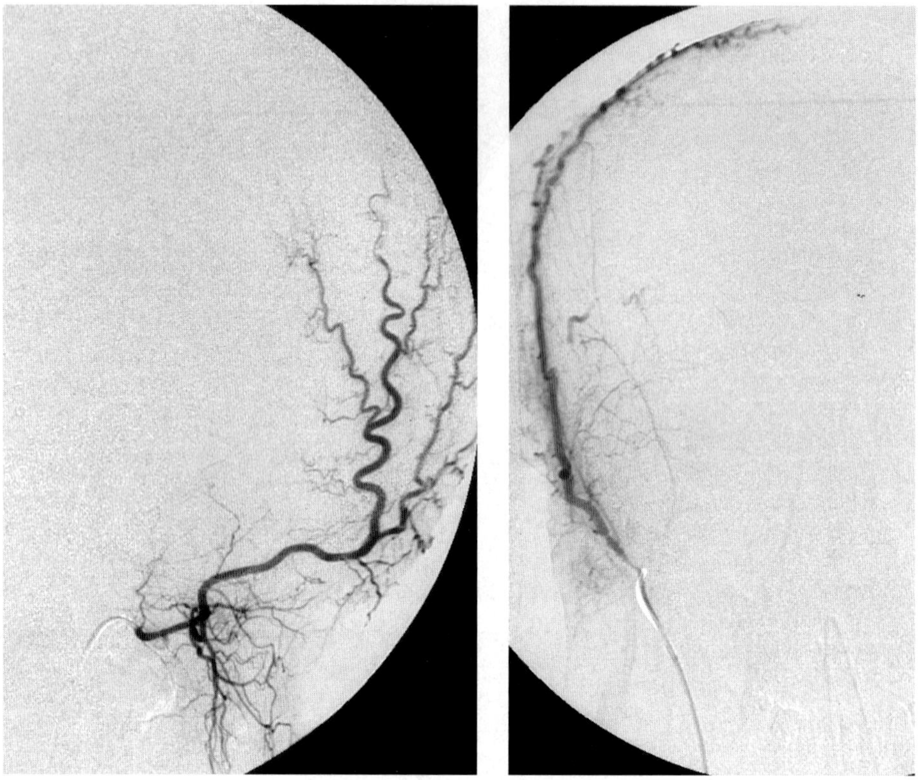

FIGURE 15-5. *Continued.* **L–N:** Left external carotid angiogram, lateral projection **(L)**; left occipital angiogram, lateral projection **(M)**; right superficial temporal arteriogram, frontal projection **(N)**: All show no evidence of arteriovenous shunting.

lies centers, is the preferred treatment [20,41–48]. Sclerotherapy usually is not curative but results in significant improvement in swelling and pain in most patients. Patients with diffuse lesions undergo an initial series of injection procedures, spaced 2 to 3 months apart, until the lesion is reduced in size as much as possible and no longer swells or refills on dependency (Fig. 15-6). Lesions involving the lips recur consistently and are best managed by contour resection after sclerotherapy [42,43]. Tracheotomy is often performed before embarking on treatment of extensive airway lesions.

Lymphatic Malformations

LMs can be classified as macrocystic (e.g., cystic hygroma) or microcystic. Those in the head and neck result from maldevelopment of the cervicofacial lymphatic system, which normally begins as paired jugular lymph sacs sprouting from the primitive jugular venous plexus in the 6-week-old embryo. The macrocystic types of LMs are believed to result from maldevelopment of the primitive jugular, subclavian, and axillary sacs, possibly by failure to reestablish venous connections. Interruption or obstruction of the peripheral lymphatic channels presumably results in diffuse or microcystic LMs. These lesions are usually evident at birth. The macrocystic lesions, most commonly located in the neck, axilla, and chest wall, may be massive, interfering with the birth process. Microcystic lesions usually appear as diffuse soft tissue thickening. The lesions typically grow proportionally with the child but undergo episodic swelling related to lymphatic congestion (e.g., with viral infections) or hemorrhage. Communication between the macrocystic LMs and adjacent veins frequently is present. Complications of cervicofacial LMs include sepsis and airway obstruction.

On physical examination, LMs have a rubbery or cystic consistency. Typically, they cannot be decompressed manually like VMs. The overlying skin or mucosa may manifest CM, vesicles, or both.

MRI findings in macrocystic LMs include cystic fluid collections, often with fluid–fluid levels, associated with rim or no contrast enhancement [49]. Evidence of blood may be present. Enlargement of adjacent veins, including the superior vena cava, are frequent in cervicofacial LMs. Microcystic LMs typically appear as diffuse areas of bright signal on T2-weighted spin-echo MRI, usually without contrast enhancement. The adjacent subcutaneous fat often has a lymphedema pattern. CT best demonstrates osseous distortion and overgrowth and shows the soft tissue component of the malformation to be of lower density than surrounding muscle.

The treatment of cervicofacial macrocystic LMs is generally by staged early surgical excision. Residual or recurrent

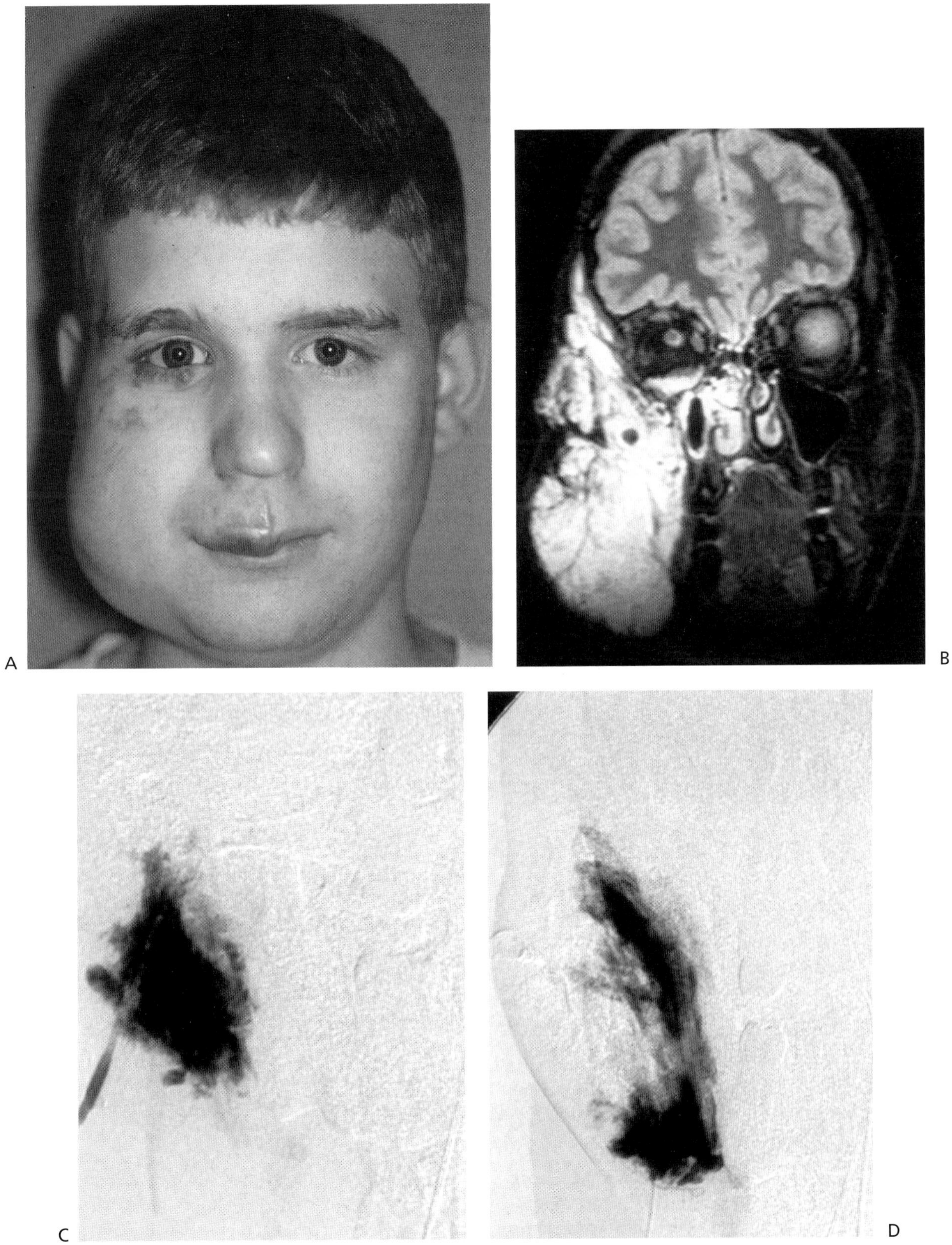

FIGURE 15-6. Diffuse VM of the right face, involves the exterior facial muscles as well as the subcutaneous soft tissues, skin, and upper lip. **A:** Patient at 17 years of age shows the right facial deformity, enlargement of the upper lip, cutaneous involvement especially on and near the lower eyelid, and a scar on the upper lip related to previous laser treatment. **B:** Coronal T2-weighted MRI shows the extensive T2 hyperintensity. The lesion on this image is mainly in the right temporalis and masseter muscle. Note the involvement of the lower eyelid and the large phlebolith. **C:** Direct contrast injection into the superficial muscular component of the right cheek, digital subtraction, frontal projection. **D:** Subsequent direct injection of the deeper masseter component following sclerosant injection into the more superficial lesion. *(Figure continues.)*

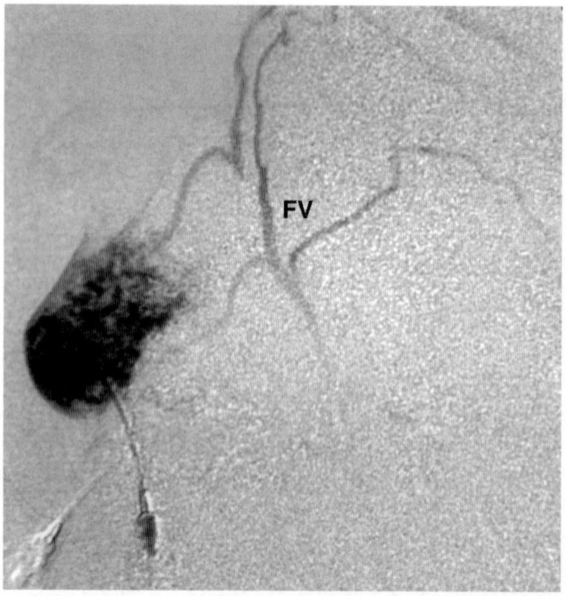

E

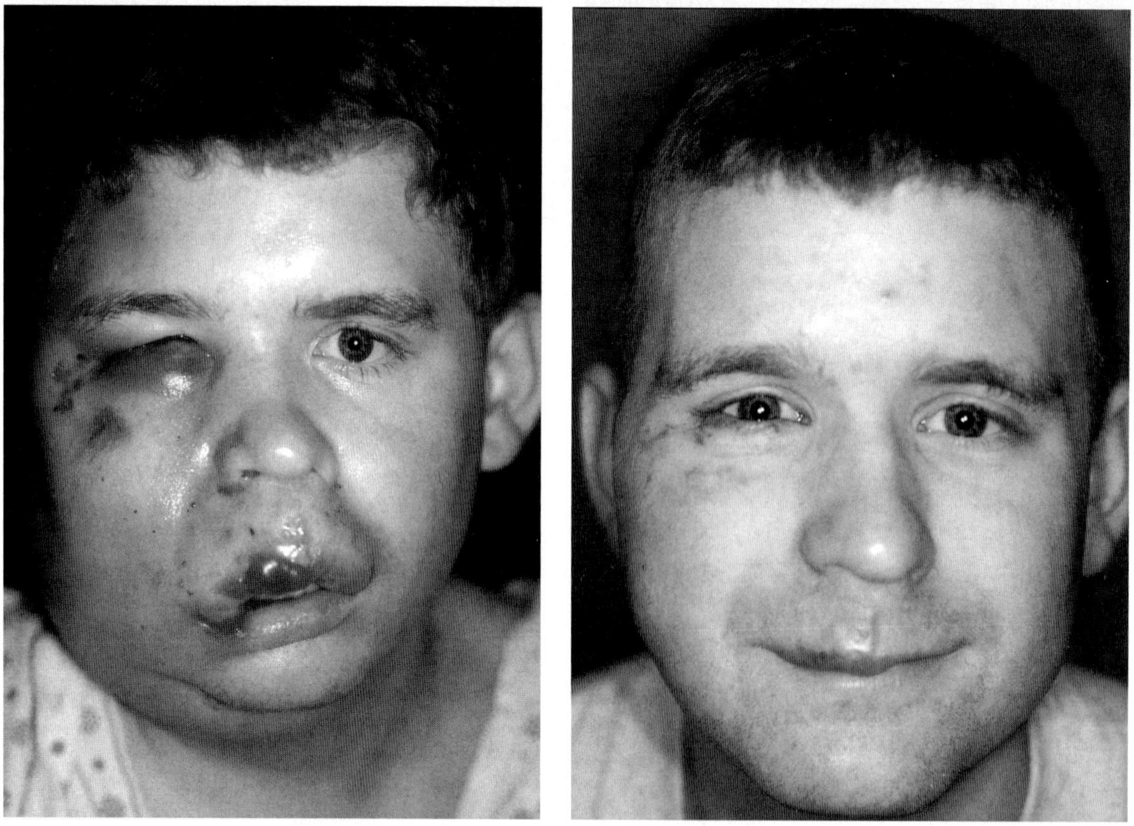

F G

FIGURE 15-6. *Continued.* **E:** Direct contrast injection into the upper lip component of the VM that drains into the facial vein, lateral projection. **F:** Patient 24 hours after sclerotherapy showing the extensive edema and blister formation on the upper lip. **G:** Patient at 21 years of age, 6 months after his last sclerotherapy and contrast sclerotherapy session and contour resection of the upper lip. Patient has retained full facial nerve function and now has only minor asymmetry of the right cheek. (From Holt PD, Burrows PE. Interventional radiology in the treatment of vascular lesions. *Facial Plast Surg Clin North Am* 2001;9, with permission.)

cysts may be treated by injection of sclerosant agents, including ethanol (Fig. 15-7), doxycycline, Ethibloc, and OK-432 [50–60]. OK-432, a suspension of killed *Streptococcus* that stimulates an immunologic reaction, appears to be an effective drug with minimal toxicity for treating macrocystic lesions. It is currently being assessed in a multicenter trial in the United States [57]. Many infants with bilateral involvement require tracheostomy. Lingual involvement is common in this disease and often necessitates partial glossectomy. Lingual artery embolization is effective in some patients with acute macroglossia who have increased flow [9]. Sclerotherapy with ethanol is useful in LMs of the tongue and floor of the mouth in patients with mild to moderate macroglossia with or without prior glossectomy, as well as those with residual mass effect in the floor of the mouth. Orbital LM frequently causes severe proptosis and

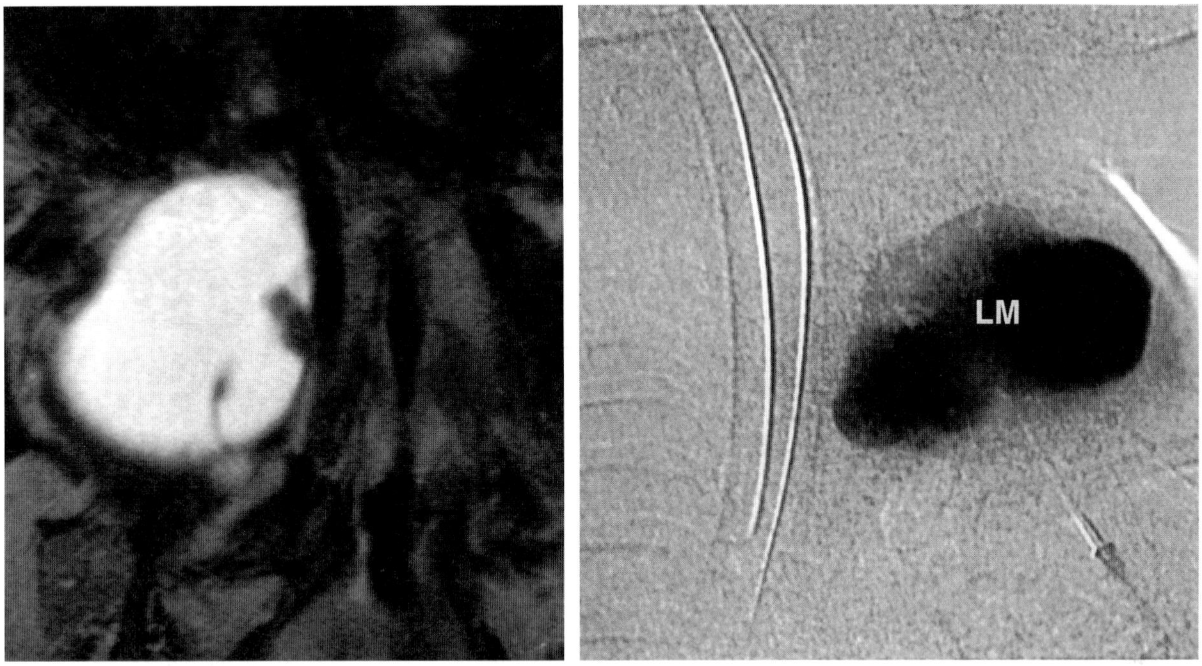

FIGURE 15-7. Sclerosant injection to treat a focal macrocystic LM of the left lower neck in a 2-year-old girl. **A:** T2-weighted MRI confirms the presence of a macrocystic LM. **B:** Direct contrast injection into the cyst (LM) confirms the unilocular nature of this lesion. The fluid and contrast medium were aspirated and a small amount of STS was injected, followed by 1 ml/kg of absolute ethanol. The lesion regressed nicely after one ethanol injection, leaving only a small rubbery collection of tissue. (From Holt PD, Burrows PE. Interventional radiology in the treatment of vascular lesions. *Facial Plast Surg Clin North Am* 2001;9, with permission.)

visual loss due to hemorrhage and infection (Fig. 15-8). Surgical treatment is difficult; residual lesions usually reexpand. Injection of OK-432 was reported to be successful in one patient in England [52].

OK-432 has shown promise in Japan and is undergoing clinical trials in the United States [53,54,56,61]. It has been suggested that this compound works by increasing endothelial permeability and accelerating lymph drainage from lymphatic spaces [58].

Combined Vascular Malformations

Combined vascular malformations are quite common and make up most of the syndromic vascular anomalies (Table 15-3). In particular, cutaneous CM (port wine stain) is often present in association with deep AVMs, VMs, LMs, or combined malformations [2,62].

Vascular malformations involving the spinal and intracranial contents are rarely seen in patients with Klippel-Trenaunay syndrome [63,64].

Patients with familial multiple VMs manifest increasing numbers of VMs during their lifetimes. Some families have associated intracranial lesions (cavernomas) and others have gastrointestinal involvement (blue rubber bleb nevus syndrome). The cutaneous lesions range in size from 1 millimeter to several centimeters. They have a rubbery consistency, possibly due to the presence of intralesional thrombus. The musculoskeletal VM may be painful. Treatment of the superficial lesions consists of sclerotherapy, excision, and laser.

Hereditary hemorrhagic telangiectasia (Rendu-Osler-Weber syndrome; AVMs, AVFs, arteriolar-venular malformations) is an autosomal dominant syndrome for which two genetic defects involving the endoglin gene have been identified [65]. Patients progressively develop cutaneous and mucosal telangiectasias, which on histologic examination are seen to be the result of venular dilatation leading to arteriovenous shunting. These lesions are most significant in the nasal area, where repeated epistaxis is a serious problem. Standard interventions for epistaxis, including embolization of the internal maxillary and facial arteries, frequently are needed. Macroscopic AVMs can occur, especially in the liver, lungs, and brain. In general, two types of pulmonary and cerebral AVMs have been described: simple AVFs, usually associated with a varix of the immediate draining vein, and complex AVM [66]. The latter, when present in the brain, may consist of a tiny collection of vessels. Symptoms from the pulmonary AVM and AVF include cyanosis with clubbing, fatigability, and cerebral infarction or abscess (related to the loss of filter function of the pulmonary vascular bed). Cerebral AVMs may manifest with hemorrhage. AVFs are generally treated by embolization.

Sturge-Weber syndrome (capillary venous malformation

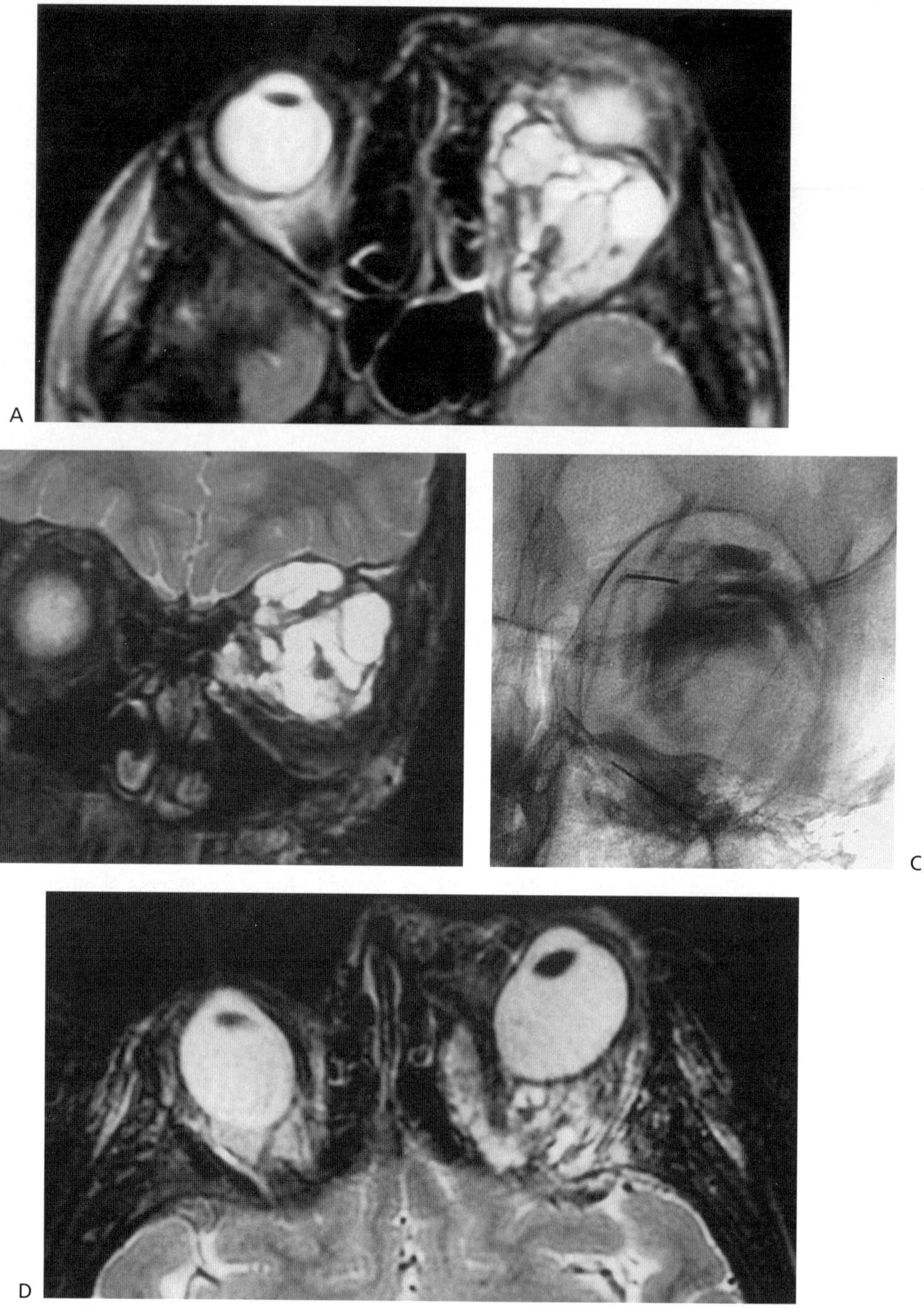

FIGURE 15-8. Lymphatic malformation of the left orbit with severe recurrent proptosis and progressive loss of ocular movement and decrease in vision in an 11-year-old girl. **A,B:** Axial and coronal T2-weighted MRIs, respectively, show the multicystic intraconal and extraconal lesion, displacing the globe anteriorly and inferiorly. Note the component of the lesion between the superior rectus muscle and the orbital roof, which was easily accessible for percutaneous injection through the upper eyelid, with ultrasonographic guidance. **C:** Direct contrast injection into the intraorbital LM, by percutaneous access with a 25-gauge butterfly needle, using ultrasonographic guidance. The contrast medium and lymphatic fluid were aspirated and a small amount of OK-432 injected. The patient underwent a second similar procedure, which markedly decreased the proptosis and improved ocular movement. Vision was preserved and was improved slightly and there have been no further episodes of acute proptosis. **D:** Axial T2-weighted image 6 months after sclerotherapy, showing the regression in the size of the lymphatic cysts. (Distortion of the image was caused by the patient's braces).

TABLE 15-3. SYNDROMES WITH VASCULAR MALFORMATIONS

Sturge-Weber (CVM)
Turner, Noonan (LM)
Blue rubber bleb nevus (VM)
Maffucci (VM and osteochondromata)
Klippel-Trenaunay (CLVM with limb overgrowth)
Parkes Weber (CVM with limb overgrowth)
Bonnet-Dechaume-Blanc (orbital and cerebral AVM)
Cobb (metameric AVM)
Proteus (progressive vascular anomalies with lipomas, etc.)

CVM, capillary venous malformation; LM, lymphatic malformation; VM, venous malformation; CLVM, capillary lymphaticovenous malformation; AVM, arteriovenous malformation.

[CVM], capillary lymphotic venous malformation [CLVM]) usually includes a facial port wine stain in the sensory cutaneous area V1 and ophthalmologic and leptomeningeal vascular anomaly [67]. The ocular involvement leads to glaucoma in one-third of patients due to the presence of a retinal vascular malformation, probably a VM or CVM. Associated intracranial vascular anomalies in Sturge-Weber syndrome usually consist of leptomeningeal capillary and venous malformations, associated with progressive ischemic cerebral atrophy with cortical calcification, resulting in seizures, focal neurologic deficits, and mental retardation. Intracranial involvement may also include AVMs and AVFs of the calvarium and meninges. The facial malformation may include LMs. Approximately 1% to 2% of patients with port wine stains have Sturge-Weber syndrome. The intracranial manifestations are generally not present in patients with port wine stains confined to V2 and V3 distribution, but they may be seen without surface vascular malformations. CT and MRI findings may be absent in the first year or two of life. Typical positive findings include gyral enhancement, with enlargement and enhancement of the ipsilateral choroid plexus. Later findings include progressive cortical atrophy and gyral calcification. Cerebral angiographic findings are variable but include parenchymal contrast stasis and abnormal cortical veins.

Laser therapy is usually effective in fading the cutaneous CM. Close ophthalmologic monitoring is important to detect glaucoma. Infants with severe seizure disorders may be evaluated for hemispherectomy. High-flow vascular malformations of the scalp or dura may require embolization, especially prior to neurosurgical procedures.

TREATMENT TECHNIQUES

Endovascular Treatment: Embolization

Endovascular treatment in the form of embolization can be used to treat hemangiomas, AVMs, and AVFs. Internal carotid angiography is usually performed prior to embolization in the external carotid arteries, to assess possible arterial supply from the internal carotid or ophthalmic branches, and to ascertain the ophthalmic artery supply to the retina. Distal catheterization of external carotid branches is facilitated by the use of general anesthesia and hypercarbia. Microcatheters are usually used with a 4-French guiding catheter. The choice of embolic agent is based on both the flow characteristics of the lesion and the desired therapeutic effect. In general, temporary occluding materials, including polyvinyl alcohol (PVA) particles, microspheres, and Gelfoam, are used for preoperative devascularization, and permanent agents, such as N-butyl-2-cyanoacrylate (NBCA) and ethanol, are reserved for primary treatment of appropriate fast-flow lesions. PVA and acrylic gelatin microspheres (Embospheres) are suspended in contrast medium and delivered by superselective catheterization of feeding arteries. The particle size is based on the size of arteriovenous shunts. The goal of embolization is for the particles to occlude the nidus, or the feeding arteries immediately adjacent to the nidus. Generally, to avoid skin necrosis and other ischemic tissue complications, the diameter of PVA particles should be more than 150 μm and that of Embospheres should be more than 300 μm. Preembolization angiograms should be examined carefully to detect intralesional macrofistulas, because these lead to migration of particulate embolic material to the venous circulation. NBCA is the best agent to use in this situation. If the catheter cannot be positioned sufficiently close to the fistula to permit safe use on NBCA, liquid coils can be used. Once the macrofistulas are closed, large particles may be appropriate to complete the preoperative embolization. Pledgets of Gelfoam may be used to occlude temporarily the feeding artery after particle embolization, to minimize the risk of early recanalization or reflux of particles. Coils should not be used to occlude feeding arteries, because they preclude successful reembolization of recurrences. Proximal arterial occlusion is contraindicated, also, because it leads to the development of collateral blood supply from surrounding vascular territories, leading to worsening of tissue ischemia and making future treatment more difficult. Following proximal occlusion of external carotid branches, there is generally an increase in collateral flow to both AVMs and normal tissue by branches of ophthalmic and internal carotid arteries (see Fig. 15-3).

Although particles are useful in providing preoperative devascularization, there is no evidence that their use provides any long-term benefit or change in the natural history of cervicofacial AVMs.

Coils and detachable balloons are useful to occlude large or medium-sized vascular channels, especially AVFs (Fig. 15-9).

Fibered platinum coils are preferable to steel, because the former are not ferromagnetic and are compatible with MRI. Fibered detachable coils are useful in lesions in which flow control is difficult and there is a high risk of device migration during placement. Large AVFs often require placement

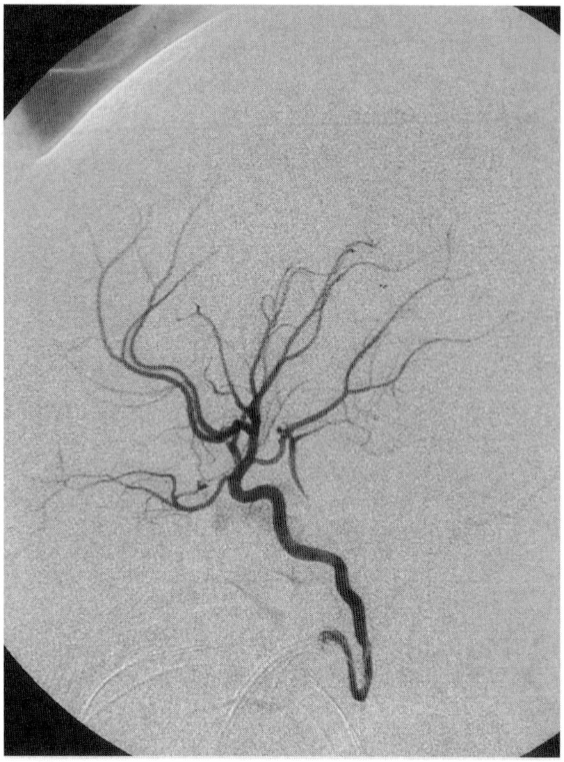

A

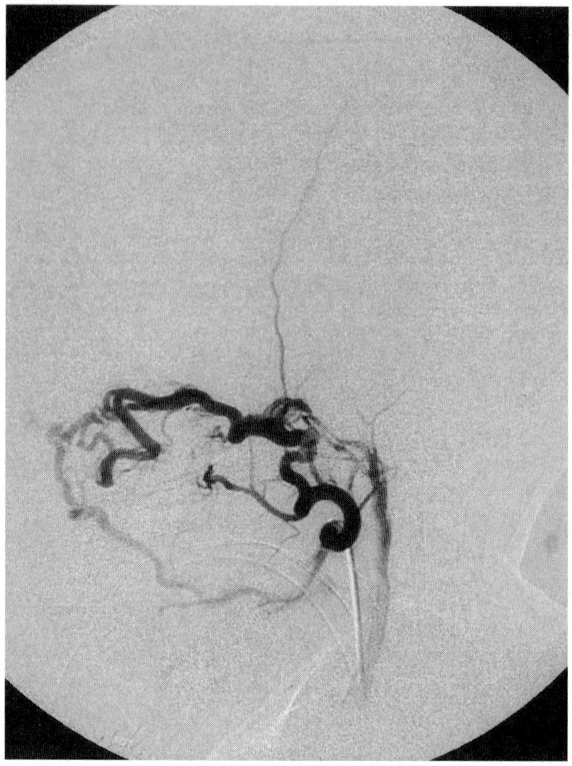

B

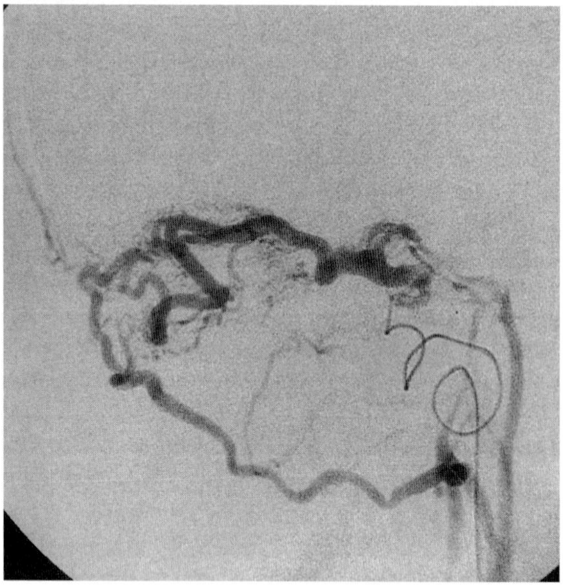

C

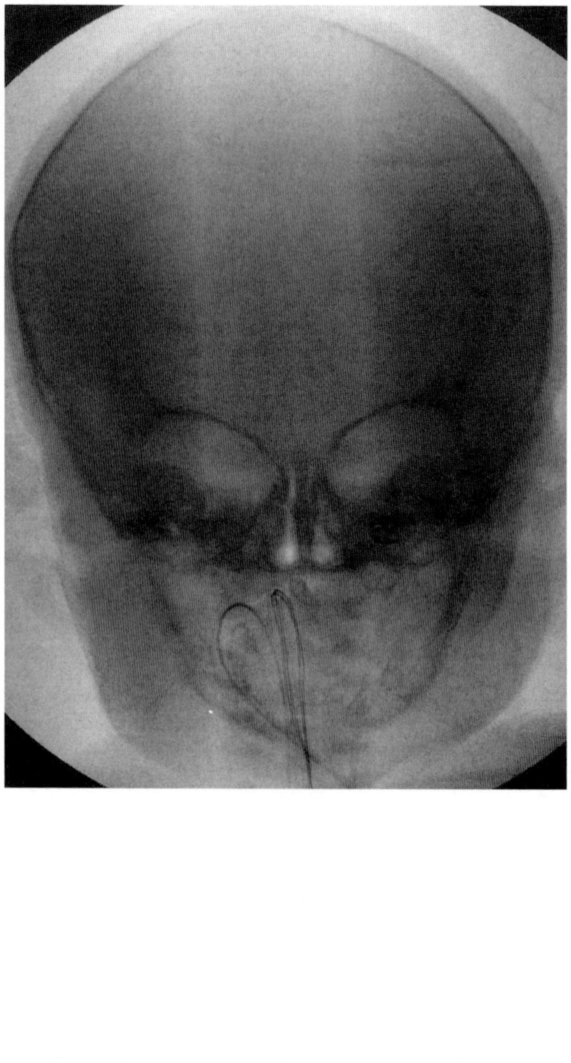

D

FIGURE 15-9. Orbital AVF in a newborn girl with left proptosis and chemosis. MRI showed dilated superior ophthalmic vein and cavernous sinus. **A:** Left internal carotid arteriogram, lateral projection, shows no arteriovenous shunts. **B:** Left distal external carotid arteriogram, lateral projection, shows a single communication between the middle meningeal artery and the superior ophthalmic vein. **C:** Selective catheter placement just proximal to the fistula. Embolization using a fibered platinum microcoil rather than liquid agent was chosen in order to avoid the risk of thrombosis of the superior ophthalmic vein. **D:** Frontal radiograph shows the coil position. *(Figure continues.)*

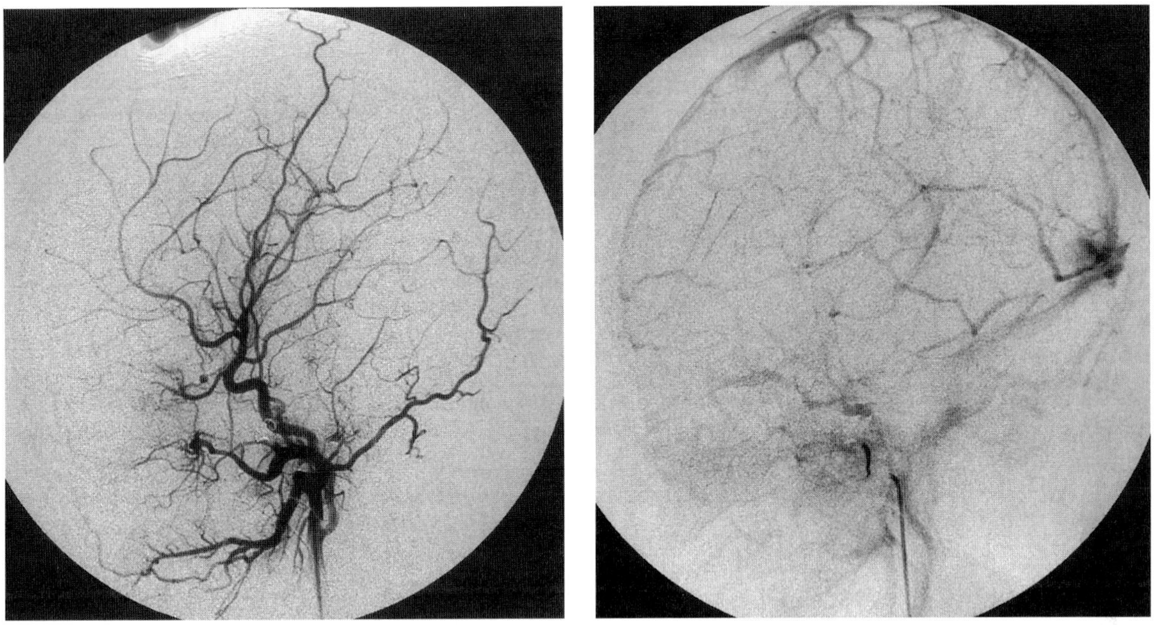

E F

FIGURE 15-9. *Continued.* **E:** Left common carotid arteriogram after coil placement confirms occlusion of the fistula. **F:** Venous phase shows normal opacification of ophthalmic and facial veins as well as the cavernous sinus.

of many coils before occlusion is achieved. The interventional radiologist should not assume that thrombosis will occur after the procedure is completed; if there is still flow around the device additional coils are probably necessary.

NBCA is often inappropriate for embolizing facial lesions, in which the nidus tends to be diffuse and composed of microfistulas. NBCA can result in a foreign body reaction and should be avoided in superficial soft tissues. Ethanol may be the most effective agent for primary treatment of AVMs, but it must be used with great caution to avoid tissue necrosis. In general, ethanol is administered intraarterially through a microcatheter that is positioned immediately adjacent to the AVM nidus. In extremely high-flow lesions, inflow or outflow occlusion is necessary for retention of the ethanol in the lesion. The ethanol should be delivered as a bolus (usually 1 to 5 ml), and the operator must then wait at least 5 minutes before checking the result. Additional ethanol should never be injected without first checking blood flow with a contrast injection, because once the shunt is occluded ethanol will reflux into normal territories, causing tissue necrosis. Likewise, contrast injection is advised after applying inflow or outflow occlusion, because these maneuvers may have changed the direction of flow. Cardiac effects must be monitored because of the potential risk of pulmonary hypertension and cardiac arrest [33]. This is frequently done by placement of a pulmonary artery catheter and continuous pressure monitoring. A drop in heart rate and oxygen saturation are ominous signs. If these occur, the ethanol injection must be stopped, at least until the parameters return to baseline. The skin surface should be inspected frequently for signs of ischemia. Soft tissue swelling is much greater after embolization with ethanol than with other agents. Corticosteroids and ice, as well as airway protection, are important postprocedure considerations. Analgesics, such as ketorolac and morphine, are usually necessary during the early recovery period.

Direct puncture of the nidus or immediate draining veins may be the most effective way of embolizing some AVMs (see Fig. 15-4). This technique has been especially useful in treating AVMs of the dental arcades. In these lesions, after controlling arterial inflow by selective embolization with the most appropriate agent, a needle is placed through the thinned mandibular or maxillary cortex into the lytic bone lesion. The intraosseous component is then occluded or sclerosed with coils, ethanol, or NBCA. There is a high rate of bony healing, obviating the need for mandibulectomy or even dental extraction [18]. Direct intranidal injection of NBCA has also been reported as part of preresection procedures for cervicofacial AVMs [15].

Percutaneous Treatment: Sclerotherapy

Sclerotherapy is performed via percutaneous access for VMs and some LMs [41,42,44,46,50]. Small, localized lesions can be injected with STS under local anesthesia [43]. Patients with extensive VMs, and those undergoing ethanol sclerotherapy, are anesthetized. The eyes are covered with adhesive plastic dressings, and the face is prepared and draped. Patients are pretreated with corticosteroids and a Foley catheter is placed in the urinary bladder. The lesion is accessed with a 20-gauge Teflon intravenous cannula, often using ultrasonographic guidance. Appropriate placement of the angiocatheter is documented by return of blood. Injection of iodinated contrast medium is imaged using low-dose digital subtraction. In the case of VMs, this injection also serves to demonstrate venous drainage of the lesion.

The appropriate sclerosant drug is then injected. Absolute ethanol is the most commonly used sclerosing agent due to its superior ability to cause endothelial damage and induce thrombosis and sclerosis. Disadvantages of ethanol include its neurolytic and cardiovascular effects, central nervous system depression, and pain on injection. Ethanol should not be used in lesions adjacent to major nerves, such as the facial nerve in the parotid region, or in cutaneous lesions. STS is a weaker sclerosing agent with no neurotoxicity or cardiovascular effects. It can be used in a very dilute form (e.g., 0.5% to 1%) in cutaneous lesions (Fig. 15-10). Patients with combined deep and superficial lesions are often treated using both agents. STS presently is not available in the United States. Some centers have begun to substitute Ethamolin, a mixture of ethanolamine and oleic acid that is approved for use in esophageal and saphenous varices.

The sclerosing agents may be opacified by adding a contrast agent if fluoroscopic guidance is important. Ethanol is best opacified with powdered (e.g., metrizamide [Amipaque]) or oily (ethiodized oil [Ethiodol]) contrast medium to minimize dilution. STS can be mixed with either oily or water-soluble liquid contrast. Opacified sclerosant is observed with fluoroscopic subtraction (roadmap) to avoid extravasation and sclerosis of draining veins. The amount of agent injected is estimated by the initial amount of contrast medium needed to opacity the lesion. Additional sclerosant is injected until the lesion is filled completely by fluoroscopic evaluation, or firm to palpation, or until there is no further blood return on aspiration of the cannula. Manual compression of the documented venous drainage is necessary to minimize egress of sclerosant. Sclerotherapy of superficial vascular malformations is performed with unopacified sclerosant. The skin color, rather than the fluoroscopic image, is observed during injection. Sclerosant injection must be terminated when ischemic changes such as pallor or duskiness become evident. Applying cold sterile saline to the surface of the skin to induce local vasoconstriction seems to minimize damage.

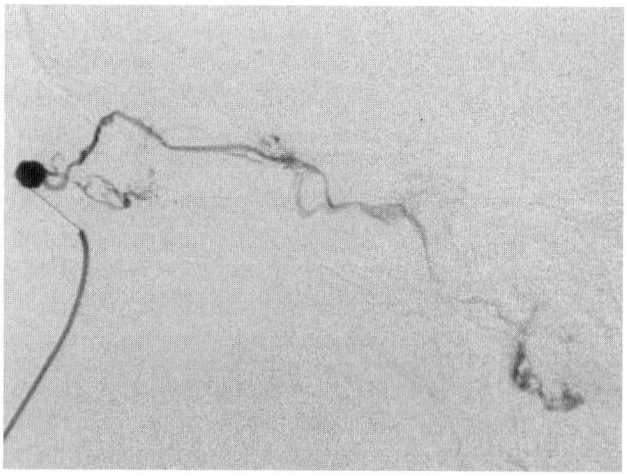

FIGURE 15-10. Venous malformation of the left upper eyelid and temple. A focal varix of the superior palpebral vein results in a focal blue area of swelling on the upper eyelid. This is part of a more extensive VM. These varices can be injected very gently with a mild sclerosant, with manual compression on the medial canthus to prevent sclerosant from entering the superior ophthalmic vein.

Thrombosis begins in about 5 to 10 minutes with ethanol and is indicated by increasing induration of the soft tissues. STS has a more subtle effect than ethanol; more time is needed before thrombosis is evident and it is important to avoid over-injecting. Ultrasonography or palpation is used to identify patent portions of the malformation and the process is repeated (Fig. 15-11). Variceal VMs do not thrombose well after simple liquid sclerosant injection. In these lesions, fibered platinum coils can be injected through the cannulas to augment thrombosis (Fig. 15-12). The maximal dose of sclerosant is limited by the weight of the patient, with an upper limit of 1 ml/kg of ethanol or 0.5 ml/kg of STS. Potential toxic effects of ethanol include respiratory depression, cardiac arrhythmias, seizures, rhabdomyolysis, hemolysis, and hypoglycemia [33]. Because pulmonary hypertension and electromechanical dissociation can develop with ethanol administration, oxygen saturation and heart rate are observed closely. Some advocate placement of a pulmonary artery catheter for pressure monitoring.

After sclerotherapy, the lesion should feel firm to palpation. Swelling is maximal 24 hours after the procedure (see Fig. 15-10). The inflammatory response is blunted by the administration of a systemic corticosteroid (dexamethasone, 1 mg/kg every 8 hours) and by applying ice packs to the lesion. Antibiotic ointment is applied to needle puncture sites. Patients should receive generous intravenous fluids (generally twice maintenance) during and after sclerotherapy, and urine output should be monitored carefully. Hemoglobinuria secondary to hemolysis is an expected effect of ethanol and STS. Gross hemoglobinuria is managed with hydration and urine alkalization. Hemoglobinuria can be monitored visually and usually clears within 6 hours.

Although patients with small facial lesions can recover after sclerotherapy in the day surgery unit, patients with malformations that are extensive or in close proximity to the airway are monitored in the hospital overnight. Oxygen saturation should be monitored. Airway protection including endotracheal intubation is mandatory for patients with intrinsic airway lesions. Ketorolac tromethamine and morphine sulfate are appropriate analgesics; older patients generally have patient-controlled analgesia. After discharge, patients receive a tapering dose of corticosteroids for 1 week, as well as analgesics. If skin injury is present, they are reevaluated frequently for evidence of infection. Otherwise, they are assessed clinically 2 months after the procedure.

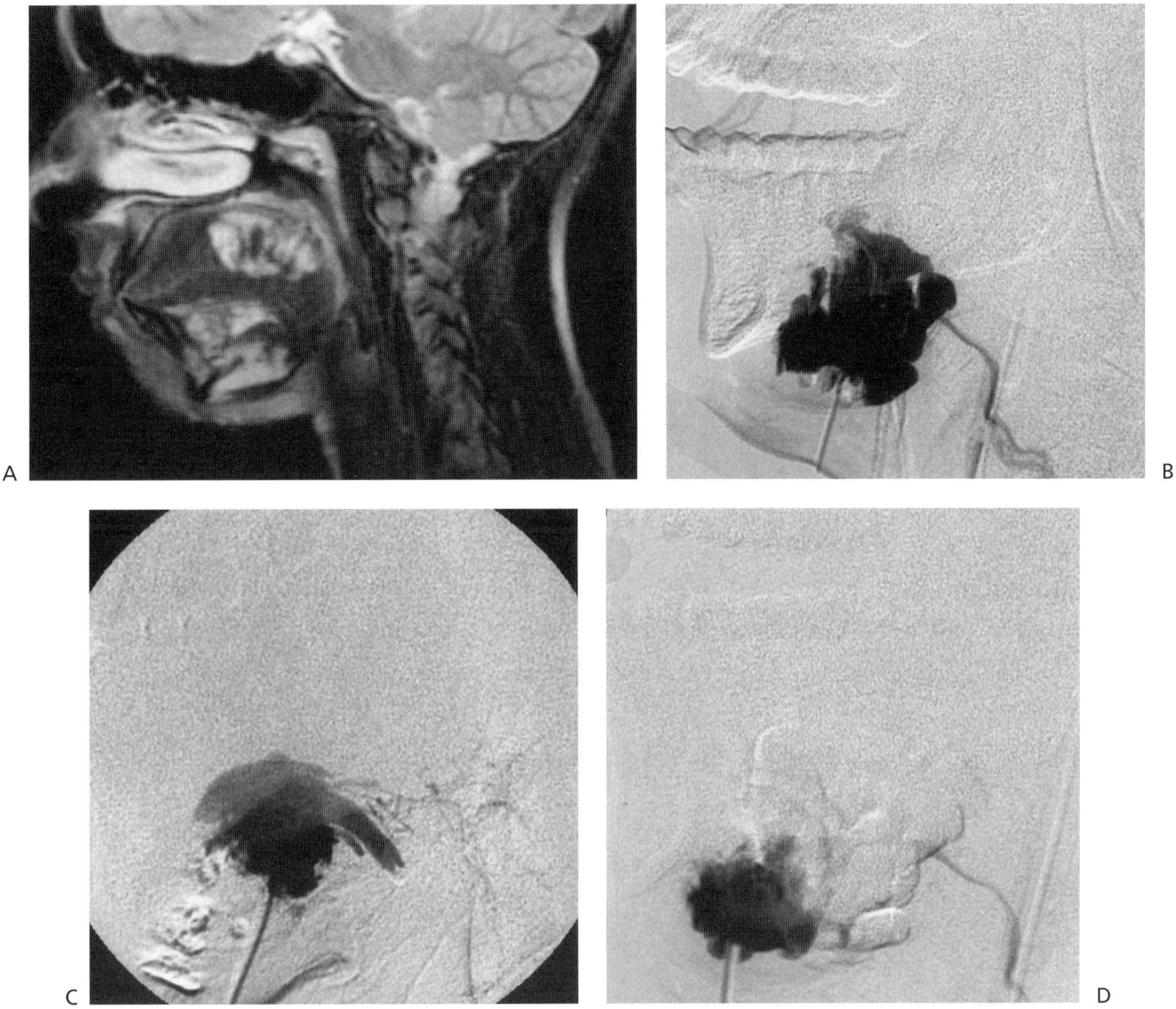

FIGURE 15-11. Percutaneous injection of sclerosant into a VM of the floor of the mouth. **A:** Sagittal T2-weighted MRI of the face shows multicompartmental VM of the floor of the mouth, illustrating the multicompartmental nature of these malformations. The contrast injections match the MRI like pieces of a jigsaw puzzle. **A:** Sagittal T2-weighted MRI of the face shows multicompartmental VM of the floor of the mouth, as well as in the dorsum of the tongue. The tongue lesion was not treated at this time. **B–D:** Digital subtraction images, lateral projection, were made during sequential cannulation and contrast injection into three components of the lesion in the floor of the mouth. Note the abnormal channels arranged parallel to the different muscle fibers and drainage into normal submental veins. Each site was injected with opacified ethanol.

Serious complications of sclerotherapy are rare when the procedure is performed by an experienced practitioner. Skin blistering is common and usually heals uneventfully with appropriate supportive care. Skin necrosis and scarring occur in about 10% to 15% of patients, usually at the site of cutaneous involvement with the malformation. In addition to airway obstruction, marked swelling can cause feeding difficulty, particularly for very young patients. Patients and parents should be warned about the swelling in advance. Severe swelling is not a complication, as long as precautions are taken to protect the patient from swelling of the airway and orbit, and is often associated with a good therapeutic response. Careful neurologic evaluation should be performed to document possible peripheral cranial nerve deficits although they are rarely permanent. In one study of 40 patients with craniofacial VMs, three developed deficits involving the facial or laryngeal nerves. Unilateral vocal cord paralysis was permanent, while the facial nerve injuries recovered within 2 to 3 months. In the same study, one-half of the patients had acute blistering, 12 experienced

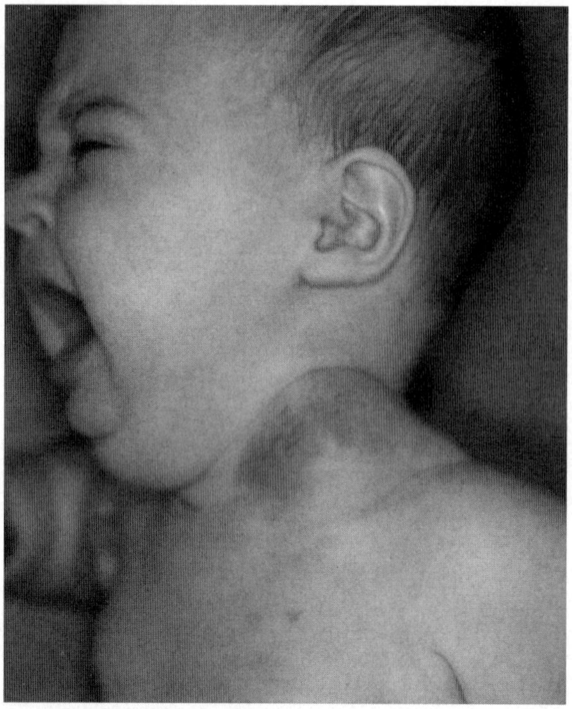

A

FIGURE 15-12. Varicocele form of VM of the left side of the neck became apparent with a rapidly enlarging mass in infancy. **A:** Patient at 9 months of age shows the lesion, with a bluish purple skin color, bulging when the child cries. The lesion was soft and compressible. **B:** Coronal T2-weighted MRI of the neck shows a large fluid-filled space representing subclavian vein varix, with some less discrete adjacent lesions, in the left supraclavicular area. **C:** Coronal T2-weighted MRI of the anterior face, shows varicocele VM, with thrombi or phlebolith, in the submental and sublingual spaces. *(Figure continues.)*

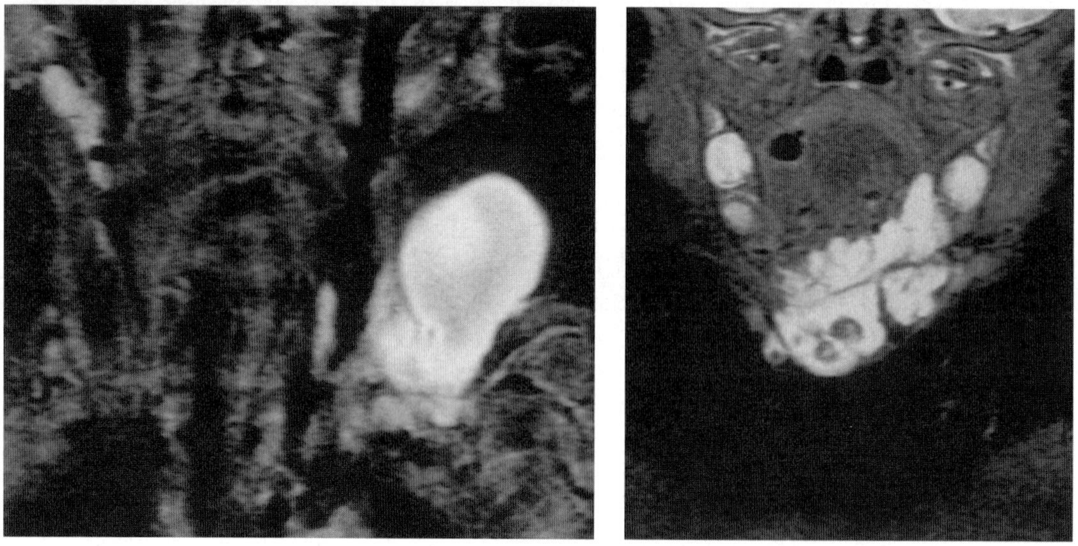

B C

hemoglobinuria, and 7 suffered deep ulceration [42]. Loss of vision has been reported following sclerotherapy of VMs near the orbit, presumably due to increased intraorbital pressure caused by swelling [41].

Objective analysis of the results of sclerotherapy is difficult, because cure is rarely achieved. Several series report the results of patient questionnaires as assessment of the outcomes. Patient satisfaction using ethanol or STS is high, with over 75% of patients reporting good or excellent results. One group reported their results first with ethanol, then with STS, and found STS to be slightly less effective [20,41,47]. We tried to determine factors predicting the result of treatment, but the only significant correlation was with the number of sclerotherapy sessions [42].

Other techniques for the treatment of head and neck VMs have been reported. Derby and Low reported treating 34 patients with facial VMs using intralesional laser photocoagulation in 63 consecutive procedures, although they also report a high rate of recurrence in as little as 2 months [68]. Others have advocated intralesional injection of other sclerosant or coagulation agents. One study describes intraoperative injection of tissue adhesive (NBCA) immediately

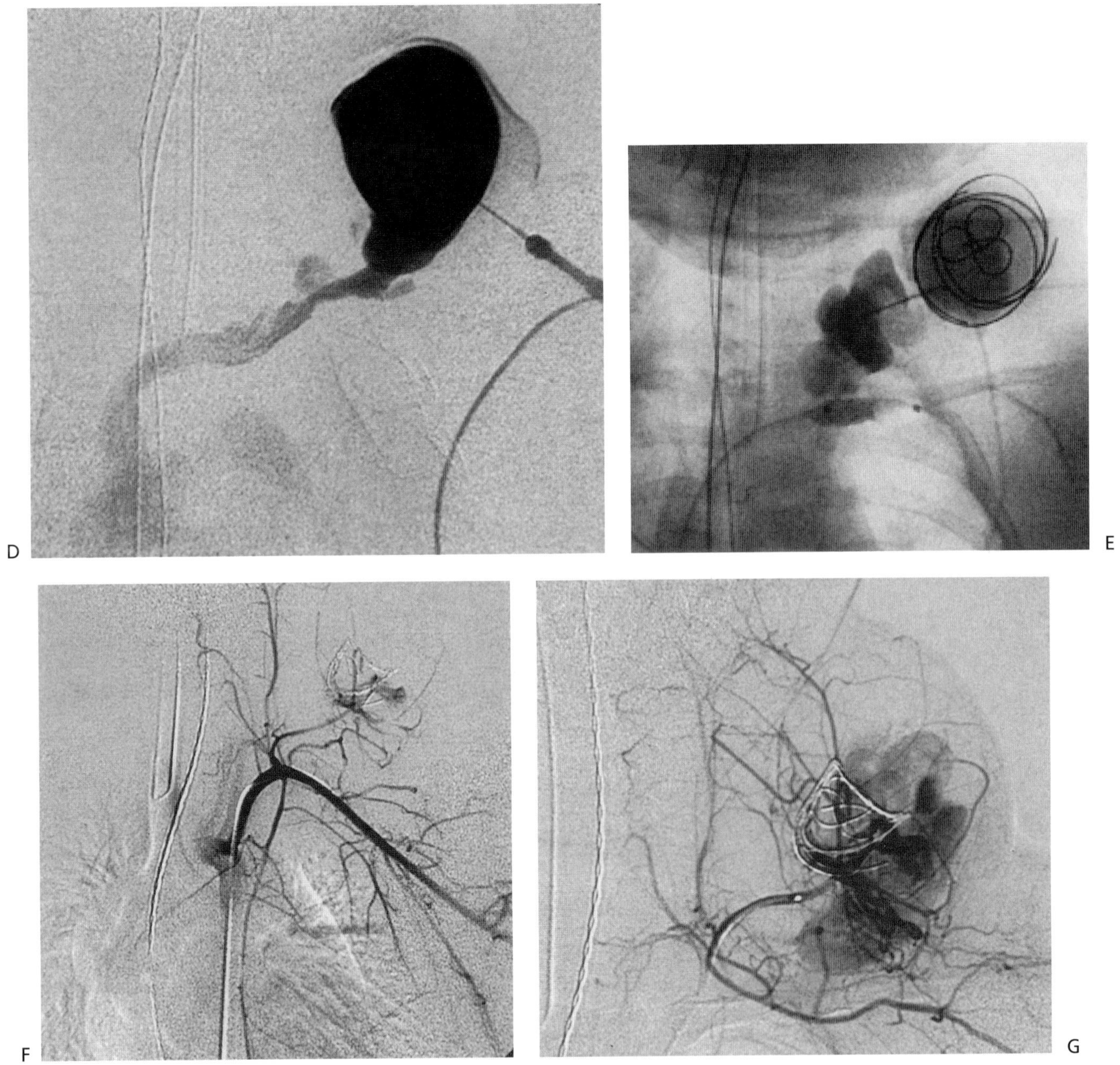

FIGURE 15-12. *Continued.* **D:** Direct contrast injection confirms the presence of a varix draining into the left subclavian vein. **E:** Using the balloon angioplasty catheter to occlude the venous egress (the infant had an atrial septal defect), two large fibered platinum microcoils were placed through a 20-gauge needle into the large varix, which was then sclerosed with ethanol. The adjacent VM was then accessed with a small butterfly needle and injected with additional ethanol. **F:** Left subclavian arteriogram carried out at the time of the second embolization procedure shows tiny arterial fistulas into the lesion, presumably accounting for its failure to regress completely after sclerotherapy. **G:** Selective angiography in the transverse cervical artery confirms the shunting. Several tiny branches were embolized with microcoils. *(Figure continues.)*

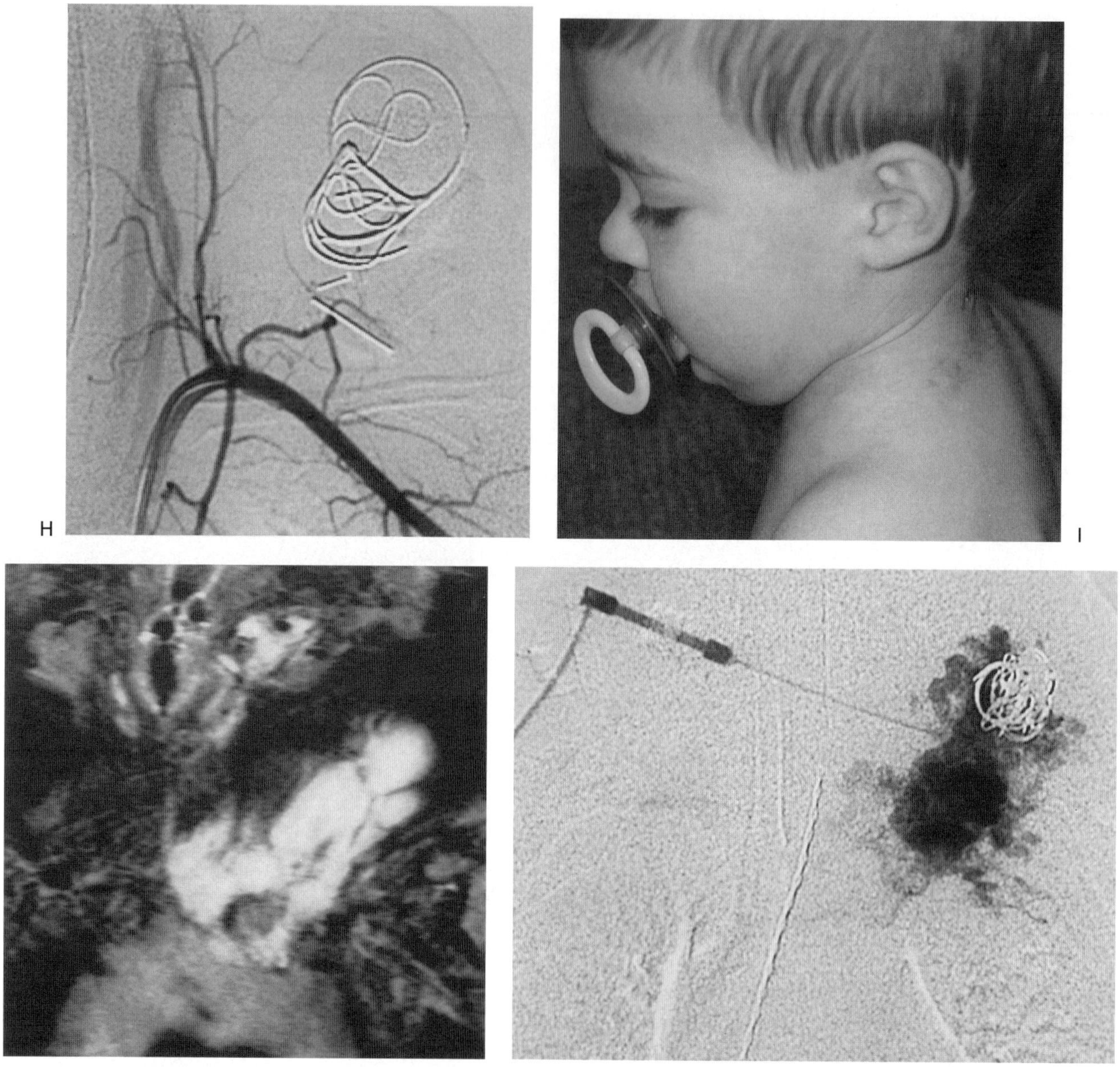

FIGURE 15-12. *Continued.* **H:** Left subclavian angiogram following arterial embolization shows control of the arterial supply to the lesion. **I:** Mass shows regression after two sclerotherapy-embolization sessions. The lesion, however, subsequently recurred in the adjacent soft tissues. **J:** Coronal T2-weighted MRI shows expansion of new channels medial to the previously treated lesion. **K:** Direct contrast injection into the residual left cervical VM. Note the compression of the coils previously placed in the large varix. This residual lesion was injected with ethanol, resulting in a Horner syndrome. The patient has undergone six therapeutic procedures by age 18 months. He continues to develop new areas of swelling.

before surgical excision of 30 VMs of the orbit while manually controlling venous outflow with pressure at the superior or inferior orbital fissure [69]. Successful treatment of a single patient with a facial VM with injection of fibrin glue was reported recently [70].

REFERENCES

1. Mulliken JB, Glowacki J. Hemangiomas and vascular malformations in infants and children: a classification based on endothelial characteristics. *Plast Reconstr Surg* 1982;69:412–420.
2. Mulliken J, Young A. *Vascular birthmarks, hemangiomas, and vascular malformations.* Philadelphia: WB Saunders, 1988:483.
3. North PE, Waner M, Mizeracki A, et al. GLUT1: a newly discovered immunohistochemical marker for juvenile hemangiomas. *Hum Pathol* 2000;31:11–22.
4. Takahashi K, Mulliken J, Kozakewich HP, et al. Cellular markers that distinguish the phases of hemangiomas during infancy and childhood. *J Clin Invest* 1994;93:2357–2364.
5. Baker LL, Dillon WP, Heishima BG, et al. Hemangiomas and vascular malformations of the head and neck: MR characterization. *AJNR Am J Neuroradiol* 1993;14:307–314.
6. Burrows PF, Robertson RL, Barnes PG. Angiography and the

evaluation of cerebrovascular disease in childhood. *Neuroimaging Clin N Am* 1996;6:561–588.

7. Burrows PE, Mulliken JB, Fellows KE, et al. Childhood hemangiomas and vascular malformations: angiographic differentiation. *AJR Am J Radiol* 1983;141:483–488.
8. Disa JJ, Chung KC, Gellad FE, et al. Efficacy of magnetic resonance angiography in the evaluation of vascular malformations of the hand. *Plast Reconstr Surg* 1997;99:136–147.
9. Lasjaunias P. *Vascular diseases in neonates, infants and children.* New York: Springer Verlag, 1997.
10. Paltiel HJ, Burrows PE, Mulliken JB. Color Doppler ultrasound of soft tissue vascular anomalies. *Radiology* 1994;193:292.
11. Rak KM, Yakes WF, Ray RL, et al. MR imaging of symptomatic peripheral vascular malformations. *AJR Am J Radiol* 1992;159:107–112.
12. Vikkula M, Boon LM, Mulliken JB, et al. Molecular basis of vascular anomalies. *Trends Cardiovasc Med* 1998;8:281–292.
13. Meyer JS, Hoffer FA, Barnes PD, et al. Biological classification of soft-tissue vascular anomalies: MR correlation. *AJR Am J Radiol* 1991;157:559–564.
14. Erdmann MW, Jackson JE, Davies DM, et al. Multidisciplinary approach to the management of head and neck arteriovenous malformations. *Ann R Coll Surg Engl* 1995;77:53–59.
15. Han MH, Seong SO, Kim HD, et al. Craniofacial arteriovenous malformation: preoperative embolization with direct puncture and injection of n-butyl cyanoacrylate. *Radiology* 1999;211:661–666.
16. Komiyama M, Khosla VK, Yamamoto Y, et al. Embolization in high-flow arteriovenous malformations of the face. *Ann Plast Surg* 1992;28:575–583.
17. Persky MS, Berenstein A, Cohen NL. Combined treatment of head and neck vascular masses with preoperative embolization. *Laryngoscope* 1984;94:20–27.
18. Rodesch G, Soupre V, Vazquez MP, et al. Arteriovenous malformations of the dental arcades. The place of endovascular therapy: results in 12 cases are presented. *J Craniomaxillofac Surg* 1998;26:306–313.
19. Seccia A, Salgarello M, Farallo E, et al. Combined radiological and surgical treatment of arteriovenous malformations of the head and neck. *Ann Plast Surg* 1999;43:359–366.
20. Svendsen P, Wikholm G, Fogdestam I, et al. Instillation of alcohol into venous malformations of the head and neck. *Scand J Plast Reconstr Surg Hand Surg* 1994;28:279–284.
21. Teitelbaum GP, Halbach VV, Fraser KW, et al. Direct-puncture coil embolization of maxillofacial high-flow vascular malformations. *Laryngoscope* 1994;104:1397–1400.
22. Smith JK, Castillo M, Wilson JD. MR characteristics of low-flow facial vascular malformations in children and young adults. *Clin Imaging* 1995;19:109–117.
23. Yuh WTC, Buehner LS, Kao SCS, et al. Magnetic resonance imaging of pediatric head and neck cystic hygromas. *Ann Otol Rhinol Laryngol* 1991;100:737–742.
24. Boon LM, Enjolras O, Mulliken JB. Congenital hemangioma: evidence for accelerated involution. *J Pediatr* 1996;128:329–335.
25. Pascual-Castroviejo I, Viano J, Moreno F, et al. Hemangiomas of the head, neck and chest with associated vascular and brain anomalies: a complex neurocutaneous syndrome. *AJNR Am J Neuroradiol* 1996;17:461–471.
26. Frieden IJ, Reese V, Cohen D. PHACE syndrome: the association of posterior fossa brain malformations, hemangiomas, arterial anomalies, coarctation of the aorta and cardiac defects, and eye abnormalities. *Arch Dermatol* 1996;132:307–311.
27. Burrows P, Robertson R, Mulliken J, et al. Cerebral vasculopathy and neurologic sequelae in infants with cervicofacial hemangioma. *Radiology* 1998;207:601–607.
28. Enjolras O, Riche MC, Merland JJ, et al. Management of alarming hemangiomas in infancy: a review of 25 cases. *Pediatrics* 1990;85:491–498.
29. Ezekowitz RAB, Mulliken JB, Folkman J. Interferon α-2a therapy for life threatening hemangiomas of infancy. *N Engl J Med* 1992;326:1456–1463.
30. Enjolras O, Wassef M, Mazoyer E, et al. Infants with Kasabach-Merritt syndrome do not have true hemangiomas. *J Pediatr* 1997;130:631–640.
31. Kohout MP, Hansen M, Pribaz JJ, et al. Arteriovenous malformations of the head and neck: natural history and management. *Plast Reconstr Surg* 1998;102:643–654.
32. Widlus DM, Murray RR, White RI Jr, et al. Congenital arteriovenous malformations: tailored embolotherapy. *Radiology* 1988;169:511–516.
33. Yakes WF, Rossi P, Odink H. Arteriovenous malformation management. *Cardiovasc Intervent Radiol* 1996;19:65–71.
34. Aoki S, Sasaki Y, Machida T. Embolization of extensive facial arteriovenous malformation via the orbital branches of the ophthalmic artery. *Radiat Med* 1991;9:98–100.
35. Hayes BH, Shore JW, Westfall CT, et al. Management of orbital and periorbital arteriovenous malformations. *Ophthalmic Surg* 1995;26:145–152.
36. Jackson JE, Mansfield AO, Allison DJ. Treatment of high-flow vascular malformations by venous embolization aided by flow occlusion techniques. *Cardiovasc Intervent Radiol* 1996;19:323–328.
37. Marotta TR, Berenstein A, Zide B. The combined role of embolization and tissue expanders in the management of arteriovenous malformations of the scalp. *AJNR Am J Neuroradiol* 1994;15:1240–1246.
38. Bradley JP, Zide BM, Berenstein A, et al. Large arteriovenous malformations of the face: aesthetic results with recurrence control. *Plast Reconstr Surg* 1999;103:351–361.
39. Vikkula M, Boon LM, Carraway KL III, et al. Vascular dysmorphogenesis caused by an activating mutation in the receptor tyrosine kinase TIE2. *Cell* 1996;87:1181–1190.
40. Boukobzka M, Enjolras O, Guichard JP, et al. Cerebral developmental venous anomalies associated with head and neck venous malformations. *AJNR Am J Neuroradiol* 1996;17:987–944.
41. Siniluoto TM, Svendsen PA, Wikholm GM, et al. Percutaneous sclerotherapy of venous malformations of the head and neck using sodium tetradecyl sulphate (Sotradecol). *Scand J Plast Reconstr Surg Hand Surg* 1997;31:145–150.
42. Berenguer B, Burrows PE, Zurakowski D, et al. Sclerotherapy of craniofacial venous malformations: complications and results. *Plast Reconstr Surg* 1999;104:1–15.
43. Gelbert F, Enjolras O, Deffrenne D, et al. Percutaneous sclerotherapy for venous malformation of the lips: a retrospective study of 23 patients. *Neuroradiology* 2000;42:692–696.
44. Suh JS, Shin KH, Na JB, et al. Venous malformations: sclerotherapy with a mixture of ethanol and lipiodol. *Cardiovasc Intervent Radiol* 1997;20:268–273.
45. de Lorimier AA. Sclerotherapy for venous malformations. *J Pediatr Surg* 1995;30:188–193.
46. Dubois JM, Sebag GH, De Prost Y, et al. Soft-tissue venous malformations in children: percutaneous sclerotherapy with Ethibloc. *Radiology* 1991;180:195–198.
47. Berthelsen B, Fogdestam I, Svendsen P. Venous malformations in the face and neck. Radiologic diagnosis and treatment with absolute ethanol. *Acta Radiol Diagn (Stockh)* 1986;27:149–155.
48. Herbreteau D, Riche MC, Enjolras O, et al. Venous vascular malformations and their treatment with Ethibloc. *J Mal Vasc* 1992;17:50–53.
49. Siegel MJ, Glazer HS, St Amour TE, et al. Lymphangiomas in children: MR imaging. *Radiology* 1989;170:467–470.
50. Dubois J, Garel L, Abela A, et al. Lymphangiomas in children:

percutaneous sclerotherapy with an alcoholic solution of zein. *Radiology* 1997;204:651–654.
51. Tovi M, Herbreteau D, Enjolras O, et al. 52 patients with cystic lymphatic vascular malformations: percutaneous sclerotherapy—simple, fast and repeatable. *Lakartidningen* 1998;95: 643–647.
52. Suzuki Y, Obana A, Gohto Y, et al. Management of orbital lymphangioma using intralesional injection of OK-432. *Br J Ophthalmol* 2000;84:614–617.
53. Brewis C, Pracy JP, Albert DM. Treatment of lymphangiomas of the head and neck in children by intralesional injection of OK-432 (Picibanil). *Clin Otolaryngol* 2000;25:130–134.
54. Luzzatto C, Midrio P, Tchaprassian Z, et al. Sclerosing treatment of lymphangiomas with OK-432. *Arch Dis Child* 2000;82: 316–318.
55. Samuel M, McCarthy L, Boddy SA. Efficacy and safety of OK-432 sclerotherapy for giant cystic hygroma in a newborn. *Fetal Diagn Ther* 2000;15:93–96.
56. Greinwald JJ, Burke DK, Sato Y, et al. Treatment of lymphangiomas in children: an update of Picibanil (OK-432) sclerotherapy. *Otolaryngol Head Neck Surg* 1999;121:381–387.
57. Smith RJ, Burke DK, Sato Y, et al. OK-432 therapy for lymphangiomas. *Arch Otolaryngol Head Neck Surg* 1996;122:1195–1199.
58. Ogita S, Tsuto T, Nakamura K, et al. OK-432 therapy for lymphangioma in children: why and how does it work? *J Pediatr Surg* 1996;31:477–480.
59. Zulfiqar MA, Zaleha AM, Zakaria Z, et al. The treatment of neck lymphangioma with intralesional injection of bleomycin. *Med J Malaysia* 1999;54:478–481.
60. Molitch HI, Unger EC, Witte CL, et al. Percutaneous sclerotherapy of lymphangiomas. *Radiology* 1995;194:343–337.
61. Ogita S, Tsuto T, Nakamura K, et al. OK-432 therapy in 64 patients with lymphangioma. *J Pediatr Surg* 1994;29:784–785.
62. Burns AJ, Kaplan LC, Mulliken JB. Is there an association between hemangioma and syndromes with dysmorphic features? *Pediatrics* 1991;88:1257–1267.
63. Oyesiku NM, Gahm NH, Goldman RL. Cerebral arteriovenous fistula in the Klippel-Trenaunay-Weber syndrome. *Dev Med Child Neurol* 1988;30:245–251.
64. Taira T, Tamura Y, Kawamura H. Intracranial aneurysm in a child with Klippel-Trenaunay-Weber syndrome: case report. *Surg Neurol* 1991;36:303–306.
65. Guttmacher AE, Marchuk DA, White RI Jr. Hereditary hemorrhagic telangiectasia. *N Engl J Med* 1995;333:918–924.
66. Sobel D, Norman D. CNS manifestations of hereditary hemorrhagic telangiectasia. *AJNR Am J Neuroradiol* 1984;5:569–573.
67. Rocco CD. *Sturge-Weber disease. Cerebrovascular diseases in children.* New York: Springer-Verlag, 1992:168–187.
68. Derby LD, Low DW. Laser treatment of facial venous vascular malformations. *Ann Plast Surg* 1997;38:371–378.
69. Lacey B, Rootman J, Marotta TR. Distensible venous malformations of the orbit: clinical and hemodynamic features and a new technique of management. *Ophthalmology* 1999;106: 1197–1209.
70. Jemec B, Sanders R. A facial low-flow venous malformation treated with fibrin glue. *Br J Plast Surg* 2000;53:73–75.

Endovascular and Percutaneous Therapy of the Brain and Spine, edited by Michael P. Marks and Huy M. Do.
Lippincott Williams & Wilkins, Philadelphia © 2002.

16

SPINAL CORD ARTERIOVENOUS MALFORMATIONS

ROBERT A. WILLINSKY

CLASSIFICATION

Since the introduction of selective spinal angiography in the 1960s, Djindjian recognized that vascular malformations consisted of arteriovenous shunts that differed in the volume of shunting and number of feeders [1]. Aminoff and Logue in 1974 studied the pathophysiology of these AVMs and introduced the concept of venous congestion of the cord [2]. Kendall and Logue in 1977 [3], and Merland et al. in 1980 [4] distinguished dural malformations from the true cord AVMs.

Spinal arteriovenous malformations (AVMs) are a heterogeneous group of congenital and acquired lesions that can impair spinal cord function. A number of classification schemes have been used based on the location and appearance of the nidus [5,6]. These schemes are difficult to use, because the criteria for the grouping is subjective and the numerical categories are not widely known. A simplified classification can be used based on the arterial supply (Table 16-1). This classification separates the AVMs into dural, perimedullary, intramedullary, extradural, and complex. Spinal dural arteriovenous fistulas (SDAVFs) are supplied via radiculomeningeal arteries and the venous drainage is into the perimedullary venous plexus. Spinal cord arteriovenous malformations (SCAVMs) are fed by anterior spinal (radiculomedullary) or posterior spinal (radiculopial) arteries, or both, and drain into the intrinsic medullary or extrinsic perimedullary venous system. These SCAVMs may have a nidus or may consist only of a single fistula. A nidus is a collection of arteries and veins with multiple shunts. Those with a nidus are referred to as intramedullary and those with a single fistula are called perimedullary. The intramedullary SCAVMs always have supply from the radiculomedullary arteries and often have additional supply from the radiculopial arteries. The perimedullary SCAVMs are either on the surface of the cord or subpial just deep to the cord surface. The term perimedullary is commonly used in the literature, but it may be misleading by suggesting that the fistula is easily accessible on the cord surface. Halbach et al. suggested the term *intradural arteriovenous fistula* to highlight those cases in which the transition from artery to vein occurs without an intervening tangle of vessels (nidus) and the fistula site is on the surface of the cord or deep to the pia [7]. The perimedullary fistulas derive their blood supply from the radiculomedullary and the radiculopial arteries. Extradural arteriovenous fistulas (EAVFs) derive their blood supply from segmental arteries, and the venous drainage is into epidural or paraspinal veins or both.

Perimedullary SCAVMs have been subclassified into three types [8]. Type I is a slow-flow fistula located on the anterior surface of the cord. There is only minimal enlargement of the feeding radiculomedullary artery and the draining anterior spinal vein. Type II perimedullary fistulas have multiple enlarged feeders, with a dominant radiculomedullary artery (anterior perimedullary) or radiculopial artery (posterior or posterolateral) that defines the location of the single shunt. The blood flow is relatively slow through the tortuous, dilated perimedullary veins. The type II fistulas are often located at the conus medullaris [7,9]. Type III fistulas are high-flow arteriovenous fistulas (AVFs) with multiple enlarged radiculomedullary and radiculopial arteries. Marked venous ectasia of the involved vein is present and there is rapid metameric drainage.

Spinal AVMs can be isolated or multiple. If multiple they may be metameric, involving soft tissues, bone, dura, and spinal cord. These metameric AVMs can be referred to as complex because the blood supply includes radiculomedullary, radiculopial, radiculomeningeal, and segmental arteries. If the skin is involved this is referred to as Cobb syndrome [10]. If there are multiple separate spinal AVMs one of the vascular syndromes should be considered (i.e., Rendu-Osler-Weber, Klippel-Trenaunay) [11–13].

SPINAL DURAL ARTERIOVENOUS FISTULAS

Clinical

SDAVFs are symptomatic due to the shunting into the perimedullary venous plexus, resulting in a venous hyperten-

R.A. Willinsky: Department of Medical Imaging, Toronto Western Hospital, Toronto, Ontario, Canada.

TABLE 16-1. CLASSIFICATION OF SPINAL ARTERIOVENOUS MALFORMATIONS

Type	Arterial Supply	Venous Outflow
Dural	Radiculomeningeal	Intradural
Perimedullary	Radiculopial (anterior spinal) or radiculomedullary (posterior spinal)	Intradural
Intramedullary	Radiculomedullary and/or radiculopial	Intradural
Extradural	Segmental	Epidural
Complex	Radiculomeningeal, radiculomedullary, radiculopial, segmental	Intradural and epidural

sion and chronic passive venous congestion of the cord [14]. This has been referred to as a *venous congestive myelopathy.* The patient's signs and symptoms usually are attributed to dysfunction in the lower thoracic cord and conus, irrespective of the location of the shunt.

SDAVFs usually become apparent in the fourth to sixth decade with a slowly progressive thoracic myelopathy. SDAVFs are more common in males (3.4:1) [15]. Berenstein and Lasjaunias analyzed the clinical findings in 172 patients from five series in the literature [16]. Leg weakness was the initial complaint in 40%. Low back or radicular pain was the initial symptom in 18%. Stocking or saddle paraesthesias often develop in association with bladder, bowel, and sexual disturbances. Activity, or maneuvers that increase intraabdominal pressure, often aggravates symptoms. Some patients develop a rapid aggravation of their myelopathy superimposed on a slowly progressive course [17]. This rapid decline has been precipitated by myelography. Cervical SDAVFs are rare and can manifest intradural hemorrhage or cervical radiculopathy [18–22].

Most SDAVFs have a relentless downhill course unless treated. This results in the Foix-Alajouanine syndrome as a result of progressive vascular thrombosis and a necrotic myelopathy [23,24]. In most patients there is a long delay between onset and diagnosis. In early reports only one-third of patients were diagnosed within 1 year of the onset of symptoms, and only two-thirds of patients had their diagnosis within 3 years [25]. With magnetic resonance (MR) technology becoming more available and MR resolution improving, there should be less delay in the diagnosis. If treatment is done early in the course of the disease, there is reversibility of the cord dysfunction that results from the venous congestion [26]. There are a few reports of spontaneous thrombosis of SDAVFs [27].

Intracranial dural AVFs with spinal venous drainage can cause a cervical or thoracic myelopathy. The venous drainage of the fistula correlates with the clinical picture [28]. The spinal venous drainage through cervical radicular veins is often not associated with a myelopathy. These patients may come to medical attention because of a hemorrhage. When the venous drainage descends along the perimedullary veins of the entire cord a myelopathy is usually present.

Patients with SDAVFs often have both upper and lower motor neuron findings in the lower limbs, suggesting a low cord or conus lesion. Power is usually grade 4. Deep tendon reflexes may be increased despite wasting of the buttocks and lower extremities. Clonus is often present. Loss of pain and temperature sensation, as well as joint position sense, is frequently seen.

Imaging

Prior to the advent of magnetic resonance imaging (MRI), myelography was critical in suggesting the diagnosis of SDAVFs. In the proper clinical setting, tortuous filling defects on the myelogram would prompt angiography in a search for a vascular lesion. It was important to assess the entire spine on the myelogram, with particular attention paid to the thoracic region. Supine myelography was done to better assess the dorsal subarachnoid space where most of the dilated veins lay. MR is now the imaging modality of choice in the investigation of a possible SDAVF. In a review of 17 patients with angiographically proven SDAVFs, MRI could suggest the diagnosis in all 17 (Table 16-2) [26]. Fourteen (82%) had enlarged perimedullary vessels, 11 (65%) had cord swelling, and 16 (94%) had a central T2 hyperintensity in the thoracic region extending down to the conus (Fig. 16-1). A peripheral T2 hypointensity outlines the T2 hyperintensity within the cord [29]. Isolated involvement of the thoracic cord with sparing of the conus is uncommon. Involvement of the cervical cord with a normal thoracic cord suggests an intracranial dural AVF or a cervical dural AVF [20,30,31]. Gadolinium administration may be useful to verify the presence of dilated vessels, and often a diffuse or patchy enhancement of the involved cord may be seen [26]. Fast three-dimensional (3-D) contrast-enhanced magnetic resonance angiography (MRA) can confirm the presence of dilated perimedullary vessels and may identify the enlarged radiculomedullary vein draining the fistula [32,33]. Identification of the fistula site on coronal or axial MR angiograms is a tremendous advantage before embarking on the spinal angiogram (Fig. 16-2). Selective spinal angiography, especially in the elderly,

TABLE 16-2. MAGNETIC RESONANCE FINDINGS IN 17 PATIENTS WITH SPINAL DURAL ARTERIOVENOUS FISTULAS

Patient No.	Sex/Age (yr)	Vessels	MR Cord Swelling	T2 Hyperintensity	Gd Vessels	Enhance	Level
1	F/28	[a]	No	T4 to conus	N/A	N/A	Left L2
2	F/68	No	No	To conus[b]	No	Diffuse	Left T7
3	M/63	Yes	Conus	T8 to conus	Same	Patchy	Left L2
4	M/64	Yes	No	T4 to conus	N/A	N/A	Right T6
5	M/66	Yes	T6 to conus	T6 to conus	N/A	N/A	Right T7
6	M/64	Yes	Conus	T5 to conus	Better	No	Right T6
7	F/62	Yes	Conus	T5 to conus	N/A	N/A	Left L2
8	M/46	Yes	Conus	T5 to conus	Same	No	Left T7
9	M/55	Yes	T7 to conus	T7 to conus	Same	No	Left T2
10	M/47	Yes	Conus	Conus	Same	Patchy	Left T3
11	M/59	Yes	Conus	T5 to conus	No	Diffuse	Left T6
12	M/74	Yes	Conus	T7 to conus	Same	No	Right L2
13	M/70	Yes	No	No	Better	Patchy	Right T7
14	M/68	[a]	No	T7 to conus	N/A	N/A	Left L4
15	M/71	Yes	Conus	T7 to conus	Better	Patchy	Left T5
16	M/76	Yes	Conus	T6 to conus	N/A	N/A	Right T7
17	M/39	Yes	No	T7 to conus	N/A	N/A	Left T4

T, thoracic; L, lumbar; Gd, gadopentetate dimeglumine; M, male; F, female; N/A, not available.
[a]Hazy margin of cord or suspicious for flow voids.
[b]Upper level not seen on imaging.
From Willinsky RA, TerBrugge K, Montanera W, et al. Posttreatment MR findings in spinal dural arteriovenous malformations. *AJNR Am J Neuroradiol* 1995;16:2063–2071, with permission.

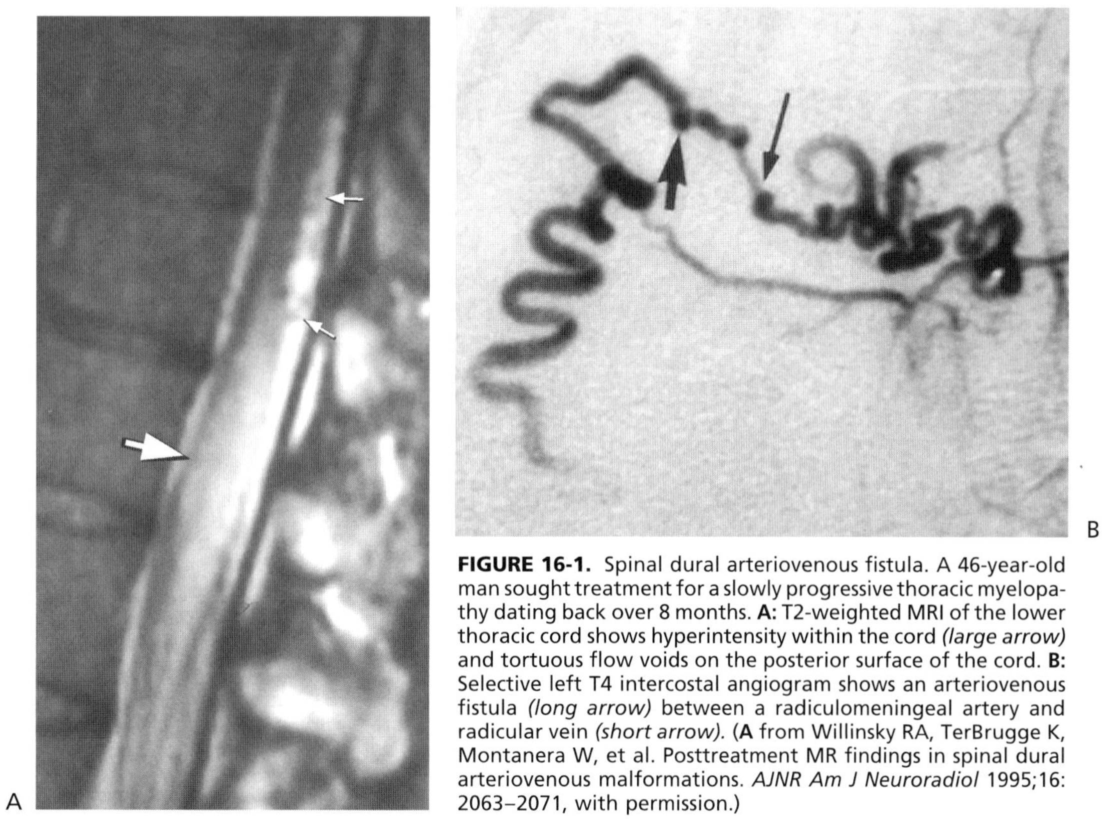

FIGURE 16-1. Spinal dural arteriovenous fistula. A 46-year-old man sought treatment for a slowly progressive thoracic myelopathy dating back over 8 months. **A:** T2-weighted MRI of the lower thoracic cord shows hyperintensity within the cord *(large arrow)* and tortuous flow voids on the posterior surface of the cord. **B:** Selective left T4 intercostal angiogram shows an arteriovenous fistula *(long arrow)* between a radiculomeningeal artery and radicular vein *(short arrow).* (**A** from Willinsky RA, TerBrugge K, Montanera W, et al. Posttreatment MR findings in spinal dural arteriovenous malformations. *AJNR Am J Neuroradiol* 1995;16: 2063–2071, with permission.)

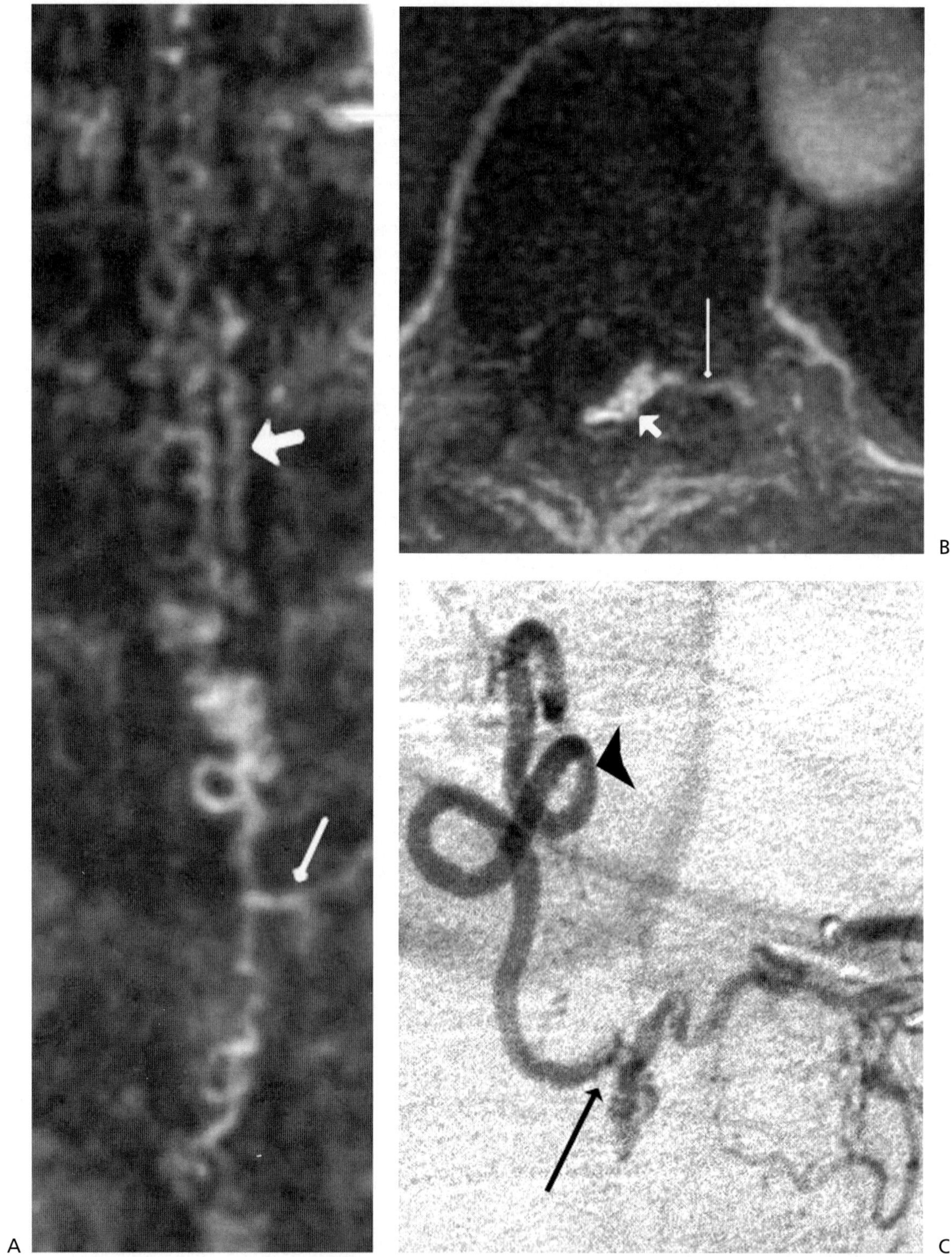

FIGURE 16-2. Gadolinium MRA localizes site of a spinal dural arteriovenous fistula. A 59-year-old man with bilateral leg weakness dating back over 1 month had an MRI that showed perimedullary flow voids and T2 hyperintensity within the central lower thoracic cord. **A:** Coronal gadolinium MRA shows the prominent perimedullary vessels *(upper arrow)* and an enlarged vessel in the left T10 foramina *(lower arrow).* **B:** Axial gadolinium MRA shows the large vessel in the T10 foramina *(long arrow)* and prominent posterior perimedullary veins *(short arrow).* **C:** Left T10 intercostal angiogram confirms the site of the fistula *(arrow)* draining into the perimedullary veins *(arrowhead).* (From R. Farb, unpublished material, with permission.)

may be a long and tedious procedure due to difficulty in catheterizing each intercostal and lumbar pedicle. At present, we use MRI in deciding if angiography is warranted when an SDAVF is suspected. If MRI reveals dilated perimedullary vessels then angiography is mandatory. If MRI with gadolinium shows only the intramedullary T2 hyperintensity, then angiography is indicated if the clinical picture suggests an SDAVF. Early in the disease it is possible for a patient to have a radiculopathy and there will be no signal change within the cord (Fig. 16-3). After treatment, MRI shows that cord swelling resolves, the T2 hyperintensity is less, and in most patients the prominent vessels are no longer evident [26].

Selective spinal angiography has been important in separating the SDAVFs from other AVMs. Identification of the radiculomedullary supply is important for treatment planning. Demonstration of a slow spinal cord circulation time is consistent with the venous congestion associated with SDAVFs [34]. It is important to recognize the common segmental origin of a dural branch supplying the fistula and a radiculomedullary artery (Fig. 16-4) [35]. SDAVFs are usually isolated dural shunts between a radiculomeningeal artery and an intradural vein. Most are at the thoracic or lumbar levels [26]. The shunt is usually located on the root sleeve and the vein follows the course of the nerve root (Fig. 16-5) [7]. Most drain into the posterior perimedullary plexus. Rarely, SDAVFs drain into the anterior spinal vein mimicking an anterior perimedullary SCAVM [36]. When

A,B 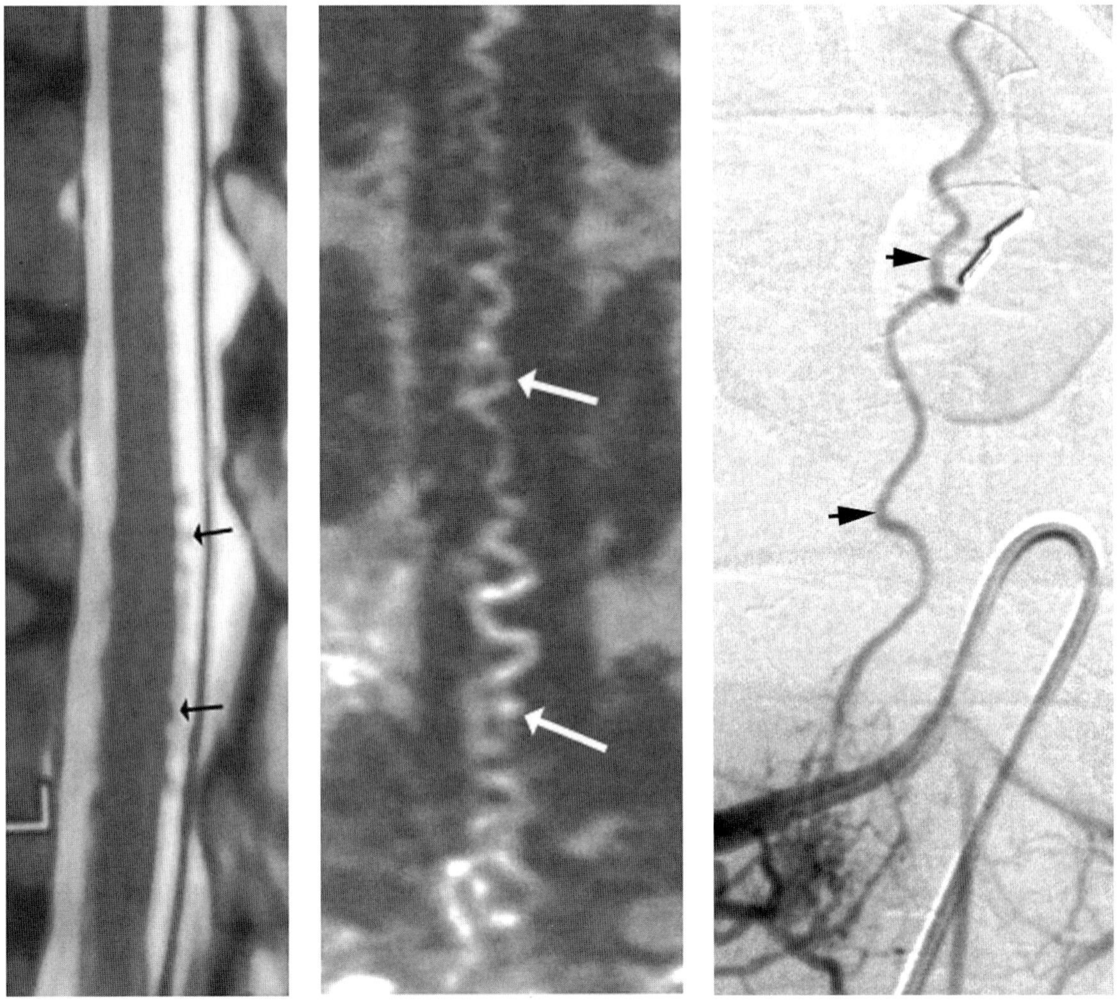 C

FIGURE 16-3. Spinal dural arteriovenous fistula caused symptoms of sciatica only in a 47-year-old man with right leg pain. **A:** T2-weighted MRI shows prominent flow voids *(arrows)* on the dorsal aspect of the lower cord but no abnormal signal within the cord. **B:** Coronal gadolinium MRA confirms the presence of the tortuous perimedullary vessels *(arrows)*. **C:** Right L3 angiogram shows reflux into the L3 radicular vein *(arrows)* and perimedullary venous plexus. (**B** from R. Farb, unpublished material, with permission.)

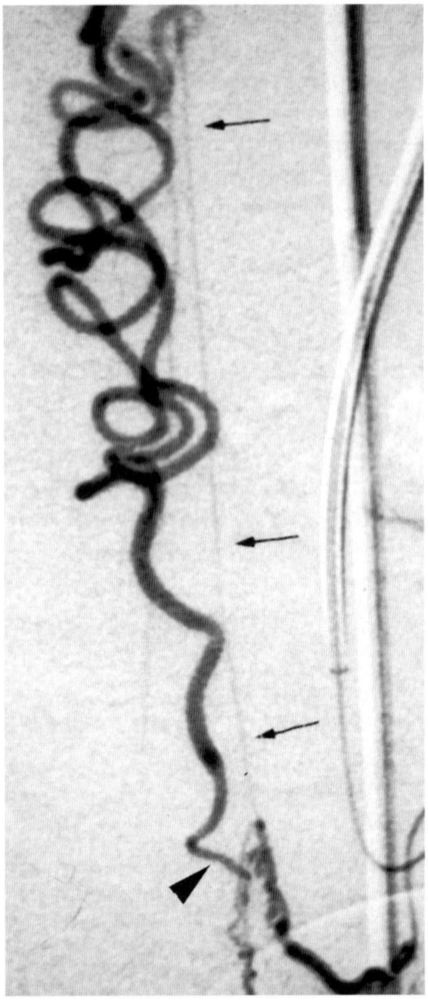

FIGURE 16-4. Common origin of a radiculomeningeal branch supplying a spinal dural arteriovenous fistula and the radiculomedullary artery. This 63-year-old man had a 3-year history of a thoracic myelopathy. Superselective angiogram of the radiculomeningeal branch at the left L2 shows an arteriovenous fistula *(arrowhead)* draining into the perimedullary veins and a radiculomedullary artery *(arrows)* arising at the same site.

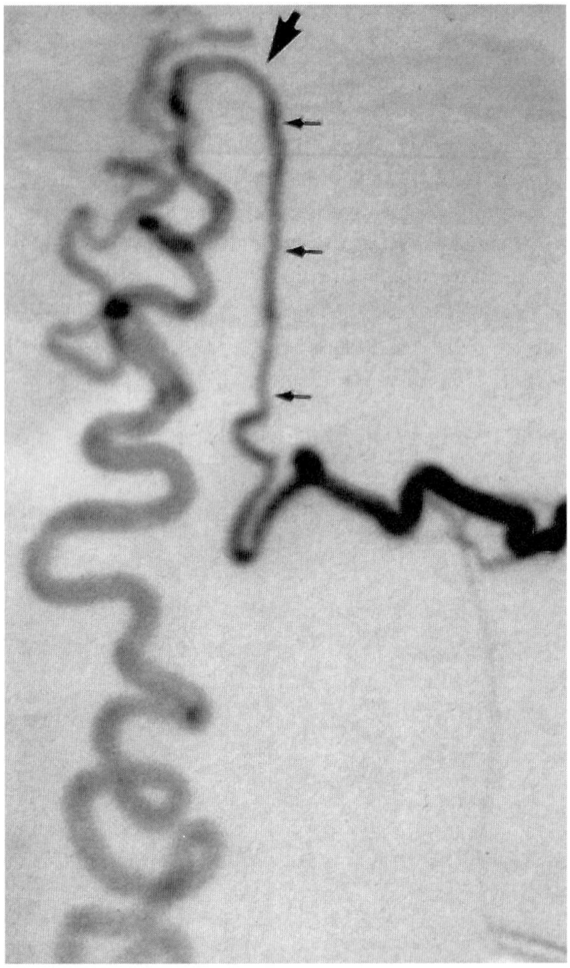

FIGURE 16-5. SDAVF remote from the root sleeve. Superselective angiogram of the left T7 intercostal shows the vertical course along the dura of the radiculomeningeal artery *(small arrows)* with the shunt *(large arrow)* far from the root sleeve. The left T6 intercostal artery also made a small contribution to the shunt (not shown). The transition between the artery and the vein at the dura distinguishes this SDAVF from a perimedullary fistula fed by radiculopial or radiculomedullary arteries.

the shunt is remote from the root sleeve, dural arterial supply from two levels (bimetameric) can be expected (Fig. 16-6). A thoracic myelopathy may be due to a fistula at any site along the spinal axis including the foramen magnum and intracranial locations (Fig. 16-7). Occasionally the shunt can drain both intradurally and extradurally (Fig. 16-8).

On magnification angiography a fine network of vessels leading to the dilated vein may be evident. McCutcheon et al. elegantly showed this arterial network in a microangiopathic study of *en bloc* resections of the involved nerve root sleeve in SDAVFs [37]. The dilated vein fills early but the flow in the perimedullary veins is sluggish, consistent with the pathophysiology of venous hypertension. Due to the prolonged circulation time it is often difficult to demonstrate the venous outflow from the involved perimedullary veins. This suggests a venous outflow obstruction that may be related to venous thrombosis in the past. The venous thrombosis may be the underlying cause of this acquired disorder. Because the proximal vein often follows the nerve root, its initial course is cranial. The direction of flow in the perimedullary venous plexus can be either cranial or caudal. The dilated perimedullary veins are usually posterior and often visualized from the upper thoracic region to the conus [26].

Treatment

The natural history of SDAVFs is that of a progressive downhill course [23]. All SDAVFs should be treated. Endovascular therapy with liquid adhesives N-butyl-2-cyanoacry-

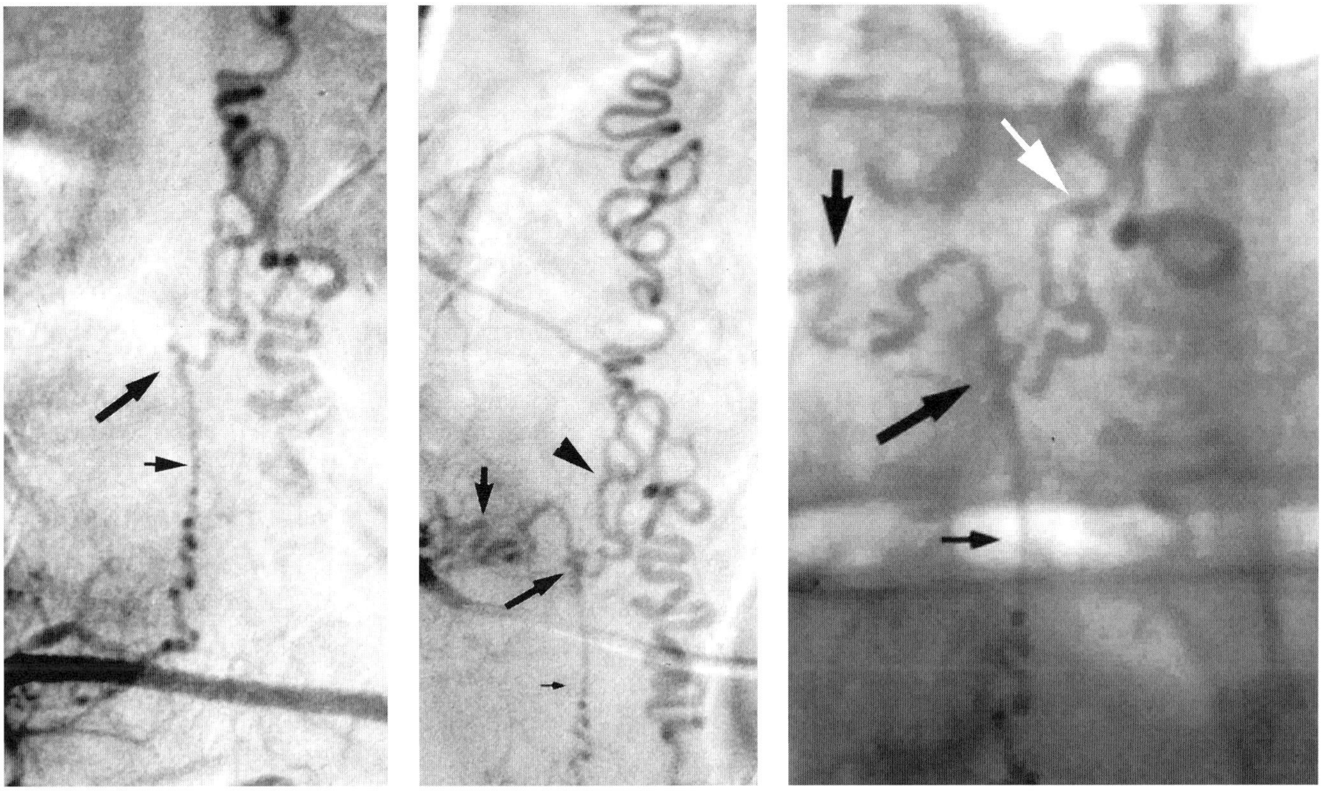

A,B C

FIGURE 16-6. Embolization of an SDAVF with bimetameric dural supply. This 76-year-old suffered from urinary incontinence, leg weakness, and low back pain dating back 4 months. Right T7 **(A)** and right T8 **(B)** intercostal angiograms show a shunt *(long arrow)* between radiculomeningeal branches of T7 and T8 *(small arrows)* and the perimedullary veins *(arrowhead)*. **C:** Cast of the liquid adhesive from the embolization outlines the arterial feeders *(black arrows)* and the proximal veins *(white arrow)*. Control angiograms confirmed the closure of the shunt.

late (NBCA) or surgical ligation of the draining vein can be effective treatment modalities. In 90% of patients closure of the fistula by either embolization or surgery results in clinical improvement [26,38]. The back or radicular pain is relieved immediately. Motor function improves early after treatment, followed by improvement in sensation. Bladder and bowel dysfunction are the last to show any improvement. Recovery is more dramatic when symptoms have been of short duration. Surgical interruption of the draining radicular vein can also be curative with SDAVF [39,40]. Excision of the fistula site is not necessary, although coagulation of the fistula site is often done [40]. If there is both intradural and extradural venous drainage, surgical interruption of the intradural vein will treat the congestive myelopathy and the extradural drainage can be left alone (see Fig. 16-8). The extradural venous drainage may regress.

Aggravation of symptoms after treatment of SDAVFs can occur after embolization or surgery. If there is angiographic proof of a cure, then the clinical deterioration may be due to venous thrombosis. Thrombosis of the perimedullary veins may be related to distal penetration of the embolic material. The deterioration usually occurs within days of the treatment. Heparinization should be given when venous thrombosis is felt to be the cause of the early posttreatment worsening. Niimi et al. proposed heparin therapy for 3 days following embolization for all patients with significantly compromised venous drainage [38]. This finding is determined by the analysis of the venous drainage of the SDAVF. The hallmark of a compromised venous drainage is marked prolongation of the circulation time.

INTRAMEDULLARY SPINAL CORD ARTERIOVENOUS MALFORMATIONS

Clinical

SCAVMs usually occur in the second or third decades. In the Rosenblum et al. series of 54 patients, 70% were male [41]. In this series, 31% experienced a subarachnoid hemorrhage, and at the time of diagnosis 52% had bled. A spinal bleed often results in severe back or radicular pain, followed by a headache and signs of meningeal irritation. This can be mistaken for an intracranial bleed. Hemorrhages are often

A,B 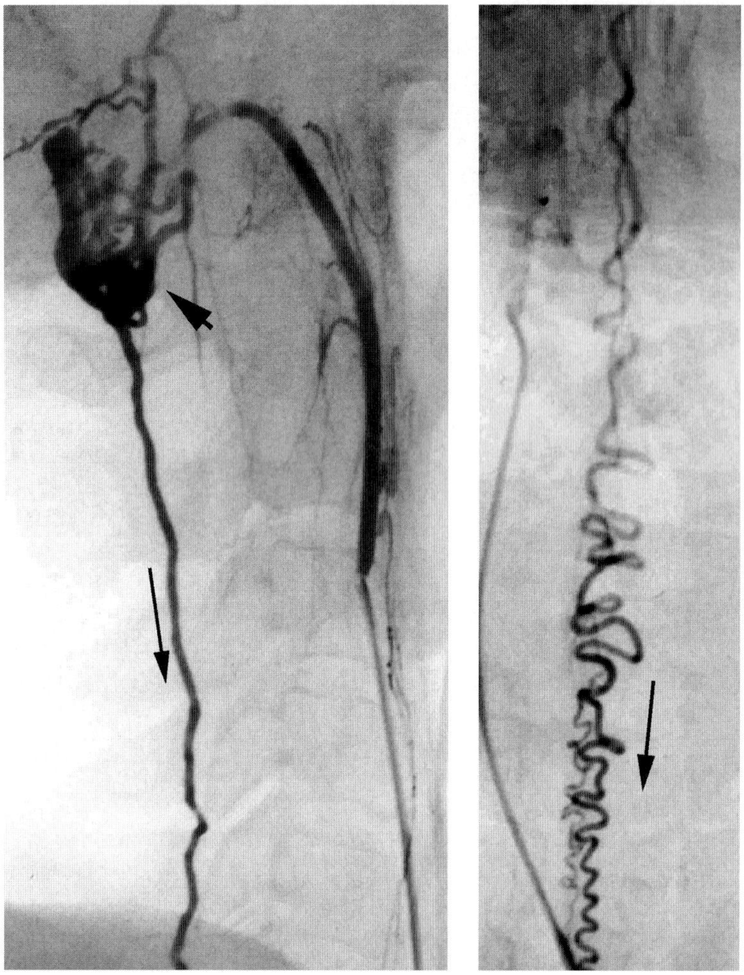

FIGURE 16-7. Intracranial DAVF manifested as a thoracic myelopathy in a 62-year-old man. Lateral **(A)** and anteroposterior **(B)** ascending pharyngeal angiogram shows a shunt at the foramen magnum *(short arrow)* draining into perimedullary veins *(long arrows)*. (**A** from Willinsky R, TerBrugge K, Lasjaunias P, et al. The variable presentations of craniocervical and cervical dural arteriovenous malformations. *Surg Neurol* 1990;34:118–123, with permission.)

multiple, and can either be subarachnoid or within the cord (hematomyelia). Hemorrhages frequently result in new deficits or aggravation of existing deficits. In the series by Berenstein and Lasjaunias, hemorrhage was more frequent in cervical SCAVMs, occurring in 78% [16]. A spastic lower limb paresis was the initial feature in 30% of patients in the report by Rosenblum et al. [41]. In 60% of these the onset was acute, however some patients have an insidious onset. Other symptoms at diagnosis included back pain, root pain, sensory change, impotence, bowel disturbance, bladder dysfunction, and spinal deformity. At the time of diagnosis most patients have motor and sensory deficits. Symptoms can be aggravated by pregnancy, and bleeding during pregnancy may be the initial symptom.

Aminoff and Logue analyzed the outcome of 53 patients who had a hemorrhage from an SCAVM [42]. The rebleed rate was 50%, and of these 50% then bled a third time. Mortality from any bleed was 4% to 11%. In an autopsy series of 27 patients with untreated SCAVMs, 30% died as a result of intraspinal hemorrhage [1].

SCAVMs can be associated with vascular malformations in other parts of the body. Telangiectasias, fistulas, and AVMs are found in brain and spinal cord in Rendu-Osler-Weber syndrome [43]. In the Halbach et al. series of perimedullary fistulas, 20% had Rendu-Osler-Weber syndrome [7]. In a series of Djindjian et al. of 24 patients with SCAVMs, three had Klippel-Trenaunay-Weber syndrome with either venous or arteriovenous malformations in the extremities [11]. SCAVMs can be associated with other diseases including neurofibromatosis, von Willebrand disease, and Parkes Weber syndrome.

Imaging

Diagnostic angiography is always required for ultimate treatment planning. However, MRI provides important noninvasive imaging information prior to angiographic evaluation. Intramedullary vessels and enlarged perimedullary veins are seen well with MRI (Fig. 16-9). In addition, evidence of intermedullary hemorrhage and gliosis or cord infarction can be seen easily (Fig. 16-10).

Intramedullary SCAVMs have a nidus and are fed by anterior spinal (radiculomedullary) or posterior spinal (radiculopial) arteries or both (see Fig. 16-10). Enlargement of

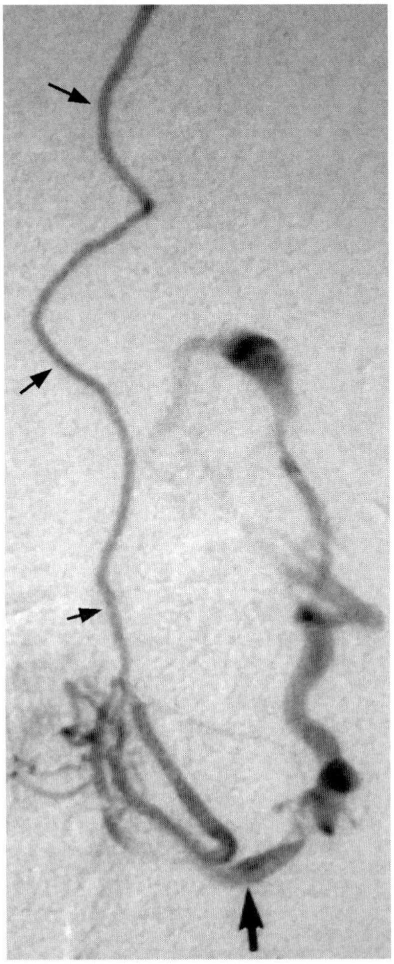

FIGURE 16-8. Spinal dural arteriovenous fistula with intradural and extradural venous drainage in a 68-year-old female who had a thoracic myelopathy. Left L3 superselective angiogram shows a shunt draining into intradural *(small arrows)* and extradural veins *(large arrow).*

feeding branches denotes a direct supply to the nidus. Participating medullary or pial branches that are not significantly enlarged indicates that their involvement is by collateral flow. Analysis of the size of these participating arteries helps in localization of the nidus within the cord.

Biondi et al. found that 14 out of 70 patients (20%) with intramedullary SCAVMs had an aneurysm on a feeding artery [44]. There were no aneurysms associated with their 44 patients with perimedullary SCAVMs or 72 patients with SDAVFs. Subarachnoid hemorrhage occurred in all their patients with aneurysms. Superselective angiography is useful in detecting these aneurysms and helps in differentiating them from venous pouches or pseudoaneurysms related to a venous rupture.

Treatment

Symptomatic SCAVMs should be treated if possible. If the treatment is unlikely to achieve a cure then the therapeutic decisions are based on clinical and angiographic criteria. A patient with repeated bleeds who is neurologically intact should be treated even if only a partial obliteration can be expected. A progressive neurologic deficit is also an indication for treatment in the hope of preventing any further deterioration. A severe, fixed deficit in the lower thoracic cord, with motor, sensory, and sphincter involvement, may not warrant a partial treatment. If there is an aneurysm on the feeding pedicle treatment should be targeted to that pedicle. SCAVMs predominantly fed by radiculopial branches are more favorable for any type of treatment than those with a dominant radiculomedullary supply. These are more favorable to treatment because the posterior location of the nidus is easier to access by surgery and the radiculopial branches are safer to embolize than the radiculomedullary arteries. The radiculopial branches supply the periphery of the spinal cord and there are multiple anastomoses between the radiculopial arteries [45].

Embolization is often the first step in the treatment of intramedullary SCAVMs [16]. Embolization may be the only treatment or may be a preoperative adjunct. Embolization should be done with liquid adhesives, because these agents are most likely to achieve a permanent result. Liquid adhesives can be used with reasonable safety in radiculopial feeders because occlusion of these feeders is usually tolerated. In the anterior spinal axis, liquid adhesives can be used when superselective catheterization of sulcocommissural branches is achieved (Fig. 16-11). Care is taken to prevent reflux, because there is a risk of a neurologic deficit if the radiculomedullary artery is occluded.

Biondi et al. reported their results of embolization using particles in 35 patients with intramedullary SCAVMs [46]. Recanalization occurred in 80%. In this series 37% were clinically unchanged after the first embolization, 57% were improved, and 6% worsened. In the long term, 31% deteriorated.

Berenstein and Lasjaunias reported their results in the embolization of 47 patients with SCAVMs [16]. A liquid adhesive (NBCA or isobutyl-2-cyanoacrylate [IBCA]) was used in 81%, particles in 11%, and 8% of the embolizations were not successful. Clinically 23 of 47 (49%) had an excellent outcome (no deficits and AVM obliterated). In addition, 13 of 47 (28%) had a good outcome (deficit was at baseline or they were better), and 90% of AVMs were obliterated. This yielded excellent or good results in a total of 36 of 47 (77%) patients, giving results that are much better than the natural history previously outlined. In addition, 91% had either complete occlusion or the morphological goal (i.e., elimination of an aneurysm) was achieved. Their permanent morbidity from embolization was 11% (two severe, two moderate, one mild) and the transient complication rate was 11%.

Embolization of aneurysms associated with intramedullary SCAVMs has gained acceptance for patients who have a bleed [47,48]. Depending on the angioarchitecture and

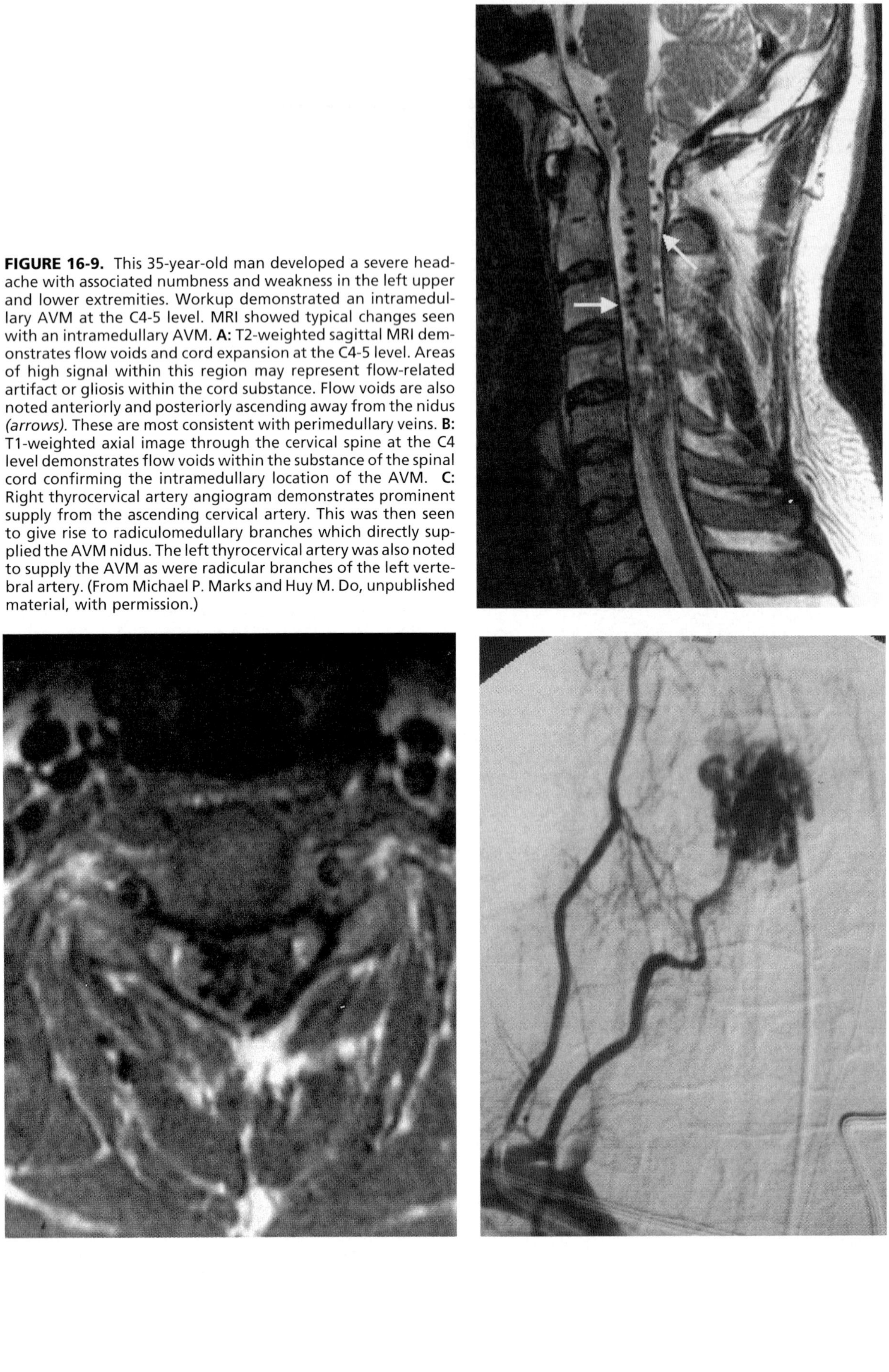

A

B

C

FIGURE 16-9. This 35-year-old man developed a severe headache with associated numbness and weakness in the left upper and lower extremities. Workup demonstrated an intramedullary AVM at the C4-5 level. MRI showed typical changes seen with an intramedullary AVM. **A:** T2-weighted sagittal MRI demonstrates flow voids and cord expansion at the C4-5 level. Areas of high signal within this region may represent flow-related artifact or gliosis within the cord substance. Flow voids are also noted anteriorly and posteriorly ascending away from the nidus *(arrows)*. These are most consistent with perimedullary veins. **B:** T1-weighted axial image through the cervical spine at the C4 level demonstrates flow voids within the substance of the spinal cord confirming the intramedullary location of the AVM. **C:** Right thyrocervical artery angiogram demonstrates prominent supply from the ascending cervical artery. This was then seen to give rise to radiculomedullary branches which directly supplied the AVM nidus. The left thyrocervical artery was also noted to supply the AVM as were radicular branches of the left vertebral artery. (From Michael P. Marks and Huy M. Do, unpublished material, with permission.)

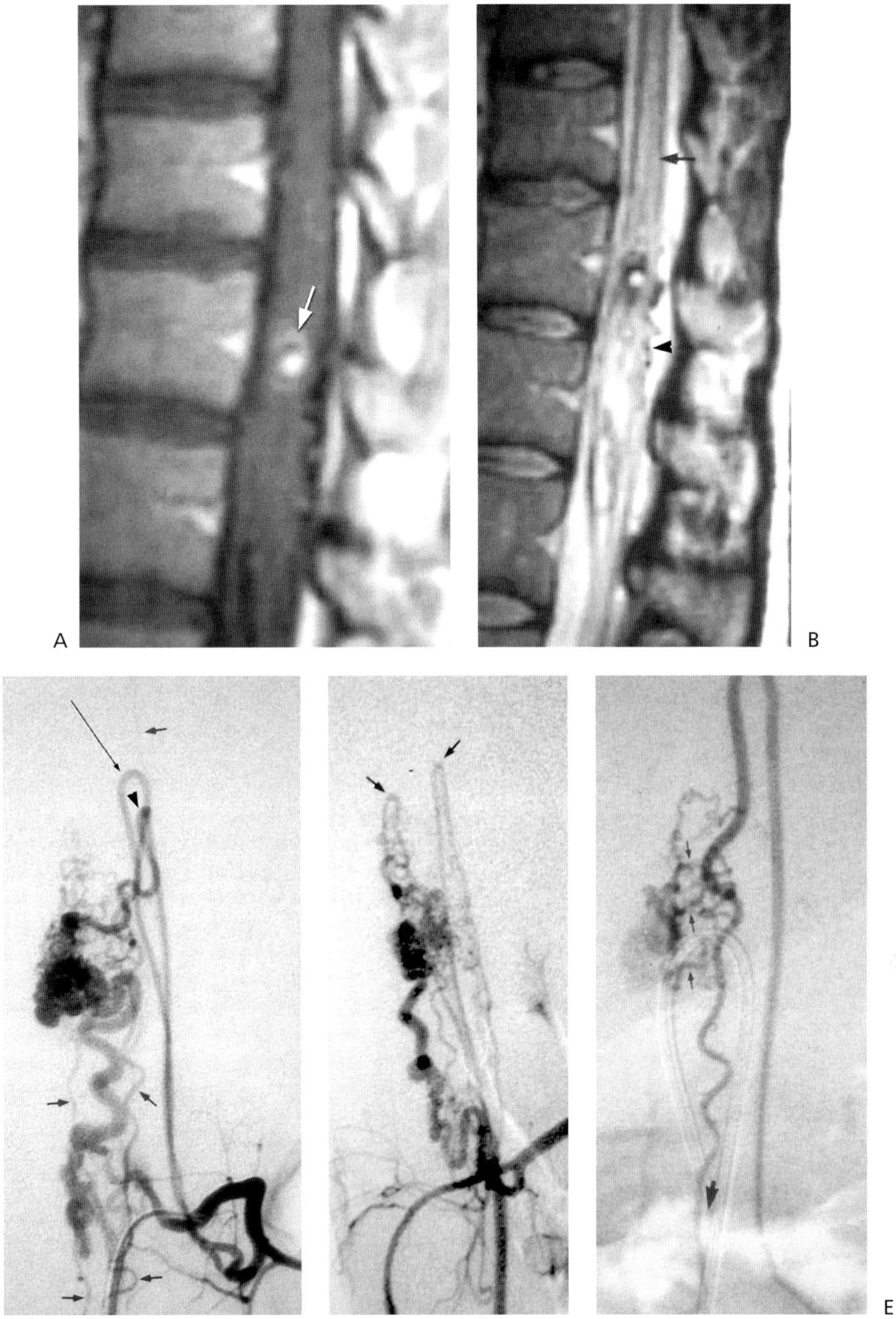

FIGURE 16-10. Intramedullary SCAVM. This 24-year-old female sought treatment for a sudden onset of pain, weakness, and incoordination in the right leg. An attempt to embolize the SCAVM was unsuccessful due to the small size of the feeders. Four years later she suddenly developed a complete paraplegia. She was then operated on. A postoperative angiogram showed no residual AVM. Initial T1-weighted **(A)** and T2-weighted **(B)** MRI show hematomyelia *(white arrow)* with cord edema *(black arrow)* and flow voids *(arrowhead)*. **C:** Left T10 intercostal angiogram shows a nidus fed by radiculomedullary *(long arrow)* and radiculopial *(arrowhead)* arteries. The continuation of the radiculomedullary artery is outlined *(small arrows)*. **D:** Lateral left T10 intercostal angiogram *(posterior to the left)* shows the separate hairpin loops *(arrows)* of the radiculomedullary and radiculopial arteries, with the bulk of the nidus posterior. **E:** Superselective angiogram of the radiculomedullary artery (AP projection) shows that its contribution is indirect through small perforators *(small arrows)* and around the conus *(large arrow)*. This confirms that the nidus is posterior within the cord.

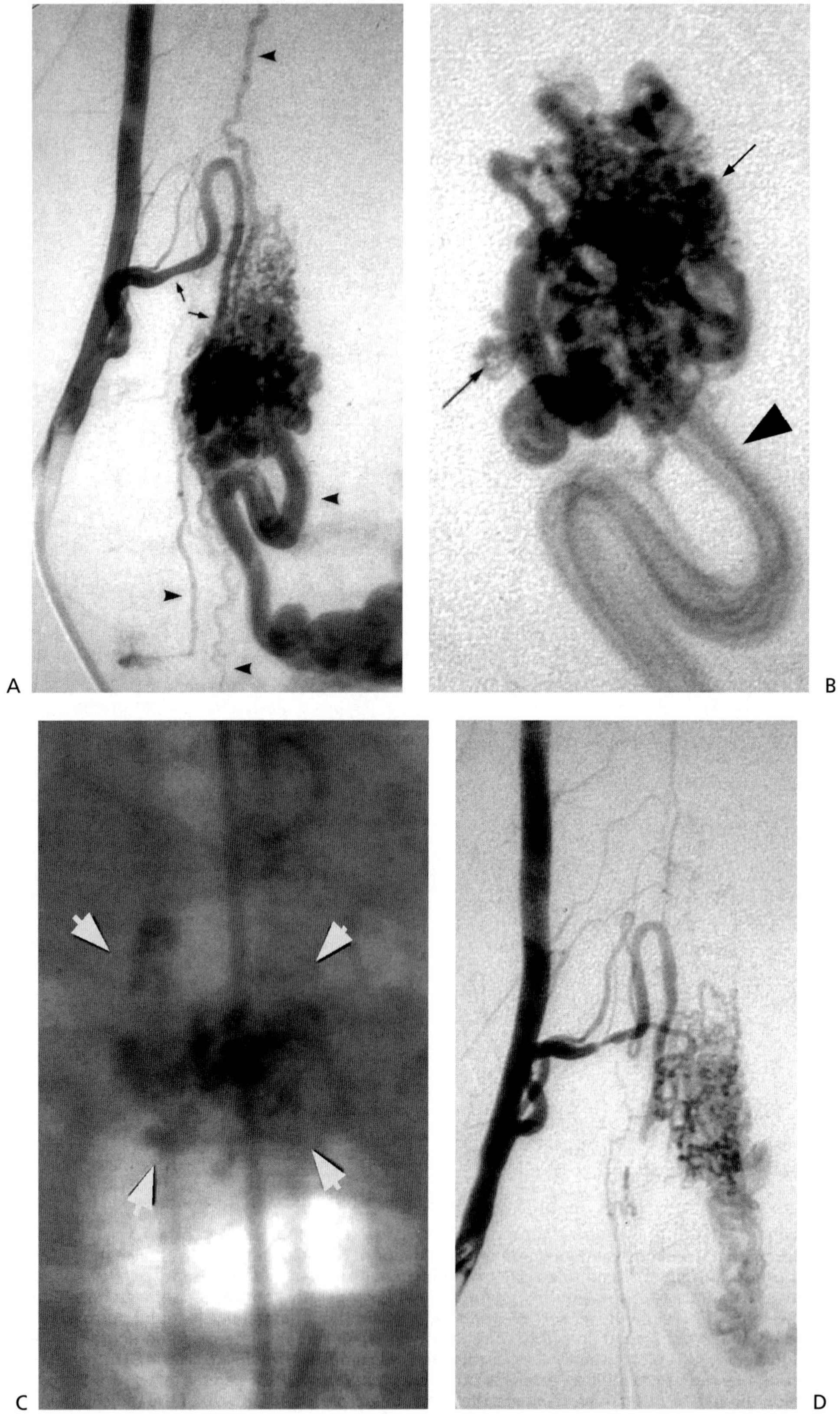
A
B
C
D

location of the AVM, this may be used as the only treatment (Fig. 16-12). In some patients this may be used as the initial treatment, to be followed by elective surgery after the patient has made some clinical recovery. In a series by Konan et al., two of the patients had subarachnoid bleeds and two had hematomyelia [48]. They embolized five aneurysms in four patients with intramedullary SCAVMs without complications. Liquid adhesives were used, and there were no rebleeds in the 17 to 37 months of follow-up.

Surgery of intramedullary SCAVMs is reserved for those lesions that are incompletely treated by embolization and when the residual malformation is accessible. Connolly et al. reported on the surgical management of 15 cases of intramedullary AVMs using a posterior approach [49]. Sixty percent had subarachnoid bleeds, and 47% had deficits related to these bleeds. Outcomes were generally good, with 40% improved, 53% stable, and 7% being worse. Martin et al. reported on a posterolateral approach with dentate ligament section and spinal cord rotation to provide exposure to the anterior spinal (radiculomedullary) artery and its sulcocommissural branches [50]. This approach avoids the more difficult anterior spinal approach.

Radiosurgery may provide a treatment alternative for those intramedullary lesions that prove inaccessible by endovascular or surgical means. It has been shown to be efficacious in the treatment of brain AVMs. The spinal cord does have a low radiation tolerance, however, and postradiation myelopathy and edema are well-documented complications [51–53]. Nevertheless, some centers are using stereotactic radiosurgery to treat intramedullary AVMs that are untreatable by conventional means (Fig. 16-13) [54].

PERIMEDULLARY SPINAL CORD ARTERIOVENOUS FISTULAS

Clinical

Perimedullary SCAVMs may appear acutely with a bleed or with a slowly progressive myelopathy usually related to venous congestion [9,55]. The clinical expression of type I slow-flow, anterior perimedullary fistulas differs from SCAVMs with a nidus [8,9,56]. These type I perimedullary fistulas occur at a later age, with a mean age of 45 years, with a slowly, progressive thoracic myelopathy similar to that of SDAVFs. The type II fistulas often are associated with a progressive neurologic deficit of the conus medullaris and cauda equina. In contrast, Halbach et al. reviewed ten type III giant perimedullary fistulas, five patients with subarachnoid hemorrhage, and the mean age for the ten patients was 19.5 years [7]. The high-flow AVFs are often discovered in children and may be associated with Rendu-Osler-Weber syndrome [7,12,57].

Imaging

Type III giant perimedullary fistulas are easy to recognize on MRI due to the marked vascular dilation. The type I and type II perimedullary SCAVMs may be difficult to distinguish on MRI from other types of spinal AVMs. Patients with a slowly progressive myelopathy often demonstrate T2 hyperintensity within a swollen spinal cord. Enlarged perimedullary vessels may or may not be evident within the subarachnoid space. The MRI findings may be indistinguishable from spinal dural AVMs. Perimedullary SCAVMs may have involvement of the cervical or high thoracic cord, a location that is unusual for the typical SDAVF.

Type 1 perimedullary SCAVMs may be difficult to recognize because the feeding radiculomedullary artery is only slightly enlarged and the shunt is slow. The fistula site is evident due to a subtle caliber change between the relatively straight feeding artery and the more tortuous anterior spinal vein that eventually drains through radicular veins (Figs. 16-14 and 16-15). Superselective angiography of the radiculomedullary feeder may show that multiple small sulcocommissural branches feed the fistula that is deep in the central sulcus of the cord (see Fig 16-14). The fistula site may be subpial and embedded within the cord substance. Type II perimedullary SCAVMs can be differentiated from intramedullary SCAVMs by the presence of a single fistula and multiple arterial feeders. In contradistinction, intramedullary SCAVMs have a nidus with a network of multiple shunts and multiple draining veins. Type III perimedullary SCAVMs have multiple, enlarged pial or medullary feeders

FIGURE 16-11. This 19-year-old man with an intramedullary SCAVM experienced a sudden onset of paraplegia related to a bleed into the lower cervical spinal cord. Two years before this bleed he had a similar spinal hemorrhage but made a complete recovery. **A:** Anteroposterior right vertebral angiogram shows an AVM fed by an enlarged radiculomedullary artery *(arrow)* and multiple draining veins *(arrowheads).* Radiculopial supply was present from the left supreme intercostal artery. **B:** Oblique superselective angiogram of a sulcocommissural feeder demonstrates the nidus *(arrows)* and draining vein *(arrowhead).* Three sulcocommissural branches were embolized with liquid adhesives (NBCA and iodized oil). **C:** Plain radiographic film postembolization demonstrates cast of the liquid adhesive *(arrows).* **D:** Right vertebral postembolization angiogram shows a significant flow reduction in the AVM. The patient has remained stable after this partial treatment during the past 7 years.

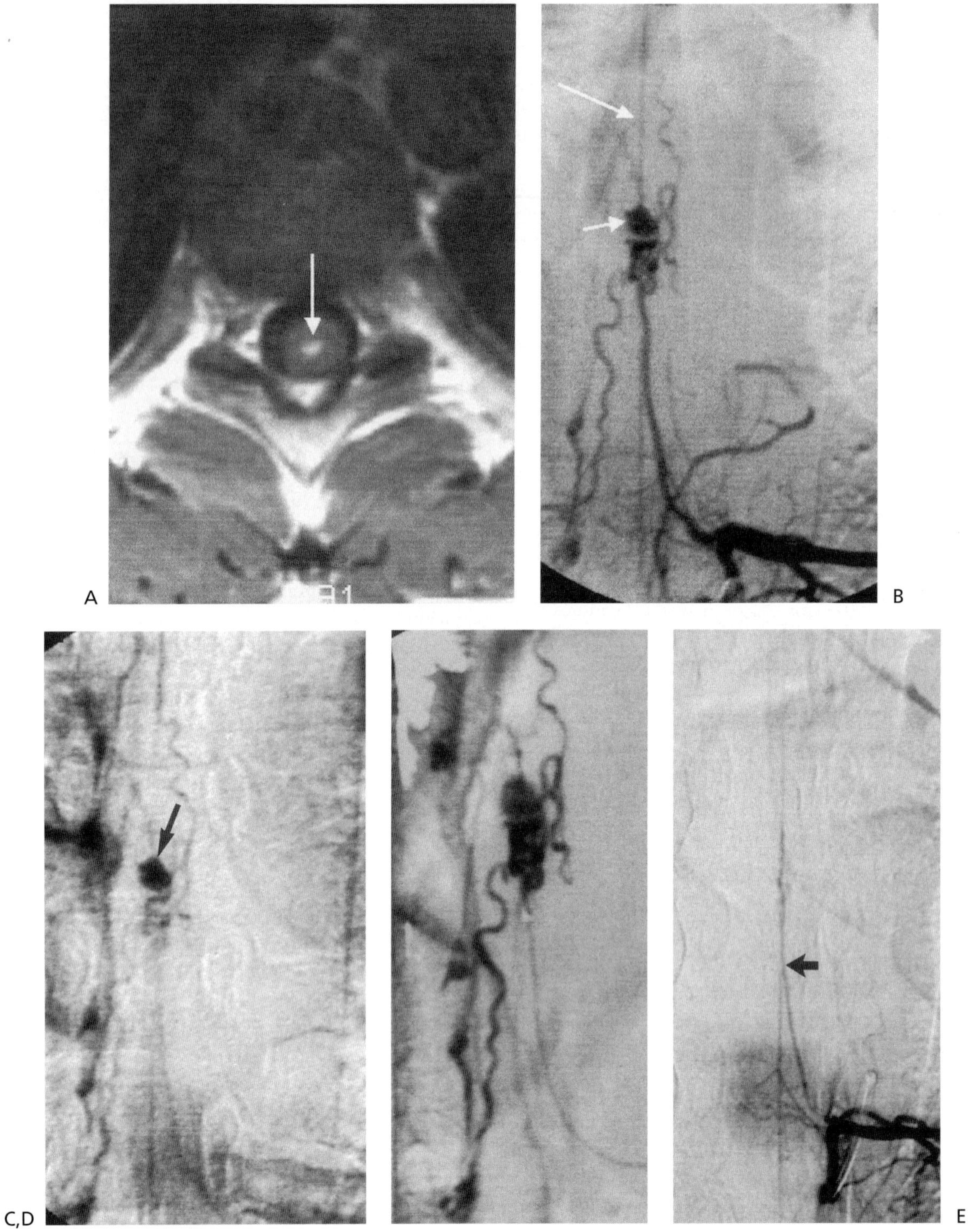

FIGURE 16-12. This 18-year-old man developed sudden onset of bilateral lower extremity weakness. Workup demonstrated an intramedullary AVM. **A:** T1-weighted axial image through the thoracic cord at approximately the T7 level demonstrates an area of high signal *(arrow)* consistent with hematomyelia. **B:** Left T9 intercostal artery angiogram demonstrates an intramedullary AVM at the T7-8 level. Note the filling of the anterior spinal artery *(long arrow)* and the presence of an intranidal aneurysm *(short arrow)*. **C:** Later image from the same left T9 intercostal artery angiogram demonstrates the intranidal aneurysm *(arrow)*. **D:** Angiogram from a microcatheter placed distally in the intercostal artery circulation demonstrates selective filling of the nidus, nidal aneurysm, and perimedullary veins. Embolization was subsequently performed through this microcatheter. **E:** Selective left T9 intercostal artery angiogram obtained 12 years following the embolization. The patient had been lost to follow-up but returned for follow-up imaging studies without any new symptoms. Angiogram demonstrates continued nidal obliteration and nonfilling of the intranidal aneurysm. There is still continued supply to the anterior spinal artery *(arrow)* from the left T9 intercostal artery. (From Michael P. Marks and Huy M. Do, unpublished material, with permission.)

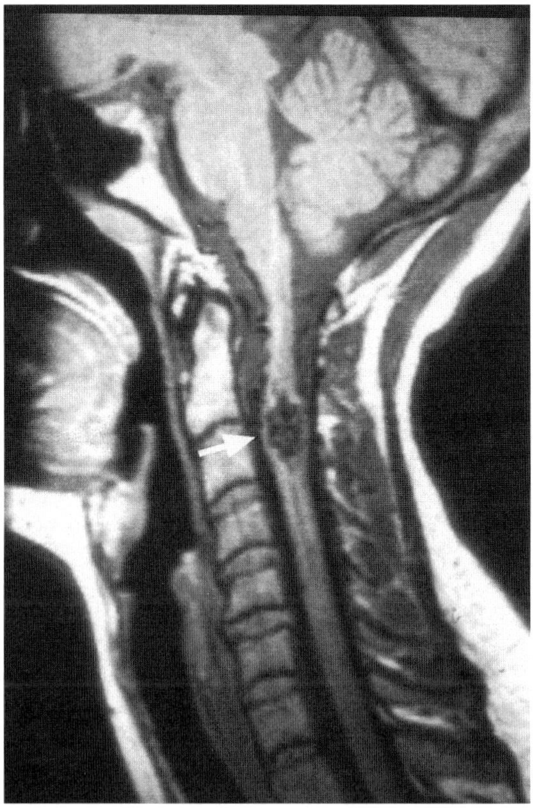

A

FIGURE 16-13. This 40-year-old woman had a history of progressive right upper and lower extremity weakness and numbness. Workup demonstrated an intramedullary AVM at the C1-2 level. Because of the size of the AVM and the complex radiculomedullary and radiculopial supply, stereotactic radiosurgery was performed. **A:** T1-weighted sagittal image demonstrates the intramedullary AVM nidus *(arrow)* with evidence of cord atrophy above and below the level of the nidus. **B,C:** Anteroposterior and lateral views from a right vertebral artery angiogram demonstrate the AVM nidus *(arrow)* with combined radiculomedullary and radiculopial supply and perimedullary drainage. The patient underwent stereotactic radiosurgery. *(Figure continues.)*

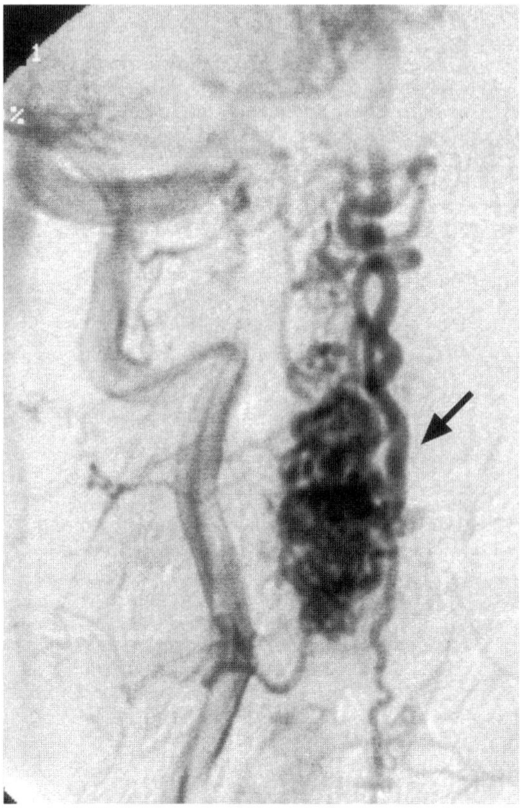

B

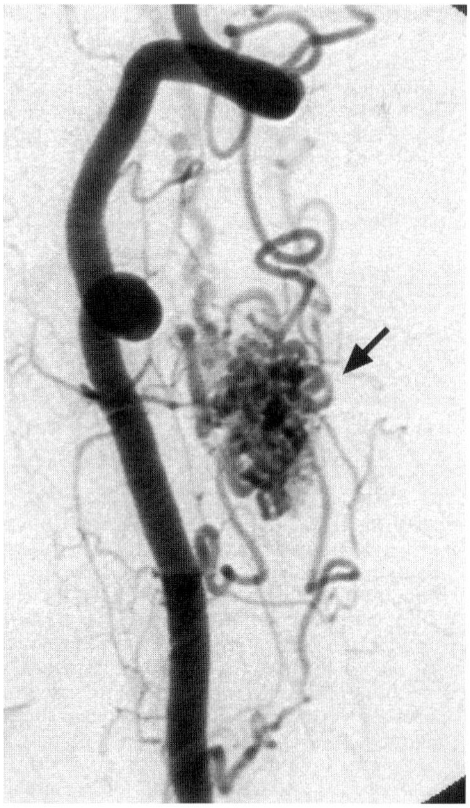

C

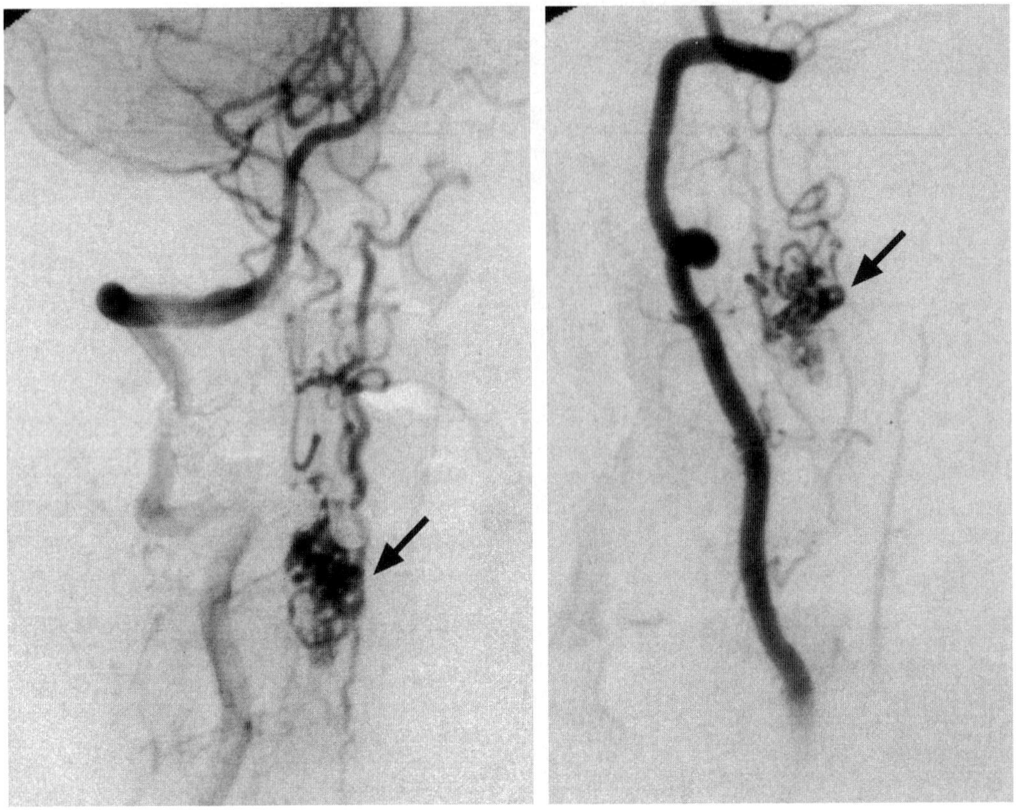

D E

FIGURE 16-13. *Continued.* **D,E:** Anteroposterior and lateral right vertebral artery angiograms obtained 4 years following stereotactic radiosurgery demonstrate continued filling of the AVM nidus *(arrows)*. However, the shunt flow and nidus size is significantly reduced, indicating extensive thrombosis within the AVM nidus. The patient had no change in her symptoms during the 4-year follow-up period. At this point she underwent further radiosurgery and is awaiting further follow-up. (From Steven Chang, Department of Neurosurgery, Stanford University Medical Center, unpublished material, with permission.)

FIGURE 16-14. Type I perimedullary fistula. A 57-year-old man had calf pain, leg weakness, and incoordination of gait for 6 years. MRI showed T2 hyperintensity in the thoracic cord with prominent perimedullary flow voids suggesting a spinal dural arteriovenous fistula. **A:** Left T8 intercostal angiogram shows a fistula *(short arrow)* supplied by the radiculomedullary artery and draining into the perimedullary venous plexus *(long arrows)*. **B:** Oblique, magnified view of the left T8 intercostal angiogram shows the radiculomedullary artery *(small arrows)*, the fistula site *(solid arrow)*, and the perimedullary veins *(open arrows)*. **C:** Superselective lateral radiculomedullary angiogram close to the fistula site *(long arrow)* shows that there are multiple sulcocommissural feeders to the shunt. The radiculomedullary artery is outlined *(small arrows)* and there is early filling of the veins *(open arrows)*. The sulcocommissural feeders could not be catheterized and therefore no embolization was done. **D:** Postoperative lateral left T8 angiogram shows the surgical clips used to occlude the fistula and preservation of the anterior spinal axis *(arrows)*. This required two surgical sessions and embolization of a dural feeder that developed after the second surgery.

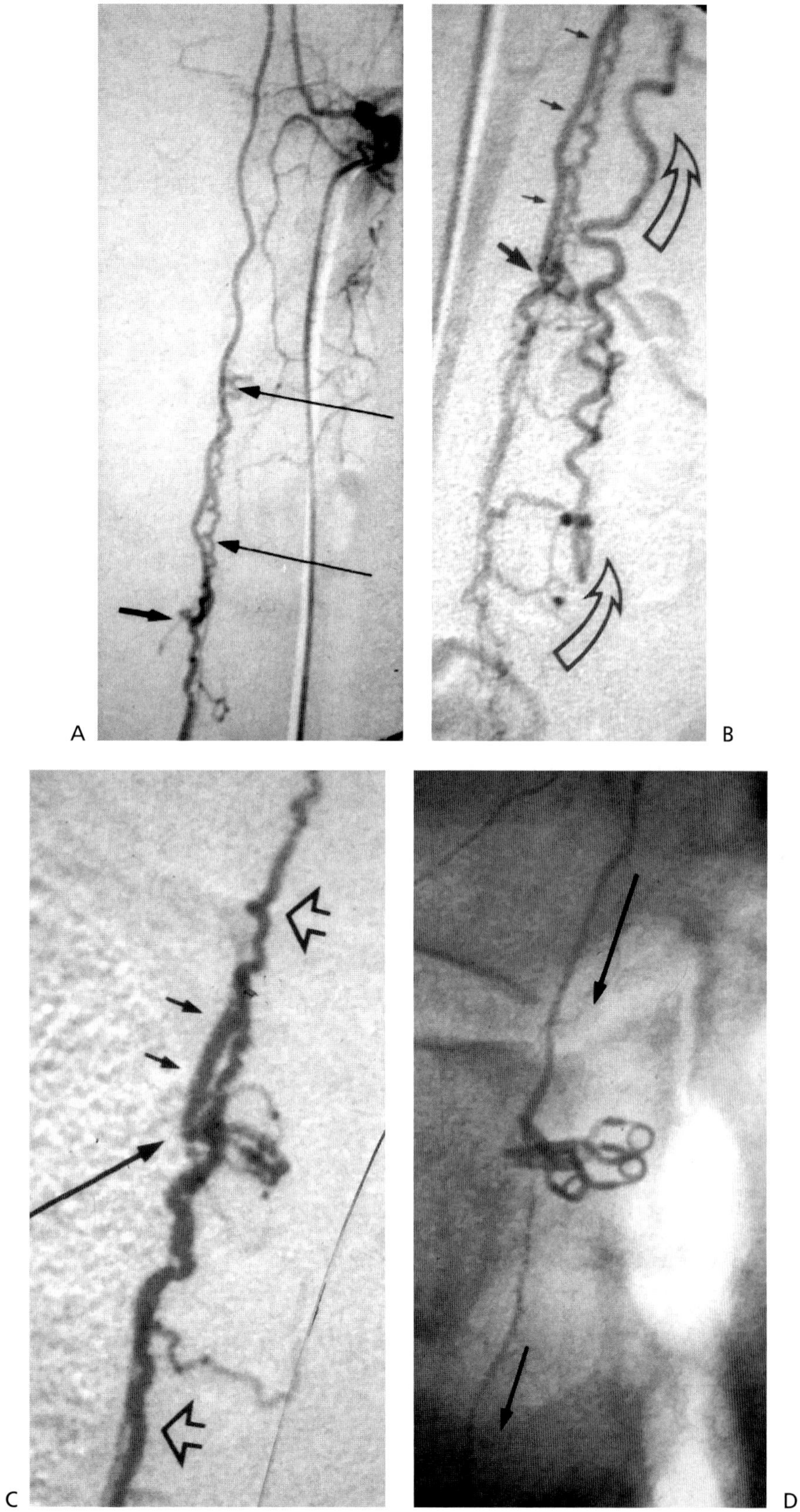
A
B
C
D

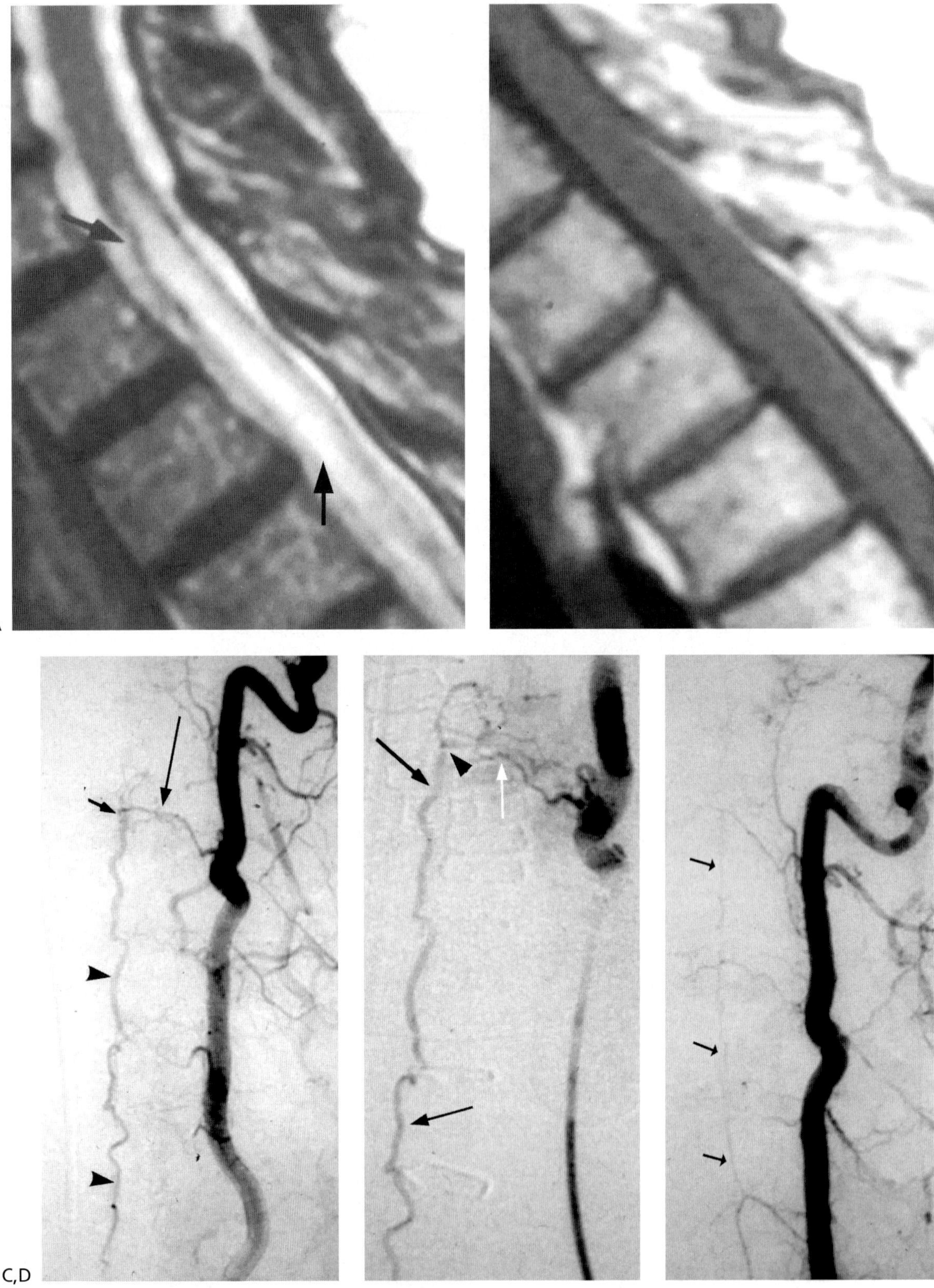
A
B
C,D
E

with rapid shunting through a single fistula into an ectatic perimedullary vein (Fig. 16-16).

Treatment

The approach to treatment of perimedullary fistula depends on the angioarchitecture. The type III giant perimedullary fistulas are well suited to endovascular treatment [7,57,58]. Type II fistulas may be treated with embolization, surgery, or a combination of embolization and surgery [9,55]. Type I fistulas usually require surgery due to the small size of the radiculomedullary feeder, and there may be multiple small sulcocommissural branches leading to the fistula site (see Figs. 16-14 and 16-15). A posterolateral approach is feasible with cutting of the dentate ligament and rotation of the cord [50]. The fistula site in these perimedullary fistulas may be subpial and therefore embedded in the cord itself. The actual fistula site may be difficult to recognize during surgery and it may be difficult to distinguish the feeders from normal sulcocommissural branches. Postoperative angiography is critical, because residual shunting after surgery is not rare and a second surgical exploration may be necessary.

In a Halbach et al. series of type II or III perimedullary fistulas, most were treated with embolization alone or with embolization and surgery [7]. If the feeding vessels are enlarged then selective catheterization can allow embolization with liquid adhesives. If there is marked enlargement of the feeder and dilation of the vein, the transarterial approach can be used to enter the vein and block it with coils, followed by an arterial embolization with a liquid adhesive [57]. Coils are used on the venous side to avoid escape of the liquid adhesive. Closure of the vein is critical if there are multiple shunts into this dilated vein. Not all arterial pedicles need to be treated if the embolic material closes the fistula. Closure of the arteries proximal to the shunt should not be done because it promotes the development of collateral flow. In the Halbach et al. series, the venous pouch was selectively catheterized by both transarterial and transvenous routes to allow direct embolization of the venous pouch [7].

Similar to all the spinal AVMs, the clinical outcome after treatment of a perimedullary SCAVM is dependent on the clinical status of the patient at the time of treatment. Surgery often results in transient worsening of the symptoms but most patients return to baseline or better [7]. Endovascular treatment of type III AVFs often results in a good clinical recovery [9]. Mourier et al. reported that none of patients deteriorated after treatment, one-half remained unchanged, and the other one-half had some clinical improvement [9].

EXTRADURAL ARTERIOVENOUS FISTULAS

Clinical

Spinal EAVFs are shunts from metameric arteries to the epidural and paravertebral veins. A number of names that have been used to describe the EAVF include paraspinal, paravertebral, and epidural. The descriptive term extradural may be the most appropriate, because these fistulas may be either in the epidural space, in the bone, or adjacent to the bone.

Spinal EAVFs are rare lesions that have diverse clinical features [59,60]. EAVFs can produce a venous congestive myelopathy similar to DAVFs (Fig. 16-17), a compressive myelopathy due to enlarged epidural veins, or they may be detected incidentally (Table 16-3). Like SDAVFs, the EAVFs rarely hemorrhage. Hui et al. described three cases of paraspinal AVMs in which one patient sought treatment for myelopathy due to the mass effect by the veins, one had a bruit, and the third patient had a congestive myelopathy related to perimedullary reflux [61]. Arnaud et al. described a case of an EAVF with a congestive myelopathy due to reflux into the perimedullary veins at two levels [62]. Extradural presacral AVFs may be associated with a congestive myelopathy due to their perimedullary venous drainage [63, 64]. Goyal et al. found that compression by large epidural veins was the cause of symptoms in three patients [65]. One patient in the series had a vascular flank mass. On imaging, an EAVF was found draining into the flank mass, probably secondary to obstruction of the azygos system (Fig. 16-18). EAVFs are associated with neurofibromatosis and spinal teratomas [59,65].

Perimedullary reflux from an EAVF is uncommon (see

FIGURE 16-15. Type I perimedullary AVF. A 78-year-old woman was evaluated for a slowly progressive cervical thoracic myelopathy dating back over 6 months. **A:** T2-weighted MRI shows hyperintensity in the cervical-thoracic cord *(arrows)* but no abnormal flow voids. **B:** Gadolinium-enhanced T1-weighted MRI shows no enhancement. **C:** Left vertebral angiogram shows a fistula *(small arrow)* between a radiculomedullary artery *(long arrow)* and the anterior spinal vein *(arrowheads).* An operation was done to clip the fistula. **D:** Postoperative selective left vertebral angiogram shows that the midline fistula remained open *(arrowhead).* It was supplied by a radiculomedullary artery *(white arrow)* and drained into the anterior spinal vein *(black arrows).* **E:** Repeat surgery was done, and the follow-up left vertebral angiogram shows that the fistula is closed and the anterior spinal axis *(arrows)* is preserved. During surgery the fistula was found to be subpial within the central sulcus.

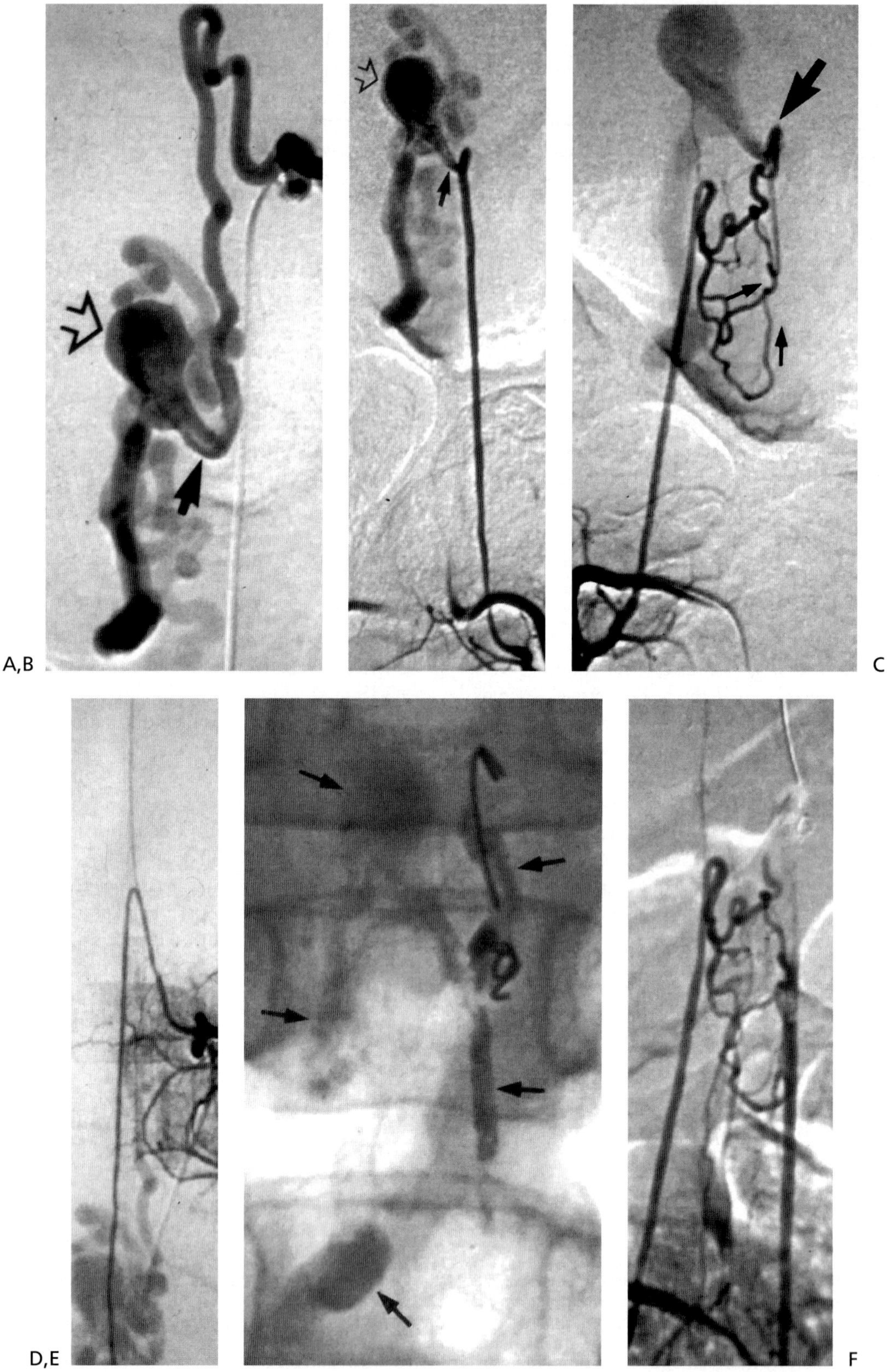
A,B
C
D,E
F

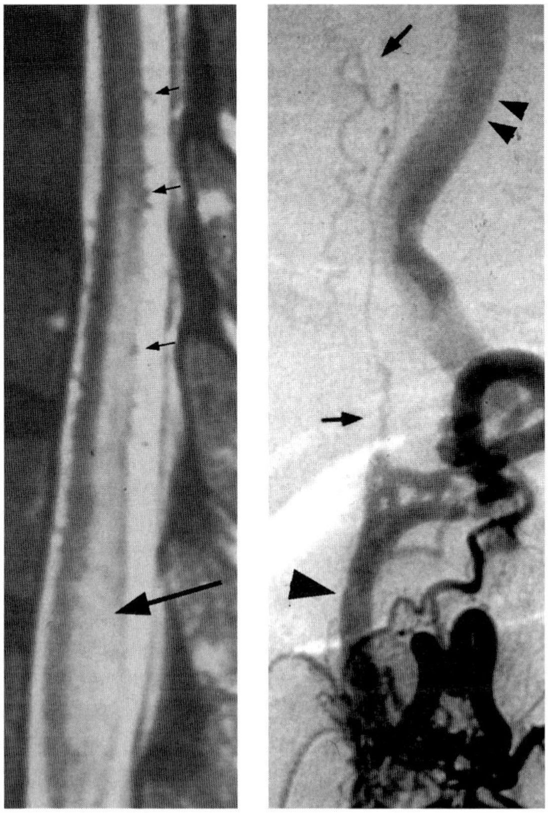

A,B

FIGURE 16-17. Extradural AVF with retrograde flow into the perimedullary venous plexus. This 72-year-old female had a thoracic myelopathy of 2 years' duration. **A:** T2-weighted MRI shows hyperintensity within the conus *(long arrow)* and prominent subarachnoid flow voids *(small arrows)* suggesting an SDAVF. **B:** Left L3 angiogram shows a high-flow shunt draining into the epidural venous plexus *(single arrowhead)* with reflux into an intradural radicular vein *(arrows).* There is also drainage into the paraspinal veins *(double arrowhead).* The patient was treated by surgical disconnection of the intradural radicular vein. The clinical status improved after surgery. (From Goyal M, Willinsky R, Montanera W, et al. Paravertebral arteriovenous malformations with epidural drainage: clinical spectrum, imaging features, and results of treatment. *AJNR Am J Neuroradiol* 1999;20:749–755, with permission.)

Fig. 16-17) [59]. Tadie et al., in histologic sections, demonstrated narrowing of the radiculospinal veins at the point where they crossed the dura [66]. They postulated that, under normal physiologic conditions, the narrowing and zigzag course of these veins oppose any blood flow from the periphery into the intradural space. Reflux into the perimedullary veins from EAVFs must be due to a failure of the antireflux mechanism, perhaps related to the presence of chronic venous hypertension in the epidural space [59].

Arteriovenous fistulas between the vertebral artery and the vertebral veins (VVAVFs) can be included in the EAVFs. Trauma was the commonest etiology in early series [16,67]. However, 59% of the VVAVFs were spontaneous in a large series by Beaujeux et al. [68], and 100% (12 of 12) VVAVFs were spontaneous in a series by Goyal et al. [69]. Fibromuscular dysplasia, neurofibromatosis, and Ehlers-Danlos syndrome are known predisposing conditions for VVAVFs [65, 70,71]. These fistulas may be congenital. In the Goyal et

FIGURE 16-16. Type III perimedullary AVF. A 10-year-old boy with a family history of Rendu-Osler-Weber syndrome had a history of three subarachnoid hemorrhages. He was neurologically intact. **A:** Left T10 intercostal angiogram shows an enlarged radiculopial artery supplying a fistula *(solid arrow)* at T12 and a venous ectasia *(open arrow)* proximal to the perimedullary veins. **B:** Left L3 angiogram shows a radiculopial feeder to the fistula *(arrow)* and the same venous pouch *(open arrow).* **C:** Right L2 angiogram shows a radiculopial feeder that contributes to the same fistula *(large arrow)* through the arterial "basket" around the conus *(small arrows).* **D:** Left T9 intercostal angiogram shows that the radiculomedullary artery does not contribute to the fistula. **E:** Plain radiographic film postembolization with coils and NBCA *(arrows).* The embolization was done by selectively catheterizing the left L3 radiculopial artery to close the contribution from the left T10 radiculopial artery. The catheter was then placed in the L3 radiculopial artery just proximal to the fistula site. The fistula was closed using liquid adhesives with penetration into the venous pouch. **F:** Postembolization right L2 angiogram shows that the fistula is occluded (compare with C). The patient was neurologically intact after the procedure. (From Emery DJ, Willinsky R, Burrows PE, et al. Pediatric spinal arteriovenous malformations: angioarchitecture and endovascular treatment. *Interv Neuroradiol* 1998;4:127–139, with permission.)

TABLE 16-3. EXTRADURAL ARTERIOVENOUS FISTULA[a]: CLINICAL FEATURES, MAGNETIC RESONANCE FEATURES, ANGIOARCHITECTURE, AND RESULTS OF TREATMENT IN TEN PATIENTS

Pt. No.	Sex/Age (yr)	Features	MR Findings	Angiogram: Feeders	Angiogram: Drainage	Pathophysiology	Tx	Outcome
1	M/73	Progressive leg weakness	↑ Cord signal on T2, ↑ vessels	Epidural fistula, lateral sacral artery; reflux to PM veins	Azygos; PM veins	Venous hypertension	Surg	Improved
2	M/68	Cervical myelopathy	Large epidural veins; cord compression	Epidural fistula; RVA, LVA, both ECA, bilateral thyrocervical & costocervical	Epidural veins to paravertebral venous plexus	Compression	Embo	Improved
3	M/34	Thoracic myelopathy	AVM: spinal cord, epidural space and vertebra	SCAVM: anterior spinal artery; metameric supply to epidural & bone AVM	Epidural: azygos SCAVM: PM	SCAVM	Embo attempt	—
4	M/70	Thoracic myelopathy	↑ Cord signal on T2, ↑ vessels; vessels in epidural at T-L junction	Epidural fistula; lt T12; reflux to PM veins	Lumbar veins; PM veins	Venous hypertension	Surg	Improved
5	M/41	NF, nocturia, pain	Epidural vein at rt T8–9 compressing cord	Epidural fistula; multiple intercostal feeders	Hemiazygos	Compression	Embo	Improved
6	F/5	Ulcerated flank mass	Not available	Epidural fistula; rt T10, lt T11	Into flank mass; hemiazygos not seen	? Thrombosis of hemiazygos	Embo	Transient limp; mass removed
7	M/7	Asymptomatic bruit: lt scapula	Prominent epidural & paraverebral veins	Epidural fistula; lt T5 & lt costocervical	Superior intercostal	Asymptomatic	Embo	Fistula cured
8	M/1	Spasticity of lower limbs	Tethered cord, cord tumor; epidural vessel: lt L5	Epidural fistula; lt L5	Azygos	Asymptomatic	Embo	Fistula cured
9	F/13	Back pain	↑ Cord signal on T2, ↑ vessels	Bone and epidural AVM; lt T11–12 & rt T11 arteries	Azygos	Venous hypertension	None	—
10	F/17	Paraparesis (arterial embolism elsewhere)	Epidural & paravertebral vessels: T9–L1 compressing cord	Paravertebral AVM; multiple intercostal & lumbar feeders	Azygos	Mass effect	Embo	Minimally improved

Pt, patient; M, male; F, female; AVM, arteriovenous fistula; SCAVM, spinal cord arteriovenous malformation; MR, magnetic resonance; NF, neurofibromatosis; PM, perimedullary; T, thoracic; L, lumbar; RVA, right vertebral artery; LVA, left vertebral artery; ECA, external carotid artery; TL, thoracolumbar; lt, left; rt, right; Tx, treatment; Embo, embolization; Surg, surgery.

[a]Excluding vertebrovertebral arteriovenous fistulas.

From Goyal M, Willinsky R, Montanera W, et al. Paravertebral arteriovenous malformations with epidural drainage: clinical spectrum, imaging features, and results of treatment. *AJNR Am J Neuroradiol* 1999;20:749–755, with permission.

FIGURE 16-18. Extradural AVF. A 7-month-old girl was evaluated for an enlarging congenital vascular mass in the left flank. Angiography revealed a high-flow extradural AVF draining into a large epidural pouch, which then drained into lumbar veins toward the flank mass. Early **(A)** and late **(B)** aortic flush angiograms show a fistula fed by segmental right T10 and left T12 branches (*short arrows* in **A**) with drainage into an epidural pouch *(long arrows)*, paraspinal veins *(curved arrow)*, and lumbar veins (*small arrows* in **B**). **C:** Right T10 angiogram shows the fistula *(open arrow)* in the wall of a large epidural pouch that drains through the foramina *(closed arrow)* into the paraspinal veins. **D:** Selective left T12 angiogram, after embolization of the epidural venous pouch with coils and liquid adhesives, shows stasis in the pouch. The right T10 feeder was closed with coils and NBCA. Coils were placed directly into the epidural pouch after catheterization from the left T12 feeder. A controlled injection of NBCA was done from the left T10 feeder after deposition of the coils. **E:** Postembolization aortogram shows that the fistula is closed. The "stumps" of the right T10 and left T12 feeders are evident *(arrows)*. (From Emery DJ, Willinsky R, Burrows PE, et al. Pediatric spinal arteriovenous malformations: angioarchitecture and endovascular treatment. *Interv Neuroradiol* 1998;4:127–139, with permission.)

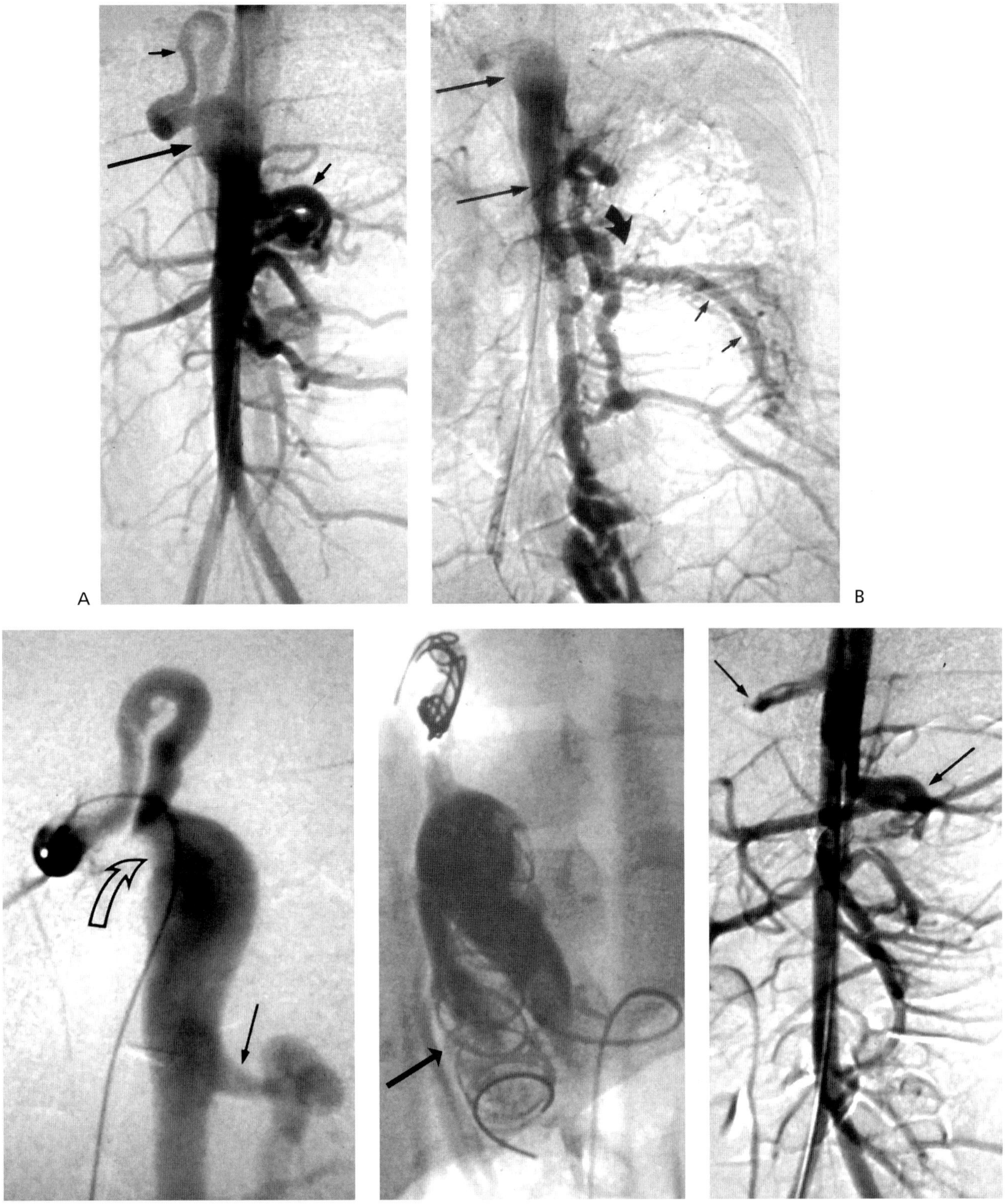

A B

C,D E

TABLE 16-4. CLINICAL FEATURES, ANGIOARCHITECTURE, AND RESULTS OF TREATMENT IN 12 PATIENTS WITH VERTEBROVERTEBRAL ARTERIOVENOUS FISTULAS

Pt. No.	Sex/Age (yr)	Features	Site	Retrograde Flow in Distal Vertebral Artery	Embolic Agent	Approach	Vertebral Artery Preserved	Complications
1	F/11	Bruit	C1	Yes	Balloons & coils	IVA	Yes	—
2	F/8	Bruit	C1	Yes	Coils	IVA + CVA	No	—
3	M/6	Bruit	C1	No	None	—	—	—
4	M/50	Bruit	C4	No	None	—	—	—
5	M/52	Myelopathy, epidural hematoma, NF-1	C4	Yes	Balloons & glue	IVA + CVA	No	—
6	F/52	Ehlers-Danlos syndrome; asymptomatic	C4,C2	No	None	—	—	—
7	F/13	Bruit	C1	Yes	Balloons	IVA + CVA	No	—
8	F/31	TIA; high-output CHF	C1	Yes	Balloons	IVA + CVA	No	alopecia, TIA
9	F/32	Bruit	T1	Yes	None	—	—	—
10	F/32	Bruit	C1	No	Balloons	IVA + CVA	Yes	—
11	M/5	Bruit	C1	Yes	Balloons & coils	IVA + CVA	No	—
12	M/3	Bruit	C7	No	Coils	IVA	Yes	—

C, cervical; NF-1, neurofibrimatosis type 1; TIA, transient ischemic attack; CHF, congestive heart failure; IVA, ipsilateral vertebral artery; CVA, contralateral vertebral artery.
From Goyal M, Willinsky R, Montanera W, et al. Spontaneous vertebrovertebral arteriovenous fistulae: clinical features, angioarchitecture and management of twelve patients. *Interv Neuroradiol* 1999;5:219–224, with permission.

al. series of VVAVFs, 6 of the 12 patients were children (Table 16-4) [69]. Most of the fistulas in children are at C1-2, and presence of a neurologic deficit is rare [69]. The most common symptom of VVAVFs is a bruit [69]. The natural history of these fistulas is not well known. Myelopathy is rare and may be due to mass effect from dilated veins in the epidural space [69]. Congestive heart failure due to volume overload is rare [69].

Imaging

The MRI features of EAVFs depend on the location of the nidus and the venous drainage pattern. If there is reflux into the perimedullary veins, MRI may show a T2 hyperintensity within the spinal cord and prominent perimedullary flow voids similar to an SDAVF (see Fig. 16-17) [59]. Additional vascular channels in the epidural space, intervertebral foramina, or paraspinal space may be evident. On computed tomography (CT) an enlarged epidural vein with its bone remodeling may be mistaken for a nerve sheath tumor [20].

Angiographic evaluation of EAVFs includes a complete spinal angiogram to determine the arterial supply to the AVM, the site of the shunt, and the venous drainage. Reflux to the perimedullary veins should be searched for, especially when the MRI shows prominent flow voids in the subarachnoid space and increased T2 signal in the cord.

EAVFs can be complex, with multiple feeders shunting into a single dilated vein (see Fig. 16-18). Ipsilateral and contralateral collaterals from adjacent metameres often contribute to the shunts. From the dilated epidural veins the drainage is into the paraspinal veins. In most cases, there is no reflux into the intradural veins, due to an antireflux mechanism described by Tadie et al. [66]. Demonstration of the normal spinal cord supply is important to support the diagnosis of an extradural location of the shunt.

Treatment

Treatment of most symptomatic EAVFs is endovascular. If the patient can tolerate the symptoms (i.e., bruit) treatment would be based on the feasibility of cure. A single fistula is technically the ideal lesion to treat. With a single fistula it may be possible to close the shunt with a balloon placed in the vein from the arterial side. Halbach et al. reported on the treatment of VVAVFs, in which the fistula was closed using balloons, with preservation of the vertebral artery, in 12 of 20 patients [67]. When the vertebral artery is interrupted completely, a large pseudoaneurysm usually develops and it is necessary to trap the transected segment.

Reports on the treatment of EAVFs are anecdotal [60, 61,71–73]. Hui et al. treated two patients with paraspinal AVMs with arterial injections of liquid adhesives, and in one patient these injections were performed after transvenous deposition of coils [61]. The diverse morphology and variable clinical effects of EAVFs necessitates an individualized approach to treatment. When a patient has a venous congestive myelopathy due to reflux into the perimedullary veins, the most appropriate treatment is surgical clipping of the radicular vein adjacent to the fistula (see Fig. 16-17). This alleviates symptoms, leaving the fistula intact. This strategy has been used in SDAVFs and intracranial dural arteriovenous fistulas (DAVFs) with cortical venous reflux [74].

Treatment of symptomatic high-flow EAVFs with multiple feeders remains a challenge. Embolization of the feeding arteries without complete obliteration of the draining vein leads to further recruitment of feeders, making subsequent treatment more difficult [60]. The intention of treatment should be to completely occlude the fistula itself and the draining vein. If there is a large fistula it may be possible to reach the venous pouch from the transarterial route to allow deposition of coils into the vein. This meshwork of coils can facilitate the safe, accurate transarterial deposition of the liquid adhesive at the site of the fistula. Alternatively, it may be necessary to deliver a meshwork of coils into the epidural venous pouch from the transvenous route (see Fig. 16-18) [60,73]. The epidural venous plexus may be accessible from the venous route in the cervical region through vertebral veins, and in the thoracolumbar region from the azygos or ascending lumbar veins [60]. A cast of liquid adhesives or the presence of coils within the involved epidural vein does not produce symptoms of cord compression [60, 61,73].

The goal of treatment in VVAVFs is occlusion of the fistula with preservation of the vertebral artery. In the high-flow fistula at the C1-2 level preservation of the vertebral artery is often not possible (see Table 16-4). Proximal vessel ligation should be avoided, because this may lead to symptoms of vertebrobasilar insufficiency caused by increased retrograde flow from the basilar artery [71]. If a trapping procedure is necessary we prefer to start with the contralateral vertebral artery. Balloons can often be positioned precisely, bridging the fistula in a dumbbell configuration. Balloons are preferred because they can be positioned precisely [68,75]. In case of incomplete occlusion by balloons, other embolic materials may be used to supplement the closure. Use of balloons may not be possible, especially from the contralateral artery, if there is marked tortuosity or arterial narrowing. From the contralateral approach coils can be used to occlude the vertebral artery just distal to the fistula. An ipsilateral approach can be used to reach the vertebral artery segment distal to the fistula. Vertebral artery sacrifice is often necessary but well tolerated.

Complex Spinal Arteriovenous Malformations

Complex SCAVMs involve both ectoderm and mesodermal derivatives along a dermatome. These have been referred to as *metameric* because they follow a dermatome distribution. These complex SCAVMs have also been referred to as juvenile SCAVMs because they often occur at a young age. The term *complex* accurately describes their diffuse nature, crossing the anatomical boundaries that define the other spinal AVMs. The spinal cord involvement can vary from a fistula to more complex malformations. The adjacent bone, paraspinal muscles, and subcutaneous tissues are involved to a varying degree. If the skin is involved this is the true Cobb syndrome [10]. The skin lesion may be separate from the spinal cord and bone involvement. Rarely, the spinal AVM may drain into a dysplastic vascular skin lesion resulting in a venous congestion of the skin abnormality (see Fig. 16-18) [59]. The skin malformation may be the initial finding and a bruit is often evident. The most common clinical feature is progressive neurologic deficit. The frequency of complex spinal AVMs was 14% in Djindjian's series, 21% in Doppman's, and 7% in Berenstein and Lasjaunias' [16]. In the Halbach et al. series of perimedullary fistulas, 20% of patients had Cobb syndrome [7].

The management of complex spinal AVMs is difficult. The treatment is targeted toward the symptomatic components. Treatment may involve embolization or surgery or a combination of the two. No treatment may be the best option if patients are stable. It may not be possible or necessary to treat the bone or extradural components of these complex lesions.

A summary of the clinical features, angioarchitecture, and treatment options of spinal AVMs and spinal AVFs is outlined in Table 16-5.

TECHNIQUE FOR EMBOLIZATION

Spinal Dural Arteriovenous Malformations

Patient Selection and Workup

The challenge with spinal dural AVMs is to make the diagnosis in a timely fashion. Often there is a delay in the referral to imaging because the early signs and symptoms may be subtle and nonspecific. CT of the lumbar region will not detect any signs of the disease. Initial MRI may be centered on the lumbar region, resulting in failure to appreciate the T2 hyperintensity within the central component of the conus or the prominent subarachnoid flow voids dorsal to the lower thoracic cord. Once the diagnosis is suggested on MRI there are a number of pitfalls possible during the search on angiography. Motion artifact from breathing or bowel activity may obscure completely the visualization of the

TABLE 16-5. ANGIOARCHITECTURE, CLINICAL FEATURES, AND TREATMENT OPTIONS OF SPINAL ARTERIOVENOUS MALFORMATIONS

Type	Typical Angioarchitecture	Age (yr)	Features	Hemorrhage	Treatment	Notes
Dural	Fistula	40–70	Progressive myelopathy	Rare (cervical)	Surg or embo	Male predominance, cervical location rare
Type I perimedullary	Fistula	30–70	Progressive myelopathy	Rare	Surg	Clinical and MR findings mimic spinal dural AVF
Type II perimedullary	Fistula	20–40	Acute neurologic deficit	Common	Embo or surg	Conus location common
Type III perimedullary	Fistula	2–30	Acute neurologic deficit	Common	Embo	Association with Rendu-Osler-Weber syndrome
Intramedullary	Nidus	10–40	Acute neurologic deficit	Common	Embo or surg	Flow-related aneurysms
Extradural	Fistula	All ages	Variable: asymptomatic to progressive myelopathy	Rare	Embo or surg	Clinical findings depend on venous drainage
Complex	Nidus	5–20	Acute or progressive neurologic deficits	Common	Embo or surg	Partial treatment often best option

Surg, surgery; Embo, embolization; MR, magnetic resonance; AVF, arteriovenous fistula.

slow-flow fistula. Failure to catheterize the contributing pedicle is common due to atherosclerotic disease in the aorta or aneurysmal dilation in the aorta. Aortic flush angiography may miss a dural fistula due to overlapping of multiple vessels.

Diagnosis of dural AVFs has been facilitated by advances in MRI. Improved resolution facilitates detection of the perimedullary flow voids. Advanced MRA techniques using gadolinium have been a major advance in confirming the presence of abnormal subarachnoid vessels and localization of the fistula site (see Fig. 16-2). These techniques involve the dynamic acquisition of the data after a bolus of gadolinium.

The search for an SDAVF requires high-resolution selective angiography under general anesthesia. Bowel peristalsis can be reduced using pharmacological measures. Digital subtraction and magnification are important parameters to facilitate detection of these fistulas. Due to the variations in the anatomy a number of catheter shapes and French sizes may be needed. We often start with a #2, 4-French (Fr.) femoral–visceral (Cobra) curve catheter to do the selective thoracic intercostals injections. The #1 and # 3 Cobra catheters may be needed, depending on the size of the aorta. Other shapes may be needed in some patients. A "spinal" curve placed on a 4-Fr. straight catheter may be useful. A preshaped 5-4 Fr. spinal medullary catheter (Nycomed, Paris) or the Mapper Chiras I (Nycomed, Paris) can be used. In some patients #1 or #2 sidewinder catheters are needed.

The angiographic protocol should begin by selectively injecting the thoracic intercostal arteries between T8 and T11 where the artery of Adamkiewicz usually arises. In 50% of patients the artery of Adamkiewicz arises from the intercostal artery at T9 or T10 on the left. If the fistula has not been localized using MRA then the rest of the intercostal branches and the lumbar arteries should be injected selectively. Both internal iliac arteries are studied to fill the lateral sacral arteries. The median sacral artery is often visualized on the lateral sacral injections or it can be injected separately. A sacral location is not rare [38,64,76,77]. In the series by Niimi et al., 9 of the 58 (15%) consecutive cases of SDAVFs were at the sacral level [38]. These sacral dural AVFs can be overlooked easily due to obscuration by bowel gas [64]. If an SDAVF is found, oblique views are often helpful to visualize the transition between the arterial network and the intradural vein. The ipsilateral and contralateral levels above and below the fistula are studied because a dual arterial supply may be present (see Fig. 16-6). If the fistula is identified and the venous drainage into the perimedullary plexus corresponds to the MR findings then the rest of the spinal axis does not need to be studied, because multiple separate

SDAVFs are rare [78,79]. If no fistula is found, the cervical cord and intracranial circulation may be studied during a second session. This includes selective injections of both vertebral arteries as well as the costocervical and thyrocervical arteries. Study of the intracranial circulation includes the vertebral, internal carotid, and external carotid arteries.

Endovascular Treatment

Embolization of SDAVFs is done when the anatomy is suitable. The patient is heparinized and a 5-Fr. catheter is used as a guide. Instability of the guide is a common problem and may prevent selective placement of the microcatheter. A braided microcatheter (i.e., Prowler-10, Cordis, Miami Lakes, FL) with a guidewire (i.e., Transend Platinum, Boston Scientific, Fremont, CA) facilitates a selective position in the feeding artery. A mixture (i.e., 17% NBCA–to–83% iodized oil [Lipiodol]) of the liquid adhesive is injected. Subtracted fluoroscopy is critical to see the delivery of the embolic material. Control angiography includes the ipsilateral and contralateral pedicles at the fistula site and the adjacent levels. If the embolic material did not reach the vein, these patients need surgery even if there is a dramatic reduction in the flow through the fistula. After successful embolization, heparin is continued for 24 to 48 hours if there is slow flow through the involved dilated perimedullary veins.

Particulate embolization should not be done because the incidence of symptomatic recurrence is high [80]. Endovascular therapy can be done during the same session as the diagnostic angiography and often is. With the endovascular tools available presently, initial success with embolization can approach 87% in selected cases when the anatomy is favorable [38]. Embolization is not attempted if catheterization of the branch to the feeding pedicle proves to be difficult on the diagnostic angiogram. A common origin of the radiculomedullary artery and the radiculomeningeal branch supplying the fistula is a contraindication to embolization (see Fig. 16-4). After embolization with liquid adhesives, recurrences may occur despite what was considered an adequate treatment [38]. These recurrences occur when the embolic material does not reach the vein, allowing collateral dural branches to keep the fistula open. This collateral flow may not be evident at the time of the embolization and therefore patients require close clinical follow-up and follow-up MRI. Patients who are partially treated may improve initially. Delayed deterioration suggests recurrence of the fistula and warrants repeat investigation.

After embolization, patients are observed in the hospital for at least 3 to 5 days. If there is any clinical deterioration, heparin therapy is initiated and warfarin (Coumadin) is prescribed for 4 to 6 months. All patients have a limited spinal angiogram before discharge. This includes the ipsilateral and contralateral levels at the fistula site and the adjacent levels. Patients continue to be followed on an outpatient basis. MRI is done 1 year after treatment. If patients have delayed deterioration, MRI is done to investigate the cause of this deterioration. MRI will often show resolution of cord swelling if the embolization is successful (Fig. 16-19). If the cord remains swollen or flow voids are still evident MRA with gadolinium is done. If the MRA confirms the presence of prominent vessels then repeat angiography of the entire spine is necessary.

Intramedullary Spinal Cord Arteriovenous Malformations

Patient Selection and Workup

The diagnosis of intramedullary SCAVMs is often not a challenge with advanced MR techniques. Often patients are young and have clear signs and symptoms of spinal cord dysfunction. The challenge lies in whom to treat and how to treat. Because the natural history of SCAVMs is poor, treatment should be done if feasible. The goals of treatment vary according to the risks involved in the therapy. A multidisciplinary approach is important during the treatment planning. Patients with repeated bleeds who are neurologically intact are generally treated even if only a partial obliteration can be done. In contradistinction, a patient with a fixed major deficit of the lower thoracic spinal cord may not warrant even partial obliteration. Embolization may be done in an attempt to cure the AVM or as an adjunct before surgery. Partial treatment by embolization is an option if complete obliteration cannot be done safely by either surgery or embolization. Partial treatment may include occlusion of prenidal or intranidal aneurysms.

MRI has limited value in treatment planning. It is useful in the detection of acute or chronic parenchymal blood (see Fig. 16-10) but does not delineate the exact location of the nidus within the cord. All patients need selective angiography to define the AVM. Superselective angiography under general anesthesia is important to delineate clearly the nidus and aneurysms on the feeding pedicle or within the nidus.

Endovascular Treatment

Endovascular treatment is done under general anesthesia with full heparinization. Liquid adhesives are the only permanent agent available. If the feeding branches are large, flow-guided microcatheters may be useful to allow superselective catheterization of branches of the radiculomedullary and radiculopial feeders. The #1.5 and #1.2 flow-guided microcatheters (i.e., Magic, Balt, Montmorency, France; Elite, Boston Scientific, Fremont, CA) have expedited catheterization of the sulcocommissural branches of the radiculomedullary arteries. We use these with a supporting guidewire, either the 0.010- or 0.007-inch guidewires (Sorcerer, Balt, Montmorency, France) depending on the catheter size. A selective position in the feeding branch allows the inter-

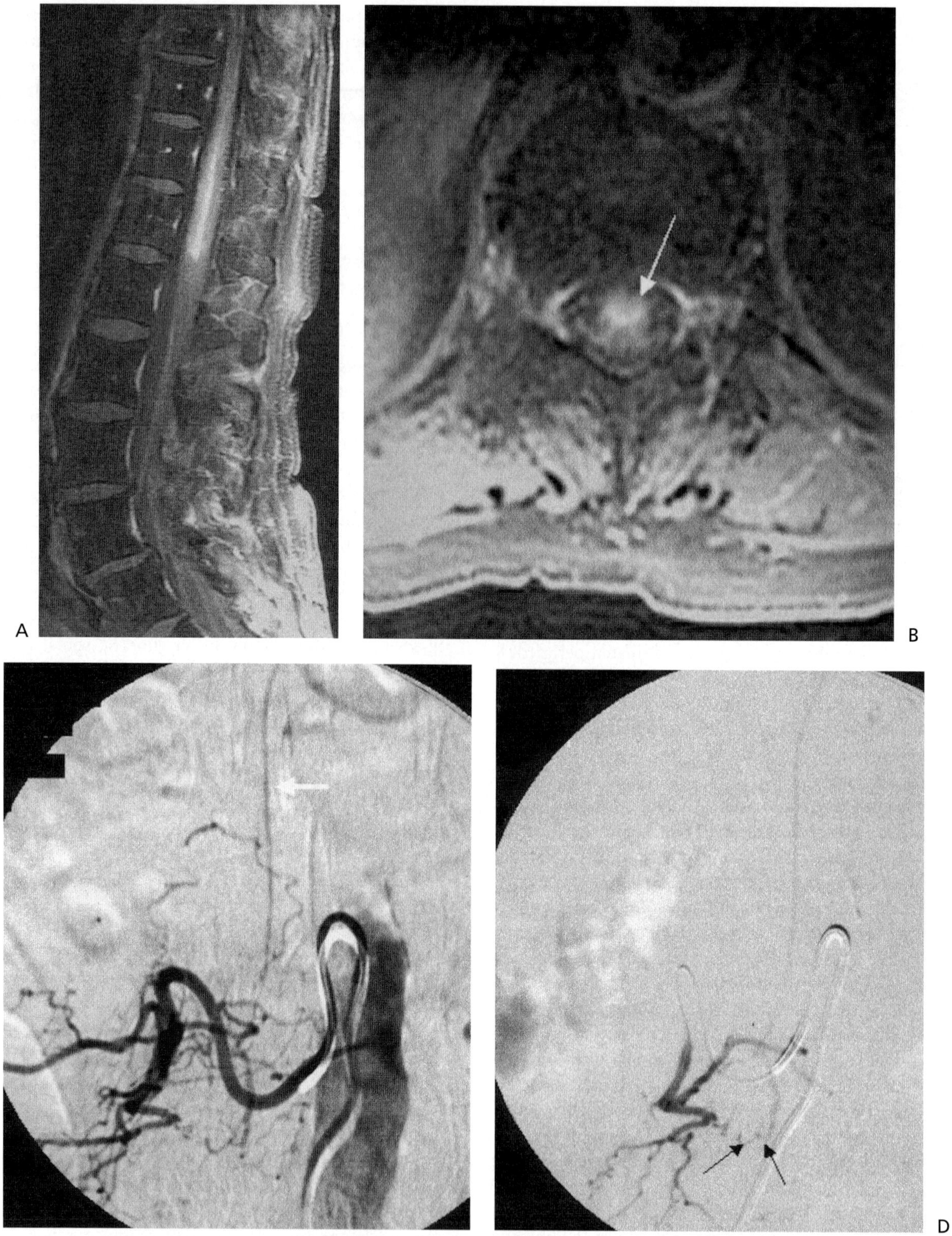

FIGURE 16-19. A 68-year-old woman experienced 2 months of low back pain and gradually worsening lower extremity paresthesia and paresis. Diagnostic workup revealed a dural arteriovenous fistula causing conus and lower spinal cord edema and enhancement consistent with venous hypertension and ischemia. Transarterial embolization resulted in a cure of this lesion with resolution of the patient's signs and symptoms. Sagittal **(A)** and axial **(B)** T1-weighted fat-saturation postcontrast images demonstrate edema and marked intramedullary enhancement of the conus and lower spinal cord (*arrow* in **B**). Right L3 selective **(C)** and superselective **(D)** arteriograms in the anteroposterior projection disclose a high-flow fistula (*black arrows* in **D**) arising from a dural artery to a single medullary vein that drains cephalad. *(Figure continues.)*

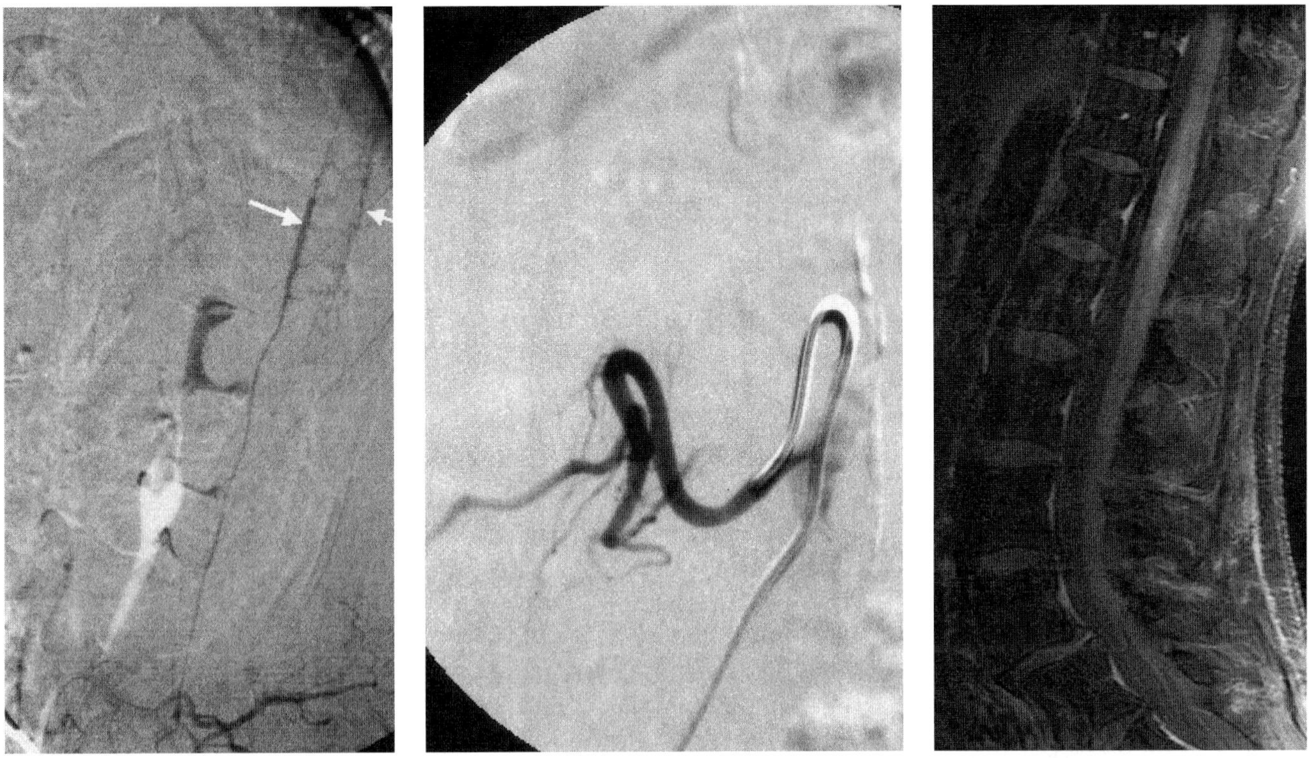

E,F G

FIGURE 16-19. *Continued.* **E:** Right L3 angiogram in lateral projection shows that the draining vein is on the anterior aspect of the thecal sac and cord, with multiple anastomoses to a posterior medullary vein as it eventually drains superiorly *(arrows)*. **F:** Postembolization angiogram shows obliteration of the fistula. **G:** One-month follow-up sagittal T1-weighted fat-saturation postcontrast image reveals decreased swelling and enhancement of the spinal cord when compared to the pretreatment scan **(A)**. (From Michael P. Marks and Huy M. Do, unpublished material, with permission.)

ventional therapist to distinguish flow to the AVM from flow to the normal cord. This requires high-quality, biplane, and magnification angiography. As previously discussed, embolization of the posterior spinal axis in the radiculopial feeders is usually of less risk (Fig. 16-20). In the anterior spinal axis, embolization should not be performed unless superselective catheterization of the sulcocommissural artery can be done (see Fig. 16-11).

Clinical and electrophysiologic monitoring can be done during embolization of SCAVMs [16]. Clinical monitoring necessitates that the patient be awake, therefore a neuroleptic anesthesia is used. Electrophysiologic monitoring can be used in conjunction with general anesthesia. Under general anesthesia patient motion is eliminated, thereby allowing excellent visualization of the angioarchitecture. Electrophysiologic monitoring is done using provocative tests and somatosensory evoked potentials. Berenstein uses 50 to 75 mg of amobarbital and then tests neurologic function and observes the somatosensory evoked potentials [16]. If provocative testing is not used, superselective magnification biplane angiography allows differentiation of the arterial supply to an AVM from the supply to the spinal cord. Embolization would be done only if the branch exclusively supplies the AVM.

After any treatment of SCAVM, patients will be monitored in the hospital for a few days. If treatment is complete a control angiogram is done before discharge. This requires the highest quality pictures and, therefore, general anesthesia is done. Patients are followed as outpatients, and if there is any delayed deterioration MRI is repeated to look for cord swelling or hemorrhage. If a patient is partially treated, repeat angiography should be considered if delayed deterioration occurs.

Perimedullary Spinal Cord Arteriovenous Malformations

Patient Selection and Workup

Most perimedullary SCAVMs are associated with bleeding or progressive neurologic deficit, and therefore treatment should be proposed if feasible. Type II fistulas have multiple enlarged feeders and a dominant anterior or posterior arterial supply defined by the location of the single shunt. The type II fistula may be suitable for embolization as a definitive treatment or as an adjunct for surgery, depending on the location and angioarchitecture of the fistula. Type I fistulas demonstrate slow flow and are usually located on the ante-

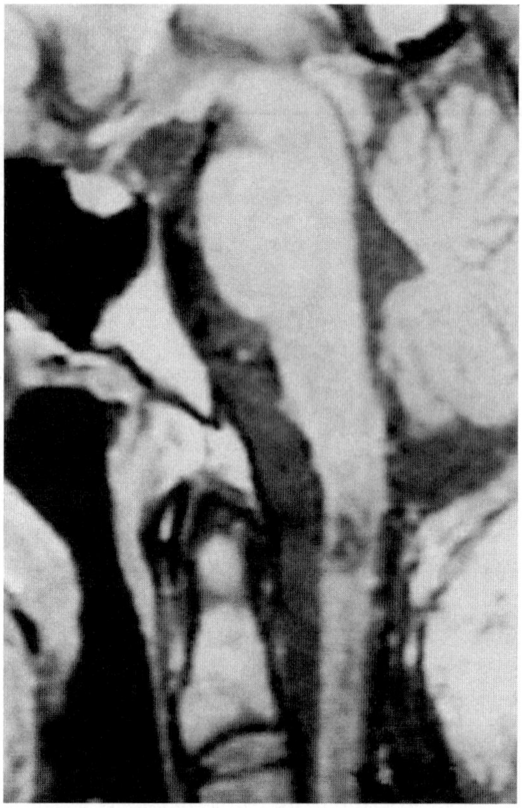

A

FIGURE 16-20. This 32-year-old man sought treatment for progressive left upper extremity weakness and numbness. Workup demonstrated an intramedullary AVM at the C1 level. The patient underwent partial embolization of the AVM nidus followed by stereotactic radiosurgery. **A:** T1-weighted sagittal image demonstrates flow voids in the upper cervical cord at the C1 level consistent with the intramedullary AVM. **B,C:** Anteroposterior and lateral views from a right vertebral artery angiogram demonstrate supply to the AVM nidus from the anterior spinal artery *(short arrow)* as well as the right posterior inferior cerebellar artery (PICA) *(long arrow)*. *(Figure continues.)*

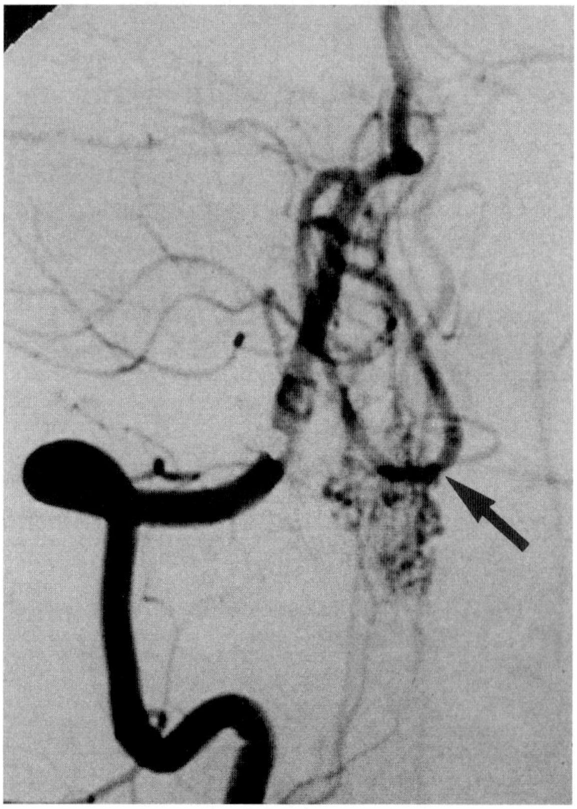

B

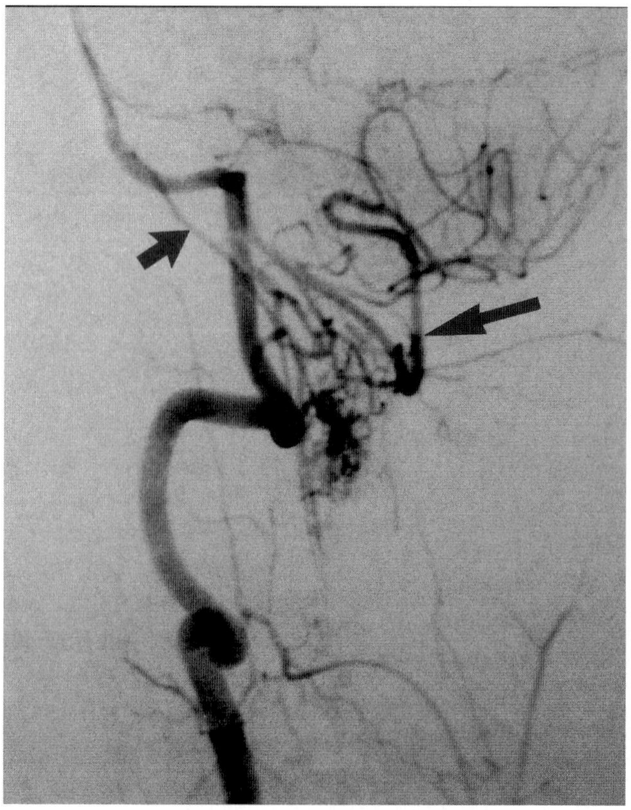

C

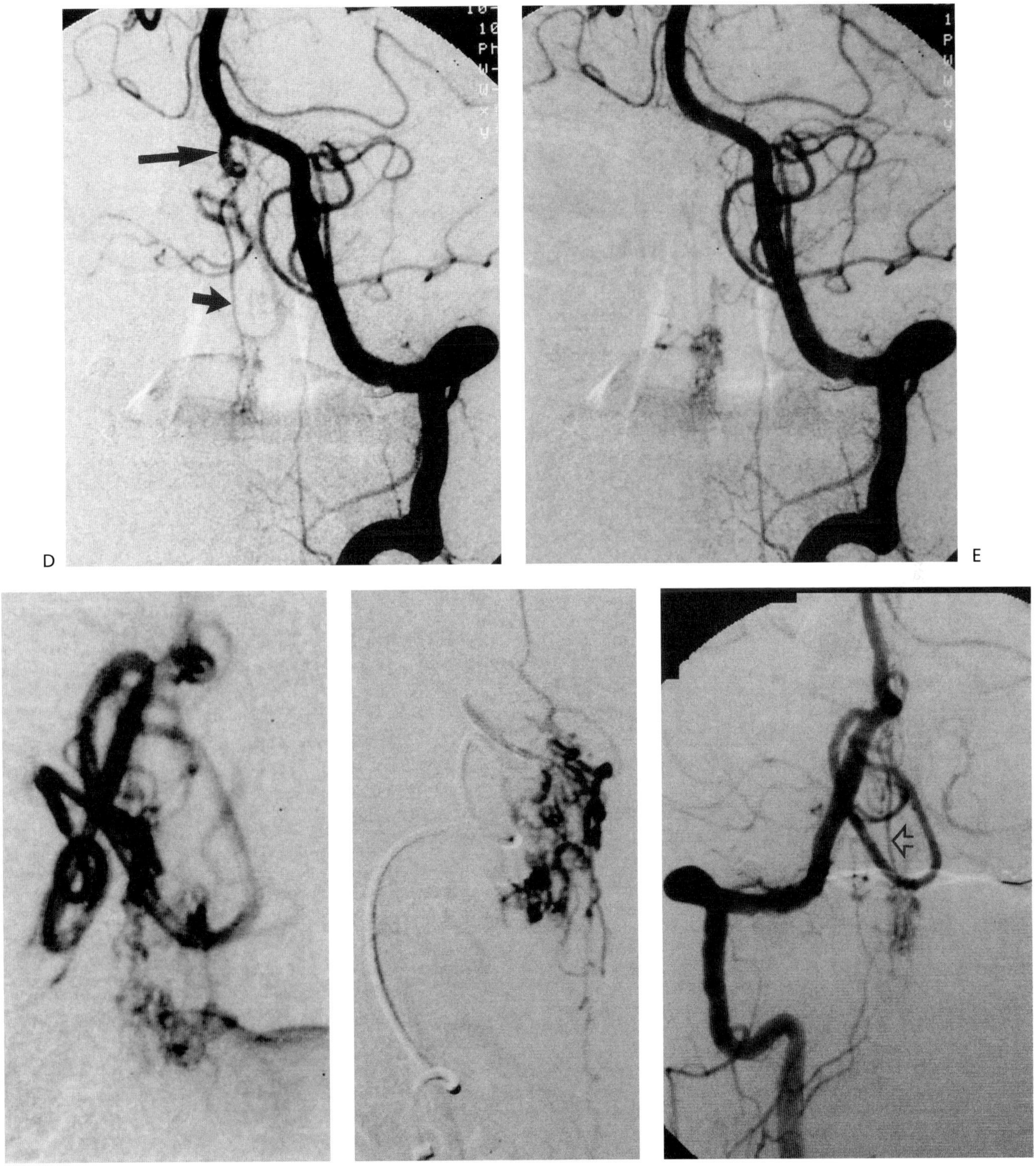

D E

F,G H

FIGURE 16-20. *Continued.* **D,E:** Anteroposterior views from the left vertebral artery angiogram, early and slightly later in the angiogram, demonstrate reflux across the vertebrobasilar junction into the distal right vertebral artery *(long arrow),* with filling of the anterior component via the anterior spinal artery *(short arrow).* The later film **(E)** demonstrates the portion of the nidus that is filling from this anterior spinal artery supply. **F:** An anterior projection of a selective right PICA injection (via microcatheter). This demonstrates filling of the radiculopial or posterior component to the AVM supplied by the right PICA. **G:** A lateral angiogram (preembolization) shows the microcatheter now advanced distally in the PICA circulation. The microcatheter is now exclusively filling the posterior component of the AVM nidus. **H:** Anterior projection of a right vertebral artery angiogram postembolization. This demonstrates continued filling of the nidus from the anterior spinal artery *(arrow),* with reduction in size of the AVM nidus. The patient had no change in symptoms. This anterior portion of the AVM then underwent stereotactic radiosurgery and the patient is awaiting follow-up. (From Michael P. Marks and Huy M. Do, unpublished material, with permission.)

rior surface of the cord. They require surgery due to the small size of the contributing radiculomedullary artery and the small sulcocommissural feeders participating in the supply to the fistula. A type III fistula is a high-flow AVF with multiple enlarged anterior and posterior feeding arteries. The type III giant perimedullary fistula is ideally suited for endovascular treatment.

Type I and II perimedullary SCAVMs may be difficult to distinguish on MRI from other spinal AVMs. Patients will have T2 hyperintensity due to cord swelling, but enlarged perimedullary vessels may or may not be present. Type III perimedullary SCAVMs are usually easier to recognize due to marked dilation of perimedullary vessels. High-quality biplane angiography is required to define clearly the shunt location and angioarchitecture of the fistula. As previously discussed, the single fistula site is identified clearly only by using angiography.

Endovascular Treatment

Endovascular treatment is done under general anesthesia. Full heparinization is performed. The guiding catheter must have a shape that results in a stable position to allow the microcatheter to be delivered to the fistula site. In high-flow fistulas, larger braided microcatheters (i.e., Prowler Plus, Cordis, Miami Lakes, FL; Renegade, Boston Scientific, Fremont, CA) are used so that either fibered coils (i.e., Vortex, Boston Scientific, Fremont, CA) or liquid adhesives can be delivered. In type II fistulas the smaller braided microcatheters or flow-guided catheters are used to achieve a selective position close to the fistula site. The goal of treatment is to close the fistula itself. Often multiple feeders lead to a single fistula that can be recognized by the transition to a dilated venous pouch (see Fig. 16-16). Closure of the arterial feeders alone only promotes collateral flow to the fistula. Therefore it is imperative that embolic material reach and close the fistula itself. The embolic material of choice is a liquid adhesive. Due to the tortuosity of the spinal arteries it is not possible to deliver a detachable balloon in most cases, with the exception of some VVAVFs. In high-flow fistulas it may be difficult to control the delivery of the liquid adhesives. It may be possible to place coils in the dilated venous sac at the fistula site, to prevent the inadvertent distal migration of the liquid adhesive which is delivered from the artery close to the fistula. The coils slow the flow and act as an umbrella to catch the liquid adhesive. The coils can be placed in the vein from either a transarterial approach or from a transvenous approach. The transarterial approach to reach the vein is preferred due its simplicity, and then the liquid adhesive can be delivered through the same catheter after it is withdrawn into the artery. Following treatment, all patients should have a spinal angiogram before discharge from the hospital to ensure that the fistula remains completely closed. After discharge, regular clinical follow-up is needed.

Extradural Spinal Arteriovenous Fistulas

Patient Selection and Workup

Treatment of the extradural AVFs depends on angioarchitecture and clinical findings. If there is a compressive myelopathy from a dilated epidural venous pouch then treatment is warranted. If there is a congestive myelopathy related to reflux into a radicular vein then disconnection of the venous reflux will treat the clinical problem and the extradural fistula can be left alone. Asymptomatic fistulas may be left untreated, especially if the angioarchitecture is not favorable.

MRI may show T2 hyperintensity and prominent perimedullary flow voids when reflux into the perimedullary veins is present. A complete spinal angiogram is needed, however, to identify the site of the shunt, and also to demonstrate normal spinal cord supply and confirm the extradural location of the shunt.

Endovascular Treatment

Identification of the exact fistula site is critical, because closure of feeding pedicles alone will only promote collateral supply. With large high-flow fistulas it may be possible to reach the venous side from the arterial side, allowing the deposition of coils. This is done with a stable guide and a larger microcatheter. If stability of the coils is a concern, GDC-18 fibered coils (Boston Scientific, Fremont, CA) should be used to build the initial basket followed by fibered "push" coils. If there is a venous ectasia at the fistula site proximal to venous narrowing, then GDC coils may not be necessary and push coils may be used exclusively. The coil mass does not need to be occlusive but should result in a significant decrease in the flow. The coils should expedite a controlled injection of the liquid adhesive from the feeding artery. If the venous side cannot be reached from the artery then a transvenous approach may be possible.

In VVAVFs with a small hole it may be possible to deliver a detachable gold valve balloon (Nycomed, Paris, France) or coils into the venous side, preserving the vertebral artery (see Table 16-4). GDC-18 fibered coils are ideal if the venous pouch is small, to avoid the inadvertent delivery of a coil into the vertebral artery. If there is a large gap in the vertebral artery at the site of the fistula then a "trapping" procedure is necessary.

In a large fistula, 8 mg of dexamethasone is given 3 times a day on the day of the treatment and the following day. This is done to reduce any swelling associated with thrombosis of the large epidural vein. Follow-up angiography is done before discharge in selected cases when there is concern that the fistula may reopen from collateral flow.

REFERENCES

1. Djindjian R. *L'angiographie de la moelle epiniere.* Paris: Masson, 1970:122–296.

2. Aminoff MJ, Logue V. Clinical features of spinal vascular malformations. *Brain* 1974;97:197–210.
3. Kendall BE, Logue V. Spinal epidural angiomatous malformations draining into intrathecal veins. *Neuroradiology* 1977;13: 181–189.
4. Merland JJ, Riche MC, Chiras J. Les fistules arterioveineuses intracanalaires extramedullaires a drainagew veineux medullaire. *J Neuroradiol* 1980;7:221–230.
5. Bao YH, Ling F. Classification and therapeutic modalities of spinal vascular malformations in 80 patients. *Neurosurgery* 1997; 40:75–81.
6. Detwiler PW, Porter RW, Spetzler RF. Spinal arteriovenous malformations. *Neurosurg Clin N Am* 1999;10:89–100.
7. Halbach VV, Higashida RT, Dowd CF, et al. Treatment of giant intradural (perimedullary) arteriovenous fistulas. *Neurosurgery* 1993;33:972–979.
8. Gueguen B, Merland JJ, Riche MC, et al. Vascular malformations of the spinal cord: intrathecal perimedullary arteriovenous fistulas fed by medullary arteries. *Neurology* 1987;37:969–979.
9. Mourier KL, Gobin YP, George B, et al. Intradural perimedullary arteriovenous fistulae: results of surgical and endovascular treatment in a series of 35 cases. *Neurosurgery* 1993;32:885–891.
10. Cobb S. Haemangioma of the spinal cord: associated with skin naevi of the same metamere. *Ann Surg* 1915;62:641–649.
11. Djindjian M, Djindjian R, Hurth M, et al. Spinal cord arteriovenous malformations and the Klippel-Trenaunay-Weber syndrome. *Surg Neurol* 1977;8:229–237.
12. Mandzia JL, TerBrugge KG, Faughnan ME, et al. Spinal cord arteriovenous malformations in two patients with hereditary hemorrhagic telangiectasia. *Child's Nerv Syst* 1999;15:80–83.
13. Nakstad PH, Hald JK, Bakke SJ. Multiple spinal arteriovenous fistulas in Klippel-Trenaunay-Weber syndrome treated with platinum fibre coils. *Neuroradiology* 1993;35:163–165.
14. Aminoff MJ, Barnard RO, Logue V. The pathophysiology of spinal vascular malformations. *J Neurol Sci* 1974;23:255–263.
15. Gilbertson JR, Miller GM, Goldman MS, et al. Spinal dural arteriovenous fistulas: MR and myelographic findings. *AJNR Am J Neuroradiol* 1995;16:2049–2057.
16. Berenstein A, Lasjaunias P. *Surgical neuroangiography: endovascular treatment of spine and spinal cord lesions.* Berlin: Springer-Verlag, 1992:1–85.
17. Niimi Y, Berenstein A. Endovascular treatment of spinal vascular malformations. *Neurosurg Clin N Am* 1999;10:47–71.
18. Cahan LD, Higashida RT, Halbach VV, et al. Variants of radiculomeningeal vascular malformations of the spine. *J Neurosurg* 1987;66:333–337.
19. Do HM, Jensen ME, Cloft HJ, et al. Dural arteriovenous fistula of the cervical spine presenting with subarachnoid hemorrhage. *AJNR Am J Neuroradiol* 1999;20:348–350.
20. Willinsky R, TerBrugge K, Lasjaunias P, et al. The variable presentations of craniocervical and cervical dural arteriovenous malformations. *Surg Neurol* 1990;34:118–123.
21. Glasser R, Masson R, Mickle JP, et al. Embolization of a dural arteriovenous fistula of the ventral cervical spinal canal in a nine-year-old boy. *Neurosurgery* 1993;33:1089–1093.
22. Morimoto T, Yoshida S, Basugi N. Dural arteriovenous malformation in the cervical spine presenting with subarachnoid hemorrhage: case report. *Neurosurgery* 1992;31:118–120.
23. Foix C, Alajouanine T. La myelite necrotique subaigue. *Rev Neurol (Paris)* 1926;33:1–42.
24. Criscuolo GR, Oldfield EH, Doppman JL. Reversible acute and subacute myelopathy in patients with dural arteriovenous fistulas: Foix-Alajouanine syndrome reconsidered. *J Neurosurg* 1989;70: 354–359.
25. Symon L, Kuyama H, Kendall B. Dural arteriovenous malformations of the spine: clinical features and surgical results in 55 cases. *J Neurosurg* 1984;60:238–247.
26. Willinsky RA, TerBrugge K, Montanera W, et al. Posttreatment MR findings in spinal dural arteriovenous malformations. *AJNR Am J Neuroradiol* 1995;16:2063–2071.
27. Meder JF, Devaux B, Merland JJ, et al. Spontaneous disappearance of a spinal dural arteriovenous fistula. *AJNR Am J Neuroradiol* 1995;16:2058–2062.
28. Brunereau L, Gobin YP, Meder JF, et al. Intracranial dural arteriovenous fistulas with spinal venous drainage: relation between clinical presentation and angiographic findings. *AJNR Am J Neuroradiol* 1996;17:1549–1554.
29. Hurst RW, Grossman RI. Peripheral spinal cord hypointensity on T2-weighted MR images: a reliable imaging sign of venous hypertensive myelopathy. *AJNR Am J Neuroradiol* 2000;21: 781–786.
30. Wrobel CJ, Oldfield EH, Di Chiro G, et al. Myelopathy due to intracranial dural arteriovenous fistulas draining intrathecally into spinal medullary veins: report of three cases. *J Neurosurg* 1988;69:934–939.
31. Gobin YP, Rogopoulos A, Aymard A, et al. Endovascular treatment of intracranial dural arteriovenous fistulas with spinal perimedullary venous drainage. *J Neurosurg* 1992;77:718–723.
32. Binkert CA, Kollias SS, Valavanis A. Spinal cord vascular disease: characterization with fast three-dimensional contrast-enhanced MR angiography. *AJNR Am J Neuroradiol* 1999;20:1785–1793.
33. Farb R, Goyal M, Kim J, et al. Novel contrast-enhanced MR angiographic technique to ascertain the level of fistula and arterial feeders in spinal dural AVM: our early experience. Proceedings of the American Society of Neuroradiology, 38th Annual Meeting, 2000 (abstr).
34. Willinsky R, Lasjaunias P, TerBrugge K, et al. Angiography in the investigation of spinal dural arteriovenous fistula: a protocol with application of the venous phase. *Neuroradiology* 1990;32: 114–116.
35. Aggarwal S, Willinsky R, Montanera W, et al. Superselective angiography of a spinal dural arteriovenous fistula having a common segmental origin with the artery of Adamkiewicz. *Neuroradiology* 1992;34:352–354.
36. Niimi Y, Setton A, Berenstein A. Spinal dural arteriovenous fistulae draining to the anterior spinal vein: angiographic diagnosis. *Neurosurgery* 1999;44:999–1003.
37. McCutcheon IE, Doppman JL, Oldfield EH. Microvascular anatomy of dural arteriovenous abnormalities of the spine: a microangiographic study. *J Neurosurg* 1996;84:215–220.
38. Niimi Y, Berenstein A, Setton A, et al. Embolization of spinal dural arteriovenous fistulae: results and follow-up. *Neurosurgery* 1997;40:675–682.
39. Afshar JK, Doppman JL, Oldfield EH. Surgical interruption of intradural draining vein as curative treatment of spinal dural arteriovenous fistulas. *J Neurosurg* 1995;82:196–200.
40. Huffmann BC, Spetzger U, Reinges M, et al. Treatment strategies and results in spinal vascular malformations. *Neurol Med Chir (Tokyo)* 1998;38[Suppl]:231–237.
41. Rosenblum B, Oldfield EH, Doppman JL, et al. Spinal arteriovenous malformations: a comparison of dural arteriovenous fistulas and intradural AVMs in 81 patients. *J Neurosurg* 1987;67: 795–802.
42. Aminoff MJ, Logue V. The prognosis of patients with spinal vascular malformations. *Brain* 1974;97:211–218.
43. Matsubara S, Manzia JL, TerBrugge K, et al. Angiographic and clinical characteristics of patients with cerebral arteriovenous malformations associated with hereditary hemorrhagic telangiectasia. *AJNR Am J Neuroradiol* 2000;21:1016–1020.
44. Biondi A, Merland JJ, Hodes JE, et al. Aneurysms of spinal arteries associated with intramedullary arteriovenous malforma-

tions. I. Angiographic and clinical aspects. *AJNR Am J Neuroradiol* 1992;13:913–922.

45. Lasjaunias P, Berenstein A. *Surgical neuroangiography: functional vascular anatomy of brain, spinal cord and spine.* Berlin: Springer-Verlag, 1990:80–87.
46. Biondi A, Merland JJ, Reizine D, et al. Embolization with particles in thoracic intramedullary arteriovenous malformations: long-term angiographic and clinical results. *Radiology* 1990;177:651–658.
47. Biondi A, Merland JJ, Hodes JE, et al. Aneurysms of spinal arteries associated with intramedullary arteriovenous malformations. II. Results of AVM endovascular treatment and hemodynamic considerations. *AJNR Am J Neuroradiol* 1992;13:923–931.
48. Konan AV, Raymond J, Roy D. Transarterial embolization of aneurysms associated with spinal cord arteriovenous malformations: report of four cases. *J Neurosurg* 1999;90[Suppl]:148–154.
49. Connolly ES Jr, Zubay GP, McCormick PC, et al. The posterior approach to a series of glomus (type II) intramedullary spinal cord arteriovenous malformations. *Neurosurgery* 1998;42:774–785.
50. Martin NA, Khanna RK, Batzdorf U. Posterolateral cervical or thoracic approach with spinal cord rotation for vascular malformations or tumors of the ventrolateral spinal cord. *J Neurosurg* 1995;83:254–261.
51. Kopelson G, Linggood R, Kleinman G. Management of intramedullary spinal cord tumors. *Radiology* 1980;135:473–479.
52. Marcus MB, Million RR. The incidence of myelitis after irradiation of the cervical spinal cord. *Int J Radiat Oncol Biol Phys* 1990;19:3–8.
53. McCuniff AJ, Liang MJ. Radiation tolerance of the cervical spinal cord. *Int J Radiat Oncol Biol Phys* 1989;16:675–678.
54. Ryu SI, Chang SD, Kim DH, et al. Image-guided frameless robotic stereotactic radiosurgery to spinal lesions. *Neurosurgery (in press).*
55. Hida K, Iwasaki Y, Goto K, et al. Results of the surgical treatment of perimedullary arteriovenous fistulas with special reference to embolization. *J Neurosurg* 1999;90[Suppl]:198–205.
56. Tomlinson FH, Rufenacht DA, Sundt TM Jr, et al. Arteriovenous fistulas of the brain and the spinal cord. *J Neurosurg* 1993;79:16–27.
57. Emery DJ, Willinsky R, Burrows PE, et al. Pediatric spinal arteriovenous malformations: angioarchitecture and endovascular treatment. *Interv Neuroradiol* 1998;4:127–139.
58. Ricolfi F, Gobin PY, Aymard AB, et al. Giant perimedullary arteriovenous fistulas of the spine: clinical and radiologic features and endovascular treatment. *AJNR Am J Neuroradiol* 1997;18:677–687.
59. Goyal M, Willinsky R, Montanera W, et al. Paravertebral arteriovenous malformations with epidural drainage: clinical spectrum, imaging features, and results of treatment. *AJNR Am J Neuroradiol* 1999;20:749–755.
60. Willinsky R, TerBrugge K, Montanera W, et al. Spinal epidural arteriovenous fistulas: arterial and venous approaches to embolization. *AJNR Am J Neuroradiol* 1993;14:812–817.
61. Hui F, Trosselo MP, Meisel HJ, et al. Paraspinal arteriovenous shunts in children. *Neuroradiology* 1994;36:69–73.
62. Arnaud O, Bille F, Pouget J, et al. Epidural arteriovenous fistula with perimedullary venous drainage: case report. *Neuroradiology* 1994;36:490–491.
63. Cognard C, Semaan H, Bakchine S, et al. Paraspinal arteriovenous fistula with perimedullary venous drainage. *AJNR Am J Neuroradiol* 1995;16:2044–2048.
64. Pirouzmand F, Wallace MC, Willinsky R. Spinal epidural arteriovenous fistula with intramedullary reflux: case report. *J Neurosurg* 1997;87:633–635.
65. Deans WR, Bloch S, Leibrock L, et al. Arteriovenous fistula in patients with neurofibromatosis. *Radiology* 1982;144:103–107.
66. Tadie M, Hernet J, Aaron C. Le dispostif protecteur anti-reflux des veins de la moelle. *Neurochirurgie* 1979;5:28–30.
67. Halbach VV, Higashida RT, Hieshima GB. Treatment of vertebral arteriovenous fistulas. *AJR Am J Roentgenol* 1988;150:405–412.
68. Beaujeux RL, Reizine DC, Casasco A, et al. Endovascular treatment of vertebral arteriovenous fistula. *Radiology* 1992;183:361–367.
69. Goyal M, Willinsky R, Montanera W, et al. Spontaneous vertebrovertebral arteriovenous fistulae: clinical features, angioarchitecture and management of twelve patients. *Interv Neuroradiol* 1999;5:219–224.
70. Hieshima GB, Cahan LD, Mehringer CM, et al. Spontaneous arteriovenous fistulas of cerebral vessels in association with fibromuscular dysplasia. *Neurosurgery* 1986;18:454–458.
71. Lasjaunias P. *Vascular diseases in neonates, infants and children.* Berlin: Springer, 1997:501–530.
72. Matsumura A, Tsuboi K, Hyodo A, et al. Lumbosacral extradural spinal arteriovenous malformation with blood supply from branches of internal iliac arteries. *Neurochirurgie* 1986;29:235–237.
73. Szajner M, Weill A, Piotin M, et al. Endovascular treatment of a cervical paraspinal arteriovenous malformation via arterial and venous approaches. *AJNR Am J Neuroradiol* 1999;20:1097–1099.
74. Davies MA, TerBrugge K, Willinsky RA, et al. The natural history and management of intracranial dural arteriovenous fistula. Aggressive lesions. *Interv Neuroradiol* 1997:3;303–311.
75. Lasjaunias P, Berenstein A. *Surgical neuroangiography: endovascular treatment of craniofacial lesions.* Berlin: Springer-Verlag, 1992:175–233.
76. Larsen DW, Halbach VV, Teitelbaum GP, et al. Spinal dural arteriovenous fistulas supplied by branches of the internal iliac arteries. *Surg Neurol* 1995;43:35–40.
77. Partington MD, Rufenacht DA, Marsh WR, et al. Cranial and sacral dural arteriovenous fistulas as a cause of myelopathy. *J Neurosurg* 1992;76:615–622.
78. Pierot L, Vlachopoulos T, Attal N, et al. Double spinal dural arteriovenous fistulas: report of two cases. *AJNR Am J Neuroradiol* 1993;14:1109–1112.
79. Thiebot J, Clavier E, Tadie M, et al. Multiple intrathecal extramedullary arteriovenous fistulae draining "freely" into the spinal veins. *J Neuroradiol* 1986;13:173–180.
80. Nichols DA, Rufenacht DA, Jack CR Jr, et al. Embolization of spinal dural arteriovenous fistula with polyvinyl alcohol particles: experience in 14 patients. *AJNR Am J Neuroradiol* 1992;13:933–940.

Endovascular and Percutaneous Therapy of the Brain and Spine, edited by Michael P. Marks and Huy M. Do.
Lippincott Williams & Wilkins, Philadelphia © 2002.

17

PERCUTANEOUS THERAPY FOR THE SPINE

HUY M. DO
RAYMOND R. GAETA
MICHAEL P. MARKS

Back pain is a highly prevalent and costly problem in industrialized societies. Pain from a spinal origin has a lifetime prevalence greater than 60%, with an annual incidence of at least 5% in most industrialized countries [1–4]. Back pain incapacitates up to 20% of workers, with estimated annual costs exceeding $24 billion in the United States [5–7]. Percutaneous treatment for pain arising from two common causes of spine pain, facet arthropathy and vertebral compression fractures, has become a widespread treatment modality. Since its introduction in 1987 [8], vertebroplasty has rapidly increased in popularity as a viable and potential standard of care for management of pain and disabilities associated with vertebral body compression fractures [9]. This chapter will review relevant pain pathways and anatomy relating to these two major diseases. It will also discuss the clinical significance, history, and indications for percutaneous treatment of facet arthropathy and vertebral compression fractures. Finally, the percutaneous techniques used to treat facet arthropathy and compression fractures will be discussed, along with pitfalls and complications associated with these techniques.

BACKGROUND

Pain Pathways

Pain is a common human experience, serving as warning of real or threatened tissue injury. This warning is transmitted via specialized pathways to the central nervous system. In response to a painful stimulus, specialized pain fibers, A-δ and C fibers, convert the stimulus into an electrical impulse signal in the process known as *transduction.* Heat, mechanical pressure, and even chemical stimuli begin a cascade of events that affect the perception of the stimulus prior to its journey along the specialized fibers. With tissue injury, neurotransmitters bradykinin, serotonin, hydrogen, and potassium ions and prostaglandins are all elaborated. These substances impact the nature of the transduction process. These postinjury events produce the hallmarks of pain and inflammation that can perpetuate the cycle of pain.

Transmission of the painful signals occurs along the fast-conducting myelinated A-δ fibers and along the slow-conducting unmyelinated C fibers. These fibers converge in the dorsal horn of the spinal cord. Cells in the dorsal horn receive input from the injured site and also from embryonically related areas. This phenomenon is responsible for referred pain. In this way, pain from the low back may be sensed in the hip region and, similarly, pain from cervical origin may radiate to the scapula and shoulder areas. This information is particularly pertinent because patients may complain of referred pain in characteristic anatomical locations that require familiarity with these syndromes in order to diagnose correctly the source of pain.

Fibers cross the midline in the cord after reaching the dorsal horn and predominately ascend in the spinothalamic tract, passing through various nuclear centers where the signal is further modified. These signals arrive at the thalamus which acts as a major relay station. Fibers extend from the thalamus to the somatosensory cortex, allowing the individual to discriminate a localized pain in a particular body region. Another set of fibers also extends from the thalamus into the area of the cingulate gyrus. These projections are responsible for the affective components of pain. These emotional components, along with the somatosensory components, give rise to the definition of pain put forth by the International Association for the Study of Pain (IASP) as "an unpleasant sensory and emotional experience associated with actual or potential tissue damage or described in terms of such damage" [10]. More plainly stated, pain is a subjec-

H.M. Do: Departments of Radiology and Neurosurgery, Stanford University School of Medicine, Stanford, California.

R.R. Gaeta: Department of Anesthesia, Division of Pain Management, Stanford University School of Medicine, Stanford, California.

M.P. Marks: Departments of Radiology and Neurosurgery, Stanford University Medical Center, Stanford, California.

tive experience requiring the medical practitioner to use great care in its diagnosis and treatment.

It is important to recognize the contribution of higher centers to the modulation of signals ascending from the spinal cord. A parallel but descending pathway provides the opportunity for descending signals to modulate the intensity of the signals in a process known as *descending noxious inhibitory control.* These pathways are used to modulate the barrage of information constantly coming from our peripheral sensors [11].

Pain can be described in terms of three separate categories that allow a better understanding of various pain syndromes and provide a useful initial paradigm for treatment. The term *nociceptive* pain is used to describe pain in response to a direct stimulus such as heat, or a mechanical or chemical phenomenon. It is the normal neurophysiologic process by which we detect stimuli such as that of an osteoporotic compression fracture of the spine. It represents the warning system that protects our body and joints from further tissue damage. That referred to as *inflammatory* pain generally accompanies nociceptive pain. It is the response of the body to tissue injury that then leads to the elaboration of substances such as prostaglandins, histamine, and bradykinins, which sensitize nociceptors and cause them to respond at a much lower threshold to painful stimuli. A classic example is that of a sprained and swollen joint such that any subsequent minor stimulus is perceived as painful and clearly is to be avoided.

The third type identified, *neuropathic* pain, is experienced similarly to other types of pain but is due to the abnormal function of the nervous system. Common examples include diabetic neuropathy and postherpetic neuralgia, wherein the stimulus is no longer present but spontaneous generation of painful impulses produces the experience of pain. Neuropathic pain generally results from injury to the nervous system from trauma, radiation, metabolic injury, and infectious etiologies. These conditions are less responsive to the classic opioid and nonsteroidal antiinflammatory agents and are more difficult to treat. Medications such as the anticonvulsants, membrane stabilizers, and antidepressants are used to treat these conditions. More aggressive therapies include the delivery of various agents into the spinal fluid as well as the use of electrical stimulation in the spinal column to produce analgesia.

The cortex and endosteum of vertebral body lack pain fibers and therefore are insensitive to pain. Pain receptors are present, however, in the periosteum and adjacent joint capsules. These give rise to pain associated with facet arthropathy. Vertebral body compression fracture pain likely arises from direct stimulation from compression or structural damage, or indirectly from release of chemical mediators associated with tissue injury. In addition, the mechanical alterations in the affected vertebrae alter the nearby joints and may result in pain [12,13].

Vertebral Compression Fractures

Vertebral collapse occurs most commonly in osteoporosis. Osteoporosis is a major health problem facing women and older people of both sexes. It is defined by the World Health Organization as a bone mineral density of more than 2.5 standard deviations below the mean in young, normal people [14]. Based on data obtained from epidemiologic studies in Rochester, Minnesota, and extrapolated to the American white population, approximately 1.5 million fractures occur each year from osteoporosis. These include about 700,000 vertebral fractures [15]. The lifetime risk of a symptomatic vertebral compression fracture is approximately 16% in white women and 5% in white men [16].

In patients over 65 years of age, vertebral compression fractures account for 150,000 hospital admissions, 161,000 physician office visits, and over 5 million restricted activities days in the United States annually [17,18]. In a report from the National Osteoporosis Foundation, Ray et al. [19] estimated the health care expenditure attributable to all osteoporotic fractures to be $13.8 billion in 1995. For osteoporotic vertebral compression fractures, the cost was estimated to be $746 million [19,20]. These already high costs will increase further with continued aging of the population.

After peak bone mass has been achieved, orderly remodeling ensures that the amount of bone resorbed by osteoclasts is balanced by the amount of new bone formed by osteoblasts. A net loss in bone mass occurs when changes in bone turnover result in increased bone resorption or decreased bone formation. With aging, a protracted slow phase of bone loss occurs in both men and women (type II osteoporosis) [12]. For most women entering menopause, trabecular bone loss is approximately 1% per year [12]. A subset of women, however, may have a phase of accelerated bone loss of up to 5% per year, beginning at menopause, which may continue for 15 to 20 years (type I osteoporosis). Type I osteoporosis results from a disproportional loss of trabecular bone that leads to an increase in painful vertebral compression fractures, distal forearm fractures, ankle fractures, and loss of teeth. Patients with vertebral body fractures actually have fewer trabecular elements rather than just thinning of the trabeculae (Fig. 17-1).

Although involutional osteoporosis from aging is the most common cause of osteoporosis, certain medical conditions, surgical procedures, and medications are associated with the development of osteoporosis in 20% of women and 40% of men who suffer vertebral or hip fractures [21]. These associated conditions include corticosteroid medications, history of early oophorectomy, hypogonadism, hyperthyroidism, chronic obstructive lung disease, hemiplegia, chronic anticonvulsant use, smoking, and ethanol use [22].

Vertebral compression fractures can be defined as the reduction in vertebral body height by 15% or greater and classified by degree and type of deformity (wedge, biconcavity, or compression) [23–25]. Vertebral collapse occurs

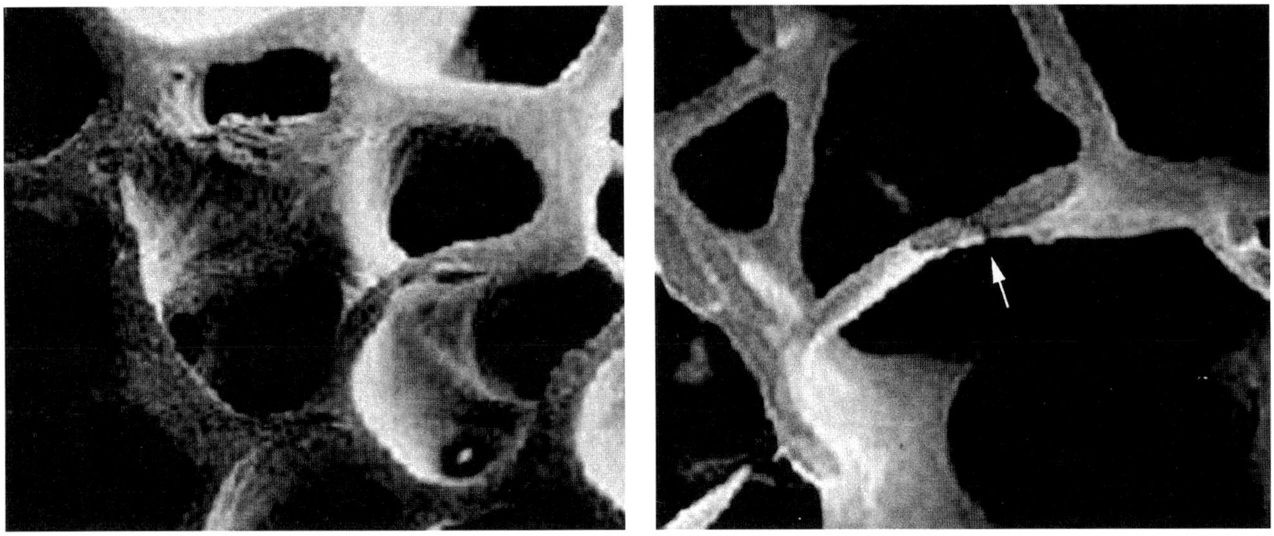

FIGURE 17-1. Scanning electron micrographs of normal **(A)** and osteoporotic **(B)** trabecular bone. In osteoporosis, the trabecular plates are fewer, thinner, and in the process of fracturing (*arrow* in **B**).

when the combined axial and lateral bending stresses on the spinal column exceed the strength of the vertebral body, which is weakened by osteoporosis or by tumor infiltration [9]. The most commonly compressed levels are T8, T12, L1, and L4. The axial stress from physiologic thoracic spine kyphosis is greatest at T8, and the thoracolumbar junction frequently is affected because of the change in mobility between the relatively restricted rib-bearing thoracic spine and the more mobile lumbar spine [23,26,27]. Most fractures occur spontaneously and are associated with trivial stress or strain such as lifting or rolling.

Symptomatic fractures usually are associated with acute pain of variable intensity [23,28]. Approximately one-third lead to physician office visits, 8% to hospitalization, and 2% to nursing care [24]. Other initial complaints besides pain are limitations in mobility and loss of independence. Risk factors associated with vertebral fractures in postmenopausal women are history of prior vertebral or nonvertebral fracture, age, height loss, and clinical diagnosis of osteoporosis [29]. Vertebral compression fractures may cause significant morbidity due to progressive loss of spinal column height, postural changes, kyphoscoliosis, and chronic pain that interferes with the activities of daily life. Self-esteem, body image, and mood may be affected in those with more severe disease [30].

Pain due to vertebral fractures typically is localized to the fracture site and described by patients as being intense and deep. It can be exacerbated by palpation over the fracture site, and sometimes it radiates to the flanks. Radiation of pain to the legs is not typical but has been reported [27]. Although some symptoms mimic lumbar disc protrusion or extrusion, disc disease can be excluded by careful examination with spinal magnetic resonance imaging (MRI), the pain radiation patterns, and leg-raising tests [13,24,28,31, 32]. Both acute pain and chronic pain caused by vertebral fractures have been described. A distinct separation between acute and chronic pain is difficult to establish because it is not often possible to determine exactly when a fracture has occurred. Pain may last from 1 to 3 months, but severe pain may persist for many years. Acute pain can respond to analgesic medications and typically lasts several weeks or months [24,28]. Chronic pain can persist for years, is usually not responsive to pain medications, but may diminish with physical therapy and exercise [33].

Facet Arthropathy

Facet arthropathy was recognized as a cause for back pain as early as 1911 by Goldthwait when he identified peculiarities of the facet joints responsible for low back pain and instability [34]. In 1927, Putti presented an article in support of this etiology [35]. Finally in 1933, Ghormley described facet symptoms with lumbosacral pain after twisting or rotational strain [36]. Unfortunately, the recognition of disc protrusions as an alternative cause of back pain was introduced in 1934 and thus pain of facet arthropathy was overshadowed for many years. Studies by Hirsch in 1963 demonstrated pain referral patterns from the intraarticular injection of hypertonic saline into the facet joints. Mooney and Robertson demonstrated the use of intraarticular facet injections for the treatment of low back pain [37–38]. More recently, Rees demonstrated that surgical denervation of the facets was a viable treatment option [39]. Shealy described a percutaneous approach that was much less invasive for the treatment of this syndrome [40]. The work of Bogduk and his group is responsible for our more recent knowledge about this syndrome and the appropriate interventions [41].

VERTEBROPLASTY

Clinical Results

Percutaneous vertebroplasty is a minimally invasive, radiologically guided, therapeutic procedure for the treatment of pain caused by a vertebral body compression fracture, symptomatic vertebral hemangiomas, multiple myeloma, or metastases. Initially described in patients suffering from painful hemangiomas, myeloma, or metastases [42–44], percutaneous vertebroplasty has gained popularity in the treatment of fractures associated with osteoporosis [23,45].

Pain control and functional improvement are the immediate goals in the treatment of symptomatic patients with vertebral compression fractures. Conservative treatment is limited to analgesics and muscle relaxants, immobilization through bed rest, and support devices such as back braces. Immobilization is potentially harmful, leading to decubitus complications, increased bone resorption, which can worsen bone demineralization, and defunctionalization of these often frail elderly patients due to loss of muscle mass. Surgical indications are rare. Unstable fractures may require surgical stabilization to prevent neurologic complications [32, 46]. Patients with vertebral compression fractures have significantly lower pulmonary vital capacity and forced expiratory volume than do control subjects [47]. A 1.23-fold higher mortality rate was found in women with compression fractures when compared with age-matched control subjects [48]. This suggests that early symptomatic relief with stabilization would lead to earlier mobilization and therefore could decrease the risks of prolonged immobilization. Percutaneous vertebroplasty can achieve this goal and is a promising treatment that may one day replace medical therapy as the standard of care for vertebral body compression fractures [9,32,46].

Review of the medical literature demonstrates many series of patients treated with vertebroplasty showing good outcomes [42–44,49–51]. Interpretation of the various results is difficult, however, due to the retrospective designs of these studies, relative short-term clinical follow-up, outcomes criteria based solely upon the patient's perception of pain or pain relief, and multiple concurrent treatment modalities.

Cotten et al. [42] measured complete or partial pain relief in 40 patients treated for metastases or multiple myeloma, using the McGill-Melzack classification, which measures patients' perception of pain relief. Patients also received radiation therapy 12 to 22 days following vertebroplasty. Pain relief was achieved in 39 patients and was not directly proportional to the percentage of lesion filling. Analgesic use was not measurable because most patients had other painful lesions requiring continued use of medication. Pain relief appeared durable. Unfortunately long-term follow-up was limited due to patient mortality from the underlying diseases.

Weill et al. [44] recorded analgesic use and mobility in 37 patients with 52 metastatic lesions. Indications for treatment included pain control or stabilization of the axial skeleton or both. Improvement was defined as decreased analgesic use and improved mobility. Twenty-three patients (73%) showed clear improvement, defined as a 50% decrease in narcotic dosage or change to a nonnarcotic drug, and ability to walk. Seven patients (21%) showed moderate improvement, defined as a decrease in pain without gain in mobility, or decrease of less than 50% in narcotic dosage. Improvement appeared durable, with 73% and 65% of patients showing persistent pain relief at 6 months and 1 year, respectively. Recurrent pain was associated with appearance of new metastases in five patients. The use of radiation and chemotherapy were complicating factors in the analysis of vertebroplasty treatment in some patients. The effect on the overall pain syndrome of these additional therapies is uncertain.

Deramond et al. [43,51] treated 80 patients. Immediate results were excellent in more than 90% of cases, with complete relief of symptoms. These patients were capable of standing up and walking 24 hours after the procedure. Percutaneous vertebroplasty was performed 3 weeks to 5 months after the onset of the initial symptoms. Jensen et al. [45] reported the first U.S. experience with vertebroplasty and noted similar benefits to patients. Twenty-nine patients with 47 painful vertebral fractures were treated over a 3-year period. Twenty-six patients (90%) reported significant pain relief immediately after treatment. Patients were treated after failing conservative therapy as directed by their primary care physicians. Conservative therapy typically consisted of narcotic analgesia and immobilization for 4 weeks. Long-term follow-up was not reported in either series. Debussche-Depriester et al. [50] reported on five treated patients with 12 to 18 months of follow-up who demonstrated complete pain relief immediately following vertebroplasty, with no or minimal residual discomfort. In another small series, Gangi et al. [52] observed four treated patients for 4 to 15 months. There was no recurrence of pain. The results of these early small-to-moderate–sized series indicate that vertebroplasty can be done safely and clinical outcomes are favorable.

Continued accumulation of data and longer-term follow-up by Jensen et al. support the long-term efficacy of vertebroplasty for patients with osteoporotic vertebral fractures [53] (Jensen ME, personal communication, 2000). Eighty-four patients with 159 fractures were treated and followed for an average of 5.6 months. Eighty-one patients (96%) underwent vertebroplasty after the referring physician deemed medical therapy ineffective, and three patients were treated for vertebral instability. Analgesic use and patient activity level were recorded. Twelve percent of patients developed additional fractures during the follow-up period and were treated more than once. Two percent of patients reported no pain medication use pretreatment as compared with 19% posttreatment ($p < 0.001$). Similarly, 3% of patients reported unrestricted activity pretreatment as compared with 34% posttreatment ($p < 0.001$).

Amar et al. [54] recently published results of functional outcome on 97 patients with 258 treated fractures. The mean age was 76 years (range 42 to 99 years). The mean duration of follow-up was 14.7 months (range 2 to 35 months). They reported that 74% of the patients had an overall improved quality of life, 26% were unchanged, and no patients had a decline in their quality of life.

Cyteval et al. [49] reported percutaneous vertebroplasty for acute osteoporotic vertebral collapse in a series of 20 patients with 23 fractures. All patients had acute pain of less than 1 month's duration that hindered ambulation and required treatment with narcotics. All patients were admitted to the hospital for pain medication and vertebroplasty. The visual analog scale (VAS) for pain was used for scoring assessment. Follow-up was obtained after 1 and 6 months. Within the first week 15 patients (75%) experienced complete pain relief or had only minimal pain. Analgesic medication was stopped in 14 patients (70%). The pain relief at the treated sites was durable at 6 months. Five patients (25%) returned with new fractures at other levels. The study did not report on the subsequent management of these patients.

Despite the excellent clinical results and safety profile reported in the above-mentioned clinical series, some physicians still have reservations regarding the effectiveness of vertebroplasty. There has not been a trial directly comparing vertebroplasty to medical therapy [55–57]. A prospective randomized trial comparing percutaneous vertebroplasty to medical therapy for acute (less than 6 weeks) osteoporotic vertebral body compression fractures is underway at Stanford University. The early results have suggested a benefit to vertebroplasty [58]. Of the 40 patients enrolled, 21 were randomized to vertebroplasty and 19 were randomized to continued medical therapy. Crossover was allowed in patients who failed medical therapy after they were 6 weeks from symptom onset. Outcomes variables measured at 6 weeks are an 11-point VAS (0 to 10), and 6-point activity and analgesic intake scales (0 to 5) (Table 17-1). Patients initially offered vertebroplasty had significant improvement in measured outcomes. For the group that was offered vertebroplasty first, the mean preoutcome and postoutcome scores are as follows: 9.5 and 3.7 (VAS), 3.7 and 1.8 (activity), 3.8 and 1.8 (analgesic) ($p < 0.001$). There was no significant improvement in outcomes of patients offered medical therapy. Only 3 of 19 (16%) patients had mild to moderate improvement in their pain score, and therefore these patients were not offered vertebroplasty. Sixteen of 19 (85%) patients who were randomly assigned to medical therapy and had either no improvement or worsening in their pain scores were offered vertebroplasty. When this group was offered vertebroplasty, their outcome scores improved significantly before and after augmentation as follows: 8.7 and 2.1 (VAS), 3.3 and 1.5 (activity), 3 and 1.1 (analgesic) ($p < 0.001$). Despite the encouraging results, criticisms regarding the placebo effect remain, and therefore larger multicenter trials with the comparison of vertebroplasty and a sham procedure may be needed for further evaluation of the clinical effectiveness of this procedure. In addition, cost-effectiveness studies are needed to compare the costs of medical therapy and vertebroplasty.

Concern has been raised over the issue that vertebroplasty may increase the risk of fracture at an adjacent level. In a study comparing a group of patients previously treated with vertebroplasty who returned with new fractures with a control group of patients who initially had multiple painful fractures, Jensen et al. found no statistically significant difference in the rates of adjacent-level fractures between the two groups [23,53]. The researchers postulate that these new fractures are more likely to be the result of the natural history of osteoporosis rather than the presence of a vertebroplasty.

Polymethylmethacrylate

No discussion of vertebroplasty would be complete without reviewing the polymeric material used for this procedure. Before its use in percutaneous vertebroplasty, polymethylmethacrylate (PMMA) was used in anterior and posterior stabilization of the spine for metastatic disease [59–61], for bone packing after curettage of giant cell tumors of the extremities [62,63], and for the surgical treatment of vertebral hemangiomas [64].

PMMA for vertebroplasty is prepared as a liquid, allowing it to be injected through needles. Starting 30 to 40

TABLE 17-1. ANALGESIC USE AND ACTIVITY LEVEL SCORING SYSTEM

Score	Medication Use	Activity Level
0	No medication	Unrestricted activity
1	Aspirin, over-the-counter NSAIDs	Ambulatory with assistance
2	Physician-prescribed nonnarcotic	Restricted to wheelchair use
3	Oral narcotic, p.r.n.	Upright in bed or chair, nonmobile
4	Oral narcotic, scheduled	Flat in bed
5	Parenteral narcotic	

NSAIDs, nonsteroidal antiinflammatory drugs; p.r.n., as needed.

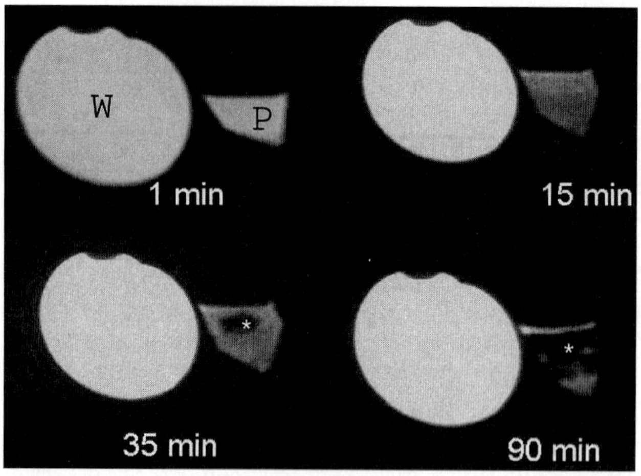

FIGURE 17-2. MRI of PMMA polymerizations. Sequential T2-weighted MR images at 1 minute, 15 minutes, 35 minutes, and 90 minutes after preparation of PMMA mixture for injection. PMMA *(P)* is hypointense to reference water signal *(W)*. Note the progressive loss of signal in a centrifugal pattern at 35 and 90 minutes *(asterisk)*.

minutes after mixing powdered PMMA polymer with the liquid PMMA monomer, the mixture undergoes progressive polymerization and slowly changes from a liquid to a solid state [31] (Fig. 17-2). MRI signal on conventional spin-echo sequences shows signal intensity alterations that reflect the physicochemical process of PMMA polymerization. PMMA liquid mixture possesses high signal intensity on T2-weighted MR sequences, which then increasingly becomes hypointense with progressive polymerization. The "cured" or "hardened" PMMA appears markedly hypointense on all sequences (Fig. 17-3).

Potential toxicities of PMMA have been described. McLaughlin et al. [65] found decreased pulmonary function in dogs only when the dosage of PMMA monomer was more than 35 times the amount liberated in humans during total hip replacement. Phillips et al. [66] described a fall in systemic arterial blood pressure after deposition of PMMA into the femoral shaft during hip arthroplasty. Wong and Vidovich [67] reported on a patient who developed acute bronchospasm on application of PMMA during cranioplasty. This patient immediately responded to nebulized albuterol. These authors speculated that the hypotension may have been due to absorption of monomer and additives

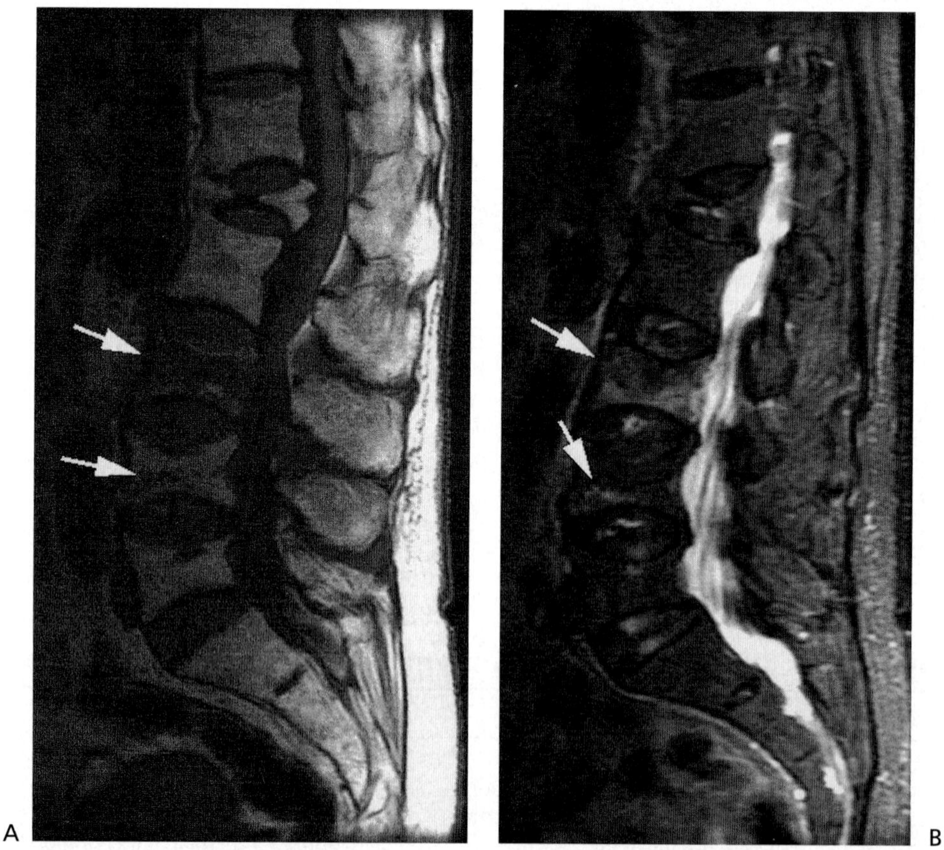

FIGURE 17-3. MRIs before and after vertebroplasty. **A,B:** Sagittal T1-weighted **(A)** and short tau inversion recovery (STIR) **(B)** images of the lumbar spine obtained during initial patient evaluation demonstrate bone marrow edema of L3 and L4 as evidenced by hypointensity on T1 and hyperintensity on STIR *(arrows)*. The chronic severe compression of L1 is asymptomatic. *(Figure continues.)*

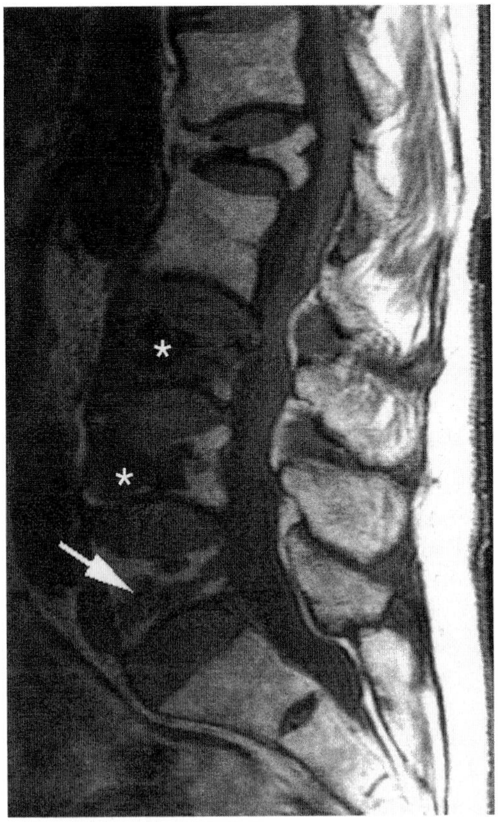

C

FIGURE 17-3. *Continued.* **C–E:** Follow-up study, performed 2 months after treatment when the patient developed new pain, reveals a new compression fracture of L5 (*arrows* in **C,E**). Note the low signal intensity of deposited PMMA at L3 and L4 on T1-weighted **(C)**, T2-weighted **(D)**, and STIR **(E)** sequences *(asterisks)*.

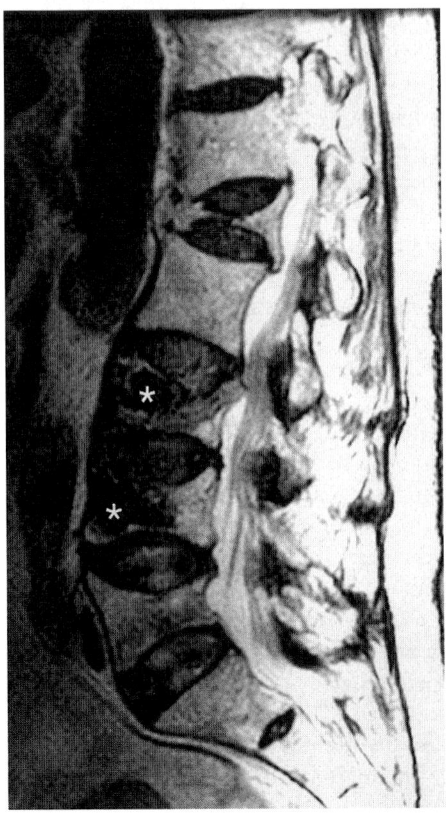

D

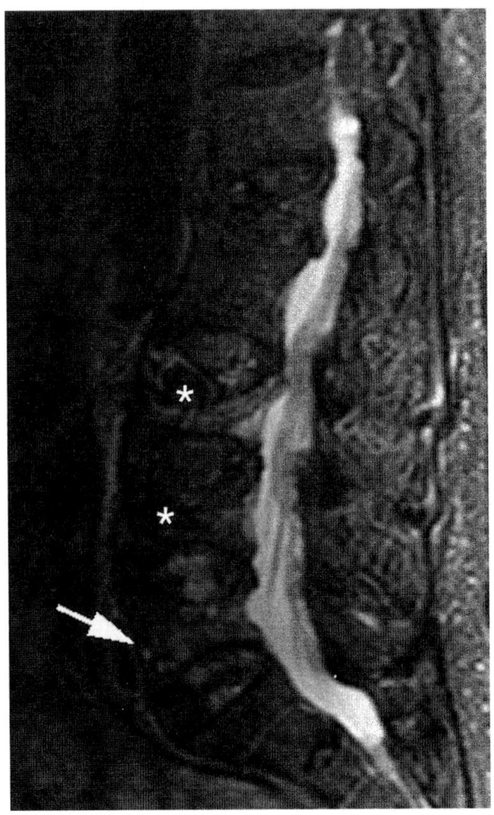

E

into the circulation. Convery et al. [68] found no evidence of pulmonary function alteration or change in liver enzyme levels that could be related to PMMA placement during total hip arthroplasty. These potential problems have not been noted with vertebroplasty.

Another potential toxicity is from thermal injury. The PMMA undergoes an intense exothermic reaction as it changes from a liquid to solid state, and the heat released could damage adjacent neural structures. However, *in vitro* work in human cadaveric spine by Deramond et al. [69] found no significant difference in peak temperature when measured at three key locations (anterior cortex, center, and spinal canal). Similarly, an *in vivo* experiment by Wang et al. [70] found no spinal cord injury occurring in dogs undergoing cervical spinal fusion with PMMA, even when gelatin sponges were not used as heat insulators. Intervening ligaments, vascular-rich dura, and cerebrospinal fluid flow may act as natural insulators and also to dissipate heat created by the polymerization process.

Operator injury from PMMA vapor exposure may be of concern to treating physicians and members of the treating staff. However, Cloft et al. have shown exposures of less than 5 parts per million (ppm) to physicians performing vertebroplasty in a standard-ventilation neuroangiography suite [71]. The occupational safety and health administration limits for personnel are set at l00 ppm per 8-hour shift.

Currently, percutaneous vertebroplasty is performed with several types of PMMA, such as Codman Cranioplastic (CMW Laboratories , Blackpool, England), Simplex P (Stryker-Howmedica-Osteonics, Rutherford, NJ), and Osteobond (Zimmer, Warsaw, IN). At present, only surgical Simplex P is approved by the U.S. Food and Drug Administration for use in pathologic fractures including those in the spine, but no commercially available PMMA is specifically approved for vertebroplasty. Therefore, patients should be informed that the materials are being used in an "off-label" manner. Simplex P and Osteobond contain 10% weight-to-volume of barium sulfate for opacification [9]. This amount of barium, however, is insufficient for easy visualization during the fluoroscopically guided procedure. Cranioplastic cement contains no barium sulfate and is not radiopaque. Therefore, all currently available PMMA cement requires the addition of an opacifying agent, most commonly barium sulfate, in large enough volume to allow for adequate visualization and safe injection under fluoroscopy. Tungsten and tantalum powder are used commonly in Europe and may be added, as well, for added opacification. The Codman Cranioplastic, type 1 (slow-setting), PMMA is probably the most suitable agent for vertebroplasty. Biomechanical testing has shown that injection of Codman Cranioplastic cement increases vertebral body strength, although it does not restore vertebral body stiffness [72]. Simplex P and Osteobond both increase strength and restore stiffness; however, they have a much shorter usable working time (5 to 7 minutes) than does Codman Cranioplastic (15 to 20 minutes). Therefore, the benefits of the longer working time of Codman Cranioplastic, especially in the injection of multiple vertebral body compression fractures, outweighs the improved biomechanics of Simplex P and Osteobond given the difference appears to be of no clinical consequence in case series [23]. Recent work has explored the possibility of substituting other bone cements for PMMA. Hitchon et al. found that hydroxyapatite (HA), an osteoconductive, biocompatible, nonexothermic cement that also undergoes remodeling, has stabilizing effects similar to those of PMMA in a cadaveric spinal compression fracture model [73].

PATIENT EVALUATION

Vertebroplasty

Clinical history and physical examination are done to establish significant focal back pain, point tenderness on palpation, and limited mobility. All patients have imaging evidence of a fracture in the immediate region of the pain. When indicated, cross-sectional imaging is obtained to exclude other causes of pain, such as intervertebral disc protrusion or extrusion or spinal stenosis. Infection is a contraindication for the procedure. The level to be treated is determined by physical examination, sometimes under fluoroscopic guidance. If necessary, ancillary tests, such as nuclear medicine bone scanning or MRI, are performed to better define or pinpoint more acute or subacute fractures [31,74].

MRI has made a significant contribution in the detection of spinal abnormalities. On T1- and T2-weighted images normal bone marrow has a characteristic signal intensity generally distinguishable from the intensity of an abnormal process such as a benign or pathologic fracture. Osteoporotic and malignant vertebral compression fractures are frequent in elderly patients. In the majority of cases, clinical evaluation, routine blood tests, and plain radiographic examinations are sufficient to distinguish a benign from a malignant condition. Nevertheless, in certain difficult cases, MRI or another additional imaging study is needed to differentiate benign from pathologic vertebral compression fractures [75,76]. Discrimination is generally possible with spin-echo sequences. Chronic benign fractures demonstrate isointense marrow signal intensity compared with that of normal vertebrae on T1- and T2-weighted sequences. Pathologic fractures show low signal intensity on T1-weighted images and high signal intensity on T2-weighted images. However, an acute or subacute benign compression fracture may demonstrate a signal intensity similar to that of pathologic fracture on spin-echo sequences. Ancillary imaging signs, or patterns such as conspicuity of lesion margins, involvement of pedicles, and enhancement pattern, are helpful in the distinction between benign and malignant causes [77]. Malignant compression fractures tend to have ill-defined margins, abnormal signal involvement of the pedicles, marked and heterogeneous MR enhancement patterns, and irregular nodular type paravertebral soft tissue components (Fig. 17-4). Diffusion-weighted MR imaging

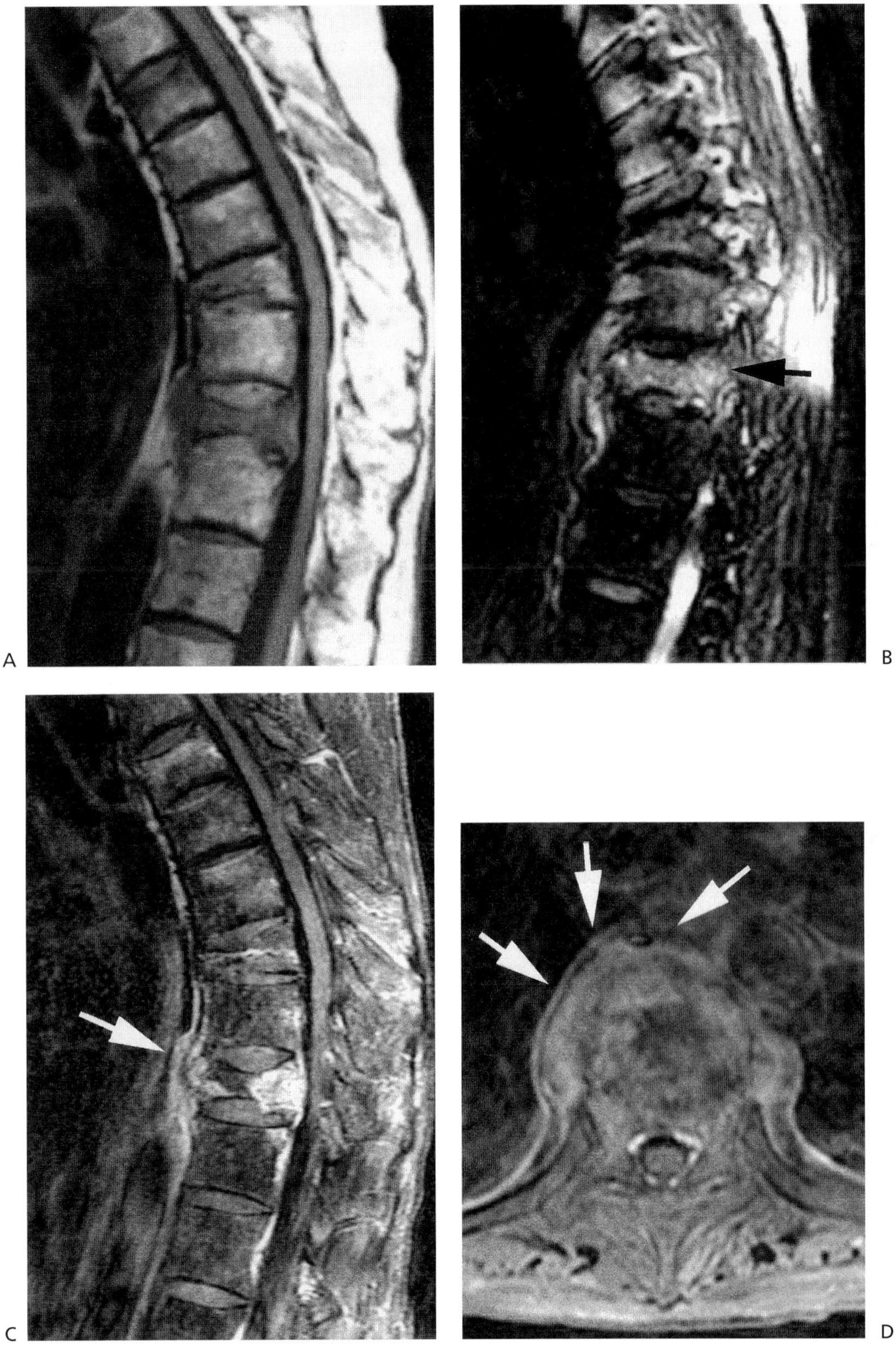

FIGURE 17-4. MRI of metastatic disease in an 80-year-old woman with history of lung carcinoma who sought treatment for new-onset midback pain. Sagittal T1-weighted **(A)** and T2-weighted **(B)** images show compression of T10 with diffuse bone marrow signal abnormality. Note abnormal hyperintense signal extending into the pedicle (*arrow* in **B**). Sagittal **(C)** and axial **(D)** T1-weighted images show intense heterogeneous enhancement of the compressed vertebra and adjacent anterior paraspinal soft tissue mass *(arrows)*. Note also heterogenous mottled enhancement of the more superior vertebrae and severe compression of T8. Biopsy was positive for metastatic disease.

(DWI) of the bone marrow was found to provide excellent distinction between pathologic and benign vertebral compression fractures [78]. Benign vertebral compression fractures are hypo- to isointense to normal vertebral bodies, indicating reduced apparent diffusion coefficient (ADC) values. Pathologic compression fractures are hyperintense to normal vertebral bodies, representing increased ADC values. Recently, however, conventional noncontrast T1-weighted images were found to be superior in quality to this same DWI sequences in the detection of vertebral metastases [79]. Tumors were all hypointense to normal marrow on the T1-weighted sequence. With DWI, 48% of tumors were hyperintense and 52% were hypointense to normal bone marrow. Increasing the diffusion weighting of DWI sequences can reduce false-positive hyperintensities of osteoporotic compression fractures, or make the hypointensities of these benign fractures more obvious and may improve the differentiation between benign and pathologic compression fractures [80]. Recent work suggests that quantitative determination of ADC values is more accurate than qualitative evaluation for the differentiation between benign and pathologic fractures [81,82]. The mean ADC values were $1.9 \pm 0.3 \times 10^{-4}$ mm^2/s for metastatic involvement versus $3.2 \pm 0.5 \times 10^{-4}$ mm^2/s for benign compression fractures [81].

For a patient with multiple compression fractures, spinal MRI and nuclear medicine bone scanning are helpful ancillary tests for better differentiation of acute or subacute fracture from chronic fractures. This differentiation can be of importance, because acute fractures generally respond more favorably to percutaneous vertebroplasty than do chronic compression fractures. Chronic fractures tend to have isointense bone marrow signal to adjacent nonfractured vertebrae, whereas acute or subacute compressions tend to have lower signal on T1-weighted images and higher signal on T2-weighted images in comparison to normal vertebrae (see Fig. 17-3). On bone scanning, the active fractures tend to have more radionuclide uptake than do more chronic fractures.

Increased activity on whole-body bone scan is highly predictive of a positive clinical response to vertebroplasty (Fig. 17-5). Maynard et al. found subjective moderate to complete pain relief (defined as pain improvement of at least 3 points on a 10-point VAS) in 93% (26 of 28) of patients who had positive pretreatment bone scans obtained during the course of evaluation for potential vertebroplasty treatment [74].

The primary indication for patient referral for percutaneous vertebroplasty evaluation is pain caused by a vertebral compression fracture [23,45,83,84]. Treatment is directed toward the patient who has failed a reasonable course of medical therapy consisting of analgesics, bed rest, physical therapy, and back bracing [23,45,49]. Some patients with acute fractures who are hospitalized for parenteral narcotic analgesics will be candidates almost immediately. Vertebroplasty is highly efficacious for relief of pain and improvement in mobility [85]. Other indications for vertebroplasty include unstable vertebral compression fractures associated with osteonecrosis or conditions in which reinforcement of the vertebral body or pedicle is desired. Examples of needed reinforcement include a planned posterior surgical destabilization procedure or interbody fusion in severely osteoporotic patients. Lack of fixation of hardware inside such osteoporotic vertebral bodies is an anticipated postsurgical problem [23,86]. Sufficient data is currently lacking to support routine prophylactic percutaneous vertebroplasty. However, patients with preexisting multiple compression fractures in whom further collapse would lead to pulmonary compromise due to ensuing severe kyphotic deformity may rarely be considered for such treatment.

Contraindications to vertebroplasty include improvement on conservative medical therapy. Some physicians advocate not treating patients with greater than 20% to 30% spinal canal compromise from retropulsed fracture fragments [23]. The severity of the vertebral collapse can also be a relative contraindication to vertebroplasty, although this is controversial. Some authors have recommended that treatment be withheld in patients with compression fractures greater than 70% [23,87]. O'Brien et al. [88], however, found vertebroplasty to be both feasible and efficacious in a small group of six patients with fractures in which the average compression was 73%.

Local palpation over the spinous process of the involved vertebra will often elicit pain and tenderness and aid in the localization of the level(s) to be treated [9,23]. This can be done under direct fluoroscopic guidance. Other causes of pain such as facet arthropathy may be revealed at this time. Diagnostic facet joint injection can be performed in selected cases as part of the screening examination.

Facet Arthropathy

Patients with pain due to facet arthropathy generally describe a deep aching sensation in a unilateral distribution. Patients may provide a history of rotation and extension injury . The pain is made worse with extension of the spine than with flexion. Therefore, activities such as going downstairs are classic for the exacerbation of lumbar facet arthropathy. In the lumbar spine, the radiation pattern is generally into the buttocks, trochanteric region, groin, hip, and thigh [89]. Distal radiation into the leg is an uncommon feature. Generally, the patients report no neuroclaudication symptoms, and thus the syndrome is distinguished from the pain of disc protrusion. In the cervical spine, radiation into the cervical and shoulder areas have been described; however, distinguishing this condition from disc protrusion is more difficult.

On examination, patients describe localized tenderness over the paraspinous region, particularly with provocative testing. Flexion is generally preserved. However, extension

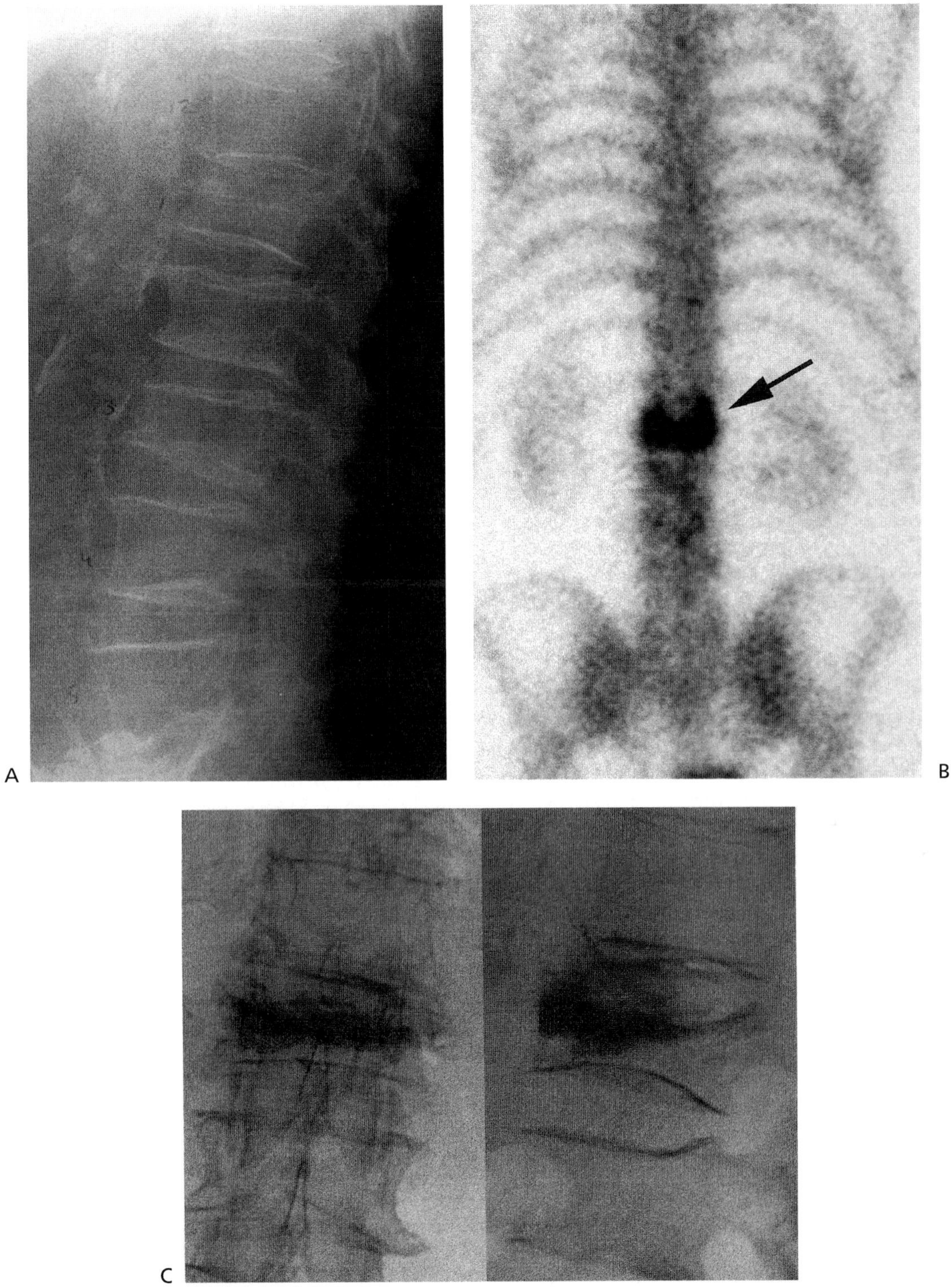

FIGURE 17-5. Positive bone scan imaging. **A:** Lateral lumbar spine radiograph shows compressions of L1, L2, and L3 vertebrae. **B:** A technitium-99m bone scan marked radionuclide uptake at L1 only *(arrow)*. **C:** This level was treated, resulting in complete pain relief during follow-up.

and side-bending rotation generally reproduce symptoms. On specific testing, segmental motion restrictions can be detected along with associated trigger points and spasm of the overlying musculature. Patients with cervical facet arthropathy generally hold their heads in an abnormal position as a compensatory mechanism to avoid pressure on the joints. Neurologic testing and straight leg–raising maneuvers are usually negative when facet arthropathy alone is responsible for the patient's condition. Laboratory data is generally not helpful except for specific imaging techniques of both CT and MRI, on which thickening of the joint capsule and facet hypertrophy are hallmarks of the disease.

After appropriate initial diagnosis, interventional techniques for facet arthropathy can help confirm the diagnosis or can be used for therapeutic purposes. From a diagnostic standpoint, two approaches for rendering the facet joint insensate, each with different therapeutic implications, have been used to distinguish back pain of facet arthropathy.

Direct injection of local anesthetic into the joint capsule allows discrete blockade of individual facet joints in order to determine whether the facet in question is the source of the pain. Using the same technique, instillation of a steroid into the joint offers the opportunity for therapeutic benefit [41].

An alternative to direct joint injection is neuroblockade of the medial branches of the posterior primary rami that provide sensory innervation to the facet joint [90]. Local anesthetic placed along the appropriate segments will effectively denervate that segment, confirming the diagnosis of facet arthropathy. As with intraarticular injection, the neuroblockade of medial branches also has therapeutic implications. Patients who respond to at least two separate injections of medial branches are candidates for percutaneous radiofrequency lesions of those same nerves. This renders the segments insensate and may provide relief for patients for an extended period [91].

The contribution of facet arthropathy to the entire clinical syndrome of low back pain has only recently been afforded proper attention. As such, controversy still exists regarding the appropriate use of diagnostic blockade and its implications for interventions including steroid injection, surgery, and radiofrequency neuroablation. Although it is clear that the pain of facet arthropathy in both the cervical and lumbar regions can be relieved temporarily with local anesthetics, well-controlled blinded studies using steroid instillation are lacking [92]. There are few studies related to the use of radiofrequency as well. Geurts et al. produced a systematic review of randomized clinical trials using radiofrequency for a variety of facet-related conditions [93]. Unfortunately, the six studies cited in the systematic review included three with low back pain and one with cervical pain, with the combination of neck and shoulder pains consistent with arthropathy in the cervical region. These studies all reported positive results, with only one study demonstrating an unequivocal clinical result. The overall conclusion of this systematic review is that moderate evidence exists that facet denervation by radiofrequency is better than placebo in the lumbar region, and that only limited evidence exists for the efficacy of radiofrequency lesions in the cervical region after whiplash. Future studies on a more homogeneous population with adequate numbers are needed to determine the utility of this technique in both the lumbar and cervical regions.

TECHNIQUE FOR PERCUTANEOUS TREATMENT

Vertebroplasty

Informed consent is obtained in all cases. The indications, risks, benefits, and possible alternatives must be explained to the patient. Risks cited should include infection, bleeding, fracture, untoward deposition or extravasation of PMMA material into the epidural or paravertebral veins, possibly resulting in worsening pain, paralysis, pulmonary compromise, and death. The potential need for immediate surgical intervention should be discussed at the same time. Blood work and laboratory testing may be indicated and often includes hemoglobin, hematocrit, creatinine, and electrolyte levels, coagulation panel, and complete blood count with differential.

Patients are treated routinely with prophylactic intravenous antibiotics, 30 minutes prior to the start of vertebroplasty or, alternatively, antibiotics may be administered in the cement. For preoperative prophylaxis, 1 g of cephazolin given intravenously 30 minutes prior to the procedure typically is used [9]. For the latter option, 1.2 g of tobramycin powder is typically added to the cement mixture [45]. These practices are empirical. Although there has not been a reported case of infection of the treated level following percutaneous vertebroplasty, the routine use of antibiotics requires further evaluation.

Conscious sedation with intravenous fentanyl and midazolam is used in most cases. In selected situations such as the patient with multiple compression fractures requiring extended operating time or the patient in whom movement is a problem, general anesthesia is indicated.

Pedicle Targeting

The vertebral body to be treated is isolated on both true anteroposterior (AP) and lateral planes, and a single image series is obtained for reference. The pedicle to be punctured, most often the left, is isolated on the lateral plane for positioning in the inferior superior plane and under AP oblique fluoroscopy for the medial lateral approach. Previously, authors have advocated a simple "bull's-eye" approach to the pedicle. This positions the needle in the midportion of the ipsilateral side of the vertebral body. However, if the pedicle is visualized in the more oblique, "scotty dog" view, then the needle track will start more lateral to the superior articular facet and pass through the pedicle in a steeper lateral-

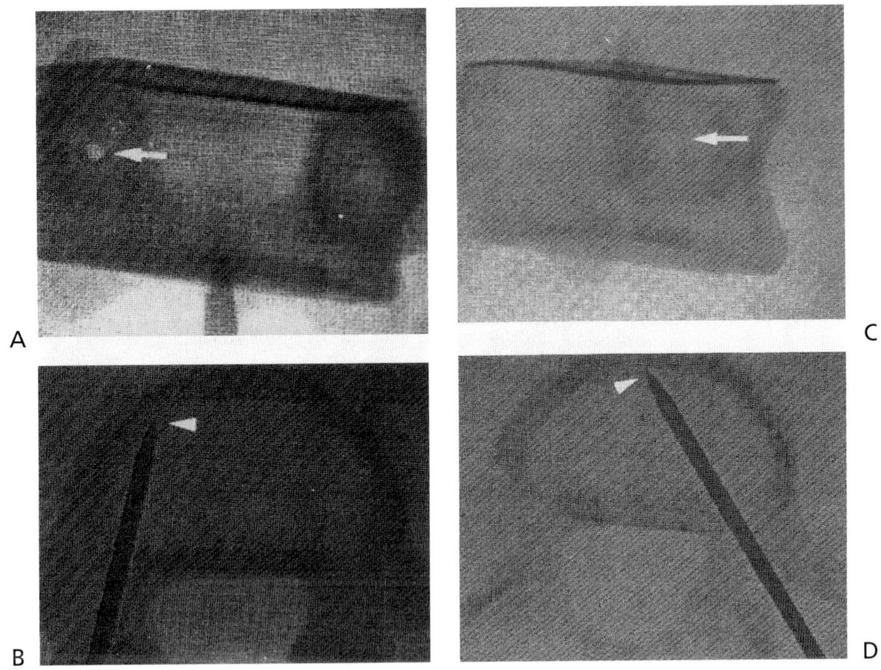

FIGURE 17-6. AP **(A)** axial **(B,D)** and AP oblique **(C)** radiographs of a spine model. In AP projection **(A)**, the outline of the pediculate cortex is distinct and the bull's-eye lucent needle track (*arrow* in **A**) is well seen. Needle advancement in the AP projection results in the needle tip in the anterior one-third and midportion of the left hemivertebra (*arrowhead* in **B**), and adequate filling of the right hemivertebra is not likely. From the AP oblique position **(C)**, the pediculate cortex is less distinct but adequate. Needle advancement guided by this projection is better for bihemispheric filling. Note midline and more anterior location of the needle tip (*arrowhead* in **D**). (From Jensen ME, Dion JE. Percutaneous vertebroplasty in the treatment of osteoporotic compression fractures. *Neuroimaging Clin N Am* 2000;10:547–568, with permission.)

to-medial course [23] (Fig. 17-6). Therefore, the final positioning of the tip of the needle will be more anterior and closer to the midline of the vertebral body. This allows for a single transpediculate injection, with cement crossing the midline and filling most of the vertebral body. This more midline positioning obviates the need for a contralateral puncture. Caution must be used in performing this technique because the pediculate cortex is not as well seen as it is on the "bull's-eye" view. If the needle is positioned too laterally, the transverse process may be fractured. Local anesthesia is applied to the skin and deep structures, including periosteum of the bone at the intended site of entry using a 11- to 13-gauge bone biopsy needle. The needle is advanced into the pedicle under biplane fluoroscopic guidance (Fig. 17-7).

Intraosseous Venography

Controversy exists regarding the utility of antecedent venography in determining improved clinical outcome or de-

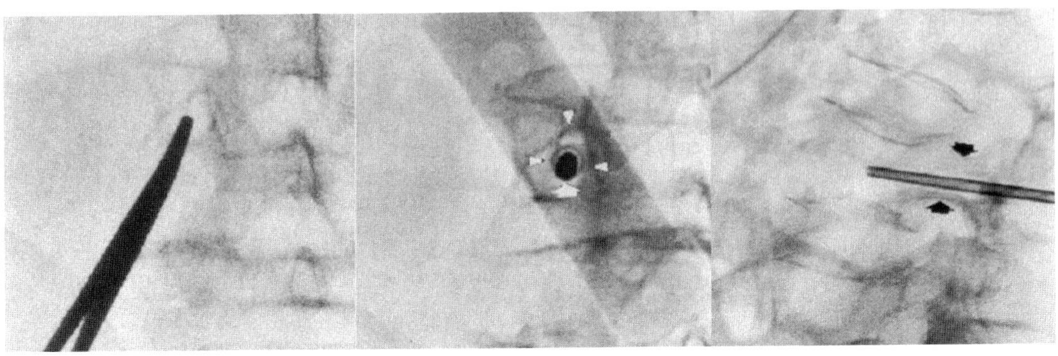

FIGURE 17-7. The left pedicle is localized under AP oblique projection *(left)*, marked, and local anesthesia is achieved from the skin to the periosteum. Frequent observation under AP oblique *(center)* and lateral *(right)* fluoroscopy planes is needed to ensure good needle positioning.

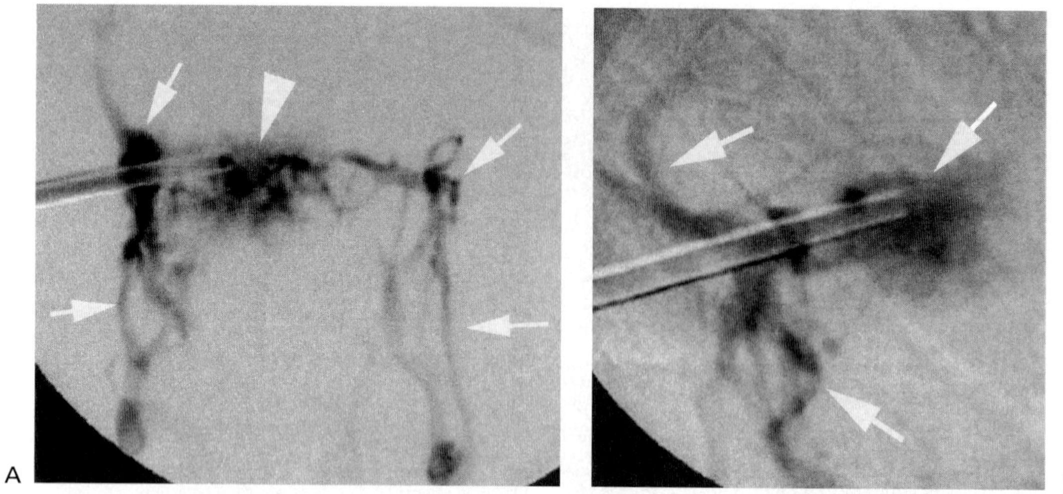

FIGURE 17-8. Intraosseous venography. AP **(A)** and lateral **(B)** lumbar venograms demonstrate mottled spongiform trabecular opacification *(arrowheads)* prior to opacification of paravertebral veins *(arrows)*.

creased number of complications during vertebroplasty (Fig. 17-8). A report by Jensen et al. in 1997 [45] advocated the use of antecedent venography in order to avoid potential complications associated with incorrect or suboptimal needle placement within the basivertebral venous plexus or in direct connection with a paravertebral vein. This is to delineate the potentially dangerous route of possible escape of PMMA cement outside the confines of the vertebral body. PMMA cement can escape posteriorly into the spinal canal causing spinal canal stenosis or cord compression, to the intervertebral foramina causing nerve root compression, or to the vena cava and pulmonary arteries causing pulmonary embolism. In the setting of a right-to-left cardiac shunt, such as patent foramen ovale or ductus arteriosus, a potential stroke may occur, although it has never been reported. Preventing cement extravasation may require needle readjustment or maneuvers such as placing Gelfoam pledgets prior to injection of PMMA. Another maneuver is the initial deposition of PMMA followed by a period of waiting to allow the cement to harden and obliterate the direct venous connection(s), and then using a second needle for injection of cement into the vertebral body. Some authors [9,44,56], however, disagree with this approach and have stated that due to the differences in viscosity and flow characteristics of contrast material and cement, venography will not be predictive of the actual flow and path of PMMA cement extravasation. Additionally, persistence of intravertebral opacifications, such as with injection into necrotic cavities in cases of vertebral osteonecrosis or Kummell disease (Fig. 17-9), or through the endplates to the intervertebral discs, could obscure visualization of cement [23,86]. Preoperative imaging with demonstration of intravertebral gas or fluid collection should alert one to the possibility of vertebral osteonecrosis. It therefore requires modification of the venogram by injecting contrast gently, using a minimal volume of contrast (1 to 2 ml).

Gaughen et al. [94] conducted a retrospective review of consecutive patients treated with percutaneous vertebroplasty for vertebral body compression fractures. The first group of patients (n = 20) had antecedent venography while the second group (n = 22) was treated without venography. The clinical outcomes were assessed through quantitative measurements of pain and mobility. The intraosseous venograms and postvertebroplasty radiographs were evaluated for extravertebral PMMA deposition, the amount of extravasation at each treated level, and correlation between venography and vertebroplasty results. The authors found that there were no differences in pain improvement and mobility improvement between the two treated groups. Similarly, there was no statistical difference in the demon-

FIGURE 17-9. This patient had pain and instability due to vertebral osteonecrosis (Kummel disease). Sagittal T1-weighted **(A)** and T2-weighted **(B)** MR images from an outside study show marked hypointense signal *(asterisks)* within a seemingly partially compressed L1 vertebra in this patient with severe back pain, especially with movement. This initially was interpreted as a chronic compression fracture with sclerosis. However, subsequent plain films in upright weightbearing **(C)** and recumbent nonweightbearing positions **(D)** reveal that the MR hypointense signal actually represents gas. Note severe compressive change of vertebra on upright films (*arrowhead* in **C**), which expands to near normal on prone films (*arrows* in **D**). **E,F:** Postvertebroplasty images in upright weightbearing position show stabilization of fracture.

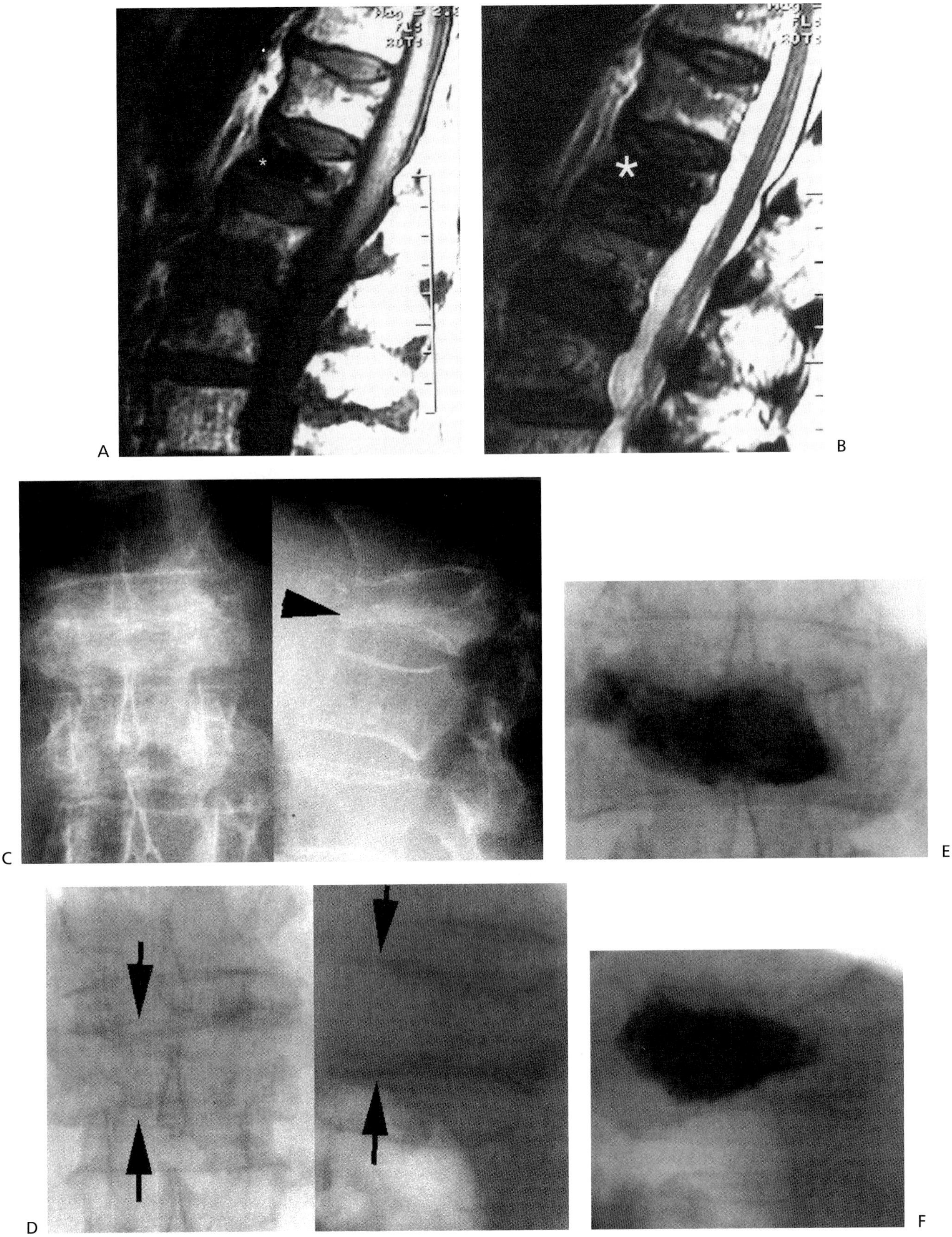
A
B
C
E
D
F

strated extravasation of PMMA cement between the two groups. Interestingly, 14 of 22 levels (64%) in the group that had antecedent venography showed a correlative extravasation on venography. The authors concluded that antecedent venography does not significantly augment the efficacy or safety of percutaneous vertebroplasty procedures performed by this group of experienced interventional neuroradiologists.

Although venography may not augment the safety of vertebroplasty by experienced operators, it may very well guide the novice or inexperienced operator to perform vertebroplasty in a safer manner. Although venography may not have absolute correlation with actual extravasation of cement, the additional information provided by delineation of the venous anatomy around the vertebral body potentially may be of benefit [94]. Percutaneous vertebroplasty is an intravascular procedure because the bony trabecula is a large venous space with connections to draining veins. PMMA cement should be considered a liquid embolic agent used with caution and full knowledge of its possible side effects. When the venography images are saved on separate monitors, these reference images may guide in the detection of early small quantities of extravasated cement. Cement extravasation will occur; however, it is the volume and amount of extravasation that will cause clinical complications. Therefore, early detection of cement extravasation is key to the performance of safe vertebroplasty. The amount of contrast used per venogram is approximately 3 to 5 ml, therefore the risk of renal failure is minimal. For those adept at the performance of vertebroplasty, venography may represent a superfluous step. Venography, however, may be extremely beneficial.

Cement Opacification

Radiopaque barium sulfate comes prepackaged in 5-g aliquots in capped graduated cylinders. We mix 1.2 g of tobramycin powder with the powdered PMMA polymer (CMW Laboratories, Blackpool, England) and fill the cylinder to the 17-ml mark. The bottle is capped and shaken to disperse the barium throughout the powder. Approximately 7.5 ml of liquid PMMA monomer is then added and the cylinder is capped securely. The materials, when mixed together, should be in a thin, cake-frosting consistency prior to injection. PMMA can be injected under fluoroscopic control using 1-ml Luer-Lok syringes or via a commercially available cement reservoir delivery system (EZ Flow Cement Delivery System, Parallax Medical, Scotts Valley, CA) (Fig. 17-10). With the delivery system, instead of using multiple syringes, the PMMA is loaded into the barrel of the injection device and the screw-type plunger is applied. The system is attached to the needle through a high-pressure tubing. Each turn of the plunger delivers approximately 0.25 ml of material. This system eliminates the need for syringes and keeps the operator's hand out of the radiation field. However, this

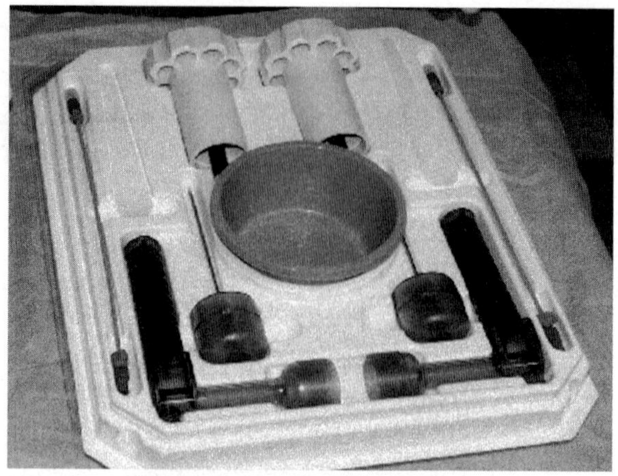

FIGURE 17-10. The EZ Flow Cement Delivery System (Parallax Medical, Scotts Valley, CA) comes with needles, reservoirs, twist-type plungers for injection, and high-pressure tubings.

system does not allow for the exquisite tactile feedback that is available with 1-ml syringes, and a steeper learning curve is required to become proficient with this delivery technique. It is important to recognize cement compaction that can be identified by the lack of movement of the opacified PMMA down the needle during injection and crowding of the suspended barium particles at the distal tip of the needle lumen. If injection is immediately difficult, the syringe or delivery system is disconnected and evaluated for plug formation at the tip of the syringe or in the injection tubing. Clearing of the needle will require a plunger or stylette to push some of the cement into the vertebra. This maneuver should be done under constant fluoroscopic control. If there is continued difficulty of delivery, the needle may need to be pulled back slightly and injection tried again. Sometimes, careful evaluation of cement flow pattern with comparison to vertebrogram will aid in the detection of early venous extravasation. If adequate cement crosses the midline to the contralateral hemivertebra, a contralateral transpediculate approach is needed (Figs. 17-11 and 17-12). Injection should be stopped when the cement reaches the posterior one-fourth of the vertebral body on the lateral projection. It should also be halted if significant amounts of cement leak across an endplate fracture, or if there is persistent filling of the epidural or paravertebral veins despite needle repositioning.

Potential Pitfalls

A number of other factors may relate to complications of vertebroplasty These include inappropriate patient selection, poor cooperation from the patient, and lack of patient monitoring. The operator may have trouble visualizing the procedure due to inadequate fluoroscopic equipment or unsatisfactory cement opacification. Operator error may be due to lack of knowledge of spinal anatomy viewed radio-

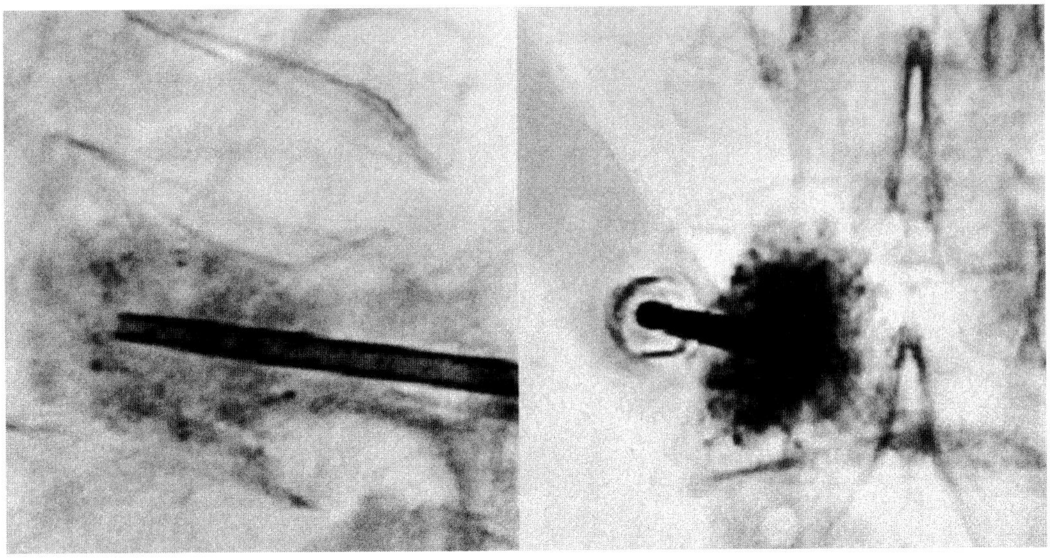

FIGURE 17-11. Left transpediculate vertebroplasty hemispheric filling. With the needle tip far lateral to the midline *(right)*, PMMA usually fills only the ipsilateral hemivertebra.

graphically, particularly the bony and venous anatomy (Fig. 17-13); poor fluoroscopic triangulation skills; unfamiliarity with equipment; poor embolization technique; and improper aseptic technique [23]. Major vertebroplasty series report complication rates from 1% to 10%. More of these complications are seen in series of pathologic compression fractures and not the osteoporotic compression population. Deramond et al. [43] noted a single transient neurologic complication in 80 patients with osteoporotic fracture. Jensen et al. [45] noted only two complications of benign rib fractures in a series of 29 patients. In a study of 38 patients, Barr et al. [84] reported a single case of cement-induced neuritis among 40 patients who responded to steroids. Two minor nonneurologic complications were also noted. Padovani et al. [95] reported a case of symptomatic pulmonary embolus in a patient treated for vertebral Langerhans cells histiocytosis. CT demonstrated cement in the pulmonary arteries from the venous extravasation and embolization to the inferior venae cava. This patient was treated with anticoagulation and responded favorably. Small asymptomatic cement leaks may be more common than realized. Cotten et al. [42] demonstrated PMMA leaks, both venous and corti-

A

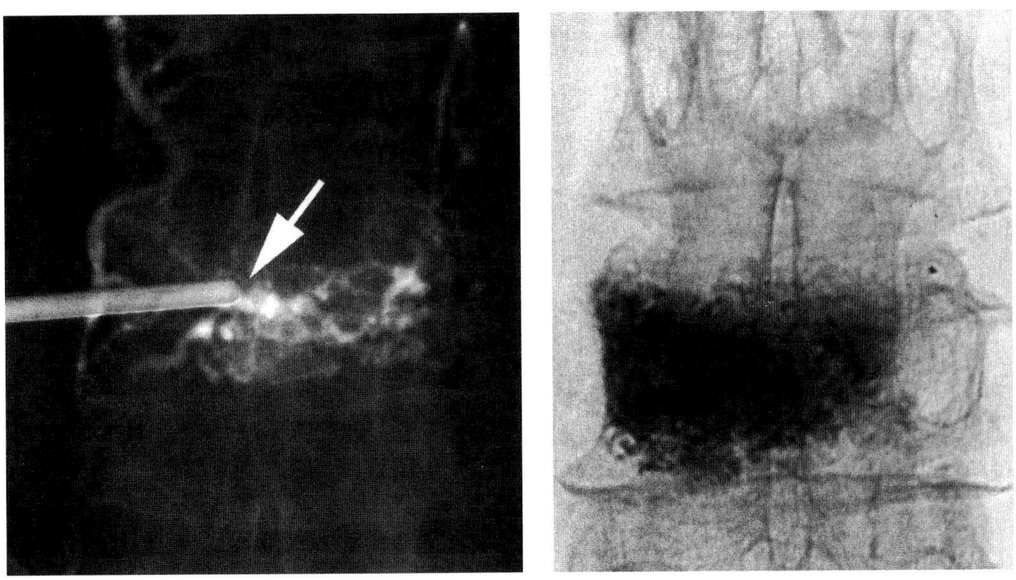

B

FIGURE 17-12. Left transpediculate vertebroplasty, bihemispheric filling. With more medial needle positioning (**A** from venogram, *arrow*), one can achieve adequate PMMA penetration and filling of the contralateral hemivertebra **(B)**.

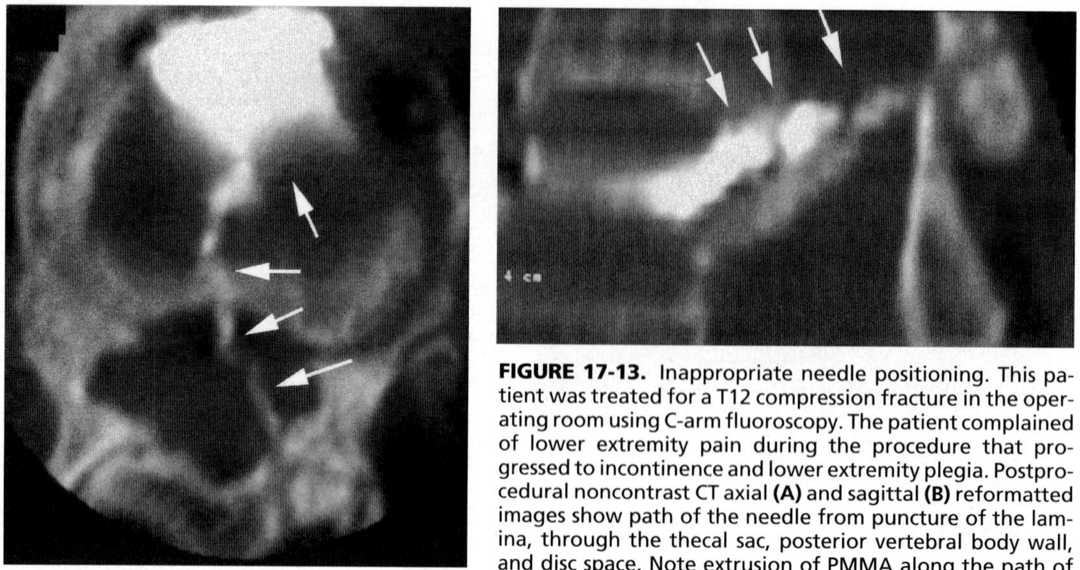

A B

FIGURE 17-13. Inappropriate needle positioning. This patient was treated for a T12 compression fracture in the operating room using C-arm fluoroscopy. The patient complained of lower extremity pain during the procedure that progressed to incontinence and lower extremity plegia. Postprocedural noncontrast CT axial **(A)** and sagittal **(B)** reformatted images show path of the needle from puncture of the lamina, through the thecal sac, posterior vertebral body wall, and disc space. Note extrusion of PMMA along the path of the needle *(arrows)*. (From M.E. Jensen, with permission.)

cal, by CT in 29 of 40 patients with osteolytic metastasis or myeloma. The majority of these extravasations were asymptomatic, but two of eight foraminal leaks produced nerve root compression that required decompressive surgery. In a larger series, Cotten et al. [96] reported that 1 patient of 258 treated experienced spinal cord compression requiring surgery. Of the 13 patients experiencing radicular pain after treatment, only 3 underwent decompression with the remaining 10 responding to a local anesthetic infiltration or medical therapy.

After the procedure, the patient is asked to remain flat for 2 hours to allow complete curing of the PMMA prior to axial loading. Activity is increased gradually as tolerated. Outpatients are discharged directly from the radiology department to home under the care of a responsible adult. Patients are instructed to contact the treating physician if there is worsening pain, fever, breathing difficulty, or neurologic change. Telephone contact with or direct observation of every patient is done within 24 to 48 hours of treatment. A CT scan of the treated vertebra is obtained in patients with worsening pain to assess for possible pedicle fractures and PMMA distribution within the vertebral body, and to detect leaks into the spinal canal, neural foramina, adjacent intervertebral disks, paravertebral tissue, and venous plexus.

Research and Future Directions

For percutaneous vertebroplasty to be widely accepted by the medical community, scientific validation through prospective randomized clinical trials comparing percutaneous vertebroplasty with conventional medical therapy is needed. Published case study series are not randomized, but they do report rapid pain control, increased mobility, and decreased medication intake in a high percentages of treated patients. The complication rates in these series have been extremely low, especially in patients with osteoporotic vertebral body compression fractures who account for the majority of the patients treated with percutaneous vertebroplasty. Studies providing scientific validation would also provide improved data regarding guidelines for appropriate use of percutaneous vertebroplasty. Such data are needed to decide what treatment is appropriate for acute fractures and chronic fractures, multiple fractures, and for the prophylactic treatment of vertebrae at higher risk for fracture.

New non-PMMA cements are currently being developed. Biomaterial testing may result in more aggressive therapy of pathologic disease by providing strengthening of the affected vertebra, as well as potential chemotherapeutic treatment of the tumor. Some authors have also started using PMMA beyond the spine, such as for metastatic involvement of the pelvis or clavicle (Fig. 17-14) [97,98]. The biomechanical efficacy of unipedicular versus bipedicular vertebroplasty has been studied by Tomeh et al. in an *in vitro* cadaveric model [99]. PMMA from a unipediculate approach (6 ml) or from a bipediculate approach (10 ml) was used to treat vertebrae. These vertebrae were then subjected to compression. The authors found no significant difference in the height changes between either group.

A competing technology is emerging in the form of balloon vertebroplasty or kyphoplasty, a procedure that purports to restore vertebral body height by inflation of a high-pressure puncture-proof balloon within the vertebral body, followed by PMMA injection into the cavity produced by inflated balloon. Clinical trials evaluating this new investigative procedure are underway and data are forthcoming.

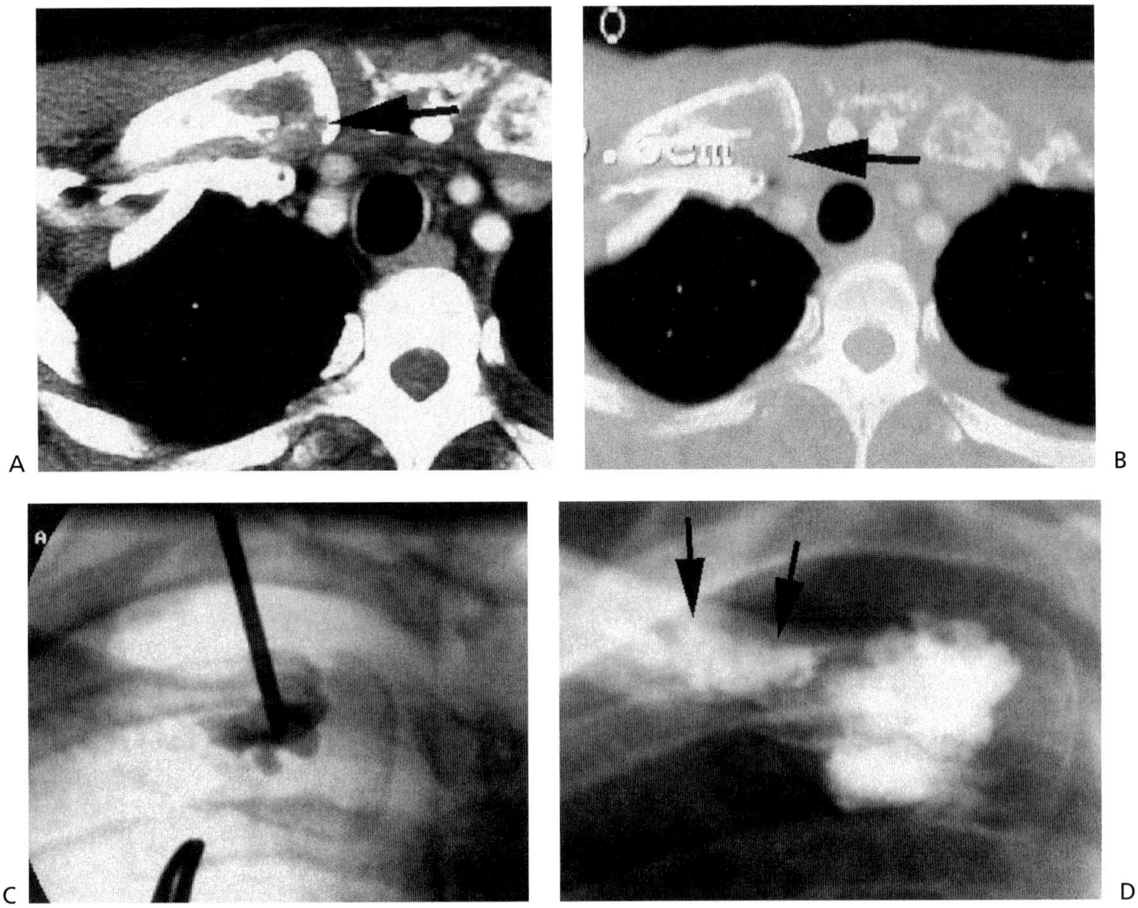

FIGURE 17-14. PMMA injection of clavicular breast metastasis. **A,B:** This 40-year-old woman had a lytic metastasis from the breast to the medial right clavicle *(arrows)*. Patient was right handed and in severe pain refractory to narcotic analgesia. She had undergone multiple cycles of chemotherapy and radiation therapy and was no longer considered a candidate for these types of therapy. The interventional neuroradiology service was consulted for pain palliation. **C:** The lytic lesion was punctured in the superior and anterior aspect of the medial clavicular head, taking care to avoid the posterior surface subjacent to the blood vessels and nerves. **D:** Posttreatment radiograph demonstrates filling of lytic cavity with some PMMA tracking along the medullary cavity of the clavicle *(arrows)*. The patient experienced immediate pain relief, was able to regain full function of her right arm, and has remained pain free for 15 months.

Facet Block

Facet injections in the lumbar and cervical regions should be performed only after appropriate patient selection to minimize unnecessary procedures and undue risk to patients. Patients with lumbar back pain primarily on extension or rotation, localized to the low back and hip region in the absence of disc injury, would be considered appropriate candidates for injection. In the case of cervical pain, patients with a history of an extension whiplash injury with radiation to the occipital, neck, and shoulder regions are candidates for facet injections. Imaging studies consistent with facet arthropathy, demonstrating facet hypertrophy or joint thickening or both, would be minimal criteria for the performance of this block.

Generally the injections are safe, but preoperatively the patient should be apprised of both common and uncommon side effects when consent is obtained. Most patients require some form of conscious sedation and consent must be obtained for this also. Patients should be counseled to discontinue agents that promote bleeding, such as oral anticoagulants and the nonsteroidal antiinflammatory drugs. The selective cyclooxygenase (COX)-2 inhibitors rofecoxib and celecoxib, and do not interfere with platelet function, can be continued in the periprocedure time frame. Indeed, the use the COX-2 inhibitors prior to the block provides an opportunity to reduce the prostaglandin effects of inflammation and peripheral nociceptor sensitization. Both effects will aid in the relief of pain after the procedure.

Pain, bleeding, infection, and nerve injury are potential complicating events. More serious events include intravas-

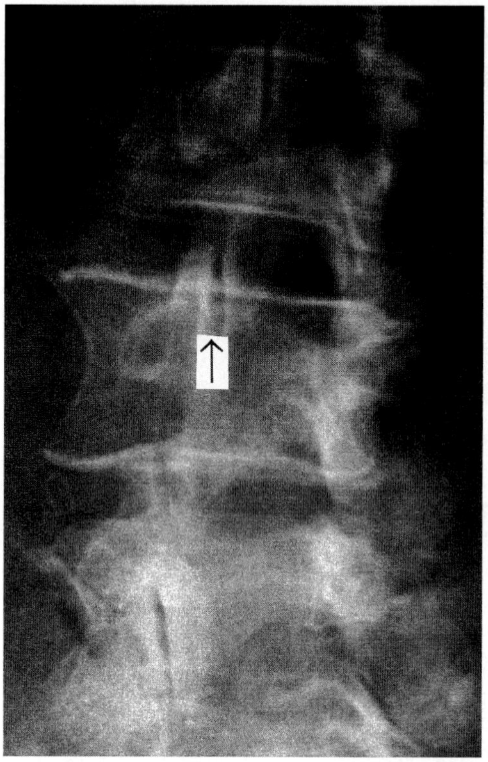

FIGURE 17-15. Fluoroscopic view of lumbosacral spine at 45-degree oblique angle. *Arrows* illustrate the appropriate needle positions for intraarticular injection of the L3-4 facet in the "scotty dog" view.

cular injection, with subsequent seizure, and intraspinal (epidural or intrathecal) injection. Spinal blockade, either partial or complete, can lead to hemodynamic instability, loss of airway reflexes, temporary paraplegia or quadriplegia, and loss of consciousness. These complications are life-threatening and thus appropriate resuscitative equipment and medications should be readily available. With proper care, expertise, and knowledge of both bony landmarks and neuroanatomy, these complications should rarely be encountered.

Performance of the lumbar intraarticular injections is accomplished with the patient in the prone position. After identifying proper levels on an AP view, the fluoroscopic unit should be tilted to approximately a 45-degree angle from the vertical in order to demonstrate an end-on view of the facet joints (Fig. 17-15). In this "scotty dog" projection, the joint space appears as parallel lines just above the superior articular process, or "ear of the scotty dog." Using aseptic technique, the tip of a 22-gauge 2-inch spinal needle is then projected at 90 degrees to the beam over the facet joint. The needle can then be rotated 90 degrees, so that it is parallel to the beam of the fluoroscopy unit, and then advanced in this parallel direction until it makes contact with the joint capsule. On occasion, the needle may impact just outside the capsule on the bony portion of the facet, and thus the needle should be manipulated slightly until the joint space is entered, with a distinct sensation similar to pushing a pin into cork board. Because the joint space is of extremely small volume, approximately 1.0 to 1.5 cc in total, small amounts of contrast, local anesthetic, and even steroids should be used. In general, 0.3 ml of Omnipaque introduced into the joint space should properly delineate the joint to establish true intraarticular placement of the needle. Subsequently, in the case of the diagnostic block, 0.5 to 0.7 ml of 0.5% bupivacaine can then be injected into the joint. The injection should continue until either the entire volume is injected or resistance is met, suggesting that the joint and capsule have reached full distention. For therapeutic blocks, 0.5 ml containing 20 mg of methylprednisolone can be injected into the site in place of the local anesthetic, or in an admixture with local anesthetic not to exceed the capacity of the joint space. Because multiple joints are usually injected, 20 mg of methylprednisolone at each joint is sufficient.

An alternative technique for temporary denervation of the lumbar facets is a blockade of the medial branches of the posterior primary rami that provide sensory innervation to the joints (Fig. 17-16). An understanding of the neuroan-

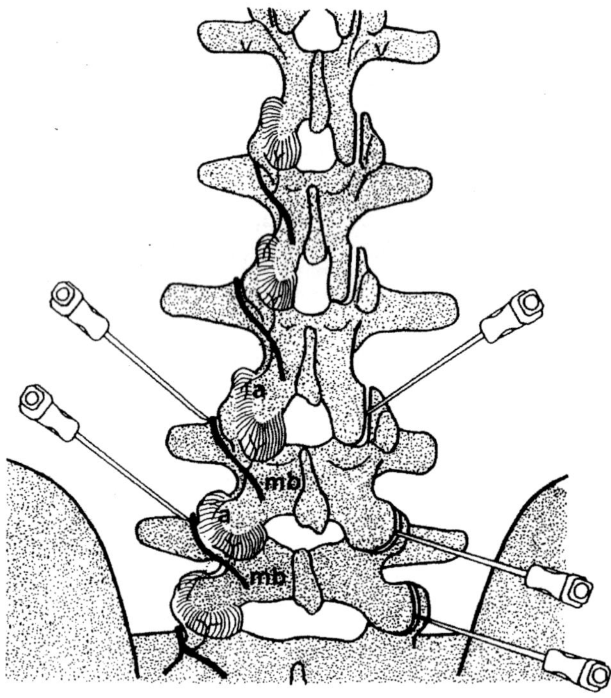

FIGURE 17-16. Sketch of the needle placements used for lumbar medial branch blocks and lumbar intraarticular zygapophysial blocks. On the left, the courses of the medial branches of the lumbar dorsal rami *(mb)* and their articular branches *(a)* are shown. Needles have been introduced onto the L3 and L4 medial branches, which would be anesthetized to block the L4-5 joint. On the right, the needle placement for intraarticular blocks of the L3-4, L4-5, and L5-S1 zygapophysial joints is depicted. (From Cousins MJ, Bridenbaugh PO, eds. *Back pain: zygapophysial blocks and epidural steroids.* London, Churchill Livingstone, 1988: 937, with permission.)

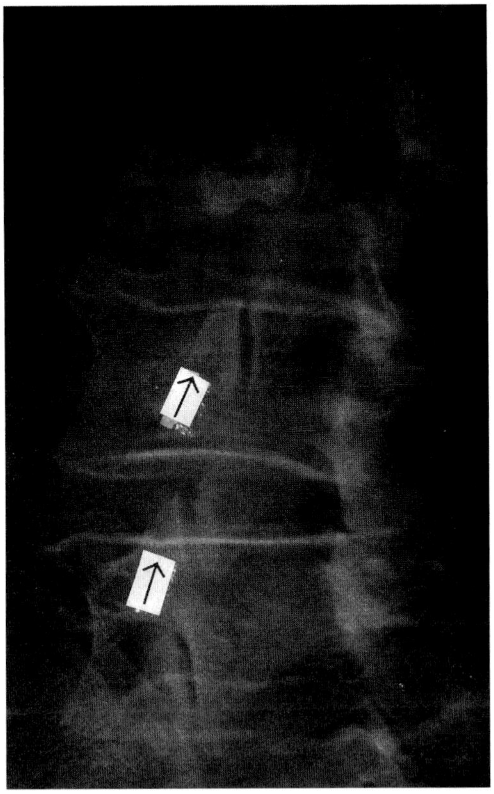

FIGURE 17-17. Fluoroscopic view of the lumbosacral spine at 45-degree oblique angle. *Arrows* illustrate the appropriate needle positions for medial branch blocks at the L3-4 and L4-5 levels in the "scotty dog" view. Note that these two blocks completely denervate the L4-5 facet and incompletely block L3-4 and L5-S1.

atomy is key, because each facet joint is innervated segmentally by the corresponding spinal level as well as the level above. For example, the L4-5 facet joint is innervated by L4 inferiorly, whereas L3 innervates the superior portion of the joint. Complete denervation requires that both contributing branches are blocked.

With the patient prone, the proper levels are identified in an AP fluoroscopic view. The fluoroscopic unit should then be tilted to approximately a 45-degree angle from the vertical in order to demonstrate an end-on view of the facet joints. In this "scotty dog" projection, the joint space appears as parallel lines just above the superior articular process, or "ear of the scotty dog." With aseptic technique, the tip of the 22-gauge 2-inch spinal needle is introduced over the junction between this superior articular process of the facet and the transverse process of that same spinal segment. In this position it is considered at the "eye of the scotty dog" on this oblique view (Fig. 17-17). The needle can then be rotated 90 degrees so that it is parallel to the beam of the fluoroscopy unit, and then advanced in this parallel direction until it makes contact with the junction of the superior articular process and the transverse process. On contact with bone, small volumes, 0.5 to 1.0 ml of 0.5% bupivacaine, can be injected to produce denervation of that segment. In the case of the L4-5 facet joint, this procedure must be repeated on the segment above to completely denervate this L4-5 facet joint.

In the cervical spine, the facet joints occupy a more horizontal position relative to the lumbar spine and thus the intraarticular injections can be accomplished from either a posterior or a lateral approach (Fig. 17-18). With the patient prone and the head in a neutral position, an AP projection can be obtained so that the facet joints are seen on-end. The fluoroscopy unit may require rotation in a caudal direction to obtain the best view of the facets. In this posterior approach, using aseptic technique, the 22-gauge 2-inch spinal needle can be advanced so the tip is over the joint at 90 degrees to the beam. The needle is then rotated 90 degrees, parallel to the beam, and advanced until the joint is entered. Similarly, a lateral approach can be taken with the patient again prone; however, the beam is directed from a lateral position. The facets generally appear as a diagonal line and can be entered similarly by placing the spinal needle perpendicular to the beam, with the tip over the projection of the joint space. The needle is then rotated 90 degrees, parallel to the beam, and advanced until the joint space is entered. In each case, volumes of contrast and local anesthetic similar to those used for lumbar intraarticular blocks can be used to provide confirmation of needle placement,

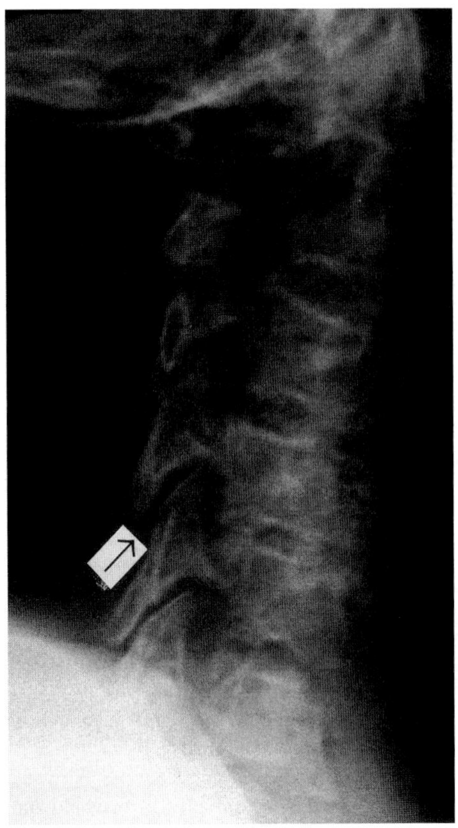

FIGURE 17-18. Lateral view of the C-spine. *Arrow* illustrates needle position for an intraarticular injection of C5-6 facet.

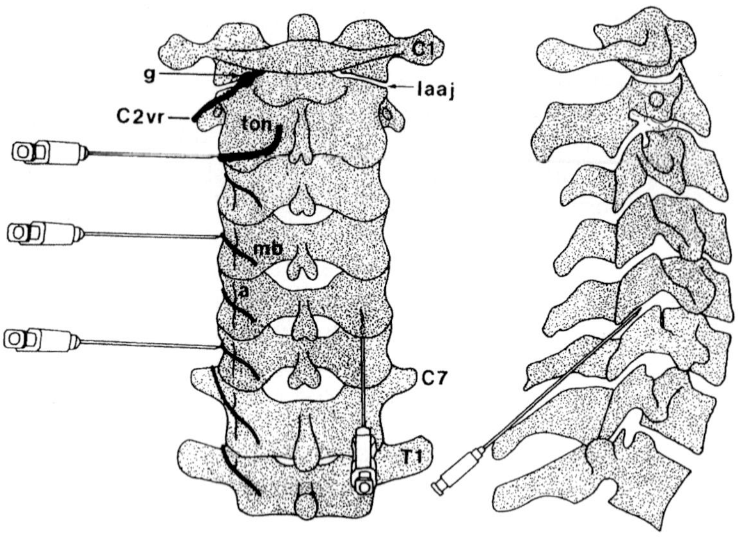

FIGURE 17-19. Illustrations of the needle placement for cervical medial branch blocks and intraarticular zygapophysial blocks. **Left:** Posterior view of the cervical spine showing the location of the C2 ganglion *(g)* behind the lateral atlantoaxial joint *(laaj)*, the C2 ventral ramus *(C2vr)*, the courses of the medial branches of the cervical dorsal rami *(mb)*, their articular branches *(a)*, and the third occipital nerve *(ton)*. Needles are shown in position as they would be used for blocks of the C4 and C6 medial branches and the third occipital nerve. The articular pillar of C7 may be obscured by the shadow of the large C7 transverse process, in which case the C7 medial branch can be located midway between the lateral convexities of the C6-7 and C7-T1 zygapophysial joints. **Right:** Lateral view of the cervical spine showing the course of a needle into the cavity of the right C5-6 zygapophysial joint. (From Cousins MJ, Bridenbaugh PO, eds. *Back pain: zygapophysial blocks and epidural steroids.* London, Churchill Livingstone, 1988:937, with permission.)

as well as for temporary blockade of the joint. This approach can be used for facets C3-4 through C6-7. The C2-3 joint may require manipulation of the fluoroscopy unit to achieve the best view of this joint, because it tends to slope more downward and medially than the lower segments.

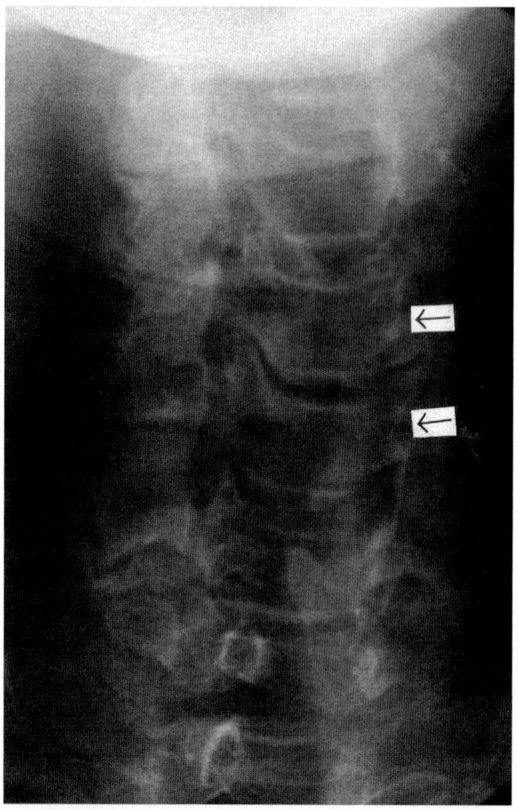

FIGURE 17-20. AP view of cervical spine. *Arrows* illustrate needle positions for a medial branch block at the C4 level and C5 levels. Note that these two blocks completely denervate the C4-5 facet and incompletely block these C3-4 and C5-6 facets.

In the cervical facets, each joint receives innervation from its corresponding segment as well as from the level above. The nerves arise from the posterior primary rami and then curve dorsally and medially about the midpoint of the articular pillars. It is at this point that the needle placement is positioned to denervate the spinal segment. In the cervical spine medial branch blocks are less difficult to perform than the intraarticular injection and should be the preferred technique (Fig. 17-19).

From a lateral view, a needle can be placed at the midpoint of the lateral mass of the vertebral body and then advanced until it makes contact with bone (Fig. 17-20). An injection of 0.5 ml of 0.5% bupivacaine applied at each segment is sufficient to anesthetize the medial branches. Extreme caution should be taken to demonstrate negative aspiration before injection, because the introduction of local anesthetic into the vertebral artery will cause instant local-anesthetic toxicity and seizure.

REFERENCES

1. Frymoyer JW. Back pain and sciatica. *N Engl J Med* 1998;318: 291–300.
2. Stein M, Elliott D, Glen J, et al. Percutaneous facet joint fusion: preliminary experiences. *J Vasc Interv Radiol* 1993;4:69–74.
3. Borenstein DG. Epidemiology, etiology, diagnostic evaluation, and treatment of low back pain. *Curr Opin Rheumatol* 1997;9: 144–150.
4. Frymoyer JW. An overview of the incidences and costs of low back pain. *Orthop Clin North Am* 1991;22:263–271.
5. Manchikanti L. Facet joint pain and the role of neural blockade in its management. *Curr Rev Pain* 1999;3:348–358.
6. El-Khoury GY, Reinfrew DL. Percutaneous procedures for the diagnosis and treatment of low back pain: diskography, facet-joint injection, and epidural injection. *AJR Am J Radiol* 1991; 157:685–691.
7. Haldeman S. Failure of pathology to predict back pain. *Spine* 1990;15:718–724.

8. Galibert P, Deramond H, Rosat P, et al. Preliminary note on the treatment of vertebral angioma by percutaneous acrylic vertebroplasty. *Neurochirurgie* 1987;33:166–168.
9. Mathis JM, Barr JD, Belkoff SM, et al. Percutaneous vertebroplasty: a developing standard of care for vertebral compression fractures. *AJNR Am J Neuroradiol* 2001;22:373–381.
10. Cousins MJ. Taxonomy of pain (Appendix A). In: Cousins MJ, Bridenbaugh PO, eds. *Neural blockade in clinical anesthesia and management of pain,* 2nd ed. Philadelphia: JB Lippincott, 1988: 752–754.
11. Brose WG, Gaeta R, Spiegel D. Neuropsychiatric aspects of pain management. In: Yudofsky SC, Hales RE, eds. *The American Psychiatric Press textbook of neuropsychiatry,* 3rd ed. Washington, DC: American Psychiatric Press, 1997:349–379.
12. Hurley DL, Khosla S. Update on primary osteoporosis. *Mayo Clin Proc* 1997;72:943–949.
13. Gennari C, Agnusdei D, Camporeale A. Use of calcitonin in the treatment of bone pain associated with osteoporosis. *Calcif Tissue Int* 1991;49:9S–13S.
14. Kanis JA, Melton LJ III, Christiansen C, et al. The diagnosis of osteoporosis. *J Bone Miner Res* 1994;9:1137–1141.
15. Riggs BL, Melton LJ III. The worldwide problem of osteoporosis: insights afforded by epidemiology. *Bone* 1995;17[Suppl]: 505S–511S.
16. Melton LJ III. Epidemiology of spinal osteoporosis. *Spine* 1997; 22:2S–11S.
17. Holbrook TL, Grazier K, Kelsey JL, et al. *The frequency of occurrence, impact, and cost of selected musculoskeletal conditions in the United States.* Chicago: American Academy of Orthopedic Surgeons, 1984.
18. Jacobsen SJ, Cooper C, Gottlieb MS, et al. Hospitalization with vertebral fracture among the aged: a national population-based study, 1986–1989. *Epidemiology* 1992;2:515–518.
19. Ray NF, Chan JK, Thamer M, et al. Medical expenditures for the treatment of osteoporotic fractures in the United States in 1995: report from the National Osteoporosis Foundation. *J Bone Miner Res* 1997;12:24–35.
20. Melton LJ III, Chrischilles EA, Cooper C, et al. How many women have osteoporosis? *J Bone Miner Res* 1992;7:1005–1010.
21. Riggs BL, Melton LJ. Involutional osteoporosis. *N Engl J Med* 1986;315:1676–1686.
22. Ross PD, Davis SW, Epstein RS, et al. Preexisting fractures and bone mass predict vertebral fracture incidence in women. *Ann Intern Med* 1991;114:919–923.
23. Jensen ME, Dion JE. Percutaneous vertebroplasty in the treatment of osteoporotic compression fractures. *Neuroimaging Clin N Am* 2000;10:547–568.
24. Ross PD. Clinical consequences of vertebral fractures. *Am J Med* 1997;103:30S–42S.
25. Eastell R, Cedel SL, Wahner HW, et al. Classification of vertebral fractures *J Bone Miner Res* 1991;6:207–215.
26. Cooper C, Atkinson EJ, O'Fallon WM, et al. Incidence of clinically diagnosed vertebral fractures: a population-based study in Rochester, Minnesota, 1985–1989. *J Bone Miner Res* 1992;7: 221–227.
27. Patel U, Skingle S, Campbell GA, et al. Clinical profile of acute vertebral compression fractures in osteoporosis. *Br J Rheumatol* 1991;30:418–421.
28. Silverman SL. The clinical consequences of vertebral compression fractures. *Bone* 1992;13:S27–S31.
29. Vogt TM, Ross PD, Palermo L, et al. Vertebral fracture prevalence among women screened for the Fracture Intervention Trial and a simple clinical tool to screen for undiagnosed vertebral fractures. *Mayo Clin Proc* 2000;75:888–896.
30. Ross PD, Ettinger B, Davis JW, et al. Evaluation of adverse health outcomes associated with vertebral fractures. *Osteoporos Int* 1991; 1:134–140.
31. Do HM. Magnetic resonance imaging in the evaluation of patients for percutaneous vertebroplasty. *Top Magn Reson Imaging* 2000;11:235–244.
32. Rapado A. General management of vertebral fractures. *Bone* 1996;3:191S–196S.
33. Gold DT. The clinical impact of vertebral fractures: quality of life in women with osteoporosis. *Bone* 1996;18:185S–189S.
34. Goldthwait JE. The lumbosacral articulation: an explanation of many cases of lumbago, sciatica, and paraplegia. *Boston Med Surg J* 1911;164:365.
35. Putti V. Lady Jones' lecture on new concepts in pathogenesis of sciatic pain. *Lancet* 1927;2:53–60.
36. Ghormley RK. Low back pain with special reference to the articular facet, with presentation of an operative procedure. *JAMA* 1933;101:1773–1777.
37. Mooney V. Facet syndrome: clinical entities. In: Weinstein JN, Wiesel SW, eds. *The lumbar spine.* Philadelphia: WB Saunders, 1990:422–441.
38. Mooney V, Robertson J. The facet syndrome. *Clin Orthop* 1976; 115:149–156.
39. Rees WES. Multiple bilateral subcutaneous rhizolysis of segmental nerves in the treatment of the intervertebral disk syndrome. *Ann Gen Pract* 1971;16:126.
40. Shealy CN. Percutaneous radiofrequency denervation of spinal facets: treatment for chronic back pain and sciatica. *J Neurosurg* 1975;43:448–451.
41. Bogduk N. International spinal injection society guidelines for the performance of spinal injection procedures. Part 1: zygapophysial joint blocks. *Clin J Pain* 1997;13:285–302.
42. Cotten A, Dewatre F, Cortet B, et al. Percutaneous vertebroplasty for osteolytic metastases and myeloma: effects of the percentage of lesion filling and the leakage of methyl methacrylate at clinical follow-up. *Radiology* 1996;200:525–530.
43. Deramond H, Depriester C, Galibert P, et al. Percutaneous vertebroplasty with polymethylmethacrylate. *Radiol Clin North Am* 1998;36:533–546.
44. Weill A, Chiras J, Simon J, et al. Spinal metastases: indications for and results of percutaneous injection of acrylic surgical cement. *Radiology* 1996;199:241–247.
45. Jensen ME, Evans AJ, Mathis JM, et al. Percutaneous polymethylmethacrylate vertebroplasty in the treatment of osteoporotic vertebral body compression fractures: technical aspects. *AJNR Am J Neuroradiol* 1997;18:1897–1904.
46. Tamayo-Orozco J, Arzac-Palumbo P, Peon-Vidales H, et al. Vertebral fractures associated with osteoporosis: patient management. *Am J Med* 1997;103:44S–48S.
47. Schlaich C, Minne HW, Bruckner T, et al. Reduced pulmonary function in patients with spinal osteoporotic fractures. *Osteoporos Int* 19988;8:261–267.
48. Kado DM, Browner WS, Palermo L, et al. Vertebral fractures and mortality in older women: a prospective study: study of Osteoporotic Fractures Research Group, *Arch Intern Med* 1999; 159:1215–1220.
49. Cyteval C, Baron Sarrabere MP, Rouz JO, et al. Acute osteoporotic vertebral collapse: open study on percutaneous injection of acrylic surgical cement in 20 patients. *AJR Am J Radiol* 1999; 173:1685–1690.
50. Debussche-Depriester C, Deramond H, Fardellone P, et al. Percutaneous vertebroplasty with acrylic cement in the treatment of osteoporotic vertebral crush fracture syndrome. *Neuroradiology* (Suppl) 1991;33:149–152.
51. Depriester C, Deramond H, Toussaint P, et al. Percutaneous vertebroplasty: indications, technique, and complications. Connors JJ III, Wojak JC, eds. *Interventional neuroradiology: strategies*

and practical techniques. Philadelphia: WB Saunders, 1999: 347–357.
52. Gangi A, Kastler B, Dietemann JL. Percutaneous vertebroplasty guided by a combination of CT and fluoroscopy. *AJNR Am J Neuroradiol* 1994;15:83–86.
53. Jensen ME, Kallmes DF, Short JG, et al. Percutaneous vertebroplasty does not increase the risk of adjacent vertebral fracture—a retrospective study. Proceedings of the ASNR 2000 paper 1:4–5.
54. Amar AP, Larsen DW, Esnaashari N, et al. Percutaneous transpedicular polymethylmethacrylate vertebroplasty for the treatment of spinal compression fractures. *Neurosurgery* 2001;49: 1105–1115.
55. Jarvik JG, Deyo RA. Cementing the evidence: time for a randomized trial of vertebroplasty. *AJNR Am J Neuroradiol* 2000;21: 1373–1374.
56. Goltra DD Jr. Vertebroplasty for osteoporotic compression fracture: effective treatment for a neglected disease. *AJNR Am J Neuroradiol* 2001;22:594–595.
57. Jarvik JG, Deyo RA. Vertebroplasty for osteoporotic compression fracture: effective treatment for a neglected disease. *AJNR Am J Neuroradiol* 2001;22:594–595.
58. Do HM, Marcellus ML, Weir RU, et al. Percutaneous vertebroplasty versus medical therapy for treatment of acute vertebral body compression fractures: a prospective randomized study. Proceedings of the ASNR 2002 paper 81 and Proceedings of the AUR 2002 paper 49.
59. Cybulski GM. Methods of surgical stabilization for metastatic disease of the spine. *Neurosurgery* 1989;25:240–252.
60. Harrington K. Anterior decompression and stabilization of the spine as a treatment for vertebral collapse and spinal cord compression from metastatic malignancy. *Clin Orthop Rel Res* 1988;233:177–197.
61. Sundaresan N, Galicich JH, Lane JM, et al. Treatment of neoplastic epidural cord compression by vertebral body resection and stabilization. *J Neurosurg* 1985;63:676–684.
62. O'Donnell RJ, Springfield DS, Motwani HK, et al. Recurrence of giant cell tumors of the long bones after curettage and packing with cement. *J Bone Joint Surg* 1994;76A:1827–1833.
63. Persson BM, Ekelund L, Lovdahl, et al. Favourable results of acrylic cementation for giant cell tumors. *Acta Orthop Scand* 1984;55:209–214.
64. Nicola N, Lins E. Vertebral hemangioma: retrograde embolization-stabilization with methyl methacrylate. *Surg Neurol* 1987; 27:481–486.
65. McLaughlin RE, DiFazio CA, Hakala M, et al. Blood clearance and acute pulmonary toxicity of methylmethacrylate in dogs after simulated arthroplasty and intravenous injection. *J Bone Joint Surg* 1973;55:1621–1628.
66. Phillips H, Cole PV, Letton AW. Cardiovascular effects of implanted acrylic bone cement. *BMJ* 1971;3:460–461.
67. Wong HY, Vidovich MI. Acute bronchospasm associated with polymethylmethacrylate cement. *Anesthesiology* 1997;87: 696–698.
68. Convery FR, Gunn DR, Hughes JD, et al. The relative safety of polymethylmethacrylate. *J Bone Joint Surg* 1975;57:57–64.
69. Deramond H, Wright NT, Belkoff SM. Temperature elevation caused by bone cement polymerization during vertebroplasty. *Bone* 1999;2:17S–21S.
70. Wang GW, Wilson CS, Hubbard SL, et al. Safety of anterior cement fixation in the cervical spine: in vivo study of dog spine. *South Med J* 1984;77:178–179.
71. Cloft HJ, Easton DN, Jensen ME, et al. Exposure of medical personnel to methylmethacrylate vapor during percutaneous vertebroplasty. *AJNR Am J Neuroradiol* 1999;20:352–353.
72. Belkoff SM, Maroney M, Fenton DC, et al. An *in vitro* biomechanical evaluation of bone cements used in percutaneous vertebroplasty. *Bone* 1999;25:23S–26S.
73. Hitchon PW, Goel V, Drake J, et al. Comparison of the biomechanics of hydroxyapatite and polymethylmethacrylate vertebroplasty in a cadaveric spinal compression fracture model. *J Neurosurg* 2001;95:215–220.
74. Maynard AS, Jensen ME, Schweickert PA, et al. Value of bone scan imaging in predicting pain relief from percutaneous vertebroplasty in osteoporotic vertebral fractures. *AJNR Am J Neuroradiol* 2000;21:1807–1812.
75. Yuh WTC, Zachar CK, Barloon TJ, et al. Vertebral compression fractures: distinction between benign and malignant causes with MR imaging. *Radiology* 1989;172:215–218.
76. Baker LL, Goodman SB, Perkash I, et al. Benign versus pathologic compression fractures of vertebral bodies: assessment with conventional spin-echo, chemical-shift, and STIR MR imaging. *Radiology* 1990;174:495–502.
77. Shih TTF, Huang KM, Li YW. Solitary vertebral collapse: distinction between benign and malignant causes using MR patterns. *J Magn Reson Imaging* 1999;9:635–642.
78. Baur A, Stabler A, Bruning R, et al. Diffusion-weighted MR imaging of bone marrow: differentiation of benign versus pathologic compression fractures. *Radiology* 1998;207:349–356.
79. Castillo M, Arbelaez A, Smith JK, et al. Diffusion-weighted MR imaging offers no advantage over routine noncontrast MR imaging in the detection of vertebral metastases. *AJNR Am J Neuroradiol* 2000;21:948–953.
80. Baur A, Huber A, Ertl-Wagner B, et al. Diagnostic value of increased diffusion weighting of a steady-state free precession sequence for differentiating acute benign osteoporotic fractures from pathologic vertebral compression fractures. *AJNR Am J Neuroradiol* 2001;22:366–372.
81. Zhou XJ, Leeds NE, McKinnon GC, et al. Characterization of benign and metastatic vertebral compression fractures with quantitative diffusion MR imaging. *AJNR Am J Neuroradiol* 2001;23: 165–170.
82. Falcone S. Diffusion-weighted imaging in the distinction of benign from metastatic vertebral compression fractures: is this a numbers game? *AJNR Am J Neuroradiol* 2001;23:5–6.
83. Murphy KJ, Deramond H. Percutaneous vertebroplasty in benign and malignant disease. *Neuroimaging Clin N Am* 2001;10: 547–568.
84. Barr JD, Barr MS, Lemley TJ, et al. Percutaneous vertebroplasty for pain relief and spinal stabilization. *Spine* 2000;25:923–928.
85. Kaufmann TJ, Jensen ME, Schweickert PA, et al. Age of fracture and clinical outcomes of percutaneous vertebroplasty. *AJNR Am J Neuroradiol* 2001;22:1860–1863.
86. Do HM, Jensen ME, Marx WF, et al. Percutaneous vertebroplasty in the treatment of patients with vertebral osteonecrosis (Kummell's disease). *Neurosurg Focus* 1999;7:Article 2(www.neurosurgery.org), 1999.
87. Mathis JM, Petri M, Naff N. Percutaneous vertebroplasty treatment of steroid-induced osteoporotic compression fractures. *Arthritis Rheum* 1998;41:171–175.
88. O'Brien JP, Sims JT, Evans AJ. Vertebroplasty in patients with severe vertebral compression fractures. l: a technical report. *AJNR Am J Neuroradiol* 2000;21:1555–1558.
89. Fukui S, Ohseto K, Shiotani M, et al. Distribution of referred pain from the lumbar zygapophyseal joints and dorsal rami. *Clin J Pain* 1997;13:303–307.
90. Kaplan M, Dreyfuss P, Halbrook B, et al. The ability of lumbar medial branch blocks to anesthetize the zygapophysial joint: a physiologic challenge. *Spine* 1998;23:1847–1852.
91. Gray DP, Bajwa ZH, Warfield CA. Facet block and neurolysis.

In: Waldman SD, ed. *Interventional pain management,* 2nd ed. 2001.
92. Lord SM, Barnsley L, Wallis BJ, et al. Percutaneous radio-frequency neurotomy for chronic cervical zygapophyseal-joint pain. *N Engl J Med* 1996;335:1721–1726.
93. Geurts JW, van Wijk RM, Stolker RJ, et al. Efficacy of radiofrequency procedures for the treatment of spinal pain: a systematic review of randomized clinical trials. *Reg Anesth Pain Med* 2001; 26:394–400.
94. Gaughen Jr. JR, Jensen ME, Schweikent PA, et al. Relevance of antecedent venography in percutaneous vertebroplasty for treatment of osteoporotic compression fractures. *AJNR Am J Neuroradiol* 2002;23:594–600.
95. Padovani B, Kasriel O, Brunner P, et al. Pulmonary embolism caused by acrylic cement: a rare complication of percutaneous vertebroplasty. *AJNR Am J Neuroradiol* 1999;20:375–377.
96. Cotten A, Boutry N, Cortet B, et al. Percutaneous vertebroplasty: state of the art. *Radiographics* 1998;18:311–320.
97. Cotten A, Demondion X, Boutry N, et al. Therapeutic percutaneous injections in the treatment of malignant acetabular osteolysis. *Radiographics* 1999;19:647–653.
98. Do HM, Wong BB. Pathologic clavicular fracture stabilization with polymethylmethacrylate. Proceedings of the ASNR 2001, paper 117:86.
99. Tomeh AG, Mathis JM, Fenton DC, et al. Biomechanical efficacy of unipedicular versus bipedicular vertebroplasty for the management of osteoporotic compression fractures. *Spine* 1999; 24:1772–1776.

Endovascular and Percutaneous Therapy of the Brain and Spine, edited by Michael P. Marks and Huy M. Do.

INDEX

INDEX

Page numbers followed by a f refer to figures; those followed by a t refer to tabular material.

I